Nursing Diagnosis Index

Nursing Diagnosis

Application to Clinical Practice

Nursing Diagnosis

Application to Clinical Practice

7th Edition

LYNDA JUALL CARPENITO, R.N., M.S.N., F.N.P.

Family Nurse Practitioner, Private Practice
Philadelphia, Pennsylvania
Nursing Consultant
Mickleton, New Jersey

with 36 additional contributors

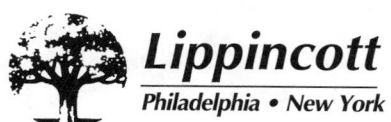 **Lippincott**
Philadelphia • New York

Acquisitions Editor: Mary Gyetvan
Assistant Editor: Susan Keneally
Project Editor: Tom Gibbons
Production Manager: Helen Ewan
Production Coordinator: Pat McCloskey
Design Coordinator: Doug Smock
Indexer: Maria Coughlin

9 8 7 6 5 4 3 2 1

Library of Congress Cataloging in Publication Data

Carpenito, Lynda Juall.
    Nursing diagnosis : application to clinical practice / Lynda Juall
Carpenito ; with 36 additional contributors. — 7th ed.
        p.   cm.
    Includes bibliographical references and index.
    ISBN 0-397-55431-1
    1. Nursing diagnosis.   2. Nursing care plans.
    [DNLM: 1. Nursing Diagnosis—outlines.   2. Patient Care Planning—
outlines.   WY 18.2 C294n 1997]
RT48.6.C386   1997
616.07′5—dc21
DNLM/DLC
for Library of Congress   96-40214
                                                                              CIP

Care has been taken to confirm the accuracy of the information presented and to describe generally accepted practices. However, the authors, editors, and publisher are not responsible for errors or omissions or for any consequences from application of the information in this book and make no warranty, express or implied, with respect to the contents of the publication.

The authors, editors and publisher have exerted every effort to ensure that drug selection and dosage set forth in this text are in accordance with current recommendations and practice at the time of publication. However, in view of ongoing research, changes in government regulations, and the constant flow of information relating to drug therapy and drug reactions, the reader is urged to check the package insert for each drug for any change in indications and dosage and for added warnings and precautions. This is particularly important when the recommended agent is a new or infrequently employed drug.

Some drugs and medical devices presented in this publication have Food and Drug Administration (FDA) clearance for limited use in restricted research settings. It is the responsibility of the health care provider to ascertain the FDA status of each drug or device planned for use in their clinical practice.

To Richard, my husband
Through bright and dark you are there, thank you again.

It was such a pretty day we decided
    to take a walk,
And we had not gone ten steps
    before I knew
That you and I are long past the point
    of no return.

Hand in hand we go.
Still close, still loving
Still looking and overlooking
The flaws we hide from others.

Side by side we move,
Sometimes closer, sometimes farther apart.
Because of ways we read and talk,
Agree and disagree.

Step by step we advance
Against the cynics
Those all-knowing unknowings who
    honestly think
Marriage is dead.

—Lois Wyse, "I Still Love You"

Contributors

Rosalinda Alfaro-LeFevre, R.N., M.S.N., President, Teaching Smart/Learning Easy, Stuart, Florida

(Risk for Altered Respiratory Function; Ineffective Airway Clearance; Ineffective Breathing Patterns; Diversional Activity Deficit; Impaired Verbal Communication; Fluid Volume Deficit; Fluid Volume Excess; Risk for Altered Body Temperature; Hyperthermia and Hypothermia)

Caroline McAlpine Alterman, R.N., M.S.N., C.N.S., Program Director, Spinal Cord Injury, Lakshore Hospital, Birmingham, Alabama

(Altered Bowel Elimination; Altered Patterns of Urinary Elimination, Sixth Edition)

Ann H. Barnhouse, R.N., M.S.N., Nurse Educator, Hudson, Ohio

(Relocation Stress)

Christine J. Brugler, R.N., M.S.N., Private Practice, Warren, Ohio

(Relocation Stress)

Judith S. Carscadden, R.N., Head Nurse, London Psychiatric Hospital, London, Ontario, Canada

(Self-Concept Disturbance; Body Image Disturbance; Chronic Low Self-Esteem; Situational Low Self-Esteem, Fifth Edition; Risk for Self-Mutilation)

Deana DeMare, P.T., B.S., Neurobehavioral Specialist, Children's Regional Hospital/Cooper Hospital University Medical Center, Camden, New Jersey

(Disorganized Infant Behavior; Potential for Enhanced Organized Infant Behavior; Risk for Altered Parent–Infant Attachment)

Nancy Eppich, R.N., M.S.N., Vice President, Clinical Services, Grace Hospital, Cleveland, Ohio

(Altered Parenting; Parental Role Conflict)

Dru Hammell, R.N., M.S.N., Nurse Manager, Newborn Services, Cooper Hospital/University Medical Center, Camden, New Jersey

(Disorganized Infant Behavior; Potential for Enhanced Organized Infant Behavior; Risk for Altered Parent–Infant Attachment)

Joan T. Harkulich, R.N., M.S.N., Director of Research and Professional Services, Care Services, Beachwood, Ohio

(Relocation Stress)

Eric Harris, R.N., Nurse Manager, Continuing Care Services, London Psychiatric Hospital, London, Ontario, Canada

(Defensive Coping)

Judy A. Hartmann, Director of Nursing, Kansas Rehabilitation Hospital, Topeka, Kansas

(Altered Patterns of Urinary Elimination; Unilateral Neglect, Third Edition)

Mark Hemmings, R.N., Nurse Manager, Continuing Care, London Psychiatric Hospital, London, Ontario, Canada

(Social Isolation; Impaired Social Interactions)

Eileen Hubler, R.N., M.S., Neonatal Clinical Nurse Specialist, Children's Regional Hospital/Cooper Hospital University Medical Center, Camden, New Jersey

(Disorganized Infant Behavior; Potential for Enhanced Organized Infant Behavior; Risk for Altered Parent–Infant Attachment)

Jean Jenny, Professor, retired from University of Ottawa, Ottawa Canada

(Dysfunctional Ventilatory Weaning Response; Risk for Dysfunctional Ventilatory Weaning Response)

Jo Logan, R.N., M.Ed., Director of Nursing Research & Professional Development, Ottawa Civic Hospital, Ottawa, Canada

(Dysfunctional Ventilator Weaning Response; Risk for Dysfunctional Ventilatory Weaning Response)

Morris A. Magnan, R.N., B.S.N., Clinical Nurse Specialist/Case Manager, Harper Hospital, Detroit Medical Center, Detroit, Michigan

(Activity Intolerance)

Jo Ann Maklebust, M.S.N., R.N., C.S., Clinical Nurse Specialist/Wound Care, Nurse Practitioner, Harper Hospital, Detroit Medical Center, Detroit, Michigan

(Impaired Tissue Integrity; Risk for Altered Health Maintenance related to lack of knowledge of ostomy care; Impaired Skin Integrity; Altered Comfort: Pruritis; Altered Oral Mucous Membrane)

Judy McElvanney, R.N., London Psychiatric Hospital, London, Ontario, Canada

(Altered Thought Process related to effects of dementia)

Janet Hoffman Mennies, R.N.C., M.S.N., Adult Nurse Practitioner Coordinator, Family Forum, Inc., Newtown Square, Pennsylvania

(Noncompliance; Altered Health Maintenance; selected sections of Altered Family Processes; Ineffective Individual Coping; Health-Seeking Behaviors)

Amy Meredith, R.N., M.S.N., F.N.P., Private Practice, Chatsworth, New Jersey

(Risk for Altered Body Temperature; Hyperthermia and Hypothermia, Seventh Edition)

Linda C. Mondoux, R.N., M.S.N., Botsford Hospital, Farmington Hills, Michigan

(Gerontologic Considerations for Activity Intolerance; Grieving; Impaired Home Maintenance Management; Spiritual Distress; Impaired Communication; Diversional Activity Deficit; Powerlessness; Impaired Tissue Integrity; selected sections of Caregiver Role Strain)

Sharon Morgan, R.N., M.N., Manager, Staff Development, Victoria Hospital, London, Ontario, Canada

(Grieving, Fifth Edition)

Kathe H. Morris, R.N., M.S.N., Educational Consultant, West Chester, Pennsylvania

(Rape Trauma Syndrome)

Nancy J. Morwessel, R.N., M.S.N., C.P.N.P., Pediatric Nurse Practitioner, Children's Hospital Medical Center, Cincinnati, Ohio

(Altered Comfort in Children; Ineffective Infant Feeding Pattern)

Nursing Diagnosis Discussion Group, Nancy A. Eppich, Chairwoman, Rainbow Babies and Childrens Hospital, University Hospitals of Cleveland, Cleveland, Ohio

(Parental Role Conflict, Third Edition)

Mary M. Owen, R.N., B.S.N., P.H.N., Associate Director, Health Outcomes, CalOptima, Orange, California

(Risk for Infection; Risk for Infection Transmission)

Rhonda Panfilli, R.N., M.S.N., Business Manager, Deborah R. Dunison, Ph.D., Bloomfield Hills, Michigan

(Altered Health Maintenance related to Increased Food Consumption)

Gayle Vandendool Parker, R.N., B.S.N., Nursing Practice Coordinator, London Psychiatric Hospital, London, Ontario, Canada

(Altered Thought Processes; Altered Thought Process related to [Specify] as evidenced by inability to evaluate reality; Powerlessness; PC: Neuroleptic Malignant Syndrome)

Cheryl Rozelle, R.N., C.R.R.N., Director of Nursing, Lakeshore Rehabilitation Hospital, Birmingham, Alabama

(Altered Bowel Elimination; Altered Patterns of Urinary Elimination, Sixth Edition)

Mary Sieggreen, M.S.N., R.N., C.S., Nurse Practitioner, Vascular Surgery, Harper Hospital, Detroit Medical Center, Detroit, Michigan

(Altered Peripheral Tissue Perfusion; Risk for Injury related to Effects Secondary to Orthostatic Hypotension)

Deborah Soholt, R.N., M.S.N., Director, Women & Children Services, McKennan Hospital, Sioux Falls, South Dakota

(Decisional Conflict)

Katsuko Tanaka, R.N., M.S., C.S., A.R.N.P., Staff Nurse, VA Puget Sound Health Care Systems, Seattle, Washington

(Post-Trauma Response; Fear; Ineffective Denial, Fifth Edition)

Carol Van Antwerp, R.N., M.S.N., Pediatric Nurse Practitioner, Rambling Road Pediatrics, Kalamazoo, Michigan

(Risk for Injury related to Maturational Age, Pediatric Considerations; Altered Growth and Development, Fifth Edition)

Julie Waterhouse, R.N., M.S., Assistant Professor, College of Nursing, University of Delaware, Newark, Delaware

(Spiritual Distress; Altered Sexuality Patterns)

Janet R. Weber, R.N., M.S.N., Ed.D., Associate Professor of Nursing, Southeast Missouri State University, Cape Girardeau, Missouri

(Hopelessness)

Anne E. Willard, R.N., M.S.N., Associate Professor, Cumberland County College, Vineland, New Jersey

(Anxiety; Risk for Violence; Ineffective Family Coping; Risk for Self-Harm; Impaired Social Interactions; Self-Esteem Disturbance; Defensive Coping; Ineffective Denial; Chronic Low Self-Esteem; Situational Low Self-Esteem; Altered Thought Processes)

Margaret Chamberlain Wilmoth, Assistant Professor, College of Nursing and Health Professions, University of North Carolina, Charlotte, North Carolina

(Altered Sexuality Patterns)

Consultants

Jane Bloom, R.N., M.S.N., Clinical Nurse Specialist, Medical Respiratory Intensive Care Unit, Thomas Jefferson Hospital, Philadelphia, Pennsylvania

Ushi Choudhry, R.N., Ph.D., Professor, School of Health Sciences, Seneca College, North York, Ontario, Canada

Michele Clements, R.N., Nurse Manager Labor and Delivery, Women's Health Care, Victoria Hospital, London, Ontario, Canada

Ann Delengowski, R.N., M.S.N., Oncology Clinical Nurse Specialist, Thomas Jefferson University Hospital, Philadelphia, Pennsylvania

Mary Ann Ducharme, R.N., M.S.N., Case Manager, Intensive Care, Harper Hospital Detroit, Michigan

Cissy Englebert-Passanza, R.N., M.S.N., Clinical Nurse Educator, Mercy Catholic Medical Center, Darby, Pennsylvania

Ann Feins, R.D., Assistant Professor, Saint Anselm College, Manchester, New Hampshire

Jamie Jolly, R.N., CIC, Infection Control, Saddleback Memorial Hospital, Orange, California

Debra J. Lynn-McHale, R.N., M.S.N., C.C.R.N., Coordinator, Staff Development, Thomas Jefferson University Hospital, Philadelphia, Pennsylvania

Kathleen A. Michalski, R.N., B.S.N., C.C.R.N., Clinical Nurse III, Surgical Cardiac Care Unit, Thomas Jefferson University Hospital, Philadelphia, Pennsylvania

Susan Ross, R.N., M.S., Assistant Professor, American International College, Springfield, Massachusetts

Ann Smith, R.N., M.S.N., C.C.R.N., Clinical Nurse Specialist, Surgical Intensive Care Unit, Thomas Jefferson University Hospital, Philadelphia, Pennsylvania

Linda H. Snow, R.N., M.S., Assistant Professor, American International College, Springfield, Massachusetts

Donna Zazworsky, R.N., M.S.N., Case Manager, Community Nursing Organization, Carondolet Health System, Tucson, Arizona

Preface

The practice of nursing often interfaces with the practices of the other health care providers.* Sometimes the nurse sees the client problems that require referral for treatment and ignores or fails to detect the problems that she can treat independently. *Nursing Diagnosis: Application to Clinical Practice* focuses on the diagnosis and treatment of client situations that the nurse can and should treat, legally and independently. It provides a condensed, organized outline of clinical nursing practice designed to communicate creative clinical nursing. It is not meant to replace textbooks of nursing, but rather to provide nurses in a variety of settings with the information they need without requiring a time-consuming review of the literature.

From assessment criteria to specific interventions, the book focuses on nursing. It will assist students in transferring their theoretical knowledge to clinical practice; it can also be used by experienced nurses to recall past learning and to intervene in those clinical situations that previously went ignored or unrecognized.

The author agrees that nursing needs a classification system to organize its functions and define its scope. Use of such a classification system would expedite research activities and facilitate communication between nurses, consumers, and other health care providers. After all, medicine took over 100 years to develop its taxonomy. Our work, at the national level, only began in 1973. It is hoped that the reader will be stimulated to participate at the local, regional, or national level in the utilization and development of these diagnoses.

Since the first edition was published, the use of nursing diagnosis has increased markedly throughout the United States, Canada, and internationally. Practicing nurses vary in experience with nursing diagnosis from just beginning to full practice integration for over 15 years. With such a variance in use, questions posed from the neophyte, such as

- What does the label really mean?
- What kinds of assessment questions will yield nursing diagnoses?
- How do I differentiate one diagnosis from another?
- How do I tailor a diagnosis for a specific individual?
- How should I intervene after I formulate the diagnostic statement?
- How do I care-plan with nursing diagnoses?

differ dramatically from such questions from experts as

- Should nursing diagnoses represent the only diagnoses on the nursing care plan?
- Can medical diagnoses be included in a nursing diagnosis statement?
- What are the ethical issues in using nursing diagnoses?
- What kind of problem statement should I write to describe a person at risk for hemorrhage?
- What kind of nursing diagnosis should I use to describe a healthy person?
- Do I need nursing diagnoses with critical pathways?

This seventh edition seeks to continue to answer these questions.

Section I begins with a chapter on the development of nursing diagnosis and the work of the North American Nursing Diagnosis Association (NANDA). The concepts of nursing diagnosis, classification, and taxonomic issues are explored. This chapter discusses the review process of NANDA and describes the evolving taxonomy of NANDA's Human Response Patterns.

Chapter 2 differentiates among actual, risk, and possible nursing diagnoses. A discussion of wellness and syndrome diagnoses also is presented. Guidelines for writing diagnostic

---

* The model of interlocking circles on the cover depicts this relationship. The common area represents those situations in which nurses and physicians collaborate; the rest denotes the dimensions for which each professional prescribes interventions to prevent or treat.

statements and avoiding errors are outlined. Chapter 2 also covers the use of non–NANDA-approved diagnoses and practice dilemmas associated with nursing diagnoses.

Chapter 3 describes the Bifocal Clinical Practice Model. This chapter includes a more detailed discussion of nursing diagnoses and collaborative problems, covering their relationship to assessment, goals, interventions, and evaluation.

Chapter 4 addresses issues and controversies. Arguments regarding the ethics and cultural implications of nursing diagnoses are explored. The implications of a consistent language for nurses as members of a multidisplinary team are discussed.

Chapter 5 focuses on assessment and diagnosis, covering data interpretation and assessment format and concluding with a case study to illustrate clinical applications.

Chapter 6 describes the process of care planning and discusses various care planning systems. Topics covered include priority identification, nursing goals versus client goals, case management and nursing accountability. Interventions for nursing diagnoses and collaborative problems are differentiated. This chapter also clarifies evaluation, distinguishing evaluation of nursing care from evaluation of the client's condition. A discussion of multidisplinary care is presented, as is a three-tiered care planning system aimed at increasing the clinical use of care plans without increasing writing. Samples of nursing records appear throughout the chapter.

Section II compiles the nursing diagnoses accepted by NANDA along with additional clinically useful diagnoses. The seventh edition includes 138 diagnoses (123 NANDA-approved and 15 added by the author).

Each nursing diagnosis group is discussed under the following subheads:

- Definition
- Defining Characteristics or Risk Factors
- Related Factors
- Author's Notes
- Errors in Diagnostic Statements
- Focus Assessment
- Key Concepts
    Generic Considerations
    Pediatric Considerations
    Gerontologic Considerations
    Transcultural Considerations

Author's Notes and Errors in Diagnostic Statements are designed to help the nurse understand the concept behind the diagnosis, differentiate one diagnosis from another, and avoid diagnostic errors. Maternal, Child, and Gerontologic Key Concepts for all relevant diagnoses provide additional pertinent information. Transcultural Considerations strive to increase the reader's sensitivity to cultural diversity without stereotyping.

New to the seventh edition is that each nursing diagnosis is addressed with generic interventions and rationale. If applicable, Maternal, Child, and Older Adult focus interventions and rationale are included. Each nursing diagnosis is then followed by one or more specific nursing diagnoses that relate to familiar clinical situations. Outcome criteria for the diagnosis are provided with the related interventions, which represent activities in the independent domain of nursing derived from the physical and applied sciences, pharmacology, nutrition, mental health, and nursing research.

Section III consists of a Manual of Collaborative Problems. In this section, each of the nine generic collaborative problems is explained under the subheads.

- Physiologic Overview
- Definition
- Diagnostic Considerations
- Focus Assessment Criteria
- Significant Laboratory Assessment Criteria

Discussed under their appropriate problems are 52 specific collaborative problems, covering:

- Definition
- High-Risk Populations

- Nursing Goals
- Interventions

Sections II and III of *Nursing Diagnosis: Application to Clinical Practice* address both types of situations that nurses are responsible for treating. The clarification of the focus of nurses is intended to assist them in addressing clients' human needs, with the expectation that—as more "nursing" is added to nursing—the profession, the nurse, and, most importantly, the client will reap the rewards.

The author invites comments or suggestions from readers. Correspondence can be directed to the publisher or to the author's address: 66 East Rattling Run Road, Mickleton, NJ 08056.

Lynda Juall Carpenito, R.N., M.S.N., F.N.P.

Acknowledgments

When immersed in a manuscript, I seem able to meet only basic needs: air, food, elimination, and safety. I am grateful for all my good friends who don't wait for me to call them. It's these friends who help me meet my other needs—love, belonging, trust—to approach self-actualization. Thank you, Ginny, Pati, and Ronnie.

My publisher, Lippincott-Raven, has provided me with professional marketing, editorial support, and creative freedom. My editor, Mary Gyetvan, nudges me to pursue new approaches with my work. Thank you also to Susan Keneally, who always helps me keep track of the work and missing items, and Tom Gibbons, for bringing confusing or conflicting text to my attention and for his unrelentingly positive approach to work and life. This book has been translated into French, Spanish, and Japanese, all due to the efforts of Alice McElhinney, who supports my work and spirit.

Since the first edition, hundreds of nurse colleagues have shared their experiences with nursing diagnoses and have challenged me to grow, learn, and change. I am grateful for their challenges. Also, thank you to those departments of nursing and schools of nursing that have shared their success stories after integration of the Bifocal Clinical Nursing Model.

At last, I would like to thank Laura Terrill for her moral and professional support while I wrote the first edition; the group in Detroit (Jo Ann Maklebust, Mary Sieggreen, Linda Mondoux) for our late-night talks; Rosalinda Alfaro-LeFevre, who recognized the need for the book and sought to make it a reality; and lastly, a very special person—my son, Olen Juall Carpenito. Of all my accomplishments, he's the one I treasure most.

Contents

Section I

Nursing Diagnosis in the Nursing Process

Introduction

Nursing is primarily assisting individuals (sick or well) with those activities contributing to health or its recovery (or to a peaceful death) that they perform unaided when they have the necessary strength, will, or knowledge; nursing also helps individuals carry out prescribed therapy and to be independent of assistance as soon as possible. *

Individuals are open systems who continually interact with the environment, creating individual interaction patterns. These patterns are dynamic and interact with life processes (physiologic, psychological, sociocultural, developmental, and spiritual) to influence the individual's behavior and health. A person becomes a client not only when an actual or potential alteration in this interaction pattern compromises his health but also when the person desires assistance to achieve a higher level of health.

The use of the term *client* in place of the term *patient* to identify the health care consumer suggests an autonomous person who has freedom of choice in seeking and selecting assistance. The client is no longer a passive recipient of services but an active participant who assumes responsibility for his choices and also for the consequences of those choices. *Family* is used to describe any person or persons who serve as support systems to the client. *Group* is used to describe support systems as well as communities, such as senior citizen centers. Societal health needs have changed in the last decade; so must the nurse's view of the consumers of health care (individual, family, community).†

Health is the state of wellness as defined by the client; it is no longer defined as whether a biologic disease is present. Health is a dynamic, ever-changing state influenced by past and present interaction patterns. The individual is an expert on himself and is responsible for seeking or refusing health care.

The Bifocal Clinical Practice Model describes the unique responsibilities of nursing in two components. *Nursing diagnoses* address the responses of clients, families, or groups to situations for which the nurse can prescribe interventions for outcome achievement. In contrast, *collaborative problems* describe certain physiologic complications that nurses manage using both nurse- and physician-prescribed interventions. No other discipline but nursing can treat nursing diagnoses and also manage collaborative problems.

The Bifocal Clinical Practice Model provides nurses with a classification system to describe the health status of an individual, family, or community and the risk for complications. Using this system, nurses can describe the health status of individuals or groups concisely and systematically, while also addressing the unique aspects of each situation.

---

* Henderson, V., & Nite, G. (1960). *Principles and practice of nursing* (5th ed.). New York: Macmillan.
† Carpenito, L. J., & Duespohl, T. A. (1985). *A guide to effective clinical instruction* (2nd ed.). Rockville, MD: Aspen Systems.

Development of Nursing Diagnosis

Nursing diagnosis provides a useful method for organizing nursing knowledge. Nightingale wrote that the purpose of nursing is "to put the patient in the best condition for nature to act upon him." In the present health delivery system, individual clients, families, and communities present with many health problems and needs. Limited resources (*e.g.*, time, money, personnel) require that the health care professional best prepared to manage the health problem or need be used. Nursing diagnosis has made it possible for the expertise of nursing to be defined and clarified.

Why Nursing Diagnoses?

Nursing needs a classification system, or taxonomy, to describe and develop a sound scientific foundation, thus fulfilling one of the criteria for professional status. The requisites commonly demanded of the occupational group seeking to claim professional status are listed by Styles (1982) as:

- An extensive university education
- A unique body of knowledge
- An orientation of service to others
- A professional society
- Autonomy and self-regulation

A classification system for nursing defines the body of knowledge for which nursing is held accountable. The relationship of nursing diagnosis to accountability and autonomy can be expressed as follows:

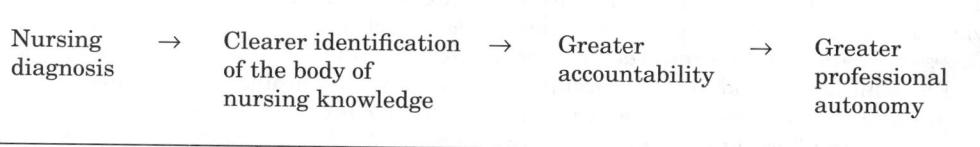

The use of a classification system to identify nursing's domain provides nurses with a common frame of reference. Historically, nurses have been educated to use medical diagnoses to describe the nursing focus. Because medical terminology provides an easy, convenient solution, some nurses have resisted other, more nursing-oriented, terminology. Many clinicians would rather use terms like "congestive heart failure," "bipolar disease," "asthma," and "placenta previa" than "social isolation," "impaired skin integrity," and "self-care deficit."

The need for a common, consistent language for medicine was identified over 200 years ago. If physicians elected to use just any words to describe their clinical situations, then:

- How could they communicate with each other? With nurses?
- How would research be organized?
- How would new practitioners be educated?
- How could quality be improved if the data could not be retrieved systematically to determine which interventions resulted in improvement of the client's condition?

For example, before the formal labeling of acquired immunodeficiency syndrome (AIDS), it was difficult or perhaps impossible to define or study the disease. Often, medical records would show various diagnoses or causes of death, such as sepsis, cerebral hemorrhage, or pneumonia, that were listed to describe the client with AIDS.

From the viewpoint of health care delivery, classification of nursing diagnoses establishes a system suitable for computerization. With the expanding potential for computer use, nursing diagnosis can

- Provide nurses with a system for retrieving client records using nursing, not medical, diagnoses
- Provide an opportunity for nurses to develop or be included in a computerized health care information system that would collect, analyze, and synthesize nursing data for practice and research
- Provide a system for the reimbursement of nursing activities related to nursing diagnoses, not medical diagnoses

Criticism of most theories and frameworks usually arises from difficulty in applying them to clinical practice. In a critique of theory development in nursing, Kritek (1978) stated that most nursing theories "describe how nursing should be, not how it is in reality." She noted that the use of poorly defined or confusing terms by theorists only limits professional application of these theories. Kritek advocated beginning with a theory that is operational in nature, one that describes "what we see and what we do," rather than with one that appears sophisticated but is obscure.

Nursing diagnosis can provide a solution by

- Defining the present art and science of nursing
- Providing a framework for the evolving science of nursing
- Emphasizing the focus of nursing for its members, students, colleagues, and consumers

Basic Concepts

The word *diagnosis* evokes many responses in nurses—some positive, some negative. Because nurses historically have linked diagnosis exclusively with medicine, some may tend to overlook the fact that many practitioners make diagnoses; for example, teachers diagnose learning disabilities, hairdressers diagnose hair problems, and mechanics diagnose automotive disorders. In addition, many nurses were taught to avoid making definitive statements when documenting and were advised to use phrases such as "seems to be" or "appears to be." This socialization process rewarded nurses for *not* diagnosing.

By definition, diagnosis is the careful, critical study of something to determine its nature. The question is not *whether* nurses can diagnose, but *what* nurses can diagnose.

In 1953, the term *nursing diagnosis* was introduced by V. Fry (1953) to describe a step necessary in developing a nursing care plan. Over the next 20 years, references to nursing diagnosis appeared only sporadically in the literature. However, from 1973 (when the first meeting of the National Group for the Classification of Nursing Diagnosis was held) to the present, attention in the literature has increased tenfold.

In 1973, the American Nurses Association (ANA) published its *Standards of Practice*; this was followed in 1980 by the ANA *Social Policy Statement*, which defined nursing as "the diagnosis and treatment of human response to actual or potential health problems" (ANA, 1980). Most state nurse practice acts describe nursing in accordance with the ANA definition.

In March, 1990, at the Ninth Conference of the North American Nursing Diagnosis Association (NANDA), the General Assembly approved an official definition of nursing diagnosis (NANDA, 1990):

> *Nursing diagnosis is a clinical judgment about individual, family, or community responses to actual or potential health problems / life processes. Nursing diagnosis provides the basis for selection of nursing interventions to achieve outcomes for which the nurse is accountable.*

Nursing Diagnosis: Process or Outcome?

A review of the literature reveals that, over time, the term *nursing diagnosis* has been used in three contexts:

1. *As the second step of the nursing process.* In this step, the nurse analyzes data collected during the assessment step and evaluates the health status. Some of the conclusions resulting from data analysis lead to nursing diagnoses, but others do not. It is important to recognize that the outcome of this process can include problems treated primarily by nurses and problems requiring treatment by several disciplines. For example, while assessing a particular client, the nurse may record observations that point to the medical problems of seizures, hypoglycemia, and hypertension, as well as the nursing diagnosis of *Risk for Injury*. Using the term *nursing diagnosis* to designate the second step of the nursing process may be confusing and may have the undesirable effect of leading nurses to try to state all conclusions or problems as nursing diagnoses.
2. *As a list of diagnostic labels or titles.* After the first conference on nursing diagnosis in 1973, the term *nursing diagnosis* was applied to specific labels describing health states that nurses could legally diagnose and treat. The purpose of establishing these labels was to define and classify the scope of nursing. These labels are concise descriptors of a cluster of signs and symptoms, such as *Anxiety* or *Altered Family Processes*, or of increased vulnerability, such as *Risk for Injury*.
3. *As a two-part or three-part statement.* Nurses use the term *nursing diagnosis* to describe a two-part or three-part statement about an individual's, a family's, or a group's response to a situation or a health problem.

Thus, it has become necessary to indicate clearly whether the term *nursing diagnosis* is being used in the context of problem identification, a classification system of diagnostic labels (such as that developed by NANDA), or an individualized statement. To avoid misuse and confusion, the author recommends using the following terms:

- For the second step of the nursing process: *diagnosis*
- For the list of diagnostic labels or titles: *diagnostic label* or *nursing diagnosis*
- For the diagnostic statement: *nursing diagnosis*

The North American Nursing Diagnosis Association

In 1973, the first conference on nursing diagnosis was held to identify nursing knowledge and establish a classification system suitable for computerization. From this conference developed the National Group for the Classification of Nursing Diagnosis, composed of nurses from different regions of the United States and Canada, representing all elements of the profession: practice, education, and research. From 1973 to the present, the National Group has met 12 times. Their most recent list of nursing diagnoses is presented in Appendix XI.

At its first meeting in 1973, the National Group also appointed a task force to

1. Gather and disseminate information on nursing diagnosis
2. Encourage educational activities at regional and state levels to promote the implementation of nursing diagnoses, including conferences to identify additional diagnostic labels and workshops to teach about nursing diagnoses
3. Promote and organize activities to continue the development, classification, and scientific testing of nursing diagnoses, including planning national conferences, identifying criteria for accepting diagnoses, surveying current research activities, and exploring varied methods for classification

A proposal from the task force for a more formal organization was approved at the fifth national conference, and the group was renamed the North American Nursing Diagnosis Association. NANDA has elected officers, a board of directors, and standing committees.

Breu, Dracup, and Walden (1987) described assimilation of scientific advances like nursing diagnosis into practice as usually a three-step process. Initially, the research question is formulated and the research conducted. Next, the research findings are disseminated at scientific meetings and in journals. Finally, the relevant findings are incorporated into clinical practice. This process is usually linear, with little feedback.

NANDA has taken a different approach to the scientific assimilation of nursing diagnosis into practice. It involves three concurrent activities: consensus development, research, and infiltration occurring in an open system (Breu et al., 1987). As new nursing diagnoses are identified, clinical research using selected designs (*e.g.*, Gordon & Sweeney, 1979; Fehring, 1987) tests and refines assumptions. Figure 1-1 contrasts the traditional method and NANDA's method of incorporating scientific advances into practice.

In 1994, NANDA convened Diagnosis Workgroups to refine or clarify ten previously accepted nursing diagnoses. Clinical experts and researchers were invited to participate in workgroups. The objectives of the sessions were (Rantz & LeMone, 1995)

- Review and make recommendations for changes in labels, definitions, and defining characteristics
- Use research findings reported in the literature
- Prepare a bibliography

Changes recommended by these workgroups have been integrated into Section II of this edition under the ten pertinent diagnoses (*i.e.*, *Grieving, Decreased Cardiac Output, Altered Thought Processes, Ineffective Breathing Pattern, Ineffective Airway Clearance, Impaired Gas Exchange, Self-Esteem Disturbance, Ineffective Individual/Family Coping, Fluid Volume Excess/Deficit, Risk for Violence*).

In 1987, the ANA officially sanctioned NANDA as the organization to govern the development of a classification system of nursing diagnoses. The ANA councils have been advised to submit proposed nursing diagnoses to NANDA. This timely and significant action by the ANA has facilitated a uniform classification system for the nursing profession.

In March 1990, the first issue of *Nursing Diagnosis*, NANDA's official journal, was published. This journal aims to promote the development, refinement, and application of nursing diagnoses and to serve as a forum for issues pertaining to development and classification of nursing knowledge.

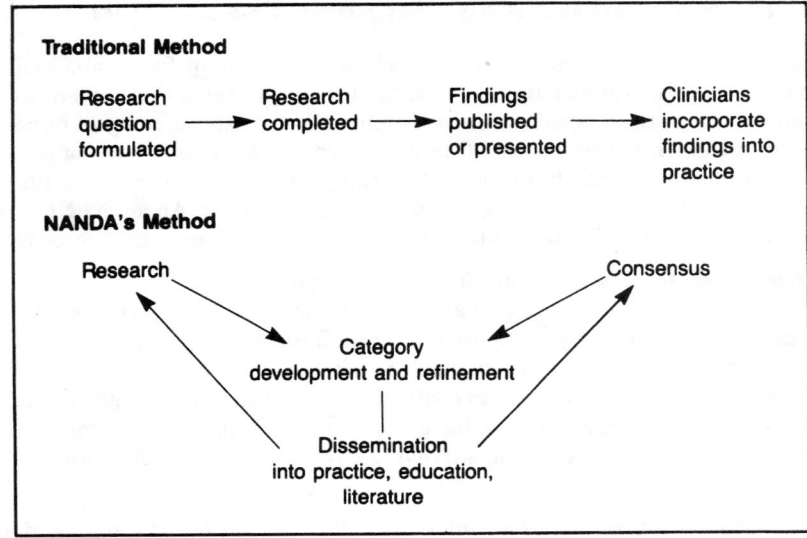

Fig. 1-1 Traditional method versus NANDA's method of incorporating scientific advances into practice.

International Classification of Nursing Practice

In December, 1986, an ANA advisory panel on Classification for Nursing Practice met with liaisons from NANDA to compile a nursing system for submission to the World Health Organization (WHO) for possible inclusion in the tenth revision of the International Code of Diseases (IDC). The document submitted represented a compilation of the work of NANDA, the Omaha Classification System, and the ANA's Psychiatric–Mental Health Council: In August 1987, as the result of collaborative work of the ANA and NANDA, a replacement document, detailing the NANDA classification system, was sent to WHO under the sponsorship of the Canadian and American nurses' associations. This submission was declined by WHO because of lack of international support.

At the International Council of Nursing (ICN) in Seoul in 1989, the Canadian and American nurses' associations proposed a resolution to the Council of National Representatives. The resolution asked that "ICN encourage member nurses' associations to become involved in developing classification systems for nursing care, nursing information management systems, and nursing data sets to provide tools that nurses in all countries could use to describe nursing and its contributions to health" (Clark & Lang, 1992, p. 110). The resolution passed, and a task force was formed to consider how ICN could best assist member associations. At the ICN meeting in Spain in June, 1993, the task force distributed a working draft of a compilation of classification systems found in the literature. NANDA's system was included. The plan is to continue to gather data for all countries and then to organize it under one classification system, titled International Classification of Nursing Practice (ibid).

Evolving Nursing Diagnoses

According to Maas, Hardy, and Craft (1990), "for the science of a practice discipline to progress, the concepts that describe subject matter of the field must be identified, defined, and empirically validated." Classification systems for other professionals (such as physicians, biologists, and pharmacists) developed over hundreds of years and continue to change and evolve. For example, AIDS did not appear in the IDC 12 years ago. But now, after the disorder was added to the IDC and given the label "AIDS," all physicians use this diagnostic label. Standardization gives users the expectation of, as Gordon (1990) states, "established usage and meaning for each diagnostic label."

Establishing usage and meaning for diagnostic labels in nursing has been an exciting and sometimes frustrating process. From 1973 to 1984, NANDA-approved nursing diagnoses were developed by groups of nurses invited to participate at the national conferences. At these conferences, nurses with various clinical and educational experience collaborated to identify and describe health problems that nurses diagnose and treat. These nurses drew on their clinical experience or related literature to identify clinical phenomena that occur in various states of health, then developed defining characteristics to describe these states.

The process for generating and accepting nursing diagnoses changed in 1984, when NANDA established a Diagnosis Review Committee (DRC) to develop a process for reviewing and approving proposed changes to the list of approved diagnoses. The documentation requirements for submitting a proposed change have increased appreciably with each subsequent review cycle, in large part because of the need for a thorough literature investigation of the proposed diagnosis. Since 1980, the number of published (and unpublished) research studies on nursing diagnosis has increased greatly. In 1990, the Cumulative Index of Nursing and Allied Health (CINAHL) began indexing all NANDA diagnosis-related articles. Currently, the index contains more than 2000 citations, including nursing dissertations, research and clinical application reports, and conference proceedings.

Avant (1990) described the need to apply both art and science in developing nursing diagnoses. First, a creative force is necessary to stimulate the exploration of concepts and the development of inventive diagnostic labels and taxonomic structures—the art. Next comes the need for systematic validation of concepts, nursing diagnoses, and the taxonomic structures—the science. In most cases, a single nurse simply is not qualified to bring both art and science to diagnosis development. As Avant (1990) explains, "teams of researchers and clinicians working together would result in much more creative, precise, and useful concepts."

Concept Development and Formalization

Each nursing diagnosis represents a concept that nurses "claim as an area of accountability for research on the phenomena" (Gordon, 1990). In nursing practice, such concepts provide a guiding structure for identifying, naming, and finally diagnosing. As Gordon (1990) explains, "we see what we are ready to see, and perceptual readiness (or cue sensitivity) depends to a large degree on the availability and accessibility of concepts within the structure of long-term memory." Ignorance of basic concepts can interfere with good nursing care. For example, a beginning student reports that a client is drinking a lot of fluid, urinating frequently, and reporting constant hunger. The student likely would recognize each symptom as abnormal, but might not know that, as a cluster, they may represent a concept (in this case, a medical disorder)—diabetes mellitus.

Unfortunately, many current NANDA-approved diagnoses are too abstract, such as *Altered Thought Processes*, or overlap unnecessarily with other diagnoses, such as *Altered Family Processes* and *Ineffective Family Coping: Compromised*. Unclear and imprecise concepts in the literature increase the risk of diagnostic error in clinical situations. As discussed earlier in this chapter, NANDA has supported the revision of ten diagnoses.

The Diagnostic Review Process

Developing a complete classification system for nursing diagnosis has proven a slow and difficult process involving extensive review and evaluation. Obviously, nursing cannot stop and wait until its classification system is complete, so practice continues while the system evolves.

NANDA's diagnostic review process from 1984 to 1994 was primarily a function of the DRC and expert reviewers. Submitted diagnoses were reviewed and decisions concerning their inclusion on NANDA's list were based on scholarship and application.

At the 11th conference in 1994, the DRC presented a new review system, which was approved by the board. A four-stage process of diagnostic development was established: comprehensive and systematic literature review, reanalysis of collected data, and field studies and collaboration of interested parties to conduct extensive field trials (*NANDA News*, 1994). Appendix I includes the new guidelines.

Diagnoses presented for the first time at a NANDA conference, as in March, 1994, are labeled "Works in Progress." The DRC, in collaboration with the Research Committee, will manage this process. Specialty organizations and other interested parties will be coopted into the process. The 19 diagnoses added to the list in 1994 were at stage I.

NANDA Taxonomy

The work of the initial theorist group at the third national conference and subsequently of the NANDA taxonomic committee has produced the beginnings of a conceptual framework for the diagnostic classification system. This framework is named NANDA Nursing Diagnosis Taxonomy I; the taxonomy comprises nine patterns of human response (Table 1-1).

A *taxonomy* is "a type of classification; the theoretical study of systematic classifications including their bases, principles, procedures, and rules" (*Taxonomy I*, p. 5). These nine patterns are for classification purposes only. They are for "behind-the-scene role for the clinician" (Fitzpatrick, 1991, p. 24). It is not necessary for clinicians, novice or expert, to understand the development of or the rules for classification. These nine patterns should not be used to organize assessment tools or curricula. Each pattern is followed by two or more levels of abstraction that are more concrete and clinically useful. The second level could become the category structure for assessment; the third and lower levels would serve as the diagnostic label for the individual or group (Kritek, 1986). The nursing diagnoses at level 4 are more clinically specific than those at level 3. For example, *Ineffective Individual Coping* still remains a useful category, but requires very specific etiologic or contributing factors to determine nursing

Table 1-1 **Human Response Patterns and Definitions**

Human Response Pattern	Definition
Choosing	To select between alternatives; the action of selecting or exercising preference in a matter in which one is a free agent; to determine in favor of a course; to decide in accordance with inclinations
Communicating	To converse; to impart, confer, or transmit thoughts, feelings, or information, internally or externally, verbally or nonverbally
Exchanging	To give, relinquish, or lose something while receiving something in return; the substitution of one element for another; the reciprocal act of giving and receiving
Feeling	To experience a consciousness, sensation, apprehension, or sense; to be consciously or emotionally affected by a fact, event, or state
Knowing	To recognize or acknowledge a thing or a person; to be familiar with by experience or through information or report; to be cognizant of something through observation, inquiry, or information; to be conversant with a body of facts, principles, or methods of action; to understand
Moving	To change the place or position of a body or any member of the body; to put or keep in motion; to provoke an excretion or discharge; the urge to action or to do something; to take action
Perceiving	To apprehend with the mind; to become aware of by the senses; to apprehend what is not open or present to observation; to take in fully or adequately
Relating	To connect, to establish a link between, to stand in some association to another thing, person, or place; to be borne or thrust in between things
Valuing	To be concerned about, to care; the worth or worthiness; the relative status of a thing, or the estimate in which it is held, according to its real or supposed worth, usefulness, or importance; one's opinion of liking for person or thing; to equate in importance

(*Taxonomy I.* [1989]. St. Louis: North American Nursing Diagnosis Association.)

prescriptions for treatment. Figure 1-2 illustrates the levels of abstraction related to one human response pattern—choosing.

Axes

NANDA's work is representative of the investigation and exploration of the submitter of the work. The work reflects submitters' origins, culture, clinical specialty, and professional experience. For example, chronic pain would have different manifestations in 18-month-old, 18-year-old, 44-year-old, and 74-year-old clients. The current defining characteristics for *Chronic Pain* do not encompass these age-related differences.

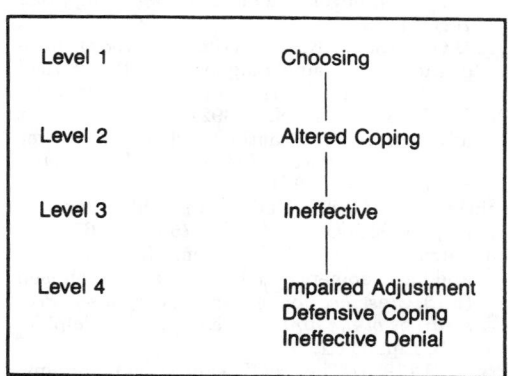

Level 1	Choosing
Level 2	Altered Coping
Level 3	Ineffective
Level 4	Impaired Adjustment Defensive Coping Ineffective Denial

Fig. 1-2 Diagram showing one set of multiple levels of abstraction associated with the human response pattern of choosing.

In response to these diagnostic dilemmas, NANDA's taxonomy committee has proposed taxonomy axes. An *axis* would be "a dimension of the human condition considered in the diagnosis" (Warren, 1991).

Examples include:

- Unit of analysis—individual, family, community
- Chronological age, fetus to elderly
- Wellness
- Illness

A diagnosis could have only one axis or several axes, for example:

Decisional conflict			
Unit of analysis (Individual)	Age (Teenager)	Wellness (Not applicable)	Illness (Level of conflict)

The wellness and illness axes are problematic if one attempts to place them at the same level as the unit of analysis or age axis. The wellness axis would not be applicable to decisional conflict, but it could apply to decision making.

The introduction of the concept of axes provides an opportunity to designate a diagnosis as representing a response for toddlers or aged adults rather than to continue to disseminate defining characteristics or risk factors as if they cross all age groups. Axes should encourage the development of age-specific diagnoses, such as "High Risk for Suicide in Adolescents." Nurses in all specialties should rise to this challenge.

Summary

The development of a classification system for nursing diagnoses has been ongoing since 1973. During this period, the initial question—"Does nursing really need a classification system?"—has been replaced by "How can such a system be developed in a scientifically sound manner?" The ANA has designated NANDA as the official organization to develop this classification system. Despite problems, through the concerted effort of many fine clinical nurses, nurse researchers, and other nursing professionals and organizations, this evolving classification system increasingly reflects both the art and science of nursing.

References

American Nurses Association. (1980). *ANA social policy statement*. Washington, DC: ANA.

Avant, K. C. (1990). The art and science in nursing diagnosis development. *Nursing Diagnosis, 1*(2), 51–56.

Breu, C., Dracup, K., & Walden, J. (1987). Integration of nursing diagnoses in the critical care literature. *Heart and Lung, 16*, 605–616.

Clark, J., & Lang, N. (1992). Nursing's next advance: An international classification for nursing practice. *International Nursing Review, 39*(4), 109–112.

Fehring, R. J. (1987). Methods to validate nursing diagnoses. *Heart and Lung, 16*(6), 62–67.

Fitzpatrick, J. J. (1991). Taxonomy II: Definitions and development. In R. M. Carroll-Johnson (Ed.), *Classification of nursing diagnoses: Proceedings of the ninth conference*. Philadelphia: J. B. Lippincott.

Fry, V. S. (1953). The creative approach to nursing. *American Journal of Nursing, 53*, 301–302.

Gordon, M. (1982). Historical perspective: The National Group for Classification of Nursing Diagnoses. In M. J. Kim & D. A. Moritz (Eds.), *Classification of nursing diagnoses*: Proceedings of the fourth national conference. New York: McGraw-Hill.

Gordon, M. (1990). Toward theory-based diagnostic categories. *Nursing Diagnosis, 1*(1), 511.

Gordon, M., & Sweeney, M. A. (1979). Methodological problems and issues identifying and standardizing nursing diagnoses. *Advances in Nursing Science, 7*(2), 1–15.

Kritek, P. (1986). Development of a taxonomic structure for nursing diagnosis. In M. Hurley (Ed.), *Classification of nursing diagnoses: Proceedings of sixth NANDA national conference*. St. Louis: C. V. Mosby.

Kritek, P. B. (1978). The generation and classification of nursing diagnoses: Toward a theory of nursing. *Image: The Journal of Nursing Scholarship, 10*(2), 33–40.

Maas, J., Hardy, M., & Craft, M. (1990). Some methodologic considerations in nursing diagnoses. *Nursing Research, 1*(1), 24–30.

NANDA News. (1994). *Nursing Diagnosis, 5*(2), 52–53.

North American Nursing Diagnosis Association. (1989). *Taxonomy I.* St. Louis: NANDA.

North American Nursing Diagnosis Association. (1990). *Taxonomy of nursing diagnoses.* St. Louis: NANDA.

Rantz, M. J., & LeMone, P. (1995). *Classification of nursing diagnoses: Proceedings of the 11th conference, NANDA.* Glendale, CA: CINAHL Information Systems.

Styles, M. M. (1982). *On nursing: Toward a new endowment.* St. Louis: C. V. Mosby.

Warren, J. J. (1991). Implications of introducing axis into a classification system. In R. M. Carroll-Johnson (Ed.), *Classification of nursing diagnoses*: Proceedings of the ninth conference. Philadelphia: J. B. Lippincott.

2

Types and Components of Nursing Diagnosis

Nursing diagnosis is both a structure and a process. The structure of a nursing diagnosis—its components—depends on its type: actual, risk, possible, wellness, or syndrome.

Actual Nursing Diagnoses

An actual nursing diagnosis represents a state that has been validated by the presence of major defining characteristics. This type of nursing diagnosis has four components: label, definition, defining characteristics, and related factors.

Label

The label should be descriptive of the diagnosis definition and defining characteristics (Gordon, 1990). The term "actual" is not part of the label in an actual nursing diagnosis.

Definition

By expressing a clear, precise meaning of the diagnosis, the definition helps differentiate a particular diagnosis from similar diagnoses. The definition should be conceptual and consistent with the label and defining characteristics (Gordon, 1990).

Defining Characteristics

In an actual nursing diagnosis, defining characteristics refer to clinical cues—subjective and objective signs or symptoms that, in a cluster, point to the nursing diagnosis.

Before 1986, all defining characteristics were listed together, without consideration for criticalness to the diagnosis. When attempts were made to differentiate critical cues from other listed cues, "critical" usually was defined as "must be present 100% of the time"—which proved to be an unworkable restriction. Researchers have found that validation of major defining characteristics as occurring 100% of the time could not be achieved. Attempts resulted in very general cues.

Defining characteristics are now separated into major and minor designations. According to NANDA, major defining characteristics are defined "as usually present when the diagnosis exists" (North American Nursing Diagnosis Association, 1992, p. 84). Minor defining characteristics are defined "as providing supporting evidence for the diagnosis, but may not be present" (NANDA, 1992, p. 84).

Some of NANDA's diagnoses have undergone content validity research using Fehring's diagnostic content validity scores. This research design differentiates major from minor defining characteristics. Major defining characteristics are defined as critical indicators present 80%–100% of the time; minor defining characteristics, as supporting indicators, occur 50%–79% of the time. For an example of this differentiation see Table 2-1, which lists major and minor defining characteristics for the nursing diagnosis *Defensive Coping*.

Not all the diagnoses accepted by NANDA have been clinically tested, and thus the 80%–100% and 50%–79% criteria are not applicable to them. For these nonresearched diagnoses, this author uses the consensus of experts to differentiate between major and minor. The consensus method is more valid if major is defined as "must be present (100%)." Thus, when clinical validation studies identify the major as between 80% and 100%, the author considers the major to be 80%–100% instead of 100%.

Table 2-1 **Frequency Scores for Defining Characteristics of Defensive Coping**

Defining Characteristics
Major (80%–100%)

Denial of obvious problems/weaknesses	88%
Projection of blame/responsibility	87%
Rationalizes failures	86%
Hypersensitive to slight criticism	84%

Minor (50%–79%)

Grandiosity	79%
Superior attitude toward others	76%
Difficulty in establishing/maintaining relationships	74%
Hostile laughter or ridicule of others	71%
Difficulty in testing perceptions against reality	62%
Lack of follow-through or participation in treatment or therapy	56%

(Norris, J., & Kunes-Connell, M. [1987]. Self-esteem disturbance: A clinical validation study. In A. McLane [Ed.], *Classification of nursing diagnoses: Proceedings of the seventh NANDA national conference.* St. Louis: C. V. Mosby.)

Related Factors

In actual nursing diagnoses, related factors are etiologic or other contributing factors that have influenced the health status change. Such factors can be grouped into four categories: pathophysiologic (biologic or psychological), treatment-related, situational (environmental, personal), and maturational. Examples of these factors include:

Pathophysiologic (biologic or psychological)

- Compromised immune system
- Inadequate peripheral circulation

Treatment-Related

- Medications
- Diagnostic studies
- Surgery
- Treatments

Situational

- Environmental
- Home
- Community
- Institution
- Personal
- Life experiences
- Roles

Maturational

- Age-related influences

Example

The following example illustrates the components of an actual nursing diagnosis—in this case, the diagnosis *Impaired Physical Mobility*.

DEFINITION

Impaired Physical Mobility: The state in which an individual experiences or is at risk of experiencing limitation of physical movement, but is not immobile.

DEFINING CHARACTERISTICS (LEVIN, KRAINOVITCH, BAHRENBURG, & MITCHELL, 1989)

Major (80%–100%)

Compromised ability to move purposefully within the environment (*e.g.*, bed mobility, transfers, ambulation)
Range-of-motion (ROM) limitations

Minor (50%–80%)

Imposed restriction of movement
Reluctance to move

RELATED FACTORS

Pathophysiologic

Related to decreased strength and endurance secondary to:
   (Neuromuscular impairment)
       Autoimmune alterations (*e.g.*, multiple sclerosis, arthritis)
       Nervous system diseases (*e.g.*, parkinsonism, myasthenia gravis)
       Muscular dystrophy
       Partial or total paralysis (*e.g.*, spinal cord injury, stroke)
       Central nervous system tumor
       Increased intracranial pressure
       Sensory deficits
   (Musculoskeletal impairment)
       Fractures
       Connective tissue disease (systemic lupus erythematosus)
       Related to edema (increased synovial fluid)

Treatment-Related

Related to external devices (casts or splints, braces, IV tubing)
Related to insufficient strength and endurance for ambulation with (specify)
   Prosthesis
   Crutches
   Walker

Situational (Personal, Environmental)

Related to:
   Fatigue
   Motivation
   Pain

Maturational

Children
   Related to abnormal gait secondary to:
       Skeletal deficiencies
       Osteomyelitis
       Congenital hip dysplasia
       Legg-Calvé-Perthes disease
Older adult
   Related to decreased motor agility
   Related to muscle weakness

Risk and High-Risk Nursing Diagnoses

As defined by NANDA, a risk nursing diagnosis is "a clinical judgment that an individual, family, or community is more vulnerable to develop the problem than others in the same or similar situation." In the past, all potential nursing diagnoses began with the phrase "Potential for," as in *Potential for Infection*. Now, however, all potential nursing diagnoses start with "Risk for."

This author recommends that nurses use "Risk for" or "High Risk for," depending on vulnerability. All clients are at risk for infection and injury in the hospital, long-term care facility, or community, but some are at higher risk than others. In light of a health care delivery system that, for financial reasons, passes on sicker clients to nurses and allows less time for interventions, high-risk nursing diagnoses provide nurses with a valuable means of identifying clients most vulnerable to problems.

The concept of "potential" or "at risk" does have clinical utility; nurses routinely prevent problems in populations who are not at high risk. For example, all postoperative clients are at risk for infection related to loss of protective barrier secondary to incision. This generic diagnosis for all surgical clients is routine; as such, it does not need to be included on the client's care plan, but instead, is part of the unit's standard of care. (See Chapter 5 for a discussion of standards of care.) In contrast, a diabetic client who has undergone emergency surgery for a perforated duodenal ulcer may have a nursing diagnosis of *High Risk for Infection related to surgical incision and impaired healing secondary to diabetes mellitus and blood loss*. Unlike the generic diagnosis, this diagnosis is included in the client's individualized care plan, because the client with diabetes is at *high* risk for infection, whereas the former client is merely at risk. The at-risk concept is also very useful for healthy people who are vulnerable because of age or a condition such as pregnancy. Pregnant women are not at high risk for injury, but they are at risk during the third trimester.

Label

In a risk nursing diagnosis, the concise description of the client's altered health status is preceded by the term "Risk for." For at-high-risk populations, the term is "High Risk for."

Definition

As in an actual nursing diagnosis, in a risk nursing diagnosis the definition expresses a clear, precise meaning of the diagnosis. It should be conceptual and consistent with the label and risk factors, to enable differentiation among similar diagnoses.

Risk Factors

Risk factors for risk and high-risk nursing diagnoses represent those situations that increase the vulnerability of a client or group. These factors differentiate high-risk clients and groups from all others in the same population who are at some risk. The validation to support an actual diagnosis is signs and symptoms—for example, *Impaired Skin Integrity related to immobility secondary to pain as evidenced by 2-cm erythematous sacral lesion*. In contrast, the validation to support a high-risk diagnosis is risk factors—for example, *High Risk for Impaired Skin Integrity related to immobility secondary to pain*.

Related Factors

The related factors for risk nursing diagnoses are the same risk factors previously explained. The components of a risk nursing diagnostic statement are discussed later in this chapter.

Possible Nursing Diagnoses

Possible nursing diagnoses are statements describing a suspected problem for which additional data are needed. It is unfortunate that many nurses have been socialized to avoid appearing tentative. In scientific decision making, a tentative approach is not a sign of weakness or indecision, but rather an essential part of the process. One must reserve judgment until all necessary information has been gathered and analyzed to arrive at a sound scientific conclusion. Physicians demonstrate tentativeness with the statement *rule out (R/O)*. Nurses should also adopt a tentative position until data collection and evaluation have been completed and they are able to confirm or rule out. The word *possible* is used in nursing diagnoses to describe problems that may be present, but that require additional data to be confirmed or ruled out. NANDA does not address possible nursing diagnoses, because they are not a classification issue, but instead, an option available for all approved NANDA diagnoses. With a possible nursing diagnosis, the nurse has some data to support a confirmed diagnosis, but they are insufficient.

Possible nursing diagnoses are two-part statements consisting of

- The possible nursing diagnosis
- The "related to" data that lead the nurse to suspect the diagnosis

An example would be: *Possible Self-Concept Disturbance related to recent loss of role responsibilities secondary to exacerbation of MS*.

When a nurse records a possible nursing diagnosis, other nurses are alerted to assess for more data to support or rule out the tentative diagnosis. After additional data collection, the nurse may take one of three actions:

- Confirm the presence of major signs and symptoms, thus labeling an actual diagnosis
- Confirm the presence of potential risk factors, thus labeling a risk diagnosis
- Rule out the presence of a diagnosis (actual or risk) at this time

A decision tree used to differentiate among actual, risk, and possible nursing diagnoses is shown in Figure 2-1.

Wellness Nursing Diagnoses

According to NANDA, a wellness nursing diagnosis is "a clinical judgment about an individual, group, or community in transition from a specific level of wellness to a higher level of wellness (1992, p. 84)." For an individual or group to have a wellness nursing diagnosis, two cues should be present:

- Desire for a higher level of wellness
- Effective present status or function

Diagnostic statements for wellness nursing diagnoses are one-part statements containing the label only. The label begins with "Potential for Enhanced," followed by the higher-level wellness that the individual or group desires—for example, *Potential for Enhanced Family Processes*.

Wellness nursing diagnoses do not contain related factors. Inherent in these diagnoses is a client or group who understands that higher-level functioning is available if desired or capable. The related goals would give direction for interventions:

Nursing Diagnosis: Potential for Enhanced Family Process
  Outcomes: The family will:
      Eat breakfast together 5 days/week
      Include children in family decisions
      Respect privacy of each member

Stolte (1996, p. 9) describes "wellness nursing diagnoses as a conclusion from assessment data which focuses on patterns of wellness, healthy responses, or client strengths." Interventions focus on attainment of health behaviors or achievement of developmental tasks (Stolte, 1996).

Wellness and Nursing Diagnosis

Since 1973, many nurses have expressed concern that the NANDA list primarily represents alteration or dysfunction (Gleit & Tatro, 1981; Popkess-Vawter, 1984; Stolte, 1996). Many nurses interact with healthy clients, such as new parents, school-aged children, and clients

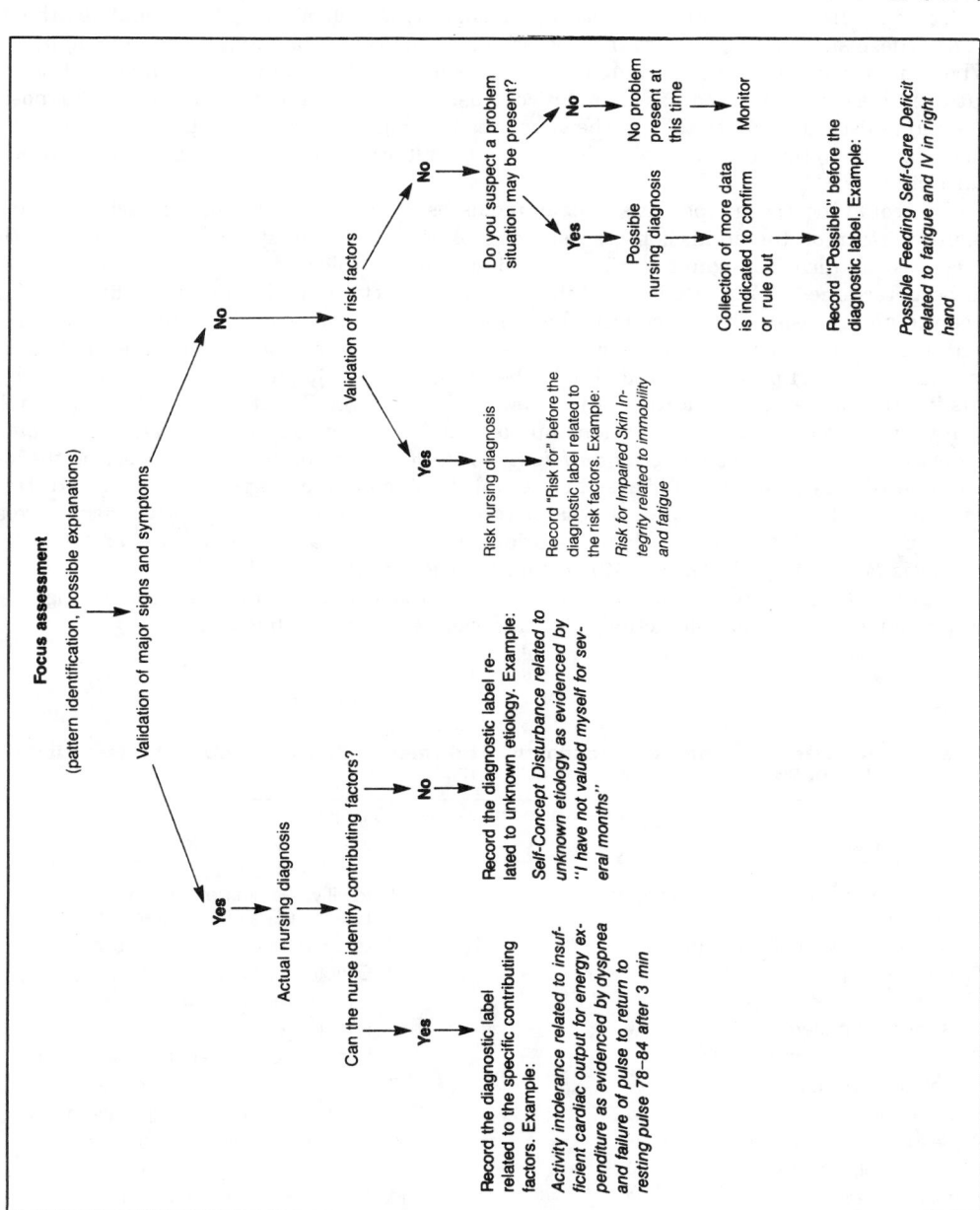

Fig. 2-1 Decision tree for differentiating among actual, risk, and possible nursing diagnoses. (© Lynda Juall Carpenito)

Focus assessment

(pattern identification, possible explanations)

Validation of major signs and symptoms

Yes — Actual nursing diagnosis

Can the nurse identify contributing factors?

Yes — Record the diagnostic label related to the specific contributing factors. Example:

Activity intolerance related to insufficient cardiac output for energy expenditure as evidenced by dyspnea and failure of pulse to return to resting pulse 78–84 after 3 min

No — Record the diagnostic label related to unknown etiology. Example:

Self-Concept Disturbance related to unknown etiology as evidenced by "I have not valued myself for several months"

No — Validation of risk factors

Yes — Risk nursing diagnosis

Record "Risk for" before the diagnostic label related to the risk factors. Example:

Risk for Impaired Skin Integrity related to immobility and fatigue

No — Do you suspect a problem situation may be present?

Yes — Possible nursing diagnosis

Collection of more data is indicated to confirm or rule out

Record "Possible" before the diagnostic label. Example:

Possible Feeding Self-Care Deficit related to fatigue and IV in right hand

No — No problem present at this time — Monitor

of college health services and well-baby clinics. Nurses also help ill clients to pursue optimal health through interventions such as stress management, exercise programs, and nutritional counseling.

It is important to distinguish the focus of nursing's accountability to a client or group in the area of health and positive functioning. For example, is the focus on assisting a client with a poor diet to achieve better nutrition, or on assisting a client with good nutrition to achieve optimal nutritional intake, or to prevent inadequate intake? It is true that almost everyone can improve his or her nutritional status; however, often the focus of nursing is not on changing effective functioning to optimal functioning, but rather on improving areas of compromised functioning. In this situation, the nurse can conclude that the client is exhibiting effective or positive functioning, without assuming the responsibility for assisting the client to achieve a higher level of functioning at this time.

Table 2-2 lists statements that describe strengths for each of the 11 functional health patterns. These statements are also incorporated into the case study application in Chapter 6. When the nurse and client conclude that there is positive functioning in a functional health pattern, this conclusion is an assessment conclusion, but by itself is not a nursing diagnosis. The nurse uses these data to help the client reach a higher level of functioning, or uses the identified strengths in planning interventions for altered functioning or at risk for altered functioning.

One could incorporate positive functioning assessment statements under each functional health pattern on the admission assessment tool. Figure 2-2 illustrates an example for the sleep–rest pattern. For example, after assessing a client's role and relationship patterns, the nurse determines that the client exhibits positive functioning. If this client has recently received a diagnosis of breast cancer, the nurse can use the client's strength to assist her in dealing with the diagnosis. Another example would be a young couple who recently became parents and report positive functioning in the role–relationship pattern. The nurse could use this information and the addition of the new baby to the family unit to assist the family in maintaining an effective role–relationship pattern. The diagnosis *Health-Seeking Behaviors related to insufficient knowledge of anticipated role change* could be used to describe the situation in which the nurse would assist the couple to plan for and adapt to new roles and stressors. Imagine that, 6 years later, this same couple reports a continued positive marital relationship and desires a higher-level relationship. In this case, the nurse could use the diagnosis *Potential for Enhanced Marital Relationship* to describe the situation.

Figure 2-3 illustrates a decision tree that the nurse can use to differentiate among positive/effective functioning and actual, risk, and wellness nursing diagnoses.

Table 2-2 **Positive Functioning Assessment Statements Grouped Under the Functional Health Patterns**

Functional Health Pattern	Positive Functioning Assessment Statements
1. Health perception–health management pattern	1. Positive health perception Effective health management
2. Nutritional–metabolic pattern	2. Effective nutritional–metabolic pattern
3. Elimination pattern	3. Effective elimination pattern
4. Activity–exercise pattern	4. Effective activity–exercise pattern
5. Sleep–rest pattern	5. Effective sleep–rest pattern
6. Cognitive–perceptual pattern	6. Positive cognitive–perceptual pattern
7. Self-perception pattern	7. Positive self-perception pattern
8. Role–relationship pattern	8. Positive role–relationship pattern
9. Sexuality–reproductive pattern	9. Positive sexuality–reproductive pattern
10. Coping–stress intolerance pattern	10. Effective coping–stress tolerance pattern
11. Value–belief pattern	11. Positive value–belief pattern

Sleep–Rest Pattern

Habits: 8 hr/night _____ <8 hr __X__ >8 hr _____ AM nap _____ PM nap

    Feel rested after sleep __X__ Yes _____ No

Problems: __X__ None _____ Early waking _____ Insomnia _____ Nightmares

    ☒ Effective Sleep–Rest Pattern

Fig. 2-2 Positive functioning statements related to sleep–rest pattern.

Syndrome Nursing Diagnoses

Syndrome nursing diagnoses are an interesting development in nursing diagnosis. McCourt (1991) presented an innovative paper on syndromes at NANDA's ninth conference. Her literature exploration revealed the following:

- *Syndrome* is derived from the Greek word "running together."
- Syndromes in medicine represent a cluster or group of signs and symptoms.
- Syndromes usually have a single cause or represent a group of coincident characteristics, the cause of which is unknown.

NANDA's Diagnosis Review Committee (DRC) explored the concept of syndrome in nursing diagnoses and found differences from medical diagnoses. Syndrome nursing diagnoses comprise a cluster of actual or high-risk nursing diagnoses that are predicted to be present because of a certain event or situation. NANDA currently has approved two syndrome diagnoses: *Rape Trauma Syndrome* and *Risk for Disuse Syndrome*.

Approved in 1980, *Rape Trauma Syndrome* does not represent a cluster of nursing diagnoses, but rather a cluster of signs and symptoms. This diagnosis could be restructured with a cluster of these nursing diagnoses:

Anxiety	*Sleep–Rest Disturbance*
Fear	*High Risk for Altered Sexuality Patterns*
Grieving	*Pain*

In 1988, *Potential Disuse Syndrome* and *Disuse Syndrome* were submitted to NANDA. The DRC approved *Potential Disuse Syndrome*, but not *Disuse Syndrome*. However, as the committee evolved its understanding of syndromes, it became apparent that syndromes cannot be potential. *Risk for Disuse Syndrome* should be revised to *Disuse Syndrome*. Table 2-3 lists the cluster of nursing diagnoses associated with *Disuse Syndrome*.

Syndrome diagnosis development should be approached carefully. The nurse must also dialogue with the client to determine the presence of other nursing diagnoses indicating the need for client–nurse interventions. The clinical advantage of a syndrome diagnosis is that it alerts the nurse that a "complex clinical condition requiring expert nursing assessments and interventions exists" (McCourt, 1991).

Syndrome nursing diagnoses usually are one-part diagnostic statements with the etiologic or contributing factors for the diagnosis contained in the diagnostic label—for example, *Rape Trauma Syndrome*.

Types of Diagnostic Statements

In describing the health status of a client or group, diagnostic statements can have one, two, or three parts. One-part statements contain only the diagnostic label, as in wellness and syndrome nursing diagnoses. Two-part statements contain the label and the factors that have contributed or could contribute to a health status change, as in possible and risk diagnoses. Used for actual nursing diagnoses, three-part statements contain the label, the contributing

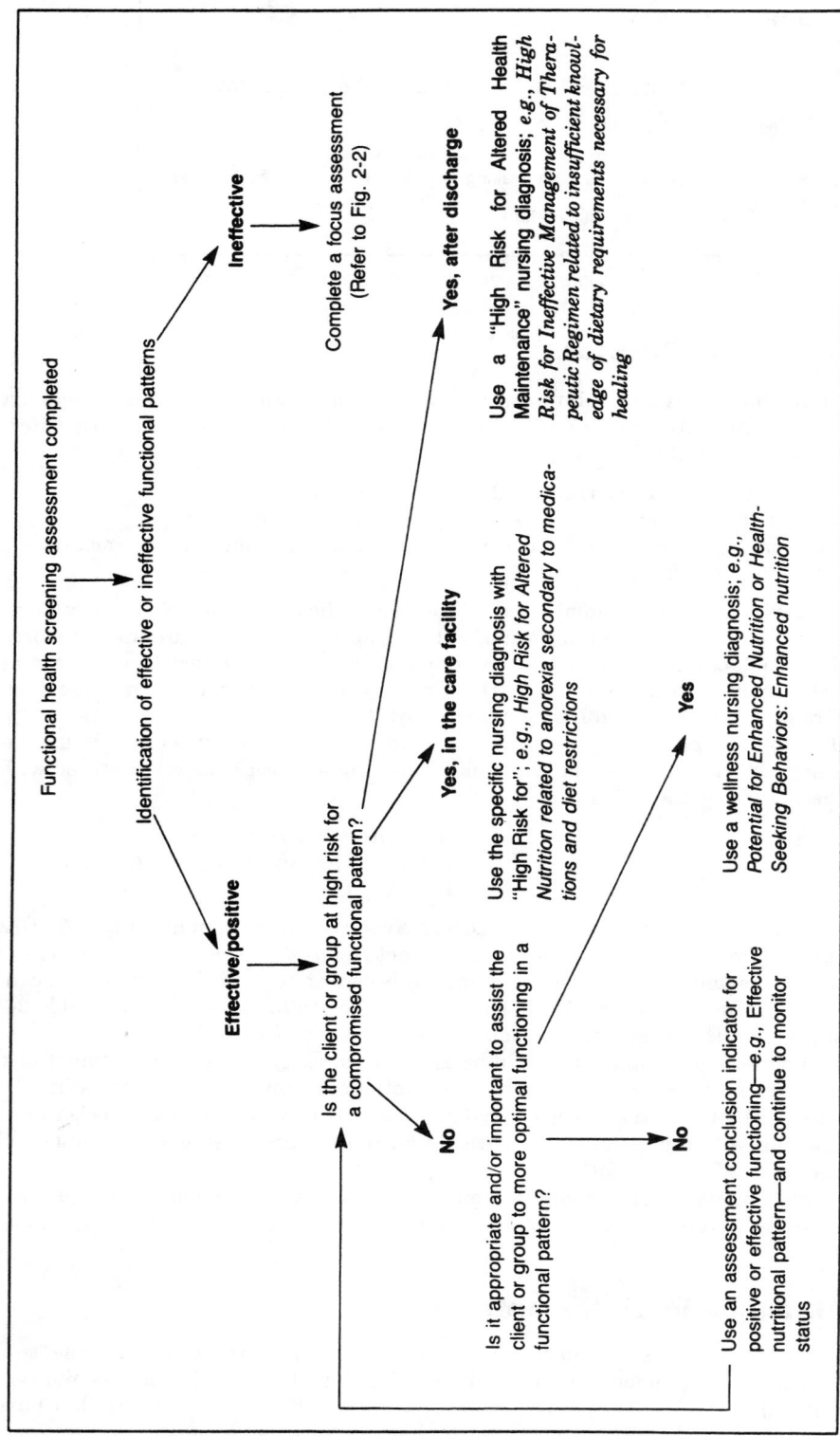

Fig. 2-3   Decision tree for differentiating among positive/effective functioning and actual, risk, and wellness nursing diagnoses.

Table 2-3 **Nursing Diagnoses Associated With *Disuse Syndrome***

Risk for Constipation
Risk for Altered Respiratory Function
Risk for Infection
Risk for Thrombosis
Risk for Activity Intolerance
Risk for Injury
Impaired Physical Mobility
Risk for Altered Thought Processes
Risk for Body Image Disturbance
Risk for Powerlessness
Risk for Impaired Tissue Integrity

factors, and the signs and symptoms of the diagnosis. Table 2-4 lists types of diagnostic statements with examples.

Writing Diagnostic Statements

Three-part diagnostic statements contain the following elements:

Problem	related to	Etiology	as evidenced by	Symptom
Diagnostic label		Contributing factors		Signs and symptoms

In two- and three-part diagnostic statements, the phrase *related to* reflects a relationship between the first and the second parts of the statement. It is important that the nurse not link the statements with words implying liability; this error could result in legal or professional difficulty. Examples of this error include:

- *Impaired Skin Integrity related to infrequent turning*
- *High Risk for Injury related to the mother's frequently leaving the children at home unsupervised*

The more specific the second part of the statement, the more specialized the interventions can be. For example, the diagnosis *Noncompliance* when stated by itself usually conveys the negative implication that the client is not cooperating. When the nurse relates the noncompliance to a factor, this diagnosis can transmit a very different message, for example:

- *Noncompliance related to the negative side effects of the drug (reduced libido, fatigue), as evidenced by "I stopped my B/P medicine."*
- *Noncompliance related to inability to understand the need for weekly blood pressure measurements, as evidenced by "I don't keep my appointments if I am busy."*

Unknown Etiology

If the defining characteristics of a nursing diagnosis are present, but the etiologic and contributing factors are unknown, the statement can include the phrase *unknown etiology*, for example:

- *Fear related to unknown etiology, as evidenced by rapid speech, pacing, and "I am worried."*

Table 2-4   **Types of Diagnostic Statements**

One-Part Statement
Wellness nursing diagnoses, *e.g.*,
  Potential for Enhanced Parenting
  Potential for Enhanced Nutrition
Syndrome nursing diagnoses, *e.g.*,
  Disuse Syndrome
  Rape Trauma Syndrome

Two-Part Statement
Risk nursing diagnoses, *e.g.*,
  Risk for Injury related to lack of awareness of hazards
Possible nursing diagnoses, *e.g.*,
  Possible Body Image Disturbance related to reports of husband of isolating behaviors postsurgery
Actual nursing diagnoses (when signs and symptoms are recorded outside the diagnostic statement, such as in a SOAP note), *e.g.*,
  Impaired Skin Integrity related to prolonged immobility secondary to fractured pelvis

Three-Part Statement
Actual nursing diagnoses, *e.g.*,
  Impaired Skin Integrity related to prolonged immobility secondary to fractured pelvis, as evidenced by a 2-cm sacral lesion

The use of *unknown etiology* alerts the nurse and other members of the nursing staff to assess for contributing factors at the same time that they intervene for the current problem.

If the nurse suspects that certain factors are present or that there is a relationship between certain factors and the nursing diagnosis, the term *possible* can be used—for example, *Anxiety related to possible marital discord*.

Syndrome diagnoses that may represent an exception to the need to use the phrase *related to* are *Rape Trauma Syndrome* and *Disuse Syndrome*. As more specific diagnoses evolve, it may become unnecessary for the nurse to write *related to* statements. Instead, many nursing diagnoses of the future may be single-part statements, such as *Functional Incontinence* or *Unilateral Neglect*.

Directions for Care

The literature has specified that the nurse direct interventions toward reducing or eliminating etiologic or contributing factors. Specifically, if the nurse cannot treat the contributing factors, then the nursing diagnosis is considered incorrect. This is problematic.

As the diagnostic labels evolve into more specific labels, the nurse may encounter nursing diagnoses with contributing factors that are not treatable by nursing. Consider, for example, the nursing diagnosis *Risk for Infection related to compromised immune system*. The nurse does not prescribe for a compromised immune system, but can prevent infection in some of these clients. It is unnecessary to force the nurse to rewrite the contributing factors to reflect the direction for treatment, such as *Risk for Infection related to susceptibility to environmental contagions secondary to compromised immune system*.

In some instances, the label directs the interventions, and the etiologic or contributing factors are not involved. Examples of such categories include:

- *Impaired Swallowing*
- *Functional Incontinence*
- *Risk for Infection*

Figure 2-4 illustrates this relationship.

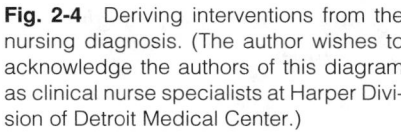

Fig. 2-4 Deriving interventions from the nursing diagnosis. (The author wishes to acknowledge the authors of this diagram as clinical nurse specialists at Harper Division of Detroit Medical Center.)

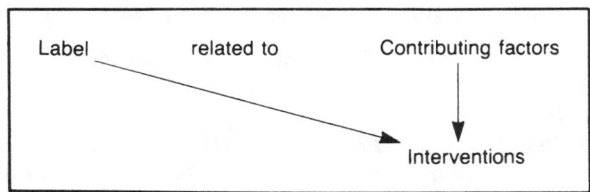

The nurse should be able to prescribe the definitive therapy for the nursing diagnosis label or the related factors. In the sample diagnosis *Sensory–Perceptual Alteration: Visual related to progressive loss of vision*, the nurse cannot prescribe the definitive interventions for the first or second parts. For this reason, the nurse should rewrite the diagnosis or reevaluate; perhaps the diagnosis is incorrect and would be better stated as *Fear related to progressive loss of vision*.

A thorough discussion of types of interventions for various types of diagnoses is presented in Chapter 3.

Non–NANDA-Approved Diagnoses

The issue of whether nurses should use only NANDA-approved diagnoses continues to spark debate. Some agencies and schools of nursing mandate use only of NANDA-approved diagnoses, whereas others do not support these restrictions.

Several authors, including Alfaro (1990), Gordon (1990), and Carpenito (1990), have made recommendations on using non-NANDA nursing diagnoses. Every agency and school of nursing should have an approved list containing all NANDA-approved nursing diagnoses as well as any other approved for use by the agency or school. This list would help nurses avoid using unknown and possibly confusing labels.

Nurses, faculty members, or students could submit a non–NANDA-approved diagnosis to be considered for inclusion on the agency or school list for further clinical development. (Of course, any proposed diagnosis should contain all its appropriate components—definition, defining characteristics, or risk factors.) Including non–NANDA-approved diagnoses on agency or school lists can help encourage orderly, scientific development of nursing diagnoses while avoiding terminologic chaos.

Avoiding Errors in Diagnostic Statements

As discussed earlier, the nursing diagnostic statement reflects some change in the client's or group's health status related to factors that have contributed to or could contribute to its development, or a healthy state that may be threatened or achieved. As with any other skill, writing diagnostic statements takes knowledge and practice. To increase the accuracy and usefulness of diagnostic statements (and also to reduce the nurse's frustration), several common errors should be avoided. Nursing diagnoses are *not* new terms for

- Medical diagnoses (*e.g.*, diabetes mellitus)
- Medical pathology (*e.g.*, decrease in cerebral tissue oxygenation)
- Treatments or equipment (*e.g.*, hyperalimentation, Levin tube)
- Medication side effects
- Diagnostic studies (*e.g.*, cardiac catheterization)
- Situations (*e.g.*, pregnancy, dying)

Nursing diagnostic statements should not be written in terms of

- Cues (*e.g.*, crying, hemoglobin level)
- Inferences (*e.g.*, dyspnea)
- Goals (*e.g.*, should perform own colostomy care)
- Client needs (*e.g.*, needs to walk every shift; needs to express fears)
- Nursing needs (*e.g.*, change dressing, check blood pressure)

The nurse should avoid legally inadvisable or judgmental statements, such as

- *Fear related to frequent beatings by husband*
- *Ineffective Family Coping related to mother-in-law's continual harassment of daughter-in-law*
- *Risk for Altered Parenting related to low IQ of mother*
- *Noncompliance related to failure to return for follow-up visits*

A nursing diagnosis should not be related to a medical diagnosis, such as *Self-Concept Disturbance related to multiple sclerosis* or *Anxiety related to myocardial infarction*. If the use of a medical diagnosis adds clarity to the diagnosis, it can be linked to the statement with the phrase *secondary to*, as follows:

Self-Concept Disturbance related to recent losses of role responsibilities secondary to multiple sclerosis, as evidenced by, "My mother comes every day to run my house," "I can no longer be the woman in charge of my house."

Even with defining characteristics and etiologic factors for each nursing diagnosis, nurses continue to have difficulty using nursing diagnoses, as is illustrated by the questions cited in the Preface:

- What does the label really mean?
- What kinds of assessment questions will yield nursing diagnoses?
- How do I tailor a nursing diagnosis for a specific client?
- How should I intervene after I formulate the diagnostic statement?
- How do I develop a care plan with nursing diagnoses?

To assist the nurse in using nursing diagnoses, Section II of this book, *Manual of Nursing Diagnoses*, has been designed so that each nursing diagnosis is described in terms of:

- Definition
- Etiologic, contributing, and risk factors (related factors)
- Defining characteristics
- Author's notes
- Errors in diagnostic statements
- Focus assessment criteria to validate diagnoses
- Key concepts

Each diagnostic label is further described in terms of one or more specific nursing diagnoses. For example, consider the diagnostic label *Impaired Tissue Integrity*. A specific diagnosis under this label would be *Impaired Skin Integrity*.

Each specific diagnosis is explained in terms of:

- Assessment data (subjective and objective)
- Outcome criteria
- Nursing interventions with rationale

Thus, Section II provides an explanation of each nursing diagnosis, along with related interventions that will assist the nurse in applying nursing diagnoses in clinical practice.

Summary

On the surface, nursing diagnosis appears to be a convenient, simple solution to some of professional nursing's problems. This impression has led many nurses to use nursing diagnoses; however, many still do not integrate diagnosis into their nursing practice. Integrating nursing diagnosis into practice is a collective and personal process. Collectively, the nursing profession has developed the structure of nursing diagnosis and continues to identify and refine specific diagnoses. Individually, each nurse struggles with diagnostic reasoning and confirmation as well as with related ethical implications. Collectively and individually, these struggles will continue.

References

Alfaro, R. (1990). *Applying nursing diagnosis and nursing process: A step-by-step guide* (2nd ed.). Philadelphia: J. B. Lippincott.

Carpenito, L. J. (1990). *Nursing diagnosis: Application to clinical practice* (4th ed.). Philadelphia: J. B. Lippincott.

Gleit, C., & Tatro, S. (1981). Nursing diagnoses for healthy individuals. *Nursing Health Care, 2,* 456–457.

Gordon, M. (1990). Towards theory-based diagnostic categories. *Nursing Diagnoses, 1*(1), 5–11.

Levin, R. F., Krainovitch, B. C., Bahrenburg, E., & Mitchell, C. A. (1989). Diagnostic content validity of nursing diagnoses. *Image—The Journal of Nursing Scholarship, 21*(1), 40–44.

McCourt, A. (1991). Syndromes in nursing. In R. M. Carroll-Johnson (Ed.), *Classification of nursing diagnoses: Proceedings of the ninth NANDA national conference.* Philadelphia: J. B. Lippincott.

North American Nursing Diagnosis Association. (1992). *Taxonomy of nursing diagnoses.* Philadelphia: Author.

Norris, J., & Kunes-Connell, M. (1987). Self-esteem disturbance: A clinical validation study. In A. McLane (Ed.), *Classification of nursing diagnoses: Proceedings of the seventh NANDA national conference.* St. Louis: C. V. Mosby.

Popkess-Vawter, S. (1984). Strength-oriented nursing diagnoses. In M. J. Kim, G. McFarland, & A. McLane (Eds.), *Classification of nursing diagnoses.* St. Louis: C. V. Mosby.

Stolte, K. M. (1996). *Wellness: Nursing diagnosis for health promotion.* Philadelphia: J. B. Lippincott.

3

The Bifocal Clinical Practice Model

The official NANDA definition of nursing diagnosis, as discussed in Chapter 1, specifically links nursing diagnosis to nursing interventions. But what about other clinical situations—those not covered by nursing diagnosis—that necessitate nursing intervention? Where do they fit in the scope of nursing practice?

Along with nursing diagnoses and interventions, nursing practice also often involves collaborative relationships with other health care disciplines. Frequently, such collaboration provides the nurse with additional interventions to add to the client's nursing care plan. As in any collaborative relationship, functions and activities sometimes overlap.

In 1983, Carpenito (1983) introduced a model for practice that describes the clinical focus of professional nurses. This *bifocal clinical practice model* identifies the two clinical situations in which nurses intervene—one as primary prescriber and the other in collaboration with other disciplines. This model not only organizes the focus of nursing practice, but helps distinguish nursing from other health care disciplines.

Nursing's theoretical knowledge derives from various fields, including the natural, physical, and behavioral sciences, the humanities, and nursing sciences. In fact, the major differences between nursing and the other health care disciplines with which it interacts lie in nursing's greater breadth of focus. Certainly, the nutritionist has more expertise in the field of nutrition, and the pharmacist in the field of therapeutic pharmacology, than any nurse has. But every nurse brings a knowledge of nutrition and pharmacology to client interactions that is sufficient for most clinical situations. (And when a nurse's knowledge is insufficient for a situation, nursing practice calls for consultation with appropriate disciplines.) No other discipline has this wide knowledge base, possibly explaining why past attempts to substitute other disciplines for nursing have proved costly and ultimately unsuccessful.

For this reason, any workable model for nursing practice must encompass all the varied situations in which nurses intervene, while also identifying situations in nursing that nonnursing personnel must address. These situations can be organized into five categories, as follows:

- Pathophysiologic (*e.g.*, myocardial infarction, borderline personality, burns)
- Treatment-related (*e.g.*, anticoagulant therapy, dialysis, arteriography)
- Personal (*e.g.*, dying, divorce, relocation)
- Environmental (*e.g.*, overcrowded school, no handrails on steps, rodents)
- Maturational (*e.g.*, peer pressure, parenthood, and aging)

Nursing prescribes for and treats client and group *responses* to situations. The bifocal clinical practice model, diagrammed in Figure 3-1, identifies these responses as either *nursing diagnoses* or *collaborative problems*. Together, nursing diagnoses and collaborative problems comprise the range of responses that nurses treat and as such define the unique nature of nursing. Table 3-1 describes the basic assumptions on which the bifocal clinical practice model rests.

Developing specific nursing diagnoses to describe all situations in which nurses intervene would result in a huge, unwieldy list. Attempting to attach a nursing diagnosis to every facet of nursing practice likewise would lead to misuse of nursing diagnoses.

The classification of certain situations as collaborative problems has helped minimize such problems while further refining the scope of nursing practice.

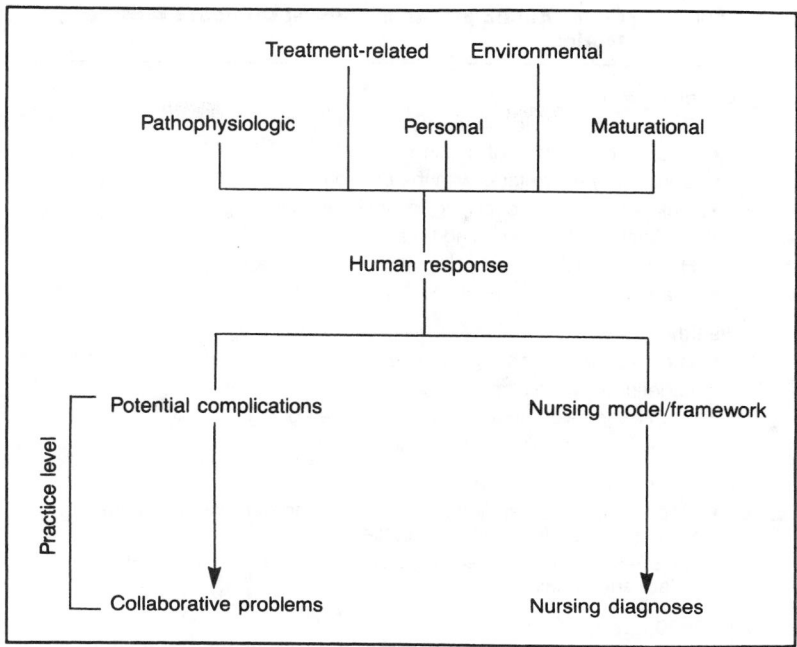

Fig. 3-1 Bifocal clinical nursing model. (© 1985, Lynda Juall Carpenito)

Understanding Collaborative Problems

Collaborative problems are certain physiologic complications that nurses monitor to detect onset or changes in status. Nurses manage collaborative problems using physician-prescribed and nursing-prescribed interventions to minimize the complications of the events.

The designation "certain" clarifies that all physiologic complications are not collaborative problems. If the nurse can prevent the onset of the complication or provide the primary treatment, then the diagnosis is a nursing diagnosis. For example:

Nurses Can Prevent	Nursing Diagnosis
Pressure ulcers	Risk for Impaired Skin Integrity
Thrombophlebitis	Risk for Altered Peripheral Tissue Perfusion
Complications of immobility	Disuse Syndrome
Aspiration	Risk for Aspiration

Nurses Can Treat	Nursing Diagnosis
Stage I or II pressure ulcers	Impaired Skin Integrity
Swallowing problems	Impaired Swallowing
Ineffective cough	Ineffective Airway Clearing

Nurses Cannot Prevent
Paralytic ileus
Bleeding

Unlike medical diagnoses, however, nursing diagnoses represent situations that are the primary responsibility of nurses, who diagnose onset and manage changes in status. When a situation no longer requires nursing management, the client is discharged from nursing care. In some cases, a collaborative problem can revert to a medical diagnosis after discharge from

Table 3-1   **Major Assumptions in Bifocal Clinical Practice Model**

Client
- Refers to an individual group, or community
- Has the power for self-healing
- Continually interrelates with the environment
- Makes decisions according to individual priorities
- Is a unified whole, seeking balance
- Has individual worth and dignity
- Is an expert on own health

Health
- Is dynamic, ever-changing state
- Is defined by the client
- Is an expression of optimum level of well-being
- Is the responsibility of the client

Environment
- Represents external factors, situations, and persons who influenced or are influenced by the client
- Includes physical and ecologic environments, life events, and treatment modalities

Nursing
- Is accessed by the client when assistance is needed to improve, restore, or maintain health or to achieve a peaceful death (Henderson & Nite, 1960)
- Engages the client to assume responsibility in self-healing decisions and practices
- Reduces or eliminates environmental factors that can or do cause compromised functioning

---

nursing care; for example, *Potential Complication: Ascites* could become a medical diagnosis of ascites. And certain physiologic complications are actually nursing diagnoses—for example, pressure ulcers (*Impaired Skin Integrity*)—because nurses can prescribe the definitive treatment.

For a collaborative problem, nursing focuses on monitoring for onset or change in status of physiologic complications and on responding to any such changes with physician- and nurse-prescribed nursing interventions. The nurse makes independent decisions for both collaborative problems and nursing diagnoses. The difference is that for nursing diagnoses, nursing prescribes the definitive treatment to achieve the desired outcome; in contrast, for collaborative problems, prescription for definitive treatment comes from both nursing and medicine.

Collaborative Problem Diagnostic Statements

All collaborative problems begin with the diagnostic label "Potential Complication" (or PC), for example:

- *Potential Complication: Hypokalemia*
- *Potential Complication: Sepsis*
- *Potential Complication: Asthma*

This label indicates that the nursing focus for collaborative problems is to reduce the severity of certain physiologic factors or events. For example, the diagnosis *Potential Complication: Hypertension* alerts the nurse that this client is either experiencing hypertension or is at high risk for hypertension. In either event, the nurse will receive a report on the status of the collaborative problem or will proceed to acquire baseline data on the client's blood pressure. Changing the terminology to distinguish whether the client is actually hypertensive or simply at risk is not necessary or realistic, given the fluctuating condition of most clients. Figure 3-2 illustrates this difference.

If the nurse is managing a cluster or group of complications, the collaborative problems may be recorded together, for example:

- *Potential Complications: Cardiac*
- *Potential Complications of pacemaker insertion*

The nurse also can word the collaborative problem to reflect a specific cause, as in *Potential Complication: Hyperglycemia related to long-term corticosteroid therapy*. In most cases, however, such a link is unnecessary.

When writing collaborative problem statements, the nurse must make sure not to omit the stem *Potential Complication*. This stem designates that nurse-prescribed interventions are required for its treatment. Without the stem, the collaborative problem could be misread as a medical diagnosis, in which case nursing involvement becomes subordinate to medicine, the discipline primarily responsible for the diagnosis and treatment of medical conditions.

Differentiating Nursing Diagnoses From Collaborative Problems

Both nursing diagnoses and collaborative problems involve all steps of the nursing process: assessment, diagnosis, planning, implementation, and evaluation. But each requires a different approach from the nurse. This section discusses some of the important differences in approach; refer to Chapters 5 and 6 for more detailed information on each aspect of the nursing process.

Assessment and Diagnosis

In nursing diagnoses, assessment involves data collection to identify signs and symptoms of actual nursing diagnoses or risk factors for high-risk nursing diagnoses. Assessment for collaborative problems focuses on determining physiologic stability or risk for instability. The nurse identifies a collaborative problem when certain situations are present that increase the client's vulnerability for the complication or when the client has experienced the complication.

Collaborative problems occur or probably will occur in association with a specific pathology or treatment. For example, all postoperative abdominal surgery clients are at some risk for certain problems, such as hemorrhage and hypoxia. Expert nursing knowledge is required to assess a particular client's specific risk for these problems and to identify problems early to prevent morbidity and mortality. Figure 3-3 illustrates the process of assessing for collaborative problems.

In contrast, nursing diagnoses sometimes can be predicted or expected with a high degree of certainty, but often require repeated assessments for validation. Because of the uniqueness

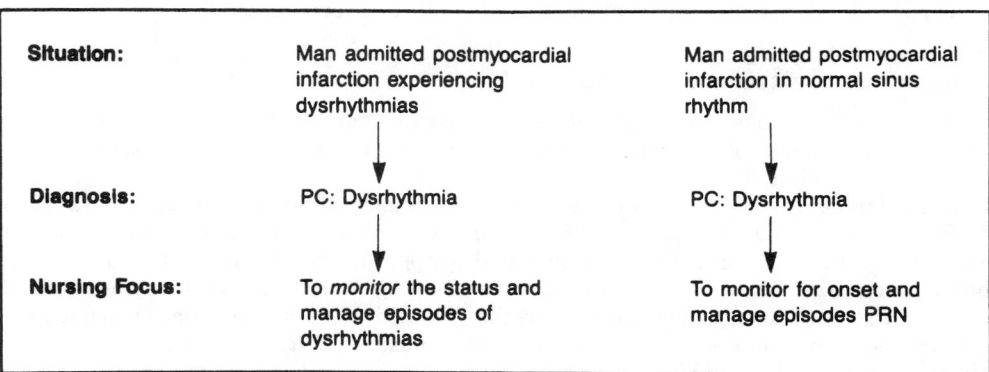

Fig. 3-2   Examples of types of collaborative problems.

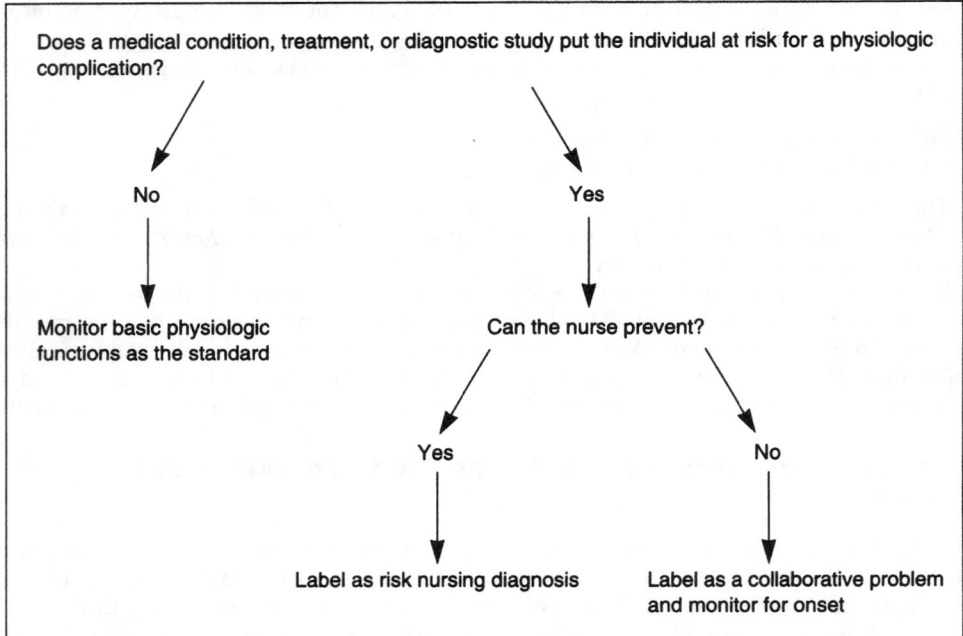

Fig. 3-3   Screening assessment.

of individual clients, identifying nursing diagnoses is often more difficult than identifying collaborative problems. This does not mean, however, that nursing diagnoses are more important. Importance is determined by each client's situation.

Goals

Nursing diagnoses and collaborative problems have different implications for expected outcomes. Bulechek and McCloskey (1985) define goals as "guideposts to the selection of nursing interventions and criteria in the evaluation of nursing interventions." These authors continue by saying that "readily identifiable and logical links should exist between the diagnoses and the plan of care, and the activities prescribed should assist or enable the client to meet the identified expected outcome." Thus, outcome criteria and interventions may be critical to differentiating nursing diagnoses from collaborative problems that nurses treat.

For example, if the diagnosis *Risk for Fluid Volume Deficit related to loss of fluid during surgery and possible hemorrhage postop* is formulated, the following client outcome may be written:

The client will demonstrate continued fluid balance, as evidenced by

- Absence of bleeding
- BP and pulse within normal limits

Client goals are used to determine the success or appropriateness of the nursing care plan. If the goals are not achieved or progress to achievement is not evident, then the nurse must revise the plan with the client.

In the foregoing example, if the client showed evidence of bleeding, would it be appropriate for the nurse to change the goals? What changes in the nursing care plan would the nurse make to stop the bleeding? Neither action would be appropriate. The nurse should confer with the physician for delegated orders to treat the bleeding. When the nurse writes client outcomes that require delegated medical orders for goal achievement, the situation is not a nursing diagnosis but a collaborative problem. Thus, for example, *Risk for Fluid Volume Deficit related to loss of fluid during surgery and possible hemorrhage postop* would be better described as *Potential Complication: Bleeding*.

Client outcome criteria are inappropriate for collaborative problems. They represent criteria that cannot be used to evaluate the effectiveness or appropriateness of nursing interventions. Outcome criteria for collaborative problems on multidisciplinary plans or critical paths are appropriate. Figure 3-4 illustrates the relationship of goals to nursing diagnoses and collaborative problems.

Intervention

According to Bulechek and McCloskey (1989), nursing interventions are "any direct care treatment that a nurse performs on behalf of a client. These treatments include nurse-initiated treatments resulting from nursing diagnoses, physician-initiated treatments resulting from medical diagnoses and performance of the daily essential functions for the client who cannot do these." By this definition, all nursing-initiated treatments are related to nursing diagnoses. This would mean that cardiac arrest, seizures, and hypokalemia should all be nursing diagnoses.

Nursing interventions can be classified as two types: nurse-prescribed and physician-prescribed (*delegated*). Regardless of type, all nursing interventions require astute nursing judgment because the nurse is legally accountable for intervening appropriately.

In 1987, Carpenito (1987) wrote that the relationship of diagnosis to nursing interventions is a critical element in defining nursing diagnosis. Many definitions of nursing diagnosis—including the 1990 NANDA definition—focus on the relationship of selected interventions to nursing diagnosis.

For both nursing diagnoses and collaborative problems, the nurse makes independent decisions concerning nursing interventions. The nature of these decisions differs, however. For nursing diagnoses, the nurse independently prescribes the primary treatment for out-

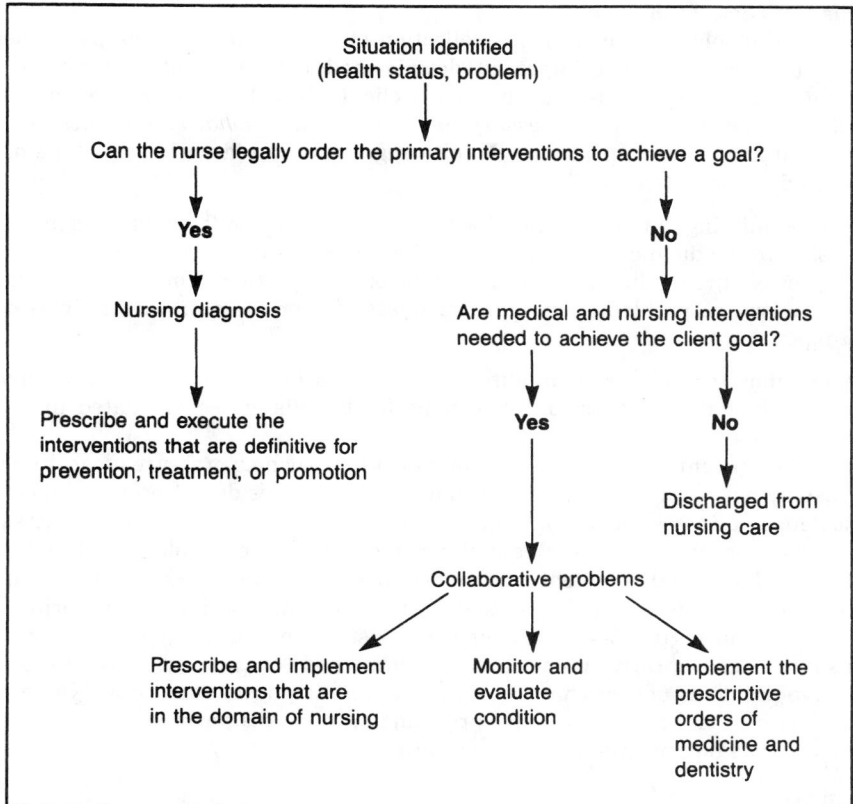

Fig. 3-4 Differentiating nursing diagnoses from collaborative problems. (© 1990, 1988, 1985, Lynda Juall Carpenito)

come achievement. In contrast, for collaborative problems, the nurse confers with a physician and implements physician-prescribed nursing interventions as well as nurse-prescribed interventions.

Primary treatment describes those interventions that are most responsible for successful outcome achievement. However, these are not the only interventions used to treat the diagnosed condition. For example, interventions for a client with the nursing diagnosis *Impaired Physical Mobility related to incisional pain* might include the following:

- Explain the need for moving and ambulation.
- Teach the client how to splint the incision before coughing, deep breathing, sitting up, or turning in bed.
- If pain relief medication is scheduled PRN, instruct the client to request medication as soon as pain returns.
- Evaluate if pain relief is satisfactory; if not, contact the physician for increased dosages or decreased time interval between doses.
- Schedule activities, bathing, and ambulation to correspond to times when the client's comfort level is highest.
- Discuss and negotiate ambulation goals with the client.

All of these are nurse-prescribed interventions. A physician-prescribed intervention for this client might be Demerol 75 mg IM q 4 h. This medication is important to manage the client's postoperative pain, but cannot be considered a primary treatment by itself.

Monitoring Versus Prevention

Is monitoring an intervention? It depends on the definition used. As previously noted, Bulechek and McCloskey define interventions as "treatments" that should directly influence the status of a client (1985).

Monitoring involves the continuous collection of selected data to evaluate whether the client's condition has changed (improved, deteriorated, not improved, or remained within a normal range). Monitoring does not improve a client's health status or prevent a problem; rather, it provides information necessary to determine *if* or *what type* of interventions are needed. Monitoring detects problems. Monitoring is associated with every type of nursing diagnosis and collaborative problem:

- For actual nursing diagnosis—monitor the client's condition for improvement
- For risk nursing diagnosis—monitor the client for signs of the problem
- For wellness nursing diagnosis—monitor the client's participation in lifestyle changes
- For collaborative problems—monitor for onset of a problem or change in status of an existing one

Although monitoring does not qualify as an intervention, it is an action. For convenience, monitoring is included with the interventions for the diagnoses presented in Sections II and III.

Nurses can prevent some physiologic complications, such as pressure ulcers and infection from invasive lines. Prevention differs from detection. Nurses do not prevent hemorrhage or paralytic ileus but, instead, monitor to detect its presence early to prevent greater severity of illness or even death. Physicians cannot treat collaborative problems without nursing's knowledge, vigilance, and judgment. For collaborative problems, nurses institute orders, such as position changes, client teaching, or specific protocols, in addition to monitoring.

The diagram in Figure 3-4 is designed to assist the nurse in differentiating a nursing diagnosis from a collaborative problem. As nursing's body of knowledge evolves, some of the collaborative problems of today may become nursing diagnoses tomorrow. Nurses are cautioned not to try to make a collaborative problem a nursing diagnosis simply because the latter is perceived as having greater value or status.

Evaluation

The nurse evaluates a client's status and progress differently for nursing diagnoses and for collaborative problems. When evaluating nursing diagnoses, the nurse

- Assesses the client's status
- Compares this response to the outcome criteria
- Concludes whether the client is progressing toward outcome achievement

The nurse can record this evaluation on a flow record or on a progress note. In contrast, to evaluate collaborative problems, the nurse

- Collects selected data
- Compares the data to established norms
- Judges whether the data are within an acceptable range

The nurse records the assessment data for collaborative problems on flow records or on progress notes if findings are significant. Nurses evaluate if the collaborative problem has improved or worsened, or is stable or unchanged. The physician is also notified if changes in treatment are indicated.

Thus, evaluation of nursing diagnoses focuses on progress toward achieving client goals, whereas evaluation for collaborative problems focuses on the client's status compared with established norms. Evaluation is discussed further in Chapter 5.

Case Study Examples

By using the criteria questions from Figure 3-4, the nurse can differentiate collaborative problems from nursing diagnoses, as illustrated in the following case studies.

Case Study 1

Mr. Smith, a 35-year-old-man, is admitted for a possible concussion after a car accident, with a physician's order for

- Clear liquid diet
- Neurologic assessment every hour

On admission the nurse records the following on a flow record:

- Oriented and alert
- Pupils 6 mm, equal, and reactive to light
- BP 120/72, pulse 84, resp 20, temp 99°F

Two hours later, the nurse records the following on the nurse's or progress note:

- Vomiting
- Restlessness
- Pupils 6 mm, equal, with a sluggish response to light
- BP 140/60, pulse 65, resp 12, temp 99°F

Problem: Possible increased intracranial pressure (ICP)
Now, apply the criteria questions to Case Study 1.

Q. Can the nurse legally order the primary interventions to achieve the client goal (which would be a reversal of the increasing ICP)?
A. No, nurses do not definitively treat or prevent increased ICP. They collaborate with the physician for definitive treatment.
Q. Are medical and nursing interventions needed for goal achievement?
A.   Yes
                                        ↓
                          Collaborative problem
                    PC: Increased Intracranial Pressure
                ↙   ↘
Prescribes and imple-   Monitors and evaluates   Implements the pre-
ments interventions   the client's condition   scriptive orders of
that are in the do-   medicine
main of nursing

In this situation, the nurse would monitor to detect increasing ICP. The nurse also prescribes interventions that reduce ICP, but these interventions are not considered primary and must be accompanied by treatments prescribed by physicians. This problem thus is the joint responsibility of medicine and nursing.

Case Study 2

Mr. Green is a 45-year-old-man with a cholecystectomy incision (10 days postop). The incision is not healing, and there is continual purulent drainage. The nursing care consists of

- Inspecting and cleansing the incision and the surrounding area q 8 h
- Applying Stomahesive and a drainage pouch to contain drainage and protect skin
- Promoting optimal nutrition and hydration to enhance healing

Problem: Adjacent skin at risk for erosion
Now apply the criteria questions to Case Study 2.

Q. Can the nurse legally order the definitive interventions to achieve the goals (which would be continued intact surrounding tissue)?
↓
A. Yes, nurses do prescribe the interventions that will prevent skin erosion from occurring as a result of wound drainage.
↓
Nursing diagnosis
↓
Risk for Impaired Skin Integrity related to draining purulent wound

In this situation, the nurse would prescribe the interventions to preserve adjacent skin. No collaboration with medicine is warranted.

Because each client is unique, it is difficult to develop exclusive criteria that will always differentiate nursing diagnoses from other client problems. Ultimately, the decision to use or not to use a diagnostic label rests with the individual nurse until more refined defining characteristics for each diagnosis are developed and tested.

Learning to formulate nursing diagnoses requires knowledge and practice. The nurse needs to familiarize herself with the nursing diagnoses and their components. Certain ones, such as *Altered Bowel Elimination* and *Altered Nutrition*, are familiar to most nurses and thus are easier to use. Section II provides specific information on each diagnosis to increase working knowledge of the various diagnosis.

Summary

According to Wallace and Ivey (1989), "understanding which nursing diagnoses are most effective and the situations in which the term collaborative problem is best applied helps group the mass of data the nurse must consider." The bifocal clinical practice model provides a structure for forming this understanding. In doing so, it uniquely distinguishes nursing from other health care professions, while providing nurses with a logical description of the focus of clinical nursing.

References

Bulechek, G., & McCloskey, J. (1985). *Nursing interventions: Treatments for nursing diagnoses*. Philadelphia: W. B. Saunders.

Bulechek, G., & McCloskey, J. (1989). Nursing interventions: Treatments for potential nursing diagnoses. In R. M. Carroll-Johnson (Ed.), *Classification of nursing diagnoses: Proceedings of the eighth national conference.* Philadelphia: J. B. Lippincott.

Carpenito, L. J. (1983). *Nursing diagnosis: Application to clinical practice*. Philadelphia, J.B. Lippincott.

Carpenito, L. J. (1987). *Nursing diagnosis: Application to clinical practice* (2nd ed.). Philadelphia: J.B. Lippincott.

Carpenito, L. J. (1989). *Nursing diagnosis: Application to clinical practice* (3rd ed.). Philadelphia: J. B. Lippincott.

Carpenito, L. J. (1995). *Nursing care plans and documentation: Nursing diagnoses and collaborative problems* (2nd ed.). Philadelphia: J. B. Lippincott.

Gordon, M. (1987). *Nursing diagnosis: Process and application* (2nd ed.). New York: McGraw-Hill.

Henderson, U., & Nite, G. (1960). *Principles and practice of nursing* (5th ed.). New York: Macmillan.

Wallace, D., & Ivey, J. (1989). The bifocal clinical nursing model: Descriptions and application to patients receiving thrombolytic or anticoagulant therapy. *Journal of Cardiovascular Nursing, 4*(1), 33–45.

4

Nursing Diagnoses:
Issues and Controversies

Nursing diagnosis arouses some emotion in almost every nurse. Responses range from apathy to excitement, from rejection to enthusiasm for scientific investigation. Despite the fact that nursing diagnoses have been an accepted part of professional nursing practice for almost 25 years, some nurses continue to resist using them. This chapter explores some of the most commonly cited reasons for doing so, including the following:

- Why can't we just use the words we've always used?
- Other disciplines will not understand our diagnoses.
- Clients will not understand our diagnoses.
- Nursing diagnoses are not needed by nurse practitioners, nurse anesthetists, or nurse midwives.
- Nursing diagnoses are not culturally sensitive.
- It is unethical to label behaviors.
- Nursing diagnoses can violate confidentiality.

Why Can't We Just Use The Words
That We've Always Used?

What are the words that nurses have always used? Diabetes mellitus? Prematurity? Pneumonia? Cystic fibrosis? For many years, nurses used only medical diagnoses to describe the client problems that they addressed. Gradually, however, nurses have learned that medical diagnoses do not describe many client problems in sufficient detail to enable other nurses to provide continuing care for clients with special needs.

Early on, Abdellah and Levine (1965, p. 25) pointed to the need for a specialized nursing language to describe nursing practice:

> *Crucial to the development of nursing science is the nurse's ability to make a nursing diagnosis and prescribe nursing actions that will result in specific responses in the client. Nursing diagnosis is a determination of the nature and extent of nursing problems presented by individual clients or families receiving nursing care. The position is taken that it is an independent function of the professional nurse to make a nursing diagnosis and to decide upon a course of action to be followed for the solution of the problem.*

Until 1973, when the first Conference for the Classification of Nursing Diagnosis convened, some attempts at classifying nursing actions were attempted, but were not sustained (*e.g.*, Henderson's needs, Abdellah's 21 nursing problems).

The fact is that nurses have always shared a common language for certain client problems with other disciplines, such as medicine, respiratory therapy, and physical therapy. Examples of terms from this language include hypokalemia, hypovolemic shock, hyperglycemia, and increased intracranial pressure. Any attempt to rename labels such as these should be viewed as foolhardy and unnecessary. For instance, dysrhythmias should not be renamed decreased cardiac output, nor should hyperglycemia be relabeled as altered carbohydrate metabolism.

This author takes the position that preestablished terminology should be used when appropriate, whether as a collaborative problem (*e.g.*, *Potential Complication: Hyperglycemia*) or as a nursing diagnosis (*e.g.*, *Risk for Pressure Ulcer*). Nursing should continue to use the terminology that clearly communicates a client situation or problem to other nurses and other disciplines.

Having said this, let us now examine the discipline-specific language of nurses. Have nurses had a common language or set of labels for client problems that they diagnose and treat in addition to the shared language previously discussed? Before the advent of nursing diagnoses, how did nurses describe client problems such as

- Inability to dress self
- Difficulty selecting among treatment options
- Risk for infection
- Breast-feeding problems
- Ineffective cough
- Spiritual dilemmas

Sometimes a nurse would use the terms listed above, but sometimes not. Often, the nurse had many options available to describe a problem. For example, a nurse may use any of the following terms to describe a client at risk for pressure ulcers:

- Immobility
- Comatose
- Decubitus ulcers
- Reddened skin
- Incontinence
- Inability to turn in bed
- Bed sores
- Paralysis

An examination of this list reveals the inconsistency of the terms; some are signs and symptoms, some are causative factors, some are risk factors, and some are problems.

Some nurses, particularly those with much experience, want to be able to describe client problems in any way they wish. Although an experienced nurse may be able to decipher inconsistent terminology, how can the nursing profession teach its science to its students if every instructor, textbook, and staff nurse uses different words to describe the same situation? Consider medicine: How could medical students learn the difference between cirrhosis and cancer of the liver if "impaired liver function" were used to describe both situations? Medicine relies on a standardized classification system to teach its science and to communicate client problems to other disciplines. Nursing needs to do likewise.

So, although nurses traditionally have had a common language for certain problems, this language has been incomplete to describe all the client responses that nurses diagnose and treat. It is also important to emphasize that some responses labeled as nursing diagnoses (e.g., *Decisional Conflict* and *Powerlessness*) were nonexistent in the nursing literature as recently as 15 years ago. The official classification of these responses as nursing diagnoses has advanced their investigation and increased their presence in the nursing literature. For example, whereas in 1982 there were 2 citations in the literature on Powerlessness, the number increased to 113 by 1994.

Other Disciplines Will Not Understand Our Diagnoses

According to Seahill (1991), the use of nursing diagnosis in a multidisciplinary inpatient child psychiatry setting proved problematic, because this setting emphasized the "whole patient" and the importance of effective information sharing among disciplines. Let us examine the validity of this assertion. For the purposes of this discussion, health care disciplines are separated into three groups: medicine, licensed health care disciplines, and nonlicensed health care personnel.

Medicine

Because it is important for nurses to understand certain aspects of medical diagnoses, nurses have committed to learning these diagnoses and to be knowledgeable about current changes in conditions and treatments. But as physicians originally defined these conditions, how often did they say: "Do you think that nurses will understand (for example) disseminated intravascular coagulation?" Most likely never.

If it is important for a physician to understand such nursing diagnoses as *Spiritual Distress* or *Decisional Conflict*, then the physician can seek the pertinent knowledge as a nurse does. The nurse also should share information with the physician concerning nursing diagnoses that the client and nurse have identified as priorities. Multidisciplinary conferences provide an opportunity for this sharing. Some nursing diagnoses may prove useful to some physicians, such as those in primary care.

Licensed Health Care Disciplines

In addition to nursing, licensed health care disciplines include physical, occupational, speech, nutritional, respiratory, and recreational therapy and social service. Each of these disciplines is involved in care planning for clients—some in their individual departments and some as part of multidisciplinary teams. These disciplines should be introduced to the nursing diagnosis language and encouraged to use those diagnoses that are applicable to their discipline. Table 4-1 lists examples of nursing diagnoses that are often useful for other disciplines.

Sharing nursing diagnosis terminology with other disciplines can only strengthen the role of nursing and emphasize a multidisciplinary approach. Keep in mind, however, that other disciplines should not use nursing diagnoses to determine interventions that nurses should perform. For example, a physical therapist using the nursing diagnosis *Impaired Physical Mobility* will write interventions only for physical therapy, not for nursing. Refer to Chapter 6 for a discussion of multidisciplinary care planning.

Nonlicensed Health Care Personnel

In most acute, long-term, and community health care settings in the United States and Canada, nursing care is provided by registered nurses, licensed practical nurses, and registered nurse assistants, nursing aides, or technicians. It is not important that all nursing team members understand nursing diagnoses—but it is important that each team member understands the interventions for which he or she is responsible. For example, an aide may be expected to explain why a client needs to be repositioned every 2 hours and why he needs to be helped to the bathroom after eating, but may not be expected to explain the difference between functional and total incontinence.

Table 4-1 **Examples of Nursing Diagnoses Useful for Other Disciplines**

Physical Therapy
Self-Care Deficits
High Risk for Injury
Impaired Physical Mobility
Noncompliance
Unilateral Neglect
Fatigue

Occupational Therapy
Diversional Activity Deficit
Fatigue
Impaired Home Maintenance
Instrumental Self-Care Deficit

Social Service
Caregiver Role Strain
Ineffective Family Coping
Decisional Conflict
Altered Family Process
Impaired Home Maintenance
Instrumental Self-Care Deficit
Social Isolation

Speech Therapy
Impaired Communication
Impaired Swallowing
Altered Thought Processes

Nutritional Therapy
Altered Nutrition
Impaired Swallowing
Feeding Self-Care Deficit

Respiratory Therapy
High Risk for Aspiration
High Risk for Altered Respiratory Function
Ineffective Airway Clearance
Dysfunctional Weaning Response

Clients Will Not Understand Our Diagnoses

It is important for the client and family to understand and agree with the nursing diagnosis and the associated goals and interventions planned. The nurse should emphasize to the client and family that the nursing diagnosis terminology is designed primarily to give nurses consistent language for communicating this information. The nurse also can explain why a medical diagnosis does not describe the client's problems or concerns from a nurse–client perspective. Keep in mind that, regardless of the specific terminology used, the nurse must tailor all explanations to the client's and family's ability and readiness to learn, cultural background, educational level, and so forth. This will help promote understanding and decision making.

Nursing Diagnoses Are Not Needed by Nurse Practitioners, Nurse Anesthetists, and Nurse Midwives*

Advanced nursing practice has been a hot topic of discussion in nursing circles and in legislative forums. Many state boards of nursing have defined or are in the process of defining advanced practice. For example, the Florida Board of Nursing defines an advanced registered nurse practitioner as "educated to perform in the monitoring and altering of drug therapies and initiation of appropriate therapies according to the established protocol and consistent with the practice setting" (1988, p. 16). The 1995–1996 annual update in the journal *Nurse Practitioner* presented the legislation for reimbursement and prescriptive authority and the source of the legal authority for nurses in advanced practice. Currently, 48 states grant nurse practitioners some form of prescriptive authority; in 15 states, nurse practitioners can prescribe independently (Pearson, 1996). In the last 10 years, prescriptive and protocol authority for certain nurses has come to be equated with advanced practice.

In reality, nurse practitioners are responsible for diagnosing medical problems and initiating treatment. For some acute conditions (*e.g.*, respiratory infection), this diagnosis may be all that is needed. If, however, a client returns with repeated infections, then the nurse practitioner needs to obtain more data to ensure that another medical diagnosis is not present or to identify poor client health habits (*e.g.*, inadequate rest or nutrition) that may be contributing to the problem.

An editorial in the *Journal of Pediatric Nurse Practitioners* described nursing diagnoses as "a separate language that is often burdensome and has the potential to be misunderstood by those not educated in the use of the language" (Nelms, 1991). The writer went on to state that "as editor of this journal, I find few [pediatric nurse practitioners] submit articles that include nursing diagnoses. Is that because we do not use them?" (Nelms, 1991).

Advanced nurses demonstrate expert nursing practice by diagnosing client responses to varied situations (*e.g.*, medical diagnoses, personal or maturational crises), which are nursing diagnoses. An advanced nurse would explore such questions as

- How has the client's ability to function changed since his cerebrovascular accident?
- How has a family system changed, or how is it vulnerable because of an ill neonate who required several months of hospitalization?

Compared with nursing, medicine has little to offer clients and families experiencing chronic disease such as multiple sclerosis or diabetes. Clients' most common complaints do not involve the medical care they receive, but rather focus on dissatisfaction with how their other problems are addressed. Nurses are in the optimum position to address such problems and increase client satisfaction with health care.

Certain complex nursing diagnoses are beyond the scope of practice of the average registered nurse. Examples of such advanced nursing diagnoses include:

* Excerpted from Carpenito, L. J. (1992, February). *Are nurse practitioners expert nurses?* Paper presented at the 11th Annual National Nursing Symposium, Advanced Practice Within a Restructured Health Care Environment, Los Angeles.

- *Risk for Caregiver Stress*
- *Powerlessness*
- *Risk for Ineffective Coping*
- *Risk for Altered Parenting*

A nurse cannot learn the diagnosis and treatment of advanced nursing diagnoses on the job. Rather, she must study the theory and concepts behind them to learn how to put them into practice. Nursing science is no less rigorous, less scientific, or less difficult to learn than medical science. If nurses in advanced practice do not use nursing diagnosis terminology, but only treat the nursing diagnosis concept, they fail to define their practice as nursing.

Nurse practitioners, nurse anesthetists, or nurse midwives who do not formulate or treat nursing diagnoses are not practicing as expert nurses. To evaluate this practice, a nurse in advanced practice should ask: Do I consult with physician colleagues for complex medical problems? Do physicians consult with me for complex nursing diagnoses? If the answer is no, the nurse should explore the reason why not. Does the problem lie with the physician's attitude, or is the nurse not overtly demonstrating diagnosis and treatment of nursing diagnoses? Or is the nurse not practicing nursing?

If nurse practitioners, nurse anesthetists, and nurse midwives do not define their practice as requiring an advanced degree in nursing, as diagnosing and treating selected medical diagnoses using protocols, and as formulating and treating nursing diagnoses, 5 years from now these nurses may still be struggling to define their roles.

Carpenito (1995) uses nursing diagnoses to differentiate the discipline-specific expertise of nurse practitioners and physicians in primary care. Figure 4-1 illustrates this relationship.

Nursing Diagnoses Are Not Culturally Sensitive

Nursing diagnoses, specifically the NANDA classifications, have been accused of being insensitive to cultural considerations. According to Leininger (1990), major concerns with the NANDA classifications are the "problems of using, promoting, and implementing the taxonomy with such limited international or transcultural data, including theoretical cultural ideas, conditions, and practices in diverse cultures." Leininger (1990) also states that there are "a host of culture-specific illnesses and culture-bound syndromes that need to be documented and understood by nurses," because expressions of health care, wellness, and illness are different in different cultures.

NANDA is the clearinghouse for nursing diagnosis work from nurses in the United States and Canada. To date, no diagnoses have been submitted by nurses from other countries. Nursing diagnoses accepted by NANDA are based primarily on the dominant Anglo-American cultural values, norms, and standards. Never has this work been portrayed or disseminated as relevant to other cultures. Clearly, North America is home to hundreds of distinctly diverse ethnic groups—but the NANDA classifications do not address this cultural diversity.

How can nursing diagnosis represent the wide cultural diversity in North America? Only those nurses who deeply understand a particular culture can develop the culture-specific defining characteristics and risk factors to make a nursing diagnosis relevant. For example, Native American nurses and non–Native American nurses who care for Native American clients can examine NANDA's work and determine its relevance to Native American culture. They can promote necessary additions and revisions to the NANDA classifications and can also develop and submit culturally specific responses currently not on the NANDA list.

Many texts on nursing diagnosis have been translated for use outside of North America. Although these translations are done by nurses from different cultures, all too often important cultural differences are not addressed. If nursing diagnosis is determined to be useful as a concept, then nurses in other countries will need to develop diagnoses relevant to their particular cultures. The following two books specifically address nursing diagnoses from different cultural perspectives: *Planification des Soins Infirmiers* (Grondin, Lussier, Phaneuf, & Riopelle, 1990) from a French-Canadian perspective, and *Diagnostico de Enfermeria* (Luis, 1995) from a Spanish perspective.

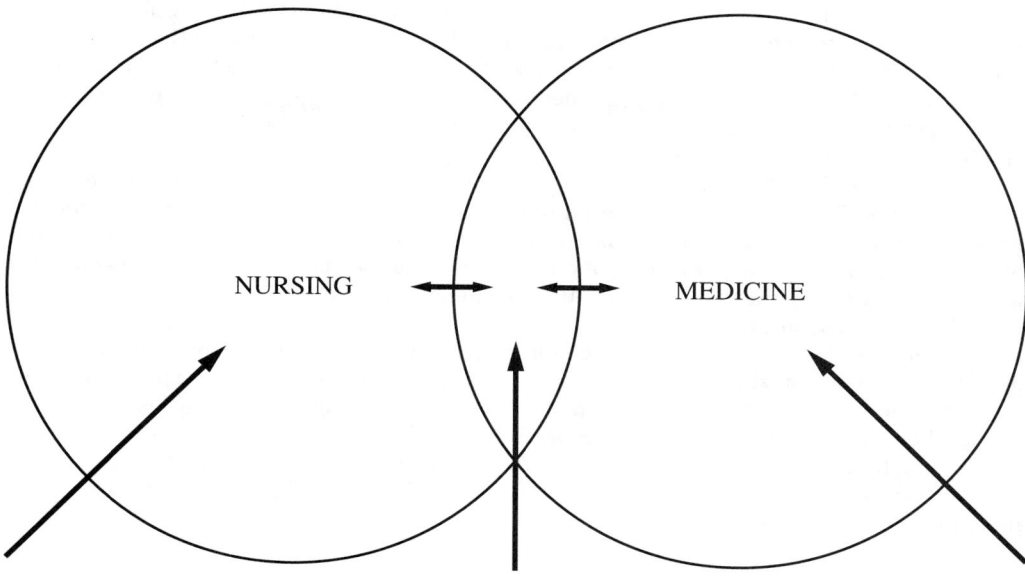

| Discipline Expertise | Shared Expertise | Discipline Expertise |

- Screens for high-risk individuals, families, or communities and teaches preventive strategies
- Diagnosis and management of complex altered functional responses of individuals, families, communities
- Utilizes a variety of intervention modalities, e.g., counseling, teaching, self-help, non-traditional therapies, negotiation
- Manages refractive health problems

- Primary prevention
- Secondary prevention
- Tertiary prevention
- Interview, history, and physical assessment
- Diagnosis of acute and chronic medical problems
- Uses prescriptions, interventions, and teaching to manage uncomplicated acute and chronic medical problems
- Seeks consultation when appropriate

- Differential diagnosing of complex medical problems
- Management of refractive acute medical problems
- Management of multisystem diseases with high morbidity or mortality

Fig. 4-1 Domains of expertise of primary care nurse practitioners and primary care physicians. (© 1995, Lynda Juall Carpenito; written permission needed to duplicate)

Keep in mind that a nursing diagnosis is not a judgment that nurses make about a client's or family's responses, values, or health based on *their own* cultural perspectives. Rather, it represents a response that the client or family finds problematic from his or their cultural perspective. For example, some cultures believe in fatalism; that is, one's fate and health are controlled by outside forces. The nurse unfamiliar with this belief may incorrectly diagnose the problem as Powerlessness. *Transcultural Considerations* are incorporated into Section II to increase the nurse's appreciation of cultural diversity.

Nursing Diagnosis Is Unethical

Nursing diagnosis has been criticized by some as emphasizing problem-based practice, encouraging professional arrogance, and requiring "value judgments by nurses about another's way of living, viewing self, being or relating with others" (Mitchell, 1991, p. 102). Case studies cited in the literature (Mitchell, 1991) of nursing diagnosis causing poor or unethical nursing care are interesting. Close examination of these cases reveals that the origin of the unacceptable nursing care rested in the nurse, not in the nursing diagnosis. Obviously, unsatisfactory, irresponsible, and unethical nursing care existed before the advent of nursing diagnosis.

According to Mitchell (1991), "when an individual's definition of health is not consistent with the nurse's, the person's health value is judged as ineffective, maladaptive, or dysfunctional" (p. 100). The nurse's determination of a client's response as ineffective, maladaptive, or dysfunctional should be based on the client's perspective of the problem and on the nurse's knowledge and expertise. A client's ineffective response is not ineffective for the nurse, but rather, is ineffective for the client.

To illustrate, let us examine the diagnosis *Dysfunctional Grieving*, with the defining characteristics of unsuccessful adaptation to loss, prolonged denial, depression, and delayed emotional reaction. How can a nurse diagnose dysfunctional grieving? What may be a sign or symptom of dysfunctional grieving in one person may not be such in another. The question is: For whom is the grieving dysfunctional? The client? The family? Or the nurse? For grieving to be dysfunctional, it must be dysfunctional for the person experiencing the grief. For example, if a mother visits the gravesite of her deceased child every day for 1 year after the child's death, is this dysfunctional? To determine if it is, the nurse should explore with this client whether these visits interfere with other necessary or enjoyable activities. What does she do when she is not visiting the gravesite? What would happen if she decreased the visits? Only through such a dialogue could the nurse and client be able to identify whether the client's grieving is dysfunctional or whether, perhaps, the client finds the visits comforting and an effective coping mechanism.

Nursing Diagnoses Can Violate Confidentiality

Nurses and other health professionals commonly are privy to significant personal concerns of clients under their care. According to the American Nurses Association Code of Ethics, "the nurse safeguards the client's right to privacy by judiciously protecting information of a confidential nature." However, the professional mandate to apply the nursing process for all clients sometimes places the nurse in a position of conflict. Certain information recorded in assessments and diagnostic statements may compromise a client's right to privacy, choice, or confidentiality. Nursing diagnostic statements should never be used to influence others to view or treat an individual, family, or group negatively. Great caution must be taken to ensure that a nursing diagnosis does no harm!

Nurses have a responsibility to make nursing diagnoses and to prescribe nursing treatments. Inherent in the diagnostic process and planning of care is the responsibility to ascertain that there is permission to write the diagnosis, treat the diagnosis, or refer the diagnosis as appropriate.

When a client shares personal information or emotions with the nurse, does this information automatically become part of the client's record or care plan? The nurse has two basic obligations to a client: to address applicable nursing diagnoses, and to protect the client's confidentiality. The nurse is *not* obligated to pass on all of a client's nursing diagnoses to other nurses, as long as the nurse can ensure that all diagnoses are addressed. Consider the following example: Ms. Jackson, age 45, is hospitalized for treatment of ovarian cancer. At one point, she states to the nurse "the God I worship did this to me, and I hate him for it." Further discussion validates that Ms. Jackson is disturbed about her feelings and changes in her previous beliefs. From these assessment data, the nurse develops the nursing diagnosis *Spiritual Distress related to conflict between disease occurrence and religious faith* for Ms. Jackson. But what should the nurse do with the information, which Ms. Jackson makes clear she considers confidential? The nurse can assist Ms. Jackson with this nursing diagnosis through several different avenues, including:

1. Apprising her of available community resources for follow-up assistance in dealing with her spiritual distress
2. Continue assisting her to explore her feelings and using the nurse's notes to reflect discussions (without using quotation marks to denote her actual words)
3. Recording the nursing diagnosis *Spiritual Distress* on the care plan and developing appropriate interventions
4. Referring her to an appropriate spiritual advisor

Analysis of Options

Option 1 returns the problem to the client for management after discharge. Sometimes the nature of a problem and its priority among the client's other problems makes providing the client or family with information on available resources for use after discharge the most appropriate option. The nurse should, however, be cautioned against using this option merely to "wash one's hands" of a problem.

Option 2 allows the nurse to continue a dialogue with the client about the problem, but without divulging the problem specifically. The problem with this option is that the client's care plan will not reflect this problem as a nursing diagnosis on the active list. As a result, should the client's nurse become unable to care for the client for some reason, this diagnosis likely would not be addressed.

Option 3 incorporates the problem, as a nursing diagnosis, into the client's care plan, where it can be addressed by the entire nursing staff. To help protect the confidentiality of very sensitive disclosed information, the nurse should make a few modifications, such as not quoting the client's statements exactly.

Documentation of the nursing diagnosis on the care plan raises another possible dilemma. What if the primary nurse whom the client or family has confided in is not able to follow the diagnosis full-time? How can the primary nurse involve others in addressing this diagnosis without violating the client's confidentiality? The primary nurse should encourage the client to allow another nurse to intervene in his or her absence. If the client refuses referral or another nurse, the nurse should document this in the progress notes, continuing to protect the client's confidentiality. For example:

> Discussed with Ms. Jackson the feasibility of another nurse intervening with her regarding her spiritual concerns in my absence. Ms. Jackson declined involvement of another nurse. Instructed her on whom to contact if she changes her mind.

This note documents the nurse's responsibility to the client as well as the nurse's accountability.

It is also important to note that, in most cases, the nurse should not share confidential information with family members without the client's permission. However, exceptions to preserving confidentiality "may be necessary if the information the client shares with the nurse contains indications of a threat to the lives of the patient or others" (Curtin & Flaherty, 1982).

Option 4 is a commonly chosen action for clients with spiritual conflicts. Before referring a client, however, the nurse should ascertain the client's receptivity to such a referral. To assume receptivity without first consulting the client can be problematic. The client chose to share very personal information with a particular nurse, who then is obligated to assist the client with the problem. If the nurse believes that a religious leader or another professional would be beneficial to the client, the nurse should approach the client with the option. An example of such a dialogue follows:

> Ms. Jackson, we've been discussing your concerns about your illness and how it has changed your spiritual beliefs. I know someone who has been very helpful for people with concerns similar to yours. I'd like to ask her to visit you. What do you think about this?

Such a dialogue clearly designates the choice as Ms. Jackson's. Just as nurses have an obligation to inform clients and families of available resources, clients have the right to accept or reject these resources.

Summary

Nursing diagnosis has sparked much debate, with some in favor and some not. Too often, those opposed to nursing diagnosis practice in isolation as primary providers and see no need for diagnoses in their nurse–client relationships. If they engage in therapeutic interventions, they are engaged in treating phenomena. They see no need for diagnoses, yet they must analyze responses, which directs them to future interventions. If intervening is not part of a nurse–client relationship, then perhaps there is no nurse–client relationship. Nursing actively assists clients, families, or communities to reduce or eliminate problems, reduce risk factors, prevent problems, and promote healthier lifestyles.

Nursing diagnosis provides nursing with a framework within which to organize its science. It is, however, each individual nurse's responsibility to apply nursing diagnoses with caution and care.

References

Abdellah, F. G., & Levine, E. (1965). *Better patient care through nursing research*. New York: Macmillan.

Carpenito, L. J. (1995). *Nurse practitioner and physician discipline specific expertise in primary care*. Unpublished manuscript.

Curtin, L., & Flaherty, M. J. (1982). *Nursing ethics*. Bowie, MD: Brady Communications.

Florida Board of Nursing. (1988). *Administrative policies pertaining to certification of advanced registered nurse practitioners*. Rule chapter 210–11, pp. 15–17.

Grondin, L., Lussier, R., Phaneuf, M., & Riopelle, L. (1990). *Planification des soins infirmiers*. Montreal: Les Editions de la Cheneliere.

Leininger, M. (1990). Issues, questions, and concerns related to the nursing diagnosis cultural movement from a transcultural nursing perspective. *Journal of Transcultural Nursing, 2*, 23–32.

Luis, M. T. (1995). *Diagnostico de enfermeria* (2nd ed.). Barcelona: Doyma.

Mitchell, G. J. (1991). Nursing diagnosis: An ethical analysis. *Image—The Journal of Nursing Scholarship, 23*, 99–103.

Nelms, B. C. (1991). Nursing diagnosis: Opinions please [editorial]. *Journal of Pediatric Health Care, 5*, 1.

Pearson, L. (1996). Annual update of how each state stands on legislative issues affecting advanced practice. *Nurse Practitioner, 21*(1), 10, 12–14, 16, 21–23.

Seahill, L. (1991). Nursing diagnosis vs. goal oriented treatment planning in inpatient child psychiatry. *Image: The Journal of Nursing Scholarship, 23*, 95–97.

5

Deriving Nursing Diagnoses: Assessment and Diagnosis

Each client is an autonomous and precious person who interacts in a unique manner with the environment and must be assessed within the context of this uniqueness. Because nursing diagnoses are derived from these assessments, and because the client is continually interacting with the environment, the nurse must apply the process in a continuous round of assessing, diagnosing, planning, implementing, and evaluating. Nursing diagnosis cannot be taken out of the nursing process context. To do so would result in a misuse of the concept and would lead to premature labeling or stereotyping. This, in turn, would interfere with accurate and careful observations and result in inappropriate nursing interventions.

Figure 5-1 illustrates the cyclic relationship of each step of the nursing process to the other steps and to the whole. Each step depends on the accuracy of the step preceding it; assessment and evaluation are related to diagnosis, planning, and implementation. For example, when implementing the plan, the nurse also is assessing the client's current condition and evaluating response to the interventions. Thus, the separation into five steps is for explanation purposes; in reality, the process is continuous and the steps are interrelated.

After a client has sought health care in his or her home, office, clinic, hospital, or institution, the nurse uses systematic assessment and problem-solving techniques to evaluate the client's functional status: Is it positive or altered, or is the client at risk for altered functioning? Does the client identify a problem with his or her health status? The nurse and client collaborate on planning and implementing appropriate interventions and on evaluating the effectiveness of these interventions. The nursing process describes this method, for through its five components—assessment, diagnosis, planning, intervention, and evaluation—it sets the practice of nursing in motion.

Assessment

The first step of the nursing process, assessment, is the deliberate and systematic collection of data to determine a client's current and past health status and functional status and to evaluate the client's present and past coping patterns. Data are obtained by five methods:

- Interview
- Physical examination
- Observation
- Review of records and diagnostic reports
- Collaboration with colleagues

    Data collection focuses on identifying the client's

- Present and past health status
- Present and past coping patterns (strengths and limitations)
- Present and past functional status
- Response to therapy (nursing, medical)
- Risk for potential problems
- Desire for a higher level of wellness

Nurses collect data to determine the need for nursing service and to assist other professionals (*e.g.*, pharmacists, nutritionists, social workers, physicians) in determining their activities. It is therefore important that health care professionals freely exchange data about their clients to increase the quality and the validity of health care. For example, a nurse assesses the signs of orthostatic hypotension in a client, then refers the client to a physician to investigate the cause and determine the treatment. The nurse plans nursing activities to help the client reduce those factors that contribute to the vertigo and also to prevent injury.

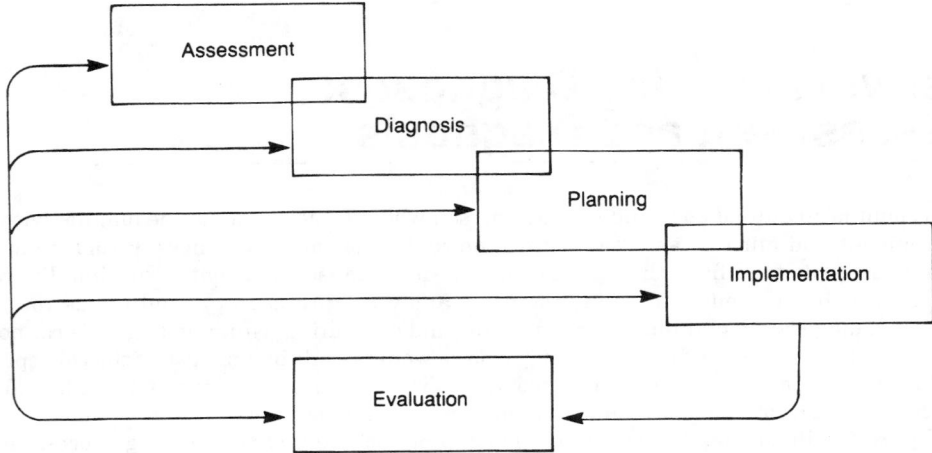

Fig. 5-1   Relationships between the steps of the nursing process. (Alfaro, R. [1990]. *Application of nursing process: A step-by-step guide.* Philadelphia: J.B. Lippincott.)

Unfortunately, many nurses gather physiologic data primarily for other professionals to use and ignore the other life processes that involve psychological, sociocultural, developmental, and spiritual considerations. From a holistic point of view, the nurse needs an understanding of the interaction patterns in all five areas to identify the client's strengths and limitations and to help him achieve optimal health. Ignoring any of the life processes can result in frustration and failure for all concerned.

Similar to the other components of the nursing process, the assessment process is dynamic and ongoing. During every nurse–client interaction, the nurse is continually processing data. The types of data gathered depend on the nurse's knowledge base, experience, and philosophy.

The Assessment Process

To perform an accurate assessment, the nurse must be able to

- Communicate effectively
- Observe systematically
- Interpret data accurately

Communicating Effectively

All nurse–client interactions are based on communication. The term *therapeutic communication* describes techniques that encourage the client or family to share views and feelings openly. The technique incorporates verbal and nonverbal skills, as well as empathy and a sense of caring. Verbal techniques include asking closed- and open-ended questions, exploring the answers, and validating responses. Nonverbal techniques include active listening and using silence, touch, and eye contact. Active listening, which is most vital in data collection, is the most difficult skill to learn. Few people listen objectively; most tend to concentrate on their own forthcoming responses, rather than on what the other person is saying. Elements of active listening include:

- Channeling attention to the sender and staying quiet within oneself
- Reducing or eliminating barriers
- Maintaining eye contact
- "Squaring off" eye-to-eye, shoulder-to-shoulder (positioning one's body in alignment with the other person's body)
- Avoiding interruptions
- Listening for feelings as well as words (Alfaro, 1994)
- Allowing pauses in conversation (Alfaro, 1994)

Barriers to active listening are always present; the professional nurse must take appropriate measures to eliminate them or their influence on an interaction. Table 5-1 lists some barriers to active listening.

Learning effective communication skills requires knowledge of self and of communication and learning theory, as well as continuous practice. Above all, it calls for the determination to retain sensitivity, which can be lost as more advanced communication skills are developed (Alfaro, 1994).

Observing Systematically

The ability to observe systematically depends on the nurse's knowledge base. Knowing what contributes to or causes a particular problem enables the nurse to explore these areas with the client. If the nurse does not know what a problem looks like, she will be unable to recognize and diagnose it. For example, if the nurse does not know the signs and symptoms of *Self-Concept Disturbance*, the presence of this response may be overlooked. Written guidelines can enhance systematic observation. Such guidelines are invaluable because they identify the specific types of data that should be collected. Once the nurse becomes familiar with the guidelines, the data can be gathered without referring to a written guide.

For each diagnosis listed in Section II, a focus assessment is presented to direct the nurse in gathering data to confirm or to rule out the nursing diagnosis.

Interpreting Data Accurately

After data collection, the nurse has large amounts of data. To interpret these data, the nurse must order them or group cues into chunks or patterns (Carnevali, 1993). These chunks are stored as a pattern representing something.

For example, the nurse learns to cluster a group of signs or symptoms that represent moderate anxiety as increased heart rate, dilated pupils, trembling, irritability, difficulty concentrating. When the nurse recognizes this cluster, an inference of moderate anxiety is made.

Cues Versus Inferences. A *cue* is information that is acquired through one or more of the five senses (taste, touch, smell, hearing, and sight). Primary sources of cues are subjective statements by the client and objective facts observed by the nurse. Secondary sources are family, other health care providers, and diagnostic studies. An *inference* is the nurse's judgment or interpretation of these cues. Inferences are always subjective and are influenced by the nurse's knowledge base, values, and experiences.

Table 5-1 **Barriers to Active Listening**

Internal

- The client's views are different from the nurse's perceptions.
- The client's appearance or accent is different or distracting.
- The client is in pain or is anxious.
- The client is telling the nurse something that he or she does not want to hear.
- The nurse feels dislike toward the client.
- The nurse is thinking of something else.
- The nurse is planning the next statement.
- The nurse is anxious or apprehensive.
- The nurse is in a hurry.

External

- There is noise from equipment, speakers, television, radio, etc.
- There is lack of privacy.
- There are physical hindrances such as desks, equipment, space, etc.
- Others make verbal remarks such as clichés, trite comments, or interruptions.

(Carnevito, L. J., & Duespohl, T. A. [1986]. *A guide to effective clinical instruction* [2nd ed.]. Rockville, MD: Aspen Systems Co.)

Cue	Corresponding Inference
Hgb 9.1	Abnormal
Crying	Possible fear, sadness
5 ft 1 in, 220 lb	Obesity

Differentiating between inferences and cues is important. Although an inference is a subjective judgment, nurses frequently report it as a fact or fail to gather sufficient cues to confirm it or rule it out. Inferences made with fewer or no supporting cues can result in inappropriate and sometimes dangerous care, especially when invalid inferences are passed on to other members of the health team.

Validating and Interpreting Data. As mentioned before, during data collection, the nurse is simultaneously validating and interpreting the data. Validating the data with the client helps the nurse avoid making incorrect inferences. If, for example, a client is observed crying in her room, the nurse familiar with the client's recent medical diagnosis of breast cancer may quite logically connect the crying (cue) with the diagnosis. That the nurse initially makes this inference is not wrong, but problems could result if the nurse does not validate this inference with the client. To validate, the nurse should say something like "I see that you're crying; would you like to talk about your feelings?" By doing so, the nurse may in fact discover that the client's crying is related to something other than her diagnosis, such as missing her loved ones.

Validation sometimes involves clarifying vague or ambiguous data with the client (Gordon, 1987). For example, a nurse assessing a client who states, "I feel drained," could interpret this statement in various ways, such as evidence of fatigue or stress. For validation, the nurse should ask the client to elaborate on the statement and provide more specific information. It is important to appreciate that in diagnosing human responses, sometimes cues are not obvious and clear (Carnevali, 1993). In addition, sometimes cues for more than one diagnosis overlap. For example, anger is a cue of several nursing diagnoses (*e.g.*, *Ineffective Coping, Anxiety, Fear, Altered Family Processes*, and *Caregiver Role Strain*).

Interpreting data involves two cognitive activities:

- Recognizing the cue or inference as significant
- Assigning meaning to the significance

A nurse recognizes the significance of data based on certain knowledge that denotes these data as abnormal or diagnostic. This knowledge can come from memory of similar experiences or from other nurses, nursing faculty, and professional books and journals. The client must be an active partner in data validation.

Past experiences or knowledge from other sources also can alert the nurse to the significance of certain cues found in preencounter data, the information available to the nurse before the initial assessment, such as age, racial or ethnic background, and medical diagnosis. Consider the following example: When assessing a 45-year-old woman with diabetes mellitus who has been admitted for abdominal surgery, the nurse finds a new lesion on the client's foot. When questioned, the client states that "It must be from my new shoes." Because of prior knowledge of the client's diabetes gained from preencounter data, the nurse would assign this assessment finding more significance than it might warrant in another client.

To summarize, data to support a nursing diagnosis must be a cluster of cues documented to represent the condition. By carefully validating observations and client complaints, the nurse can avoid or minimize potentially harmful inaccuracies in data interpretation.

Data Collection Formats

Data collection usually consists of two formats: the nursing baseline or screening assessment and the focus assessment. Each of these can be used either alone or in conjunction with the other.

Historically, the assessment forms used by nurses were organized under a body system format. Information collected under a body system model is useful to nursing, but is incomplete, because it does not include data on the areas of sleep, activity, spirituality, and so on. In an attempt to focus data collection on concerns that are more relevant to nursing, the body system model was discarded and replaced by a nursing model. Unfortunately, the nursing model alone failed to provide the nurse with complete data about physiologic functioning.

As was discussed in Chapter 3, nurses encounter, diagnose, and treat two types of responses: those that can be described by nursing diagnoses and those that represent collaborative problems. Each type requires a different assessment focus.

Initial Screening Assessment

An initial, baseline, or screening assessment involves collecting a predetermined set of data during the initial contact with the client, for example, on admission or first home visit. This assessment serves as a tool for "narrowing the universe of possibilities"(Gordon, 1987). During this assessment, the nurse interprets data as significant or insignificant. This process is explored later in this chapter.

Assessment Framework

As discussed earlier, nursing assessment should focus on collecting data that validate nursing diagnoses. Gordon's system of functional health patterns provides an excellent, relevant format for nursing data collection.

Functional Health Patterns. To direct the nurse in collecting data to determine an individual's or group's health status and functioning, Gordon developed a system for organizing a nursing assessment based on function (1987). After data collection is complete, the nurse and client can determine positive functioning, altered functioning, or at-risk status for altered functioning. Altered functioning is defined as functioning that is perceived as a negative change or as undesirable by the client (individual or group). These functional health patterns include:

1. Health Perception–Health Management Pattern
   - Perceived pattern of health, well-being
   - Knowledge of lifestyle and relationship to health
   - Knowledge of preventive health practices
   - Adherence to medical, nursing prescriptions
2. Nutritional–Metabolic Pattern
   - Usual pattern of food, fluid intake
   - Types of food, fluid intake
   - Actual weight, weight loss or gain
   - Appetite, preferences
3. Elimination Pattern
   - Bowel elimination pattern, changes
   - Bladder elimination pattern, changes
   - Control problems
   - Use of assistive devices
   - Use of medications
4. Activity–Exercise Pattern
   - Pattern of exercise, activity, leisure, recreation
   - Ability to perform activities of daily living (self-care, home maintenance, work, eating, shopping, cooking)
5. Sleep–Rest Pattern
   - Patterns of sleep, rest
   - Perception of quality, quantity
6. Cognitive–Perceptual Pattern
   - Vision, learning, taste, touch, smell
   - Language adequacy
   - Memory
   - Decision-making ability, patterns
   - Complaints of discomforts
7. Self-Perception–Self-Concept Pattern
   - Attitudes about self, sense of worth
   - Perception of abilities
   - Emotional patterns
   - Body image, identity

8. Role–Relationship Patterns
   - Patterns of relationships
   - Role responsibilities
   - Satisfaction with relationships and responsibilities
9. Sexuality–Reproductive Pattern
   - Menstrual, reproductive history
   - Satisfaction with sexual relationships, sexual identity
   - Premenopausal or postmenopausal problems
   - Accuracy of sex education
10. Coping–Stress Tolerance Patterns
    - Ability to manage stress
    - Knowledge of stress tolerance
    - Sources of support
    - Number of stressful life events in last year
11. Value–Belief Pattern
    - Values, goals, beliefs
    - Spiritual practices
    - Perceived conflicts in values

These functional health patterns are interrelated, interactive, and interdependent. When assessing functional health status, the nurse should encourage the client to share current and previous patterns of functioning.

Keep in mind that this standardization of assessment data should not interfere with the nurse's theoretical or philosophical beliefs. It simply directs the nurse to the initial data that should be collected, not to the approach that should be used in interpreting the data or determining interventions.

The initial assessment presented in Figure 5-2 is organized according to functional health patterns. It is designed to assist the nurse in gathering subjective and objective data. Should questions arise concerning a pattern, the nurse would gather more data about the diagnosis by using the focus assessment under the diagnosis.

When collecting data under the functional health patterns, the nurse questions, observes, and evaluates the client or family. For example, under the Cognitive–Perceptual Pattern, the nurse asks the client if she has difficulty hearing, observes if she is wearing a hearing aid, and evaluates if she understands English.

Physical Assessment. In addition to functional pattern assessment, the nurse also collects data related to body system functioning. Physical assessment, the collection of objective data concerning the client's physical status, incorporates head-to-toe examination, with a focus on the body systems. The techniques used include inspection, palpation, percussion, and auscultation.

What does a staff nurse do with the data acquired from physical assessment? If the answer is to report the findings only to a physician, perhaps the nurse should leave that portion of the examination to the physician. The important thing is to stress the assessment skills that are crucial for the nurse generalist. For example, the nurse needs to be able to identify signs of increased intracranial pressure, but not necessarily perform an entire neurologic examination. However, this does not mean that advanced skills should not be learned by nurses who routinely screen, case-find, and treat selected problems, such as staff nurses, neurology unit nurses, nurse practitioners, or clinical specialists.

Figure 5-2 lists those areas of physical assessment in which nurse generalists should be proficient. Physical assessment by nurses should be clearly "nursing" in focus. The individual nurse must decide how important it is to her own practice to learn to palpate livers, auscultate murmurs, or use an ophthalmoscope. By examining her philosophy and definition of nursing, the nurse should seek to develop expertise in those areas that will enhance her nursing practice.

Keep in mind that separation of functional health patterns from physical assessment is done for organizational purposes only. No useful nursing assessment framework can restrict actual data collection in such a manner. Because humans are open systems, positive or

(text continues on page 54)

NURSING ADMISSION DATA BASE

Date _____ Arrival Time _____ Contact Person _____ Phone _____

ADMITTED FROM: ___ Home alone   ___ Home with relative   ___ Long-term care
                  ___ Homeless   ___ Home with _____   facility
                  ___ ER   ___   (Specify)   ___ Other _____

MODE OF ARRIVAL: ___ Wheelchair   ___ Ambulance   ___ Stretcher

REASON FOR HOSPITALIZATION: _____
_____
_____

LAST HOSPITAL ADMISSION: Date _____ Reason _____
_____

PAST MEDICAL HISTORY: _____
_____

MEDICATION (Prescription/Over-the-Counter)	DOSAGE	LAST DOSE	FREQUENCY

HEALTH MAINTENANCE–PERCEPTION PATTERN

USE OF:

Tobacco: ___ None ___ Quit (date) ___ Pipe ___ Cigar ___ <1 pk/day
           ___ 1–2 pks/day ___ >2 pks/day Pks/year history _____

Alcohol: ___ Date of last drink ___ Amount/type
         ___ No. of days in a month when alcohol is consumed

Other Drugs: ___ No ___ Yes Type _____ Use _____

Allergies (drugs, food, tape, dyes): _____ Reaction _____
_____

ACTIVITY–EXERCISE PATTERN

SELF-CARE ABILITY:

0 = Independent   1 = Assistive device   2 = Assistance from others
3 = Assistance from person and equipment   4 = Dependent/Unable

	0	1	2	3	4
Eating/Drinking					
Bathing					
Dressing/Grooming					
Toileting					
Bed Mobility					
Transferring					
Ambulating					
Stair Climbing					
Shopping					
Cooking					
Home Maintenance					

ASSISTIVE DEVICES: ___ None ___ Crutches ___ Bedside commode ___ Walker
                   ___ Cane ___ Splint/Brace ___ Wheelchair ___ Other

CODE: (1) Not applicable (2) Unable to acquire
      (3) Not a priority at this time   (4) Other (specify in notes)

Side One

Fig. 5-2   Assessment form. (© 1990, 1988, Lynda Juall Carpenito)

NUTRITION–METABOLIC PATTERN
Special Diet/Supplements _____
Previous Dietary Instruction: ___ Yes ___ No
Appetite: ___ Normal ___ Increased ___ Decreased ___ Decreased taste sensation
___ Nausea___ Vomiting ___ Stomatitis
Weight Fluctuations Last 6 Months: ___ None _____ lbs. Gained/Lost
Swallowing difficulty (Dysphagia): ___ None ___ Solids ___ Liquids
Dentures: ___ Upper (_ Partial _ Full) ___ Lower (_ Partial _ Full)
With Person ___ Yes ___ No
History of Skin/Healing Problems: ___ None ___ Abnormal Healing ___Rash
___ Dryness ___ Excess Perspiration

ELIMINATION PATTERN
Bowel Habits: ___ # BMs/day ___ Date of last BM ___ Within normal limits
___ Constipation ___ Diarrhea ___ Incontinence
___ Ostomy: Type: ___ Appliance ___ Self-care ___ Yes ___ No
Bladder Habits: ___ WNL ___ Frequency ___ Dysuria ___ Nocturia ___ Urgency
___ Hematuria ___Retention
Incontinency: ___ No ___ Yes ___ Total ___ Daytime ___ Nighttime
___ Occasional ___ Difficulty delaying voiding
___ Difficulty reaching toilet
Assistive Devices: ___ Intermittent catheterization
___ Indwelling catheter ___ External catheter
___ Incontinent briefs ___ Penile implant type _____

SLEEP–REST PATTERN
Habits: ___ hrs/night ___ AM nap ___ PM nap
Feel rested after sleep ___ Yes ___ No
Problems: ___None ___ Early waking ___Insomnia ___ Nightmares

COGNITIVE–PERCEPTUAL PATTERN
Mental Status: ___Alert ___ Receptive aphasia ___ Poor historian
___ Oriented ___ Confused ___ Combative ___ Unresponsive
Speech: ___ Normal ___Slurred ___Garbled ___ Expressive aphasia
Spoken language _____ Interpreter _____
Language Spoken: ___ English ___ Spanish ___ Other _____
Ability to Read English: ___ Yes ___ No _____
Ability to Communicate: ___Yes ___ No _____
Ability to Comprehend: ___ Yes ___ No _____
Level of Anxiety: ___ Mild ___ Moderate ___ Severe ___ Panic
Interactive Skills: ___ Appropriate ___ Other _____
Hearing: ___ WNL ___ Impaired (_ Right _ Left) ___ Deaf (_ Right _ Left)
___ Hearing Aid ___ Tinnitus
Vision: ___ WNL ___ Eyeglasses ___ Contact lens
___ Impaired ___ Right ___ Left
___ Blind ___ Right ___ Left
___ Prosthesis ___ Right ___ Left
Vertigo: ___ Yes ___ No memory intact ___Yes ___ No
Discomfort/Pain: ___ None ___ Acute ___ Chronic ___ Description _____
_____
Pain Management: _____

COPING–STRESS TOLERANCE/SELF-PERCEPTION/SELF-CONCEPT PATTERN
Major concerns regarding hospitalization or illness (financial, self-care): _____
_____
Major loss/change in past year: ___ No ___ Yes _____
Fear of Violence ___ Yes ___ No Who_____
Outlook on Future _____ (rate 1–poor–to 10–very optimistic)

CODE: (1) Not applicable (2) Unable to acquire
(3) Not a priority at this time (4) Other (specify in notes)

Side Two

Fig. 5-2 (Continued)

SEXUALITY–REPRODUCTIVE PATTERN

LMP: _____ Gravida _____ Para _____
Menstrual/Hormonal Problems: ___ Yes ___ No _____
Last Pap Smear: _____ Hx of Abnormal PAP _____
Monthly Self-Breast/Testicular Exam: ___ Yes ___ No
Sexual Concerns R/T Illness: _____
_____

ROLE–RELATIONSHIP PATTERN

Marital status: _____
Occupation: _____
Employment Status: ___ Employed ___ Short-term disability
                   ___ Long-term disability ___ Unemployed
Support System: ___ Spouse ___ Neighbors/Friends ___ None
                ___ Family in same residence ___ Family in separate residence
                ___ Other _____
Family concerns regarding hospitalization: _____
_____

VALUE–BELIEF PATTERN

Religion: ___
Religious Restrictions: ___ No ___ Yes (Specify) _____
Request Chaplain Visitation at This Time: ___ Yes ___ No

PHYSICAL ASSESSMENT (Objective)

1. CLINICAL DATA
    Age _____ Height _____ Weight _____ (Actual/Approximate)
    Temperature _____
    Pulse: ___ Strong ___ Weak ___ Regular ___ Irregular
    Blood Pressure: Right Arm ___ Left Arm ___ Sitting ___ Lying ___

2. RESPIRATORY/CIRCULATORY
    Rate _____
    Quality: ___ WNL ___ Shallow ___ Rapid ___ Labored ___ Other _____
    Cough: ___ No ___ Yes/Describe _____
    Auscultation:
        Upper rt lobes ___ WNL ___ Decreased ___ Absent ___ Abnormal sounds ___
        Upper lt lobes ___ WNL ___ Decreased ___ Absent ___ Abnormal sounds ___
        Lower rt lobes ___ WNL ___ Decreased ___ Absent ___ Abnormal sounds ___
        Lower lt lobes ___ WNL ___ Decreased ___ Absent ___ Abnormal sounds ___
    Right Pedal Pulse: ___ Strong ___ Weak ___ Absent
    Left Pedal Pulse: ___ Strong ___ Weak ___ Absent

3. METABOLIC–INTEGUMENTARY
    SKIN:
        Color: ___ WNL ___ Pale ___ Cyanotic ___ Ashen ___ Jaundice ___ Other ___
        Temperature: ___ WNL ___ Warm ___ Cool
        Turgor: ___ WNL ___ Poor
        Edema: ___ No ___ Yes/Description/location _____
        Lesions: ___ None ___ Yes/Description/location _____
        Bruises: ___ None ___ Yes/Description/location _____
        Reddened: ___ No ___ Yes/Description/location _____
        Pruritus: ___ No ___ Yes/Description/location _____
        Tubes: Specify _____
        Changes _____ None, If Yes/Description/location _____
    MOUTH:
        Gums: ___ WNL ___ White plaque ___ Lesions ___ Other _____
        Teeth: ___ WNL ___ Other _____
    ABDOMEN:
        Bowel Sounds: ___ Present ___ Absent
                        Side Three

Fig. 5-2 (Continued)

4. NEURO/SENSORY

Pupils: ____ Equal ____ Unequal

    Left: • • • • • • • •

    Right: • • • • • • • •

Reactive to light:

    Left: ____ Yes ____ No/Specify _____

    Right: ____ Yes ____ No/Specify _____

Eyes: ____ Clear ____ Draining ____ Reddened ____ Other _____

5. MUSCULAR–SKELETAL

Range of Motion: ____ Full ____ Other _____

Balance and Gait: ____ Steady ____ Unsteady

Hand Grasps: ____ Equal ____ Strong ____ Weakness/Paralysis (__ Right __ Left)

Leg Muscles: ____ Equal ____ Strong ____ Weakness/Paralysis (__ Right __ Left)

DISCHARGE PLANNING

Lives: Alone ____ With _____ No known residence _____

Intended Destination Post Discharge: ____ Home ____ Undetermined ____ Other ____

Previous Utilization of Community Resources:

    ____ Home care/Hospice ____ Adult day care ____ Church groups ____ Other _____

    ____ Meals on Wheels ____ Homemaker/Home health aide ____ Community support group

Post-discharge Transportation:

    ____ Car ____ Ambulance ____ Bus/Taxi

    ____ Unable to determine at this time

Anticipated Financial Assistance Post-discharge?: ____ No ____ Yes _____

Anticipated Problems with Self-care Post-discharge?: ____ No ____ Yes _____

Assistive Devices Needed Post-discharge?: ____ No ____ Yes _____

Referrals: (record date)

    Discharge Coordinator _____ Home Health _____

    Social Service _____ V.N.A. _____

Other Comments: _____

SIGNATURE/TITLE _____ Date _____

Side Four

Fig. 5-2   (Continued)

altered functioning in one functional health pattern invariably influences body system functioning or functioning in another functional health pattern. The following case study illustrates this concept.

Mr. Gene, aged 61, is admitted for neurologic surgery. He has a history of peripheral vascular disease and Parkinson's disease. The nurse's initial assessment reveals the findings on page 55 under the functional health pattern Activity–Exercise Pattern and physical assessment of musculoskeletal function.

Depending on associated findings, these data could support various nursing diagnoses, such as *Self-Care Deficit, Risk for Disuse Syndrome*, and *Risk for Injury*. Two of these diagnoses—*Self-Care Deficit* and *Risk for Disuse Syndrome*—are grouped under the functional health pattern Activity–Exercise, whereas *Risk for Injury* is listed under Health Perception–Health Maintenance Patterns.

Abnormal or otherwise significant physical assessment data can support various nursing diagnoses or collaborative problems. For example, if inspection of Mr. Gene's feet revealed a lesion on his left instep, the nurse would assign the primary nursing diagnosis of *Impaired Skin Integrity*. If further questioning reveals that Mr. Gene does not understand why his feet are vulnerable and why daily foot care and inspection are necessary, the nurse would identify another nursing diagnosis for him: *Ineffective Management of Therapeutic Regimen related to insufficient knowledge of peripheral vascular disease and its effects on the feet.*

ACTIVITY–EXERCISE PATTERN

SELF-CARE ABILITY:

0 = Independent	1 = Assistive device
3 = Asssistance from person and equipment	

2 = Assistance from others	
4 = Dependent/Unable	

	0	1	2	3	4
Eating/Drinking	✓				
Bathing			✓		
Dressing/Grooming			✓		
Toileting			✓		
Bed Mobility			✓		
Transferring			✓		
Ambulating		✓			
Stair Climbing	✓				
Shopping					✓
Cooking					✓
Home Maintenance					✓

ASSISTIVE DEVICES: ____ None ____ Crutches ____ Bedside commode _✓_ Walker
____ Cane ____ Splint/Brace ____ Wheelchair ____ Other ____

PHYSICAL ASSESSMENT

MUSCULAR–SKELETAL

Range of Motion: _✓_ Full ____ Other _____

Balance and Gait: ____ Steady _✓_ Unsteady

Hand Grasps: _✓_ Equal _✓_ Strong ____ Weakness/Paralysis (____ Right ____ Left)

Leg Muscles: ____ Equal ____ Strong _✓_ Weakness/Paralysis (_✓_ Right ____ Left)

Assessment Format

Initial assessment should be organized to permit systematic, efficient data collection. The assessment form in Figure 5-2 illustrates checking or circling options, which can help save time when documenting findings. The nurse can always elaborate with additional questions and comments. Certain functional areas are better assessed using open-ended questions. A printed data assessment form should be viewed as a guide for the nurse, not a mandate. Before requesting information from a client, the nurse should ask herself, "What am I going to do with the data?" If certain information is useless or irrelevant for a particular client, then its collection is unnecessary and may be distressing to the client. Asking a terminally ill client how much he smokes or drinks, for example, is inexcusable unless the nurse has a specific goal. If a client will be NPO for an unlimited time, it is probably unnecessary to collect data on eating habits. This assessment will be indicated when the client resumes a diet.

If the client is extremely stressed, the nurse should collect only necessary data and defer the collection of functional patterns to another time or day. A stressed client may not be the best source of data because stress may cloud the memory.

The admission interview form can be structured to allow for deferring or not collecting certain data. (Answer code appears on bottom of pages in Figure 5-2.) If desired, the admission assessment form can be marked to indicate selected items that must always be assessed (unless, of course, the information cannot be acquired). When each question on the assessment form has either an answer or an answer code of 1, 3, or 4, the form should be viewed as complete. When the answer code of 2 is used, the form can be viewed as incomplete. If the information is collected later, the nurse should enter it on the form, then date and initial it, as shown in the following sample:

HEALTH MAINTENANCE–PRESCRIPTION PATTERN

USE OF: *7/8 ℒℊC*
2 Tobacco: ✓ None ____ Quit (date) ____ Pipe ____ Cigar ____ <1 pk/day
                     ____ 1–2 pks/day ____ >2 pks/day Pks/year history _____
2 Alcohol: *7/8* ✓ None ____ Type/amount ____ /day ____ /wk ____ /month
2 Other Drugs: *7/8* ✓ No ____ Yes Type _____ Use _____
2 Allergies (drugs, food, tape, dyes): *none known* Reaction _____
                   7/8 ℒ ℊC

In an acute care setting, initial assessment should be completed as soon as possible after admission, preferably within 8 hours. In other care settings (such as community health, rehabilitation, mental health, and extended-care facilities), performing a baseline assessment may be more appropriate at later client contacts, rather than on initial contact. Obviously, a nurse–client relationship that evolves over weeks or months allows a more detailed baseline assessment than can be obtained in an acute care setting. Keep in mind, however, that if a complete baseline assessment is delayed, the nurse still should perform an abbreviated initial assessment of critical functions, such as elimination, self-care ability, and respiratory status. See Appendices II, III, IV, V, and XII for sample screening assessment forms appropriate for mental health care settings, pediatric clients, extended care settings, and maternal and oncology clients, respectively.

Focus Assessment

Focus assessment, which can take a few minutes or longer, is the acquisition of selected or specific data as determined by the nurse and the client or family, or by the client's condition. The nurse who assesses the condition of a new postoperative client (vital signs, incision, hydration, comfort) is performing a focus assessment.

A focus assessment can also be performed during the initial interview if the data collected suggest a possible problem area that needs to be validated or ruled out. For example, during the baseline interview, the nurse suspects that certain data (S_1, S_2) may represent a nursing diagnosis. The nurse considers a possible or tentative diagnosis. The nurse then collects additional data (focus assessment) to confirm or rule out the tentative diagnosis. This process can be depicted as:

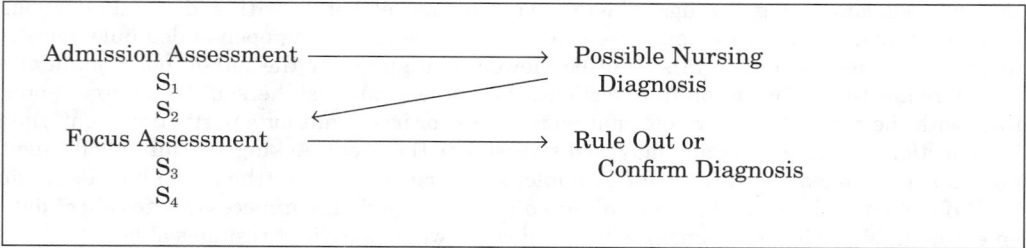

In a focus assessment, the nurse asks additional questions or performs further physical examination aimed at uncovering more cues to form an inference.

Designating data as a diagnostic cue is a complex cognitive activity; grouping a set of cues as a diagnosis is even more difficult (Gordon, 1987). For example, a client's unkempt hair, dirty fingernails, and shabby clothes could be clustered as "poor grooming," an inference that, with other cues, could support a nursing diagnosis of *Self-Care Deficit*. Although a nurse may be able to infer that these assessment data reflect poor grooming, she may not understand the possible relation between the client's poor grooming and the inability to perform self-grooming, lack of desire to perform self-grooming, or a lifelong habit of poor grooming. In some cases, apparently significant data may, in fact, have no diagnostic significance, such as if the client stated, "I'm sorry for my appearance. I rushed here from my work at the gas station." Interpreting data is discussed later in this chapter.

In Section II, each nursing diagnosis is described in terms of focus assessment criteria to identify specific data that may need to be collected. Some questions confirm or rule out defining characteristics or risk factors. Other questions seek to identify related factors. These focus assessment criteria can be used in conjunction with the baseline interview or in an isolated situation requiring additional information. Focus assessments can yield either collaborative problems or nursing diagnoses.

Diagnosing

Nurses make judgments concerning various assessment data, aimed at assisting the client to achieve or maintain the health status he desires. Some of these judgments are nursing diagnoses, some are not. When a nurse concludes that a certain ECG pattern is abnormal, or labels certain tonic–clonic movements a seizure, she has made a diagnosis. In both of these situations the nurse diagnosed something, but neither one is a nursing diagnosis. Both of these situations require nursing and medical interventions for achievement of successful outcomes. (See Chapter 3 for an in-depth discussion of nursing diagnoses and collaborative problems.)

Diagnosis involves complex thinking about the data gathered from the client, family records, and other health care providers. This thinking, combined with relevant clusters stored in the nurse's memory, is used to generate possible explanations for the data. These cognitive activities are difficult to teach and learn; many nurses who acquire expertise in assessment often flounder when asked to synthesize the data and identify a pattern. Aspinall and Tanner (1981) found that nurses take various approaches to problem identification, ranging from systematic testing of several possible explanations to the quick generation of one explanation. However, if the nurse does not take an approach that considers more than one explanation, the validity and effectiveness of the care plan are jeopardized. According to Aspinall and Tanner (1981), potential problems that can result when alternative explanations are not considered and tested include

- Overvaluing one explanation over other possible explanations
- Failing to include the accurate diagnosis in the initial hypothesis
- Failing to consider all the data because of the narrow focus
- Reaching an incorrect diagnosis because of speed, bias, or assumptions based on experience

To assist in identifying alternative explanations and in confirming or ruling out alternatives, the nurse should supplement her own memory-stored information by consulting the client or family, references on the subject, or other health team members. Unfortunately, nurses do not always use the most valuable resource available—other nurses.

Nursing staff conferences on client care are a nonthreatening and productive method for helping staff members identify alternative solutions to problems and interventions. After the background of the problem has been shared with the group, members are asked to think of possible explanations for the data. These explanations are then written on a blackboard, after which the group considers what data are needed to confirm or rule out each possibility. Explanations that have been ruled out are crossed off. The nurse caring for the client then proceeds to confirm or rule out the remaining explanations while caring for the client.

As the nurse gains more knowledge and experience, she needs less time to think of alternative explanations. However, this step should never be eliminated. Identifying alternatives is also important when determining interventions, to avoid failure, stereotyping, and monotony.

Identifying Nursing Diagnoses

During assessment, the nurse elicits data that reflect the client's past and present functional patterns. As discussed earlier, the nurse must be careful not to diagnose patterns with isolated data. Isolated data may be important in the content of the usual pattern, but the usual pattern must be determined before analysis can take place.

As mentioned earlier, to cluster or group data for analysis and diagnosis, the nurse must be knowledgeable about the signs and symptoms that represent the diagnosis. Using this knowledge, the nurse then

- Reviews the data collected during a screening or focus assessment.
- Examines each functional health pattern and determines if there is optimal functioning in the pattern, or a problem with functioning in the pattern
- Identifies risk factors present that increase the vulnerability of the person to development of a functional pattern problem

The following questions may help in analysis of data: Does the person have a problem with _____, or is he at risk for development of a problem with _____

1. Health Perception–Health Management
    Health practices?
    Compliance?
    Injuries?
    Unhealthy life-style?
2. Nutritional–Metabolic
    Nutrition?
    Fluid intake?
    Peripheral edema?
    Infection?
    Oral cavity health?
3. Elimination
    Bowel elimination?
    Incontinence?
4. Activity–Exercise
    Activities of daily living?
    Leisure activities?
    Home care?
    Respiratory function?
5. Sleep–Rest
    Sleep?
6. Cognitive–Perceptual
    Decisions?
    Comfort?
    Knowledge?
    Sensory input?
7. Self-Perception–Self-Concept
    Anxiety/fear?
    Control?
    Self-concept?
8. Role–Relationship
    Communication?
    Family?
    Loss?
    Parenting?
    Socialization?
    Violence?
    Responsibilities?
9. Sexuality–Reproductive
    Problems?
10. Coping–Stress tolerance
    Coping?
11. Value–Belief
    Spirituality?

The following is an example of this error.

Mrs. F. is a 33-year-old woman. In response to a 24-hour recall of her diet, she reports:

- Breakfast: coffee (1 cup)
- Morning break: coffee (1 cup)
- Lunch: yogurt
- Afternoon break: pound cake (1 slice)
- Dinner: pizza, salad, coffee (2 cups)

The inference drawn from this data could be inadequate intake of the basic four food groups. The nurse should ask Mrs. F., "Is this your usual daily intake?" Mrs. F.'s response will help the nurse determine the reason for the diet, such as financial factors, lack of knowledge of nutrition, or unusual circumstances.

If the nurse determines a diagnosis of *Possible Altered Nutrition*, she then should look to other assessment data to validate the existence of the altered state, for example, skin, bowel elimination, weight/height ratio. If the nurse is uncertain about what data are needed to confirm the nursing diagnosis, she can refer to the specific diagnosis in Section II for the focus assessment criteria and the defining characteristics.

The nurse should also try to determine whether the client's usual pattern may contribute to an altered functional pattern. In the case of Mrs. F., if her diet recall is her usual state, the nurse can infer that this diet is nutritionally deficient and can elicit contributing factors with additional questions. When the nurse diagnoses the state of risk, she uses the diagnosis of *Risk for Altered Health Maintenance related to lack of knowledge of implications of inadequate diet and daily nutritional requirements and the inconvenience of preparing meals for one person.*

The following questions may be applied to each area of functioning to assist the nurse in formulating a conclusion about the data collected for that diagnosis:

- Is there a problem (actual), or is there a high risk for developing a problem in this area of functioning?
- Do the data collected lead one to suspect a problem (possible) in this area?
- Is there an area in which a higher level of wellness is desired?*

Identifying Collaborative Problems

During assessment, the nurse acquires data on medical history and treatment. With this information, the nurse can identify physiologic complications that are present or predict those for which the client is at risk and for which the nurse must monitor. For example, a client admitted for elective surgery who also has diabetes mellitus is monitored for blood sugar fluctuations under the collaborative problem *Potential Complication: Hypo/hyperglycemia*. (See Chapter 3 for a complete discussion of collaborative problems.)

To help identify collaborative problems, the nurse may ask the following question: In any of the following body systems, is a physiologic complication present, or is there a *high* risk for one developing because of a disease, treatment, diagnostic study, or medication that requires monitoring and joint management by a nurse and physician?

- Cardiac, vascular
- Metabolic immune, hematopoietic
- Respiratory
- Renal, urinary
- Neurologic, sensory
- Muscular, skeletal
- Reproductive
- Gastrointestinal, hepatic, biliary

Thus, the nurse must analyze data using functional health patterns and physiologic complications or risks.

* © 1985, Lynda Juall Carpenito.

Summary

Assessment encompasses data collection, interpretation, clustering, and analysis. This complex cognitive activity requires knowledge gained from theory, personal experience, and other sources. At some point, assessment data become diagnostic cues that support diagnostic statements—nursing diagnoses and collaborative problems.

The nurse must approach this first step of the nursing process cautiously to reduce the risk of erroneous assumptions and interpretations. Errors in assessment result in invalid diagnoses and ineffective interventions, which can be detrimental to clients and lead to inefficient use of nursing resources.

References

Alfaro, R. (1994). *Applying nursing process: A step-by-step guide* (3rd ed.). Philadelphia: J. B. Lippincott.

Aspinall, M. J., & Tanner, C. (1981). *Decision-making in patient care*. New York: Appleton-Century-Crofts.

Bellack, J. P. (1984). *Nursing assessment: A multidimensional approach*. Monterey, CA: Wadsworth.

Block, G. J., & Nolan, J. W. (1986). *Health assessment for professional nursing: A developmental approach* (2nd ed.). New York: Appleton-Century-Crofts.

Carnevali, D., & Thomas, M. (1993). *Diagnostic reasoning and treatment decision making in nursing*. Philadelphia: J. B. Lippincott.

Fuller, J., & Schaller-Ayres, J. (1990). *Health assessment: A nursing approach*. Philadelphia: J. B. Lippincott.

Gordon, M. (1987). *Nursing diagnosis: Process and application* (2nd ed.). St. Louis: McGraw-Hill.

Gordon, M. (1990). Toward theory-based diagnostic categories. *Nursing Diagnosis, 1*(1), 5–11.

Miskowski, C., & Nielson, B. (1985). A cancer nursing assessment tool. *Oncology Nursing Forum, 12*(6), 37–42.

Smith, V. N., & Bass, T. (1979). *Communication for health professionals*. Philadelphia: J. B. Lippincott.

6

Nursing Diagnosis and Care Planning

Nurses practicing in many settings must rely on other nurses and nonlicensed nursing personnel to achieve outcomes of care. This reliance necessitates a system of communication. For over 25 years, the system of communication consisted of handwritten care plans; as originally designed, this system was unwieldy and not very useful. This chapter addresses the purpose of care plans and their utility today.

Care Plan Defined

Care plans have two professional purposes—administrative and clinical. The administrative purposes of care plans are to

- Define the focus of nursing care for the client or group
- Differentiate the accountability of the nurse from that of other members of the health team
- Provide criteria for reviewing and evaluating care (quality improvement)
- Provide criteria for classification and financial reimbursement

Care plans serve the following clinical purposes:

- Represent the priority set of diagnoses (collaborative problems and nursing diagnoses) for a client
- Provide blueprints to direct charting
- Communicate to the nursing staff what to teach, what to observe, and what to implement
- Provide outcome criteria and nursing goals for reviewing and evaluating care
- Direct specific interventions for the client, family, and other nursing staff members to implement

To direct and evaluate nursing care, the care plan should include the following elements:

- Diagnostic statement (collaborative problems, nursing diagnoses)
- Outcome criteria (client goals) or nursing goals
- Nursing actions or interventions
- Evaluation (status of plan)

Nurses need a system for recording the nursing actions that address problems not described by nursing diagnoses. Because nurses often find it difficult to separate the collaborative dimension from the independent dimension of nursing, it would be best to use a system that designates and includes both collaborative problems and nursing diagnoses. In such a system, the nurse could record complex collaborative problems and nursing diagnoses with the related interventions on the care plans, and address routine problems on the standard of care. This type of documentation is explained later in this chapter.

Are Care Plans Necessary?

Traditionally, care plans have been defined as handwritten documents addressing the problem, goal, and interventions. As mentioned earlier, care plans are a method of communicating the care of a client to the nurse providing the care.

Most clients require care that is predicted to be needed because of the primary condition present. For example, all postoperative clients require monitoring of fluid volume and pain management. Most of the nursing interventions would be standardized. The care for predicted nursing diagnoses and collaborative problems associated with the primary condition can be read from a standard of care. It is unnecessary to write this care on a care plan.

Critical pathways reflect a condensed version of the care predicted to be needed for a condition. They can serve to direct nurses in providing routine care. Because a critical pathway is not specific, the nurse must be experienced in the care. An inexperienced nurse cannot provide care based only on a critical pathway. Later in this chapter, case management is discussed, using critical pathways and standards of care.

If, however, the nurse has no format for a care plan, how can that nurse direct another nurse to provide interventions that are not on the critical path or standardized care plan? Furthermore, what if the client has additional nursing diagnoses or collaborative problems that need nursing attention that are not part of the standard or critical path? Reliance on verbal communication to pass on care of a client to the next nurse is problematic. There will be no record of the problem in the chart, and the quality of the care will depend on the memory of the last nurse. Thus, in settings when more than one nurse cares for the client, a mechanism for communicating nonstandard care is necessary.

The Care Planning Process

After identifying the actual or high-risk problems, the nurse formulates the nursing activities to monitor, prevent, reduce, or eliminate the problems. Care plans represent the planning of care, not the delivery of care. This planning phase of the nursing process has three components:

1. Establishing a priority set of diagnoses
2. Designating outcome criteria and nursing goals
3. Prescribing nursing interventions

Establishing a Priority Set of Diagnoses

Realistically, a nurse cannot hope to address all, or even most, of the nursing diagnoses and collaborative problems that can apply to an individual, family, or community. By identifying a priority set—a group of nursing diagnoses and collaborative problems that take precedence over other nursing diagnoses or collaborative problems—the nurse can best direct resources toward goal achievement. It is useful to differentiate priority diagnoses from those that are important, but not priority.

Priority diagnoses are those nursing diagnoses or collaborative problems that, if not managed now, will deter progress to achieve outcomes or will negatively affect the client's functional status.

Important diagnoses are those nursing diagnoses or collaborative problems for which treatment can be delayed to a later time without compromising present functional status.

As discussed in Chapter 2, the concept of risk nursing diagnoses versus high-risk nursing diagnoses should be clarified. Risk diagnoses represent vulnerability that all clients in a given situation share, as in Risk for Injury or Risk for Infection. It is not clinically useful to add risk diagnoses to a priority list of diagnoses unless they are from a standard. Instead, the nurse should determine if the person is at higher risk than other clients in the same situation. Only high-risk diagnoses should be included on the list. Later in this chapter, a case study is used to illustrate this difference.

How does the nurse identify a priority set? Figure 6-1 summarizes the process. In an acute care setting, the client enters the hospital for a specific purpose, such as surgery or other treatments for acute illness. In such a situation, certain nursing diagnoses or collaborative problems requiring specific nursing interventions often apply. Carpenito (1995) uses the term diagnostic cluster to describe such a group. Thus, for example, different clients recovering from abdominal surgery share the same diagnostic cluster. Each of their problem lists contains the diagnostic cluster diagnoses, along with additional (addendum) diagnoses added to the priority set on the problem list.

What are the nursing diagnoses or collaborative problems associated with the primary condition (*e.g.*, surgery)?

Are there additional collaborative problems associated with coexisting medical conditions that require monitoring (*e.g.*, hypoglycemia)?

Are there additional nursing diagnoses that, if not managed or prevented now, will deter recovery or affect the client's functional status (*e.g.*, *High Risk for Constipation*)?

What problems does the client perceive as priority?

Fig. 6-1 Questions to establish a priority set of diagnoses.

How are other diagnoses not on the diagnostic cluster selected for a client's problem list? Limited nursing resources and increasingly reduced client care time mandate that nurses identify important, but not priority, nursing diagnoses that can be addressed at a later time and do not need to be included on the client's problem list. For example, for a client hospitalized after myocardial infarction who is 50 lb overweight, the nurse eventually would want to explain the effects of obesity on cardiac function and refer the client to community resources for a weight reduction program after discharge. The discharge summary record would reflect the teaching and the referral; a nursing diagnosis related to weight reduction would not need to appear on the client's problem list.

With use of the questions in Figure 6-1, consider the following client:

Mr. Gene is a 76-year-old man admitted for emergency gastric surgery for repair of a bleeding ulcer. Mr. Gene also has diabetes mellitus and peripheral vascular disease. After completing a functional assessment, the nurse identifies

Compromised gait
Occasional incontinence
Wife complaining of many caregiver responsibilities and an unmotivated husband

Figure 6-2 provides the priority set of diagnoses for Mr. Gene. Because of the presence of *Functional Incontinence* and *Caregiver Role Strain*, a referral to a community nursing service is needed.

Mr. Gene and his wife probably have many other nursing diagnoses that are important; however, because of the limited length of stay, nursing resources must be directed toward those problems that will deter progress at this time. Important diagnoses can be discussed with the client and family, with recommendations for future attention (*e.g.*, referral to a community agency).

Numbering the diagnoses on a problem list does not indicate priority, but rather the order in which the nurse entered them on the list. Assigning absolute priority to nursing diagnoses or collaborative problems can create the false assumption that number 1 is automatically the first priority. As you know, in the clinical setting, priorities can change rapidly as the client's condition changes. For this reason, the nurse must view the entire problem list as the priority set, with priorities shifting within the list periodically.

Designating Outcome Criteria and Nursing Goals

Sometimes referred to as objectives, expected outcomes, or outcomes, goals of care planning are based on client criteria or nursing criteria. They are predicted.

Client goals and nursing goals are standards or measures used to evaluate the client's progress (outcome) or the nurse's performance (process). According to Alfaro (1994), client goals are statements describing a measurable behavior of the client, family, or group that denotes a favorable status (changed or maintained) after nursing care has been delivered. Nursing goals, on the other hand, are statements describing measurable actions that denote the nurse's accountability for the situation or diagnosis. As discussed in Chapter 3, nursing diagnoses have client goals and collaborative problems have nursing goals.

PC: Urinary retention
PC: Hemorrhage
PC: Hypovolemia/shock
PC: Pneumonia (stasis)
PC: Peritonitis
PC: Thrombophlebitis
PC: Paralytic ileus
PC: Evisceration
PC: Dehiscence

Risk for infection related to destruction of first line of
    defense against bacterial invasion
Risk for Altered Respiratory Function related to
    postanesthesia state, postoperative immobility, and pain
Impaired Physical Mobility related to pain and weakness
    secondary to anesthesia, tissue hypoxia, and insufficient
    fluids/nutrients
Risk for Altered Nutrition: Less Than Body Requirements
    related to increased protein/vitamin requirements for
    wound healing and decreased intake secondary to pain,
    nausea, vomiting, and diet restrictions
Risk for Ineffective Management of Therapeutic Regimen
    related to insufficient knowledge of home care, incisional
    care, signs and symptoms of complications, activity
    restriction, and follow-up care

From postoperative standard of care

PC: Hypo/Hyperglycemia

From medical history of diabetes mellitus

Possible Functional Incontinence
    related to reports of occasional
    incontinence when walking to bathroom

From nursing admission assessment

High Risk for Caregiver Role
    Strain (wife) related to multiple
    caregiver responsibilities and
    progressive deterioration of husband

From nursing admission assessment

High Risk for Injury related to
    altered gait and deconditioning
    secondary to peripheral vascular
    disease and decreased motivation

From medical history of peripheral vascular disease and reports of prolonged immobility

Fig. 6-2   Mr. Gene's priority list.

Client Goals

Bulechek and McCloskey (1985) define client goals as "guideposts to the selection of nursing interventions and criteria in the evaluation of nursing interventions." These authors go on to state that "readily identifiable logical links should exist between the diagnosis and the plan of care, and the activities prescribed should assist or enable the client to meet the identified expected outcome."

Thus, client goals serve as the criteria for measuring the effectiveness of a care plan. Because these outcome criteria for nursing diagnoses represent favorable statuses that can be achieved or maintained through nursing-prescribed (independent) interventions, they can help differentiate nursing diagnoses from collaborative problems. Outcomes for nursing diagnoses do not serve to evaluate the effectiveness of nursing interventions if physician-initiated interventions are also needed.

Certain situations may call for involvement of several disciplines. For example, for a client experiencing extreme anxiety, the physician may prescribe an antianxiety medication, an occupational therapist may provide diversional activities, and a nurse may institute non-pharmacologic anxiety-reducing measures, such as relaxation exercises and more effective problem-solving strategies. According to Gordon (1987), "saying a nursing diagnosis is a health problem a nurse can treat does not mean that non-nursing consultants cannot be used. The critical element is whether the nurse-prescribed interventions can achieve the outcome established with the client."

Client goals should be specific and realistically achievable. In the literature, client outcomes with nursing diagnoses are sometimes problematic. Table 6-1 provides selected examples of these. Examine the goals outlined in the table and imagine caring for a client with one or more of the listed goals, such as "Will not experience cardiac dysrhythmias" or "Vital signs within normal limits for the client." What if premature ventricular contractions or a decrease in blood pressure or pulse rate developed in this client—how should the nurse respond? Should the nurse add or correct any nursing orders to address the problem? Should the nurse change a goal because it proves unachievable? No, the nurse should do neither, but rather should either initiate delegated orders from medicine (protocols, standing orders) or contact the physician for delegated orders. Changing nursing orders will not address the client's problem.

If a client goal is not achieved, or if progress toward achievement is not evident, the nurse must reevaluate the attainability of the goal or review the nursing care plan, asking the following questions (Carpenito, 1995):

- Is the diagnosis correct?
- Has the goal been set mutually? Is the client participating?
- Is more time needed for the plan to work?
- Does the goal need to be revised?
- Does the plan need to be revised?
- Are physician-prescribed interventions needed?

Table 6-1 **Literature Examples of Client Goals**

ABGs are within the client's normal limits (p. 26)

Blood sugar/electrolytes are within acceptable limits (p. 243)

Blood loss from mediastinal or pleural tubes is within acceptable limits (p. 23) (Doenges, Moorhouse, & Geissler, 1994)

Vital signs remain stable

Hemoglobin and hematocrit return to normal

Electrolytes within normal range

No evidence of arrhythmias

Cardiac output remains adequate (Sparks, Taylor, & Dyer, 1996)

Blood pressure will not increase more than 30 mm Hg systolic or 15 mm Hg diastolic (p. 112)

The causative organism will respond to treatment (p. 116)

Will progress through labor and delivery without incident or severe fluid deficit, hemorrhage and/or shock (p. 124) (Aukamp, 1984)

Cardiac rhythm and rate are within normal limits (p. 45)

Hypoxemia is resolved or improved (Kim, McFarland, & McLane, 1995)

Goals for Collaborative Problems

As discussed earlier, identifying client goals for collaborative problems is inappropriate and can imply erroneous accountability for nurses. Rather, collaborative problems involve nursing goals that reflect nursing accountability in situations requiring physician-prescribed and nurse-prescribed interventions. This accountability includes:

- Monitoring for physiologic instability
- Consulting standing orders and protocols or a physician to obtain orders for appropriate interventions
- Performing specific actions to manage and reduce the severity of an event or situation
- Evaluating client responses

Nursing goals for collaborative problems can be written as either "The problem will be managed and minimized" or "The nurse will manage and minimize the problem." Table 6-2 presents examples of collaborative problems and corresponding nursing goals.

If the plan or critical pathway includes nursing and medical interventions, then goals can be written for collaborative problems as

PC: Dysrhythmias: The client will demonstrate NSR or a non–life-threatening dysrhythmia.

Goals for Nursing Diagnoses

Client goals can represent predicted resolution of a problem, evidence of progress toward resolution of a problem, progress toward improved health status, or continued maintenance of good health or function. These goals are used to

- Direct interventions to achieve the desired changes or maintenance
- Measure the effectiveness and validity of the interventions

Goals or outcome criteria can be formulated to direct and measure positive and negative outcomes. *Positive outcome criteria* seek to direct interventions to provide the client with

1. Improved health status by increasing comfort (physiologic, psychological, social, spiritual) and coping abilities—for example: The client will discuss relationship between activity and carbohydrate requirements and walk unassisted to end of hall four times a day.
2. Maintenance of present optimal level of health—for example: The client will continue to share her fears.
3. Optimal levels of coping with significant others—for example: The client will relate an intent to discuss with her husband her concern about returning to work.
4. Optimal adaptation to deterioration of health status—for example: The client will visually scan the environment while walking, to prevent injury.
5. Optimal adaptation to terminal illness—for example: The client will compensate for periods of anorexia and nausea.
6. Collaboration and satisfaction with health care providers—for example: The client will ask questions concerning the care of his colostomy.

Negative outcome criteria seek to direct interventions to prevent negative alterations in the client, such as

Table 6-2　**Collaborative Problems With Corresponding Nursing Goals**

Potential Complication: Dysrhythmias
The nurse will manage and minimize dysrhythmic episodes.

Potential Complication: Fluid/Electrolyte Imbalances
Fluid and electrolyte imbalances will be managed and minimized.

1. Complications—for example: The client will not experience the complications of imposed bed rest.
2. Disabilities—for example: The client will elevate left arm on pillow and exercise fingers on sponge ball to reduce edema.
3. Unwarranted death—for example: The infant will be attached to an apnea monitor at night.

Components of Outcome Criteria. The essential characteristics of outcome criteria are as follows: Outcome criteria should

- Be long-term or short-term
- Have measurable behavior
- Be specific in content and time
- Be attainable

Client goals can be *long-term* or *short-term* goals. These may be defined as follows:

- Long-term: An objective expected to be achieved over weeks or months
- Short-term: An objective expected to be achieved as a stepping stone to reach a long-term goal (Alfaro, 1994)

Sometimes short-term goals are called objectives for care.

Previously, when hospital stays were frequently longer than a week, it was appropriate to formulate short-term and long-term goals. With current schedules, this is no longer necessary for most hospitalized clients.

Long-term goals are appropriate for all clients in long-term care facilities and some clients in rehabilitation units, mental health units, community nursing settings, and ambulatory services.

The following represents a long-term goal with the associated short-term goals for a client with *Risk for Suicide* (Townsend, 1994):

- Short-term goals
  1. Patient will seek out staff when feeling urge to harm self during shift.
  2. Patient will make short-term verbal (or written) contract with nurse not to harm self during shift.
- Long-term goal
  Patient will not harm self while in the hospital.

Measurable verbs are verbs that describe the exact action or behavior of the client that the nurse expects will occur when the goal has been met. The action or behavior must be such that the nurse can validate it by seeing or hearing. (The other senses—touch, taste, and smell—can also be used to measure goal achievement, but their use is infrequent.)

If the verb used does not describe a result that can be seen or heard (*e.g.*, the client *will experience* less anxiety), the nurse can change it to a behaviorally measurable one (*e.g.*, the client *will report* less anxiety).

Examples of verbs that are *not* measurable by sight or sound are

- Accepts
- Knows
- Appreciates
- Understands

Examples of verbs that are measurable include

- States
- Performs
- Identifies
- Exhibits decreased
- Exhibits increased
- Reports absence of
- Specifies
- Administers

Measurement of goal achievement can be made easier by

- Using the phrase *as evidenced by* to introduce measurable evidence of a reduction in signs and symptoms; for example: The client will experience less anxiety, as evidenced by a reduction in pacing and rapid pulse >90; or the client will demonstrate tolerance to activity, as evidenced by a return to resting pulse 76 3 minutes postactivity.
- Adding the expression *within normal limits* (WNL); for example: The client will demonstrate healing WNL.

The process of writing measurable goals is shown in Figure 6-3.

The outcome criteria should describe the *specific response* planned. Three elements add to the specificity of a goal: content, modifiers, and achievement time. The *content* indicates what the client is to do, experience, or learn (usually a verb)—for example: drink, walk, cough, or verbalize.

Associated with the verb are *modifiers*, which add the specifics or individual preferences to the goal. Modifiers are usually adjectives or adverbs. They explain what, where, when, and how, such as: drink (what and when), walk (where and when), learn (what), and cough (how and when).

The *time for achievement* of a goal can be added to the goal using one of three options:

- By discharge (*e.g.*, the client will relate an intent to discuss fears regarding diagnosis with wife at home)
- Continued (*e.g.*, the client will demonstrate continued intact skin)
- By date (*e.g.*, the client will walk half the length of the hallway with assistance by Friday morning)

Often, the nurse has limited data when initial care plans are formulated. As a result, the goals and interventions may lack specificity. As the nurse interacts with the client, more data are collected. The longer the nurse–client interaction, the more specific the plan would be.

For each nursing diagnosis in Section II, outcome criteria are stated in measurable terms, but they must be made specific to each client by adding modifiers. These outcome criteria guide the nurse in the areas that need to be observed and measured. The following is an example of outcome criteria for the diagnosis *Pain* that have been rewritten to reflect the goal for a particular client on a rehabilitation unit:

Outcome Criteria

The client will report reduced pain and improved mobility by discharge.

Individualized Outcome Criteria

The client will:
1. Complete his bath without assistance
2. Report reduced pain (<5 on 0–10 scale)
3. Remain out of bed from 11 A.M. to 2 P.M. and 5 P.M. to 9 P.M.

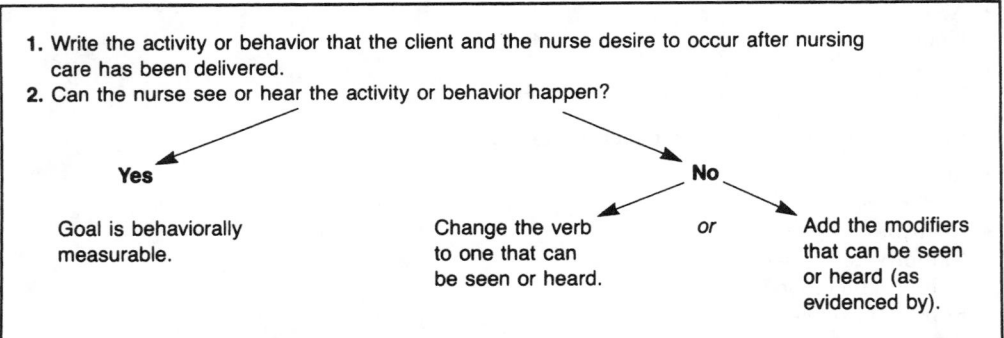

1. Write the activity or behavior that the client and the nurse desire to occur after nursing care has been delivered.

2. Can the nurse see or hear the activity or behavior happen?

Yes

Goal is behaviorally measurable.

No

Change the verb to one that can be seen or heard.

or

Add the modifiers that can be seen or heard (as evidenced by).

Fig. 6-3 Steps to formulate behaviorally measurable goals.

The nurse must ask: How will I measure that the client is experiencing less pain and has increased mobility? For this particular client, the previously stated goals will serve as measurements. As the client's mobility increases, the nurse may have to revise the goals to reflect the client's changing status.

Goals for Possible Nursing Diagnoses. Many students and nurses have been instructed to write only client goals (outcome criteria) for all the problem statements on the care plan. Because outcome criteria refer to the expected changes in the client's status after he has received nursing care, it is inappropriate for the nurse to formulate outcome criteria for collaborative problems and for possible nursing diagnoses. Consider the following sample nursing diagnosis and associated outcome criteria:

- Nursing diagnosis: *Possible Feeding Self-Care Deficit related to IV in right hand*
- Outcome criteria: The client will feed himself.

As one can easily see, this goal is problematic. How can the nurse write a client goal for a possible nursing diagnosis if it is not known whether the client actually has the problem? Thus, goals for possible nursing diagnosis are omitted because they are not indicated.

Prescribing Nursing Interventions

As previously discussed (see Chapter 3), there are two types of nursing interventions: nurse prescribed and physician prescribed (delegated). Nurse-prescribed interventions are those prescriptions formulated by nurses for themselves or other nursing staff to implement. Delegated interventions are prescriptions for clients formulated by physicians for nursing staff to implement. Physicians' orders are not orders for nurses, but rather, are orders for clients that nurses implement if indicated.

Both types of interventions require independent nursing judgment, because legally the nurse must determine whether it is appropriate to initiate the action, regardless of whether it is independent or delegated. Table 6-3 shows a sample nursing care plan with both types of interventions.

It is important to note that nurses can and should consult with other disciplines, such as social workers, nutritionists, and physical therapists, as appropriate. However, this relationship is consultative only; if interventions for nursing diagnoses result from this consultation, the nurse writes these orders on the nursing care plan for other nursing staff to implement. (A discussion of other disciplines and their role in nursing care plans is included later in this chapter.)

Bulechek and McCloskey (1989) define nursing interventions as "any direct care treatment that a nurse performs on behalf of a client. These treatments include nurse-initiated treatments resulting from nursing diagnoses, physician-initiated treatments resulting from medical diagnoses, and performance of essential daily functions for the client who cannot do these." Their definition links all nursing interventions with nursing diagnoses. This author links all nursing interventions with nursing diagnoses and collaborative problems. Figure 6-4 lists the six basic types of nursing interventions identified by Bulechek and McCloskey (1989), with this author's changes.

As discussed in Chapter 3, the major focus of interventions differs for actual, risk, and possible nursing diagnoses and collaborative problems.

For *actual nursing diagnoses*, interventions seek to

- Reduce or eliminate contributing factors or the diagnosis
- Promote higher-level wellness
- Monitor status

For *risk nursing diagnoses*, interventions seek to

- Reduce or eliminate risk factors
- Prevent occurrence of the problem
- Monitor for onset

Table 6-3 **Nurse-Prescribed and Delegated Interventions**

Standard of Care

Potential Complication: Increased Intracranial Pressure

NP　　1. Monitor for signs and symptoms of increased intracranial pressure
- Pulse changes: Slowing rate to 60 or below; Increasing rate to 100 or above
- Respiratory irregularities: Slowing rate with lengthening periods of apnea
- Rising blood pressure or widening pulse pressure with moderately elevated temperature
- Temperature rising
- Level of responsiveness: Variable change from baseline (alert, lethargic, comatose)
- Pupillary changes (size, equality, reaction to light, movements)
- Eye movements (doll's eyes, nystagmus)
- Vomiting
- Headache: Constant, increasing in intensity; aggravated by movement/standing
- Subtle changes: Restlessness, forced breathing, purposeless movements and mental cloudiness
- Paresthesia, paralysis

NP　　2. Avoid:
- Carotid massage
- Prone position
- Neck flexion
- Extreme neck rotation
- Valsalva maneuver
- Isometric exercises
- Digital stimulation (anal)

NP　　3. Maintain a position with slight head elevation

NP　　4. Avoid rapidly changing positions

NP　　5. Maintain a quiet, calm environment (soft lighting)

NP　　6. Plan activities to reduce number of interruptions

NP　　7. Intake and output; use infusion pump to ensure accuracy

NP　　8. Consult for stool softeners

Del　　9. Maintain fluid restrictions as ordered (may be restricted to 1000 mL/day for a few days)

Del　10. Administer fluids at an even rate as prescribed

Del　11. Administer medications (osmotic diuretics, *e.g.*, mannitol; and corticosteroids, *e.g.*, dexametha-sone, methylprednisolone if administered)

(Del = Delegated; NP = Nurse-prescribed)

For *possible nursing diagnoses*, interventions seek to

- Collect additional data to rule out or confirm the diagnosis

For *collaborative problems*, interventions seek to

- Monitor for changes in status
- Manage changes in status with nurse- and physician-prescribed interventions
- Evaluate response

The specific directions for nursing—*nursing orders*—are composed of the following:

- Date
- Directive verb
- What, when, how often, how long, where
- Signature (Carnevali, 1983)

The objective of the nursing order is to direct individualized care to a client. Nursing orders differ from nursing actions, which are standard interventions that can apply to any number of clients sharing a similar problem. Examples of nursing actions include:

- Increase fluid intake
- Ambulate the client
- Monitor for dysrhythmias

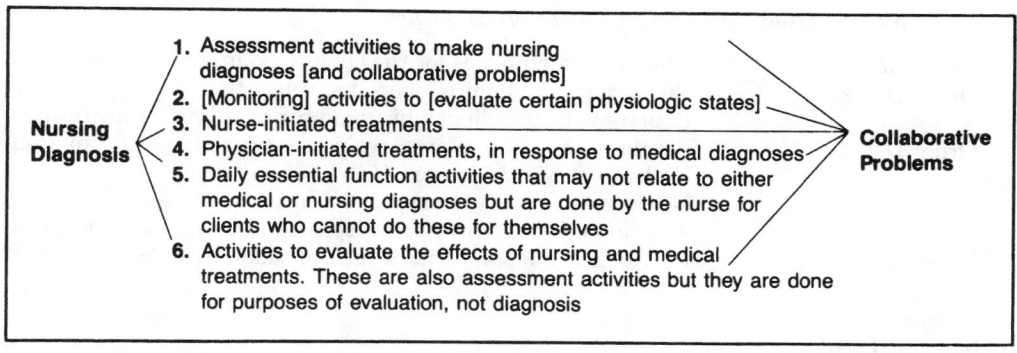

Fig. 6-4 Relationship of nursing interventions to nursing diagnosis and collaborative problems. (Bulechek, G., & McCloskey, J. Nursing interventions: Treatments for potential nursing diagnoses. In Carroll-Johnson, M. [Ed.]. *Classification of nursing diagnoses: Proceedings of the eighth national conference.* Philadelphia: J.B. Lippincott. Brackets indicate changes made by author.)

To translate some nursing actions into nursing orders, the nurse must have data from the client to answer the following: what, when, how often, how long, and where? The following example illustrates translation of a nursing action to a nursing order:

Nursing Action	Nursing Order
Increase fluid intake	Increase fluids to at least 2500 mL/24 hr:
	1000 mL 7 A.M.–3 P.M.
	700 mL 3 P.M.–11 P.M.
	100 mL 11 P.M.–7 A.M.
	Client likes oranges and apple juice; dislikes carbonated beverages.
	Do not count coffee or tea in the 2500 mL.

This nursing order reflects the need to hydrate a client with tenacious secretions, considers preferences, and indicates that coffee and tea are permitted, although not as part of the measured increase, because they act as diuretics.

The nursing interventions outlined in Section II for each nursing diagnosis provide guidelines for the nurse. If necessary, the nurse can rewrite the interventions considering the components of a nursing order. The following example illustrates rewriting a nursing intervention from Section II as a nursing order:

Nursing Diagnosis: *Sleep Pattern Disturbance related to daytime sleeping secondary to decreased daytime activity level, as evidenced by reports of frustration over inability to sleep at night*

Nursing Action	Individualized Nursing Order
Promote a well-scheduled daytime program of activity	Assist the client to dining room for each meal
	Have another resident accompany him on a daily afternoon walk around the grounds

As with outcome criteria, the nurse must have specific knowledge of the client to write nursing orders. Student nurses can write care plans for clients they are yet to meet based on information from their instructors, but they must understand that they are writing guidelines for care, not nursing orders. After caring for a client, the student can revise the plan with specific orders if needed.

As a nurse increases her knowledge about a client, she may need to revise the nursing orders to reflect changes or make them more specific. The following example illustrates a nursing order that underwent such revisions.

Nursing Diagnosis: *Fear related to uncertain future*

Initial order (Day 1)   Provide opportunities for the client to ventilate her concerns
Order Day 2   Encourage the client to share her concerns
                        Explore with the client's husband his concerns for his future
Order Day 4   Reinforce the need to preserve present function (refer to prob-
                          lem *Impaired Physical Mobility*)
                        Discuss a plan for increasing self-care activities
                        Assess the communication pattern between husband and wife
                        Provide the husband with a time to talk outside wife's room

Implementation

The implementation component of the nursing process involves applying the skills needed to implement the nursing interventions. The skills and knowledge necessary for implementation usually focus on

- Performing the activity for the client or assisting the client
- Performing nursing assessments to identify new problems or to monitor the status or existing problems
- Performing teaching to help clients gain new knowledge concerning their own health or the management of a disorder
- Assisting clients to make decisions about their own health care
- Consulting with and referring to other health care professionals to obtain appropriate direction
- Providing specific treatment actions to remove, reduce, or resolve health problems
- Assisting clients to perform activities themselves
- Assisting clients to identify risks or problems and to explore options available (Alfaro, 1994)

The nurse not only must possess these skills but must assess, teach, and evaluate them in all nursing personnel she manages. Often, the nurse is responsible for planning care, but not for actually implementing it. This requires the nurse to have the management skills of delegation, assertion, evaluation, and knowledge of change and motivational theory. The nurse should consult the appropriate literature on these topics.

Evaluation

Evaluation involves three different considerations:

- Evaluation of the client's status
- Evaluation of the client's progress toward goal achievement
- Evaluation of the care plan's status and currentness

The nurse is responsible for evaluating the client's status regularly. Some clients require daily evaluation; others, such as those with neurologic problems, need hourly or continuous evaluation. The nurse approaches evaluation differently for nursing diagnoses and collaborative problems.

Evaluating Nursing Diagnoses

Outcome criteria or client goals are needed to evaluate a nursing diagnosis. After the nurse and client mutually set client goals, the nurse will

- Assess the client's status
- Compare this response to the outcome criteria
- Conclude whether the client is progressing toward outcome achievement

Figure 6-5 presents a decision tree for evaluating nursing diagnoses and collaborative problems. The following example illustrates the evaluation process for a nursing diagnosis:

Goal: The client will walk unassisted half the length of the hall by 6/5.

Evaluation: The nurse observes the client's response to interventions, asking "How far did the client walk?" and "Was assistance needed?" The nurse then compares the client's response after interventions with the established outcome criteria.

The nurse can record the client's response on flow charts or progress notes. Flow charts record clinical data, such as vital signs, skin condition, presence or absence of side effects, and wound assessments. Progress notes record specific responses that are not appropriate for flow charts, such as response to counseling, response of family members to the client, and any unusual responses.

Evaluating Collaborative Problems

Because collaborative problems do not have client goals, the nurse evaluates them differently from nursing diagnoses. For collaborative problems, the nurse will

- Assess the client's status
- Compare the data to established norms
- Judge whether the data fall within acceptable ranges
- Conclude if the client is stable, improved, unimproved, or worse

For example, for the collaborative problem *Potential Complication: Hypertension*, the nurse takes a blood pressure reading and compares it with the normal range for blood pressures. If it falls within the range, the nurse concludes that the client exhibits normal blood pressure. If the blood pressure is higher than the normal range, the nurse checks the client's previous blood pressure readings. If readings have been high, this latest reading is not as significant as if they had not been high. If the client is not showing improvement despite a new treatment regimen, then the high blood pressure reading would be more significant.

The nurse can record the assessment data for collaborative problems on flow records and use progress notes for significant or unusual findings, along with nursing management of the situation.

Evaluating the Care Plan

This type of evaluation depends on the conclusions derived from the evaluation of the client's progress or condition. After examining the client's response, the nurse should ask the following questions:

Nursing Diagnosis

> Does the diagnosis still exist?
> Does a risk or high-risk diagnosis still exist?
> Has the possible diagnosis been confirmed or ruled out?
> Does a new diagnosis need to be added?

Goals

> Have they been achieved?
> Do they reflect the present focus of care?
> Can more specific modifiers be added?
> Are they acceptable to the client?

Interventions

> Are they acceptable to the client?
> Are they specific to the client?
> Do they provide clear instructions for the nursing staff?

Collaborative Problems

> Is continuing monitoring indicated?

In reviewing the problems and interventions, the nurse records one of the following decisions in the evaluation column, or in the progress notes at the time prescribed for evaluation:

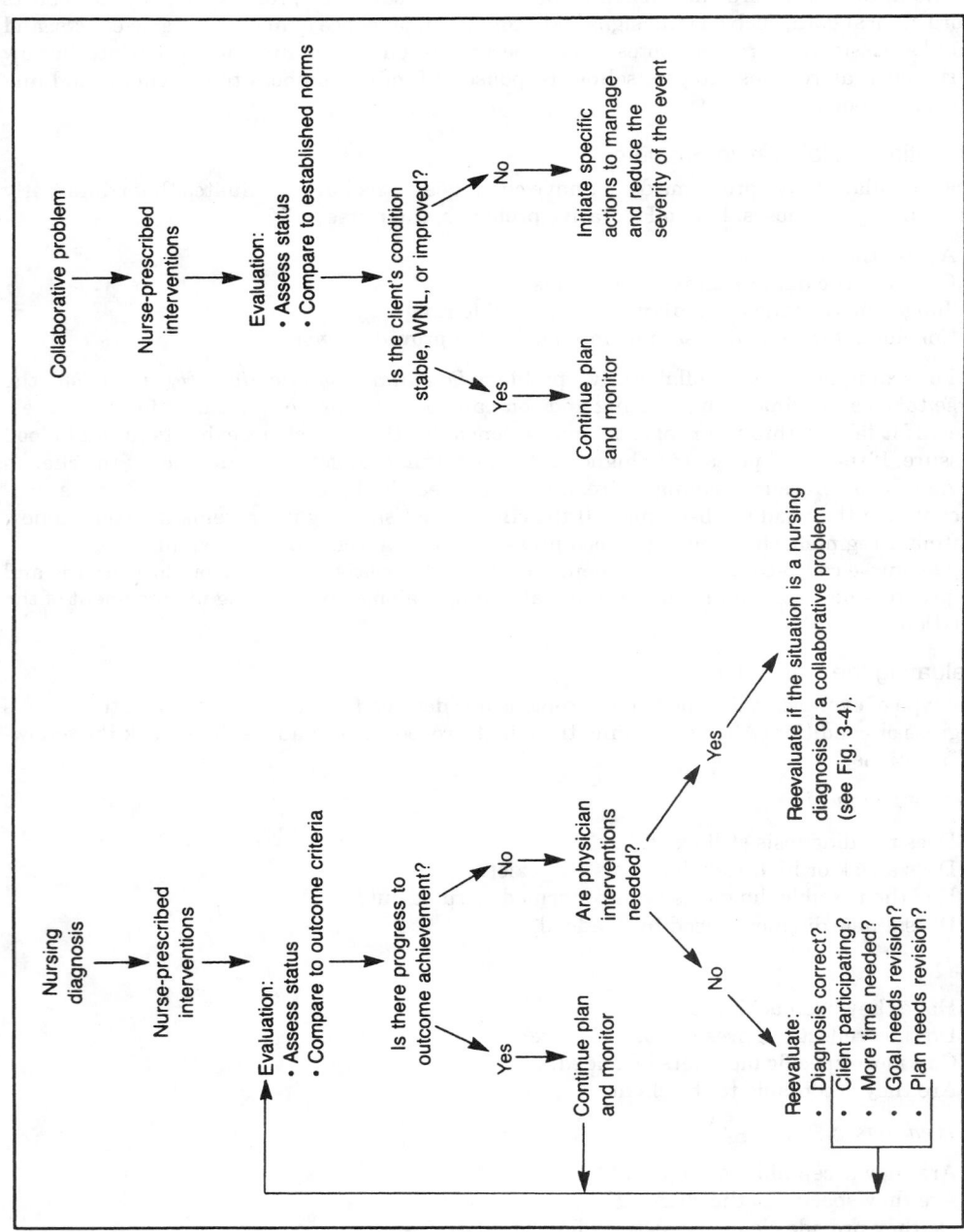

Fig. 6-5   Decision trees representing the evaluation processes for nursing diagnoses and collaborative problems.

- *Continue:* The diagnosis is still present, and the goals and interventions are appropriate.
- *Revised:* The diagnosis is still present, but the goals or nursing orders require revision. The revisions are then recorded.
- *Ruled out/confirmed:* A possible diagnosis has been confirmed or ruled out by additional data collection. Goals and nursing orders are written.
- *Achieved:* The goals have been achieved, and that portion of the care plan is discontinued.
- *Reinstate:* A diagnosis that had been resolved returns.

A care plan representing a short-term nurse–client relationship should have a status column instead of an evaluation column to reflect goals that have been achieved or discontinued. The nurse can then indicate when sections of the plan are no longer active. An example of a status column is presented later in this chapter.

Students who care for clients for only a short time (less than 2 weeks) usually incorporate this evaluation into the evaluation of the client's response. Both can then be recorded on the care plan in the evaluation section. It is, however, important that students recognize that practicing nurses record client responses on the flow record or nursing note, not on the care plan.

Minor revisions can be made daily on a care plan by the nurse caring for or directing the client care. A yellow felt-tip marker (Hi-Liter) can be used to mark those areas no longer being used. Because it is still possible to read through the yellow marking, the nurse can always refer to what was planned previously. In addition, the marking will not interfere with photocopying. Examples of evaluation documentation are presented later in this chapter.

Care Planning Conferences

Client care conferences are an excellent way to help nurses with diagnosing, planning, and evaluating care. These conferences can be held daily and should be restricted to 15 to 20 minutes. It is sometimes advantageous to begin with weekly sessions and move gradually to daily or three-times-a-week sessions. Planning conferences should not be restricted to the day shift, but should also be conducted on evening and night shifts. The client or clients discussed can be those who are new admissions, those who have complex problems or conflicts with the staff, or those who are difficult to diagnose from a nursing diagnosis standpoint. The conference time provides nurses with an opportunity to share assessment data, feelings, problems, and knowledge (theory and practice). It can provide nurses who are reluctant to formulate plans of care with an opportunity for collaboration.

Planning conferences should include all levels of nursing staff. Other members of the health team (therapists, social workers) may attend when appropriate, but it is not appropriate for other health care professionals to coordinate or conduct these conferences. The planning of nursing care, such as discharge planning, should be coordinated by the professional nurse, who can consult other disciplines as indicated.

The success of conferences can be influenced positively if the following guidelines are considered:

- Manage the conference time judiciously by starting and ending on time.
- Include all levels of nursing personnel and encourage their participation when appropriate.
- Have personnel rotate to cover the unit during conferences.
- Discourage interruptions.
- Select an experienced group leader for beginning sessions.
- Introduce inexperienced group leaders only after the conferences are firmly established.

Multidisciplinary Care Planning

Care of individuals, families, or groups commonly is provided by at least two disciplines, sometimes more. Good coordination of this care is critical to promote optimum use of resources and to prevent duplication of care. Given overall knowledge level and time spent with clients, the nurse typically is in the best position to coordinate this care. The case management model subscribes to this philosophy (Cronin & Maklebust, 1989).

Agencies take various steps to promote coordinated multidisciplinary planning. Strategies include

- Conducting regular multidisciplinary planning conferences
- Creating multidisciplinary problem lists
- Creating multidisciplinary care plans

Some of these strategies can be problematic for nurses, however. As discussed earlier in this chapter, care plans serve as directions for nursing staff in providing client care. Should staff from other disciplines—physical therapy, social services, nutrition, and others—write on nursing care plans? If so, should they write interventions for nurses to follow or write interventions specific to their discipline?

When the services of another discipline are needed, the physician orders a consultation or the services. Staff from the needed discipline then create a plan of care with goals and interventions relating specifically to their discipline, not to nursing. Should this plan be part of a multidisciplinary client care plan? Yes, but only if the plan clearly designates which sections apply only to specific disciplines.

By law, there are two types of nursing interventions: nurse prescribed and physician prescribed. Physician-prescribed interventions are transferred from the chart to appropriate documents, such as medication administration records, treatment records, and Kardexes. It is not necessary to enter physician-prescribed interventions on nursing care plans.

A nurse is accountable for following the interventions prescribed by other professional nurses. If a nurse disagrees with another nurse's care plan, the two nurses should consult and discuss the disagreement. If this is impossible, then the disagreeing nurse can delete or revise the existing nursing orders. Professional courtesy dictates that this nurse leave a note to the previous nurse explaining the change, if it could be problematic.

Should other disciplines add interventions for nursing staff to the nursing care plan? When a discipline other than nursing or medicine has suggestions for nursing management of a nursing diagnosis, the nurse should view these suggestions as expert advice. The nurse may or may not incorporate these suggestions into the nursing care plan. This situation is similar to that of a consulting physician, who may make recommendations but does not write medical orders for another physician's client.

When a nurse enters an intervention on the care plan based on a suggestion from another discipline, professional courtesy mandates that the nurse credit the order to that discipline. For example:

Gently perform passive ROM to arms after meals and at 8–9 P.M., as suggested by C. Levy, RPT.

Historically, nursing diagnoses and collaborative problems have been used exclusively by nurses to describe the focus of nursing care. But nursing diagnoses and collaborative problems can also describe the focus of care for other nonphysician disciplines, such as physical therapy, respiratory therapy, social service, occupational therapy, nutritional therapy, and speech therapy.

Other disciplines could add their discipline-specific interventions to standardized care plans with the designation that the interventions are prescribed by and provided by that discipline (not nursing). These disciplines would also be encouraged to revise or add to care plans for their interventions. Table 6-4 illustrates a multidisciplinary care plan. Note that all nursing diagnoses or collaborative problems do not have non–nursing-prescribed interventions.

Multidisciplinary conferencing provides an excellent way to review and evaluate a client's, family's, or group's status and progress. In some facilities, such conferencing is required for all applicable clients.

Care Planning Systems

For years, practicing nurses have held an ambivalent view of care planning. Staff nurses' common oppositions to written care plans include the following:

- Most nurses do not have enough time to write them.
- They are not necessary except for accreditation.
- They are not used after they are written.

Table 6-4 **Sample Multidisciplinary Care Plan for a Client After Total Hip Replacement**

Nursing diagnosis: Impaired Physical Mobility related to pain, stiffness, fatigue, restrictive equipment, and prescribed activity restrictions

Outcome criterion: The client will increase activity to a level consistent with abilities

Interventions:

PT	1. Establish an exercise program tailored to the client's ability.
	2. Implement exercises at regular intervals.
PT/Nsg	3. Teach body mechanics and transfer techniques.
	4. Encourage independence.
PT/Nsg	5. Teach and supervise use of ambulatory aids.

Supporters of care planning in nursing cite these benefits:

- Care plans provide written directions to nursing staff rather than relying on verbal communication.
- They help ensure continuity of care for a client.
- They direct nurses to intervene in the priority set of diagnoses for a particular client.
- They provide a means of reviewing or evaluating care.
- They demonstrate the complex role of professional nurses to validate their positions in health care settings.

Because care plans usually contain only routine interventions, nurses often do not use them. Obviously, a care plan that is not used is not revised. As a result, the care plan that a nurse reads often does not represent the most current plan for the client. To update the staff on the care that the client requires, the nurse then uses oral communication. This type of communication makes the delivery of nursing care very inefficient and costly. An efficient, professional, and useful care planning system encompasses standards of care, client problem lists, and standardized and addendum care plans.

Standards of Care

Standards of care are detailed guidelines that represent the predicted care indicated in specific situations. They do not direct nurses to provide medical interventions, but, rather, provide an efficient method for retrieving predicted generic nursing interventions. Standards of care identify a set of problems (actual or at risk) that typically occur in a particular situation—a diagnostic cluster.

Keep in mind that standards of care should represent the care that nurses are responsible for providing, not an ideal level of care. As discussed earlier, the nurse cannot hope to address all—or, usually, even most—of the problems that a client may have. Rather, the nurse must focus on the client's most serious or most important problems. Problems that will not be addressed in the health care facility should be referred to both the client and family for interventions after discharge. Referrals to community agencies, such as weight loss or smoking cessation programs and psychological counseling, may be indicated after discharge. Nurses must create realistic standards based on client acuity, length of stay, and available resources. Unrealistic, ideal standards merely frustrate nurses and hold them legally accountable for care that they cannot provide.

A care planning system can be structured with three tiers or levels of care:

- Level I—generic unit standard of care
- Level II—diagnostic cluster or single-diagnosis standardized care plan
- Level III—addendum care plans

Level I—Unit Standards of Care

Level I standards of care represent the predicted generic care required for all or most clients on a unit. These standards contain nursing diagnoses or collaborative problems (the diagnostic cluster) applicable to the specific situation. Table 6-5 presents a sample diagnostic cluster for standards of care in a general medical unit. Each unit—orthopedics, oncology,

Table 6-5   **Generic Diagnostic Cluster for Hospitalized Adults With Medical Conditions**

Collaborative Problems
Potential Complication: Cardiovascular
Potential Complication: Respiratory

Nursing Diagnosis
Anxiety related to unfamiliar environment, routines, diagnostic tests and treatments, and loss of control
Risk for Injury related to unfamiliar environment and physical/mental limitations secondary to condition, medications, therapies, and diagnostic test
Risk for Infection related to increased microorganisms in environment, the risk of person-to-person transmission, and invasive tests and therapies
Self-Care Deficit related to sensory, cognitive, mobility, endurance, or motivation problems
Risk for Altered Nutrition: Less Than Body Requirements related to decreased appetite secondary to treatments, fatigue, environment, and changes in usual diet, and increased protein/vitamin requirements for healing
Risk for Constipation related to change in fluid/food intake, routine and activity level, effects of medications, and emotional stress
Sleep Pattern Disturbance related to unfamiliar, noisy environment, change in bedtime ritual, emotional stress, and change in circadian rhythm
Risk for Spiritual Distress related to separation from religious support system, lack of privacy, or inability to practice spiritual rituals
Altered Family Process related to disruption of routines, change in role responsibilities, and fatigue associated with increased workload and visiting hour requirements

---

pediatrics, surgical, postanesthesia, neonatal, emergency, mental health, and so on—should have a generic unit standard of care.

Level I standards can be laminated and placed in each client care area as a reference for nurses. Because these standards apply to all clients, the nurse does not have to write the nursing diagnoses or collaborative problems associated with the generic standard of care on an individual client's care plan. Instead, institutional policy can specify that the generic standard will be implemented for all clients if indicated.

The concept of high risk is not useful at the unit standard level. At this level, all or most clients are at risk, but not at *high* risk. For example, after surgery all individuals are at risk for infection but not all are at high risk. Table 6-5 illustrates the use of *risk* instead of *high risk*.

To document Level I standards of care, the nurse should use flow chart notations unless unusual data are found or significant incidents occur. Although standards of care do not have to be part of the client's record, the record should specify what standards have been selected for the client. The problem list, representing the priority set of nursing diagnoses and collaborative problems for an individual client, can serve this purpose.

Level II—Standardized Care Plans

Preprinted care plans that represent care to be provided for a client, family, or group in addition to the Level I unit standards of care, Level II standardized care plans are supplements to the generic unit standard. Thus, a client admitted to a medical unit will receive nursing care based on both Level I unit standards and the Level II standardized care plan for the specific condition that led to admission.

PC: Hemorrhage
PC: Evisceration
PC: Urinary retention
PC: Paralytic ileus
Risk for Infection
Impaired Physical Mobility
Risk for Altered Nutrition
Risk for Colonic Constipation
Risk for Ineffective Management of Therapeutic Regimen

} From Level I Generic Standard of Care (do not appear on problem list)

A Level II standardized care plan contains either a diagnostic cluster or a single nursing diagnosis or collaborative problem, such as *High Risk for Impaired Skin Integrity* or *PC: Fluid/electrolyte imbalances*. Figure 6-6 presents a Level II standardized care plan for the collaborative problem *PC: Hypo/Hyperglycemia*.

A diagnostic cluster Level II standard would contain additional nursing diagnoses and collaborative problems that are predicted to be present and prior because of a medical condition, surgical intervention, or therapy. For example, the following presents a problem list of the client who is 1 day after total hip replacement surgery, and the source of the care.

PC: Dislocation of joint
PC: Neurovascular compromise
PC: Emboli (fat, blood)
Impaired Physical Mobility
High Risk for Impaired Skin Integrity
High Risk for Injury
High Risk for Ineffective Management of Therapeutic Regimen

Client's problem list
from Level II
Standard—Post
Total Hip
Replacement

If this client also had diabetes mellitus, the following single diagnosis standard would be added to her problem list: *PC: Hypo/Hyperglycemia*.

After the nursing staff are well oriented to the details of the unit standard, the diagnoses on the Level I unit standard could be omitted from individual client problem lists or care plans. Policy would indicate that this standard would apply to all the clients on the unit.

Level III—Addendum Care Plans

An addendum care plan lists additional interventions beyond the Level I and II standards that an individual client requires. These specific interventions may be added to a standardized care plan or may be associated with additional priority nursing diagnoses or collaborative problems not included on the Level II standardized care plan or Level I unit standards.

POTENTIAL COMPLICATION: HYPO/HYPERGLYCEMIA

Nursing Goal: The nurse will manage and minimize hypo- or hyperglycemia episodes.

1. Monitor for signs and symptoms of hypoglycemia:
   a. Blood glucose <70 mg/dL
   b. Pale, moist, cool skin
   c. Tachycardia, diaphoresis
   d. Jitteriness, irritability
   e. Headache, slurred speech
   f. Incoordination
   g. Drowsiness
   h. Visual changes
   i. Hunger, nausea, abdominal pain
2. Follow protocols when indicated, *e.g.,* concentrated glucose (oral, IV).
3. Monitor for signs and symptoms of ketoacidosis:
   a. Blood glucose >300 mg/dL
   b. Positive plasma ketone, acetone breath
   c. Headache, tachycardia
   d. Kussmaul's respirations, decreased BP
   e. Anorexia, nausea, vomiting
   f. Polyuria, polydipsia
4. If ketoacidosis occurs, follow protocols, *e.g.,* initiation of IV fluids, insulin IV.
5. If episode is severe, monitor vital signs, urine output, specific gravity, ketones, blood sugar, electrolytes q 30 mins or PRN.
6. Document blood glucose findings and other assessment data on flow record. Document unusual events or responses on progress notes.

Fig. 6-6   Level II standardized care plan for *Potential Complication: Hypo/Hyperglycemia*.

For many hospitalized clients, the nurse can direct initial care responsibility using standards of care. Assessment information obtained during subsequent nurse–client interactions may warrant specific additions to the client's care plan to ensure outcome achievement. The nurse can add or delete from standardized plans or handwrite or free-text (by computer) an addendum diagnosis with its applicable goals and interventions.

Problem List/Care Plan

As discussed earlier, a problem list represents the priority set of nursing diagnoses and collaborative problems that the nursing staff will manage for a particular client. When appropriate, the term *diagnostic* can be used in place of *problem* (*i.e.*, diagnostic list/care plan) to accommodate wellness diagnoses.

The problem list is a permanent chart record that identifies both the nursing diagnoses and collaborative problems receiving nursing management and also the source for interventions: standard of care, standardized care plan, or addendum care plan. Figure 6-7 illustrates a sample nursing problem list/care plan for a client with a history of insulin-dependent diabetes mellitus who is admitted to a medical unit for treatment of pneumonia. This sample includes the client's priority set of diagnoses as well as the addendum interventions that the nurse has added to the standardized care plan under the diagnosis *Altered Comfort*.

The Concept of Standardization

Like any concept or system, standardized care planning forms have both advantages and disadvantages. Their advantages include:

- Eliminate the need to write routine nursing interventions
- Illustrate to new employees or part-time personnel the unit standard of care
- Direct nursing staff to selected documentation requirements
- Provide the criteria for a quality improvement program and resource management
- Allow the nurse to spend more time delivering care than documenting care

    The disadvantages are:

- May take the place of a needed individualized intervention
- May encourage nurses to focus on predictable problems instead of additional ones

Some nurses experienced these disadvantages when standardized care plans were introduced into their clinical setting.

When these problems were experienced, the solution was to eliminate standardized care plans. When they were eliminated, care plan audits revealed that the nurses were writing what previously was contained on the standard of care, for example, turn q 2 hr or administer pain relief medication.

Nurses have also been socialized to view standardization as mediocre nursing—unprofessional care. Standards of care or standardized care plans should represent responsible nursing care that is predicted to be needed in certain situations. Nurses should view these predictions as scientific. When problems arise with the use of standardized forms, the solution is not to change the forms, but to address the nurse's misuse of the forms.

To minimize the disadvantages of standardized care plans, certain strategies can be implemented. The nurse who initiates the plan crosses out all sections that do not apply to her particular client. However, with clinical use, in time it may prove unnecessary to require additions to all standardized care plans. The staff may find it more efficient to use the Kardex to communicate minor variations, such as in frequency or quantities. Other interventions not appropriate for a Kardex can be entered on an addendum care plan to indicate that additional interventions have been added to a standardized plan. This prevents the experienced nurse from having to read through known standardized interventions to find addendum interventions.

The documentation of implementation does not take place on a care plan but on flow charts, graphic charts, or nursing progress notes, depending on the types of data being recorded. Figure 6-8 illustrates the nursing process with the related documentation.

Flow charts are excellent formats for recording treatments, activities of daily living, selected teaching, and observations. Figure 6-9 is an example of a flow chart. Flow charts should be used cautiously to record interactions in the spiritual, cultural, social, and psycho-

NURSING PROBLEM LIST/CARE PLAN

NURSING DIAGNOSIS/ COLLABORATIVE PROBLEM	STATUS	STAND -ARD	ADDENDUM	EVALUATION OF PROGRESS					
Med Unit Standard	7/28 A	✓		7/21 P /LfC	7/22 P /PW	7/23 P -GA			
PC· Hyperthermia	7/20			S /LfC	S /fw	S -GA			
PC· Hyper/Hypoglycemia	7/20 P	✓							
Altered Comfort	7/20 A	✓	✓						

STATUS CODE: A=Active   R=Resolved   RO=Ruled-out
EVALUATION CODE: S=Stable, I=Improved, *W=Worsened, U=Unchanged
*P=Not Progressing, P=Progressing

Reviewed With Client/Family 9/21 LfC , _____ , _____ , (Date)

ADDENDUM CARE PLAN

Nsg Dx/ Coll Prob	Client/Nursing Goals	Date/ Initials	Interventions
Altered Comfort	—	7/23 LfC	1. Provide a gentle back rub in evening 2. leave blanket at foot of bed for easy access

Initials/Signature			
1. LfC Lyndal Carpenter		5.	7.
2. PW Poti Wrychliff	4. 6. Arcangelo	6.	8.

Abridged

Fig. 6-7 Sample problem list/care plan.

logical domains. These responses may need to be recorded in the progress notes, as in explanations and counseling given to clients and families and unusual or unexpected situations (*e.g.*, injuries, clinical emergencies). If the nurses are recording the same data over and over in the progress notes, it may be possible to adapt a flow sheet to accommodate these data more frequently.

Critical Pathways

Critical pathways are a management tool introduced into health care in 1985 by Bower and Zander. Critical pathways "are based on the process of anticipating and describing *in advance* the care clients, within the specific case types, require and then comparing the actual status of the client to that anticipated" (Bower, 1993, p. 10). Critical paths are simple, direct timelines that focus on an episode of illness. They are not standards of care or care plans; they cannot focus care over a continuum.

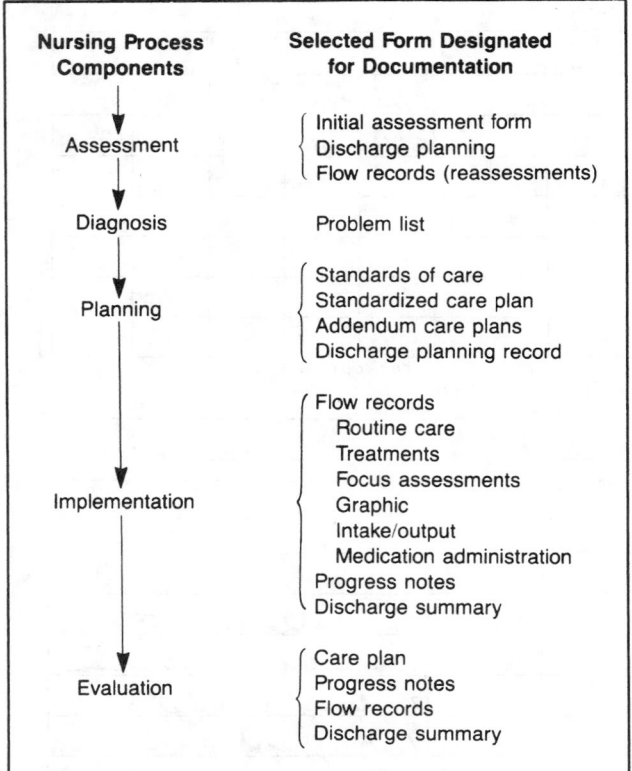

Fig. 6-8 Nursing process components with corresponding form of documentation.

Critical pathways should represent an at-a-glance reminder of the standard of care. In other words, the critical pathways should be drawn from the standard of care. Table 6-6 represents a portion of a critical pathway for clients undergoing a total hip replacement. On this pathway, the nursing diagnoses and collaborative problems are linked with outcomes and intermediate goals. A corresponding standard of care would provide the nurse with specific, detailed interventions for nursing care.

As discussed, critical paths offer an at-a-glance timeline to evaluate the progression of a client in a population. Critical pathways cannot accommodate additional nursing diagnoses or collaborative problems (addendum diagnoses) that are present and need nursing interventions. These addendum diagnoses, if not addressed, can delay client progress. For example, a woman scheduled for a hip replacement also has been on steroids for 2 years. This would necessitate monitoring for the collaborative problem—*PC: Hypo/Hyperglycemia and adrenal insufficiency*. How will the nurse communicate this problem to other nurses with a critical path? One option is to write this additional problem under the problem list in the critical path and to insert the monitoring of blood glucose levels under the assessment section. This would work if the interventions were brief, such as "monitor blood glucose levels." However, what if this woman is also confused before surgery? This would necessitate the addition of *Chronic Confusion* to the problem list. The interventions for this addendum diagnosis are not brief. A problem list/care plan can provide the solution. A detailed explanation of problem lists can be found earlier in this chapter.

Case Study Applications of Care Planning

The following two case studies and related documentation illustrate care planning for the individuals discussed. Functional health patterns are used in organizing the assessment and the analysis of the data.

(text continues on page 86)

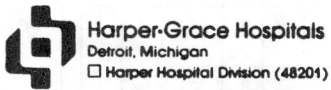

Harper-Grace Hospitals
Detroit, Michigan
☐ Harper Hospital Division (48201)

NURSING SHIFT ASSESSMENT

CODE: LOC = LEVEL OF CONSCIOUSNESS + = POSITIVE
NA = NOT APPLICABLE − = NEGATIVE
NP = NO PROBLEM x = TIMES

INITIAL ASSESSMENT	2300-0700	0700-1500	1500-2300
NUTRITION/ METABOLIC PATTERN	Skin: ☐ NP ☐ Edema ☐ Pressure Areas: _____ Other: _____	Skin: ☐ NP ☐ Edema ☐ Pressure Areas: _____ Other: _____	Skin: ☐ NP ☐ Edema ☐ Pressure Areas: _____ Other: _____
RESPIRATION/ CIRCULATION PATTERN	Breath Sounds: ☐ Normal ☐ Abnormal _____ ☐ NA Cough ☐ YES ☐ NO ☐ Productive ☐ Non-productive Peripheral Pulses: ☐ NA ☐ + ☐ − Other: _____	Breath Sounds: ☐ Normal ☐ Abnormal _____ ☐ NA Cough ☐ YES ☐ NO ☐ Productive ☐ Non-productive Peripheral Pulses: ☐ NA ☐ + ☐ − Other: _____	Breath Sounds: ☐ Normal ☐ Abnormal _____ ☐ NA Cough ☐ YES ☐ NO ☐ Productive ☐ Non-productive Peripheral Pulses: ☐ NA ☐ + ☐ − Other: _____
ELIMINATION PATTERN	☐ Nausea ☐ Vomiting ☐ Diarrhea ☐ NP Abdomen: ☐ Distended ☐ Non-Distended Bowel Sounds ☐ + ☐ − ☐ NA Other: _____	☐ Nausea ☐ Vomiting ☐ Diarrhea ☐ NP Abdomen: ☐ Distended ☐ Non-Distended Bowel Sounds ☐ + ☐ − ☐ NA Other: _____	☐ Nausea ☐ Vomiting ☐ Diarrhea ☐ NP Abdomen: ☐ Distended ☐ Non-Distended Bowel Sounds ☐ + ☐ − ☐ NA Other: _____
COGNITIVE/ PERCEPTUAL PATTERN	LOC: ☐ Person ☐ Place ☐ Time Responds appropriately to questions: ☐ Yes ☐ No Discomfort ☐ + ☐ − Type: _____ Location: _____ Other: _____	LOC: ☐ Person ☐ Place ☐ Time Responds appropriately to questions: ☐ Yes ☐ No Discomfort ☐ + ☐ − Type: _____ Location: _____ Other: _____	LOC: ☐ Person ☐ Place ☐ Time Responds appropriately to questions: ☐ Yes ☐ No Discomfort ☐ + ☐ − Type: _____ Location: _____ Other: _____
ONGOING ASSESSMENT	Time:	Time:	Time:
HEALTH PERCEPTION/ HEALTH MANAGEMENT PATTERN	Safety: Siderails x _____ ☐ Equipment _____ ☐ Restraints _____ ☐ Special Precautions _____ Other _____	Safety: Siderails x _____ ☐ Equipment _____ ☐ Restraints _____ ☐ Special Precautions _____ Other _____	Safety: Siderails x _____ ☐ Equipment _____ ☐ Restraints _____ ☐ Special Precautions _____ Other _____
NUTRITION/ METABOLIC PATTERN	Supplement/Tube Feeding _____ ☐ NPO Other _____	Diet Breakfast ☐ 100% ☐ 75% ☐ 50% ☐ 25% ☐ Refused ☐ NPO Lunch ☐ 100% ☐ 75% ☐ 50% ☐ 25% ☐ Refused ☐ NPO Supplement _____ Other _____	Diet Dinner ☐ 100% ☐ 75% ☐ 50% ☐ 25% ☐ Refused ☐ NPO Supplement _____ Other _____
ELIMINATION PATTERN	Bowel Movement X _____ ☐ Incontinent of stool Urine ☐ NP ☐ Incontinent of Urine Devices _____ Other _____	Bowel Movement X _____ ☐ Incontinent of stool Urine ☐ NP ☐ Incontinent of Urine Devices _____ Other _____	Bowel Movement X _____ ☐ Incontinent of stool Urine ☐ NP ☐ Incontinent of Urine Devices _____ Other _____
ACTIVITY/EXERCISE PATTERN	Hygiene ☐ Complete ☐ Partial ☐ Self-Care ☐ NA Skin Products _____ Mouth Care _____ Ambulated x _____ Chair x _____ ☐ Bedrest Positioned x _____ Other _____	Hygiene ☐ Complete ☐ Partial ☐ Self-Care ☐ NA Skin Products _____ Mouth Care _____ Ambulated x _____ Chair x _____ ☐ Bedrest Positioned x _____ Other _____	Hygiene ☐ Complete ☐ Partial ☐ Self-Care ☐ NA Skin Products _____ Mouth Care _____ Ambulated x _____ Chair x _____ ☐ Bedrest Positioned x _____ Other _____
SLEEP/REST PATTERN	☐ Restless ☐ Sleeping at intervals ☐ Awake ☐ None Other _____	☐ Restless ☐ Sleeping at intervals ☐ Awake ☐ None Other _____	☐ Restless ☐ Sleeping at intervals ☐ Awake ☐ None Other _____
SIGNATURE & TITLE			

300955 (3/90)

Fig. 6-9 Sample flow chart. (Courtesy of Harper Hospital, Detroit, Michigan.)

Harper-Grace Hospitals
Detroit, Michigan
☐ Harper Hospital Division (48201)

NURSING TREATMENTS/PROCEDURES

TREATMENTS

Start Date		Date:	Time/Initials			Date:	Time/Initials			Date:	Time/Initials		
			2300-0700	0700-1500	1500-2300		2300-0700	0700-1500	1500-2300		2300-0700	0700-1500	1500-2300

SPECIMENS

Date													

PROCEDURES: TO OTHER DEPARTMENTS

Initials	Date	Department	Mode of Transportation	Time

Signature & Title	Initials	Signature & Title	Initials	Signature & Title

Fig. 6-9 (Continued)

Table 6-6 Critical Pathways—Total Hip Replacement

| Nsg Dx/Coll Prob | Intermediate Goals | | Outcomes |
	Day 1	Day 2	Day 8
Pot Comp: • Fat emboli • Compartmental syndrome • Hemorrhage • Joint displacement • Sepsis • Thrombosis	The nurse will manage and minimize vascular and joint complications	→	State signs and symptoms that must be reported to health care professional
Risk for Infection		Will exhibit wound healing free of infection	Will demonstrate healing with approximated wound edges on
Impaired Physical Infection	Will relate the purpose of strengthening exercises	Will do strengthening exercises	Regain mobility while adhering to weight-bearing restrictions using walker
Acute Pain	Will report satisfactory relief of pain	→	Will report progressive reduction of pain and an increase in activity
Risk for Injury	Identify factors that increase his risk of injury; describe appropriate safety measures	→	Describe risk factors for injury in home
Risk for Impaired Skin Integrity	Demonstrate skin integrity free of pressure ulcers	→	Demonstrate skin integrity free of pressure ulcers
Risk for Ineffective Management of Therapeutic Regimen	Communicates questions and concerns	→	Describe activity restrictions Describe a plan for resuming activities of daily living (ADLs)

	/OR DAY	/POD #1	/POD #2	/POD #3
Consults		OT PT Homecare		
Tests	Postop x-ray Hct; SMA6 PT/PTT	→	→	
Treatments	Hemovac drain IV	→	D/C Hemovac	D/C staples
Medication	Antibiotic preop	Antibiotic IM pain meds Anticoagulant	po pain meds.	Prescription D/C anticoagulant
Diet	As ordered	→	→	
Activity	Bed rest with abduction pillow; maintain alignment	OOB/Chair	Weight bear as tolerated; transfer/assist Ambulate/walker	→
Assessments	Postop assessments	Assess Ace Wrap Monitor neurovascular status Monitor tissue integrity	→	→
Teaching	S/S neurovascular compromise; reinforce activity and safety measures	Postop exercises	→	Written instructions
Discharge Planning			Social work prn Home care prn	Written instructions

(Carpenito, L.J. [1995]. *Nursing care plans and documentation* [2nd ed.]. Philadelphia: J.B. Lippincott, used with permission.)

Case Study 1

Mrs. Gates, a 42-year-old woman, is recently diagnosed with metastatic carcinoma of the breast.

Medical History

Mrs. Gates went to see her medical doctor because of a lump she discovered under her left arm. After a biopsy confirmed a diagnosis of metastatic carcinoma of the breast, a mammogram revealed a lesion in the left breast. Mrs. Gates is scheduled for a left lower quadrant resection of the breast and node dissection on Thursday (3 days away).

Medical Plan

Present

    Schedule for surgery on Thursday 9/20

        Schedule bone scan, liver scan, chest x-ray

        Complete blood count and urinalysis

        SMA 24 blood studies

        ECG

Future

    Dr. Drong discussed with Mrs. Gates that approximately 3 weeks after surgery she will begin a course of chemotherapy to last 8 months.

Admission Data Base	Assessment Conclusions:
	• Positive Functioning
	• Collaborative Problems
	• Nursing Diagnoses (actual, risk, possible)

Health History

Past unusual childhood diseases
Appendectomy at age 21
Menarche at age 13 with a 28-day cycle

Health Perception–Health Management Pattern

Does not smoke	Altered Health Maintenance related to insufficient exercise
Drinks 1 glass of wine with dinner	
Does not exercise regularly	
States she "just signed up for an exercise dance class but will have to cancel now"	

Nutritional–Metabolic Pattern

(24-hr diet recall)	Effective nutritional pattern
Breakfast: 2 eggs, 1 slice toast, orange juice, coffee	Inadequate fluid intake
Lunch: Yogurt or cottage cheese with fruit, water	
Dinner: Meat, potatoes, vegetable, salad, water, 1 glass wine	
Other: 2–3 cups coffee, 1–2 pieces fruit, 1 serving ice cream/cake, cookies	
Water: 2 glasses/day	

Elimination Pattern

Chronic constipation, which she treats with over-the-counter laxatives	Colonic Constipation related to inadequate water intake, insufficient exercise as evidenced by reports of BM q 3–4 days
Bowel movement q 3–4 days	

Activity–Exercise Pattern

Works full-time as a librarian
Spends most of her free time sewing, gardening, and in activities with husband (plays, day trips)

Refer to Health Perception Pattern

Sleep–Rest Pattern

Sleeps 7–8 hours a night
Retires at 11 P.M., awakens at 6 A.M.
Falls asleep easily

Effective sleep-rest pattern

Cognitive–Perceptual Pattern

Master's degree

Effective cognitive-perceptual pattern

Self-Perception Pattern

States she "hoped that their relationship would not change after the surgery."

High Risk for Self-Concept Disturbance related to change in appearance from surgery

Role–Relationship Pattern

Married 22 years
Relies on husband for daily support
Married sister with 2 children (ages 12 and 14) lives 20 minutes away; they talk q.o.d. (every other day) on telephone and usually have Saturday or Sunday dinner together

Positive role–relationship pattern

Sexuality–Reproductive Pattern

No children: "I never got pregnant, so we both accepted it as God's will."
States that both she and her husband are very happy and satisfied with their sex life
Engages in intercourse approximately 5 times/month

Positive sexuality pattern

Coping–Stress Management Pattern

Is worried what her husband will do without her at home (e.g., meals)
Expressed concern about getting sick with chemotherapy
Related that her cousin, who had chemotherapy for leukemia, vomited all the time and lost all her hair but has been doing well for 5 years now

Fear related to cancer diagnosis, uncertainty about treatments and future
High Risk for Impaired Home Maintenance Management related to uncertainty about husband's ability to manage household

Value–Belief Pattern

Is active in her church (Lutheran)
Teaches Sunday school each week

Positive value–belief pattern

Present Medical Status

Left lower quadrant resection of left breast and node dissection surgery 9/20

Postoperative Potential Complications:
Bleedings
Paralytic ileus

Figure 6-10 is the problem list for Mrs. Gates 1 day after surgery. It contains the priority nursing diagnoses and collaborative problems for this client and the status of each.

The two diagnoses, *Colonic Constipation* and *Fear*, have both standardized and addendum interventions, as indicated by a check in each column (Standard, ACP). The diagnosis *High Risk for Self-Concept Disturbance* has interventions that are represented exclusively on the addendum care plan.

Case Study 2

While wrestling with her 15-year-old brother, 11-year-old JS sustained a fracture of her left tibia. She was admitted to the pediatric floor and placed in Buck's extension traction with a boot.

Medical Plan

Continuous traction for 5 weeks
Diazepam (Valium) 2 mg PO q 8 hr
Meperidine (Demerol) 50 mg PO q 4 hr p.r.n.
Regular diet

Medical Diagnosis

Pathologic fracture due to a benign cyst
Plan to discharge in 5 weeks in body cast; duration of body cast approximately 10 weeks

Medical History

Systems review unremarkable
1–2 episodes of upper respiratory infection each winter

Health Maintenance–Health Perception Pattern

Up-to-date with immunizations
Dental checkup q 6 months

Nutritional–Metabolic Pattern

Reports a usual daily intake of:
Breakfast: Pancakes or cereal, orange juice

Nursing Diagnosis/ Collaborative Problem	Status	Standard of Care	ACP (Addendum Care Plan)
1. Surgical Unit Standard	A 9/20	√	
2. High Risk for Fluid Volume Excess: left arm related to effects of mastectomy and dependent positions	A 9/20	√	
3. Colonic Constipation related to possible inadequate water intake, insufficient exercise as evidenced by reports of bowel movements q 3–4 days	A 9/20	√	√
4. High Risk for Self-Concept Disturbance related to fears that change in appearance will influence relations with spouse	A 9/21		√
5. Fear related to cancer diagnosis, uncertainty about treatments and future as evidenced by expressions of concern about chemotherapy and its success	A 9/21	√	√
6. High Risk for Ineffective Management of Therapeutic Regimen related to lack of knowledge of arm exercises, self-breast exams, hazards to affected arm, community services	A 9/20	√	

Fig. 6-10 Nursing problem list/care plan for Mrs. Gates 1 day postoperatively, showing priority nursing diagnoses and collaborative care problems, and the status of each.

Lunch: Sandwich, hot dog or pizza, ice cream, milk
Dinner: Meat, potatoes, vegetables (carrots, peas, corn only)
Snacks: Cookies, popcorn
Water: 4 glasses

Elimination Pattern

Reports a soft, formed BM q.d.

Activity–Exercise Pattern

Reports:
She is well liked in school
Enjoys sports (soccer)
Likes to cook
Likes school (excels in math and science, has to work at her reading skills)
States she is bored in the hospital

Sleep–Rest Pattern

Retires at 9:00 P.M. on weekdays
Awakens at 7:00 A.M.
Bedtime ritual: Bath, oral hygiene, reads a short story

Cognitive–Perceptual Pattern

Three days postadmission:
JS experiences intermittent leg spasms that were visible the first 2 days. She continues to complain of spasms that are no longer visible. She responds to the spasms by screaming.
JS is placed in private room at the end of the hall, and the door is kept closed to muffle her screams.
JS's mother arrives at 10:30 A.M. and remains until 6:30 P.M. Her husband arrives at 6:30 P.M. and stays until 8:30 or 9:00 P.M.
JS spends her day watching TV, conversing with her mother, and experiencing spasms. Her contact with the nursing staff is limited to hygiene needs and medications.
JS complains that her pain meds are often late, and then her spasms are "really bad."

Self-Perception Pattern

Reports she is well liked in school
Expects to be "as good as before, after the fracture heals"

Role–Relationship Pattern

Has a 15-year-old brother
Mother is a former librarian
Father is a pharmacist who teaches at the local university
Reports her family has a good time together

Sexuality–Reproductive Pattern

Reports she learned about sexuality, pregnancy, and menses "from her mom and dad before the health teacher had a class"

Coping–Stress Management Pattern

Says when she is sad, she talks to her mother, father, or brother, depending on the reason

Value–Belief Pattern

Attends Catholic church every Sunday
Believes in God and prays for assistance and to say, "Thank you"

You are a part-time nurse caring for JS today.

1. Examine the preceding data. For each of the following functional patterns, are there data to support:
   Positive functioning?
   Altered functioning?
   At high risk for altered functioning?*
   A. Health Perception–Health Management Pattern
      Health practices
      Compliance?
      Injuries?
      Unhealthy lifestyle?
   B. Nutritional–Metabolic Pattern
      Nutrition?
      Fluid intake?
      Peripheral edema?
      Infection?
      Oral cavity health?
   C. Elimination Pattern
      Bowel elimination?
      Incontinence?
   D. Activity–Exercise Pattern
      Activities of daily living?
      Leisure activities?
      Home care?
      Respiratory function?
   E. Sleep–Rest Pattern
      Sleep?
   F. Cognitive–Perceptual Pattern
      Comfort?
      Knowledge?
      Sensory input?
   G. Self-Perception Pattern
      Anxiety/fear?
      Control?
      Self-concept?
   H. Role–Relationship Pattern
      Communication?
      Family?
      Loss?
      Parenting?
      Socialization?
      Violence?
   I. Sexuality–Reproductive Pattern
      Knowledge of?
      Sexuality?
   J. Coping–Stress Tolerance Pattern
      Coping?
   K. Value–Belief Pattern
      Spirituality?

2. Is there a physiologic complication present, or is there a *high* risk for one developing because of a disease, treatment, diagnostic study, or medication that requires monitoring and joint management by you and a physician?
      Cardiac, circulatory
      Immune, hematopoietic

* Copyright 1985, Lynda Juall Carpenito

Respiratory
Renal
Neurologic
Muscular, skeletal
Reproductive
Endocrine, metabolic
Gastrointestinal, hepatic, biliary

3. After you have determined which functional patterns are altered or at risk for altered functioning, review the list of nursing diagnoses under that pattern and select the appropriate diagnosis.*
   A. If you select an actual diagnosis
      Do you have signs and symptoms to support its presence? (Refer to Section II, *Manual of Nursing Diagnoses,* under the selected diagnosis.)
      Write the actual diagnosis in three parts:
         (1) label, (2) related to contributing factors, (3) as evidenced by signs and symptoms
   B. If you select a risk or high-risk diagnosis
      Do you have risk factors present?
      Write the diagnosis in two parts:
         (1) High Risk (label), (2) related to risk factors
   C. Check each nursing diagnosis with the following review questions:*
      1. Is the statement clearly stated?
      2. Is the terminology correct?
      3. Is there a two-part statement?
      4. Does the second part of the statement reflect the specific factors that have contributed or may contribute to the development of the nursing diagnosis?
      5. Is there documentation of validation (signs and symptoms) for actual diagnoses?
      6. Does the nursing diagnosis statement reflect a situation for which a nurse can order the definitive interventions to treat or prevent?
      7. *Do you need additional client contact to individualize the diagnostic statement?*
4. After you have identified which physiologic complications should be monitored for, list them as:
   Potential Complications: (list here)
5. A. Write short-term outcome (client goals) or each actual and high-risk nursing diagnosis. Write nursing goals for collaborative problems.
   B. Check each client goal with the following review questions:*
      1. Is the goal a client goal or a nursing goal?
      2. Is the goal realistic and attainable?
      3. Is it measurable? (Can the nurse validate it by seeing or hearing?)
      4. Are the verbs measurable (states, demonstrates) or not measurable (knows, understands, experiences)?
      5. Has the content been clearly specified (how much, when, where)?
      6. Can a time for achievement be realistically identified?
      7. *Do you need additional client contact to individualize the goals?*
6. A. Write interventions for both the nursing diagnoses and the collaborative problems.
   B. Check each intervention with the following review questions:*
      1. Are the nursing orders clear (what, when, how often, how long, and where)?
      2. Do the nursing orders reflect creativity (and current practice)?
      3. *Do you need additional client contact to individualize the interventions?*

Now review the following care plan (Fig. 6-11), which represents the priority problems for JS.

* Copyright 1985, Lynda Juall Carpenito

(text continues on page 97)

NURSING DIAGNOSIS/ COLLABORATIVE PROBLEM	STATUS	STAND - ARD	ADDENDUM	EVALUATION OF PROGRESS				
Pediatric Unit Standard	5-1 A	✓						
Pain related to ineffective relief of muscle spasms	5-1 A	✓	✓					
High Risk for impaired skin integrity r.t. –imposed bedrest –Traction equipment	5-1 A	✓						
High Risk for Colonic Constipation r.t. – Dietary patterns (low fiber) – Embarrassment	5-1 A	✓						
High Risk for Peripheral Neurovascular Comp.	5-1 A	✓						
Diversional Activity Deficit r.t. Imposed bedrest and isolation	5-2 A		✓					

STATUS CODE: A=Active   R=Resolved   RO=Ruled-out
EVALUATION CODE: S=Stable, I=Improved, *W=Worsened, U=Unchanged
     *P=Not Progressing, P=Progressing

Reviewed With Client/Family 5/1 xjc , 5/4 xjc ____ , (Date)

Fig. 6-11 Care plan for Case Study 2.

NURSING PROBLEM LIST/CARE PLAN

NURSING DIAGNOSIS/ COLLABORATIVE PROBLEM	STATUS	STAND -ARD	ADDENDUM	EVALUATION OF PROGRESS				
High Risk for Impaired Home Maintenance Management r.t. discharge with body cast to home for 10 weeks.	5-4 A		✓					

STATUS CODE: A=Active R=Resolved RO=Ruled-out
EVALUATION CODE: S=Stable, I=Improved, *W=Worsened, U=Unchanged
*P=Not Progressing, P=Progressing

Reviewed With Client/Family _____ , _____ , _____ , (Date)

Fig. 6-11 (Continued)

ADDENDUM CARE PLAN

Nsg Dx/ Coll Prob	Client/Nursing Goals	Date/ Initials	Interventions
Pain r.t. ineffective relief of muscle spasm as manifested by frequent reports of inadequate relief	1. Report less pain 2. Practice selected distraction techniques during pain episodes	5- JW	1. Teach her rhythmic abdominal breathing to practice during muscle spasms. 2. Coach her to practice breathing during episodes of spasms 3. Administer pain med on time q 4 hrs. 4. Encourage her to use her radio with earphones during episodes of spasm and to increase the volume as pain increases
Diversional Activity Deficit r.t. imposed bedrest, isolation as manifested by statements of boredom	1. occupy her time with activities other than TV viewing	5-2 PW	1. Consult with recreational therapist for appropriate activities 2. Encourage other children on floor to visit and play cards with her. 3. Encourage her to read stories to small children

Initials/Signature			
1. Joann Woolsey RN	3.	5.	7.
2. Peti Wyckoff RN	4.	6.	8.

Fig. 6-11 (Continued)

ADDENDUM CARE PLAN

Nsg Dx/ Coll Prob	Client/Nursing Goals	Date/ Initials	Interventions
			on unit in her room
			4. Arrange for Tutoring with school district
			5. Try to stimulate her to do something other than watching T.V e.g. Hook rug, electronic games.
			6. Allow her opportunities to share her feelings of loneliness
W. Ro/impaired home maintenance r.t. discharge with body cast To home for 10 weeks (approx discharge date 6/10)		5/4 PW	1. Allow parents to share their concern about care of daughter after discharge.
			2. Assure them that they will have an opportunity to care for daughter under supervision in hospital.
			3. Discuss and Teach each of the following when indicated.
Initials/Signature 1.	3.	5.	7.
2.	4.	6.	8.

Fig. 6-11 (Continued)

ADDENDUM CARE PLAN

Nsg Dx/ Coll Prob	Client/Nursing Goals	Date/ Initials	Interventions
			Cast care
			Hygienic measures
			Nutrition (↑ calcium reqts)
			Elimination
			Diversional activities
			Tutoring
			Relief periods for parents from care.

Initials/Signature			
1.	3.	5.	7.
2.	4.	6.	8.

Fig. 6-11 (Continued)

References

Alfaro, R. (1994). *Applying nursing diagnosis and nursing process: A step-by-step guide* (3rd ed.). Philadelphia: J. B. Lippincott.

Aukamp, V. (1984). *Nursing care plans for the childbearing family*. Norwalk, CT: Appleton-Century-Crofts.

Bower, C. (1993, September). *Patient outcomes and nursing diagnosis: Expanding the value of critical paths*. Workshop. Pasadena, California.

Bulechek, G., & McCloskey, J. (1989). *Nursing interventions: Treatments for nursing diagnoses* (2nd ed.). Philadelphia: W. B. Saunders.

Carnevali, D. L. (1983). *Nursing care planning: Diagnosis and management* (3rd ed.). Philadelphia: J. B. Lippincott.

Carpenito, L. J. (1995). *Nursing care plans and documentation: Nursing diagnoses and collaborative problems* (2nd ed.). Philadelphia: J. B. Lippincott.

Cronin, C. J., & Maklebust, J. (1989). Case-managed care: Capitalizing on the CNS. *Nursing Management, 20*(3), 38–47.

Doenges, M., Moorhouse, M., & Geissler, A. (1994). *Nursing care plans* (3rd ed.). Philadelphia: F. A. Davis.

Gordon, M. (1987). *Nursing diagnosis: Process and application* (2nd ed.). New York: McGraw-Hill.

Kim, M. J., McFarland, G. K., & McLane, A. M. (1995). *Pocket guide to nursing diagnoses* (6th ed.). St. Louis: C. V. Mosby.

Sparks, S., Taylor, C., & Dyer, J. (1996). *Nursing diagnoses pocket manual*. Springhouse, PA: Springhouse Corp.

Townsend, M. C. (1994). *Nursing diagnoses in psychiatric nursing* (3rd ed.). Philadelphia: F. A. Davis.

Section II

Manual of Nursing Diagnoses

Introduction

The *Manual of Nursing Diagnoses* consists of 138 nursing diagnoses. The diagnoses are described with the three NANDA-required elements first, followed by four additional components:

- Definition
- Defining characteristics, signs and symptoms, or risk factors of the diagnosis
- Related factors, organized accoding to pathophysiologic, treatment-related, situational, and maturational factors that may contribute to or cause the actual diagnosis
- Author's Note, containing a discussion of the diagnosis to clarify its concept and clinical use
- Focus assessment criteria, subjective and objective, which serve to guide the nurse to specific data collection to help confirm or rule out the diagnosis
- Key Concepts—scientific explanations about the diagnosis and interventions presented under Generic Considerations, Specific Age-Related Considerations (subdivided into Child, Maternal, and Older Adult), and Transcultural Considerations.

Each diagnosis has one group of interventions that focuses on the treatment associated with the diagnostic label, regardless of the etiologic and contributing factors, with outcome criteria. Interventions specifically direct the nurse to:

- Clarification of causative and contributing factors
- Reduction or elimination of the factors
- Promotion of selected activities
- Health teaching and referrals

Some diagnoses are further explained by one or more specific nursing diagnoses. These specific diagnoses were selected because of their frequency in nursing and do not in any respect represent exclusive categories. For example, *Activity Intolerance* has specific contributing factors:

- Related to Insufficient Knowledge of Adaptive Techniques Needed secondary to Chronic Obstructive Pulmonary Disease
- Related to Insufficient Knowledge of Adaptive Techniques Needed secondary to Impaired Cardiac Function
- Related to Bed Rest Deconditioning

Some diagnoses have population-specific interventions for children, pregnant women, and older adults.

Each diagnosis concludes with a bibliography containing books and periodicals. Pertinent literature and organizations for the consumer are also cited when appropriate. Several of the diagnoses represent broad categories under which more specific diagnoses fall. As the taxonomic work of NANDA continues, more specific diagnoses will evolve, making the broader diagnoses no longer clinically useful. For example, the addition of the seven diagnoses (six NANDA-approved) related to incontinence—*Functional Incontinence, Reflex Incontinence, Stress Incontinence, Total Incontinence, Urge Incontinence, Urinary Retention,* and *Maturational Enuresis*—has made *Altered Patterns of Urinary Elimination* too broad for clinical use.

Readers of this manual are encouraged to become familiar with all of the nursing diagnoses and collaborative problems in order to incorporate them into their nursing practice. Until you become familiar with the nursing diagnoses and their defining characteristics or risk factors and collaborative problems, the following guidelines are suggested:

1. Collect data, both subjective and objective, from client, family, other health care professionals, and records.
2. Examine the data described above. For each of the following functional patterns, are there data to support

   positive functioning?

altered functioning?

at risk for altered functioning?*

   Health perception–health management pattern
      Health management?
      Compliance?
      Injuries?
      Self-care?
   Nutritional–metabolic pattern
      Nutrition?
      Fluid intake?
      Peripheral edema?
      Infection?
      Oral cavity health?
   Elimination pattern
      Bowel elimination?
      Incontinence?
   Activity–exercise pattern
      Activities of daily living?
      Leisure activities?
      Home care?
      Respiratory function?
   Sleep–rest pattern
      Sleep
   Cognitive–perceptual pattern
      Decisions?
      Comfort?
      Knowledge?
      Sensory input?
   Self-perception pattern
      Anxiety/fear?
      Self-concept?
   Role–relationship pattern
      Communication?
      Family?
      Loss?
      Parenting?
      Socialization?
      Violence?
   Sexuality–reproductive pattern
      Knowledge of?
      Sexuality?
   Coping–stress tolerance pattern
      Coping?
   Value–belief pattern
      Spirituality?

3. After you have selected which functional patterns are altered or present a risk for altered functioning, review the list of nursing diagnoses under that pattern and select the appropriate diagnosis (see Appendix I).
4. If you select an actual diagnosis:

   Do you have signs and symptoms to support its presence? (Refer to Section II under the selected diagnosis.)

   Write the actual diagnosis in three parts: Label; related to (contributing factors); as evidenced by (signs and symptoms)
5. If you select a risk diagnosis,

   Are risk factors present?

   Write the risk diagnosis in two parts: *Risk for (specify label) related to (risk factors)*

6. If you need assistance in writing the nursing diagnosis, refer to Chapters 2 and 4 for guidelines.

7. If you suspect a problem but have insufficient data, refer to the focus assessment data under the diagnosis and gather the additional data to confirm or rule out the diagnosis. If this additional data collection needs to be done at a later time or by other nurses, label the diagnosis *Possible* . . . on the care plan. (Refer to Chapter 2 for a discussion of possible nursing diagnoses.)

8. For the nursing diagnoses that you have validated, refer to that diagnosis and review the outcome criteria. Rewrite the outcome criteria adding the individualized criteria for the specific client. (Refer to Chapter 5 for specific guidelines.)

9. Review the interventions under the diagnosis and select those that are appropriate. Rewrite the interventions, adding individualization when needed. Add other interventions as indicated.

10. Is a physiologic complication present, or is there a high risk of one developing because of a disease, treatment, diagnostic study, or medication that you want to monitor for? (collaborative problem)
    a. Cardiac, circulatory
    b. Metabolic, hematopoietic
    c. Respiratory
    d. Renal
    e. Genitourinary
    f. Neurologic
    g. Muscular
    h. Skeletal
    i. Endocrine, immune
    j. Gastrointestinal, hepatic, biliary
    k. Reproductive

11. After you have selected which physiologic complications or collaborative problems are indicated to be monitored for or managed, list them as *Potential Complication: (Specify)*.

12. Initiate a standard care plan or write the collaborative problem on the care plan and add the appropriate interventions that direct nurses to monitor for the problems and intervene accordingly. (Refer to Section III, *Manual of Collaborative Problems,* for more information.)

Activity Intolerance

DEFINITION

Activity Intolerance: A reduction in one's physiologic capacity to endure activities to the degree desired or required (Magnan, 1987).

DEFINING CHARACTERISTICS
Major (Must Be Present)

An altered physiologic response to activity (*e.g.*)
    Respiratory
        Dyspnea
        Excessive increase in rate
        Shortness of breath
        Decrease in rate
    Pulse
        Weak
        Decrease
        Excessive increase
        Rhythm change
        Failure to return to preactivity level after 3 minutes
    Blood pressure
        Failure to increase with activity
        Increase in diastolic >15 mm Hg

Minor (May Be Present)

Weakness   Confusion
Fatigue   Vertigo
Pallor or cyanosis

RELATED FACTORS

Any factors that compromise oxygen transport, lead to physical deconditioning, or create excessive energy demands that outstrip the person's physical and psychological abilities can cause activity intolerance. Some common factors are listed below.

Pathophysiologic

Related to compromised oxygen transport system secondary to:
    (Cardiac)
        Idiopathic hypertrophic subaortic stenosis   Angina
        Congenital heart disease   Myocardial infarction
        Cardiomyopathies   Valvular disease
        Congestive heart failure
        Dysrhythmias
    (Respiratory)
        Chronic obstructive pulmonary disease
        Atelectasis
        Bronchopulmonary dysplasia
    (Circulatory)
        Anemia   Hypovolemia
        Peripheral arterial disease

Related to increased metabolic demands secondary to:
(Acute or chronic infections)

Viral infection	Hepatitis
Mononucleosis	Endocrine or metabolic disorders

(Chronic diseases)

Renal	Musculoskeletal
Hepatic	Neurological
Inflammatory	

Related to inadequate energy sources secondary to:

Obesity	Inadequate diet
Malnourishment	

Treatment-Related

Related to increased metabolic demands secondary to:

Malignancies	Diagnostic studies
Surgery	Treatment schedule/treatments (frequency)

Related to compromised oxygen transport secondary to:

Hypovolemia	Prolonged bed rest

Situational (Personal, Environmental)

Related to inactivity secondary to:

Depression	Sedentary life-style
Lack of motivation	

Related to increased metabolic demands secondary to:
Assistive equipment (walkers, crutches, braces)
Extreme stress
Pain
Environmental barriers (*e.g.*, stairs)
Climatic extremes (especially hot, humid climates)
Air pollution (*e.g.*, smog)
Atmospheric pressure (*e.g.*, recent relocation to high-altitude living)

Maturational

The older adult may experience decreased muscle strength and flexibility, as well as sensory deficits. All of these can undermine body confidence and may contribute directly or indirectly to Activity Intolerance.

Author's Note

Activity Intolerance is a diagnostic judgment that describes a person with compromised physical conditioning. This person can engage in therapies that increase strength and endurance. *Activity Intolerance* differs from *Fatigue* in that it is relieved by rest. In *Activity Intolerance*, moreover, the goal is to increase tolerance to activity; with *Fatigue*, in contrast, the goal is to assist the person to adapt to the fatigue, not to increase endurance.

Errors in Diagnostic Statements

Activity Intolerance related to dysrhythmic episodes in response to increased activity secondary to recent MI

The goal for this client at this time would not be to increase tolerance to activity, but rather to monitor cardiac response to activity and to prevent decreased cardiac output. This situation would be more appropriately labeled as a collaborative problem: *Potential Complication: Decreased Cardiac Output.*

Activity Intolerance related to fatigue secondary to chemotherapy

The fatigue associated with chemotherapy is not improved by rest and is not amenable to interventions to increase endurance. The following diagnosis would be correct: *Fatigue related to anemia and chemical changes secondary to toxic effects of chemotherapy.*

Key Concepts

1. Nursing interventions are planned to facilitate engagement in activity based on an understanding of the person's knowledge of activity demands, valuation of activity, beliefs about activity, and perceived capability for activity.
2. The ability to continue a specified task is known as *endurance*; the inability to continue a specified task, *fatigue*. Conceptually, fatigue is the reciprocal of endurance (DeLateur, 1987). Nursing interventions are directed at delaying the onset of task-related fatigue by maximizing the efficient use of muscles that control motion, movement, and locomotion. Work simplification is an important strategy for delaying onset of task-related fatigue.
3. The ability to maintain a given level of performance depends on personal factors: strength, coordination, reaction time, alertness, and motivation; and on activity-related factors: frequency, duration, and intensity of activity.
4. In normal persons, the work of breathing is very limited. In persons with COPD, however, the work of breathing may be increased five to ten times above normal. Under such conditions, the amount of oxygen required *just for breathing activities* may be a large fraction of total oxygen consumption.
5. The effects of bed rest deconditioning develop rapidly and may take weeks or months to reverse. All persons confined to bed are at risk for activity intolerance as a result of bed rest–induced deconditioning.

🐚 Key Concepts—*Child*

1. Children at special risk for activity intolerance include those with respiratory conditions, cardiovascular conditions, anemia, and chronic illnesses, such as nephrosis (Scipien, Chard, Howe, & Barnard, 1990).
2. Recent research findings show that supervised exercise training at moderate intensity is safe and produces significant beneficial changes in hemodynamics and exercise time in children with cardiac disease (Balfour, 1991, p. 627).

🏛 Key Concepts—*Older Adult*

1. Decreases in cardiac output in the elderly have been attributed to disease-related processes, not age-related changes (Miller, 1990). Fleg (1986) found no age-related changes in resting cardiac output in a study of healthy people between the ages of 30 and 80 years.
2. Studies have demonstrated an average age decline of 5%–10% per decade in maximum oxygen consumption (VO_2max) from age 25 to age 75, or approximately 0.28 mL/kg/yr. Individuals who have been very athletic still have declines in VO_2max; however, it is only half of the 10% decade decline that is exhibited in less athletic individuals. There seems to be either decreased efficiency in mobilizing blood to exercising muscles or increased difficulty for muscles in extracting and using oxygen because of decreased muscle mass. (*Note:* VO_2max is very difficult to obtain in older adults because of multiple subjective factors such as muscle fatigue, perceived exhaustion, and motivation to be tested. Often, leg muscles fail the individual before VO_2max can be achieved [Fleg, 1986; Gerber, 1990; Posner, Gorman, Klein, & Woldow, 1986].)
3. By age 75 years, only 10% of the pacemaker cells in the SA node remain, which could account for the slowed conduction during exercise (Gerber, 1990).
4. Aging brings a general decline in physical activity, which has a significant effect on cardiac performance both at rest and during exercise (Fleg, 1986; Abrams & Berkow, 1990).
5. Prolonged immobility and inactivity through self-imposed restrictions, mental status changes, and/or pathophysiologic changes can result in decreased tolerance to activity (Bortz, 1982; Matteson & McConnell, 1988).
6. Decreased muscle mass leads to decreased strength which, in turn, leads to decreased endurance. Muscle strength, which is maximal between ages 20 and 30 years, drops to 80% of that value by age 65 (Fleg, 1986; Matteson & McConnell, 1988).
7. Increased chest wall rigidity with aging leads to decreased lung expansion, resulting in decreased tissue oxygenation. This has immediate effects on activity tolerance.

Focus Assessment Criteria

Assessing for activity intolerance is a dynamic process that starts before the onset of activity, proceeds continuously throughout the activity, and terminates in a postactivity evaluation. During preactivity assessment, the nurse establishes baseline "at rest" measurements of blood pressure, pulse, and respiration. The nurse also assesses incentives for activity and the person's perceived capabilities for activity, as well as factors that may decrease tolerance for activity. If a known pathology exists in a particular organ system, then assessment during activity focuses on signs and symptoms indicating intolerance in that system (*e.g.*, exertional dyspnea or cyanosis in pulmonary disease, angina in cardiac disease, increased spasticity or decreased coordination in neuromuscular disease). During postactivity assessment, the nurse assesses recovery time, which provides an index for judging physiologic tolerance for activity.

Subjective Data

A. Assess for defining characteristics
　　1. Weakness
　　2. Fatigue
　　3. Dyspnea
　　4. Lack of sleep or rest

B. Assess for related factors
　　1. Lack of incentive
　　2. Disinclination to participate in activities
　　3. Lack of confidence in ability to perform activity
　　4. Fear of injury or aggravating disease as a result of participating in activity
　　5. Difficulty performing activities of daily living because of decreased energy or a lack of strength
　　6. Pain that interferes with performance of activities

Objective Data

A. Assess for defining characteristics
　　1. Assess strength and balance, evaluate person's ability to:
　　　　Reposition self in bed
　　　　Maintain body alignment
　　　　Assume and maintain sitting position
　　　　Rise to standing position
　　　　Maintain erect posture
　　　　Perform Romberg test
　　　　Ambulate
　　　　Perform activities of daily living
　　2. Assess response to activity.
　　　　Take resting vital signs (Table II-1)
　　　　　　Pulse (rate, rhythm, quality)　　Respirations (rate, depth, effort)
　　　　　　Blood pressure
　　　　Have person perform the activity
　　　　Take vital signs immediately after the activity
　　　　Have person rest for 3 minutes; take vital signs again
　　　　Assess for presence of:
　　　　　　Pallor　　　　Cyanosis
　　　　　　Confusion　　Vertigo

B. Assess for related factors
　　1. Situational
　　　　Personal
　　　　　　Coping strategies focusing on avoidance
　　　　　　Inadequate social support

Table II-1   **Physiologic Response to Activity (Expected and Abnormal)**

	Pulse	Blood Pressure	Respiration
Resting			
Normal	60–90	<140/90	<20
Abnormal	>100	>140/90	>20
Immediately After Activity			
Normal	↑Rate	↑Systolic	↑Rate
	↑Strength	Decrease or no change in systolic	↑Depth
Abnormal	↓Rate		Excessive
	↓Strength		↓Rate
	Irregular rhythm		
3 Minutes After Activity			
Normal	Within 6 beats of resting pulse		
Abnormal	>7 beats of resting pulse		

Environmental
  Social isolation   Sensory deprivation
  Sensory overload   Climatic extremes
  Insufficient rest and sleep periods
2. Disease-related
  Cardiopulmonary disorders   Neurologic disorders
  Nutritional deficiencies   Fluid/electrolyte imbalance
  Musculoskeletal disorders   Chronic diseases
3. Treatment-related
  Bed rest/imposed immobility Diet
  Diagnostic studies   Surgery
  Medications   Caregivers' expectations
  Treatment schedule   Assistive equipment that requires strength

---

Outcome Criteria

The person will
• Identify factors that aggravate activity intolerance
• Identify methods to reduce activity intolerance
• Progress activity to (specify level of activity desired/required)
• Maintain blood pressure, pulse, and respirations within predetermined ranges during activity

---

Interventions

A. Monitor the individual's response to activity
  1. Take resting pulse, blood pressure, and respirations.
  2. Consider rate, rhythm, and quality (if signs are abnormal—*e.g.*, pulse above 100—consult with physician about advisability of increasing activity).
  3. Have person perform the activity.
  4. Take vital signs immediately after activity. (Strenuous activity may increase the pulse by 50 beats. Such a rate is still satisfactory, as long as it returns to the resting pulse within 3 minutes.)
  5. Have person rest for 3 minutes; take vital signs again.
  6. Discontinue the activity if the individual responds to the activity with:
    a. Complaints of chest pain, vertigo, or confusion

   b. Decrease in pulse rate
   c. Failure of systolic blood pressure to increase
   d. Decrease in systolic blood pressure
   e. Increase in diastolic blood pressure by 15 mm Hg
   f. Decrease in respiratory response
7. Reduce the intensity or duration of the activity if:
   a. The pulse takes longer than 3–4 minutes to return to within six beats of the resting pulse rate
   b. The respiratory rate increase is excessive after the activity

B. Progress the activity gradually

1. Increase the person's tolerance for activity by having him perform the activity more slowly, or for a shorter period of time with more rest pauses, or with more assistance.
2. Minimize the deconditioning effects of prolonged bed rest and imposed immobility:
   a. Begin range of motion (ROM) at least b.i.d.
        If the person is unable, the nurse should perform passive ROM.
        If the person is able, have him perform active ROM.
   b. Encourage isometric exercise.
   c. Encourage the person to turn and lift himself actively unless contraindicated.
3. Promote optimal sitting balance and tolerance by increasing muscle strength.
   a. Gradually increase sitting tolerance by starting with 15 minutes for the first time out of bed.
   b. Have the person get out of bed three times a day, increasing the time out of bed by 15 minutes each day.
   c. Practice transfers. Have the person do as much active movement as possible during transfers.
4. Promote ambulation with or without assistive devices.
   a. Provide support when the person begins to stand.
   b. If the person is unable to stand without buckling his knees, he is not ready for ambulation; have him practice standing in place with assistance.
   c. Choose a gait that is safe for the individual. (If his gait appears awkward but he has stability, allow him to continue; stay close by and give clear coaching messages, *e.g.*, "Look straight ahead, not down.")
5. Allow the person to gauge the rate of ambulation.
6. Provide sufficient support to ensure safety and prevent falling.
7. Encourage the person to wear comfortable walking shoes (slippers do not support the feet properly).

C. Discuss with the person his perceptions of his condition and the effects it will have on role responsibilities, occupation, and finances

D. Determine adequacy of sleep (refer to Sleep Pattern Disturbance for additional information).

1. Plan rest periods according to the person's daily schedule. (Rest periods should occur throughout the day and between activities.)
2. Encourage person to rest during the first hour after meals. (Rest can take many forms: napping, sitting and watching TV, or sitting with legs elevated.)

E. Promote a sincere "can do" attitude to provide a positive atmosphere that encourages increased activity; convey the belief that increasing level of activity and tolerance for activity is possible.

1. Identify factors that undermine person's confidence (*e.g.*, fear of falling, perceived weakness, visual impairment).
2. Explore possible incentives with the person and the family; consider what the person values (*e.g.*):

Playing with grandchildren	Going fishing
Returning to work	Performing a task, such as a craft

3. Allow person to set activity schedule and functional activity goals. If his goal is too low, contract with him (*e.g.*, "your goal of walking 25 feet seems low. Let's increase it to 50 feet and I'll walk with you.").

4. Plan a purpose for the activity, such as sitting up in a chair to eat lunch, walking to a window to see the view, or walking to the kitchen to get some juice.

5. Help person to identify progress made. Do not underestimate the value of praise and encouragement as an effective motivational technique. In selected cases, it may be helpful to have the client keep a written record of his activities to demonstrate progress.

F. Provide family with an opportunity to share their concerns

1. Assess their knowledge of the condition, treatment, and prognosis.
2. Encourage them to share their concerns about the future and about role responsibilities.

Rationale

- A person's response to activity can be evaluated by comparing preactivity blood pressure, pulse, and respiration with postactivity blood pressure, pulse, and respiration. These, in turn, are compared with recovery time—the amount of time required for blood pressure, pulse, and respiration to return to preactivity levels.

- Tolerance for activity develops cyclically through adjusting frequency, duration, and intensity of activity until the desired level is achieved. Increasing activity frequency precedes increasing duration and intensity (work demand). Increased intensity is offset by a reduction in duration and frequency. As tolerance for more intensive activity of short duration develops, frequency is once again increased.

- The reliability of self-reports of activity has been called into question (Klesges, Eck, Mellon, Fulliton, Somes, & Hanson, 1989). Keeping a record of actual activities and responses to activity provides a more reliable means of demonstrating progress.

- The symptoms of activity intolerance are relieved by rest. The daily schedule is planned to allow for alternating periods of activity and rest and coordinated to reduce periods of excess energy expenditure.

- Nursing interventions for activity intolerance promote participation in activities to achieve a level of activity desired by the person for the therapeutic regimen.

- A person's decision to engage in a particular activity is influenced by knowledge, values, beliefs, and perceived capability for action (Magnan, 1987).

■ Activity Intolerance
Related to Insufficient Knowledge of Adaptive Techniques Needed Secondary to Chronic Obstructive Pulmonary Disease

---

Outcome Criteria

The person will
- Maintain/achieve optimal activity level (specify level)
- Demonstrate methods of controlled breathing to conserve energy
- Demonstrate ability to coordinate controlled breathing with activity

---

Interventions

The following interventions apply to people experiencing activity intolerance due to a known cause: chronic obstructive pulmonary disease. These interventions are used in conjunction with the interventions identified for general cases of activity intolerance (see Interventions, pp. 107 through 109.)

A. Assess adequacy of:
1. Knowledge of the therapeutic regimen
2. Pulmonary hygiene
3. Breathing techniques
4. Activity level
5. Nutritional intake
6. Health-related behaviors

B. Eliminate or reduce contributing factors
1. Lack of knowledge
   a. Assess person's understanding of the prescribed therapeutic regimen; proceed with health teaching using simple, clear instructions and including family members.
   b. Specifically assess knowledge of:
      Pulmonary hygiene   Adaptive breathing techniques
2. Inadequate pulmonary hygiene routine
   a. Explain the importance of adhering to daily coughing schedule for clearing the lungs and that this is a lifetime commitment.
   b. Teach the proper method of controlled coughing:
      Breathe deeply and slowly while sitting up as upright as possible.
      Use diaphragmatic breathing.
      Hold the breath for 3–5 seconds and then slowly exhale as much of this breath as possible through the mouth. (Lower rib cage and abdomen should sink down with exhaling.)
      Take a second deep breath, hold, and cough forcefully from deep in the chest (not from the back of the mouth or throat); use two short, forceful coughs.
      Rest after coughing sessions.
   c. Instruct person to practice controlled coughing four times a day, 30 minutes before meals and at bedtime. Allow 15–30 minutes rest after coughing session and before meals.

    d. Consider use of inhaled humidity, postural drainage, and chest clapping before coughing session. Assess for use of prescribed aerosol bronchodilators to dilate airways and thin secretions.

3. Suboptimal breathing techniques
   a. Encourage conscious controlled breathing techniques (pursed-lip and diaphragmatic breathing) for use during periods of increased activity and emotional and physical stress.
   b. It often is helpful to initiate instruction in physical and mental relaxation techniques before teaching controlled breathing (see Appendix X).
   c. Instruct the person by demonstrating the desired breathing technique, then directing the person to mimic your breathing pattern.
   d. For pursed-lip breathing, the person should breathe in through the nose, then breathe out slowly through partially closed lips while counting to 7 and making a "pu" sound. (Often, this is learned naturally by people with progressive lung disease.)
   e. For diaphragmatic breathing:

      Place your hands on the person's abdomen below the base of the ribs and keep them there while the person inhales.

      To inhale, the person relaxes the shoulders, breathes in through the nose, and pushes the stomach outward against your hands. The person holds the breath for 1–2 seconds to keep the alveoli open, then exhales.

      To exhale, the person breathes out slowly through the mouth while you apply slight pressure at the base of the ribs.

      Have the person practice this breathing technique several times with you; then, the person should place his own hands at the base of the ribs to practice on his own.

      Once the person has learned the technique, have him practice it a few times each hour.

4. Insufficient level of activity
   a. Assess the person's current activity level. Consider:

      Current pattern of activity/rest

      Distribution of energy demand over course of day

      Person's perceptions of most demanding required activities

      Person's perceptions of areas where increased participation is desired or required

      Efficacy of current adaptive techniques
   b. Identify physical barriers at home and at work (*e.g.*, number of stairs) that seem insurmountable or limit participation in activities.
   c. Identify ways of reducing the work demand of frequently performed tasks (*e.g.*, sitting, rather than standing, to prepare vegetables; keeping frequently used utensils on a counter top to avoid unnecessary overhead reaching or bending).
   d. Identify ways of alternating periods of exertion with periods of rest to overcome barriers (*e.g.*, place a chair in the bathroom near the sink so the person can rest during daily hygiene).
   e. Keep in mind that a plan including frequent short rest periods during an activity is less demanding and more conducive to completing the activity than a plan that calls for a burst of energy followed by a long period of rest.

5. Inadequate nutritional intake
   a. Recommend that the person brush teeth and use mouthwash before meals (and especially after coughing session, because there is frequently an associated bad taste in the mouth, causing decreased appetite and sense of taste).

    b. Encourage smaller, more frequent meals. (Large portions require more oxygen/energy to digest and also limit the downward movement of the diaphragm during inspiration.)

    c. Choose foods that are easy to chew and swallow. (Food that must be chewed extensively requires more work, causing fatigue.)

    d. Assist in food preparation (*e.g.*, cutting meat) if person is prone to fatigue easily.

    e. Avoid gas-producing foods or liquids.

    f. Discourage talking while eating; encourage thorough chewing and slow eating.

    g. Encourage drinking 2–3 quarts of liquid a day (minimum) if fluids are unrestricted. (Consult physician for desired daily fluid intake.)

6. Health-related behaviors

    a. Teach person to avoid factors that aggravate symptoms and advance disease (excessive allergens, pollution).

    b. Discourage smoking. Smoking cessation should be considered of highest priority in any program of comprehensive care of COPD clients (American Thoracic Society, 1987).

    c. If person chooses to smoke, discourage smoking before meals and activity.

    d. If person wishes to reduce or stop smoking, see further interventions under *Altered Health Maintenance related to tobacco use.*

C. Monitor the individual's response to activity

1. See Interventions, p. 107.
2. While monitoring the response to activity, observe for signs and symptoms of respiratory intolerance:

    a. Aggravated dyspnea

    b. Markedly increased respiratory rate

    c. Pallor

    d. Cyanosis

    e. Loss of ability to maintain rhythmic, controlled breathing

    f. Use of accessory muscles

D. Gradually increase activity

1. Reassure person that some increase in daily activity is possible.
2. Instruct person in controlled breathing techniques.
3. Encourage the person to use controlled breathing techniques to decrease the work of breathing during activities.
4. After the person masters controlled breathing in relaxed positions, begin to increase activity.
5. Teach person to maintain controlled breathing pattern while sitting or standing.
6. Progress person to maintaining controlled breathing during bed-to-chair transfers and walking.
7. Many patients can learn to maintain rhythmic breathing during walking by using a simple 2:4 ratio: two steps during inspiration and four steps during expiration.
8. Do not progress the person to more demanding activity until breathing is well controlled during less demanding activities.

E. Provide opportunities for the person to discuss the impact of limited activity tolerance on sexuality

Refer to *Altered Sexuality Patterns.*

F. Initiate health teaching

   1. Teach person to observe his sputum, note changes in color, amount, and odor, and seek professional advice if sputum changes.

   2. Explain that the person with COPD is susceptible to infection and must detect symptoms early and consult with physician for treatment (frequently, early antibiotic therapy is necessary).

   3. Discuss the need for annual immunizations against flu. (The usefulness of one-time-only pneumococcal vaccinations has recently been questioned; therefore, administration should be on an individual basis.)

   4. Instruct person to wear warm, dry clothing; avoid crowds, heavy smoke, fumes, and irritants; avoid exertion in cold, hot, or humid weather; and balance work, rest, and recreation to regulate energy expenditure.

   5. Emphasize the importance of maintaining a good, wholesome diet (high calorie, high vitamin C, high protein, and 2–3 quarts of liquid a day, unless on fluid restriction).

   6. Evaluate the person's knowledge of the care, cleansing, and use of inhalator equipment.

   7. If using oxygen therapy, especially at home, evaluate awareness of fire hazards; explain need for home extinguisher.

   8. Teach the importance of supporting arm weight to reduce the need for respiratory muscles to stabilize the chest wall (Breslin, 1992).

   9. Teach how to increase unsupported arm endurance with lower extremity exercises performed during the exhalational phase of respiration (Breslin, 1992).

G. Make referrals as indicated

   1. Refer to community nurse for follow-up.

   2. Consult physical therapist for a more comprehensive exercise program tailored to the needs of people with obstructive pulmonary disease.

   3. Refer to community support groups (*e.g.*, Better Breathers) and pertinent literature for people with lung disorders.

Rationale

- People with COPD can increase their ability to withstand breathlessness, participate in the therapeutic regimen, and perform activities of daily living.
- Tolerance for activity is maximized through an integrated program that incorporates the principles of physical relaxation, pulmonary hygiene, controlled breathing, and adequate nutrition and hydration, energy conservation through work simplification, and smoking cessation (American Thoracic Society, 1986; Make, 1986).
- People with COPD are instructed in techniques of physical relaxation to minimize muscle tension. Relaxation is an essential preliminary step in teaching controlled breathing to eliminate wasteful and unproductive motions of the upper chest, shoulders, and neck.
- Clearing and defense of the airways are of utmost importance in meeting tissue demands for increased oxygen during periods of rest and periods of increased activity.
- People with pulmonary disease can benefit from specific breathing exercises, which involve retraining of breathing patterns, and from general exercise programs that support normal daily activities (Sinclair, 1984).
- Therapeutic efforts directed at improving respiratory muscle function need to be tailored to each person, according to the muscle group most likely to benefit. In early stages of obstructive disease, treatment should focus on the diaphragm, whereas for people with more advanced disease, the focus must shift to the inspiratory muscles of the rib cage and the muscles of exhalation (Martinez, Couser, & Celli, 1990).

- Symptom-limited endurance training has been shown to be effective for improving performance and reducing perceived breathlessness (Punzal, Ries, Kaplan, & Prewitt, 1991). To be effective, the minimal duration and frequency of exercise required to improve performance appears to be 20–30 minutes three to five times per week (American Thoracic Society, 1987). However, not all people are candidates for exercise reconditioning. A pulmonologist should be consulted.
- The physiologic demands of unsupported arm tasks lead to both exercise-induced increases in respiratory muscle work and nonventilatory recruitment of respiratory muscles to maintain chest wall position (Breslin, 1992). Research has shown that arm support during performance of arm tasks reduces diaphragmatic recruitment (Martinez, Couser, & Celli, 1989), increases respiratory endurance (Banzett, Topulos, Leith, & Nations, 1988) and increases arm exercise endurance (Celli, Criner, & Rassulo, 1988). Providing arm support (*e.g.*, resting elbows on a table top while shaving or eating) may enhance independence and improve functional capacity.
- A person's response to activity can be evaluated by comparing preactivity blood pressure, pulse, and respiration with postactivity blood pressure, pulse, and respiration. These, in turn, are compared with recovery time—the amount of time required for blood pressure, pulse, and respiration to return to preactivity levels.

■ Activity Intolerance
Related to Insufficient Knowledge of Adaptive Techniques Needed Secondary to Impaired Cardiac Function

Outcome Criteria

The person will
- Identify factors that increase cardiac workload
- Describe adaptive techniques needed to perform activities of daily living
- Demonstrate tolerance for increased activity by maintaining pulse, respirations, and blood pressure within predetermined ranges
- Identify cues for stopping activity: fatigue, shortness of breath, chest pain

Interventions

A. Assess for causative/contributing factors
  1. Knowledge of the therapeutic regimen
  2. Activity level
  3. Smoking
  4. Overweight/obesity

B. Eliminate or reduce contributing factors if possible
  1. Specifically assess knowledge and behavior related to the four "Es":

Eating	Exposure
Exertion	Emotional stress (adapted from Day, 1984)

a. Eating

> Assess knowledge of restricted diet.
>
> Explain importance of adhering to prescribed salt-restricted diet.
>
> Explore alternatives for seasoning foods to taste using natural herbs and spices.
>
> Encourage a light meal in the evening to promote a more comfortable night's rest.
>
> Initially provide easily digestible and chewable foods.
>
> Schedule meals to avoid interfering with other activities.
>
> Offer food preferences, avoiding dislikes.
>
> Consider sociocultural influences.

b. Exertion

> Teach person to modify approaches to activities to regulate energy expenditure and reduce cardiac workload (*e.g.*, take rest periods during activities, at intervals during the day, and for 1 hour after meals; sit rather than stand when performing activities, unless this is not feasible; when performing a task, rest every 3 minutes for 5 minutes to allow the heart to recover; stop an activity if exertional fatigue or signs of cardiac hypoxia, such as markedly increased pulse rate, dyspnea, or chest pain, occur).
>
> Instruct person to avoid certain types of exertion: isometric exercises (*e.g.*, using arms to lift himself, carry objects) and Valsalva maneuver (*e.g.*, bending at the waist in a sit-up fashion to rise from bed, straining during a bowel movement).

c. Exposure

> Instruct person to avoid unnecessary exposure to environmental extremes.
>
> Exertion during hot, humid weather or extreme cold weather places additional demands on the heart and should be avoided.
>
> Instruct person to dress warmly during cold weather (*e.g.*, create a barrier to cold weather by wearing layers of clothing).

d. Emotional stress

> Assist person to identify emotional stressors (*e.g.*, at home, at work, social).
>
> Discuss his usual response to emotional stress (*e.g.*, anger, depression, avoidance, discussion).
>
> Explain the effects of emotional stress on the cardiovascular system (*e.g.*, increased heart rate, increased blood pressure, increased respirations).
>
> Discuss various methods for stress management/reduction (*e.g.*, deliberate problem-solving [see Appendix VII], relaxation techniques [see Appendix X], yoga or meditation, biofeedback, regular exercise).

2. Activity level

a. Assess person's current activity level; consider:

> Current pattern of activity/rest
>
> Distribution of energy demand over course of day
>
> Person's perceptions of most demanding required activities
>
> Person's perceptions of areas where increased participation is desired or required

b. Identify person's symptoms of cardiac intolerance.

  c. Evaluate effectiveness of adaptive techniques to manage symptoms (*e.g.,* pacing activities, frequent rest pauses, use of nitrates before planned exertion).

  d. Organize in-hospital care to allow periods of undisturbed rest.

 3. Smoking

  a. Discuss with person the effects of smoking on the cardiovascular system (*e.g.,* vasoconstriction increases workload of the heart).

  b. Teach person when not to smoke: before an activity and immediately after an activity.

  c. Discuss methods that can help reduce the number of cigarettes smoked (see *Altered Health Maintenance related to tobacco use*).

 4. Overweight/obesity

  a. Assess whether the person is overweight or obese by measuring height and weight and comparing findings with a standardized height–weight chart, or use anthropometric measurements (see *Altered Nutrition: More than Body Requirements* for charts of weight for height and anthropometric norms).

C. **Monitor the individual's response to activity (see Interventions, p. 107) and teach him self-monitoring techniques**

 1. Take resting pulse

 2. Take pulse during activity or immediately after

 3. Take pulse 3 minutes after cessation of activity

 4. Instruct person to stop activity and report:

  a. Decreased pulse rate during activity

  b. Pulse rate >112 beats/min

  c. Irregular pulse

  d. Pulse rate that does not return to within six beats of resting pulse after 3 minutes

  e. Dyspnea

  f. Chest pain

  g. Palpitations

  h. Perceptions of exertional fatigue

D. **Gradually increase activity**

 1. Allow for periods of rest before and after planned periods of exertion, such as treatments, ambulation, meals.

 2. Encourage gradual increases in activity and ambulation to prevent a sudden increase in cardiac workload.

 3. Assess person's perceived capability for increased activity.

 4. Assist person in setting short-term activity goals that are realistic and achievable.

 5. Reassure person that even small increases in activity will have the effect of lifting his spirits and restoring his self-confidence.

E. **Provide opportunities for the person to discuss the impact of limited activity tolerance in relation to sexuality**

 Refer to *Altered Sexuality Patterns*.

F. **Provide the family with an opportunity to share their concerns**

 1. Assess their knowledge of the condition, treatment, and prognosis.

 2. Encourage them to share their concerns about the future and about role responsibilities.

G. Initiate health teaching and referrals as indicated

1. Instruct the person to consult his physician and physiatrist for a long-term exercise program or to contact the American Heart Association for available local cardiac rehabilitation programs.

2. Explain dietary restrictions to the person and family. Give them written instructions or refer them to pertinent literature on preparation of food for restricted diets.

3. Explain prescribed drug therapy (*e.g.*, diuretics, vasodilators): dosage, side effects, administration, and storage.

Rationale

- People with impaired cardiac function often are able to increase both level of activity and tolerance for activity through adaptations in life-style, modifications in approach to activities, and careful monitoring of response to activity.
- Tolerance for activity is maximized through an integrated program of medically supervised exercise, dietary restriction, stress management, and limited exposure to environmental extremes.
- People with impaired cardiac function can achieve some immediate gains in activity tolerance by modifying their approach to activities (*e.g.*, pacing activities, avoiding isometric work, and limiting the duration of dynamic work by taking frequent rests).
- Required reduction in the level of personal activity may result in role identification conflict and disruption of divisions of labor within the family unit.
- A person's response to activity can be evaluated by comparing preactivity blood pressure, pulse, and respiration with postactivity blood pressure, pulse, and respiration. These, in turn, are compared with recovery time—the amount of time required for blood pressure, pulse, and respiration to return to preactivity levels.
- Tolerance for activity develops cyclically through adjusting frequency, duration, and intensity of activity until the desired level is achieved. Increasing activity frequency precedes increasing duration and intensity (work demand). Increased intensity is offset by a reduction in duration and frequency. As tolerance for more intensive activity of short duration develops, frequency is once again increased.

■ Activity Intolerance
Related to Bed Rest Deconditioning

Outcome Criteria

The person will
- Identify factors that contribute to deconditioning
- Participate in planned therapies to minimize or reverse the effects of deconditioning
- Demonstrate sufficient energy and strength to participate in and complete desired or required activities

Interventions

The nursing interventions for this diagnosis focus on overcoming the deleterious effects of bed rest–induced deconditioning through a planned program of reconditioning. These interventions are used in conjunction with the interventions identified for general cases of activity intolerance (see pp. 107 through 109).

A. Assess for causative/contributing factors:

1. Prolonged or recurrent confinement to bed rest
2. Disturbances of motor function
3. Adequacy of positioning, repositioning, and ROM regimens
4. Orthostatic intolerance
5. Adequacy of nutritional intake

B. Eliminate or reduce contributing factors if possible

1. Prolonged or recurrent confinement to bed rest
   a. Assess history of bed or bed–chair confinement (*e.g.*, short-term, long-term, repeated).
   b. Is bed or chair confinement prescribed by the medical plan of care, self-imposed, or imposed by expectations/limitations of caregivers?
   c. Evaluate bed mobility. (People without independent bed mobility may be more accurately diagnosed with *Disuse Syndrome*.)

2. Assess for motor function disturbances. (*Note:* A comprehensive motor assessment includes evaluation of muscle bulk, muscle tone, muscle strength, coordination, and involuntary movements [Bates, 1994]. What constitutes a minimally acceptable assessment depends on the extent and severity of involvement and the judgment of the nurse.)

   a. Muscle atrophy and strength

   When assessing for muscle atrophy, inspect the pelvic and shoulder girdles, hands, and extremities. Muscle wasting in the extremities may give the appearance of excessively large joints. Measuring the circumference of an extremity does not provide reliable information about muscle atrophy because it is unclear what is being measured. Comparable body parts can be compared for symmetry; however, the dominant extremities are often larger than their nondominant counterparts.

   Assess muscle strength around each major joint. Strength is conventionally expressed using the Lovett 6-grade scale (Bates, 1994):

   0 (Zero) No contraction
   1 (Trace) Some contraction; no motion
   2 (Poor) Unable to move against gravity
   3 (Fair) Can move against gravity only
   4 (Good) Moves against moderate resistance
   5 (Normal) Moves against full resistance

   b. Spasticity

   Determine the degree of spasticity or abnormally increased muscle tone.

   Spasticity increases the energy costs of activities, can seriously limit functional independence, and interferes with gait training, orthotic prescription, and contracture prevention.

   The extent and severity of spasticity often vary in a given individual, depending on time of day, previous activity, posture, and tactile and kinesthetic stimuli.

   Designate spasticity as mild, moderate, or severe.

It is often helpful to relate spasticity to functional aspects of the patient's activities (*e.g.*, mild spasticity of lower extremities that progresses to severe spasticity after walking 20 feet on a level grade).

c. Coordination

Impaired motor coordination may interfere with completion of many tasks (*e.g.*, feeding or sitting and standing) due to poor balance.

By convention, two tests of coordination are usually performed: rapid alternating movements and point-to-point testing.

Assess coordination of both upper and lower extremities.

The most effective therapy for improving coordination is repeated practice, beginning with simple exercises and progressing to more complex tasks. Patients who are confused, inattentive, or have poor memory may have considerable difficulty in acquiring coordination skills necessary for completion of therapeutic and self-care activities.

3. Assess adequacy of positioning, repositioning, and ROM regimens.

a. Positioning for comfort and pressure relief should be done at least every 2 hours.

b. If not contraindicated, the repositioning regimen should include periods of upright positioning (*e.g.*, high Fowler's position or up in chair).

c. Periods of therapeutic positioning where muscles are fully stretched should be included in the repositioning regimen, to prevent muscle shortening, because shortened muscles atrophy more quickly.

d. Prolonged stretching for 20 minutes using moderate force is much more effective than application of brief, vigorous stretches to prevent muscle shortening and contractures.

e. Evaluate need for dorsiflexion orthotics to protect plantar flexors of lower extremities from shortening and accelerated atrophy.

f. Evaluate ROM of all major joints; express ROM in degrees.

g. Assess adequacy of ROM exercises. Consider thoroughness, frequency, and resistance (*e.g.*, passive or active).

4. Assess for orthostatic intolerance.

a. Refer to *Risk for Injury related to vertigo secondary to postural hypotension*.

5. Assess adequacy of nutritional intake.

a. Evaluate calorie–nitrogen intake. Nitrogen intake must be sufficient for protein synthesis. Enough nonnitrogen calories must also be taken in to ensure that protein calories are not metabolized to meet energy needs. A malnourished or stressed client requires almost double the amount of nitrogen as a healthy individual.

b. If inadequate nutritional intake is suspected, keep a daily record of foods eaten and consult a dietitian.

c. See *Altered Nutrition: Less Than Body Requirements* for specific interventions.

C. Monitor response to activity

1. See Interventions, p. 107.

2. Rapid onset of task-related fatigue is an early indicator of intolerance in deconditioned individuals.

3. While monitoring the response to activity, assess for signs and symptoms of orthostatic intolerance (tachycardia, nausea, diaphoresis, and syncope). (See *Risk for Injury related to orthostatic hypotension* for specific interventions.)

D. Gradually increase activity
   1. Plan strategies to increase bed mobility (*e.g.*, use of overhead trapeze).
   2. Implement a planned exercise program that includes lower extremity exercises against resistance.
   3. Progress patient to exercise in upright positions against gravitational strain as early as possible.
   4. Begin weight-bearing at earliest possible date to minimize atrophy of plantar flexors in lower legs.
   5. Promote independence in activities of daily living. Activities that the person can perform independently should be performed by the patient, rather than the nurse or caregiver.

E. Initiate health teaching and referrals
   1. Instruct patient and caregivers in ROM and therapeutic exercises.
   2. Consult physical therapist for an exercise program tailored to the individual's needs.
   3. Consult dietitian for dietary evaluation and nutritional counseling.

Rationale

- Repeated confinement to bed rest and advanced age (older than 65 years) are thought to have an additive effect on the deconditioning process (Bortz, 1982; LeBlanc, Gogia, & Schneider, 1988), which may predispose the chronically ill and the elderly to activity intolerance as result of bed rest deconditioning.
- Loss of skeletal muscle mass, changes in neurohumoral mechanisms, and associated general decreases in body metabolic needs are major contributors to the deconditioning process of bed rest (LeBlanc et al., 1988).
- The deconditioning effects of bed rest lead to a decreased physical capacity for work in the supine position, as a result of changes occurring in the cardiac, circulatory, and musculoskeletal systems. The lack of exposure to orthostatic stress during bed rest leads to further decreases in the physical capacity for work in the upright position (Hung, Goldwater, & Convertino, 1983).
- Some muscle groups seem to be more vulnerable to the deconditioning effects of bed rest than others, resulting in differences in the rate and degree of muscle atrophy (LeBlanc et al., 1988). During bed rest, leg muscles tend to lose strength about twice as fast as arm muscles (Greenleaf, Wade, & Leftheriotis, 1989).
- A onefold loss of muscle mass in plantar flexors of the lower legs (*e.g.*, gastrocnemius and soleus muscles) is associated with a twofold loss in muscle strength (LeBlanc et al., 1988).
- Exercises targeted at muscle groups that are more susceptible to bed rest deconditioning may be a more effective countermeasure for deconditioning than general exercise regimens (LeBlanc et al., 1988).
- Exercises performed in an upright position, against gravitational strain, are of greater value in overcoming the effects of bed rest deconditioning than exercises performed in a supine position.
- A person's response to activity can be evaluated by comparing preactivity blood pressure, pulse, and respiration with postactivity blood pressure, pulse, and respiration. These, in turn, are compared with recovery time—the amount of time required for blood pressure, pulse, and respiration to return to preactivity levels.

🌀 Interventions—*Child Focus*

1. Provide age-appropriate games and activities that are quiet and challenging (Wong, 1993).
   a. Sensory adventures (what does the hospital smell, sound, or look like?).
   b. Story telling, story writing, collages, puppets, play acting.

Rationale

- A child's response to activity can be evaluated through physiologic parameters and engagement in age-appropriate activities. For example, the nurse should assess the infant's sleep–rest cycle, motor activities, and eating behavior (Daberkow, 1989). The nurse should assess these parameters in a toddler, preschooler, and school-aged child, as well as the child's involvement in play activities.
- Play activities are important, even for the hospitalized child with activity intolerance. Play normalizes the child's experience in the hospital and reduces stress. The nurse must continually assess the child's fatigue or readiness to engage in more vigorous activity (Wong, 1995).

Interventions—*Maternal Focus*

1. Explain the causes of fatigue and dyspnea in mid- to late pregnancy.
2. Teach energy conservation methods (see Interventions, p. 115).

Rationale

- Changes in center of gravity and increased weight and pressure of the enlarging uterus on the diaphragm contribute to fatigue and breathlessness.

References/Bibliography

General

Abrams, W. B., & Berkow, R. (Eds.). (1990). *The Merck manual of geriatrics.* Rahway, NJ: Merck & Co.

Adams, C. E., & Leverland, M. B. (1985). Environmental and behavioral factors that can affect blood pressure. *Nurse Practitioner, 10*(11), 39–50.

Aistars, J. (1987). Fatigue in the cancer patient: A conceptual approach to a clinical problem. *Oncology Nursing Forum, 14*(6), 25–30.

Balfour, I. C. (1991). Pediatric cardiac rehabilitation. *American Journal of Diseases of Children, 145,* 627–630.

Basmajian, J. V. (1984). *Therapeutic exercise* (4th ed.). London: Williams & Wilkins.

Bortz, W. M. (1982). Disuse and aging. *JAMA, 248*(10), 1203–1208.

Bulechek, G. M., & McCloskey, J. C. (Eds.). (1985). *Nursing interventions: Treatments for nursing diagnoses.* Philadelphia: W. B. Saunders.

Daberkow, E. (1989). Nursing strategies: Altered cardiovascular function. In R. L. Foster, M. M. Hunsberger, & J. J. T. Anderson (Eds.). *Family-centered nursing care of children.* Philadelphia: W. B. Saunders.

DeLateur, B. J. (1987). Exercise for strength and endurance. In J. V. Basmajian (Ed.). *Therapeutic exercise.* Baltimore: Williams & Wilkins.

Fitzmaurice, J. B. (1987). Nurse's use of cues in the clinical judgment of activity intolerance. In A. M. McLane (Ed.). *Classification of nursing diagnosis: Proceedings of the seventh conference.* St. Louis: C. V. Mosby.

Fleg, J. L. (1986). Alterations in cardiovascular structure and function with advancing age. *American Journal of Cardiology, 5*(7), 33C–44C.

Gerber, R. M. (1990). Coronary artery disease in the elderly. *Journal of Cardiovascular Nursing, 4*(4), 23–34.

Gordon, M. (1976). Assessing activity tolerance. *American Journal of Nursing, 76*(1), 72–75.

Gordon, M. (1987). *Manual of nursing diagnosis.* New York: McGraw-Hill.

Gordon, M. (1987). *Nursing diagnosis: Process and application* (2nd ed.). New York: McGraw-Hill.

Gortner, S. R., Miller, N. G., & Jenkins, L. S. (1988). Self-efficacy: A key to recovery. In C. R. Jillings (Ed.). *Cardiac rehabilitation nursing.* Rockville, MD: Aspen Publications.

Gould, M. T. (1983). Nursing diagnoses concurrent with multiple sclerosis. *Journal of Neurosurgical Nursing, 15*(6), 339–345.

Hagberg, J. M., Graves, J. E., Limacher, M., et al. (1989). Cardiovascular responses of 70- to 79-year-old men and women to exercise training. *Journal of Applied Physiology, 66*(6), 2589–2594.

Halfman, M. A., & Hojnacki, L. G. (1981). Exercise and maintenance of health. *Topics in Clinical Nursing, 3,* 1–10.

Kim, M. J., McFarland, G. K., & McLane, A. M. (1984). *Classification of nursing diagnoses: Proceedings of the fifth national conference.* St. Louis: C. V. Mosby.

Kreuger, D. W. (Ed.). (1984). *Emotional rehabilitation of physical trauma and disability.* New York: SP Medical & Scientific Books.

Louis, M. C., & Pouse, S. M. (1980). Aphasia and endurance: Considerations in the assessment and care of the stroke patient. *Nursing Clinics of North America, 15*(2), 265–282.

Magnan, M. A. (1987, September). *Activity intolerance: Toward a nursing theory of activity.*

Paper presented at the Fifth Annual Symposium of the Michigan Nursing Diagnosis Association, Detroit, Michigan.

Matteson, M. A., & McConnell, E. S. (1988). *Gerontological nursing: Concepts and practices.* Philadelphia: W. B. Saunders.

McLean, S. L. (1989). Activity intolerance: Cues for diagnosis. In R. M. Carroll-Johnson (Ed.). *Classification of nursing diagnosis: Proceedings of the eighth conference.* Philadelphia: J. B. Lippincott.

Miller, C. (1990). *Nursing care of older adults.* Glenview, IL: Scott, Foresman.

Mitchell, C. A. (1986). Generalized chronic fatigue in the elderly: Assessment and intervention. *Journal of Gerontological Nursing, 12*(4), 19–23.

Muir, B. L. (1988). *Pathophysiology: An introduction to the mechanisms of disease* (2nd ed.). New York: John Wiley & Sons.

Piper, B. F. (1986). Fatigue. In V. K. Carrieri, A. M. Lindsey, & C. M. West (Eds.). *Pathophysiological phenomena in nursing: Human responses to illness.* Philadelphia: W. B. Saunders.

Posner, J. D., Gorman, K. M., Klein, H. S., & Woldow, A. (1986). Exercise capacity in the elderly. *American Journal of Cardiology, 57:*52C–58C.

Potempa, K., Lopez, M., Reid, C., & Lawson, L. (1986). Chronic fatigue. *Image—The Journal of Nursing Scholarship, 18*(4), 165–169.

Price, S. A., & Wilson, L. M. (1982). *Pathophysiology: Clinical concepts of disease processes* (2nd ed.). New York: McGraw-Hill.

Schlant, R. C. (1982). Physiology of exercise. In G. F. Fletcher (Ed.). *Exercise in the practice of medicine.* Mount Kisco, NY: Futura Publishing.

Scipien, G. M., Chard, M. A., Howe, J., & Barnard, M. U. (1990). *Pediatric nursing care.* St. Louis: C. V. Mosby.

Sculco, C. D. (1978). The need for activity. In H. Yura & M. Walsh (Eds.). *Human needs and the nursing process.* New York: Appleton-Century-Crofts.

Wong, D. L. (1993). *Essentials of pediatric nursing* (4th ed.). St. Louis: C. V. Mosby.

Pulmonary

American Thoracic Society. (1987). Standards for the diagnosis and care of patients with chronic obstructive pulmonary disease (COPD) and asthma. *American Review of Respiratory Disease, 136,* 225–244.

Banzett, R. B., Topulos, G. P., Leith, D. E., & Nations, C. S. (1988). Bracing arms increases the capacity for sustained hyperpnea. *American Review of Respiratory Disease, 126,* 5–8.

Breslin, E. H. (1992). Dyspnea-limited response in chronic obstructive pulmonary disease: Reduced unsupported arm activities. *Rehabilitation Nursing, 17,* 12–20.

Celli, B. R., Criner, G., & Rassulo, J. (1988). Ventilatory muscle recruitment during unsupported arm exercise in normal subjects. *Journal of Applied Physiology, 64,* 1936–1941.

Hodgkin, J. E., & Petty, T. L. (1987). *Chronic obstructive pulmonary disease: Current concepts.* Philadelphia: W. B. Saunders.

Klesges, R. C., Eck, L. H., Mellon, M. W., Fulliton, W., Somes, G. W., & Hanson, C. L. (1989). The accuracy of self-reports of physical activity. *Medicine and Science in Sports and Exercise, 22,* 690–697.

Make, B. J. (1986). Pulmonary rehabilitation: Myth or reality? *Clinics in Chest Medicine, 7,* 519–540.

Martinez, F. K., Couser, J. I., & Celli, B. R. (1989). Respiratory mechanics and ventilatory muscle recruitment during arm elevation in subjects with severe chronic airflow obstruction. *American Review of Respiratory Disease, 139,* A292.

Martinez, F. K., Couser, J. I., & Celli, B. R. (1990). Factors influencing ventilatory muscle recruitment in patients with chronic airflow obstruction. *American Review of Respiratory Disease, 142,* 276–282.

Nett, L. M., & Petty, T. L. (1985). Managing the COPD patient and family at home. In T. L. Petty (Ed.). *Chronic obstructive pulmonary disease.* New York: Marcel Dekker.

Punzal, P. A., Ries, A. L., Kaplan, R. M., & Prewitt, L. M. (1991). Maximum intensity exercise training in patients with chronic obstructive pulmonary disease. *Chest, 100,* 618–623.

Selecky, P. A. (1987). Sexuality and the COPD patient. In J. E. Hodgkin & T. L. Petty (Eds.). *Chronic obstructive pulmonary disease* (2nd ed.). Philadelphia: W. B. Saunders.

Sinclair, J. D. (1984). Exercise in pulmonary disease. In J. V. Basmajian (Ed.). *Therapeutic exercise.* Baltimore: Williams & Wilkins.

Toshima, M. T., Kaplan, R. M., & Ries, A. L. (1990). Experimental evaluation of rehabilitation in chronic obstructive pulmonary disease: Short-term effects on exercise endurance and health status. *Health Psychology, 9,* 237–252.

Williams, J. H. (1986). Pneumococcal vaccine and patients with chronic lung disease. *Annals of Internal Medicine, 104,* 106–109.

Cardiac

Cantwell, J. D. (1984). Exercise and coronary heart disease: Role in primary prevention. *Heart and Lung, 13,* 6–13.

Day, N. R. (1984). *After your heart attack.* Daly City, CA: Krames Communications.

Ellestad, M. H. (1986). *Stress testing: Principles and practice* (3rd ed.). Philadelphia: F. A. Davis.

Ewart, C. K., Stewart, K. J., Gillilan, R. E., & Keleman, M. H. (1986). Self-efficacy mediates strength gains during circuit weight training in men with coronary artery disease. *Medicine and Science in Sports and Exercise, 18,* 531–540.

Ewart, C. K., Stewart, K. J., Gillilan, R. E., Keleman, M. H., Valenti, S. A., Manley, J. D., & Kaleman, M. D. (1986). Usefulness of self-efficacy in predicting overexertion during programmed exercise in coronary artery disease. *American Journal of Cardiology, 57,* 557–561.

Froelicher, V. F. (1987). *Exercise and the heart: Clinical concepts.* Chicago: Year Book Medical Publishers.

Gulanick, M. (1991). Is phase 2 cardiac rehabilitation necessary for early recovery of patients with cardiac disease? A randomized, controlled study. *Heart and Lung, 20,* 9–15.

Guyatt, G. H., Sullivan, M. J., & Thompson, P. J. (1985). The 6-minute walk: A new measure of exercise capacity in patients with chronic heart failure. *Canadian Medical Association Journal, 132,* 919–923.

Jenkins, L. S. (1987). Self-efficacy: New perspectives in caring for patients recovering from myocardial infarction. *Progress in Cardiovascular Nursing, 2,* 32–35.

Jillings, C. R. (Ed.). (1988). *Cardiac rehabilitation nursing.* Rockville, MD: Aspen Publications.

Kavanagh, T. Exercise and coronary artery disease. In J. V. Basmajian (Ed.). *Therapeutic exercise.* Baltimore: Williams & Wilkins.

Lemanski, K. M. (1990). The use of self-efficacy in cardiac rehabilitation. *Progress in Cardiovascular Nursing, 5,* 114–117.

McAuley, E., Courneya, K. S., & Lettunich, J. (1991). Effects of acute and long-term exercise on self-efficacy responses in sedentary, middle-aged males and females. *The Gerontologist, 31,* 534–542.

Parmley, W. W. (1986). Position report on cardiac rehabilitation. *Journal of the American College of Cardiology, 7,* 451–453.

Sanderson, R. G., & Kurth, C. L. (1983). *The cardiac patient: A comprehensive approach.* Philadelphia: W. B. Saunders.

Deconditioning

Bates, B. (1994). *A guide to physical examination and history taking* (6th ed.). Philadelphia: J. B. Lippincott.

Bortz, W. M. (1982). Disuse and aging. *JAMA, 248,* 1203–1208.

Brandstater, M. E., & Basmajian, J. V. (Eds.). (1987). *Stroke rehabilitation.* Baltimore: Williams & Wilkins.

Corcoran, P. J. (1991). Use it or lose it—The hazards of bed rest and inactivity. *Western Journal of Medicine, 154,* 536–538.

Fisher, S. V., & Gullickson, G. (1978). The energy costs of ambulation in health and disability: A literature review. *Archives of Physical Medicine and Rehabilitation, 59*(3), 124–133.

Greenleaf, J. E., Wade, C. E., & Leftheriotis, G. (1989). Orthostatic responses following 30-day bed rest deconditioning with isotonic and isokinetic exercise training. *Aviation, Space and Environmental Medicine, 6,* 537–542.

Harper, C. M., & Lyles, Y. M. (1988). Physiology and complications of bed rest. *Journal of the American Geriatric Society, 36,* 1047–1054.

Hung, J., Goldwater, D., & Convertino, V. A. (1983). Mechanisms for decreased exercise capacity after bed rest in normal middle-aged men. *American Journal of Cardiology, 51,* 344–348.

LeBlanc, A., Gogia, P., & Schneider, V. (1988). Calf muscle area and strength changes after five weeks of horizontal bed rest. *American Journal of Sports Medicine, 16,* 624–629.

Rubin, M. (1988). The physiology of bed rest. *American Journal of Nursing, 88*(1), 50–58.

Sandler, H., Popp, R. L., & Harrison, D. (1988). The hemodynamic effects of repeated bed rest exposure. *Aviation, Space and Environmental Medicine, 11,* 1047–1054.

Adaptive Capacity, Intracranial: Decreased

DEFINITION

Decreased Adaptive Capacity: Intracranial: A clinical state in which intracranial fluid dynamic mechanisms that normally compensate for increases in intracranial volumes are compromised, resulting in repeated disproportionate increases in intracranial pressure (ICP) in response to a variety of noxious and nonnoxious stimuli.

DEFINING CHARACTERISTICS
Major

Repeated increases in ICP of >10 mm Hg for more than 5 minutes after any of a variety of external stimuli

Minor

Disproportionate increase in ICP after a single environmental or nursing maneuver stimulus

Elevated P2 ICP waveform

Volume–pressure response test variation (volume–pressure ratio >2; pressure–volume index <10)

Baseline ICP ≥10 mm Hg

Wide-amplitude ICP waveform

Author's Note

This diagnosis represents increased intracranial pressure. It is a collaborative problem because it requires two disciplines to treat—nursing and medicine. In addition, it requires invasive monitoring for diagnosis. The collaborative problem *Potential Complication: Increased Intracranial Pressure* represents this clinical situation. Refer to Section III for interventions for which nurses are responsible.

Adjustment, Impaired

DEFINITION

Impaired Adjustment: The state in which the individual is unwilling to modify his or her lifestyle/behavior in a manner consistent with a change in health status.

DEFINING CHARACTERISTICS
Major (Must Be Present)

Verbalization of nonacceptance of health status change or inadequate capacity to be involved in problem solving or goal setting.

Minor (May Be Present)

Lack of movement toward independence; extended period of shock, disbelief, or anger regarding health status change; lack of future-oriented thinking.

Author's Note

This diagnosis has presented problems in clinical use because of its lack of specificity. Generally speaking, are not most diagnoses a problem with adjustment? It is not clinically useful to have such a general diagnosis. The responses to illness and disabilities are varied, and it is important that the nurse clarify the response so that it will be most helpful with treatment. Responses can be *Grieving, Anxiety, Fear,* and *Ineffective Coping.*

If a client is attempting to manage the changes the illness or disability has caused, but is having difficulty, the diagnosis *Ineffective Management of Therapeutic Regimen* would be more useful. This author recommends not using this diagnosis.

Anxiety

DEFINITION

Anxiety: A state in which the individual/group experiences feelings of uneasiness (apprehension) and activation of the autonomic nervous system in response to a vague, nonspecific threat.

DEFINING CHARACTERISTICS
Major (Must Be Present)

Manifested by symptoms from each category—physiologic, emotional, and cognitive. Symptoms vary according to the level of anxiety.

Physiologic

Increased heart rate	Diarrhea
Elevated blood pressure	Insomnia
Increased respiratory rate	Fatigue and weakness
Diaphoresis	Flushing or pallor
Dilated pupils	Dry mouth
Voice tremors/pitch changes	Body aches and pains (especially chest, back, neck)
Trembling	Restlessness
Palpitations	Faintness/dizziness
Nausea or vomiting	Paresthesias
Frequent urination	Hot and cold flashes

Emotional

Person states that he has feelings of

Apprehension	Losing control
Helplessness	Tension or being "keyed up"
Nervousness	Inability to relax
Lack of self-confidence	Anticipation of misfortune

Person exhibits

Irritability/impatience	Criticism of self and others
Angry outbursts	Withdrawal
Crying	Lack of initiative
Tendency to blame others	Self-deprecation
Startle reaction	

Cognitive

Inability to concentrate
Lack of awareness of surroundings
Forgetfulness
Rumination
Orientation to past rather than to present or future
Blocking of thoughts (inability to remember)
Hyperattentiveness

RELATED FACTORS
Pathophysiologic

Any factor that interferes with the basic human needs for food, air, comfort, and security

Situational (Personal, Environmental)

Related to actual or perceived threat to self-concept secondary to:

Change in status and prestige   Loss of valued possessions
Lack of recognition from others   Ethical dilemma
Failure (or success)

Related to actual or perceived loss of significant others secondary to:

Death   Moving
Divorce   Temporary or permanent separation
Cultural pressures

Related to actual or perceived threat to biologic integrity secondary to:

Dying   Invasive procedures
Assault   Disease

Related to actual or perceived change in environment secondary to:

Hospitalization   Safety hazards
Moving   Environmental pollutants
Retirement

Related to actual or perceived change in socioeconomic status secondary to:

Unemployment   Promotion
New job

Related to transmission of another person's anxiety to the individual

Maturational

Infant/child

Related to separation
Related to unfamiliar environment, people
Related to changes in peer relationships

Adolescent

Related to threat to self-concept secondary to:

Sexual development
Peer relationships changes

Adult

Related to threat to self-concept secondary to:

Pregnancy   Career changes
Parenting   Effects of aging

Older adult

Related to threat to self-concept secondary to:

Sensory losses   Financial problems
Motor losses   Retirement changes

Author's Note

The nursing diagnoses of *Anxiety* and *Fear* have been examined by several researchers (Jones & Jacob, 1984; Taylor-Loughran, O'Brien, LaChapelle, & Rangel, 1989: Yokom, 1984). Differentiation of these diagnoses focuses on whether the threat can be identified. If identification is possible, the diagnosis is fear; if not, it is anxiety (NANDA, 1989). This differentiation has not proved useful for clinicians, however (Taylor-Loughran et al., 1989).

Anxiety involves a vague feeling of apprehension and uneasiness in response to threat to one's value system or security pattern (May, 1977). The person may be able to identify the situation (*e.g.*, surgery, cancer), but actually the threat to self relates to the uneasiness and apprehension enmeshed in the situation. In other words, the situation is the source of the threat, but is not itself the threat. In contrast, fear refers to the feelings of apprehension related to a specific threat or danger to which one's security patterns respond (*e.g.*, flying, heights, snakes). When the threat is removed, the fearful feelings dissipate (May, 1977).

Anxiety and fear produce a similar sympathetic response, involving cardiovascular excitation, pupillary dilation, sweating, tremors, and dry mouth. Anxiety also involves a parasympathetic response of increased gastrointestinal (GI) activity; in contrast, fear is associated with decreased GI activity. Behaviorally, the fearful person exhibits increased alertness and concentration, with a response of avoidance, attack, or decreasing the risk of threat. The anxious person, on the other hand, experiences increased tension, general restlessness, insomnia, worry, and feelings of helplessness and vagueness concerning a situation that cannot be easily avoided or attacked.

Clinically, both anxiety and fear may coexist in a person's response to a situation. For example, a person facing surgery may be fearful of pain and anxious about a possible cancer diagnosis. According to Yokom (1984), "Fear can be allayed by withdrawal from the situation, removal of the offending object, or by reassurance. Anxiety is reduced by admitting its presence and by being convinced that the values to be gained by moving ahead are greater than those to be gained by escape."

Errors in Diagnostic Statements

Fear related to upcoming surgery

Anticipated surgery can be a source of many threats, including threats to one's security patterns, health, values, self-concept, role functioning, goal achievement, relationships, and security. These threats can produce vague feelings ranging from mild uneasiness to panic. Identifying the threat as merely surgery is too simplistic; these personal threats also are involved. Moreover, although some of the person's uneasiness may be attributed to fear (which can be eliminated by teachings), the remaining feelings relate to anxiety. Because this situation is inescapable, the nurse must assist the person with coping mechanisms for managing anxiety.

Key Concepts

1. Anxiety refers to feelings aroused by a nonspecific threat to a person's self-concept that impinge on health, assets, values, environment, role functioning, needs fulfillment, goal achievement, personal relationships, and sense of security (Miller, 1995). Anxiety varies in intensity depending on the severity of the perceived threat and the success or failure of efforts to cope with the feelings.

2. A person uses both interpersonal and intrapsychic mechanisms to reduce or relieve anxiety. The effectiveness of coping strategies depends on the individual and the situation, not on the behavior itself.

   Interpersonal patterns of coping include:
   a. Acting-out: converting anxiety into anger that is either overtly or covertly expressed
   b. Paralysis or retreating behaviors: withdrawing or being immobilized by one's own anxiety
   c. Somatizing: converting anxiety into physical symptoms
   d. Constructive action: using anxiety to learn and problem solve (includes goal setting, learning new skills, and seeking information)

   Intrapsychic mechanisms, often called defense mechanisms, lower anxiety and protect self-esteem. Examples include repression, sublimation, regression, displacement, projection, denial, conversion, rationalization, suppression, and identification.

3. Individuals develop a range of coping behaviors, both adaptive and maladaptive. Maladaptive coping mechanisms are characterized by the inability to make choices, conflict, repetition and rigidity, alienation, and secondary gains.

4. Anxiety refers to both a person's response to a particular situation—*state anxiety*—and the differences among people's interpretation of threatening situations—*trait anxiety*. People with relatively high levels of trait anxiety tend to perceive greater danger in situations that threaten self-esteem than do people with lower levels, who respond with higher levels of state anxiety (Spielberger & Sarason, 1975).

5. The anxious person tends to overgeneralize and assume and anticipate catastrophe. Resulting cognitive problems include difficulty with attention and concentration, loss of objectivity, and vigilance (Taylor & Arnow, 1988).
6. The effects of anxiety on a person's abilities vary with degree:

   Mild

   Perception and attention heightened; alert
   Able to deal with problem situations
   Can integrate past, present, and future experiences
   Uses learning; can consensually validate; formulates meanings
   Curious, repeats questions
   Sleeplessness

   Moderate

   Perception somewhat narrowed; selectively inattentive, but can direct attention
   Slightly more difficult to concentrate; learning requires more effort
   Views present experiences in terms of past
   May fail to notice what is happening in a peripheral situation; will have some difficulty in adapting and analyzing
   Voice/pitch changes
   Increased respiratory and heart rates
   Tremors, shakiness

   Severe

   Perception greatly reduced; focuses on scattered details; cannot attend to more even when instructed to
   Learning severely impaired; highly distractible, unable to concentrate
   Views present experiences in terms of past; almost unable to understand current situation
   Functions poorly; communication difficult to understand
   Hyperventilation, tachycardia, headache, dizziness, nausea

   Panic

   Perception distorted; focuses on blown-up detail; scattering may be increased
   Learning cannot occur
   Unable to integrate experiences; can focus only on present; unable to see or understand situation; lapses in recall of thoughts
   Unable to function; usually increased motor activity or unpredictable responses to even minor stimuli; communication not understandable
   Feelings of impending doom
Dyspnea	Dizziness/faintness
Palpitations	Trembling
Choking	Paresthesia
Hot/cold flashes	Sweating

7. People experiencing panic attacks report that a physical feeling most commonly precipitated episodes of anxiety. Their thoughts are related to loss of control, death, and illness (Taylor & Arnow, 1988).
8. Catastrophic misinterpretation of normal body sensations may lead to a learned response in people suffering from generalized anxiety disorders and panic attacks (Barlow & Cerny, 1988).

🌑 *Key Concepts—Child*

1. Signs of anxiety in children vary greatly depending on developmental stage, temperament, past experience, and parental involvement (Wong, 1993). The most common sign of anxiety in children and adolescents is increased motor activity. Signs of anxiety can be viewed developmentally and may be reflected in the following ways:

   Birth to 9 months: disruption in physiologic functioning (*e.g.*, sleep disorders, colic)

9 months to 4 years: Major source is loss of significant others and loss of love; therefore, anxiety may be seen as anger when parents leave, somatic illnesses, motor restlessness, regressive behaviors (thumb sucking, head banging, rocking), regression in toilet training

4–6 years: Major source is fear of body damage; belief that his bad behavior causes bad things to happen (*e.g.*, illness); somatic complaints of headache, stomachache

6–12 years: Excessive verbalization, compulsive behavior (*e.g.*, repeating a task over and over)

Adolescence: Similar to 6–12 years plus types of negativistic behavior

2. Children's anxiety may be heightened by separation from parents, change in usual routines, strange environments, painful procedures, and parental anxiety (Wong, 1993). The nurse should assess for alterations in the functional health patterns to detect the presence of anxiety.
3. Sources of anxiety for children and adolescents are related to school-associated factors (*e.g.*, performance, social), separation, social situations, peers, and family (Oski, 1994)
4. Individuals who manifest disorders of avoidance, overanxiousness, separation anxiety, and school phobia should be referred to mental health experts (Jackson & Saunders, 1993).

Key Concepts—Maternal

1. Expectant mothers experience a degree of emotional lability (May & Mahlmeister, 1994).
2. Multiple sources of anxiety are fear for personal or fetal well-being, anticipated labor, responsibilities of parenthood, and her relationship with partner (Reeder, Martin, & Koniak, 1992).

Key Concepts—Older Adult

1. Older adults may manifest anxiety with complaints of nervousness, "nerve trouble," or feelings of uneasiness (Johnson, 1993).
2. Additional signs and symptoms of anxiety are pacing, fidgeting, changes in sleeping or eating patterns, and complaints of fatigue, pain, insomnia, or GI upsets (Miller, 1995).

TRANSCULTURAL CONSIDERATIONS

1. Individuals and families from different cultures may face many challenges when they seek health care in the dominant culture's health care delivery systems. In addition to usual sources of anxiety (e.g., unfamiliar people, routines, unknown prognosis), people from other cultures may be anxious about language difficulties, privacy, separation from support systems, and cost (Boyle & Andrews, 1995; Giger & Davidhizar, 1991).
2. Members of cultures that depend on their kin for caring will expect more humanistic kinds of nursing care and less scientific–technologic care (Boyle & Andrews, 1995).

Focus Assessment Criteria

Subjective Data

A. Assess for defining characteristics

1. History of unusual sensations (e.g., palpitations, tingling, dyspnea, dry mouth, nausea, diaphoresis)

Precipitating factors	Routine time of occurrence
Frequency	Description in individual's own words
Duration	

2. Assess for feelings of
   Extreme sadness and worthlessness
   Guilt for past actions
   Apprehension

> Rejection or isolation
> Living in an unreal world
> Mistrust or suspiciousness of others
> Manipulation by others
> Harm from others
> Mind being controlled by external agents
> Being unable to cope
> Falling apart
> Thoughts racing
> Being held prisoner

B. Assess for related factors

    1. History of the individual from client and significant others

        Life-style

            Interests

            Work history

            Coping patterns (past, present)

            Strengths, limitations

            Previous level of functioning, handling stress

        Support system

            Availability

            Quality of support

        History of medical problems/treatments

            Alcohol and drug abuse

            Medications

        Activities of daily living

            Ability to perform

            Desire to perform

    2. Usual coping behavior (refer to *Ineffective Individual Coping* for further assessment criteria)

        "How do you usually handle a particular situation (*i.e.*, anger, disappointment, loss, rejection, etc.)?"

        "What did you usually do when you were faced with similar situations in the past?"

        "What happens when you do that?" (relevant coping mechanism)

        Assess for:

            Level of awareness of behavior

            Range of coping behavior

            Adaptive/maladaptive

            Secondary gains

Subjective and Objective Data

A. Assess for defining characteristics

    1. General appearance

        Facial expression (*e.g.*, sad, hostile, expressionless)

        Dress (*e.g.*, meticulous, disheveled, seductive, eccentric)

    2. Behavior during interview

        Withdrawn   Cooperative

        Hostile   Quiet

        Apathetic

    3. Communication pattern

        Content

            Appropriate

            Rambling

            Suspicious

            Denial of problem

Homicidal plans

Suicidal ideas

Sexually preoccupied

Delusions (of grandeur, persecution, reference, influence, control, or bodily sensations)

Hallucinations (visual, auditory, gustatory, olfactory, tactile)

Flow of thought

Appropriate

Blocking of ideas (unable to finish idea)

Circumstantial (unable to get to point)

Ideas loosely connected

Jumps from one topic to another

Unable to come to conclusion, be decisive

Difficulty concentrating

States he is unable to follow what is being said

Difficulty grasping circumstances or events

Rate of speech

Appropriate   Reduced

Excessive   Pressured

Nonverbal behavior

Affect appropriate/inappropriate to verbal content

Gestures, mannerisms, facial grimaces

Posture

4. Interaction skills

With a nurse

Inappropriate   Shows dependency

Relates well   Demanding/pleading

Withdrawn/preoccupied with self   Hostile

With significant others

Relates with all family members or with some

Hostile toward one member/all members

Does not seek interaction

Does not have visitors

5. Nutritional status

Appetite   Eating patterns

Weight (within normal limits, decreased, increased)

6. Sleep–rest pattern

Recent change   Early wakefulness

Sleeps too much/too little   Insomnia

7. Personal hygiene

Cleanliness (body, hair, teeth)   Grooming (clothes, hair, makeup)

Clothes (condition, appropriateness)

8. Motor activity

Within normal limits   Agitated

Increased   Repetitive

Decreased

9. Present coping behavior

"Acting-out" behaviors

Derogating   Manipulation of others to do tasks he is

Fighting   capable of

Arguing   Resentfulness

Intimidating   Motor restlessness

Ritualistic behavior   Pacing

Smoking, alcohol, drugs   Physical exertion

Paralysis and retreating behaviors

Withdrawal   Avoids talking about self

Depression | Minimizes signs and symptoms
Denial | Dissociation
Diverts attention | Ritualistic behavior
Sleeping | Blocking
Somatizing
  Headache | Anorexia
  Dyspnea | Colitis
  Muscle tension | Syncope
  Hives, eczema | Menstrual disturbance

Outcome Criteria

The person will
- Describe his own anxiety and coping patterns
- Relate an increase in psychological and physiologic comfort
- Use effective coping mechanism in managing anxiety, as evidenced by (specify)

Interventions

The nursing interventions for the diagnosis *Anxiety* can apply to any individual with anxiety regardless of the etiologic and contributing factors.

A. Assist the person to reduce his present level of anxiety
  1. Assess level of anxiety (see Key Concepts)
    a. Mild
    b. Moderate
    c. Severe
    d. Panic
  2. Provide reassurance and comfort
    a. Stay with the person.
    b. Do not make demands or ask him to make decisions.
    c. Support present coping mechanisms (*e.g.*, allow client to walk, talk, cry); do not confront or argue with his defenses or rationalizations.
    d. Speak slowly and calmly.
    e. Be aware of your own concern and avoid reciprocal anxiety.
    f. Convey a sense of empathic understanding (*e.g.*, quiet presence, touch, allowing crying, talking, and the like).
    g. Provide reassurance that a solution can be found.
    h. Reorient to reality as required.
    i. Respect the person's personal space.
  3. Decrease sensory stimulation
    a. Provide a quiet, nonstimulating environment; soft lighting.
    b. Use short, simple sentences.
    c. Give concise directions.
    d. Focus on the here and now.
    e. Remove excess stimulation (*e.g.*, take person to quieter room); limit contact with others—patients or family—who are also anxious.
    f. Share an activity with the person. Plan a schedule that can be accomplished.
    g. Provide physical measures that will aid in relaxation such as warm baths, back massage.
    h. Consult physician for possible pharmacologic therapy, if indicated.

4. If person is hyperventilating or experiencing dyspnea (DeVito, 1990)

    a. Demonstrate breathing techniques and have the client initiate the technique with the nurse.

    b. Acknowledge his fear and give positive reinforcement for his efforts. Acknowledge when dyspnea is worse than usual.

    c. Acknowledge feelings of helplessness. Avoid suggesting "take control" or "relax." Do not leave alone.

    d. Provide assistance with all tasks during acute episodes of shortness of breath.

    e. During acute episode, do not discuss preventive measures.

    f. During nonacute episodes, teach relaxation techniques (*e.g.*, tapes, guided imagery).

B. **When anxiety is diminished enough for learning to take place, assist person in recognizing his anxiety to initiate learning or problem solving**

    1. Request validation of your assessment of anxiety (*e.g.*, "Are you uncomfortable now?").

    2. If person can say yes, continue with the learning process; if he is not able to acknowledge anxiety, continue supportive measures until he is able (refer to A).

    3. When able to learn, determine usual coping mechanisms: "What do you usually do when you get upset?" (*i.e.*, reading, discussing problems, avoiding, distancing, wishful thinking, substance use, self-isolation, self-blame, seeking social support).

    4. Assess for unmet needs or expectations; encourage recall and description of what the person experienced immediately before feeling anxious.

    5. Assist in reevaluation of the perceived threat by discussing the following:

        a. Were expectations realistic?

        b. Was it possible to meet his expectations?

        c. Where in the sequence of events was change possible?

    6. Encourage to recall and analyze similar instances of anxiety.

    7. Explore what alternative behaviors might have been used if coping mechanisms were maladaptive.

    8. Teach anxiety interrupters to use when stressful situations cannot be avoided:

        a. Look up

        b. Control breathing

        c. Lower shoulders

        d. Slow thoughts

        e. Alter voice

        f. Give self directions (out loud, if possible)

        g. Exercise

        h. "Scruff your face"—change facial expression

        i. Change perspective: imagine watching the situation from a distance (Grainger, 1990)

C. **Reduce or eliminate problematic coping mechanisms**

    1. Depression, withdrawal (see *Ineffective Individual Coping*)

    2. Violent behavior (see *Risk for Violence*)

    3. Denial*

        a. Develop an atmosphere of empathic understanding.

        b. Assist in lowering level of anxiety.

        c. Focus on present situation.

        d. Give feedback about current reality; identify positive achievements.

        e. Have person describe events in detail; focus on getting specifics of who, what, when, and where.

    4. Numerous physical complaints with no known organic base

        a. Encourage expression of feelings.

---

* Denial serves a protective function and is not always maladaptive.

    b. Give positive feedback when the person is symptom free.

    c. Acknowledge that the symptoms must be burdensome.

    d. Encourage interest in external environment (*e.g.*, outside activity, volunteering, helping others).

    e. Listen to the complaints.

    f. Evaluate the secondary gains the person receives and attempt to interrupt cycle; see the person on a regular basis, not simply in response to somatic complaints.

    g. Discuss how others are reacting to him; attempt to have him identify his behavior when others react negatively (withdrawal? anger?).

    h. Avoid "doing something" to each complaint; set limits when appropriate (*e.g.*, may refuse to call physician in response to a request for headache medication).

    i. When setting limits, provide an alternative outlet (*e.g.*, redirect to use relaxation technique) (see Appendix X).

  5. Anger* (*e.g.*, demanding behavior, manipulation) (with adults refer to *Ineffective Individual Coping*)

D. Initiate health teaching and referrals as indicated

  1. For people identified as having chronic anxiety and maladaptive coping mechanisms, refer for ongoing psychiatric treatment.

  2. Instruct in nontechnical, understandable terms regarding his illness and associated treatments. Repeat explanations, because anxiety may interfere with learning.

  3. Instruct in maintenance of physical well-being (*i.e.*, nutrition, exercise, elimination).

  4. Instruct (or refer) person for assertiveness training.

  5. Instruct in use of relaxation techniques (see Appendix X).

  6. Instruct in constructive problem-solving (see Appendix VII).

  7. Provide telephone numbers for emergency intervention:

    a. Hotlines

    b. Psychiatric emergency room

    c. On-call staff if available

Rationale

- Nursing strategies differ depending on the level of anxiety (Tarsitano, 1992).
- Participating in decision making can help give a client a sense of control, which enhances his coping ability. Perception of loss of control can result in a sense of powerlessness, then hopelessness.
- Providing emotional support and encouraging sharing may help a client clarify and verbalize his fears, allowing the nurse to give realistic feedback and reassurance.
- An anxious client has a narrowed perceptual field with a diminished ability to learn. The client may experience symptoms caused by increased muscle tension and disrupted sleep patterns. Anxiety tends to feed on itself, trapping the client in a spiral of increasing anxiety, tension, and emotional and physical pain.
- Some fears are based on inaccurate information and can be relieved by providing accurate information. A client with severe anxiety or panic does not retain learning.
- Verbalization allows sharing and provides the nurse with an opportunity to correct misconceptions.
- Praising the client for effective coping can reinforce future positive coping responses.
- Relaxation techniques enhance the client's sense of control over his body's response to stress.
- Providing emotional support and encouraging the client to share allows him to clarify his fears and permits the nurse to provide realistic feedback and reassurance.
- Modifiable contributing factors to anxiety include incomplete and inaccurate information. Providing accurate information and correcting misconceptions may help eliminate fears and reduce anxiety (Redman & Thomas, 1992).

---

* Anger is a response to frustration and anxiety. Not all anger is problematic. It can be used for problem solving.

- Research has shown that involving family members in care results in increased client cooperation and positive adjustment to the experience (Leske, 1993)
- Helping the client to understand his anxiety and its sources provides an opportunity to work through it (Tarsitano, 1992).

🌀 Interventions—*Child Focus*

1. Explain events using simple, age-appropriate terms and illustrations, puppets, dolls, and sample equipment.
2. Allow to wear underwear and have familiar toys or objects.
3. Assist parents/caregivers to manage their anxiety when with child.
4. Children can be assisted in coping with anxiety through the following nursing interventions (Wong, 1993):
    a. Establish a trusting relationship
    b. Minimize separation from parents.
    c. Encourage expression of feelings.
    d. Involve the child in play.
    e. Prepare the child for new experiences (*e.g.*, procedures, surgery).
    f. Provide comfort measures.
    g. Allow for regression.
    h. Encourage parental involvement in care.
    i. Allay parental apprehension and provide them information.
5. Assist a child with anger.
    a. Encourage the child to share his anger (*e.g.*, "How did you feel when you had your injection?," "How did you feel when Mary would not play with you?").
    b. Tell the child that being angry is okay (*e.g.*, "I sometimes get angry when I can't have what I want.").
    c. Encourage and allow the child to express anger in acceptable ways (*e.g.*, loud talking, hitting a play object, or running outside around the house).

Rationale

- Children need opportunities and encouragement to express anger in a controlled, acceptable manner (*e.g.*, choosing not to play a particular game, choosing not to play with a particular person, slamming a door, or voicing anger). Unacceptable expressions of anger include throwing an object, hitting a person, and breaking an object. Children who are not permitted to express their anger may develop hostility and perceive the world as unfriendly.
- The presence of parents provides a familiar, stabilizing support.
- Parental anxiety influences the child's anxiety (Johnson, 1995).

🌀 Interventions—*Maternal Focus*

1. Discuss with woman her expectations and concerns regarding pregnancy and parenthood. Discuss these concerns with the woman alone, her partner alone, and then together as indicated.
2. Help her identify unrealistic expectations.
3. Acknowledge her anxieties and their normality.

Rationale

- Providing emotional support and encouraging sharing may help a client clarify and verbalize her fears, allowing the nurse to give realistic feedback and reassurance.
- Some fears are based on inaccurate information and can be relieved by providing accurate information.

🏛 Interventions—*Older Adult Focus*

1. Use consistent caregivers when possible.
2. Maintain a calm, unhurried manner by allowing person to set pace.
3. Evaluate the effects of medical conditions, medications, and caffeine intake on the individual's anxiety level (Miller, 1995).

Rationale

- Anxiety can be precipitated or exacerbated by pathologic processes (*e.g.*, decreased cerebral oxygen, hyperthyroidism) (Miller, 1995).
- Medications or chemicals that stimulate the central nervous system can cause or increase anxiety (Miller, 1995).

■ # Anxiety
Related to Insufficient Knowledge of Preoperative Routines, Postoperative Exercises/Activities, Postoperative Alterations/Sensations

Outcome Criteria

The person will
- Verbalize, if asked what to expect (routines, environment)
- Demonstrate postoperative exercises, splinting, and respiratory regimen
- Relate less anxiety after teaching

Interventions

1. Before surgery the person's physician should explain
   a. Nature of surgery needed
   b. Reason for and anticipated outcomes of surgery
   c. Risks involved
   d. Type of anesthesia
   e. Expectations for length of recovery and limitations imposed during the recovery period
2. Determine level of understanding of surgical procedure.
   a. Reinforce physician's explanation of surgical procedure. Notify physician if additional explanations are indicated.
3. Evaluate the anxiety level of client and family:
   a. Low (expected)
   b. Moderate (narrowed perception, difficult to concentrate, will have some difficulty analyzing, shakiness)
   c. High (perception greatly reduced, highly distractible, unable to concentrate, learning severely impaired)
4. Notify the physician if the client exhibits severe anxiety or panic.
5. If anxiety is moderate, assist the person to gain insight into their anxiety and reason. Help to reappraise the threat and to learn a new way to deal with it (Tarsitano, 1992).
6. For morning admissions or same-day surgery clients:
   a. Provide access to general information pertaining to need for active participation, routines, equipment, environment, personnel, postoperative sensations, and care before day of surgery:
      Group classes

>   Printed materials
>   Audio or video tapes
>   b. Establish a system of follow-up to educational program (*e.g.*, telephone call day before).
> 7. For hospitalized individual:
>   a. Give bedside instruction concerning specific type of surgery and sensations and appearances (*e.g.*, presence of machines, tubes) that client and family may encounter postoperatively.
>   b. Explain all procedures, the reasons for them, and their importance:
>   1. Preoperative
>   NPO
>   Medications
>   Laboratory work
>   2. Postoperative
>   Parenteral fluids
>   Vital signs
>   Dressings
>   Nasogastric and other tubes
>   Indwelling bladder catheter
>   Pain and availability of medications
>   3. Explain the importance of and teach using return demonstration:
>   To turn, cough, and breathe deep, depending on surgical procedure
>   To support incision during coughing
>   To deep breathe hourly postoperatively
>   To exercise actively and how passive ROM exercises will be done
>   To sit up, get up, and ambulate—sitting in a chair should be avoided
>   Importance of progressive care
>   Early ambulation
>   Self-care, as soon as able
>   4. Explain the rationale for leg exercises, demonstrate, and have client return demonstrate (Tarsitano, 1992).
>   With heels on bed, push the toes of both feet toward the foot of the bed until the calf muscles of the leg tighten. Relax both feet. Pull toes toward the chin, until calf muscles tighten. Relax feet.
>   With heels on bed, circle both ankles, first to the right and then to the left. Repeat three times. Relax.
>   Bend each knee alternately, sliding foot up along the bed. Relax.
>   5. Explain the rationale of deep breathing, demonstrate, and have client return demonstrate (Tarsitano, 1992).
>   Place one hand over abdomen and other where incision will be.
>   Inspire and expand abdomen.
>   Expire slowly and deeply.
>   6. Explain the rationale of coughing, demonstrate, and have client return demonstrate. Cough on expiration only to prevent elevation of pleural pressure (Huddleston, 1990).
> 8. Discuss purpose of recovery room with patient and family.
>   a. Visiting policies
>   b. Type of care
>   c. Length of stay, if applicable
>   d. Possibility of placement in intensive care unit if needed or indicated.
> 9. Explain other hospital policies as indicated
>   a. Visiting hours
>   b. Number of visitors

c. Location of waiting rooms

d. How physician will contact them after operation

10. Evaluate

   a. Person's/family's ability to meet preset, mutually planned learning goals (behaviors)

   b. Need for further teaching and support

Rationale

- The physician is responsible for explaining the surgery to the client and family; the nurse, for determining their level of understanding and then notifying the physician of the need to provide more information.
- Preoperative teaching provides the client with information, which can help decrease anxiety and fear associated with the unknown and enhance his sense of control over the situation.
- Explaining the importance and purpose of all preoperative procedures can help relieve anxiety and fear associated with lack of knowledge of necessary preoperative activities and routines.
  - Enemas are sometimes given to empty the bowel of fecal material, which can help reduce the risk of postoperative bowel obstruction as peristalsis resumes.
  - Eliminating oral fluids preoperatively reduces the risk of aspiration postoperatively.
  - Tests and studies establish baseline values and help detect any abnormalities before surgery.
  - Preoperative sedatives reduce anxiety and promote relaxation, which increases the effectiveness of anesthesia and decreases secretions in response to intubation.
- Explaining postoperative routines and sensations can help reduce fears associated with the unknown and unexpected (Christman & Kirchhoff, 1992).
  - Parenteral fluids replace fluids lost from NPO state and blood loss.
  - Careful vital sign monitoring is needed to determine status and track any changes.
  - Until wound edges heal, the wound must be protected from contaminants by dressing changes and checks.
  - A nasogastric tube promotes drainage and reduces abdominal distention and tension on the suture line.
  - A Foley catheter drains the bladder until muscle tone returns as anesthesia is excreted.
  - Nausea and vomiting are common side effects of preoperative medications and anesthesia; other contributing factors include certain types of surgery, obesity, electrolyte imbalance, rapid position changes, and psychological and environmental factors. Pain commonly occurs as medications lose their effectiveness.
- Exercises and movement promote lung expansion and mobilization of secretions. Incentive spirometry promotes deep breathing by providing a visual indicator of the effectiveness of the breathing effort (Litwack, Saleh, & Schaltz, 1991).
- Leg exercises increase venous return and prevent stasis (Caswell, 1993).

✋ Interventions—*Child Focus (Bolig, 1991; Smallwood, 1988)*

1. Organize tours for children about 5–7 days before the surgery.
2. Group children with similar problems together.
3. Encourage the participation of parents and siblings to provide added security for the child.

4. Involve as many senses as possible. Explain how it feels and smells and whether it will hurt.

5. Using a doll, demonstrate the OR garments, blood sample acquisition.

6. Using a volunteer child, demonstrate the taking of blood pressure, temperature, and heart and respiration rate.

7. Take children on OR cart to show them where their parents will be waiting while they are in surgery.

8. Have an OR nurse (fully dressed) explain:

> The reasons for OR attire
> Anesthesia machine
> Anesthesia as "hospital air" or "hospital sleep" to avoid confusion
> Postanesthesia recovery room
> Explain/demonstrate on doll or child:
>> Straps on OR table
>> Monitoring devices (ECG, pulse)
>> Anesthesia mask (on each child, or on parent if child is frightened)
>> Intravenous lines (inserted after induction; removed after child is eating and drinking)

9. Increase the effectiveness of the teaching program and promote security by:

> Using name tags so children can be addressed by name.
> Involving children in discussion (*e.g.*, ask them the colors of objects; ask them to point to their nose).
> Not forcing any child to do anything.
>> If a child resists, have parent perform the activity and encourage child to help. Allow child to handle equipment.
> Avoiding calling anesthesia gas. It may be confused with gas in a car or gas used in euthanasia of animals.
> Explaining that anesthesia does not affect memories.
> Allowing children to take home masks, hats, and ECG buttons.
> Encouraging child to bring a favorite toy when returning for surgery.

10. If tours are not feasible or child cannot attend, consider using or developing a book for parents to use at home with child that they can receive from their surgeon's office (*e.g., Your Operation Day,* by Margary Doroshow and Deborah London [1984]).

Rationale

- Tours of the facilities with opportunities to see and handle some of the equipment and meet with personnel can help to lessen anxiety (Wong, 1993).
- Playing with equipment allows the child to act out feelings, to establish familiarity, and to question procedures (Jackson & Saunders, 1993).

References/Bibliography

Barlow, D., & Cerny, J. (1988). *Psychiatric treatment of panic.* New York: Guilford.

Bolig, R., et al. (1991). Medical play and preparation: Questions and issues. *Children's Health Care, 20,* 225–229.

Boyle, A., Grap, M., Younger, J., & Thornby, D. (1991). Personality hardiness, ways of coping, social support and burnout in critical care nurses. *Journal of Advanced Nursing, 16,* 850–857.

Boyle, J., & Andrews, M. (1995). *Transcultural concepts in nursing.* Philadelphia: J. B. Lippincott.

Broome, M. E. (1990). Preparation of children for painful procedures. *Pediatric Nursing, 16,* 537–541.

Caswell, D. (1993). Thromboembolic phenomena. *Critical Care Nursing Clinics of North America, 5*, 489–497.

Christman, N., & Kirchhoff, K. (1992). Preparatory sensory information. In G. Bulechek & J. McCloskey (Eds.), *Nursing interventions.* Philadelphia: W. B. Saunders.

DeVito, A. (1990). Dyspnea during hospitalization for acute phase of illness as recalled by patients with chronic obstructive pulmonary disease. *Heart and Lung, 19*, 186–191.

Freeman, M. (1991). Therapeutic use of storytelling for older children who are critically ill. *Children's Health Care, 20*, 208–215.

Giger, J., & Davidhizar, R. (1991). *Transcultural nursing: Assessment and intervention.* St. Louis: Mosby Yearbook.

Grainger, R. (1990). Anxiety interrupters. *American Journal of Nursing, 90*(2), 14–15.

Grainger, R. (1990). Anger within ourselves. *American Journal of Nursing, 90*(7), 12.

Huddleston, V. B. (1990). Pulmonary problems. *Critical Care Nursing Clinics of North America, 2*, 527–536.

Jackson, D. B., & Saunders, R. (1993). *Child health nursing.* Philadelphia: J. B. Lippincott.

Johnson, B. S. (1993). *Psychiatric–mental health nursing: Adaptation and growth.* Philadelphia: J. B. Lippincott.

Johnson, B. S. (1995). *Child, adolescent and family psychiatric nursing.* Philadelphia: J. B. Lippincott.

Jones, P. E., & Jakob, D. F. (1984). Anxiety revisited from a practice perspective. In M. J. Kim, G. K. McFarland, & A. M. McLane (Eds.). *Classification of nursing diagnoses: Proceedings of the fifth national conference.* St. Louis: C. V. Mosby.

Krietemeyer, B. C., & Heiney, S. P. (1992). Storytelling as a therapeutic technique in a group for school-aged oncology patients. *Children's Health Care, 21*, 14–19.

Leske, J. (1993). Anxiety of elective surgical patients, family members. *AORN Journal, 57*, 1091–1103.

Litwack, K., Saleh, D., & Schaltz, P. (1991). Postoperative pulmonary complications. *Critical Care Nursing Clinics of North America, 3*(1), 77–82.

May, K. A., & Mahlmeister, L. R. (1994). *Maternal and neonatal nursing: Family-centered care* (3rd ed.). Philadelphia: J. B. Lippincott.

May, R. (1977). *The meaning of anxiety.* New York: W. W. Norton.

Miles, M., Funk, S., & Kasper, M. (1991). The neonatal intensive care unit environment: Sources of stress for parents. *Clinical Issues in Critical Care Nursing, 2*, 346–353.

Miller, C. A. (1995). *Nursing care of the older adult* (2nd ed.). Glenview, IL: Scott Foresman.

North American Nursing Diagnosis Association. (1989). *Taxonomy I.* St. Louis: Author.

Nyamathi, A., Jacoby, A., Constancia, P., & Ruvevich, S. (1992). Coping and adjustment of spouses of critically ill patients with cardiac disease. *Heart and Lung, 21*, 160–165.

Oski, F. (1994). *Principles and practice of pediatrics.* Philadelphia: J. B. Lippincott.

Redman, B., & Thomas, S. (1992). Patient teaching. In G. Bulechek & J. McCloskey (Eds.). *Nursing interventions: Essential nursing interventions* (2nd ed.). Philadelphia: W. B. Saunders.

Reeder, S. J., Martin, L. L., & Koniak, D. (1992). *Maternity nursing: Family, newborn and women's health care* (17th ed.). Philadelphia: J. B. Lippincott.

Rukoholm, E., Bailey, P., Coutu-Wakulczyk, G., & Bailey, W. (1991). Needs and anxiety levels in relatives of intensive care unit patients. *Journal of Advanced Nursing, 16*, 920–928.

Smallwood, S. (1988). Preparing children for surgery. *AORN Journal, 47*, 177–182.

Spielberger, C., & Sarason, I. (Eds.). (1975). *Stress and anxiety* (Vol. I). Washington, DC: Hemisphere.

Tarsitano, B. P. (1992). Structured preoperative teaching. In G. Bulechek & J. McCloskey (Eds.). *Nursing interventions: Essential nursing interventions.* Philadelphia: W. B. Saunders.

Taylor, C. B., & Arnow, B. (1988). *The nature and treatment of anxiety disorders.* New York: Free Press.

Taylor-Loughran, A., O'Brien, M., LaChapelle, R., & Rangel, S. (1989). Defining characteristics of the nursing diagnoses fear and anxiety: A validation study. *Applied Nursing Research, 2*, 178–186.

Thomas, D. O. (1991). How to deal with children in the emergency department. *Journal of Emergency Nursing, 17*(1), 49–50.

Wong, D. L., (1993). *Essentials of pediatric nursing* (4th ed.). St. Louis: C. V. Mosby.

Yokom, C. J. (1984). The differentiation of fear and anxiety. In M. J. Kim, G. K. McFarland, & A. M. McLane (Eds.). *Classification of nursing diagnoses: Proceedings of the fifth national conference.* St Louis: C. V. Mosby.

Body Temperature, Risk for Altered

Hyperthermia

Hypothermia

Thermoregulation, Ineffective

Body Temperature, Risk for Altered

DEFINITION

Risk for Altered Body Temperature: The state in which the individual is at risk for failing to maintain body temperature within normal range (36°–37.5°C or 98°–99.5°F) (Smeltzer & Bare, 1992).

RISK FACTORS

Presence of risk factors (see Related Factors)

RELATED FACTORS
Pathophysiologic

Related to impaired temperature control secondary to:
    Coma/increased intracranial pressure
    Brain tumor/hypothalamic tumor/head trauma
    Cerebrovascular accident
    Infection/inflammation
    Integument (skin) injury
Related to decreased circulation secondary to:
    Anemia
    Neurovascular disease/peripheral vascular disease
    Vasodilation/shock
Related to decreased ability to sweat secondary to (specify)

Treatment-Related

Related to cooling effects of:
    Parenteral fluid infusion/blood transfusion   Cooling blanket
    Dialysis   Operating suite

Situational (Personal, Environmental)

Related to:
    Exposure to cold, rain, snow, wind/exposure to heat, sun, and humidity extremes
    Inappropriate clothing for climate
    Inability to pay for shelter, heat, or air conditioning
    Extremes of weight
    Consumption of alcohol
    Dehydration/malnutrition

Maturational

Related to ineffective temperature regulation secondary to extremes of age (*e.g.*, newborn, older adult)

Author's Note

Risk for Altered Body Temperature includes those at risk for *Hyperthermia, Hypothermia*, and/or *Ineffective Thermoregulation*. If the person is at risk for only one of the diagnoses (*e.g., Hypothermia* but not *Hyperthermia*), then it is more useful to label the problem with the more specific diagnosis (*Risk for Hypothermia*). If the person is at risk for two or more of the diagnoses, then *Risk for Altered Body Temperature* is more appropriate. The focus of nursing care for these diagnoses is that of preventing abnormal body temperatures by identifying and treating those with a normal temperature who demonstrate risk factors that can be controlled by nursing-prescribed interventions (*e.g.*, by removing or adding blankets, by controlling environmental temperature). If the alteration in body temperature is related to a pathophysiologic complication that requires nursing and medical interventions, then the problem should be labeled as a collaborative problem (*e.g., Potential Complication: Severe Hypothermia related to hypothalamus injury*). The focus of concern then becomes monitoring to detect and report significant temperature fluctuations and implementing collaborative interventions (*e.g.*, a warming or cooling blanket) as ordered. See also Author's Notes for *Hyperthermia* and *Hypothermia*.

Key Concepts

1. The body has two major compartments, the *shell* (consisting of skin and subcutaneous tissue) and the *core* (consisting of vital internal organs, the intestinal tract, and large muscle groups). Heat transfer involves the shell and the core; it is possible that the shell may be warm while the core may be cold, and vice versa.
2. Regulation of body temperature is a dynamic process involving four mechanisms (Phillips & Skov, 1988):
   Conduction: Direct transfer of heat from the body to cooler objects without motion (*e.g.*, from cells and capillaries to skin and onto clothing)
   Convection: Transfer of heat by circulation (*e.g.*, from warmer core areas to peripheral areas and from air movement next to the skin)
   Radiation: Transfer of heat between the skin and the environment
   Evaporation: Transfer of heat when skin or clothing is wet and heat is lost through moisture into the environment
3. Heat production occurs in the core, which is innervated by thermoreceptor stimulation from the hypothalamus.
4. Normothermia is defined as a core temperature of 36.6°–37.5°C or 98°–99.5°F (Smeltzer & Bare, 1992).
5. Heat loss and gain vary in individuals and are influenced by body surface area, peripheral vasomotor tone, and quantity of subcutaneous tissue.
6. Shivering, the body's physiologic attempt to create more heat, produces profound physiologic responses:
   Increased oxygen consumption to two to five times the normal rate
   Increased metabolic demand to as much as 400%–500%
   Increased myocardial work, carbon dioxide production, cutaneous vasoconstriction, and eventual lactic acid production
7. The reliability of temperature depends on accurate temperature-taking technique, minimization of variables affecting the temperature measurement device, and the site chosen for measurement.
8. Oral temperature readings may be unreliable (owing to many variables, such as poor contact between the thermometer and mucosa, air movement, and smoking or drinking before temperature taking); oral temperatures measure 0.5° below core temperature.

9. Rectal temperature readings, which have fewer affecting variables and are more reliable than oral temperatures, measure 0.5°C above core temperature at normothermia, and at temperatures less than 36.5°C measure *peripheral* temperature, rather than *core* temperature. Rectal temperatures measure 1° *higher* than oral temperature readings.
10. Axillary temperature readings are reliable only for skin temperature; they measure 1° *lower* than oral temperature readings.

Key Concepts—Hyperthermia

1. The body responds to hot environments by increasing heat dissipation through
   a. Increased sweat production
   b. Dilation of peripheral blood vessels
2. Increased metabolic rate increases body temperature, and vice versa (increase in body temperature causes an increased metabolic rate).
3. Fever is a major sign of onset of infection, inflammation, and disease: treatment with aspirin or acetaminophen without medical consultation may mask important symptoms that should receive medical attention.
4. Blood is the cooling fluid of the body: low blood volume owing to dehydration predisposes to fever.

Key Concepts—Hypothermia

1. The body responds to cold environments with mechanisms aimed at preventing heat loss and increasing heat production:
   a. Muscle contraction
   b. Peripheral vasoconstriction
   c. Increased heart rate
   d. Dilation of blood vessels in muscles
   e. Shivering and vasodilation
   f. Release of thyroxine and corticosteroids
2. Severe hypothermia can cause life-threatening cardiac dysrhythmias and must be referred to a physician.
3. Hypothermia (a core temperature <35°C [95°F]) in the postoperative period has many profound negative effects (decreased myocardial and cerebral functions, respiratory acidosis, impaired hematologic and immunologic functions, and cold diuresis) in the absence of safe and effective rewarming (Howell, Macrae, Sanjines, Burke, & DeStefano, 1992). Hypothermia also reduces blood pressure and contributes to shock.
4. Vasodilation promotes heat loss and predisposes to hypothermia.

🌳 *Key Concepts—Child*

1. Almost every child experiences a fever of 100°–104°F at some time. Normal children usually are not harmed by fever; only approximately 4% of febrile children are susceptible to convulsions (Hunsberger, 1989). Children younger than 18 years of age with fever accompanied by flu symptoms should never be medicated with aspirin or products containing aspirin because of the risk of development of potentially fatal Reye's syndrome.
2. The neonate is vulnerable to heat loss because of (May & Mahlmeister, 1994):
   a. Large body surface area relative to body mass
   b. Increased basal metabolism rate
   c. Less adipose tissue for insulation
   d. Environmental conditions (delivery room, nursery)
3. Nonshivering thermogenesis is a heat production mechanism located in brown fat (highly vascular adipose tissue), which is found only in infants. When skin temperature begins to drop, thermal receptors transmit impulses to the central nervous system (May & Mahlmeister, 1994). The following sequence illustrates this mechanism:

   Central nervous system → Stimulates sympathetic nervous system → Release of norepinephrine from adrenal gland and at nerve endings in brown fat → Heat production
4. It is not necessary to treat all fevers in children. Fevers related to heat stroke can be treated with tepid or cold sponging. Fevers (<104°F or 40°C) in previously well children

with no history of febrile convulsions and without a threatening illness can be left untreated or, if desired, treated with acetaminophen. Sponging increases the child's discomfort (Lorin, 1995).

5. Tepid sponging instead of antipyretic drugs is indicated for very young infants and children with severe liver disease or a history of hypersensitivity to antipyretic drugs (Lorin, 1995).

🏛 *Key Concepts—Older Adult*

1. Older adults can become hypothermic or hyperthermic in moderately cold or hot environments, compared with younger adults, who require exposure to severe cold or hot temperatures (Miller, 1995).
2. Age-related changes that interfere with the body's ability to adapt to cold temperature include inefficient vasoconstriction, decreased cardiac output, decreased subcutaneous tissue, and delayed and diminished sweating (Miller, 1995).
3. Older adults have a higher threshold for the onset of sweating and decreased efficiency of sweating when it occurs.
4. Older adults have a dulled perception of cold and warmth and thus may lack the stimulus to initiate protective actions.
5. The thirst mechanism becomes less efficient with aging, as does the kidney's ability to concentrate urine, increasing the risk of heat-related dehydration.
6. Inactivity and immobility increase susceptibility to hypothermia by suppressing shivering and reducing heat-generating muscle activity.
7. Seventy percent of all heat stroke victims are older than 60 years of age (Robbins, 1989).

Focus Assessment Criteria

Subjective Data

A. Assess for defining characteristics
1. Assess history of symptoms (abnormal skin temperature, altered mentation, headaches, nausea, lethargy, vertigo).
   Onset?

B. Assess for related factors
1. Hyperthermia
   Dehydration
   Recent exposure to communicable disease without known immunity (*e.g.*, measles without vaccine or previous illness)
   Recent overexposure to sun, heat, humidity
   Recent overactivity
   Radiation/chemotherapy/immunosuppression
   Alcohol use
   Impaired judgment
   Home environment:
       Adequate ventilation?
       Air conditioning?
       Room temperature?
   Medications:
       Diuretics
       Anticholinergics
       Central nervous system depressants
       Antidepressants
       Vasoconstrictors?
       How often taken? Last dose taken when?

2. Hypothermia
> Recent exposure to cold/dampness
> Inactivity
> Impaired judgment
> Medications:
>> Vasodilators
>> Central nervous system depressants
> Home environment:
>> Adequate heating, blankets
>> Adequate clothing (*e.g.*, socks, hat, gloves)
>> Adequate shelter, heat

3. Clothing appropriate for environment
4. Problems that may contribute to hyperthermia or hypothermia
> Smoking
> Diabetes
> Repeated infections
> Circulatory problems (specify)
> Cardiovascular disorders/peripheral vascular disease
> Mobility problems
> Neurologic disorders
> History of frostbite

Objective Data

A. Assess for defining characteristics

1. Vital signs
> Normal baseline temperature:
>> Present temperature
>> Abnormal heart rate, rhythm
>> Abnormal respiratory rate
>> Abnormal blood pressure

2. Mental status
> Alert/drowsy/confused/oriented/comatose

3. Skin and circulation
> Intact?
> Burned (specify degree and site)?
> Injured (specify)?
> Rash (specify type and site)?
> Bites (specify site)?
> Turgor: normal/dehydrated
> Temperature/feel: hot/warm/cold/damp/dry
> Color: flushed/pale/bluish
> Frostbite (specify site)
> Quality of peripheral pulses (radial, pedal)

4. Signs of dehydration
> Parched mouth/furrowed tongue/dry lips
> Increased urine specific gravity

Hyperthermia

DEFINITION
Hyperthermia: The state in which an individual has or is at risk of having a sustained elevation of body temperature greater than 37.8°C (100°F) orally or 38.8°C (101°F) rectally due to external factors.

DEFINING CHARACTERISTICS
Major (Must Be Present)
Temperature higher than 37.8°C (100°F) orally or 38.8°C (101°F) rectally

Minor (May Be Present)
Flushed skin

Warm to touch

Increased respiratory rate

Tachycardia

Shivering/goose pimples

Dehydration

Specific or generalized aches and pains (*e.g.*, headache)

Malaise/fatigue/weakness

Loss of appetite

RELATED FACTORS
Treatment-Related
Reduced ability to sweat secondary to (specify medication):

Situational (Personal, Environmental)
Related to:
  Exposure to heat, sun
  Inappropriate clothing for climate
  No access to air conditioning
Related to decreased circulation secondary to:
  Extremes of weight
  Dehydration
Related to insufficient hydration for vigorous activity

Maturational
Related to ineffective temperature regulation secondary to age

---

Author's Note
The nursing diagnoses *Hypothermia* and *Hyperthermia* represent people with temperature below and above normal, respectively. These abnormal temperature states are treatable by nursing interventions, such as correcting the external causes (*e.g.*, inappropriate clothing, exposure to elements [heat or cold], or dehydration). The nursing focus centers on preventing or treating mild hypothermia and hyperthermia. As life-threatening situations that require medical and nursing interventions, severe hypothermia and hyperthermia represent collaborative problems and should be labeled *Potential Complication: Hypothermia* or *Potential Complication: Hyperthermia*.

Temperature elevation due to infections, other disorders (*e.g.*, hypothalamic), or treatments (*e.g.*, hypothermia units) requires collaborative treatment. If desired, the nurse could use the nursing diagnosis *Altered Comfort* and the collaborative problem *Potential Complication: Hypothermia* or *Potential Complication: Hyperthermia*.

Errors in Diagnostic Statements

Hyperthermia related to intraoperative pharmacogenic hypermetabolism

This situation describes malignant hyperthermia, a life-threatening, inherited disorder resulting in a hypermetabolic state related to the use of anesthetic agents and depolarizing muscle relaxants. The collaborative problem *Potential Complication: Malignant Hypertension* would more appropriately describe this situation, which necessitates rapid detection and cotreatment by nursing and medicine.

Hyperthermia related to effect of circulating endotoxins on hypothalamus secondary to sepsis

Nursing care for people with elevated temperature in an acute care setting focuses on monitoring and managing the fever with nursing and physician orders or promoting comfort through nursing orders. The nursing diagnosis *Altered Comfort* would more appropriately describe a situation that nurses treat, with the collaborative problem *Potential Complication: Sepsis* representing the physiologic complication that nurses monitor for and manage with nursing- and physician-prescribed interventions.

Focus Assessment Criteria

See *Risk for Altered Body Temperature*.

Outcome Criteria

The person will
- Identify risk factors for hyperthermia
- Reduce risk factors for hyperthermia
- Maintain normal body temperature

Interventions

A. Assess for the presence of contributing risk factors
   1. Dehydration
   2. Environmental warmth/exercise

B. Monitor body and environmental temperature

C. Remove or reduce contributing risk factors
   1. For dehydration:
      a. Monitor intake and output and provide favorite fluids to maintain a balance between intake and output.
      b. Teach the importance of maintaining an adequate fluid intake (at least 2000 mL a day of cool liquids unless contraindicated by heart or kidney disease) to prevent dehydration. Explain the importance of not relying on thirst sensation as an indication of the need for fluid.
      c. See also *Fluid Volume Deficit*.
   2. For environmental warmth/exercise:
      a. Assess whether clothing or bedcovers are too warm for the environment or planned activity.
      b. Remove excess clothing or blankets (remove hat, gloves, or socks, as appropriate) to promote heat loss. Encourage wearing loose cotton clothing.
      c. Provide air conditioning, dehumidifiers, fans, or cool baths or compresses as appropriate.

    d. Teach the importance of increasing fluid intake during warm weather and exercise. Advise against exercising in hot weather.

    e. Teach the need to wear a hat or use an umbrella during sun exposure.

D. Initiate health teaching as indicated

    1. Explain that children and older adults are more at risk for hyperthermia.

    2. Teach the early signs of hyperthermia or heat stroke:

Flushed skin	Headache/confusion
Fatigue	Loss of appetite

    3. Teach to take cool baths several times a day in hot temperatures, avoiding soap to prevent skin drying.

    4. Teach to apply ice packs or cool, wet towels to the body, especially on the axillae and groin.

    5. Explain the need to avoid alcohol, caffeine, and large, heavy meals during hot weather.

    6. Stress the need to report persistent elevated temperature.

Rationale

- Body temperature is greatly affected by activity level and environmental temperature; high humidity increases the effect of cold or heat on the body.
- Exposure of the head, face, hands, and feet can affect body temperature greatly. These are vascular areas where heat is conducted from the blood vessels to the skin and from the skin to the air, and where cold is conducted from the air to the skin and from the skin to the blood vessels.
- Cooling of a hyperthermic individual and rewarming of a hypothermic individual must be done with great care to avoid overcooling or overwarming; in the acute care setting cooling and rewarming are often problems that require close collaboration with the physician.
- Adding clothes or blankets to a person inhibits the body's natural ability to reduce body temperature; removing clothes or blankets enhances the body's natural ability to reduce body temperature.
- Increased calories and fluids are required to maintain metabolic functions when fever is present.
- Axillary temperatures should be measured for 5 minutes (Hunter, 1991).
- Electronic or tympanic thermometers give rapid, accurate readings in neonates, children, and adults.

Hypothermia

DEFINITION

Hypothermia: The state in which an individual has or is at risk of having a sustained reduction of body temperature of below 35.5°C (96°F) rectally because of increased vulnerability to external factors.*

---

* Temperatures below 35°C (95°F) rectally should be reported to the physician for collaborative management of rewarming.

DEFINING CHARACTERISTICS*
Major (80%–100%)
Reduction in body temperature below 35.5°C (96°F) rectally*
  Cool skin   Shivering (mild)
  Pallor (moderate)

Minor (50%–79%)
  Mental confusion/drowsiness/restlessness   Cachexia/malnutrition
  Decreased pulse and respiration

RELATED FACTORS
Situational (Personal, Environmental)
  Related to:
    Exposure to cold, rain, snow, wind
    Inappropriate clothing for climate
    Inability to pay for shelter or heat
  Related to decreased circulation secondary to:
    Extremes of weight   Dehydration
    Consumption of alcohol   Inactivity

Maturational
  Related to ineffective temperature regulation secondary to age (*e.g.*, neonate, older adult)

Author's Note
Because more serious hypothermia (temperatures below 35°C or 95°F rectally) can cause severe pathophysiologic consequences, such as decreased myocardial and respiratory function, the nurse is cautioned to report these low readings to the physician. Nurses most often initiate nurse-prescribed interventions for mild hypothermia (temperatures between 35°C [95°F] and 36°C [97°F] rectally) to prevent more serious hypothermia. Nurses are commonly responsible for identifying and treating *Risk for Hypothermia*. See also diagnostic considerations for *Risk for Altered Body Temperature*.

Errors in Diagnostic Statements
  See *Risk for Altered Body Temperature* and *Hyperthermia*.

Focus Assessment Criteria

See *Risk for Altered Body Temperature*.

Outcome Criteria

The person will
- Identify risk factors for hypothermia
- Reduce risk factors for hypothermia
- Maintain body temperature within normal limits

* Adapted from Carroll, S. M. (1989). Nursing diagnosis: Hypothermia. In R. M. Carroll-Johnson (Ed.). *Classification of nursing diagnosis: Proceedings of the eighth conference.* Philadelphia: J. B. Lippincott.

Interventions

A. Assess for the presence of risk factors

   1. Prolonged exposure to cold environment (either at home or outside)
   2. Poverty/inability to pay for adequate heat/shelter
   3. Extremes of age (*e.g.*, newborn, elderly)
   4. Neurovascular/peripheral vascular disease
   5. Malnutrition/cachexia
   6. Perioperative experience

B. Monitor body and environmental temperatures

C. Reduce or eliminate causative or contributing factors, if possible

   1. For prolonged exposure to cold environment:
      a. Assess room temperatures at home.
      b. Teach to keep room temperatures at 70°–75°F or to layer clothing with sweaters.
      c. Explain the importance of wearing a hat, gloves, and warm socks and shoes to prevent heat loss.
      d. Encourage limiting going outside when temperatures are very cold.
      e. Acquire an electric blanket, warm blankets, or down comforter and flannel sheets for bed.
      f. Provide a hot bath before the person is cold.
      g. Teach to wear close-knit undergarments to prevent heat loss.
      h. Explain that more clothes may be needed in the morning, when body metabolism is lowest.
   2. For poverty/inability to pay for heat:
      a. Consult with social service to identify sources of financial assistance/warm clothing/blankets, shelter.
      b. Teach the importance of preventing heat loss before body temperature is actually lowered.
      c. Acquire warm socks, sweaters, gloves, and hats.
   3. For neurovascular/peripheral vascular disease:
      a. Keep room temperature between 70°–74°F.
      b. Assess for adequate circulation to extremities (*i.e.*, satisfactory peripheral pulses).
      c. Instruct to wear warm gloves and socks to reduce heat loss.
      d. Teach the person to take a warm bath if he is feeling unable to get warm.
   4. Initiate health teaching if indicated.
      a. Explain the relationship of age as a risk for hypothermia.
      b. Teach the early signs of hypothermia:
         Cool skin
         Pallor, blanching, redness
      c. Explain the need to drink 8–10 glasses of water daily and to consume frequent, small meals with warm liquids.
      d. Explain the need to avoid alcohol during periods of very cold weather.

Rationale

- Significant heat losses can be prevented by reducing heat loss by evaporation, convection, conduction, and radiation (Puterbough, 1991)

🖐 🏛 Interventions—*Child and Older Adult*

1. For extremes of age (newborn, older adults):
   a. Maintain room temperature at 70°–74°F.
   b. Instruct to wear hat, gloves, and socks if necessary to prevent heat loss.
   c. Explain to family members that newborns, infants, and older adults are more susceptible to heat loss (see also *Ineffective Thermoregulation*).

2. For children and older adults during intraoperative experience, unless hypothermia is desired to reduce blood loss, consider the following interventions (Burkle, 1988):
   a. Increase ambient temperature of OR before case.
   b. Use a portable radiant heating lamp to provide additional heat during surgery.
   c. Cover with warm blankets when arriving in OR.
   d. When possible, use a warming mattress.
   e. During prepping and surgery, keep as much of body surface covered as possible.
   f. Warm prep set, blood, fluids, anesthesia, irrigants.
   g. Replace wet gowns and drapes with dry ones.
   h. Keep head well covered.
   i. Continue heat-conserving interventions postoperatively.

Rationale

- Children and older adults can become hypothermic in moderately cold OR environments (Miller, 1995; Wong, 1996).
- During the immediate postoperative period, clients are prone to hypothermia related to prolonged exposure to cold in the operating room and the infusion of large quantities of cool intravenous fluids.

References/Bibliography

Andrews, A. (1990). Inadvertent hypothermia: A complication of postoperative cholecystectomy patients. *AORN Journal, 52*, 987–991.

Burkle, N. (1988). Inadvertent hypothermia. *Journal of Gerontologic Nursing, 14*(6), 26–29.

Carroll, S. M. (1989). Nursing diagnosis: Hypothermia. In R. M. Carroll-Johnson (Ed.). *Classification of nursing diagnoses: Proceedings of the eighth conference*. Philadelphia: J. B. Lippincott.

Erickson, R., & Yount, S. (1991). Comparison of tympanic and oral temperatures in surgical patients. *Nursing Research, 40*(2), 90–93.

Howell, R., Macrae, L., Sanjines, S., Burke, J., & DeStefano, P. (1992). Effects of two types of head coverings in the rewarming of patients after coronary artery bypass graft surgery. *Heart and Lung, 21*, 1–6.

Howie, J. (1991). Hypothermia and rewarming after cardiac operation. *Focus, 18*, 414–417.

Hunsberger, M. (1989). Principles and skills adapted to the care of children. In R. L. Foster, M. M. Hunsberger, & J. J. T. Anderson (Eds.). *Family-centered nursing care of children*. Philadelphia: W. B. Saunders.

Johnson, S. (1989). Alteration in temperature regulation: Hypothermia. In R. M. Carroll-Johnson (Ed.). *Classification of nursing diagnoses: Proceedings of the eighth conference*. Philadelphia: J. B. Lippincott.

Lorin, M. (1995). Pathogenesis of fever and treatment. In F. Oski (Ed.). *Principles and practices of pediatrics* (2nd ed.). Philadelphia: J. B. Lippincott.

May, K. A., & Mahlmeister, L. R. (1994). *Maternal and neonatal nursing: Family-centered care* (3rd ed.). Philadelphia: J. B. Lippincott.

Miller, C. A. (1995). *Nursing care of older adults* (2nd ed.). Glenview, IL: Scott, Foresman.

Miller, C. (1991). Driving the temperature up—and down. *Geriatric Nursing, 12*(1), 44, 48.

Moddeman, G. (1991). The elderly surgical patient—a high risk for hypothermia. *AORN Journal, 53*, 1270–1272.

Phillips, R., & Skov, P. (1988). Rewarming and cardiac surgery: A review. *Heart and Lung, 17*(5), 511–520.

Porth, C. (1992). *Pathophysiology* (4th ed.) Philadelphia: J. B. Lippincott.

Puterbough, C. (1991). Hypothermia related to exposure and surgical interventions. *Today's OR Nurse, 13*(7), 32–33.

Reeves-Swift, R. (1990). Rational management of a child's acute fever. *American Journal of Maternal–Child Nursing, 15*(2), 82–85.

Robbins, A. S. (1989). Hypothermia and heat stroke: Protecting the elderly patient. *Geriatrics, 44*(1), 73–79.

Smeltzer, S., & Bare, B. (1992). *Brunner and Suddarth's textbook of medical–surgical nursing* (7th ed.). Philadelphia: J. B. Lippincott.

Staff. (1994). Clinical news: Ear's a good way to take temps. *American Journal of Nursing, 94*(3), 10.

Summers, S., Dudgeon, N., Byram, K., & Zingsheim, K. (1991). Validation of the nursing diagnosis hypothermia. In R. M. Carroll-Johnson (Ed.). *Classification of nursing diagnoses: Proceedings of the ninth conference*. Philadelphia: J. B. Lippincott.

Wong, D. L. (1996). *Clinical manual of pediatric nursing* (4th ed.). St. Louis: C. V. Mosby

Thermoregulation, Ineffective

DEFINITION

Ineffective Thermoregulation: The state in which an individual experiences or is at risk of experiencing an inability to maintain a stable core normal body temperature in the presence of adverse or changing external factors.

DEFINING CHARACTERISTICS
Major (Must Be Present)

Temperature fluctuations related to limited metabolic compensatory regulation in response to environmental factors

RELATED FACTORS
Situational (Personal, Environmental)

Related to:
>Fluctuating environmental temperatures
>Cold or wet articles (clothes, cribs, equipment)
>Inadequate housing
>Wet body surface
>Inadequate clothing for weather (excessive, insufficient)

Maturational

>Related to limited metabolic compensatory regulation secondary to age (*e.g.*, neonate, older adult)

Author's Note

Ineffective Thermoregulation is a useful diagnosis for people who have difficulty maintaining a stable core body temperature over a wide range of environmental temperatures. This diagnosis most commonly applies to older adults and neonates. Thermoregulation involves the balancing of heat production and heat loss. The nursing focus centers on manipulating external factors (*e.g.*, clothing and environmental conditions) to maintain body temperature within normal limits, and on teaching prevention strategies.

Errors in Diagnostic Statements

Ineffective Thermoregulation related to effects of a hypothalamic tumor

Tumors of the hypothalamus can affect the temperature-regulating centers, resulting in body temperature shifts. This situation requires constant surveillance and rapid response to changes with appropriate nursing and medical treatments. Thus, this situation would be better described as a collaborative problem: *Potential Complication: Hypo / hyperthermia.*

Ineffective Thermoregulation related to temperature fluctuations

Temperature fluctuations represent a manifestation of the diagnosis, not a related factor. If the fluctuations result from age-related limited compensatory regulation, the diagnosis would be written: *Ineffective Thermoregulation related to decreased ability to acclimatize to heat or cold secondary to age, as evidenced by temperature fluctuations.*

Focus Assessment Criteria

Objective Data

A. Assess for defining characteristics

    1. Skin

        Color

        Nailbeds

        Temperature

        Rashes

    2. Temperature

        Environment (home, infant [ambient, radiant, Isolette])

        Body (adult, child [rectal, oral], newborn [axillary])

    3. Respiratory (rate, rhythm, presence of retractions, breath sounds)

    4. Heart rate

■ Ineffective Thermoregulation
Related to Newborn Transition to Extrauterine Environment

Outcome Criteria

The infant will
- Have a temperature between 36.4° and 37°C

The parent will
- Explain techniques to avoid heat loss at home

Interventions

A. Assess for contributing factors

    1. Environmental sources of heat loss

    2. Lack of knowledge (caregivers, parents)

B. Reduce or eliminate the sources of heat loss

    1. Evaporation

        a. In the delivery room, quickly dry skin and hair with a heated towel and place infant in a heated environment.

        b. When bathing, provide a warm environment.

        c. Wash and dry infant in sections to reduce evaporation.

        d. Limit time in contact with wet diapers or blankets.

    2. Convection

        a. Reduce drafts in delivery room.

        b. Avoid drafts on infant (air conditioning, fans, windows, open portholes on Isolette).

    3. Conduction

        a. Warm all articles for care (stethoscopes, scales, hands of caregivers, clothes, bed linens, cribs).

        b. Place infant very close to mother to conserve heat (and foster bonding).

4. Radiation
   a. Place infant next to mother in the delivery room.
   b. Reduce objects in the room that absorb heat (metal).
   c. Place crib or Isolette as far away from walls (outside) or windows as possible.
   d. Preheat incubator

C. Monitor temperature of newborn (Waechter, Phillips, & Holaday, 1985)
   1. Assess axillary temperature initially q 30 min until stable, then q 4–8 hr.
   2. If temperature is less than 36.3°C:
      a. Wrap infant in two blankets.
      b. Put stockinette cap on.
      c. Assess for environmental sources of heat loss.
      d. If hypothermia persists over 1 hour, notify physician.
      e. Assess for complications of cold stress: hypoxia, respiratory acidosis, hypoglycemia, fluid and electrolyte imbalances, weight loss.
   3. If temperature is greater than 37°C:
      a. Loosen blanket.
      b. Remove cap, if on.
      c. Assess environment for thermal gain.
      d. If hyperthermia persists over 1 hour, notify physician.
   4. Assess for signs and symptoms of sepsis every shift:
      a. Respiratory function (rate, rhythm, pattern)
      b. Skin (tone, color, perfusion)
      c. Poor feeding
      d. Irritability
      e. Signs of localized infections (skin, umbilicus, circumcision, eyes, birth lacerations)

D. Initiate health teaching
   1. Teach caregiver why infant is vulnerable to temperature fluctuations (cold and heat).
   2. Explain sources of environmental heat loss (see B).
   3. Demonstrate how to conserve heat during bathing.
   4. Instruct that it is not necessary routinely to check temperature at home.
   5. Teach to check temperature if infant is hot, sick, or irritable, as follows:
      a. Shake down the thermometer
      b. Place in femoral fold
      c. Hold in place for 11 minutes
      d. Read at eye level
      e. Report temperature greater than 37.5°C to health care professional

Rationale

- The newborn loses heat through (May & Mahlmeister, 1994)
  - Evaporation (loss of heat when water on skin changes to vapor)
  - Convection (loss of heat when cool air flows over skin)
  - Conduction (transfer of heat when skin surface is in direct contact with a cool surface)
  - Radiation (transfer of heat from infant to cooler surfaces without direct contact)
- Caloric requirements are high for newborns (approximately 117 cal/kg body weight per day).

- An increased metabolic rate for heat production results in increased demands for oxygen and glucose. With prolonged cold stress or in compromised neonates, acidosis can result (May & Mahlmeister, 1994).
- Premature or low–birth-weight infants are more susceptible to heat loss because of the reduced metabolic reserves available (*e.g.*, glycogen).
- The newborn can also experience overheating from excessive clothing in hot weather. The full-term infant can sweat in response to overheating, but the premature infant cannot.
- Significant heat losses the first few moments after birth can drop the newborn's temperature 1°–3°C. Drying, heated blankets, and swaddling can reduce these losses (Mayfield, Uauy, & Warshaw, 1995).

References/Bibliography

Hunter, L. (1991). Measurement of axillary temperature in neonate. *Western Journal of Nursing Research, 13*(3), 324.

Lorin, M. (1995). Pathogenesis of fever and treatment. In F. Oski (Ed.). *Principles and practices of pediatrics* (2nd ed.). Philadelphia: J. B. Lippincott.

May, K. A., & Mahlmeister, L. R. (1994). *Maternal and neonatal nursing: Family-centered care* (3rd ed.). Philadelphia: J. B. Lippincott.

Mayfield, S., Uauy, R., & Warshaw, J. (1995). The premature newborn. In F. Oski (Ed.). *Principles and practices of pediatrics* (2nd ed.). Philadelphia: J. B. Lippincott.

Waechter, E., Phillips, J., & Holaday, B. (1985). *Nursing care of children*. Philadelphia: J. B. Lippincott.

Bowel Incontinence

DEFINITION

Bowel Incontinence: A state in which an individual experiences a change in normal bowel habits characterized by involuntary passage of stool.

DEFINING CHARACTERISTICS
Major (Must Be Present)

Involuntary passage of stool

RELATED FACTORS
Pathophysiologic

Related to impaired rectal sphincter secondary to:
Diabetes mellitus
Anal or rectal surgery
Anal or rectal injury
Related to cognitive impairment
Related to overdistention of rectum secondary to chronic constipation

Related to lack of voluntary sphincter control secondary to:
    Progressive neuromuscular disorder
    Spinal cord injury
    Spinal cord compression
    Multiple sclerosis
    Cerebral vascular accident
Related to impaired reservoir capacity secondary to:
    Inflammatory bowel disease
    Chronic rectal ischemia

Treatment-Related

Related to impaired reservoir capacity secondary to:
    Colectomy
    Radiation proctitis

Situational (Personal, Environmental)

Related to inability to recognize, interpret, or respond to rectal cues secondary to:
    Depression
    Cognitive impairment

Errors in Diagnostic Statements

Bowel Incontinence related to oozing of stool

Oozing of stool is not the cause of bowel incontinence, but rather evidence of bowel incontinence. If the etiology is not known, the diagnosis should be written: *Bowel Incontinence related to unknown etiology, as evidenced by oozing of stool.*

When the etiology is known, the diagnosis should reflect this (*e.g., Bowel Incontinence related to relaxed anal sphincter secondary to S4 lesion*).

Keys Concepts

1. Bowel incontinence has three major causes: underlying disease of the colon, rectum, or anus; long-standing constipation or fecal impaction; and neurogenic changes in the rectum (McLane & McShane, 1992)
2. Complete spinal cord injury, spinal cord lesions, neurologic disease, or congenital defects causing an interruption of the sacral reflex arc (at the sacral segments S2, S3, S4) result in an areflexic (autonomous) or flaccid bowel. Flaccid paralysis at this level, known as an LMN lesion, results in loss of the defecation reflex, loss of sphincter control (flaccid anal sphincter), and absence of the bulbocavernosus reflex.
3. Because of an interrupted sacral reflex arc and a flaccid anal sphincter, bowel incontinence can occur without rectal stimulation whenever stool is present in the rectal vault. The stool may leak out if too soft or remain (if not extracted), predisposing the person to fecal impaction or constipation. Some intrinsic contractile abilities of the colon remain, but peristalsis is sluggish, leading to stool retention with contents present in the rectal vault.
4. Complete central nervous system lesions or trauma occurring above sacral cord segments S2, S3, S4 (T12–L1–L2 vertebral level) result in a reflexic neurogenic bowel. The ascending sensory signals between the sacral reflex center and the brain are interrupted, resulting in the inability to feel the urge to defecate. Descending motor signals from the brain are also interrupted, causing loss of voluntary control over the anal sphincter. Because the sacral reflex center is preserved, it is possible to develop a stimulation–response bowel evacuation program using digital stimulation or digital stimulation devices.

Focus Assessment Criteria

See *Constipation*.

> **Outcome Criteria**
>
> The person will
> • Evacuate a soft formed stool every other day or every third day

Interventions

A. Assess contributing factors

1. Lack of routine evacuation schedule
2. Lack of knowledge of bowel elimination techniques
3. Insufficient fluid and fiber intake
4. Insufficient physical activity
5. Constipation
6. Use of elimination aids (*e.g.*, laxatives)

B. Assess individual's ability to participate

1. Neurologic status
2. Functional ability

C. Plan a consistent, appropriate time for elimination

1. Institute a daily bowel program for 5 days or until a pattern develops, then move to an alternate-day program (morning or evening).
2. Provide privacy and a nonstressful environment.
3. Provide reassurance and protection from embarrassment while establishing the bowel program.

D. Teach effective bowel elimination techniques

1. Position a functionally able person in an upright or sitting position. If the person is not functionally able (*e.g.*, quadriplegic), position in left side-lying position.
2. For a functionally able person, use assistive devices (*e.g.*, dil stick, digital stimulator, raised commode seat, and lubricant and gloves), as appropriate.
3. For a person with upper extremity mobility and abdominal musculature innervation, teach bowel elimination facilitation techniques as appropriate:
   a. Valsalva maneuver
   b. Forward bends
   c. Sitting push-ups
   d. Abdominal massage
   e. Pelvic floor exercises
4. Assist with or provide equipment needed for hygiene measures, as necessary.
5. Maintain an elimination record or a flow sheet of the bowel schedule that includes time, stool characteristics, assistive methods used, and number of involuntary stools, if any.

E. Explain fluid and dietary requirements for good stool consistency.

1. 8–10 glasses of water daily
2. Diet high in bulk and fiber
3. Refer to *Colonic Constipation* for specific dietary instructions.

F. Explain the effects of activity on peristalsis. Assist in determining the appropriate exercises for person's functional ability

G. Initiate health teaching, as indicated

1. Explain the hazards of using stool softeners, laxatives, suppositories, and enemas.
2. Explain the signs and symptoms of fecal impaction and constipation. (Refer to *Dysreflexia* for additional information.)

3. Initiate teaching of a bowel program before discharge. If the client is functionally able, encourage independence with the bowel program; if not, incorporate assistive devices or attendant care, as needed.

Rationale

- To maintain bowel continence, a person must be motivated, have an intact anorectal sensation, be able to store feces consciously, be able to contract puborectalis and external anal sphincter muscles, and have access to toileting facility (McLane & McShane, 1991).
- Stool consistency and volume are important for continence. Large volumes of loose stool overwhelm the continence mechanism. Small, hard stools that do not distend or stimulate the rectum do not alert the person to the need to defecate (McLane & McShane, 1991).
- Exercise increases gastrointestinal motility and hastens bowel function.
- Pelvic floor exercises can increase the strength of the puborectalis and external anal sphincter muscles.
- Digital stimulation results in reflex peristalsis and evacuation.
- Laxatives cause unscheduled bowel movements, loss of colon tone, and inconsistent stool consistency. Enemas can overstretch the bowel and decrease tone. Stool softeners are not needed with adequate food or fluid intake (Alterman, 1995).
- Bowel elimination is enhanced by techniques that facilitate gravity and increase intraabdominal pressure to pass stool (Alterman, 1995).
- Long-standing constipation or fecal impaction causes overdistention of the rectum by feces. This causes continuous reflex stimulation, which results in reduced sphincter tone. Incontinence will either be diarrhea leaking around the impaction or leaking of feces because of a full rectum (Maas & Specht, 1991).
- Bowel incontinence is a common problem for institutionalized older adults or for those who have chronic illnesses. Cognitive impairments can impede recognition of bowel cues. Long-standing constipation can cause leaking around the impaction. Another cause of bowel incontinence is rectal sphincter abnormalities.

References/Bibliography

Alterman, C. (1995). Spinal cord injury. In L. J. Carpenito (Ed.). *Nursing care plans and documentation* (2nd ed.). Philadelphia: J. B. Lippincott.

Maas, M., & Specht, J. (1991). Bowel incontinence. In M. Maas, K. Buckwalter, & M. Hardy (Eds.). *Nursing diagnoses and interventions for the elderly*. Redwood City, CA: Addison-Wesley Nursing.

McLane, A., & McShane, R. (1991). Constipation. In M. Maas, K. Buckwalter, & M. Hardy (Eds.). *Nursing diagnoses and interventions for the elderly*. Redwood City, CA: Addison-Wesley Nursing.

McLane, A., & McShane, R. (1992). Bowel management. In G. Bulechek & J. McCloskey (Eds.). *Nursing interventions* (2nd ed.). Philadelphia: W. B. Saunders.

Effective Breast-feeding

DEFINITION

Effective Breast-feeding: The state in which a mother–infant dyad exhibits adequate proficiency and satisfaction with the breast-feeding process.

DEFINING CHARACTERISTICS

Major (Must Be Present)

Mother's ability to position infant at breast to promote a successful latch-on response
Infant content after feeding
Regular and sustained suckling/swallowing at the breast
Infant weight patterns are appropriate for age
Effective mother–infant communication patterns (infant cues, maternal interpretation and response)

Minor (May Be Present)

Signs or symptoms of oxytocin release (let-down or milk ejection reflex)
Adequate infant elimination patterns for age
Eagerness of infant to nurse
Maternal verbalization of satisfaction with the breast-feeding process

Author's Note

This diagnosis reportedly represents a newly proposed NANDA wellness diagnosis, defined as "a clinical judgment about an individual, family, or community in transition from a specific level of wellness to a higher level of wellness" (NANDA Guidelines, Appendix VIII). The definition for this diagnosis does not describe a mother–infant dyad seeking higher-level breast-feeding, but rather "adequate proficiency and satisfaction with the breast-feeding process."

In the management of breast-feeding experience, the nurse will encounter three situations covered by the following nursing diagnoses:

Ineffective Breast-feeding
Risk for Ineffective Breast-feeding
Potential for Enhanced Breast-feeding

Effective Breast-feeding would be used to describe an evaluation judgment of a mother's and infant's breast-feeding session for both ineffective and potentially ineffective breast-feeding. This evaluation is the result of the nurse observing or the mother reporting those signs and symptoms listed as defining characteristics. These signs and symptoms do not describe higher-level breast-feeding.

If the nurse cares for a mother reporting proficiency and satisfaction with the breast-feeding process and desiring additional teaching to achieve even greater proficiency and satisfaction, the nursing diagnosis of *Potential for Enhanced Breast-feeding* would be appropriate. The focus of this teaching and continued support would not be on preventing ineffective breast-feeding or maintaining adequate proficiency and satisfaction, but rather on promoting higher-quality breast-feeding.

This diagnosis is not useful in its present form; instead, the nurse should use *Ineffective Breast-feeding* or *Risk for Ineffective Breast-feeding*. Nurses desiring to use a wellness nursing diagnosis could use *Risk for Enhanced Breast-feeding*. Because this diagnosis is not on the NANDA list, nurses using it should send their experiences to NANDA.

Ineffective Breast-feeding

DEFINITION

Ineffective Breast-feeding: The state in which a mother, infant, or child experiences or is at risk of experiencing dissatisfaction or difficulty with the breast-feeding process.

DEFINING CHARACTERISTICS
Major (Must Be Present)

Unsatisfactory breast-feeding process
>   Actual or perceived inadequate milk supply
>   Infant inability to attach onto maternal breast correctly
>   No observable signs of oxytocin release
>   Observable signs of inadequate infant intake
>   Nonsustained suckling at the breast
>   Persistence of sore nipples beyond the first week of breast-feeding
>   Infant exhibiting fussiness and crying within the first hour after breast-feeding; unresponsive to other comfort measures
>   Infant arching and crying at the breast, resisting latching on

RELATED FACTORS
Physiologic

>   Related to difficulty of neonate to attach or suck secondary to:
>   Cleft lip/palate
>   Prematurity
>   Previous breast surgery
>   Inverted nipples, inadequate let-down reflex

Situational (Personal, Environmental)

>   Related to maternal fatigue
>   Related to maternal anxiety
>   Related to maternal ambivalence
>   Related to multiple birth
>   Related to inadequate nutrition intake
>   Related to inadequate fluid intake
>   Related to history of unsuccessful breast-feeding
>   Related to nonsupportive partner/family
>   Related to lack of knowledge
>   Related to interruption in breast-feeding secondary to:
>   Ill mother, ill infant

Author's Note

In managing the breast-feeding experience, the nurse strives to reduce or eliminate factors that contribute to *Ineffective Breast-feeding* or to reduce risk factors that can increase vulnerability for a problem using the diagnosis *At Risk for Ineffective Breast-feeding*.

In the acute setting after delivery, too little time will have elapsed for the nurse to conclude that there is no problem in breast-feeding, unless the mother is experienced. For many mother–infant dyads, the nursing diagnosis *At Risk for Ineffective Breast-feeding related to inexperience with the breast-feeding process* would represent a nursing focus on preventing problems in breast-feeding. *Risk* would not be indicated for all mothers.

Errors in Diagnostic Statements

Ineffective Breast-feeding related to reports of no symptoms of let-down reflex

When a mother reports or the nurse observes no signs of let-down reflex, the nursing diagnosis *Ineffective Breast-feeding* is validated. If the contributing factors are unknown, the diagnosis could be written as: *Ineffective Breast-feeding related to unknown etiology, as evidenced by reports of no signs of let-down reflex and mother's anxiety regarding feeding.*

If the nurse has validated contributing factors, she can add them. The nurse should assess for various possible contributing factors, rather than prematurely focusing on a common etiology that may be incorrect for the specific situation.

Key Concepts

1. Lactation is the result of a complex process of interacting factors of the health and nutrition status of the mother, the health status of the infant, and breast tissue development under the influence of estrogen and progesterone.
2. Milk production and the let-down reflex are controlled by the pituitary hormones, prolactin and oxytocin, and are stimulated by infant sucking and maternal emotions.
3. Many medications are excreted in breast milk. Some are harmful to the infant. Advise the mother to consult with a health care professional (nurse, physician, pharmacist) before taking a medication (prescribed or over-the-counter).
4. The advantages of breast-feeding are:
   To infant
      Easier to digest
      Meets nutritional needs
      Reduces allergies
      Provides antibodies and macrophages for early immunization
      Fewer gastrointestinal infections, almost no constipation
      Improves tooth alignment
      Reduces childhood infections throughout childhood if nursing continues for 1 year
      In juvenile diabetes, breast-feeding can significantly stall the onset of diabetes, perhaps even into adulthood
      Fewer incidents of sudden infant death syndrome in breast-fed infants
      Bowel movements have a pleasant odor
      Vomitus does not smell sour or stain clothing
   To mother
      Hastens uterine involution and postpartum resolution
      Reduces risks for breast cancer
      Allows more time to rest during feedings
      Less preparation, less cost
      Faster bonding
5. The disadvantages of breast-feeding are:
   Someone cannot substitute
   Breast-feeding is a learned process for mother and infant
   On average, 2–3 weeks of commitment to adjust to and learn the skills of nursing are required
   Breast milk is nearly completely digested—intestinal emptying is faster and newborn may need to feed more often than with formula

Key Concepts—Child

1. An adolescent's eating habits are influenced by physical and psychosocial pressure. This may put the teenage mother and her infant at risk during the breast-feeding period (National Academy of Sciences,1991).

Focus Assessment Criteria

Subjective Data

A. Assess for related factors

    1. History of breast-feeding (self, sibling, friend)

    2. Supportive people (partner, friend, sibling, parent)

    3. Source of information on breast-feeding

    4. Daily intake:

Calories	Basic food groups
Calcium	Fluids
Vitamin supplements	Medications

Objective Data

A. Assess for defining characteristics

    1. Breast condition (soft, firm, engorgement)

        Engorged   Soft

    2. Nipples

        Cracks   Sore

        Inverted

Outcome Criteria

The mother will

- Make an informed decision related to method of feeding infant (breast or bottle)
- Identify activities that deter or promote successful breast-feeding

---

Interventions

A. Assess for causative or contributing factors

    1. Lack of knowledge

    2. Lack of role model

    3. Lack of support (partner, physician, family)

    4. Discomfort

        a. Leaking

        b. Engorgement

        c. Loss of control of bodily fluid

        d. Nipple soreness

    5. Embarrassment

    6. Client's mother's attitudes and misconceptions

    7. Social pressure against nursing

    8. Change in body image

    9. Change in sexuality

    10. Feelings of being tied down

    11. Presence of stress

    12. Lack of conviction regarding decision to nurse

    13. Sleepy, unresponsive infant

    14. Fatigue

    15. Separation from infant (premature or sick infant, sick mother)

B. Promote open dialogue

    1. Assess knowledge.

        a. Has woman taken a class in breast-feeding?

        b. Has she read anything on the subject?

    c. Does she have friends who are nursing their babies?

    d. Did her mother nurse?

  2. Explain myths and misconceptions.

    a. Ask her to list difficulties she is anticipating.

    b. Common myths:

        My breasts are too small.

        My breasts are too large.

        My mother couldn't nurse.

        How do I know my milk is good?

        How do I know the baby is getting enough?

        The baby will know that I'm nervous.

        I have to go back to work, so what's the point of nursing for a short time?

        I'll never have any freedom.

        Nursing will cause my breasts to sag.

        My nipples are inverted, so I can't nurse.

        My husband wouldn't like my breasts any more.

        I'll have to stay fat if I nurse.

        I can't nurse if I have a cesarean section.

  3. Build on mother's knowledge.

    a. Clarify misconceptions.

    b. Explain process of nursing.

    c. Offer literature.

    d. Show video.

    e. Discuss advantages and disadvantages.

    f. Bring nursing mothers together to talk about nursing and their concerns.

  4. Support her decision to breast-feed or bottle-feed.

C. Assist mother during first feedings

  1. Promote relaxation.

    a. Position comfortably.

    b. Use pillows for positioning (especially cesarean-section mothers).

    c. Use foot stool or phone book to bring knees up while sitting.

    d. Use relaxation breathing techniques.

  2. Demonstrate different positions.

    a. Sitting

    b. Lying

    c. Cradle hold: Instruct to place supporting hand on baby's bottom and turn his body toward mother's (this promotes security in infant)

    d. Cradle hold:

        Will stabilize head

        Will reduce force of initial let-down to reduce choking

  3. Demonstrate and explain rooting reflex and show how it can be used to help infant latch on.

    a. Show how to grasp breast with fingers under breast and thumbs on top; this way she can point nipple directly at baby's mouth (avoid scissors hold because it constricts milk flow).

    b. Make sure baby grasps a good portion of areola and not just the nipple.

  4. Advise to increase feeding times gradually, to start at 10 minutes per side and build up over next 3–5 days.

    a. More important than time at the breast is the latch-on. Make sure the infant has a portion of the areola as well as the nipple in his mouth.

    b. Observe gliding action of jaw, indicates proper latch-on and suck.

    c. Infant should not be chewing or simply sucking with lips.

    d. Observe for bruising after feeding.

  5. Instruct to offer both breasts at each feeding, alternating the beginning side each time.

6. Demonstrate:
   a. How to use a finger to keep breast tissue from obstructing infant's nose
   b. Use of finger in infant's mouth to break seal before removing from breast
   c. Ways to awaken infant (may be necessary before offering the second breast)
7. Inform that burping may not be necessary with breast-fed infants, but if infant grunts and seems full between breasts she should attempt to burp infant, then continue feeding.

D. Provide follow-up support during hospital stay
   1. Develop care plan so that other health team members are aware of any problems or needs. Try to establish a consistent plan so the nursing mother does not receive mixed and opposing opinions from her health care providers.
   2. Allow for flexibility of feeding schedule; avoid scheduling feedings. Strive for 10–12 feedings/24-hour period according to the infant's size and need. (Frequent feedings help prevent or reduce breast engorgement.)
   3. Promote rooming in.
   4. Allow for privacy during feedings.
   5. Be available for questions.
   6. Be positive even if experience is difficult.
   7. Reassure that this is a learning time for her and the infant and they will develop together as the days go by.

E. Assist with specific nursing problems (may need assistance of lactation consultant)
   1. Engorgement
      a. Wear well-fitting support brassiere day and night.
      b. Apply warm compresses for 15–20 minutes before nursing.
      c. Nurse frequently.
      d. Use hand expression, hand pump, or electric pump to tap off some of the tension before putting infant to breast.
      e. Massage breasts
   2. Sore nipple
      a. Apply warm, moist compress for 5–10 minutes after nursing.
      b. Decrease nursing time to 5–10 minutes per side. Start baby on nontender side first. Allow for more frequent, short feedings. Suggest alternate positions to rotate infant's grasps. Allow breasts to dry after each feeding.
      c. Keep nursing pads dry.
      d. Coat nipples with breast milk (which has healing properties) and allow to air-dry.
      e. Use breast shield as last measure and remove after milk has let down.
   3. Difficulty with baby grasping nipple
      a. Cup breast with fingers underneath.
      b. Position baby for mother's and infant's comfort (turn baby's abdomen toward mother's body).
      c. Stroke infant's cheek for rooting reflex.
      d. Hand-express some milk into infant's mouth.
      e. Roll nipples to bring them out before feeding.
      f. Use a nipple shell between feedings to help extend inverted nipples. Remove shield after let-down occurs.
      g. Assess infant's suck—may need assistance in development of suck. Use lactation consultant if indicated.
   4. Separation (after cesarean section for stressed infants, premature infants, jaundiced infants)
      a. Encourage visits and bonding as much as possible.
      b. Provide comfortable, private location for nursing during visit.
      c. Provide supportive atmosphere (*e.g.*, freedom to ask questions).
      d. Provide breast pump or make patient aware of availability.
         Rental of electric pump
         Battery-operated pump

Cylinder-type hand pump (do not use bicycle horn pump)

Provide instruction in use of pump and assist mother to integrate breast-feeding into life-style

e. Many hospitals have a lactation educator or consultant on hand to assist with instruction and support.

F. Explore feelings regarding changes in body

1. Encourage verbal expression of feelings.
   a. Many women dislike leaking and lack of control. Explain that this is temporary.
      Demonstrate use of nursing pad.
      With a disposable pad, should not use waterproof backing, to prevent irritation; cotton (washable) seems to reduce occurrence of irritation.
   b. Changes breasts from "sexual objects" to implements of nutrition. This can affect sexual relationship. Husband gets milk if he sucks on nipples. Milk is released with orgasm. Infant suckling is "sensual" feeling—this causes guilt or confusion in woman. Encourage discussion with other mothers. Include partner in at least one discussion to assess his feelings and how they most affect the nursing experience.
   c. Self-consciousness during feedings. Explore woman's feelings about nursing.
      Where?
      Around whom?
      What is husband's reaction to when and where she nurses?
      Demonstrate use of shawl for modesty, allowing nursing in public.
      Remind her that what she is doing is normal and natural and the best for her child.

G. Assist the family with

1. Sibling reaction
   a. Explore feelings and anticipation of problems. Older child may be jealous of contact with baby. Mother can use this time to read to older child. Older child may want to nurse.
   b. Allow him to try—usually does not like it.
   c. Stress older child's attributes—freedom, movement, and choices.
2. Fatigue and stress
   a. Explore situation.
   b. Encourage mother to make herself and infant a priority.
   c. Encourage to limit visits from relatives for first 4 weeks.
   d. Needs support and assistance during first 4 weeks.
   e. Encourage support person to help as much as possible.
   f. Explain to mother not to try to be "superwoman," but to ask directly for help from friends or relations, or hire someone.
3. Feelings of being enslaved
   a. Allow to express feelings.
   b. Seek assistance.
   c. Pump milk to allow others to feed baby.
      Can store harvested breast milk for 8 hours at room temperature, 3 days in refrigerator, 6 months in freezer.
      (*Note:* Never microwave frozen breast milk, which will destroy its immune properties.)
   d. Husband can change baby and bring to bed to nurse.
   e. Remember that time between feedings will get longer (every 2 hours for 4 weeks, then every 3–4 hours by 3 months).

H. Initiate referrals, as indicated

1. Refer to lactation consultant if indicated by:
   a. Lack of confidence
   b. Ambivalence

    c. Problems with infant suck and latch-on
    d. Infant weight drop or lack of urination
    e. Prolonged soreness
    f. Hot, tender spots on breast
  2. Refer to La Leche League.
  3. Refer to childbirth educator and childbirth class members.
  4. Refer to other breast-feeding mothers.

Rationale

- Listening to the mother's and partner's concerns can help the nurses focus on priority concerns (Jackson & Saunders, 1993).
- The decision to breast-feed an infant is a very personal one and should not be made without adequate information (May & Mahlmeister, 1994).
- Successful breast-feeding depends on both physical and emotional support. Physical support includes promotion of comfort and proper technique (May & Mahlmeister, 1994).
- Constant positive feedback is essential for an inexperienced mother (May & Mahlmeister, 1994).
- Lactation has two mechanisms, the secretion of milk and milk-ejection reflex (Reeder, Martin, & Koniak, 1992). Mothers are taught techniques to increase milk production (*e.g.*, sufficient emptying).
- Inadequate let-down reflex can be the result of a tense or nervous mother, pain, insufficient milk, engorgement, or inadequate sucking position or motions (Reeder et al., 1992).
- Nipple shields should not be routinely recommended. The newborn may develop a nipple shield preference, and milk supply is diminished (Auerback, 1990).
- Engorgement can be prevented by not limiting feeding time and providing enough time for adequate milk removal (Moon & Humernick, 1989).
- The infant at the breast must be in a relaxed, correct alignment, have correct tongue and areolar placement, have sufficient motion for areolar compression, and demonstrate audible swallowing (Shirago & Bocar, 1990).
- Referrals to community resources can provide the mother with continued support and information at home.

Interrupted Breast-feeding

DEFINITION

Interrupted Breast-feeding: A break in the continuity of the breast-feeding process as a result of inability or inadvisability to put baby to breast for feeding.

DEFINING CHARACTERISTICS
Major (Must Be Present)

Infant does not receive nourishment at the breast for some or all of feedings

Minor (May Be Present)

Maternal desire to maintain lactation and provide (or eventually provide) her breast milk for her infant's nutritional needs

Separation of mother and infant
Lack of knowledge regarding expression and storage of breast milk

RELATED FACTORS

Maternal or infant illness
Prematurity
Maternal employment
Contraindications to breast-feeding (*e.g.*, drugs, true breast milk jaundice)
Need to wean infant abruptly

Author's Note

This diagnosis represents a situation, not a response. Nursing interventions do not treat the interruption but, instead, the effects of the interruption. The situation is interrupted breast-feeding; the responses can be varied. For example, if continued breast-feeding or use of a breast pump is contraindicated, the nurse focuses on the loss of this breast-feeding experience using the nursing diagnosis of *Grieving*.

If breast-feeding is continued with expression and storage of breast milk, teaching, and support, the diagnosis will be *Risk for Ineffective Breast-feeding related to continuity problems secondary to (e.g., maternal employment)*, or if difficulty is experienced, the diagnosis would be *Ineffective Breast-feeding related to interruption secondary to (specify) and lack of knowledge*.

References/Bibliography

American Academy of Pediatrics. (1989). Transfer of drugs and other chemicals into human milk. (Supplement C) *Pediatrics, 84,* 23.

Auerbach, K. G. (1990). Assisting the employed breastfeeding mother. *Journal of Nurse Midwifery, 35*(11), 26–34.

Briggs, G. G., Freeman, R. K., & Yaffe, S. J. (1990). *Drugs in pregnancy and lactation* (3rd ed.). Los Angeles: Williams & Wilkins.

Coates, M. M. (1990). *The lactation consultant's topical review and bibliography of the literature on breastfeeding.* Franklin Park, IL: La Leche League International.

Jackson, D. B., & Saunders, R. B. (1993). *Child health nursing.* Philadelphia: J. B. Lippincott.

Jenks, M. (1991). Latch assessment documentation in the hospital nursery. *Journal of Human Lactation, 7*(1), 19–20.

Jordan, P. L. (1990). Breastfeeding and fathers: Illuminating the darker side. *Birth, 17,* 210–213.

La Leche League International. (1978). *The womanly art of breast-feeding.* Franklin Park, IL: Author.

Lawrence, R. (1989). *Breastfeeding: A guide for the health professional.* St. Louis: C. V. Mosby.

May, K. A., & Mahlmeister, L. R. (1994). *Maternal and neonatal nursing: Family-centered care* (3rd ed.). Philadelphia: J. B. Lippincott.

Moon, J. L., & Humernick, S. S. (1989). Breast engorgement: Contributing variables and variables amenable to nursing interventions. *Journal of Obstetric, Gynecologic and Neonatal Nursing, 18,* 309–315.

National Academy of Sciences, Food and Nutrition Board. (1991). *Nutrition during lactation.* Washington, DC: National Academy Press.

Neville, M. C., & Neifert, M. R. (1983). *Lactation, physiology, nutrition and breast-feeding.* New York: Plenum Press.

Reeder, S., Martin, L., & Koniak, D. (1992). *Maternity nursing* (17th ed.). Philadelphia: J. B. Lippincott.

Renfrew, M. J. (1989). Positioning the baby at the breast: More than a visual skill. *Journal of Human Lactation, 5*(1), 13–15.

Shirago, L., & Bocar, D. (1990). The infant's contribution to breastfeeding. *Journal of Obstetric, Gynecologic and Neonatal Nursing, 19,* 209–215.

Resources for the Consumer

Dana, N., & Price, A. (1985). *The working woman's guide to breastfeeding.* New York: Simon & Schuster.

Michaelson, K. R. (1986). *Breastfeeding basics for busy moms and dads: A training manual for lactation educators.* Santa Barbara, CA: Therapeutic Media, Inc.

Mohnrbacher, N., & Stock, J. (1991). *The breastfeeding answer book.* Franklin Park, IL: La Leche League International.

Renfrew, M., Fisher, C., & Arms, S. (Eds.). (1990). *Bestfeeding: Getting breastfeeding right for you.* Berkeley, CA: Celestial Arts.

Decreased Cardiac Output

DEFINITION

Decreased Cardiac Output: A state in which the individual experiences a reduction in the amount of blood pumped by the heart, resulting in compromised cardiac function.

DEFINING CHARACTERISTICS

Low blood pressure	Dyspnea	Fatigability
Rapid pulse	Angina	Vertigo
Restlessness	Dysrhythmia	Edema (peripheral, sacral)
Cyanosis	Oliguria	

Author's Note

This nursing diagnosis represents a situation in which nurses have multiple responsibilities. People experiencing decreased cardiac output may display various responses that disrupt functioning (such as activity intolerance, sleep–rest disturbances, and anxiety or fear) and/or may be at risk for development of physiologic complications such as dysrhythmias, cardiogenic shock, and congestive heart failure.

When *Decreased Cardiac Output* is used clinically, the associated outcome criteria are usually written:

Systolic blood pressure is >100

Urine output is >30 mL/hr

Cardiac output is >5

Cardiac rate, rhythm are within normal limits

These outcome criteria do not represent parameters for evaluating nursing care, but rather for evaluating the person's status. Because they are monitoring criteria that the nurse uses to guide implementation of nursing-prescribed and physician-prescribed interventions, *Decreased Cardiac Output* is not appropriate as a nursing diagnosis. Not using this nursing diagnosis allows the nurse to describe more specifically the related situations that nurses treat as nursing diagnoses or cotreat as collaborative problems. (Refer to *Activity Intolerance related to insufficient knowledge of adaptive techniques needed secondary to impaired cardiac function* and to *Potential Complication: Cardiac/Vascular* [Section III] for more information.)

Errors in Diagnostic Statements

Decreased Cardiac Output related to dysrhythmias

This diagnosis necessitates continuous monitoring, early detection of changes in physiologic status, rapid initiation of medical and nursing interventions, and evaluation of response. Because the nurse manages this situation with nurse-prescribed and physician-prescribed interventions, it is a collaborative problem: *Potential Complication: Decreased Cardiac Output related to dysrhythmias*.

Decreased Cardiac Output related to vasodilation and bradycardia secondary to spinal shock

As with the previous example, this situation represents a situation for which nurses cannot write outcomes that can be used to measure the effectiveness of nursing interventions. For this reason, this situation should be written as a collaborative problem: *Potential Complication: Spinal Shock*.

A nurse reading this collaborative problem on a care plan knows that this client either is experiencing spinal shock or is at risk for it. Shift reports or initial assessment will determine present status.

Caregiver Role Strain

Caregiver Role Strain, Risk for

Caregiver Role Strain

DEFINITION

Caregiver Role Strain: A state in which an individual is experiencing physical, emotional, social, and/or financial burden(s) in the process of caregiving to another.

DEFINING CHARACTERISTICS

Reports insufficient time or physical energy
Difficulty performing caregiving activities required
Caregiving responsibilities interfere with other important roles (*e.g.*, work, spouse, friend, parent)
Apprehension about the future for the care receiver's health and ability to provide care
Apprehension about care receiver's care when caregiver is ill or deceased
Depressed feelings, anger

RELATED FACTORS
Pathophysiologic

Related to unrelenting or complex care requirements secondary to:
 Debilitating conditions (acute, progressive)
 Progressive dementia
 Addiction
 Chronic mental illness
 Unpredictable illness course
 Disability

Treatment-Related

Related to 24-hour care responsibilities
Related to time-consuming activities (*e.g.*, dialysis, transportation)

Situational (Personal, Environmental)

Related to unrealistic expectations of caregiver by care receiver
Related to pattern of ineffective coping
Related to compromised physical health
Related to unrealistic expectations of self
Related to history of poor relationship
Related to history of family dysfunction
Related to unrealistic expectations for caregiver by others (society, other family members)
Related to duration of caregiving required
Related to isolation
Related to insufficient respite
Related to insufficient recreation
Related to insufficient finances
Related to no or unavailable support

Maturational

Infant, child, adolescent
Related to unrelenting care requirements secondary to:
Mental disabilities (specify)
Physical disabilities (specify)

Author's Note

There are 2.2 million unpaid home caregivers in the United States.* These caregivers provide care for individuals of all ages, some across their entire life span (*e.g.*, children with permanent disabilities). The care receivers have physical or mental disabilities, or both. These disabilities can be temporary or permanent. Some disabilities are permanent, but stable (*e.g.*, blind child), whereas others signal progressive deterioration (*e.g.*, Alzheimer's disease).

Caring and caregiving are intrinsic to all close relationships. It is "found in the context of established roles such as wife–husband, child–parent" (Pearlin, Mullan, Semple, & Skaff, 1990, p. 583). Caregiving, under some circumstances, is "transformed from the ordinary exchange of assistance among people standing in close relationship to one another to an extraordinary and unequally distributed burden" (ibid.). Caregiving becomes a dominant, overriding component, which occupies the entirety of the situation (ibid.).

Caregiver Role Strain represents the burden of caregiving on the physical and emotional health of the caregiver and its effects on the family and social system of the caregiver and care receiver. *Risk for Caregiver Role Strain* can be a very significant nursing diagnosis, for nurses can identify high-risk individuals and assist them to prevent this grave situation.

Error in Diagnostic Statements

Caregiver Role Strain related to depression and anger at family, as evidenced by unrealistic expectations of caregiver for self and by others

Too often, caregivers with multiple, unrelenting responsibilities find themselves reluctant to admit they need help. This reluctance may be interpreted by others as not needing help. The caregiver is further isolated, feeling no one really cares or appreciates the amount of work, which can result in depression and anger. Thus, this diagnosis must be rewritten to reflect the unrealistic expectations as the related factors and the resulting symptoms as evidence. It is helpful to quote the data if relevant.

Caregiver Role Strain related to unrealistic expectations of caregiver for self and by others, as evidenced by depressed feelings and anger at family "who don't understand my burden"

Key Concepts

1. One hundred and ten million people require some form of home care; one million of these individuals are children (O'Connor, Vander Plaats, & Betz, 1992).
2. The cost of caring for a person at home produces substantial savings for society. For example, Wong (1991) found that the cost of caring for a ventilator-dependent child in the home was $40,000 less per month than hospital care.
3. As the aging population grows and with advances in medicine increasing the longevity of chronically ill people, the need for health care escalates. This health care is predominantly home care provided primarily by one family member. Seventy percent of these caregivers are women (*e.g.*, spouse, daughter, daughter-in-law, niece).
4. Caregiving tasks fall into four major categories (Clark & Rakowski, 1983):
   a. Direct care of elder
   b. Personal tasks, concerns

* Stone, R., Cafferata, G., & Sang, L. J. (1987). Caregivers of the frail elderly: A national profile. *The Gerontologist, 27*, 616–626.

c. Interactions with other family members
d. Social, societal, health care networks
5. Smith, Smith, and Toseland (1991) reported the following problems (by priority) identified by family caregivers:
   a. Improving coping skills (*e.g.*, time management, stress management)
   b. Family issues (sibling conflict, other role conflicts)
   c. Responding to care receiver's needs (emotional, physical, financial)
   d. Eliciting formal, informal support
   e. Guilt and feelings of inadequacy
   f. Long-term planning
   g. Quality of relationship with care receiver
6. Caregiving to a chronically ill family member or friend, who is not independent for all or part of the daily activities needed to function, is the most stressful situation one can encounter (Pearlin et al., 1990).
7. House (1981) describes four basic types of social support:
   a. Emotional (concern, trust)
   b. Appraisal (affirms self-worth)
   c. Informational (useful advice, information for problem-solving)
   d. Instrumental (caregiving) assistance or tangible goods (money, help with chores)
8. The stress process related to caregiver role strain arises from four domains (Pearlin et al., 1990). Table II-2 illustrates the domains and examples.

Table II-2　**Domains of the Stress Process of Caregiving**

Background/Content of Stress
Caregiver characteristics (age, education, financial, and social status)
Caregiving history
Networks
Resources available

Stressors (Primary, Secondary)
Primary (directly related to needs of care receiver)
　Impaired cognitive status
　Problematic behavior (*e.g.*, verbal abuse, wandering)
　Extent of dependency
　Resistance to caregiver's help
　Fatigue of caregiver
　Relational deprivation (spouse, parent)
Secondary (derived from primary stressors)
　Family conflicts about care receiver's condition or care
　Economic strain
　Constriction of social life
　Intrapsychic strain (loss of self, loss of control, feelings of inadequacy)

Mediators of Stressors
Efficacy of coping
Social support

Outcomes of Stressors
Depression
Anxiety
Cognitive disruptions
Physical problems
Yielding of role

　(Adapted from Pearlin, L., Mullan, J., Semple, S., & Skaff, M. [1990]. Caregiving and the stress process: An overview of concepts and their measures. *The Gerontologist*, *45*[5], 192–195.)

9. Caregiver stress is not an event but "a mix of circumstances, experiences, responses and resources that vary considerably among caregivers and that consequently vary in their impact on caregivers' health and behavior" (Pearlin et al., 1990, p. 584). A change in one of the components listed in Table II-2 results in a change in other components.

10. The number of secondary, informal caregivers assisting the primary caregiver is influenced by the number of persons in the household. Spouse primary caregivers are less likely to have secondary caregivers helping them with care activities. Older people cared for by spouses received "about 15%–20% fewer person-days of help than those cared for by adult children" (Miller & McFall, 1991).

11. "Health care policy makers must recognize that while caring for a frail or disabled member is both a family choice, an obligation, even a normative experience, it may be detrimental to the overall emotional and physical health of the caregiver" (Gaynor, 1990).

Key Concepts—Child

1. Children considered candidates for home care services are those (U.S. Congress Office of Technology Assessment, 1987)
   > Dependent on mechanical ventilation
   > Needing prolonged intravenous nutritional or drug therapy
   > With terminal illness
   > Requiring nutritional (*e.g.*, tube feedings) or respiratory support (*e.g.*, tracheostomy, suctioning)
   > Needing daily or near-daily nursing care for apnea monitoring, dialysis, urinary catheters, or colostomy pouches

2. The child and family provide the basis for home care and collaborate with the nurse to provide direction for care (Jackson & Saunders, 1993).

Focus Assessment Criteria

Subjective Data

A. Assess for defining characteristics
   1. How well do you manage your
      Caregiving responsibilities?
      Household responsibilities?
      Work responsibilities?
      Family responsibilities?
   2. On a scale from 0–10 (0 = not tired, peppy, to 10 = total exhaustion), rate the fatigue you usually feel. Does it change during the day or week? If so, why does it change?
   3. What are you most concerned about?
      For present
      For future

B. Assess for related factors
   1. Caregiver history
      Life-style
         Describe a typical day
         Work history
         Weekly hobbies, leisure activities
         Satisfaction with time spent in leisure activities
      Health
         Ability to perform activities of daily living
         Chronic conditions
      Family members
         Parents, spouse
         Children, siblings
         In-laws

Economic resources
Sources
Adequacy (present, future)

2. Care receiver characteristics
Cognitive status (*e.g.*, memory, speech)
Problematic behaviors (Pearlin et al., 1990)

Wandering	Cries easily
Threatening	Repeats questions, requests
Foul language	Clings
Incontinence	Depressed
Suspicious	Up at night
Sexually inappropriate	

3. What activities does the care receiver need assistance with:

Bathing	Medicines
Dressing, grooming	Transportation
Eating	Laundry
Toileting	Shopping
Mobility	

4. Caregiver–care receiver relationship
Past
Strengths
Limitations
Role responsibilities
Present
How has it changed?

5. Family relationship
How do they help?
What do you disagree on?
Do they understand your situation?
Do they view you a good caregiver?
Do you think you are a good caregiver?

6. Support system
Who? (family, friends, clergy, agency, group)
What? (visits, respite, chores, empathy)
How often?
What have you lost because of your caregiver responsibilities?

7. What do you do when you are very stressed?

Eat	Take a medication
Smoke	Call someone
Drink alcohol	Go out
Watch TV	Spend time alone
Exercise	Read

8. Care issues related to chronically ill child
Parenting issues

Discipline of ill child	Discipline of well siblings

Family adaptations

Living arrangements	Day-to-day management
Vacations	

Support systems

Relatives	Community
Neighbors	Religious

School issues
Siblings

Participation	Peers
Responsibility	Future
Feelings	

Outcome Criteria

The person will
- Share frustrations regarding caregiving responsibilities
- Identify one source of support
- Identify two changes that, if made, would improve daily life

The family will
- Relate an intent to listen without giving advice
- Convey empathy to caregiver regarding daily responsibilities
- Establish a plan for weekly support or help

Interventions

A. Assess for causative or contributing factors
    1. Poor insight into situation
    2. Unrealistic expectations (caregiver, family)
    3. Reluctance or inability to access help
    4. Unsatisfactory caregiver–care receiver relationship
    5. Insufficient resources (*e.g.*, help, financial)
    6. Social isolation
    7. Insufficient leisure
    8. Competing roles (spouse, parenting, work)

B. Provide empathy and promote a sense of competency
    1. Allow to share her feelings
    2. Emphasize the difficulties of the caregiving responsibilities
    3. Convey your admiration of the caregiver's competency

C. Promote realistic appraisal of the situation
    1. Ask to describe her future life in 3 months, 6 months, 1 year
    2. Discuss the effects of present schedule and responsibilities on:
        a. Physical health
        b. Emotional status
        c. Relationships
    3. Discuss the positive outcomes of caregiving responsibilities (for self, care receiver, family)

D. Promote insight into the situation
    1. Ask to describe "a typical day":
        a. Caregiving tasks
        b. Household tasks
        c. Work outside the home
        d. Role responsibilities
    2. Ask to describe:
        a. At-home leisure activities (daily, weekly)
        b. Outside-the-home social activities (weekly)
    3. Engage other family members in discussion, as appropriate.
    4. Discuss the danger of viewing helpers as less competent or less essential.

E. Assist to identify for which activities assistance is desired
    1. Care receiver's needs (hygiene, food, treatments, mobility)
    2. Laundry
    3. House cleaning
    4. Meals

5. Shopping, errands
6. Transportation
7. Appointments (doctor, hairdresser)
8. Yard work
9. House repairs
10. Respite (number of hours a week)
11. Money management

F. Engage the family (separate from caregiver) in appraisal of situation (Shields, 1992)

1. Allow to share frustrations.
2. Share the need for the caregiver to feel appreciated.
3. Discuss the importance of regularly acknowledging the burden of the situation for the caregiver.
4. Discuss the benefits of listening without giving advice.
5. Differentiate the types of social support (emotional, appraisal, informational, instrumental [refer to Key Concept 8]).
6. Emphasize the importance of emotional and appraisal support.
   a. Regular phone calls
   b. Cards, letters
   c. Visits
7. Stress "that in many situations, there are no problems to be solved, only pain to be shared" (Shields, 1992, p. 31).
8. Discuss the need to give caregiver "permission" to enjoy self (*e.g.*, vacations, day trips).
9. Allow caregiver opportunities to respond to "How can I help you?"

G. Assist with accessing informational and instrumental support

1. Role play how to ask for help with activities identified in item E, for example:
   a. "I have three appointments this week, could you drive me to one?"
   b. "I could watch your children once or twice a week in exchange for you watching my husband."
2. Identify all possible sources of volunteer help.
   a. Family (siblings, cousins)
   b. Friends, neighbors
   c. Church, community groups
3. Discuss how most people feel good when they provide a "little help."

H. If appropriate, discuss if and when an alternative source of care (*e.g.*, nursing home, senior housing) may be indicated

1. Options
2. Advantages
3. Disadvantages

I. Initiate health teaching and referrals, if indicated

1. Emphasize the need for caregiver to protect his or her health, with a balance of work, sleep, leisure, and good nutrition.
2. Explain the benefits of sharing with other caregivers.
   a. Support group
   b. Telephone buddy system with another caregiver
3. Identify community resources available.
   a. Counseling
   b. Social service
   c. Transportation
   d. Home-delivered meals
   e. Day care
4. Engage others to work actively to increase state, federal, and private agencies' financial support for resources to enhance caregiving in the home.

Rationale

- Coping with the burdens of caregiving requires "constantly changing cognitive and behavioral efforts to manage specific external and/or internal demands that are appraised as taxing or exceeding the resources of the person" (Lazarus & Folkman, 1984).
- Lazarus and Folkman (1984) have identified the resources needed for successful coping as energy, beliefs, commitments, health, social skills, social support, and material resources.
- Lindgren (1990) reported that burnout in caregivers was related to emotional exhaustion and a low sense of accomplishment. Caregivers who were commended for their accomplishments reported lower levels of burnout.
- Numerous researchers have identified consistent social supports as the single most significant factor that reduces or prevents caregiver role strain (Clipp & George, 1990; Given, Collins, & Given, 1988; Lindgren, 1990; Pearlin et al., 1990; Shields, 1992).
- Shields (1992) reported a primary source of conflict among family members and the caregiver as unsatisfied needs. The caregiver wishes for others to affirm the burden, when in fact the family responds to the caregiver's complaints with problem-solving techniques. The caregiver appears to reject suggestions, which annoys the family. The results are a "caregiver feeling unappreciated, unsupported and depressed and family members feeling angry and rejecting toward the caregiver" (Shields, 1992).
- Gonyea (1989) found that support groups were most effective with informational support (*e.g.*, nature of disease, community resources), but were less successful in addressing the caregivers' emotional needs and the effects on family system.
- Pruchno, Kleban, Michaels, and Dempsey (1990) reported that in female caregiving spouses, depression predicts a decline in physical health over a 6-month period. The amount of care provided by the caregiver had little effect on levels of depression, feelings of burden, or health.
- Institutionalization of a family member has many admission-related stressors (*e.g.*, financial constraints, transferring belongings, emotional strain, feelings of failure [Dellasega, 1991]). Dellasega (1991) reported that caregivers who institutionalize their care recipient experienced the same levels of emotional stress as caregivers who have not.
- The most critical period for caregiver stress is the 2- to 4-year period (Gaynor, 1990).
- Respite and the sharing of care responsibilities are vital to prevent the caregiver–care recipient dyad from becoming the center of the universe, with all others viewed as less competent or less essential (Boland & Sims, 1996).

🕑 Interventions—*Child Focus*

1. Determine parent's understanding of and concerns about child's illness, course, prognosis, and related care needs.
2. Discuss parenting skills and issues for ill child.
3. Elicit the effects of caretaking responsibility on
   a. Personal life (work, rest, leisure)
   b. Marriage (time alone, communication, decisions, attention)
4. Assist the parents in meeting the well siblings' needs for (Siemon, 1984)
   a. Knowledge of sibling's illness and relationship to own health
   b. Sharing feelings of anger, unfairness, embarrassment
   c. Discussions of future of ill sibling and self (*e.g.*, family planning, care responsibilities)
5. Discuss strategies to help siblings adapt (Siemon, 1984):
   a. Include in family decisions when appropriate.
   b. Keep informed about ill child's condition.
   c. Maintain routines (*e.g.*, meals, vacations).
   d. Prepare for changes in home life.
   e. Promote activities with peers.
   f. Avoid making the ill child the center of the family.
   g. Determine what daily assistance in caregiving is realistic.
   h. Plan for time alone.
   i. Advise teachers of home situation.
   j. Address developmental needs. See *Altered Growth and Development* for specific needs.

Rationale

- Helping the family identify predictable stressors can assist them to plan coping strategies.
- The developmental tasks of the ill child and the well siblings must be addressed to provide opportunities to grow, develop, gain independence, and master effective coping skills (Jackson & Saunders, 1993).
- Strategies to promote family cohesiveness and individual family needs can enhance effective stress management (Jackson & Saunders, 1993).
- All family members are encouraged to learn specific skills to balance the responsibilities.
- Strategies to promote family cohesiveness can reduce feelings of isolation or aloneness (Boland & Sims, 1996).

Caregiver Role Strain, Risk for

DEFINITION

Risk for Caregiver Role Strain: A state in which an individual is at high risk to experience physical, emotional, social, and/or financial burden(s) in the process of care giving to another.

RISK FACTORS

Presence of Risk Factors (refer to Related Factors)

RELATED FACTORS

Primary caregiver responsibilities for a recipient who requires regular assistance with self-care or supervision because of physical or mental disabilities

    In addition to one or more of the following:

    Related to unrelenting or complex care requirements secondary to:

        Care receiver characteristics

            Unable to perform self-care activities

            Not motivated to perform self-care act

            Cognitive problems

            Psychological problems

            Unrealistic expectations of caregiver

        Caregiver/spouse characteristics

            Pattern of ineffective coping

            Compromised physical health

            Unrealistic expectations of self

    Related to history of poor relationship

    Related to history of family dysfunction

    Related to unrealistic expectations for caregiver by others (society, other family members)

    Related to duration of caregiving required

    Related to isolation

    Related to insufficient respite

    Related to insufficient recreation

    Related to insufficient finances

    Related to no or unavailable support

Author's Note

See *Caregiver Role Strain*

Errors in Diagnostic Statements

See *Caregiver Role Strain*

Key Concepts

See *Caregiver Role Strain*

Focus Assessment Criteria

See *Caregiver Role Strain*

Outcome Criteria

The person will
- Identify activities that are important for self
- Relate a plan on how these activities can continue despite caregiving responsibilities
- Relate an intent to enlist the help of at least two people

Interventions

A. Explain the causes of caregiver role strain
  1. Refer to Table II-2 in Key Concepts

B. Explain the four types of social support to all involved
  1. Emotional
  2. Appraisal
  3. Informational
  4. Instrumental

C. Discuss the implications of daily responsibilities with the primary caregiver (Baldwin, 1988)
  1. Emphasize that the care receiver has needs as well as the care recipient.
  2. Encourage to set realistic goals for self and for care recipient.
  3. Discuss the need for respite and short-term relief.
     a. Encourage to accept offers of help.
     b. Practice asking for help; avoid "they should know I need help" thinking and martyrdom behavior.
     c. Caution on viewing others as not "competent enough."
  4. Discuss that past conflicts will not disappear. Try to work on resolution and emphasize the present.
  5. Stress the importance of daily health promotion activities:
     a. Rest/exercise balance
     b. Effective stress management
     c. Low-fat, high–complex carbohydrate diet
     d. Supportive social networks
     e. Appropriate screening practices for age
     f. See *Health-Seeking Behaviors* for specific interventions
  6. Maintain a good sense of humor. Associate with others who laugh.

7. Caution about spending too much time complaining, which is depressing for all involved and may lead to avoidance.
8. Advise to initiate phone contacts or visits with friends or relatives rather than "waiting for others to do it."

D. Assist those involved with appraisal of the situation

1. What is at stake? Encourage family to have a realistic perspective by providing accurate information and answers to questions.
2. What are the choices? Assist family to reorganize roles at home and set priorities to maintain family integrity and reduce stress.
3. Initiate discussions concerning stressors of home care (physical, emotional, environmental, financial).
4. Emphasize the importance of respites to prevent isolating behaviors that foster depression.
5. Discuss with the nonprimary caregivers their responsibilities in caring for the primary caregiver.
6. Where is there help? Direct family to community agencies, home health care organizations, and sources of financial assistance as needed. (See *Impaired Home Maintenance Management* for additional interventions.)

E. Discuss the implications of caring for ill family member with all household members; cover

1. Available resources (finances, environmental)
2. 24-Hour responsibility
3. Effects on other household members
4. Likelihood of progressive deterioration
5. Sharing of responsibilities (with other household members, siblings, neighbors)
6. Likelihood of exacerbation of long-standing conflicts
7. Impact on life-style
8. Alternative or assistive options (*e.g.*, community-based health care providers, life care centers, group living, nursing home)

F. Assist to identify for which activities assistance is desired

1. Care receiver's needs (hygiene, food, treatments, mobility)
2. Laundry
3. House cleaning
4. Meals
5. Shopping, errands
6. Transportation
7. Appointments (doctor, hairdresser)
8. Yard work
9. House repairs
10. Respite (number of hours a week)
11. Money management

G. Assist with accessing informational and instrumental support

1. Role play how to ask for help with activities identified in item F, such as
   a. "I have three appointments this week, could you drive me to one?"
   b. "I could watch your children once or twice a week in exchange for you watching my husband."
2. Identify all possible sources of volunteer help
   a. Family (siblings, cousins)
   b. Friends, neighbors
   c. Church, community groups
3. Discuss how most people feel good when they provide "a little help."

H. Initiate health teaching and referrals, if indicated

1. Emphasize the need for caregiver to protect his or her health with a balance of work, sleep, leisure, and good nutrition.

2. Explain the benefits of sharing with other caregivers.
   a. Support group
   b. Telephone buddy system with another caregiver
3. Identify community resources available.
   a. Counseling
   b. Social service
   c. Transportation
   d. Home delivered meals
   e. Day care
4. Engage others to work actively to increase state, federal, and private agency financial support for resources to enhance care giving in the home.

Rationale

See *Caregiver Role Strain*

References/Bibliography

Baldwin, B. (1988). Community management of Alzheimer's disease. *Nursing Clinics of North America, 23*(1), 47–55.

Boland, D., & Sims, S. L. (1996). Family care giving at home as a solitary journey. *Image—The Journal of Nursing Scholarship, 28,* 55–58.

Clark, N. M., & Rakowski, W. (1983). Family caregivers of older adults: Improving helping skills. *The Gerontologist, 23,* 637–642.

Clipp, E., & George, L. (1990). Caregiver needs and patterns of social support. *Journal of Gerontology, 45*(3; Suppl), 102–111.

Dellasega, C. (1991). Care giving stress among community caregivers for the elderly: Does institution make a difference. *Journal of Community Health Nursing, 8,* 197–205.

Gaynor, S. (1990). The effects of home care on caregivers. *Image—The Journal of Nursing Scholarship, 22,* 208–212.

Given, C., Collins, C., & Given, B. (1988). Sources of stress among families caring for relatives with Alzheimer's disease. *Nursing Clinics of North America, 23*(1), 69–82.

Gonyea, J. G. (1989). Alzheimer's disease support groups: An analysis of their structure, format and perceived benefits. *Social Work in Health Care, 14*(1), 61–72.

Hileman, J., Lackey, N., & Hassanein, R. (1992). Identifying the needs of home caregivers of patients with cancer. *Oncology Nursing Forum, 19,* 771–777.

House, J. S. (1981). *Work stress and social support.* Reading, MA: Addison-Wesley.

Jackson, D. B., & Saunders, R. B. (1993). *Child health nursing.* Philadelphia: J. B. Lippincott.

Lazarus, R. S., & Folkman, S. (1984). *Stress, appraisal and coping.* New York: Springer.

Lindgren, C. (1990). Burnout and social support in family caregivers. *Western Journal of Nursing Research, 12,* 469–481.

Miller, B., & McFall, S. (1991). Stability and change in the informal task support network of frail older persons. *The Gerontologist, 31,* 735–745.

O'Connor, P., Vander Plaats, S., & Betz, C. L. (1992). Respite care services to caretakers of chronically ill children in California. *Journal of Pediatric Nursing, 7,* 269–275.

Pearlin, L., Mullan, J., Semple, S., & Skaff, M. (1990). Caregiving and the stress process: An overview of concepts and their measures. *The Gerontologist, 30,* 583–594.

Pruchno, R., Kleban, M., Michaels, J. E., & Dempsey, N. (1990). Mental and physical health of care giving spouses: Development of a causal model. *Journal of Gerontology, 45*(5), 192–199.

Shields, C. (1992). Family interaction and caregivers of Alzheimer's disease patients: Correlates of depression. *Family Process, 31*(3), 19–32.

Siemon, M. (1984). Siblings of the chronically ill child. *Nursing Clinics of North America, 19,* 302.

Smith, G., Smith, M., & Toseland, R. (1991). Problems identified by family caregivers in counseling. *The Gerontologist, 31*(1), 15–22.

Stone, R., Cafferata, G., & Sang, L. J. (1987). Caregivers of the frail elderly: A national profile. *The Gerontologist, 27,* 616–626.

U.S. Congress Office of Technology Assessment. (1987). *Technology dependent children: Hospitals vs home care—A technical memorandum* (OT-TM-H-38). Washington, DC: U.S. Government Printing Office.

Wong, D. L. (1991). Transition from hospital to home for children with complex medical care. *Journal of Pediatric Oncology, 8*(1), 3–9.

Resources for the Consumer

Alzheimer's Disease and Related Disorders, Inc., National Headquarters, 70 East Lake Street, Chicago, IL 60601-5997 (800-621-0379).

American Association of Retired Persons, 1909 K Street NW, Washington, DC 20049.

Children of Aging Parents (CAPS), 2761 Trenton Road, Levittown, PA 19056.

National Association for Home Care, 519 C Street, NE, Stanton Park, Washington, DC 20002.

National Association of Area Agencies on Aging, 600 Maryland Avenue, SW, Suite 208, Washington, DC 20024.

The National Council on the Aging, Inc., PO Box 7227, Ben Franklin Station, Washington, DC 20044.

Comfort, Altered*

Acute Pain

Chronic Pain

Comfort, Altered

DEFINITION

Altered Comfort: The state in which an individual experiences an uncomfortable sensation in response to a noxious stimulus.

DEFINING CHARACTERISTICS
Major (Must Be Present)

The person reports or demonstrates a discomfort

Minor (May Be Present)

Autonomic response in acute pain
    Blood pressure increased   Diaphoresis
    Pulse increased   Dilated pupils
    Respirations increased
Guarded position
Facial mask of pain
Crying, moaning
Abdominal heaviness
Nausea
Vomiting
Malaise
Pruritus

RELATED FACTORS

Any factor can contribute to altered comfort. The most common are listed below.

Biopathophysiologic

(Pregnancy)
    Related to uterine contractions during labor
    Related to trauma to perineum during labor and delivery
    Related to involution of uterus and engorged breasts
Related to tissue trauma and reflex muscle spasms secondary to:
    Musculoskeletal disorders)
        Fractures   Arthritis
        Contractures   Spinal cord disorders
        Spasms

* This diagnosis is not currently on the NANDA list but has been included for clarity and usefulness.

(Visceral disorders)

Cardiac   Intestinal
Renal   Pulmonary
Hepatic
Cancer
(Vascular disorders)
Vasospasm   Phlebitis
Occlusion   Vasodilation (headache)
Related to inflammation of:
Nerve   Joint
Tendon   Muscle
Bursa   Juxtaarticular structures
Related to fatigue, malaise, and/or pruritus secondary to contagious diseases
Rubella
Chicken pox
Hepatitis
Mononucleosis
Pancreatitis
Related to effects of cancer on (specify)
Related to abdominal cramps, diarrhea, and vomiting secondary to:
Gastroenteritis
Influenza
Gastric ulcers
Related to inflammation and smooth muscle spasms secondary to:
Renal calculi
Gastrointestinal infections

Treatment-Related

Related to tissue trauma and reflex muscle spasms secondary to:
Surgery
Accidents
Burns
Diagnostic tests
Venipuncture
Invasive scanning
Biopsy
Related to nausea and vomiting secondary to:
Chemotherapy
Anesthesia
Side effects of (specify)

Situational (Personal, Environmental)

Related to fever
Related to immobility/improper positioning
Related to overactivity
Related to pressure points (tight cast, elastic bandages)
Related to allergic response
Related to chemical irritants
Related to unmet dependency needs
Related to severe repressed anxiety

Maturational

Infancy: Colic
Infancy and early childhood: Teething, ear pain
Middle childhood: Recurrent abdominal pain, growing pains
Adolescence: Headaches, chest pain, dysmenorrhea

Author's Note

A diagnosis not on the current NANDA list, *Altered Comfort* can represent various uncomfortable sensations, such as pruritus, immobility, and NPO status. For a person experiencing nausea and vomiting, the nurse should assess whether *Altered Comfort, Risk for Altered Comfort,* or *Risk for Altered Nutrition: Less Than Body Requirements* is the appropriate diagnosis. Short-lived episodes of nausea and/or vomiting (*e.g.,* postoperatively) can be best described with *Altered Comfort related to effects of anesthesia or analgesics.* When nausea/vomiting may compromise nutritional intake, the appropriate diagnosis may be *Risk for Altered Nutrition: Less Than Body Requirements related to nausea and vomiting secondary to (specify).*

Altered Comfort also can be used to describe a cluster of discomforts related to a condition or treatment, such as radiation therapy.

Errors in Diagnostic Statements

Altered Comfort related to immobility

Although immobility can contribute to an altered state of comfort, the nursing diagnosis *Disuse Syndrome* describes a cluster of nursing diagnoses that apply or are at high risk to apply owing to immobility. *Altered Comfort* can be included in *Disuse Syndrome*; thus, the diagnosis should be written as *Disuse Syndrome*.

Altered Comfort related to nausea and vomiting secondary to chemotherapy

Nausea and vomiting represent signs and symptoms of an altered comfort state, not contributing factors. *Altered Comfort* can be used to describe a cluster of discomforts associated with chemotherapy, such as, *Altered Comfort related to the effects of chemotherapy on bone marrow production and irritation of emetic center, as evidenced by complaints of nausea, vomiting, anorexia, and fatigue.*

Key Concepts

1. Pruritus (itching) is the most common skin alteration. It can be a response of the skin to an allergen, or it can be a sign or symptom of a systemic disease, such as cancer, liver or renal dysfunction, or diabetes mellitus.
2. Pruritus, described as a tickling or a tormenting situation, originates exclusively in the skin and provokes the urge to scratch (Branov, Epstein, & Grayson, 1989a).
3. Although the same neurons are likely to transmit signals for itching as those for pressure, pain, and touch, each of these sensations is perceived and mediated differently (Branov et al., 1989b).
4. Pruritus arises as a result of subepidermal nerve stimulation by proteolytic enzymes. These enzymes are released from the epidermis as a result of either primary irritation or secondary allergic responses (Callen, Starviski, & Voorhees, 1980).
5. The same unmyelinated nerves that act for burning pain also serve for pruritus (Callen et al., 1980). As a pruritic sensation increases in intensity, the sensation may become burning (Baer, 1990).
6. The areas immediately surrounding body openings are most susceptible to itching. This apparently is related to a concentration of sensory nerve endings and vulnerability to external contamination (Branov et al., 1989a).
7. Nausea and vomiting, when determined to have emotional origins, may be the result of developmental adjustment and adaptation. A child learns that vomiting is unacceptable and thus learns to control vomiting. The child receives approval for not vomiting. Should childhood situations or conflicts resurface, the adult may experience nausea and vomiting.

Key Concepts—Older Adult

1. Asteatosis (excessive skin dryness) is the most common cause of pruritus in the elderly. Its incidence is anywhere from 40% to 80%, with this wide range accounted for by varying criteria and climate differences. With scratching, small breaks in the epidermis can increase the risk of infection owing to age-related changes in the immune system (Miller, 1995).

TRANSCULTURAL CONSIDERATIONS

1. Pain is a universally recognized experience. "Pain is a very private experience that is greatly influenced by cultural heritage" (Ludwig-Beymer, 1989, p. 283).
2. Nurses in the United States are preponderantly white, middle-class women, who are socialized to believe "that in any situation self-control is better than open displays of strong feelings" (Ludwig-Beymer, 1989, p. 294).
3. It is important that the nurse not stereotype members of a particular culture, but instead accept a wide range of pain expressions (Ludwig-Beymer, 1989).
4. Cultural norms relative to the pain experiences are transmitted to children by the family (Ludwig-Beymer, 1989).
5. Zborowski (1952), in his classic studies on the influence of culture on the pain experience, found that the pain event, its meaning, and responses are culturally learned and culturally specific.
6. Zborowski (1952) reported the following cultural variations in interpretation and responses to pain:
   Third-generation Americans: unexpressive, concerned with implications, controlled emotional response
   Jewish: concerned about the implication of the pain, readily seek relief, frequently express pain to others
   Irish: see pain as a private event, nonexpressive, unemotional
   Italian: concerned with immediate pain relief, oriented to present experience
   Japanese: values self-control, will not express pain or ask for relief
   Hispanic: present oriented, folk medicine frequently used; suffering is viewed as a positive experience spiritually
   Chinese: may ignore symptoms, use alternative health practices
   Black Americans: may respond stoically because of dominant culture pressure or belief that pain is God's will

Focus Assessment Criteria

This nursing assessment of pain is designed to acquire data for assessing a person's adaptation to pain, not for determining the cause of pain or whether it exists.

Subjective Data

A. Assess for defining characteristics
   1. Pain assessment
      a. "Where is your discomfort located; does it radiate?" (Ask child to point to place).
      b. "When did it begin?"
      c. "Can you relate the cause of this discomfort?" or "What do you think is the cause of your discomfort?"
      d. Ask person to describe the discomfort and its pattern.

      | Time of day | Frequency (constant, intermittent, transient) |
      | Duration | Quality/intensity |

      e. Ask person to rate the pain: at its best, after pain relief measures, and at its worst. Use consistent scale, language, or set of behaviors to assess pain.
         For adults, use a numeric scale of 0 to 10 (0 = no pain, 10 = worst pain ever experienced) orally or visually.
         For children, select a scale appropriate for *developmental* age: can use scale for assessed age or younger; include child in selection. Wong and Baker (1988) found that the favorite scale from age 3 to adolescent was the faces scale.
            3 years and older: use drawings of faces or photographs of faces (Oucher scale) ranging from smiling to frowning to crying with numeric scale (Beyer, 1984).
            4 years and older: use four white poker chips to ask child how many pieces of hurt he is feeling (no hurt = no chips) (Hester, 1979).

6 years and older: use a numeric scale, 0–5 or 0–10 (verbally or visually); use blank drawing of body, front and back, and ask child to use three colors of crayons to color where a little bit of pain, a medium amount of pain, and a lot of pain is present (Eland Color Tool).

    f. "How do you usually react to pain (crying, anger, silence)?"

    g. "Are there any other symptoms associated with your discomfort (nausea, vomiting, numbness)?"

2. Effects of pain

    a. "Do you talk to others about your discomfort (spouse, friends, doctor, nurse)?" "Who do you talk to?"

    b. Have person indicate the effect of each of the following factors on his discomfort by noting if there is an increase, a decrease, or no effect.*

Liquor	Vibration	Defecation
Stimulants (*e.g.*, caffeine)	Pressure	Tension
Eating	No movement	Bright lights
Heat	Movement/activity	Loud noises
Cold	Sleep, rest	Going to work
Damp	Lying down	Intercourse
Weather changes	Distraction (*e.g.*, TV)	Mild exercise
Massage	Urination	Fatigue

    c. Ask person what effect pain has had on the following areas or what effect is anticipated.

        Work/activity pattern (work/home activities, leisure/play)

        Relationships/relating (wanting to be alone, with people)

        Sleep pattern (difficulty falling asleep/staying asleep)

        Eating pattern (appetite, weight gain/loss)

        Elimination patterns (bowel, constipation/diarrhea, bladder)

        Menses

        Sexual pattern (libido, function)

3. Assessment of pruritus

Onset	Relieved by what
Precipitated by what	History of allergy (individual, family)
Site(s)	

4. Assessment of nausea/vomiting

    Onset, duration

    Frequency

    Vomitus (amount, appearance)

    Associated with?

Medications	Activity
Meals (specific foods)	Time of day
Position	Pain

    Relief measures?

Objective Data (Acute/Chronic Pain)

A. Assess for defining characteristics

1. Behavioral manifestations

Mood	*Eye Movements*
Calmness	Fixed
Moaning	Searching
Crying	Open
Grimacing	Closed
Pacing	Perceptions
Restlessness	Oriented to time and place
Withdrawn	

* Adapted from the McGill Pain Questionnaire.

2. Musculoskeletal manifestations

Mobility of Painful Part	Muscle Tone
Full	Spasm
Limited/guarded	Tenderness
No movement	Tremors (in effort to hide pain)

3. Dermatologic manifestations

Color (redness)	Moisture/diaphoresis
Temperature	Edema

4. Cardiorespiratory manifestations

Cardiac	Respiratory
Rate	Rate
Blood pressure	Rhythm
Palpations present	Depth

5. Sensory alterations
   Paresthesia
   Dysesthesias

6. Thought processes

Appropriate	Combative
Inappropriate	Confused
Cooperative	

7. Developmental manifestations

Infant: Irritability, changes in eating or sleeping, inconsolability, generalized body movements

Toddler: Irritability, changes in eating or sleeping, aggressive behavior (kicking, biting), rocking, sucking, clenched teeth

Preschool: Irritability, changes in eating or sleeping, aggressive behavior, verbal expressions of pain

School-age: Changes in eating or sleeping, change in play patterns, verbal expressions of pain, denial of pain

Adolescent: Mood changes, behavior extremes ("acting out"), verbal expressions of pain when asked, changes in eating or sleeping

---

Outcome Criteria

The individual will
- Report decreased symptoms
- Describe measures to improve comfort

Interventions

A. Assess for sources of discomfort
   1. Pruritus
   2. Nausea and vomiting
   3. Fever
   4. Prolonged bed rest

B. Reduce pruritus and promote comfort
   1. Maintain hygiene without producing dry skin.
      a. Baths should be given frequently.
      b. Use cool water when acceptable (Baer, 1990).
      c. Use mild soap (castile, lanolin) or a soap substitute.
      d. Blot skin dry; do not rub.

   e. Apply cornstarch lightly to skin folds by first sprinkling on hand (to avoid caking of powder); for fungal conditions, use antifungal or antiyeast powder preparations [Mycostatin (nystatin)], or clotrimazole (Lotrimin) cream.
2. Prevent excessive dryness.
   a. Lubricate skin with a moisturizer unless contraindicated; pat on by hand or with gauze.
   b. Apply lubrication after bath, before skin is dry, to help moisture retention.
   c. Apply wet dressings continuously or intermittently to relieve itching and remove crusts and exudate.
   d. Provide 20- to 30-minute tub soaks with temperature of 32°–38°C; water can contain oatmeal powder, Aveeno, cornstarch, or baking soda (Branov et al., 1989b).
3. Promote comfort and prevent further injury.
   a. Advise against scratching; explain the scratch–itch–scratch cycle.
   b. Secure order for topical corticosteroid cream for local inflamed pruritic areas; apply sparingly and occlude area with plastic wrap at night to increase effectiveness of cream and prevent further scratching (Baer, 1990).
   c. Secure an antihistamine order if itching is unrelieved.
   d. Use mitts (or cotton socks) if necessary on children and confused adults.
   e. Maintained trimmed nails to prevent injury; file after trimming.
   f. Remove particles from bed (food crumbs, caked powder).
   g. Use old, soft sheets and avoid wrinkles in bed; if bed protector pads are used, place draw sheet over them to eliminate direct contact with skin.
   h. Avoid using perfumes and scented lotions (Branov et al., 1989b).
   i. Avoid contact with chemical irritants/solutions.
   j. Wash clothes in a mild detergent and put through a second rinse cycle to reduce residue; avoid use of fabric softeners (Branov et al., 1989b).
   k. Prevent excessive warmth by use of cool room temperatures and low humidity, light covers with bed cradle; avoid overdressing.
   l. Apply ointments with gloved or bare hand, depending on type, to lightly cover skin; rub creams into skin.
   m. Use frequent, thin applications of ointment, rather than one, thick application.

C. Proceed with health teaching, when indicated
1. Explain causes of pruritus and possible methods to avoid causative factors.
2. Explain interventions that relieve symptoms.
3. Explain factors that increase symptoms.
4. Advise about exposure to sun and heat and protective products.
5. Teach person to avoid fabrics that irritate skin (wool, coarse textures).
6. Teach person to wear protective clothing (rubber gloves, apron) when using chemical irritants.
7. Refer for allergy testing, if indicated.
8. Provide opportunity to discuss frustrations.
9. For further interventions, refer to *Ineffective Individual Coping* if pruritus is stress related.

D. Promote comfort during nausea and vomiting episodes
1. Protect people at risk for aspiration (immobile clients, children).
2. Address the cleanliness of the person and environment.
3. Provide opportunity for oral care after each episode.
4. Apply cool, damp cloth to person's forehead, neck, and wrists.

E. Reduce or eliminate noxious stimuli
1. Pain
   a. Plan care so that unpleasant or painful procedures do not take place before meals.
   b. Medicate individual for pain one-half hour before meals according to physician's orders.

      c. Provide pleasant, relaxed atmosphere for eating (no bedpans in sight; do not rush); try a "surprise" (*e.g.*, flowers with meal).

      d. Arrange plan of care to decrease or eliminate nauseating odors or procedures near mealtimes.

  2. Fatigue

      a. Teach or assist individual to rest before meals.

      b. Teach individual to spend minimal energy in food preparation (cook large quantities and freeze several meals at a time; request assistance from others).

  3. Odor of food

      a. Teach person to avoid cooking odors—frying foods, brewing coffee—if possible (take a walk; select foods that can be eaten cold).

      b. Suggest using foods that require little cooking during periods of nausea.

F. Decrease the stimulation of the vomiting center

1. Reduce unpleasant sights and odors. Restrict activity.
2. Provide good mouth care after vomiting.
3. Teach person to practice deep breathing and voluntary swallowing to suppress the vomiting reflex.
4. Instruct person to sit down after eating, but not to lie down.
5. Encourage individual to eat smaller meals and eat slowly.
6. Restrict liquids with meals to avoid overdistending the stomach; also avoid fluids 1 hour before and after meals.
7. If possible, avoid the smell of food preparation.
8. Try eating cold foods, which have less odor.
9. Loosen clothing.
10. Sit in fresh air or use a fan to circulate air.
11. Avoid lying down flat for at least 2 hours after eating (an individual who must rest should sit or recline so head is at least 4 inches higher than feet).

G. Promote foods that stimulate eating and increase protein consumption

See *Altered Nutrition related to anorexia*

H. For excessive warmth, provide comfort measures as indicated

1. Keep the room cool; remove blankets as needed.
2. Offer a cool washcloth for forehead; change frequently to maintain coolness.
3. Provide tepid sponge baths or alcohol rubs; finish with powder to minimize moisture.
4. Monitor bed linens (especially pillow case) for dampness; change linens whenever they are moist.
5. Encourage wearing absorbent cotton bedclothes rather than silk or nylon.
6. Flip pillows and straighten linens frequently; assist with frequent repositioning.
7. Provide for periods of uninterrupted rest.
8. If requested, provide distractions (*e.g.*, TV, magazines, visitors).
9. Consult with physician about the use of aspirin and acetaminophen on an alternating basis (aspirin 4 hr with acetaminophen 4 hr in between).

I. For discomfort related to feeling cold

1. Apply socks, gloves, or head covering as needed.
2. Monitor room temperature; keep thermostat at 75°–80°F and monitor patient's temperature for response.
3. If possible, encourage taking a warm tub bath; offer hot liquids.
4. Provide warmed blankets.
5. Consult with a physician for use of a rewarming device.

J. For a person on bed rest, vary the position at least every 2 hours unless other variables necessitate more frequent changes

1. Use small pillows or folded towels to support limbs.

   2. Vary positions with flexion and extension, abduction or adduction.

   3. Use prone position if tolerable.

Rationale

- Pruritus is aggravated by excessive warmth, excessive dryness, rough fabrics, fatigue or stress, and monotony (lack of distractions) (DeWitt, 1990).
- Methods that interrupt pain also will interrupt pruritus. Local anesthetics, cold, or peripheral nerve resection eliminate both pain and pruritus (Baer, 1990).
- Gastric distention from fluid ingestion can trigger the vagal visceral afferent pathways that stimulate the medulla oblongata (vomiting center in brain) (Rhodes, 1990).
- Vomiting serves as a first-line defense against injurious agents ingested. Nausea may precede vomiting. Nausea and vomiting may be a signal of disease, injury, or the normal physiologic adjustment to pregnancy.
- Unpleasant sights or odors can stimulate the vomiting center.
- Coolness reduces vasodilatation.
- Dryness increases skin sensitivity by stimulation of nerve endings.
- Scratching stimulates histamine release, producing more pruritus.

Interventions—*Child Focus*

1. Explain to children why they should not scratch.
2. Dress child in long sleeves, long pants, or a one-piece outfit to prevent scratching.
3. Avoid overdressing child, which will increase warmth.
4. Give child a tepid bath before bedtime; add two cups of cornstarch to bath water.
5. Apply Caladryl lotion to weeping pruritic lesions; apply with small paint brush.
6. Use cotton blankets or sheets next to skin.
7. Remove furry toys that may increase lint and pruritus.
8. Teach child to press area that itches, but not to scratch, or to put cool cloth on the area if permitted.

Rationale

See Rationale for generic Interventions

Interventions—*Maternal Focus*

1. Teach that a variety of interventions have been reported to be helpful to control nausea when pregnant.
    a. Avoidance of fatigue
    b. High-protein meals and snack before retiring
    c. Carbohydrates (crackers) on arising
    d. Carbonated beverages, coke syrup, orange juice, ginger ale, and herbal teas
    e. Lying down to relieve symptoms
2. Instruct the pregnant woman to try one food- or beverage-type relief measure at a time (*e.g.*, high-protein meals/bedtime snack); if nausea is not relieved, try another measure.

Rationale

- From 50% to 80% of all pregnant women experience "morning sickness" (Ieioro, 1988). Fatigue has been reported to precipitate nausea/vomiting in pregnant women (Voda & Randall, 1982).
- Voda and Randall (1982) reported that eating a high-protein snack before going to bed at night decreases morning nausea in some pregnant women.

Acute Pain

DEFINITION

Acute Pain: The state in which an individual experiences and reports the presence of severe discomfort or an uncomfortable sensation, lasting from 1 second to less than 6 months.

DEFINING CHARACTERISTICS

Subjective Data

Communication (verbal or coded) of pain descriptors

Objective Data

Guarding behavior, protective
Self-focusing
Narrowed focus (altered time perception, withdrawal from social contact, impaired thought processes)
Distraction behavior (moaning, crying, pacing, seeking out other people or activities, restlessness)
Facial mask of pain (eyes lackluster, "beaten look," fixed or scattered movement, grimace)
Alteration in muscle tone (may span from listless to rigid)
Autonomic responses not seen in chronic stable pain (diaphoresis, blood pressure and pulse change, pupillary dilation, increased or decreased respiratory rate)

RELATED FACTORS

See *Altered Comfort*

Author's Note

Nursing management of pain presents specific challenges. Is acute pain a response that nurses treat as a nursing diagnosis or as a collaborative problem? Is acute pain the etiology of another response that better describes the condition that nurses treat? Does some cluster of nursing diagnoses represent a pain syndrome or chronic pain syndrome (*e.g., Fear, Risk for Ineffective Family Coping, Impaired Physical Mobility, Social Isolation, Altered Sexuality Patterns, Risk for Colonic Constipation, Fatigue*)? McCafferty and Beebe (1989) cite 18 nursing diagnoses that can apply to people experiencing pain. Viewing pain as a syndrome diagnosis can provide nurses with a comprehensive nursing diagnosis for people in pain for whom many related nursing diagnoses could apply.

Errors in Diagnostic Statements

Pain related to surgical incision

Viewing incisional pain as an etiology rather than a response may better relate to nursing's focus. For a surgical client, the nurse focuses on reducing pain to permit increased participation in activities and to reduce anxiety, as described by the nursing diagnosis *Impaired Physical Mobility related to fear of pain and weakness secondary to anesthesia and insufficient fluids and nutrients.*

Pain related to cardiac tissue ischemia

The nurse has several responsibilities for a person experiencing chest pain, including evaluating cardiac status, reducing activity, administering PRN medication, and reducing anxiety. Before discharge, the nurse teaches self-monitoring, self-medication, signs and symptoms of complications, follow-up care, and necessary life-style modifications. Because nursing management of chest pain involves nurse-prescribed and physician-prescribed interventions, this situation should be described as the collaborative problem *Potential Complication: Cardiac.*

This collaborative problem would encompass a variety of cardiac complications (*e.g.,* dysrhythmias, decreased cardiac output, angina). In addition, two nursing diagnoses would apply: *Anxiety related to present situation, unknown future, and perceived effects on self and significant others*, and *Altered Health Maintenance related to insufficient knowledge of condition, signs and symptoms of complications, risk factors, activity restrictions, and follow-up care.*

Key Concepts

1. "Pain has been described as an experience that overwhelms the individual and consumes every aspect of life" (Ferrell, 1995, p. 609).
2. Pain is inevitable; life cannot be pain free. A person must learn to live with pain, to control it, rather than be controlled by it (R. Carpenito, personal communication, 1987). Each individual experiences and expresses pain in his own manner, using various sociocultural adaptation techniques.
3. All pain is real, regardless of its causes. Pure psychogenic pain is probably rare, as is pure organic pain. Most bodily pain is a combination of mental events (psychogenic) and physical stimuli (organic).
4. Pain has two components: a sensory component, which is neurophysiologic, and a perceptual or experiential dimension with cognitive and emotional origins. The interaction of these two components determines the amount of suffering (Schechter, 1989a).
5. Pain tolerance is the duration and intensity of pain that an individual is willing to endure. Pain tolerance differs in individuals and may vary in one individual in different situations. Pain threshold is the point at which an individual reports that a stimulus is painful (McCafferty & Beebe, 1989).
6. Personal factors that influence pain tolerance are
   Knowledge of pain and its cause   Energy level (fatigue)
   Meaning of pain   Stress level
   Ability to control pain
7. Social and environmental factors that influence pain are
   Interactions with others   Sensory overload or deprivation
   Response of others (family, friends)   Stressors
   Secondary gains
8. Studies have shown that diagnosed physiologic pain does respond to placebos, so a positive response to placebos cannot be used to diagnose pain as psychogenic (Perry & Heidrich, 1981).
9. Pain can be classified as acute or chronic, according to cause and duration, not intensity.
10. Acute pain is an episode of pain that has a duration of 1 second to less than 6 months. The cause is usually organic disease or injury. With healing, the pain subsides and eventually disappears.
11. Chronic pain is a pain experience that lasts for 6 months or longer. Chronic pain can be described as limited, intermittent, or persistent. *Limited pain* is pain caused by known physical lesion, and an end of the pain will come (*e.g.,* burns). *Intermittent pain* is pain that provides the person with pain-free periods. The cause may or may not be known (*e.g.,* headaches). *Persistent pain* is pain that usually occurs daily. The cause may or may not be known and is usually not a threat to life (*e.g.,* low back pain).
12. The visible signs of pain (physical and behavioral) are determined by the individual's pain tolerance and the duration of the pain, not the pain intensity.
13. The person may respond to acute pain physiologically and behaviorally: physiologically by diaphoresis, an increased heart rate, an increased respiratory rate, and increased blood pressure; behaviorally by crying, moaning, or showing anger.
14. The person with chronic pain usually has adapted to pain, both physiologically and behaviorally, so that visible signs of pain may not be present.

15. The inability to manage pain produces feelings of frustration and inadequacy in the health care providers.
16. Nurses' fears of precipitating respiratory depression often make them reluctant to use intravenous medications. Yet a study reported that only 3 of 3263 patients experienced respiratory depression from narcotics during an acute hospitalization (Miller, 1995).
17. Nurses' fear of precipitating addiction often makes them reluctant to administer narcotics. Porter and Jick (1980) identified that 4 addicts of 11,000 reported they received Demerol in the hospital.
18. Drug tolerance is a physiologic phenomenon in which, after repeated doses, the prescribed dose begins to lose its effectiveness.
19. Drug dependence is a physiologic state that results from repeated administration of a drug. Withdrawal is experienced if the drug is abruptly discontinued. Tapering down the drug dosage manages the withdrawal symptoms.

🌀 Key Concepts—Child

1. Several studies reported that when adults and children undergo the same surgery, the children are undermedicated (Beyer, 1984; Eland & Anderson, 1977). In one study, 52% of the children received no analgesic postoperatively, whereas the remaining 48% received preponderantly aspirin or acetaminophen.
2. The child's response to pain is influenced by developmental age, procedure or condition causing pain, coping style, parental response to pain, culture, past experiences with pain, and whether it is acute or chronic pain.
3. The child's maturational and chronologic age influences this response to pain.
    Infant: Association of environment with painful experience
        Loud crying and verbal protest long after the stimulus is withdrawn
    Toddler: Fear of body intrusion
        No understanding of rationale for pain or ability to conceptualize the duration of experience, even if told
        Seeking out parental figures as a source of comfort
    Preschool: Magical thinking or fantasies (*e.g.*, something they thought or did caused the pain experience)
        Increased verbal skills to communicate pain
        Limited understanding of time
        After pain passes, talking to toys or other children about the pain experience
        Denial of pain, especially if associated with adverse consequences (*e.g.*, injection, ridicule if not brave)
    School-age: Fear of body injury
        Ability to describe the cause, type, quality, and severity of pain
        Ability to rate the severity of pain
        Attempts to relate the pain experience to previous events and gain control over actions
        Denial of pain, especially if associated with adverse consequences (see foregoing)
        Possible influence of presence of parents on child's expression of pain
    Adolescent: Importance of body image
        Overconfidence compensating for fear
        Behavioral responses to pain more "socially acceptable" than younger child's, but fear and anxiety *not* less
        Possible influence of presence of parent on child's expression of pain

🌀 Key Concepts—Maternal

1. The discomforts of labor are varied from backaches, to leg cramps, imposed immobility, and labor contractions.
2. Chapman (1991) reported that expectant fathers assumed that one of their roles during labor is to be coach, teammate, or witness.
3. Prolonged latent phase of labor (>20 hours for primigravida or 14 hours for the multipara) is usually the result of an unripe cervix. Other causes are abnormal fetal position,

dysfunctional labor, cephalopelvic disproportion, or sedation or analgesia use too early in labor (May & Mahlmeister, 1994).

Key Concepts—*Older Adult*

1. Pain is omnipresent in the elderly and may be accepted by elders and professionals as a normal and unavoidable accompaniment to aging. Unfortunately, many chronic diseases that are common in the elderly, such as osteoarthritis and rheumatoid arthritis, may not be adequately managed for pain.
2. Older adults may not demonstrate objective signs and symptoms of pain because of years of adaptation and increased pain tolerance. The individual may eventually accept the pain, thereby lowering expectations for comfort and mobility. Pain-coping mechanisms cultivated throughout life are important to identify and reinforce in pain management. Effective pain management can greatly improve the overall physical functioning and emotional well-being of the individual (Clinton & Eland, 1991).
3. The effects of narcotic analgesics are prolonged in older adults because of decreased metabolism and clearance of the drug. Also, side effects seem to be more frequent and pronounced in the elderly, especially anticholinergic effects, extrapyramidal effects, and sedation. It is advised that drugs be started at a lower dosage, and because older adults often take multiple drugs, drug interactions should be monitored (Malseed, 1990).

Focus Assessment Criteria

See *Altered Comfort*

Outcome Criteria

The person will
- Convey that others validate that the pain exists
- Relate relief after a satisfactory relief measure as evidenced by (specify)

Interventions

A. Assess for factors that decrease pain tolerance

  1. Disbelief on the part of others
  2. Lack of knowledge
  3. Fear (*e.g.*, of addiction or loss of control)
  4. Fatigue
  5. Monotony

B. Reduce or eliminate factors that increase the pain experience

  1. Disbelief on the part of others
      a. Relate to the individual your acceptance of his response to pain.
          Acknowledge the presence of his pain.
          Listen attentively to him concerning his pain.
          Convey to him that you are assessing his pain because you want to understand it better (not determine if it is really present).
      b. Assess the family for the presence of misconceptions about pain or its treatment.
          Explain the concept of pain as an individual experience.
          Discuss the reasons why an individual may experience increased or decreased pain (*e.g.*, fatigue [increased] or presence of distractions [decreased]).
          Encourage family members to share their concerns privately (*e.g.*, fear that the person will use his pain for secondary gains if they give him too much attention).

Assess whether the family doubts the pain and discuss the effects of this on the person's pain and on the relationship.

Encourage the family to give attention also when pain is not exhibited.

2. Lack of knowledge
   a. Explain causes of the pain to the person, if known.
   b. Relate how long the pain will last, if known.
   c. Explain diagnostic tests and procedures in detail by relating the discomforts and sensations that will be felt and approximate the length of time involved (*e.g.*, "During the intravenous pyelogram you might feel a momentary hot flash through your entire body").
   d. Allow person to see and handle equipment if possible.

3. Fear
   a. Provide accurate information to reduce fear of addiction.
      Explore with him the reasons for the fear.
      Explain the difference between drug tolerance and drug addiction (see Key Concepts).
   b. Assist in reducing fear of losing control.
      Provide him with privacy for his pain experience.
      Attempt to limit the number of health care providers who provide care to him.
      Allow him to share how intense his pain is and express to him how well he tolerated the pain.
   c. Provide information to reduce fear that the medication will gradually lose its effectiveness.
      Discuss drug tolerance with him.
      Discuss the interventions for drug tolerance with the physician (*e.g.*, changing the medication, increasing the dose, decreasing the interval).
      Discuss the effect of relaxation techniques on medication effects.

4. Fatigue
   Determine the cause of fatigue (sedatives, analgesics, sleep deprivation).
   Explain that pain contributes to stress, which increases fatigue.
   Assess the person's present sleep pattern and the influence of his pain on his sleep.
   Provide him with opportunities to rest during the day and with periods of uninterrupted sleep at night (must rest when pain is ↓).
   Consult with physician for an increased dose of pain medication at bedtime.
   Refer to *Sleep Pattern Disturbance* for specific interventions to enhance sleep.

5. Monotony
   a. Discuss with the person and family the therapeutic uses of distraction, along with other methods of pain relief.
   b. Emphasize that the degree an individual can be distracted from his pain is not at all related to the existence of or the intensity of the pain.
   c. Explain that distraction usually increases pain tolerance and decreases pain intensity, but after the distraction ceases the individual may experience increased awareness of pain and fatigue.
   d. Vary the environment if possible. If on bed rest:
      Encourage personnel to wear seasonal pins and bright-colored apparel.
      Encourage family to decorate room with flowers, plants, pictures.
      Provide the person with music.
      Consult with recreational therapist for an appropriate task.
   e. If at home:
      Encourage individual to plan an activity for each day, preferably outside the home.
      Discuss the possibility of learning a new skill (*e.g.*, a craft, a musical instrument).
   f. Teach a method of distraction during an acute pain (*e.g.*, painful procedure) that is not a burden (*e.g.*, count items in a picture, count anything in the room, such as patterns on wallpaper or count silently to self); breathe rhythmically; listen to music and increase the volume as the pain increases.

C. Collaborate with the individual to determine what methods could be used to reduce the intensity of pain

    1. Consider the following before selecting a specific pain relief method:

        a. The individual's willingness to participate (motivation), ability to participate (dexterity, sensory loss), preference, support of significant others for method, contraindications (allergy, health problem)

        b. The method's cost, complexity, precautions, and convenience

    2. Explain the various noninvasive pain relief methods to the individual and his family and why they are effective (see Appendix VI).

D. Collaborate with the individual to initiate the appropriate noninvasive pain relief measures (refer to Appendix VI for specific instructions on each method)

    1. Relaxation

        a. Instruct on techniques to reduce skeletal muscle tension, which will reduce the intensity of the pain.

        b. Use pillows and blankets to support the painful part to reduce the amount of muscle tension.

        c. Promote relaxation with a back rub, massage, or warm bath (*e.g.*, for a person with a fractured limb, rub the opposite limb over the fractured site).

        d. Teach a specific relaxation strategy (*e.g.*, slow, rhythmic breathing or deep breath–clench fists–yawn).

        e. Enlist the aid of the family as coaches.

    2. Counterirritant cutaneous stimulation

        a. Discuss with the person the various methods of skin stimulation and their effects on pain (see Appendix VI).

        b. Discuss the use of heat applications,* their therapeutic effects, and when indicated.

        c. Discuss each of the following methods and the precautions:

            Hot water bottle
            Electric heating pad
            Warm tub
            Moist heat pack
            Hot summer sun
            Thin plastic wrap over painful area to retain body heat (*e.g.*, knee, elbow)

        d. Discuss the use of cold applications,* their therapeutic effects, and when indicated.

        e. Discuss each of the following methods and the precautions of each:

            Cold towels (wrung out)
            Cold water immersion for small body parts
            Ice bag
            Cold gel pack
            Ice massage

        f. Explain the therapeutic uses of menthol preparations, massage, and vibration.

E. Provide with optimal pain relief with prescribed analgesics

    1. Determine preferred route of administration: oral, IM, IV, rectal.

    2. Assess vital signs, especially respiratory rate, before administering medication.

    3. Consult with pharmacist for possible adverse interactions with other medications (*e.g.*, muscle relaxants, tranquilizers).

    4. Use a preventive approach.

        a. Medicate before an activity (*e.g.*, ambulation) to increase participation, but evaluate the hazard of sedation.

---

* May require a primary care provider's order.

    b. Instruct to request PRN pain medication before the pain is severe.

    c. Collaborate with physician to order medications on a 24-hour basis rather than PRN.

F. Assess the response to the pain relief medication

    1. After administering a pain relief medication, return in one-half hour to assess effectiveness.

    2. Ask to rate the severity of pain, before the medication, and the amount of relief received.

    3. Ask person to indicate when the pain began to increase.

    4. Consult with physician if a dosage or interval change is needed; the dose may be increased by 50% until effective (Agency for Health Care Policy and Research [AHCPR], 1992).

G. Reduce or eliminate common side effects of narcotics

    1. Sedation

       a. Assess whether the cause is the narcotic, fatigue, sleep deprivation, or other drugs (sedatives, antiemetics).

       b. Inform person that drowsiness usually occurs the first 2–3 days and then subsides.

       c. If drowsiness is excessive, consult with physician to try a slight dose reduction.

    2. Constipation

       a. Explain the effect of narcotics on peristalsis.

       b. Consult with physician on the use of a stool softener with long-term drug use.

       c. Refer to *Constipation* for additional interventions.

    3. Nausea and vomiting (see also *Nausea/Vomiting*)

       a. Instruct person that nausea usually subsides after a few doses.

       b. Refrain from withholding narcotic doses because of nausea; rather, secure an order for an antiemetic.

       c. Instruct individual to take deep breaths and to swallow voluntarily to decrease vomiting reflex.

       d. If nausea persists, consult with physician for the appropriate antiemetic or for a change of narcotic that produces less nausea (*e.g.*, morphine).

    4. Dry mouth

       a. Explain that narcotics decrease saliva production.

       b. Instruct person to rinse mouth often, suck on sugarless sour candies, eat pineapple chunks or watermelon, if permissible, and drink liquids often.

       c. Explain the necessity of good oral hygiene and dental care.

H. Assist the family to respond positively to the individual's pain experience

    1. Assess the family's knowledge of and response to the pain experience.

    2. Give accurate information to correct family misconceptions (*e.g.*, addiction, doubts about pain).

    3. Provide individuals with opportunities to discuss their fears, anger, and frustrations in private; acknowledge the difficulty of the situation.

    4. Incorporate family members in the pain relief modality, if possible (*e.g.*, stroking, massage).

    5. Praise their participation and their concern.

I. Assist with the aftermath of pain

    1. Inform person when the cause of the pain has been removed or decreased (*e.g.*, spinal tap).

    2. Encourage person to discuss the pain experience.

    3. Praise person for his endurance and convey to him that he handled his pain well, regardless of how he behaved.

    4. Allow person to keep souvenir of his pain, if desired (*e.g.*, gallstones), or a record of repeated procedures (*e.g.*, venipunctures).

J. Assist with phantom limb pain

1. Advise that 80% of amputees experience phantom limb sensations during the first year after surgery (Sherman, 1989).
2. Explain that the exact cause of phantom limb pain is not agreed on. Stimulus of peripheral nerves proximal to the amputation is thought to be a cause. Another explanation is that severed nerves may send impulses that are perceived by the brain as abnormal (Rounseville, 1992).
3. Explain the sensations that may be present, including feeling limb is still present, limb is floating, tight band below amputation, warm, tingling feeling (Rounseville, 1992).
4. Explain that psychological stresses do not cause phantom pain, but can trigger or increase it (Sherman, 1989).
5. Explain measures that have been effective in alleviating phantom limb pain (Sherman, 1989).
   a. Applying heat to stump
   b. Applying pressure to stump (*e.g.*, elastic bandages)
   c. Distraction, diversion techniques, relaxation exercises
   d. Massage therapy (after 2 weeks postoperatively)
6. Explain that narcotics are ineffective for phantom limb pain but are effective for surgical stump pain (Sherman, 1989).
7. Advise client to consult with physician if phantom limb pain is unmanageable (Sherman, 1989).

K. Initiate health teaching, as indicated

1. Discuss with the person and the family noninvasive pain relief measures (relaxation, distraction, massage).
2. Teach the techniques of choice to the person and his family.
3. Explain the expected course of the pain (resolution) if known (*e.g.*, fractured arm, surgical incision).

Rationale

- If a person must try to convince health care providers that he has pain, he will experience increased anxiety that increases the pain. Both of these are energy depleting.
- People who are prepared for painful procedures by explanations of the actual sensations that will be felt experience less stress than those who receive vague explanations of the procedure.
- Studies have shown that the human brain secretes endorphins, which have opiate-like properties that relieve pain. The release of endorphins may be responsible for the positive effects of placebos and noninvasive pain relief measures (McCafferty & Beebe, 1989).
- Studies have shown that diagnosed physiological pain does respond to placebos, so a positive response to placebos cannot be used to diagnose pain as psychogenic (Perry & Heidrich, 1981).
- The use of noninvasive pain relief measures (*e.g.*, relaxation, massage, distraction) can enhance the therapeutic effects of pain relief medications.
- Adults and children who are experiencing pain feel their bodies and their lives are out of control. Attempts must be made to provide some choice or control during their day (Lubkin, 1995).
- Inadequate sleep decreases one's ability to tolerate pain and depletes the energy needed to participate in social activities (Eland, 1988).
- Pain management should be aggressive and individualized to eliminate any unnecessary pain, with the administration of drugs on a regular time schedule, rather than as needed in the early postoperative period (AHCPR, 1992).
- The preventive approach may reduce the total 24-hour dose compared with PRN approach; it provides a constant blood level of the drug, it reduces craving for the drug, and it reduces the anxiety of having to ask and wait for PRN relief (AHCPR, 1992).

- The oral route of administration is preferred when possible. Liquid medications can be given to individuals who have difficulty swallowing (AHCPR, 1992).
- If frequent injections are necessary, the IV route is preferred because it is not painful and absorption is guaranteed, but the side effects (↓ respirations, ↓ blood pressure) may be more profound.
- Addiction is a psychological syndrome characterized by compulsive drug-seeking behavior generally associated with a desire for drug administration to produce euphoria or other effects, not pain relief. Addiction is believed to be rare, and there is no evidence that adequate administration of opioids for pain produces addiction.
- Nurses' fears of precipitating respiratory depression often make them reluctant to use intravenous medications. Yet, a study reported that only 3 of 3263 patients experienced respiratory depression from narcotics during an acute hospitalization (Miller, 1995).
- Nonpharmacologic interventions provide a major treatment approach for pain, specifically chronic pain (McGuire & Sheidler, 1993).
- Nonpharmacologic interventions provide the client with an increased sense of control, provide for active involvement, reduce stress and anxiety, elevate mood, and raise pain threshold (McGuire & Sheidler, 1993).
- Cognitive interventions for pain try to modify thought processes to relieve pain. The cognitive activity distracts from the perception of pain. Examples are distraction (*e.g.*, counting, word games, conversation, breathing exercises), imagery, and educational programs about pain management (McGuire & Sheidler, 1993).
- Behavioral methods attempts to modify physiologic reactions to pain. Examples of behavioral methods are relaxation, meditation, music therapy, hypnosis, and biofeedback (McGuire & Sheidler, 1993).
- Information given in advance of a potentially stressful event reduces fear of the unknown and assists the person to adapt (Hymovich & Hagopian, 1992).
- Relaxation and guided imagery are effective in management of pain by increasing sense of control, reducing feelings of helplessness and hopelessness, providing a calming diversion, and disrupting the pain–anxiety–tension cycle (Sloman, 1995).

Interventions—*Child Focus*

A. Assess for pain experience

1. Assess the child's pain experience.
   a. Determine the child's concept of the cause of pain, if feasible.
   b. Ask child to point to the area that hurts. See Focus Assessment under *Altered Comfort*.
   c. Determine the intensity of the pain at its worst and best.
   d. Use a pain assessment scale appropriate for the child's developmental age. Use the same scale the same way each time, and encourage its use by parents and other health care professionals. Indicate on the care plan which scale to use and how (introduction of scale, language specific for child); attach copy if visual scale. (See p. 184 for a description of pain scales.)
   e. Ask the child what makes the pain better and what makes it worse.
   f. Include the parents' rating of their child's pain in assessment. Parents and nurses can rate a child's pain differently. The parents' observation of pain is often more accurate than the nurse's.
   g. Assess whether fear, loneliness, or anxiety are contributing to pain.
   h. Assess effect on sleep and play. *Note:* A child who sleeps and/or plays can be a child in pain (sleep and play can be a type of distraction) or a child adequately medicated for pain.
   i. With infants, assess crying, facial expressions, body postures, and movements. Infants exhibit distress from environmental stimuli (light, sound) as well as from touch and treatments. Use tactile and vocal stimuli to comfort infants, but assess the effect of comfort measures (does it increase or decrease distress?) and individualized intervention.

2. Assess the child and family for the presence of misconceptions about pain or its treatment.
   a. Explain the pain source to the child using verbal and sensory (visual, tactile) explanations (*e.g.,* allow child to handle equipment or perform treatment on doll; refer to Appendix IX for specific techniques of play therapy).
   b. Explicitly explain and reinforce to the child that he is not being punished.
   c. Explain to the parents the necessity of good explanations to promote trust.
   d. Explain to the parents that the child may cry more openly when they are present, but that their presence is important for promoting trust.
   e. Parents and older children may have misconceptions about pain and analgesia, and may be fearful of narcotic use/abuse. Emphasize that narcotic use for moderate or severe pain does not lead to addiction (Schechter, 1989b). Discuss with parents and older children that "say no to drugs" does not apply to analgesia for pain prescribed by physicians and monitored by physicians and nurses.

B. Promote security with honest explanations and opportunities for choice
   1. Promote open, honest communications
      a. Tell the truth; explain
         How much it will hurt
         How long it will last
         What will help the pain
      b. Do not threaten (*e.g., do not* tell the child, "If you don't hold still you won't go home").
      c. Explain to the child that the procedure is necessary so he can get better and it is important to hold still so it can be done quickly.
      d. Discuss with the parents the importance of truth-telling; instruct parents to
         Tell child when they are leaving and when they will return
         Relate to the child that they cannot take away his pain, but that they will be with him (except in circumstances when parents are not permitted to remain)
      e. Allow the parents opportunities to share their feelings about witnessing their child's pain and their helplessness.
   2. Prepare the child for a painful procedure.
      a. Discuss the procedure with the parents; determine what they have told the child.
      b. Explain the procedure in words suited to the child's age and developmental level (see *Altered Growth and Development* for age-related needs).
         Allow a 2-year-old to watch you taking out sutures from a doll or stuffed animal.
         Permit the child to hold instruments.
      c. Relate the discomforts that will be felt (*e.g.,* what the child will feel, taste, see, or smell).
         "You will get an injection that will hurt for a little while and then it will stop."
         Be sure to explain when an injection will cause two discomforts: the prick of the needle and the absorption of the drug.
      d. Encourage the child to ask questions before and during the procedure; ask the child to share with you what he thinks is going to happen and why.
      e. Share with the child (who is old enough—older than 3½ years) that:
         You expect that he will hold still and that it will please you if he can.
         It is all right to cry or squeeze your hand if it hurts.
      f. Find something to praise after the procedure, even if child was not able to hold still.
      g. Arrange to have parents present for procedures (especially for children younger than 10 years); describe what to expect to parents before procedure, and give them a role during procedure (*e.g.,* hold the child's hand, talk to the child).

3. Reduce the pain during treatments when possible.
   a. If restraints must be used, have sufficient personnel available so that the procedure is not delayed.
   b. If injections are ordered, try to obtain an order for oral or intravenous analgesics instead. If injections must be used:
      Expect the child (older than 2½ or 3 years) to hold still
      Have the child participate by holding the Band-Aid for you
      Tell the child how pleased you are that he helped
      Pull the skin surface as taut as possible (for IM)
      Comfort the child after the procedure
      Tell child step-by-step what is going to happen right before it is done
   c. Offer the child the option of learning distraction techniques for use during the procedure. (The use of distraction without the child's knowledge of the impending discomfort is not advocated because the child will learn to mistrust.)
      Tell a story with a puppet
      Ask the child to name or count objects in a picture
      Ask the child to look at the picture and to locate certain objects ("Where is the dog?")
      Ask child to tell you about his pet
      Ask child to count your blinks
   d. Avoid rectal temperatures in preschoolers; if possible, use electronic oral or ear probes.
   e. Provide the child with privacy during the painful procedure; use a treatment room rather than the child's bed.
      The child's bed should be a "safe" place.
      No procedures should be done in the playroom or schoolroom.
4. Provide the child optimal pain relief with prescribed analgesics.
   a. Medicate child before painful procedure or activity (*e.g.*, ambulation).
   b. Consult with physician for a change of the IM route to the IV route.
   c. Assess appropriateness of medication, dose, and schedule for cause of pain, child's weight, and child's response.
   d. Besides using pain scales to assess pain, observe for behavioral signs of pain (because the child may deny pain); if possible, identify specific behaviors that indicate pain in an individual child.
   e. Assess the potential for use of patient-controlled analgesia (PCA). PCA provides intermittent controlled doses of IV analgesia (with/without continuous infusion) as determined by the child's need for analgesia. PCA can be used effectively by children as young as 5 years of age and by parents of children physically unable to use the device. It has been found to be safe and to provide superior pain relief compared with conventional demand analgesia.
   f. Consult with physician about the use of epidural infusion of morphine for treatment of postoperative pain. Epidural morphine infusion has been used safely in both adults and children in nonintensive care settings.
5. Reduce or eliminate the common side effects of narcotics.
   a. Sedation
      Assess whether the cause is the narcotic, fatigue, sleep deprivation, or other drugs (sedatives, antiemetics).
      If drowsiness is excessive, consult with physician to try a slight dose reduction.
   b. Constipation
      Explain to older children why pain medications cause constipation.
      Increase roughage in diet (*e.g.*, ask child which fruits he likes; sprinkle 1 teaspoon of bran on cereal).
      Encourage to drink 8–10 (8-oz) glasses of liquids each day.
      Teach how to do abdominal isometric exercises if activity is restricted (*e.g.*, "Pull in your tummy; now relax your tummy; do this ten times each hour during the day").

Instruct child to keep a record of his exercises (*e.g.*, make a chart with a star sticker placed on it whenever the exercises are done).

Refer to *Constipation* for additional interventions.

c. Dry mouth

Explain to older children that narcotics decrease saliva production.

Instruct to rinse mouth often, suck on sugarless sour candies, eat pineapple chunks and watermelon, drink liquids often.

Explain the necessity of brushing teeth after every meal.

6. Assist the child with the aftermath of pain.
   a. Tell the child when the painful procedure is over.
   b. Pick up the small child to indicate it is over.
   c. Encourage to discuss pain experience (draw or act out with dolls).
   d. Encourage to perform the painful procedure using the same equipment on a doll under supervision (see Appendix IX for specific interventions).
   e. Praise the child for his endurance and convey to him that he handled the pain well regardless of how he behaved (unless he was violent to others).
   f. Give the child a souvenir of his pain (Band-Aid, badge for bravery).
   g. Teach to keep a record of painful experiences and to plan a reward each time he achieves a behavioral goal, such as a gold star (reward) for each time he holds still (goal) during an injection. Encourage achievable goals; holding still during an injection may not be possible for every child, but counting or blowing may be possible.

7. Collaborate with child to initiate appropriate noninvasive pain relief modalities.
   a. Encourage mobility as much as indicated, especially when pain is at its lowest level.
   b. Discuss with child and parents activities that are liked and incorporate them in daily schedule (*e.g.*, clay modeling, painting).
   c. Discuss with the child (older than 7 years) that the pain can be less if the child thinks about something else, and demonstrate the effects.

      Ask child to count to 100 (or count your eye blinks).

      As child is counting, apply gentle pressure to Achilles tendon (pinch back of heel).

      Gradually increase the pressure.

      Ask to stop counting but keep pressure on heel.

      Ask if he can feel the discomfort in his heel now and if he felt it when he was counting.

   d. Consider the use of transcutaneous electrical nerve stimulation (TENS) for procedural, acute, and chronic pain. TENS has been studied and used effectively in children with postoperative pain, headache, and procedural pain, without adverse effects.
   e. Refer to guidelines for noninvasive pain relief measures (Appendix VI).

8. Assist the family to respond optimally to the child's pain experience.
   a. Assess the family's knowledge of and response to the pain experience (*e.g.*, does the parent support the child who has pain?).
   b. Assure the parents that they can touch or hold their child, if feasible (*e.g.*, demonstrate that touching is possible even in the presence of tubes and equipment).
   c. Give accurate information to correct misconceptions (*e.g.*, the necessity of the treatment even though it causes pain).
   d. Provide parents with opportunities to discuss their fears, anger, frustrations in private.
   e. Acknowledge the difficulty of the situation.
   f. Incorporate the parents in the pain relief modality if possible (*e.g.*, stroking, massage, distraction).
   g. Praise their participation and their concern.
   h. Negotiate goals of pain management plan and reevaluate regularly (*e.g.*, pain-free, decrease in pain).

C. Promote coping behaviors
  1. Observe for coping behaviors that assist the child to prepare for and recover from pain experiences.
      a. Tension reduction strategies (keep as still as possible, think about other things, sing, talk, listen to others talk, music, TV)
      b. Self-talk (telling themselves that they are OK, that the procedure is going well, that they are getting better, rephrasing the experience in terms of its benefits)
      c. Information-seeking behaviors (asking questions about both detailed and broad aspects of the experience, immediate and future data)
      d. Controlling behaviors (verbal suggestions, rules, who does what when, how things are done)
      e. Hand-holding, comforting touch
      f. Stalling strategies (drink of water, TV program, time)
      g. Body stiffening or muscle relaxation
      h. Silent or audible cursing
      i. Laughter (usually after pain is relieved)
  2. Along with the child and parents, identify and promote coping behaviors that are effective for that child. Children are able to cope more effectively with pain when they are able to use the coping behaviors that they prefer.

D. Initiate health teaching and referrals, if indicated
  1. Provide child and family with ongoing explanations.
  2. Use the care plan to promote continuity of care for hospitalized child.
  3. Use available mental health professionals, if needed, for assistance with guided imagery, progressive relaxation, and hypnosis.
  4. Use available pain service (pain team) at pediatric health care centers for an interdisciplinary and comprehensive approach to pain management in children.
  5. Refer parents to pertinent literature for themselves and children (see Bibliography).

Rationale

- Assessment of pain in children should never be made only on the basis of behavior. Assessment of pain consists of three parts: the nature of the pain-producing pathology involved, the autonomic responses of acute pain, and the child's behaviors (Jackson & Saunders, 1993).
- Toddlers in pain may be hyperactive in an attempt to escape the pain. Screams are expressions of their pain and outrage.
- School-aged children are capable of understanding why a procedure needs to be done. Assessment tools can be used (Jackson & Saunders, 1993).
- Anxiety, fear, and separation can increase the pain sensation (Jackson & Saunders, 1993).
- Pharmacologic measures in combination with noninvasive techniques provide the most effective means of treating pain in children (Jackson & Saunders, 1993).
- Consistent pain assessment criteria (*e.g.*, assessment scale, specific behaviors) should be identified and used by nurses, physicians, and parents to assess pain in a child.
- Verbal communication is usually not sufficient or reliable for explaining pain or painful procedures to children younger than 7 years of age. The nurse can explain by demonstrating with pictures or dolls. The more senses that are stimulated in the explanations to children, the greater the communication. When possible, include parents in preparation.
- Because a child may respond more openly to pain when parents are present, the parents' presence should be encouraged to facilitate pain assessment, provide support, and promote trust.
- The weight of the child, not the age, should be considered when calculating analgesic relief.
- Children and adolescents often deny pain to avoid injections (Eland & Anderson, 1977). Although oral administration of analgesia is the route of choice for children, followed by intravenous administration (Berde, 1989), O'Brien and Konsler (1988) found that 40% of medications for postoperative pain were administered intramuscularly.

Interventions—*Maternal Focus*

1. Determine the role the expectant father chooses for the labor and birth experience: coach, teammate, or witness (Chapman, 1991).
2. Provide the expectant parents with the level of support assessed to be needed (Chapman, 1991).
3. Explain all procedures before initiation.
4. Provide comfort techniques as desired (*e.g.*, walking, massage, shower, sponge back).
5. Instruct not to use breathing techniques too early.
6. As labor progresses to active stage:
   a. Evaluate effectiveness of breathing techniques.
   b. If pain or anxiety is not reduced, consult with midwife or physician for a new plan of management.
   c. Evaluate fatigue level.
   d. Assess how well labor partner is anticipating the woman's needs.
   e. Encourage ambulation and position changes every 20–30 minutes.
   f. Approach the woman in an unhurried, gentle manner.

Rationale

- Depending on the choice of roles by the expectant father, the nurse supplements, supervises, or provides the supportive care (Chapman, 1991).
- Fear and anxiety can be reduced by providing calm explanations.
- Sensory overload can contribute to anxiety and fear.
- Walking promotes less frequent, more efficient contractions (May & Mahlmeister, 1994).
- Position changes can prevent or correct malpositions of the fetus, promote rotation and labor progress, and reduce lower back pain (May & Mahlmeister, 1994).
- If prolonged latent labor is expected, a new plan of care is needed to prevent sleep deprivation, maternal exhaustion, and increased anxiety.
- Maternal exhaustion can occur if breathing techniques are used too early.

Chronic Pain

DEFINITION

Chronic Pain: The state in which an individual experiences pain that is persistent or intermittent and lasts for more than 6 months.

DEFINING CHARACTERISTICS
Major (Must Be Present)

The person reports that pain has existed for more than 6 months (may be the only assessment data present)

Minor (May Be Present)

Discomfort	Guarded movement
Anger, frustration, depression because of situation	Muscle spasms
Facial mask of pain	Redness, swelling, heat
Anorexia, weight loss	Color changes in affected area
Insomnia	Reflex abnormalities

RELATED FACTORS

See *Altered Comfort*

Author's Note

See *Altered Comfort*

Errors in Diagnostic Statements

See *Altered Comfort*

Key Concepts

Refer to *Acute Pain*

Focus Assessment Criteria

See *Altered Comfort*

Outcome Criteria

The person will
- Relate that others validate that the pain exists
- Practice selected noninvasive pain relief measures to manage his pain
- Relate improvement of pain and an increase in daily activities as evident by (specify)

The child will
- Communicate improvement in pain verbally, by pain assessment scale, or by behavior (specify)
- Maintain usual family role and relationships throughout pain experience, as evidenced by (specify)
- Demonstrate coping mechanisms for pain, methods of controlling pain, and the pain cause/disease, as evidenced by an increase in play and usual activities of childhood, and (specify)

Interventions

A. Assess the person's pain experience; determine the intensity of the pain at its worst and best

    1. Ask person to rate his pain using a scale of 0–10 (0 = absence of pain; 10 = worst pain), or a 0–5 scale.
        a. Rate it at its best
        b. Rate it after a pain relief measure
        c. Rate it at its worst
    2. Collaborate to determine what methods could be used to reduce the intensity.

B. Assess for factors that decrease pain tolerance

    1. Disbelief on the part of others
    2. Fear
    3. Fatigue
    4. Monotony

C. Reduce or eliminate factors that increase the pain experience

See *Acute Pain*

D. Assess the effects of chronic pain on the individual's life, using the person and family (Ferrell, 1995)

1. Physical well-being (fatigue, strength, appetite, sleep, function, constipation, nausea)
2. Psychological well-being (anxiety, depression, coping, control, concentration, sense of usefulness, fear, enjoyment)
3. Spiritual well-being (religiosity, uncertainty, positive changes, sense of purpose, hopefulness, suffering, meaning of pain, transcendence)
4. Social well-being (family support, family distress, sexuality, affection, employment, isolation, financial burden, appearance, roles, relationships)

E. Assist the person and family to reduce the effects of depression on life-style

1. Encourage verbalization of individual and family concerning difficult situations.
2. Listen carefully.
3. Explain the relationship between chronic pain and depression.
4. See *Ineffective Individual Coping* for additional interventions.

F. Consult with the individual to determine what methods could be used to reduce the intensity of pain

1. Before selecting a specific noninvasive pain relief method, consider the person's
   a. Willingness to participate (motivation)
   b. Ability to participate (dexterity, sensory loss)
   c. Preference
   d. Support of significant others for method
   e. Contraindications (allergy, health problem)
2. Consider the method's cost, complexity, precautions, and convenience.
3. Explain the various noninvasive pain relief methods to the individual and his family and why they are effective (see Appendix VI).

G. Collaborate with the individual to initiate the appropriate noninvasive pain relief measures (refer to Appendix VI for specific instructions on each method)

See *Acute Pain*

H. Provide the individual pain relief with prescribed analgesics*

1. Determine preferred route of administration: oral, IM, IV, rectal (refer to Key Concepts).
2. Assess the response to the medication.
   a. For admitted people
      After administering a pain relief medication, return in one-half hour to assess effectiveness.
      Ask person to rate the severity of pain before the medication and the amount of relief received.
      Ask individual to indicate when the pain began to increase.
      Consult with the physician if a dosage or interval change is needed.
   b. For outpatients
      Ask person to keep a record of when he takes his medication and what kind of relief was received.
      Instruct person to consult physician with questions concerning medication dosage.

* May require a primary care provider's order.

3. Encourage the use of oral medications as soon as possible.
   a. Consult with physician for a schedule to change from IM to oral.
   b. Explain to individual and family that oral medications can be as effective as IM.
   c. Explain how the transition will occur:
      Begin oral medication at a larger dose than necessary (loading dose).
      Continue PRN IM medication.
      Gradually reduce IM medication dose.
      Use the person's account of pain to regulate oral doses.
   d. Consult with physician for the possibility of adding aspirin or acetaminophen to the medication regimen.

I. **Reduce or eliminate common side effects of narcotics**
See *Acute Pain*

J. **Assist the family to respond optimally to the individual's pain experience**
   1. Assess the family's knowledge of pain and of responses to the pain experience.
   2. Give accurate information to correct family misconceptions (*e.g.*, addiction, doubt about pain).
   3. Provide individuals with opportunities to discuss their fears, anger, frustrations in private; acknowledge the difficulty of the situation.
   4. Incorporate the family in the pain relief method if possible (*e.g.*, coaching relaxation, massaging).
   5. Encourage family to seek assistance if needed for specific problems, such as coping with chronic pain: family counselor; financial and service agencies (*e.g.*, American Cancer Society).

K. **Promote optimal mobility**
   1. Discuss the value of exercise to strengthen and stretch muscles, decrease stress, and promote sleep.
   2. Assist to plan daily activities when pain is at its lowest level.

L. **Initiate health teaching and referrals as indicated; discuss with the individual and family the various treatment modalities available**
   1. Family therapy
   2. Group therapy
   3. Behavior modification
   4. Biofeedback
   5. Hypnosis
   6. Acupuncture
   7. Exercise program

Rationale

- See Rationale for *Acute Pain*
- Ferrell (1995) has validated that pain affects quality of life. Assessment of the specific effects is essential.
- Nursing care that improves pain also improves aspects of well-being (*e.g.*, physical, psychological, social, spiritual; Ferrell, 1995).
- Pain is an intense experience for the individual and family members. Interventions are focused on helping families understand the effects on roles and relationships (Lubkin, 1995).
- Nonpharmacologic interventions provide a major treatment approach for pain, specifically chronic pain (McGuire & Sheidler, 1993).
- The person with chronic pain may respond with withdrawal, depression, anger, frustration, and dependency, all of which can affect the family in the same way.

😃 Interventions—*Child Focus*

1. Assess pain experiences by using developmentally appropriate assessment scales and by assessing behavior. Incorporate child and family in ongoing assessment. Identify potential for secondary gain for reporting pain (*e.g.*, companionship, attention, concern, caring, distraction) and include strategies for meeting identified needs in plan of care.
2. Set goals for pain management with child and family (short- and long-term) and evaluate regularly (*e.g.*, totally relieve pain, partially relieve pain, control behavior or anxiety associated with pain).
3. Promote normal growth and development; involve family and available resources, such as occupational, physical, and child life therapists.
4. Promote the "normal" aspects of the child's life: play, school, relationships with family, physical activity.
5. Promote a trusting environment for child and family.
   a. Believe the child's pain.
   b. Encourage child's perception that interventions are attempts to help.
   c. Have child, family, and nurse participate in controlling pain.
6. Provide continuity of care and pain management by health care providers (nurse, physician, pain team) and in different settings (inpatient, outpatient, emergency department, home).
7. Use interdisciplinary team for pain management as necessary (*e.g.*, nurse, physician, child life therapist, mental health therapist, occupational therapist, physical therapist, nutritionist).
8. Identify myths and misconceptions about pediatric pain management (*e.g.*, IM analgesia, narcotic use and dosing, assessment) in attitudes of health care professionals and child and family; provide accurate information and opportunities for effective communication.
9. Provide parents and siblings with opportunities to share their experiences and fears.

Rationale

- See Rationale for *Acute Pain*.
- Parents of a child with pain report unendurable pain, helplessness, total commitment, feeling the pain physically, being unprepared, agony, terror, and wishing for death in cases of terminal illnesses (Ferrell, 1995). Interventions attempt to bring forth these feelings and experiences.
- It is important to assess the cognitive level and age of the child to provide appropriate explanations (Lubkin, 1995).
- Preschoolers assume their pain is the result of bad deeds. Attempts are made to reduce their sense of personal blame (Lubkin, 1995).

References/Bibliography

Agency for Health Care Policy and Research. (1992). *Acute pain management: Operative or medical procedures and trauma*. Rockville, MD Author.

Agency for Health Care Policy and Research. (1994). *Management of cancer pain*. Rockville, MD: Author.

Baer, R. L. (1990). Poison ivy dermatitis. *Cutis, 46*, 34–36.

Beyer, J. E. (1984). *Ultra: A user manual and technical report*. Evanston, IL: Hospital Play Equipment Co.

Branov, C. H., Epstein, J. H., & Grayson, L. D. (1989a). When pruritus is a diagnostic puzzle. *Patient Care, 23*(15), 41–44, 50–54.

Branov, C. H. Epstein, J. H., & Grayson, L. D. (1989b). How to relieve persistent itching. *Patient Care, 23*(16), 107.

Clinton, P., & Eland, J. A. (1991). Pain. In M. Maas, K. Buckwalter, & M. Hardy (Eds.). *Nursing diagnoses and interventions for the elderly*. Redwood City, CA: Addison-Wesley Nursing.

Coyle, N. (1987). Analgesics and pain: Current concepts. *Nursing Clinics of North America, 22*, 727–741.

DeWitt, S. (1990). Nursing assessment of skin and dermatological lesions. *Nursing Clinics of North America, 25*(1), 235–245.

Eland, J. (1988). Pain management and comfort. *Journal of Gerontology Nursing, 14*(4), 10–15.

Eland, J. M. (1981). Minimizing pain associated with prekindergarten intramuscular injections: Issues in comprehension. *Pediatric Nursing, 5*, 361–372.

Ferrell, B. R. (1995). The impact of pain on quality of life. *Nursing Clinics of North America, 30*, 609–624.

Hester, N. (1979). The preoperational child's reaction to immunization. *Nursing Research, 28*, 250–255.

Ieiorio, C. (1988). The management of nausea and vomiting in pregnancy. *Nurse Practitioner, 13*(5), 23–28.

Lubkin, I. M. (1995). *Chronic illness: Impact and interventions*. Boston: Jones & Bartlett.

Ludwig-Beymer, P. (1989). Transcultural aspects of pain. In J. Boyle & M. Andrews (Eds.). *Transcultural concepts in nursing*. Glenview, IL: Scott, Foresman.

Malseed, R. (1990). *Pharmacology: Drug therapy and nursing considerations*. Philadelphia: J. B. Lippincott.

McCafferty, M. (1980). *Nursing management of the patient with pain* (2nd ed.). Philadelphia: J. B. Lippincott.

McCafferty, M., & Beebe, A. (1989). *Pain: Clinical management for nursing practice*. St. Louis: C. V. Mosby.

McGuire, D., & Sheidler, V. (1993). Pain. In S. Groenwald, M. Frogge, M. Goodman, & C. Yarbo (Eds.). *Cancer nursing: Principles and practice*. Boston: Jones and Bartlett.

Miller, C. A. (1995). *Nursing care of older adults* (2nd ed.). Glenview, IL: Scott, Foresman.

Perry, S., & Heidrich, G. (1981). Placebos. *American Journal of Nursing, 81*, 721–725.

Porter, J., & Jick, H. (1980). Addiction rate in patients treated with narcotics. *New England Journal of Medicine, 302*, 123.

Rhodes, V. (1990). Nausea, vomiting and retching. *Nursing Clinics of North American, 24*, 885–890.

Rounseville, C. (1992). Phantom limb pain: The ghost that haunts the amputee. *Orthopedic Nursing, 11*(2), 67–71.

Sherman, R. (1989). Stump and phantom limb pain. *Neurological Clinics, 1*, 249–263.

Sloman, R. (1995). Relaxation and relief of cancer pain. *Nursing Clinics of North America, 30*, 697–709.

Vitale, M., Fields-Blache, C., & Luterman, A. (1991). Severe itching in the patient with burns. *Journal of Burn Care Rehabilitation, 12*(4), 33–36.

Voda, A., & Randall, M. (1982). Nausea and vomiting of pregnancy. In C. Norris (Ed.). *Concept clarification in nursing*. Rockville, MD: Aspen Systems.

Zborowski, M. (1952). Cultural components in response to pain. *Journal of Social Issues, 8*, 16–30.

Children

Berde, C. (1989). Pediatric postoperative pain management. *Pediatric Clinics of North America, 36*, 921–940.

Callen, J. P., Sturviski, M. A., & Voorhees, J. J. (1980). Cutaneous manifestations of systemic illness. In *Manual of dermatology* (pp. 129–161). Chicago: Year Book.

Chapman, L. (1991). Searching: Expectant father's experiences during labor and birth. *Journal of Perinatal and Neonatal Nursing, 4*(4), 21–29.

Eland, J. M., & Anderson, J. (1977). The experience of pain in children. In A. K. Jacox (Ed.). *Pain: A source book for nurses and other health professionals*. Boston: Little, Brown.

Hymovich, D. P., & Hagopian, G. A. (1992). *Chronic illness in children and adults: A psychological approach*. Philadelphia: W. B. Saunders.

Jackson, D. B., & Saunders, R. B. (1993). *Child health nursing*. Philadelphia: J. B. Lippincott

May, K. A., & Mahlmeister, L. R. (1994). *Maternal and neonatal nursing: Family-centered care* (3rd ed.). Philadelphia: J. B. Lippincott.

O'Brien, S., & Konsler, G. (1988). Alleviating children's postoperative pain. *Maternal-Child Nursing Journal, 13*, 183–186.

Schechter, N. (Ed.). (1989a). Acute pain in children. *Pediatric Clinics of North America, 36*, 781–1045.

Schechter, N. (1989b). Undertreatment of pain in children: An overview. *Pediatric Clinics of North America, 36*, 781–794.

Wong, D., & Baker, C. (1988). Pain in children: Comparison to assessment scales. *Pediatric Nursing, 14*(1), 9–17.

Communication, Impaired

Communication, Impaired Verbal

Communication, Impaired*

DEFINITION
Impaired Communication: The state in which the individual experiences, or is at high risk to experience, a decreased ability to send or receive messages (*i.e.*, has difficulty exchanging thoughts, ideas, or desire).

DEFINING CHARACTERISTICS
Major (Must Be Present)
    Inappropriate or absent speech or response
    Impaired ability to speak

Minor (May Be Present)
    Incongruence between verbal and nonverbal messages
    Stuttering
    Slurring
    Problem in finding the correct word when speaking
    Weak or absent voice
    Statements of not understanding or being misunderstood
    Dysarthria
    Aphasia

RELATED FACTORS
Pathophysiologic
    Related to disordered, unrealistic thinking secondary to:

Schizophrenic disorder	Psychotic disorder
Delusional disorder	Paranoid disorder

    Related to impaired motor function of muscles of speech secondary to:
    or
    Related to ischemia of temporal frontal lobe secondary to:
        Expressive or receptive aphasia
        Cerebrovascular accident
        Oral trauma
        Facial trauma
        Brain damage (*e.g.*, birth/head trauma)
        Central nervous system (CNS) depression/increased intracranial pressure
        Tumor (of the head, neck, or spinal cord)
        Chronic hypoxia/decreased cerebral blood flow
        Quadriplegia

   * Note: This diagnosis was developed by Rosalinda Alfaro-LeFevre and is not currently on the NANDA list, but is here for clarity and usefulness.

Nervous system diseases (*e.g.*, myasthenia gravis, multiple sclerosis, muscular dystrophy)

Vocal cord paralysis

Related to impaired ability to produce speech secondary to:

Respiratory impairment (*e.g.*, shortness of breath)

Laryngeal edema/infection

Oral deformities

Cleft lip or palate   Missing teeth

Malocclusion or fractured jaw   Dysarthria

Related to auditory impairment

Treatment-Related

Related to impaired ability to produce speech secondary to:

Endotracheal intubation

Tracheostomy/tracheotomy/laryngectomy

Surgery of the head, face, neck, or mouth

Pain (especially of the mouth or throat)

Lethargy secondary to CNS depressants, anesthesia

Situational (Personal, Environmental)

Related to decreased attention secondary to:

Fatigue (affecting ability to listen)

Anger

Anxiety (severe, panic)

Pain

Related to no access to hearing aid/malfunction of hearing aid

Related to psychological barrier (*e.g.*, fear, shyness)

Related to lack of privacy

Related to loss of recent memory recall

Related to unavailable interpreter

Maturational

Infant / child

Related to inadequate sensory stimulation

Older adult (auditory losses)

Related to hearing impairment

Related to cognitive impairments secondary to (specify):

Author's Note

Impaired Communication and *Impaired Verbal Communication* are diagnoses describing people who desire to communicate, but are encountering problems. *Impaired Communication* may not be useful to describe a person in whom communication problems are a manifestation of a psychiatric illness or a coping problem. If nursing interventions focus on reducing hallucinations, fear, or anxiety, the diagnosis *Fear* or *Anxiety* would be more appropriate.

Errors in Diagnostic Statements

Impaired Communication related to failure of staff to use effective communication techniques

The diagnostic statement should not be used as a vehicle to reveal a problem resulting from incorrect or insufficient nursing intervention. Instead, the nurse should write the diagnosis as *Impaired Verbal Communication related to effects of tracheotomy on ability to talk*. The care plan would specify the communication techniques to be used. Failure to use the techniques would be a nursing management issue, not a care plan problem.

Key Concepts

1. Effective communication is an interactive process involving the *mutual exchange* of information (thoughts, ideas, feelings, and perceptions) between two or more people. This process can be hampered by problems with *sending* or *receiving* messages, or both.

2. Communication is transmitted by body cues (55%), paralinguistic cues (*e.g.*, tone of voice; 38%), and words (7%) (Meharabian, 1972).

3. After survival, perhaps the most basic human need is to communicate with others. Communication provides a sense of security to clients by reinforcing that they are not alone and that there are people who will listen. Poor communication can cause feelings of frustration, anger, hostility, depression, fear, confusion, and isolation.

4. Speech represents humans' fundamental way of expressing needs, desires, and feelings. However, if only one person expresses information, without any feedback from the listener, effective communication cannot be said to have taken place.

5. Problems with *sending* information can be caused by any of the following (Braverman, 1990):
   a. Inability or failure to send messages that can be clearly understood by the listener (*e.g.*, because of language problems, word-meaning problems, failure to speak when the listener is ready to listen)
   b. Fear of being overheard, judged, or misunderstood (*e.g.*, owing to lack of privacy, confidentiality, trust, or nonjudgmental attitude)
   c. Concern over the response to what is being said (*e.g.*, "I don't want to hurt anyone's feelings or make anyone angry at me.")
   d. Use of words that "talk down" to the individual receiving the message (*e.g.*, talking to an elderly or handicapped person as if he were a child)
   e. Failure to allow sufficient time for listening to or providing feedback
   f. Physical problems that interfere with the ability to see, talk, or move

6. Problems with *receiving* information can be caused by
   a. Language or vocabulary problems
   b. Fatigue, pain, fear, anxiety, distractions, attention span problems
   c. Not realizing the importance of the information
   d. Problems that interfere with the ability to see or hear

7. The meaning of messages is affected not only by the choice of words, but by the loudness and intonation of voice, the proximity of the communicators, and the use of body language, eye contact, and gestures. Words that express *approval or acceptance* can be negated by body language, facial expressions, and eye contact that express *disapproval* (Braverman, 1990).

8. Mutual understanding of communication can be enhanced by the use of both verbal *and* written messages. Important information should be written down, mutually discussed, and made readily available for later reference.

9. Good communicators are also good listeners, who listen for both facts and feelings.

10. "Presencing," or just being present and available, even if little is said or done, can be an effective way of communicating caring for another individual (Benner, 1984).

11. Therapeutic communication begins with
    a. Offering *unconditional positive regard*, a genuine feeling of warmth for the person being helped.
    b. Caring about the other person and being free of judgment of what he thinks or feels (Barry, 1989).

12. Ongoing therapeutic communication requires
    a. A capacity for empathic understanding of the client's *internal frame of reference*. This means working to understand how the person really feels and maintaining an unbiased attitude (Barry, 1989).
    b. The ability to be genuine, human, and *real* (Barry, 1989). Jouard (1971) labels this quality *authenticity;* Brammer and Shostrom (1985) label it *transparency*.

13. Knowledge of a foreign language depends on four elements: the knowledge of how to speak the language in conversation, the ability to understand the language in conversation, the ability to read the language, and the ability to write the language.

14. Dysarthria is a disturbance in the voluntary muscular control of speech caused by conditions such as Parkinson's disease, multiple sclerosis, myasthenia gravis, cerebral palsy, and CNS damage. The same muscles are used in eating and swallowing. People with dysarthria usually do not have problems with comprehension.
15. Aphasia is an altered ability to communicate because of cerebral damage. The alterations can be verbal, gestural, visual, or graphic.
16. Expressive aphasia is a disturbance in the ability to speak, write, or gesture understandably. Receptive aphasia is a disturbance in the ability to comprehend written and spoken language.
17. The person with receptive aphasia may have intact hearing, but cannot process or is unaware of his own sounds.
18. Emotional lability (swings between crying and laughing) is common to people with aphasia. This behavior is not intentional and declines with recovery.

🌀 *Key Concepts—Child*

1. Communication with children must take into account developmental stage, language abilities, and cognitive level (Hunsberger, 1989a; Wong, 1995).
2. Communication with children involves verbal and nonverbal aspects. Although most of the verbal communication occurs between the nurse and parents, the child's verbal input should not be ignored. Writing, drawing, play, and using body language (facial expressions, gestures) are forms of nonverbal communication used by the child (Wong, 1995).
3. Play therapy can be an invaluable tool for establishing rapport and communicating true feelings.
4. In children, receptive language is always more advanced than expressive language; children understand more than they can articulate (Hunsberger, 1989a). (See Table II-11 in the diagnostic category *Growth and Development, Altered,* under Language/Cognition.)
5. Communication impairment may result from learning disability, speech impairment, or hearing loss (Wong, 1995).
6. The child with hearing loss may exhibit alterations in the following responses.
   a. Orientation response (*e.g.*, lack of startle reflex to a loud sound)
   b. Vocalizations and sound production (*e.g.*, lack of babbling by age 7 months)
   c. Visual attention (*e.g.*, responding more to facial expression than verbal explanation)
   d. Social/emotional behavior (*e.g.*, becomes irritable at inability to make self understood [Hunsberger, 1989b]).
7. Numerous screening tests are available to assist the nurse in detecting communication impairment. Appropriate referrals should be made (Wong, 1995).

🏛 *Key Concepts—Older Adult*

1. Hearing loss is the third most prevalent condition affecting institutionalized older adults, exceeded only by arthritis and hypertension (Lindblade & McDonald, 1995). Unfortunately, Medicare does not pay for hearing aids, and only 18% of elderly clients with hearing loss own hearing aids. Many deny hearing loss because of fear of pressure to buy a hearing aid.
2. Table II-3 illustrates age-related changes affecting hearing (Miller, 1995).
3. Older adults people are at higher risk for presbycusis, a progressive bilateral, symmetric hearing loss of high-pitched frequencies. This difficulty can begin in the middle years; however, most people wait for 5–10 years before seeking medical evaluation (Matteson & McConnell, 1988; Rappaport, 1984).
4. About 40% of people older than 65 years of age have a significant hearing impairment that interferes with communication in general. Prevalence data probably overestimate hearing impairment because of problems with testing; however, prevalence from 31% to 87% has been documented in the well elderly. About 90% of all nursing home residents older than 65 years have a hearing impairment (Matteson & McConnell, 1988; Voeks, Gallagher, Langer, & Drinka, 1990).
5. Reduced auditory acuity has a positive correlation with social isolation. Understanding speech in group conversations has been identified as a prime area of hearing difficulty for older individuals. Some older individuals choose to withdraw from social gatherings

Table II-3 **Age-Related Changes Affecting Hearing**

Change	Consequence
External Canal	
• Longer, thicker hair	Potential for impacted
• Thinner, drier skin	cerumen with impaired
• Increased keratin	sound conduction
Middle Ear	
• Diminished resiliency of tympanic membrane	
• Calcified, hardened ossicles	Impaired sound conduction
• Weakened and stiff muscles and ligaments	
Inner Ear and Nervous System	
• Diminished neurons, endolymph, hair cells, and blood supply	
• Degeneration of spiral ganglion and arterial blood vessels	
• Decreased flexibility of basilar membrane	**Presbycusis:** diminished ability to hear high-pitched sounds
• Narrowing of auditory meatus	especially in the presence of background noise
• Degeneration of central processing systems	

(Miller, C. A. [1995]. *Nursing care of older adults* [2nd ed.]. Glenview, IL: Scott, Foresman.)

because of the frustration they feel in asking people to repeat what has been said. Likewise, some friends and family refrain from entertaining hearing-impaired individuals because they have labeled them as distant because they do not participate in dialogue or turn their heads away during conversation. Others are thought to have mental impairments because of inappropriate comments during conversation and irritability and inattention (Vaughn, Lightfoot, & Teter, 1988; Voeks et al., 1990).

6. Many older adults were exposed to high noise levels in occupational settings before the Occupational Safety and Health Administration (OSHA) requirements for ear protection were implemented. Certain medications used in past years have since been found to produce ototoxicity and have been virtually eliminated as treatment regimens, or else now require careful dosing and monitoring. Before immunization was available against measles, many people suffered resultant hearing loss (Moon, 1990).

7. Older adults have a higher prevalence of chronic conditions that can interfere with speech or understanding of speech. Some of these conditions are Parkinson's disease (1% of individuals older than 60 years in the United States), Alzheimer's disease (15% of those older than 65 years), cerebrovascular accidents (75% of all strokes occur in individuals older than age 65 years), structural changes owing to head and neck cancer, and functional voice disorders of inadequate loudness or quality owing to vocal abuse (Matteson & McConnell, 1988).

TRANSCULTURAL CONSIDERATIONS

1. The dominant American culture has a tendency to conceal feelings and is considered a low-touch culture (Giger & Davidhizar, 1995). Difficulties can occur if the person or family does not communicate in the way or manner expected by the nurse.

continued

2. Certain gestures in the American culture have specific meanings, such as a nod or smile to indicate understanding. In some cultures, a nod is a polite response meaning I heard you, but I do not necessarily understand or agree (Giger & Davidhizar, 1995).
3. Touch is a strong form of communication. It has many meanings and can be interpreted differently. Cultural uses of touch vary, with touch between same-gender persons taboo in some cultures and expected in others (Giger & Davidhizar, 1995).
4. English, German, and American cultures do not encourage touching. Some highly tactile cultures are Spanish, Italian, French, Jewish, and South American (Giger & Davidhizar, 1995).
5. All cultures have rules about who touches whom, when, and where. The nurse should touch deliberatively, with purpose and empathy (Giger & Davidhizar, 1995).
6. In the dominant American culture, eye contact is viewed as an indication of a positive self-concept, openness, and honesty. Lack of eye contact can be viewed as low self-esteem, guilt, or lack of interest (Giger & Davidhizar, 1995).
7. Some cultures are not accustomed to eye contact, including Filipino, Oriental, American Indian, and Vietnamese (Giger & Davidhizar, 1995).
8. With people from a different culture, "humor must be used in limited and well-thought-out situations, since humor can be misinterpreted" (Giger & Davidhizar, 1995, p. 22).
9. The client and family should be encouraged to communicate their interpretations of health, illness, and health care (Giger & Davidhizar, 1995)
10. African Americans speak English with varied geographic dialects. Some African Americans pronounce certain syllables or consonants differently (*e.g., th* may be pronounced as *d,* such as "*des*" for "these"). These different pronunciations should not be viewed as substandard or ungrammatical. In addition, some slang words may have different meanings—for example, "the birth of my daughter was a real bad experience." The person may mean it was unique and positive (Dillard, 1973).
11. Mexican-Americans speak Spanish, which has more than 50 dialects; thus, a nurse who speaks Spanish may have difficulty understanding a different dialect. Both men and women are very modest, and self-disclosure is restricted to those whom they know well. Direct confrontation and arguments are considered rude; thus, agreeing may be a courtesy, not a commitment. A folk illness called *malojo* (evil eye) is thought to harm a child when the child is admired, but not touched, by a person thought to have special powers. When interacting with children, touch them lightly to avoid malojo. Kidding can be viewed as rude and deprecating (Murillo, 1978).
12. The Chinese value silence and avoid disagreeing or criticizing. Raising one's voice is associated with anger and loss of control. Americans naturally raise their voice to make a point. "No" is rarely used, and "yes" can mean "perhaps" or "no." Touching someone's head is a serious breach of etiquette. Chinese speech is dominated by hesitation, ambiguity, and subtlety (Giger & Davidhizar, 1995).

Focus Assessment Criteria

Subjective Data

A. Assess for defining characteristics
   1. Note the usual pattern of communication as described by the person or family

Very verbal	Responds inappropriately
Sometimes verbal	Does not speak/respond
Uses sign language	Speaks only when spoken to
Writes only	Gestures only

   a. Does the person feel he is communicating normally today?
   b. If not, what does he feel may help him to communicate better?
   c. Is there a specific person he would like to talk with or have present to help him express ideas?
   2. Do you have trouble hearing?

Describe your hearing problem	Have you ever tried a hearing aid?
Both ears or one	Family history of hearing loss?
How long? gradual? sudden?	History of exposure to loud noises

3. How does the person/family describe ability to communicate in the past?
   Usually communicated well
   Sometimes had difficulty communicating
   Frequently had difficulty communicating
   Needed assistance (specify)

B. Assess for related factors
   1. Does the person feel there are barriers hindering his ability to communicate?
      Lack of privacy
      Fear of uncertain origin
      Fear of being inappropriate or "stupid"
      Not enough time to gather thoughts and ask questions
      Need for presence of significant other or familiar face
      Language, dialect, or cultural barrier (specify)
      Lack of knowledge of subject being discussed
      Pain, stress, or fatigue

Objective Data
A. Assess for defining characteristics
   1. Describe ability to form words
      Not able   Fair   Good
   2. Specify problems:
      Slurred speech   Voice weakness (whisper)
      Lisping   Language barrier
      Stuttering
   3. Describe the person's ability to comprehend
      Follows simple commands or ideas
      Able to follow complex instructions or ideas
      Sometimes able to follow instructions or ideas
      Not able to follow simple instructions or ideas
      Follows commands and ideas only if hearing aid is working
      Follows commands and ideas only if he can see your mouth (lip-reads)
      Talks, rather than listens
   4. What is the person's developmental age?
      Child   Adult
      Adolescent   Aged
   5. Describe ability to make sentences
      Good   Nonsensical or confused
      Slow   Can make short, simple sentences
      Not able   Language barrier
      Unclear ideas
   6. Does the person maintain eye contact?
      Yes   Rarely
      No   Blind/impaired vision
      Occasionally
   7. Hearing loss (check each ear separately)
      External ear: deformities, lesions, lumps or tenderness
      Middle and inner ear: cerumen, discharge, redness, swelling
      Auditory acuity: Can hear ticking watch or whispered words
      With decreased hearing: Weber and Rinne test results

B. Assess for related factors
   1. Barriers:
      Difficulty swallowing
      Tracheostomy
      Endotracheal tube

2. How does the person's affect or manner appear to you?

Nervous   Flat
Anxious   Angry
Attentive   Uncomfortable
Fearful   Comfortable
Withdrawn

3. Are there contributing factors that may inhibit the person's ability to communicate (see Related Factors)?

Outcome Criteria

The person will
• Demonstrate increased ability to understand
• Demonstrate improved ability to express himself
• Relate decreased frustration with communication

Interventions

A. Identify a method the person can use to communicate basic needs

1. Assess ability to comprehend, speak, read, and write.
2. Provide alternative methods of communication.
   a. Use pad and pencil, alphabet letters, hand signals, eye blinks, head nods, bell signals.
   b. Make flash cards with pictures or words depicting frequently used phrases (*e.g.,* "Wet my lips," "Move my foot," glass of water, bedpan).
   c. Encourage person to point, use gestures, and pantomime.
   d. Consult with speech pathologist for assistance in acquiring flash cards.

B. Identify factors that promote communication

1. Create atmosphere of acceptance and privacy.
2. Provide a nonrushed environment.
   a. Use normal loudness level and speak slowly in short phrases.
   b. Encourage to take time talking and to enunciate words carefully with good lip movements.
   c. Decrease external distractions.
   d. Delay conversation when the person is tired.
3. Assess the individual's frustration level and do not push beyond it.
   a. Estimate 30 seconds of passed time before providing the individual with the word he may be trying to find (except when the person is frustrated or needs the request immediately, *e.g.,* bedpan).
   b. Provide cues through pictures or gestures.
4. Use techniques to increase understanding.
   a. Face the individual and establish eye contact if possible.
   b. Use uncomplicated one-step commands and directives.
   c. Have only one person talk (it is more difficult to follow a multisided conversation).
   d. Encourage the use of gestures and pantomime.
   e. Match words with actions; use pictures.
   f. Terminate conversation on a note of success (*e.g.,* move back to an easier item).
   g. Validate that message is understood.

C. Initiate health teaching and referrals, if needed

1. Seek consultation with a speech or audiology specialist.

Rationale

- Using an alternative form of communication can help decrease anxiety and feelings of isolation and alienation, promote a sense of control over the situation, and enhance safety (Sawyer & Brugd, 1990).
- Communication is the core of all human relations. Impaired ability to communicate spontaneously is frustrating and embarrassing. Nursing actions should focus on decreasing the tension and conveying an understanding of how difficult the situation must be for the client (Boss, 1991).
- The nurse should make every attempt to understand the client. Each success, regardless of how minor, decreases frustration and increases motivation (Boss, 1991).

Interventions—*Child Focus*

1. Use age-appropriate words and gestures (see *Altered Growth and Development*, Table II-11).
2. Initially talk to parent and allow child to observe. Gradually include child.
   a. Approach the child slowly and speak in a quiet, unhurried, confident voice.
   b. Assume an eye-level position.
   c. Use simple words and short sentences.
   d. Talk about something not related to present situation (*e.g.*, school, toy, hair, clothes).
3. Offer choices when possible.
4. Encourage to share concerns and fears.
5. Allow children an opportunity to touch and use articles (*e.g.*, stethoscope, tongue blade).
6. Do not use analogies with small children (*e.g.*, "The injection will feel like a little stick in your arm.").
7. With adolescents (Wong, 1995)
   a. Provide for time alone.
   b. Avoid criticizing or judging.
   c. Don't overreact.
   d. Use techniques that promote sharing.
      "What if?" (*e.g.*, what if a friend of yours told you he was going to kill himself?)
      What do you like best (least) about yourself?
      Reflect back the feelings and content of their statements.
      Listen more than talk.

Rationale

- Listening carefully will allow cues to be picked up about what are issues for the child or adolescent.
- The initial interaction sets the tone for the rest of the interactions with the child and family (Johnson, 1995).
- Use of open-ended, nonjudgmental style can reduce suspicions (Johnson, 1995).
- Criticizing or lecturing does not promote an understanding of risk behaviors (Joffe, 1994).
- Successful communication depends on the ability of the nurse to involve the adolescent in discussions (Jackson & Saunders, 1993).
- Adolescents need opportunities to demonstrate their independence and to appraise options accurately (Wong, 1995).

■ Impaired Communication
Related to Effects of Hearing Loss

Outcome Criteria

The person will
- Wear a hearing aid (if appropriate)
- Receive messages through alternative methods (*e.g.*, written communication, sign language, speaking distinctly into "good" ear)
- Relate/demonstrate an improved ability to communicate

Interventions

A. Elicit what mode of communication is desired and record on care plan the method to be used by staff and by person
   1. Writing
   2. Speech-reading (or lip-reading)
   3. Speaking
   4. Sign language

B. Assess ability to receive verbal messages
   1. If he can hear with a hearing aid, make sure that it is on and functioning.
      a. Check batteries by turning volume all the way up until it whistles. (If it does not whistle, new batteries should be inserted.)
      b. Make sure volume is at a level that enhances hearing. (Many people with hearing aids turn the volume down from time to time for peace and quiet.)
      c. Make a special effort to have the person wear his hearing aid on off-the-unit visits (*e.g.*, special studies, or the operating room).
   2. If he can hear with only one ear, speak slowly and *clearly* directly into the good ear. (It is more important to speak *distinctly* than to speak loudly.)
      a. If the person is admitted to the hospital, place him so that his good ear faces the door.
      b. Approach the person from the side on which he hears best (*e.g.*, if he hears better with his left ear, approach him from the left).
   3. If the person can speech-read:
      a. Look directly at the person and talk slowly and clearly.
      b. Avoid standing in front of light—have the light on your face so that the person can see your lips.
      c. Minimize distractions that may inhibit the person's concentration.
         Minimize conversations if the person is fatigued or use written communication.
         Reinforce important communications by writing them down.
   4. If he can read and write, provide pad and pencil at all times (even when he goes to the radiology department, and so forth).
   5. If he can understand only sign language, have an interpreter with him as much as possible. Address all communication to the person, not to the interpreter (*e.g.*, do not say "ask Mrs. Jones . . ."). Record name and phone number of interpreter(s) on the care plan.
   6. If the person is in a group (*e.g.*, diabetes class), place him in the front of the room near the instructor or send interpreter with him.

C. Use factors that promote hearing and understanding
1. Talk distinctly and clearly, facing the person.
2. Minimize unnecessary sounds in the room:
   a. Have only one person talk.
   b. Be aware of background noises (*e.g.*, close the door, turn off the television or radio).
3. Repeat, then rephrase a thought, if the person does not seem to understand the whole meaning.
4. Use touch and gestures to enhance communication.
5. Encourage the person to maintain contact with other deaf people to minimize feelings of social isolation.
6. Write as well as speak all important messages.
7. Validate the person's understanding by asking questions that require more than "yes" or "no" answers. Avoid asking "Do you understand?"

D. Initiate referrals as needed
1. Seek consultation with a speech or audiology specialist.

Rationale

- People who suffer from deafness are prone to social isolation because of their difficulty in communicating with people who can hear normally.
- Hearing aids magnify *all* sounds. Therefore, extraneous sounds (*e.g.*, rustling of papers, minor squeaks) can inhibit understanding of voiced messages.
- Deafness can disrupt the reciprocal relationship necessary in the health care process.
- Many deaf people do not know their medical histories or medical terminology. It has been reported that 32.9% of deaf respondents reported that they only understood some or very little of what hospital staff said.
- Speech-reading is difficult and fatiguing in the hospital. Unfamiliar terminology, anxiety, and poor lighting all can contribute to errors.
- Writing messages is slow, causing a tendency to abbreviate content. Moreover, expressing emotions in writing is difficult.
- The following are available or will soon be available to the hearing impaired:
  - DEAFNET, a computer system under development that will allow clients to type messages that will be received by a computer at the phone company, which translates the messages into a verbal message by a voice synthesizer (Lindblade & McDonald, 1995)
  - Telecommunication devices (known as TDD) that operate by communicating electronically messages that are typed, infrared systems, computers, voice amplifiers, amplified telephones, low-frequency doorbells and telephone ringers, closed-caption TV decoders, flashing alarm clocks, flashing smoke detectors, hearing aids, and lip reading and signing instruction (Lindblade & McDonald, 1995)
  - Deaf service centers available in most communities to help with housing, job seeking, travel arrangements, recreation, and adult education opportunities
  - Hearing Access 2000, a national program to promote access to communications options for the hearing impaired
- Only 18%–20% of older adults with hearing impairments wear hearing aids. Those who wear hearing aids must be encouraged to use them consistently, clean and maintain them, and replace batteries. They should be assertive in letting significant others know about situations and environmental areas in which they experience difficulty with enhancement of background noise while wearing the aid (Ayers, 1990; Moon, 1990).

■ Impaired Communication
Related to Effects of Aphasia on Expression or Interpretation

Aphasia is a communication impairment—a difficulty in expressing, a difficulty in understanding, or a combination of both—resulting from cerebral impairments.

Outcome Criteria

The person will
- Demonstrate increased ability to understand
- Demonstrate improved ability to express himself
- Relate decreased frustration with communication

Interventions

A. Use techniques that enhance verbal expression
1. Make a concerted effort to understand when the person is speaking.
    a. Allow enough time to listen if the person speaks slowly.
    b. Rephrase messages aloud to validate what was said.
    c. Acknowledge when you understand, and do not be concerned with imperfect pronunciation at first.
    d. Ignore mistakes and profanity.
    e. Do not pretend you understand if you do not.
    f. Observe nonverbal cues for validation (*e.g.*, he answers yes and shakes his head no).
    g. Allow the person time to respond; do not interrupt; supply words only occasionally.
2. Teach techniques to improve speech.
    a. Ask to slow speech down and say each word clearly, while providing the example.
    b. Encourage to speak in short phrases.
    c. Explain that his words are not clearly understood (*e.g.*, "I can't understand what you are saying.").
    d. Suggest a slower rate of talking, or taking a breath before beginning to speak.
    e. Ask to write down his message, or to draw a picture, if verbal communication is difficult.
    f. Focus on the present; avoid topics that are controversial, emotional, abstract, or lengthy.
3. Explain the benefits of daily speech improvement. Consult with speech therapist for specific exercises.

B. Acknowledge the individual's frustration
1. Verbally address the problem of frustration over inability to communicate, and explain that patience is needed for both the nurse and the person who is trying to talk.
2. Maintain a calm, positive attitude (*e.g.*, "I can understand you if we work at it.").
3. Use reassurance (*e.g.*, "I know it's hard, but you'll get it"); use touch if acceptable.

4. Maintain a sense of humor.

5. Allow tears (*e.g.*, "It's OK. I know it's frustrating. Crying can let it all out.").

6. For the person who has a limited ability to talk (*i.e.*, can make simple requests, but not lengthy statements), encourage writing letters or keeping a diary to ventilate feelings and share concerns.

7. Give the person opportunities to make decisions about his care (*e.g.*, "Do you want a drink? Would you rather have orange juice or prune juice?").

8. Provide alternative methods of self-expression
   a. Humming/singing
   b. Dancing/exercising/walking
   c. Writing/drawing/painting/coloring
   d. Helping (tasks such as opening mail, choosing meals)

C. Identify factors that promote comprehension

1. Assess hearing ability and use of functioning hearing aids.

2. Assess ability to see, and encourage the person to wear his glasses.
   a. Explain to the person that seeing better will increase understanding of what is happening around him.
   b. Even if the person is blind, look at him when talking to "throw" voice in his direction.

3. Provide sufficient light and remove distractions (see *Sensory-Perceptual Alterations*).

4. Speak when the person is ready to listen.
   a. Achieve eye contact, if possible.
   b. Gain the person's attention by a gentle touch on the arm and a verbal message of "Listen to me" or "I want to talk to you."

5. Modify your speech.
   Speak slowly, enunciate distinctly.
   Use common adult words.
   Do not change subjects or ask multiple questions in succession.
   Repeat or rephrase requests.
   Do not increase volume of voice unless person has a hearing deficit.
   Match your nonverbal behavior with your verbal actions to avoid misinterpretation (*e.g.*, do not laugh with a coworker while performing a task).
   Try to use the same words with the same task (*e.g.*, bathroom vs. toilet, pill vs. medication).
   Keep a record at bedside of the words to maintain continuity.
   As the person improves, allow him to complete your sentences (*e.g.*, "This is a . . . [pill]").

6. Use multiple methods of communication.
   a. Use pantomime
   b. Point
   c. Use flash cards
   d. Show him what you mean (*e.g.*, pick up a glass)
   e. Write key words on a card, so he can practice them while you show the object (*e.g.*, paper, toilet)

D. Show respect when providing care

1. Avoid discussing the person's condition in his presence; assume he can understand despite his deficits.

2. Monitor other health care providers.

3. Talk to the person whenever you are with him.

E. Initiate health teaching and referrals, if indicated
   1. Teach communication techniques and repetitive approaches to significant others.
   2. Encourage the family to share feelings concerning communication problems.
      a. Explain the reasons for labile emotions and profanity.
      b. Explain the need to include the person in family decision making.
   3. Seek consultation with a speech pathologist early in treatment regimen.

Rationale

- Communication is the core of all human relations. Impaired ability to communicate spontaneously is frustrating and embarrassing. Nursing actions should focus on decreasing the tension and conveying an understanding of how difficult the situation must be for the client (Boss, 1991).
- The nurse should make every attempt to understand the client. Each success, regardless of how minor, decreases frustration and increases motivation (Boss, 1991).
- Deliberate actions can be taken to improve speech. As speech improves, confidence increases and more attempts at speaking are made.
- Improving the client's comprehension can help decrease frustration and increase trust. Tone of voice can be correctly interpreted by aphasic clients (Boss, 1991).
- Daily exercises help improve the efficiency of speech musculature and increase rate, volume, and articulation.

■ Impaired Communication
Related to Foreign Language Barrier

Outcome Criteria

The person will
- Be able to communicate needs and concerns
- Relate feelings of acceptance, reduced frustration, and isolation

---

Interventions

A. Assess ability to communicate in English*
   1. Assess what language the person speaks best.
   2. Assess the person's ability to read, write, speak, and comprehend English.
   3. Do not evaluate understanding based on "yes" or "no" responses.

B. Identify factors that promote communication through a language barrier when a translator is not present
   1. Face the person and give a pleasant greeting, in a normal tone of voice.
   2. Talk clearly and somewhat slower than normal (do not overdo it).

* English will be used as an example of the dominant language.

3. If the person does not understand or speak (respond), use an alternative method of communication.
   a. Try writing down message.
   b. Use gestures or actions.
   c. Use pictures or drawings.
   d. Make flash cards that translate words or phrases.
4. Encourage the person to teach others some of the words or greetings of his own language (this helps to promote a feeling of acceptance and a willingness to learn).
5. Do not correct a client's or family's pronunciation.
6. Clarify the exact meaning of a word that is unclear.
7. Use medical terms and the slang word when indicated (*e.g.*, vomiting/throwing up).

C. Be cognizant of possible cultural barriers
   1. Be careful when touching the person, for it may not be appropriate in some cultures.
   2. Be aware of the different ways that men and women are expected to be treated (cultural differences may influence whether a man speaks to a woman about certain matters, or vice versa).
   3. Make a conscious effort to be nonjudgmental about another's cultural differences.
   4. Make note of what seems to be a comfortable distance from which to speak.

D. Initiate referrals, when needed
   1. Use a *fluent* translator when discussing matters of importance (such as taking a health history or signing an operation permit).
   2. If possible, allow the translator to spend as much time as the person wishes (be flexible with visitors' rules and regulations).
   3. If a translator is not available, try to plan a daily visit from someone who has some knowledge of the person's language (many hospitals and social welfare offices keep a "language" bank with names and phone numbers of people who are willing to translate).
   4. Use AT&T telephone translating system when necessary.

Rationale

- An answer of "yes" from a foreigner may be an effort to please, rather than a sign of understanding what has been said.
- Even though the nurse cannot speak another's language, she can convey a climate of acceptance by talking in a pleasant tone of voice and using actions to demonstrate meaning (*e.g.*, smiling and motioning to sit down, while saying, "Sit down, please.")
- An attempt on the nurse's part to communicate over a language barrier encourages a foreign individual to do the same.
- People should overcome the human tendency either to ignore or shout at people who do not speak the dominant language.
- Be aware that when one learns a language, one usually learns only one meaning for a word. Some words have more than one meaning, such as "discharge" and "pupil."
- During the initial assessment start with general questions. Allow time for the person to talk even if it is not related. Use nondirect, open-ended questions when possible. Delay asking very personal questions, if possible.
- "An interpreter must have transcultural sensitivity, understand how to impart knowledge, and understand how to be a patient advocate to represent the

patient's needs to the nurse. Interpreting with cultural sensitivity is much more complex than simply putting words in another language" (Giger & Davidhizar, 1995, p. 26).

- Appropriate distance between communicators varies from culture to culture. Some may normally stand face to face, whereas others must stand several feet apart to be comfortable.
- Communicating through the use of touch or holding varies from culture to culture. For example, some cultures view touching as an extremely familiar gesture, some cultures shy away from touching a given part of the body (a pat on the head may be offensive), and some cultures consider it appropriate for men to kiss each other and for women to hold hands.

Communication, Impaired Verbal

DEFINITION

Impaired Verbal Communication: The state in which the individual experiences, or is at high risk to experience, a decreased ability to speak but can understand others.

DEFINING CHARACTERISTICS
Major (One Must Be Present)

Inability to speak words but can understand others
Articulation or motor planning deficits

Minor (May Be Present)

Shortness of breath

RELATED FACTORS

See *Impaired Communication*

Key Concepts
See *Impaired Communication*

Focus Assessment Criteria

See *Impaired Communication*

Outcome Criteria

The person will
- Demonstrate improved ability to express self
- Relate decreased frustration with communication

Interventions

A. Identify a method by which person can communicate basic needs

  1. Assess ability to comprehend, speak, read, and write.
  2. Provide alternative methods of communication.
     a. Use pad and pencil, alphabet letters, hand signals, eye blinks, head nods, bell signals.
     b. Make flash cards with pictures or words depicting frequently used phrases (*e.g.*, "Wet my lips," "Move my foot," glass of water, bedpan).
     c. Encourage to point, use gestures, and pantomime.
     d. Consult with a speech pathologist for assistance in acquiring flash cards.

B. Identify factors that promote communication

  1. For individuals with dysarthria
     a. Reduce environmental noise to increase the caregiver's ability to listen to words (*e.g.*, radio, TV).
     b. Do not alter your speech or messages, because person's comprehension is not affected; speak on an adult level.
     c. Encourage the person to make a conscious effort to slow down his speech and to speak louder (*e.g.*, "Take a deep breath between sentences.").
     d. Ask him to repeat words that are unclear; observe for nonverbal cues to help understanding.
     e. If he is tired, ask questions that require only short answers.
     f. If speech is unintelligible, teach the person to use gestures, written messages, and communication cards.
  2. For individuals who cannot speak (*e.g.*, endotracheal intubation, tracheostomy)
     Reassure that his speech will return, if it will.
     If not, explain what alternatives are available (*e.g.*, esophageal speech, sign language).
     Do not alter your speech, tone, or type of message, because the person's ability to understand is not affected; speak on an adult level.
     Read lips for cues.

C. Promote continuity of care to reduce frustration

  1. Observe for signs of frustration or withdrawal.
     a. Verbally address the problem of frustration over inability to communicate, and explain that patience is needed for both the nurse and the person who is trying to talk.
     b. Maintain a calm, positive attitude (*e.g.*, "I can understand you if we work at it.").
     c. Use reassurance (*e.g.*, "I know it's hard, but you'll get it").
     d. Maintain a sense of humor.
     e. Allow tears (*e.g.*, "It's OK. I know it's frustrating. Crying can let it all out.").
     f. For the person who has a limited ability to talk (*e.g.*, can make simple requests, but not lengthy statements), encourage writing letters or keeping a diary to ventilate feelings and share concerns.
     g. Anticipate needs and ask questions that need a simple yes or no answer.
  2. Maintain a specific care plan.
     a. Write the method of communication that is used (*e.g.*, "Uses word cards," "Points to night stand for bedpan").
     b. Record directions for specific measures to reduce communication problems (*e.g.*, allow him to keep urinal in bed).

D. Initiate health teaching and referrals, as indicated

  1. Teach communication techniques and repetitive approaches to significant others.
  2. Encourage the family to share feelings concerning communication problems.
  3. Seek consultation with a speech pathologist early in the treatment regimen.

Rationale

See *Impaired Communication*

🎗 Interventions—*Child Focus*

1. Establish a method of communication appropriate for age.
2. If a young child is deprived of vocalization, teach sign language to the child, caregivers, and staff (Hall & Weatherly, 1989).
3. Focus on basic signs initially (time, food, family relationships, emotions, animals, numbers, frequent requests).
4. Consult with a speech pathologist for assistance.
5. Discuss with parents or caregivers the importance of providing the child with a method of communication.

Rationale

- Children who cannot vocalize are at risk for delays in receptive and expressive language development (*i.e.*, vocal speech, voice production [Hall & Weatherly, 1989]).
- Communication promotes bonding and attachment with the child's caregiver as the primary social reinforcer (Hall & Weatherly, 1989).
- The ability to communicate with people in their environment increases the child's independence, self-esteem, and self-actualization (Hall & Weatherly, 1989).

References/Bibliography

Ayers, R. E. (1990). Getting the job done: Helping hands in geriatric primary care. *Geriatrics, 45*(2), 78.

Barry, P. (1989). *Psychosocial nursing* (2nd ed.). Philadelphia: J. B. Lippincott.

Benner, P. (1984). *From novice to expert*. Menlo Park, CA: Addison-Wesley.

Boss, B. (1991). Managing communication disorder in stroke. *Nursing Clinics of North America, 26*, 985–996.

Brammer, L., & Shostrom, E. (1985). *Therapeutic psychology: Fundamentals of actualization counseling and psychotherapy* (2nd ed.). Englewood Cliffs, NJ: Prentice-Hall.

Braverman, B. (1990). Eliciting assessment data from the patient who is difficult to interview. *Nursing Clinics of North America, 25*, 743–750.

Connolly, M., & Shekleton, M. (1991). Communicating with ventilator dependent patients. *Dimensions of Critical Care Nursing, 10*, 115–122.

Cunliffe, P. (1989). Communicating with children in the intensive care unit . . . triadic relationship of child/parent/nurse. *Intensive Care Nurse, 3*(2), 71–77.

Dillard, J. L. (1973). *Black English*. New York: Vintage Books.

Dugan, D. (1989). Symbolic expressions of dying patients: Communication, not hallucination. *Nursing Forum, 24*(2), 18–27.

Ebersole, P., & Hess, P. (1990). *Toward healthy aging: Human needs and nursing response*. St. Louis: C. V. Mosby.

Foster, S. (1988). When the message gets garbled. *American Journal of Maternal–Child Nursing, 13*, 367.

Geissier, E. (1995). Culture and the nurse-patient dyad. *MEDSURG Nursing, 4*, 4, 55–56.

Giger, J. N., & Davidhizar, R. E. (1995). *Transcultural nursing: Assessment and interventions* (2nd ed.). St. Louis: Mosby Year Book.

Hall, S., & Weatherly, K. S. (1989). Using sign language with tracheotomized infants and children. *Pediatric Nursing, 15*, 362–367.

Hunsberger, M. (1989a). Communicating with children and families. In R. L. Foster, M. M. Hunsberger, & J. J. T. Andreson (Eds.). *Family-centered nursing care of children*. Philadelphia: W. B. Saunders.

Hunsberger, M. (1989b). Nursing strategies: Sensory and communication alterations. In R. L. Foster, M. M. Hunsberger, & J. J. T. Andreson (Eds.). *Family-centered nursing care of children*. Philadelphia: W. B. Saunders.

Jackson, D. B., & Saunders, R. B. (1993). *Child health nursing*. Philadelphia: J. B. Lippincott.

Johnson, B. (1995). *Child, adolescent, and family psychiatric nursing*. Philadelphia: J. B. Lippincott.

Joffe, A. (1994). Adolescent medicine. In F. Oski (Ed.). *Principles and practice of pediatrics* (2nd ed.). Philadelphia: J. B. Lippincott.

Jouard, S. (1971). *The transparent self*. New York: Van Nostrand Reinhold.

Kuster, J. (1993). Experience a day of conductive hearing loss. *Journal of School Health, 65*, 235–237.

Lindblade, D., & McDonald, M. (1995). Removing communication barriers for the hearing-impaired elderly. *MEDSURG Nursing, 4*, 379–385.

Magilvy, J. K. (1985). Quality of life of hearing-impaired older women. *Nursing Research, 34*, 140–144.

Marr, J. (1991). The experience of living with Parkinson's disease. *Journal of Neuroscience Nursing, 23*, 325–329.

Matteson, A. M., & McConnell, E. S. (1988). *Gerontological nursing: Concepts and practice.* Philadelphia: W. B. Saunders.

Meharabian, A. (1972). *Nonverbal communication.* Chicago: Aldine.

Miller, C. A. (1995). *Nursing care of older adults* (2nd ed.). Glenview, IL: Scott, Foresman.

Moon, E. (1990). Otology. In C. K. Cassel, D. E. Riesenberg, L. B. Sorensen, & J. R. Walsh (Eds.). *Geriatric medicine* (2nd ed.). New York: Springer-Verlag.

Murillo, N. (1978). The Mexican-American family in California. In M. J. Hernandez & N. N. Wagner (Eds.). *Chicanos: Social and psychological perspectives.* St. Louis: C. V. Mosby.

Padgett, R. (1995). Registered nurses' perceptions of their communication with Spanish speaking migrant farm workers in North Carolina: An exploratory study. *Public Health Nurse, 9*(3), 193–197.

Rappaport, B. Z. (1984). Audiology. In C. K. Cassel & J. R. Walsh (Eds.). *Geriatric medicine: Medical, psychiatric and pharmacological topics.* New York: Springer-Verlag.

Sawyer, D. L., & Brugd, M. (1990). Care of the patient having radical neck dissection or permanent laryngostomy: A nursing diagnostic approach. *Focus on Critical Care, 17,* 166–173.

Vaughn, G. R., Lightfoot, R. K., & Teter, D. L. (1988). Assistive listening devices and systems enhance the lifestyles of hearing impaired persons. *American Journal of Otology, 9*(Suppl), 101–106.

Voeks, S. K., Gallagher, C. M., Langer, E. H., & Drinka, P. J. (1990). Hearing loss in the nursing home: An institutional issue. *Journal of the American Geriatrics Society, 38,* 141–145.

Wong, D. L. (1995). *Nursing care of infants and children* (5th ed.). St. Louis: Mosby.

Resources for the Consumer

Agency for Hearing Loss. Write: Alexander Graham Bell Association, 3417 Volta Place NW, Washington, DC 20007.

American Annals of Deaf, 814 Thayer Ave, Silver Spring, MD 20910.

Faber, A., & Malish, E. (1980). *How to talk so kids will listen and listen so kids will talk.* New York: Rawson, Wade.

Resource Guide for Persons with Speech, Language or Hearing Impairments, P.O. Box 2150, Atlanta, GA 30301-2150.

Confusion

Acute Confusion

Chronic Confusion

Confusion*

DEFINITION

Confusion: The state in which the individual experiences or is at risk of experiencing a disturbance in cognition, attention, memory and orientation, of an undetermined origin or onset.

DEFINING CHARACTERISTICS
Major (Must Be Present)

Disturbances of:

Consciousness	Memory
Attention	Orientation
Perception	Thinking
Sleep–wake cycle	

Psychomotor behavior (reaction time, speed of movement, flow of speech, involuntary movements, handwriting)

Minor (May Be Present)

Misperceptions
Hypervigilance
Agitation

Author's Note

This author has added *Confusion* to the diagnostic list to provide the nurse with an option when the origins, onset, or duration of the confusion is unknown. By providing this diagnostic option, the nurse can refrain from too quickly labeling the confusion as acute or chronic. Careful assessment is indicated. Until data collection is complete, the diagnosis can be written as *Confusion related to unknown etiology as evidenced by* (specify supporting data).

---

* This diagnosis is not currently on the NANDA list but has been included for clarity and usefulness.

Acute Confusion

DEFINITION

Acute Confusion: The state in which there is an abrupt onset of a cluster of global, fluctuating disturbances in consciousness, attention, perception, memory, orientation, thinking, sleep–wake cycle, and psychomotor behavior (American Psychiatric Association [APA], 1994).

DEFINING CHARACTERISTICS
Major (Must Be Present)

Abrupt onset of a cluster of fluctuating disturbances of:

Consciousness	Orientation
Attention	Thinking
Perception	Sleep–wake cycle
Memory	

Psychomotor behavior (reaction time, speed of movement, flow of speech, involuntary movements, handwriting)

Minor (May Be Present)

Hypervigilance
Hallucinations
Illusions

RISK FACTORS

Presence of risk factors (see Related Factors)

RELATED FACTORS

Related to cerebral hypoxia or disturbance in cerebral metabolism secondary to (Miller, 1995):

(Fluid and electrolyte disturbances)

Dehydration	Hypokalemia
Volume depletion	Hyponatremia/hypernatremia
Acidosis/alkalosis	Hypoglycemia/hyperglycemia
Hypercalcemia	

(Nutritional deficiencies)

Folate or vitamin B_{12} deficiency	Niacin deficiency
Anemia	Magnesium deficiency

(Cardiovascular disturbances)

Myocardial infarction	Heart block
Congestive heart failure	Temporal arteritis
Dysrhythmias	

(Respiratory disorders)

Chronic obstructive pulmonary disease	Tuberculosis
Pulmonary embolism	Pneumonia

(Infections)

Sepsis	Urinary tract infection
Meningitis, encephalitis	

(Metabolic and endocrine disorders)

Hypothyroidism/hyperthyroidism	Postural hypotension
Hypopituitarism/hyperpituitarism	Hypothermia/hyperthermia
Parathyroid disorders	Hepatic or renal failure
Hypoadrenocorticism/hyperadrenocorticism	

(Central nervous system disorders)

Multiple infarctions	Head trauma
Parkinson's disease	Tumors
Neurosyphilis	Seizures and postconvulsive states
Alzheimer's disease	Normal pressure hydrocephalus

(Collagen and rheumatoid disease)

Polymyalgia rheumatica	Periarteritis nodosa
Temporal arteritis	Lupus erythematosus

Treatment-Related

Related to a disturbance in cerebral metabolism secondary to:
  Surgery
  Therapeutic drug intoxication
    Neuroleptics
    Narcotics
  General anesthesia
  Side effects of medication

Diuretics	Phenothiazines
Digitalis	Barbiturates
Propranolol	Methyldopa
Atropine	Disulfiram
Oral hypoglycemics	Lithium
Antiinflammatory agents	Phenytoin
Anticholinergics	Antianxiety agents
Over-the-counter cold, cough, and sleeping preparations	

Situational (Personal, Environmental)

Related to disturbance in cerebral metabolism secondary to:
  Withdrawal from alcohol
  Withdrawal from sedatives, hypnotics
  Heavy metal or carbon monoxide intoxication
Related to:

Pain	Immobility
Bowel impaction	Depression

Related to chemical intoxications (specify):

Alcohol	Opiates
Cocaine	Barbiturates
Amphetamines	Hallucinogenics

Author's Note

The addition of *Acute Confusion* and *Chronic Confusion* to the NANDA list provides the nurse with more diagnostic clarity than using *Altered Thought Processes. Acute Confusion* has an abrupt onset with fluctuations of symptoms; *Chronic Confusion* describes long-standing or progressive degeneration. *Altered Thought Processes* is also a disruption of cognitive processes; however, the causes are coping problems or personality disorders.

Errors in Diagnostic Statement

Acute Confusion related to advanced age

   This diagnosis does not represent an understanding of confusion, aging, and its effects on cognition. An aged person who is confused could have a variety of reasons for confusion (*e.g.*, electrolytic imbalance, fever, cerebral infarctions, or Alzheimer's disease). This individual needs a medical and nursing assessment. Before the causes are known, this diagnosis can be stated as *Chronic Confusion related to unknown etiology.*

Key Concepts

1. "Confusion" is a term frequently used by nurses to describe an array of cognitive impairments. "Identifying a person as confused is just an initial step" (Rasin, 1990).
2. Confusion is a physiopsychological concept that indicates a disturbance in cerebral metabolism. A reduction in cerebral metabolism reduces neurotransmitter levels in the brain, especially acetylcholine and epinephrine. Acetylcholine is necessary for attention, learning, memory, and information processing (Rasin, 1990).
3. Confusion is defined as a disturbance in consciousness, attention, perception, memory, orientation, thinking, sleep–wake cycle, and psychomotor ability. Confusion is classified as acute (reversible, fluctuating, transient) or chronic (irreversible, long-standing, progressive) (APA, 1994).
4. Acute confusion can be caused by transient biochemical imbalances, by a stress response to environment, or by a loss of pattern or meaning.
5. Chronic confusion is caused by progressive degeneration of the cerebral cortex. The diseases causing degeneration of the cerebral cortex are varied but manifest similar behavioral disturbances. Alzheimer's disease causes about 60% of chronic confusion, whereas multiple infarctions or strokes cause about 10% of the pathology labeled multiinfarct disease (MID). Another 17% of dementing illness is caused by a combination of senile dementia of Alzheimer's type (SDAT) and MID. The remaining 13% of chronic confusion is caused by rare and occasionally reversible conditions such as Pick's disease, Creutzfeldt-Jakob disease, and chronic chemical intoxication (*e.g.*, alcohol, lead, opioids, cocaine) (Hall, 1991).
6. People with progressive dementia exhibit three types of behaviors (Hall, 1991; Hall & Bookwalter, 1987):
    a. *Baseline:* is cognitively accessible, calm, socially accessible. Can communicate needs and responds to others.
    b. *Anxious:* occurs when person feels stress. Eye contact is lost. Increase in psychomotor activity occurs as person attempts to avoid offending stimuli.
    c. *Dysfunctional:* if stress level is increased or allowed to continue, catastrophic behavior results (*e.g.*, confusion, purposeful wandering, panic, agitation, combativeness).
7. As the disease progresses, baseline behavior is replaced increasingly with anxious and dysfunctional behavior (Hall, 1991).

Key Concepts—Older Adult

1. Thinking ability, arithmetic ability, memory, judgment, and problem solving are measured in older adults to give a general index of overall cognitive ability. Short-term memory may decline somewhat, but long-term memory often remains intact (Miller, 1995).
2. Intelligence does not alter, perhaps until the very later years, but the person needs more time to process information. Reaction time increases as well. There may be some difficulty in learning new information because of increased distractibility, decrease in concrete thinking, and difficulty solving new problems. However, older adults usually compensate for these deficiencies by taking more time to process the information, screening out distractions, and using extreme care in making decisions. Marked cognitive decline is usually attributed to disease processes such as atherosclerosis, loss of neurons, and other pathologic changes (Miller, 1995).
3. Older adults are vulnerable to acute confusion when their ability to compensate for stressors, physiologically or psychologically, is compromised. Failure to adapt to changes in the external and internal environment results in confusion. Adaptation can be assessed in the following categories:
    a. Compromised brain function (congestive heart failure, anemia, pneumonia, hypoglycemia, fluid and electrolyte imbalance, hypotension, toxic drug reactions)
    b. Sensory–perceptual problems (decreased vision, hearing, information processing)
    c. Disruption in pattern and meaning (unable to cope with chronic stress-producing situations)
    d. Altered normal physiologic states (*e.g.*, problems in eating, sleeping, or elimination, pain)
    e. True dementias (*e.g.*, SDAT, MID [Wolanin & Phillips, 1981])

4. Most older adults exhibit no cognitive impairment. Severe cognitive impairment, a consequence of disease process, occurs in only 1% of people older than age 65 and 20% of people older than age 85 years (Katzman, 1988).
5. Age-related changes can influence medication actions and produce negative consequences. Table II-4 illustrates the age-related changes that influence medication actions.
6. Dementia describes impairments of intellectual functioning, not behavioral functioning. Dementia refers to a group of symptoms, not a disease (Miller, 1995). Alzheimer's disease, the fourth leading case of death in adults, is one type of dementia.
7. Blazer (1986) reported depressive symptoms in 27% of community-living older adults. According to Parmelee, Katz, and Lawton (1989), 12% of older adults living in nursing homes met the criteria for major depression, whereas 30% were identified with minor depressive symptoms.
8. Blazer (1986) describes a multiple causation theory for late-life depression, which emphasizes the complex interactions between several or many causative factors. Factors identified include poor economic resources, decreased social support, and decreased physical health functioning. These factors negatively affect self-esteem and motivation, which increases feelings of guilt and anger. The resulting negative emotions depress affect and increase ruminations. The person reduces social contact or is shunned, which starts the cycle again.
9. Suicide is always a possibility, especially in the early stage of dementia, for numerous reasons: depression, loss of self-worth, and impaired judgment.

Focus Assessment Criteria

Acquire data from client and significant others.

Subjective Data

1. History of the individual
   Life-style
Interests	Strengths and limitations
Work history	Previous level of functioning and
Coping patterns (past and present)	handling stress
Education	Use of alcohol/drugs

   Support system (availability)
   History of medical problems and treatments (medications)
   Activities of daily living (ability and desire to perform)
2. History of symptoms (onset and duration)
Acute or chronic	Time of day
Sudden or gradual	Downward progression with plateaus of function
Continuous or intermittent	
3. Assess for presence of
Feelings of
Extreme sadness and worthlessness	Mistrust or suspiciousness of others
Guilt for past actions	Others making him do and say things

Table II-4 **Age-Related Changes That May Influence Medications**

Age-Related Change	Effect on Some Medications
Decreased body water, decreased lean tissue, increased body fat	Increased or decreased serum concentration
Decreased serum albumin	Increased amount of the active portion of protein-bound medications
Decreased renal and liver functioning	Increased serum concentration
Decreased gastric acid, increased gastic pH	Altered absorption of medications that are sensitive to stomach pH
Altered homeostatic mechanisms	Increased potential for adverse effects
Altered receptor sensitivity	Increased or decreased therapeutic effect

(Miller, C. [1995]. *Nursing care of older adults* [2nd ed.]. Glenview, IL: Scott, Foresman.)

Apprehension in various situations   Excessive self-importance
Being rejected or isolated   Depersonalization
Living in an unreal world

Fears

That others will harm him   Of thoughts racing
That mind is being controlled by external agents   Of being held prisoner
Of being unable to cope   Body is rotting or not there
Of falling apart

Hallucinations (visual, auditory, gustatory, olfactory, tactile—includes an objective component)

Dementia

Gradual onset of impaired memory, labile affect
Alert
Evasive
Denial of symptoms
Inappropriate dress
Cognitive deficits (aphasia, apraxia, agnosia, agraphia)
Delusions used to explain deficits (*e.g.*, theft, spouse infidelity, fears)

Depression (APA, 1994)

See *Ineffective Individual Coping*, Focus Assessment Criteria

Delusions

Fixed or fleeting
Thought broadcasting (others can hear their thoughts)
Thought insertion (others putting thoughts into their mind)
Physical complaints of fatigue, anorexia, constipation, insomnia, dysphagia
Delusions of foreboding gloom, diminished self-esteem, money, death, guilt

4. Orientation

Person

"What is your name?"
"What is your birth date?"
"What is your occupation?"

Time

"What season is it?"
"What month is it?"

Place

"Where are you?"
"Where do you live?"

5. Problem-solving ability

"What would you do if the phone rang?"
"What is the difference between the doctor and the president?"

6. Memory

"Who was the last U.S. President?"
"Name three objects quickly."
Ask person to repeat them after you have said them. Repeat them until all three are learned.

7. Language

Ask person to identify a pencil and a watch.
Ask person to read and obey the following:
"Close your eyes."
"Write a sentence."

8. Recall

Ask for the names of the three objects learned previously.

9. Reality testing

Degrees of realness person feels regarding the experiences in relation to actual reality
Extent to which person will act on these experiences

Objective Data (Includes a Subjective Component)

1. General appearance
   Facial expression (alert, sad, hostile, expressionless)
   Dress (meticulous, disheveled, seductive, eccentric)
2. Behavior during interview

Withdrawn	Level of anxiety
Hostile	Cooperative
Apathetic	Quiet
Level of attention/concentration	Negativism

3. Communication pattern
   Content

Appropriate	Obsessions
Rambling	Sexual preoccupations
Suspicious	Delusions (grandeur, persecution, reference, influence,
Denying problem	control, or bodily sensations)
Homicidal plans	Religiousness
Suicidal ideas	Worthlessness
Lacking content	

   Pattern of speech

Appropriate	Jumps from one topic to another
Blocking (unable to finish idea)	Unable to come to conclusion, be
Circumstantial (unable to get to point)	decisive
Neologisms	Clang association
Word salad	Echolalia
Loose connection of ideas	

   Rate of speech

Appropriate	Reduced
Excessive	Pressured

   Affect

Blunted	Affect congruent with content of speech
Bright	Affect appropriate to verbal content
Flat	Affect inappropriate to verbal content
Sad	Gestures, mannerisms, facial grimaces
Posture	

4. Interaction skills
   With nurse

Inappropriate	Shows dependency
Relates well	Demanding/pleading
Withdrawn/preoccupied	Hostile

   With significant others

Relates with all (some) family members	Does not seek interaction
Hostile toward one (all) members	Does not have visitors

5. Activities of daily living
   Capable of self-care (observed, reported)
6. Nutritional–hydration status

Appetite	Weight (within normal limits, decreased, increased)
Eating patterns	

7. Sleep–rest pattern

Sleeps too much or too little	Early wakefulness
Cycle reversed	Insomnia
Fragmented sleep	

8. Personal hygiene

Cleanliness (body, hair, teeth)	Clothes (condition, appropriateness)
Grooming (clothes, hair, makeup)	

9. Motor activity

Within normal limits	Waxy flexibility
Agitated	Echopraxia
Decreased/stuporous	Stereotyped behavior

> **Outcome Criteria**
>
> The person will
> • Have diminished episodes of confusion

Interventions

A. Assess for causative and contributing factors

    1. Ensure that a thorough diagnostic workup has been completed.

        a. Laboratory

CBC and electrolytes	Serum thyroxine and serum-free
Vitamin B_{12} and folate, thiamine	thyroxine
VDRL	Calcium and phosphate
NA and K	Creatinine, BUN
SGOT, SGPT, and bilirubin	Serum glucose and fasting blood sugar
Urinalysis	Chest x-ray
EKG	

        b. Diagnostic

            EEG

            CT scan

        c. Psychiatric evaluation

    2. Evaluate if depression is present. (See Focus Assessment Criteria in *Ineffective Individual Coping*).

B. Promote communication that contributes to the person's sense of integrity

    1. Examine attitudes about confusion (in self, caregivers, significant others).

        a. Provide education to family, significant others, and caregivers regarding the situation and methods of coping.

    2. Maintain standards of empathic, respectful care.

        a. Be an advocate when other caregivers are insensitive to the individual's needs.

        b. Function as a role model with coworkers.

        c. Provide other caregivers with up-to-date information on confusion.

        d. Expect empathic, respectful care and monitor its administration.

    3. Attempt to obtain information that will provide useful and meaningful topics for conversations (likes, dislikes; interests, hobbies; work history). Interview early in day.

    4. Encourage significant others and caregivers to speak slowly with a low voice pitch and at an average volume (unless hearing deficits are present), as one adult to another, with eye contact, and as if expecting person to understand.

    5. Provide respect and promote sharing.

        a. Pay attention to what person is saying.

        b. Pick out meaningful comments and continue talking.

        c. Call person by name and introduce yourself each time a contact is made; use touch if welcomed.

        d. Use name the person prefers; avoid "Pops" or "Mom," which can increase confusion and is unacceptable.

        e. Convey to person that you are concerned and friendly (through smiles, an unhurried pace, humor, and praise; do not argue).

        f. Focus on feeling behind the spoken word or action.

    6. Use memory aids, if appropriate.

C. Provide sufficient and meaningful sensory input

    1. Keep person oriented to time and place.

        a. Refer to time of day and place each morning.

        b. Provide person with a clock and calendar large enough to see.

    c. If dementia is severe, remove all visible mirrors.

    d. Use night lights or dim lights at night.

    e. Use indirect lighting.

    f. Turn lights on before it gets dark.

    g. Provide person with opportunity to see daylight and dark through a window or take person outdoors.

    h. Single out holidays with cards or pins (*e.g.*, wear a red heart for Valentine's Day).

    i. Use adaptive devices to diminish sensory impediments (*e.g.*, lighting, glasses, hearing aids).

2. Encourage family to bring in familiar objects from home (*e.g.*, photographs with nonglare glass, Afghan).

    a. Ask person to tell you about the picture.

    b. Focus on familiar topics.

3. Discuss current events, seasonal events (snow, water activities); share your interests (travel, crafts).

4. Assess if person can perform an activity with his hands (*e.g.*, latch rugs, wood crafts).

    a. Provide reading materials, audio tapes, puzzles (manual, computer, crossword).

    b. Encourage person to keep his own records if possible (*e.g.*, intake and output).

    c. Provide tasks to perform (addressing envelopes, occupational therapy).

5. In teaching a task or activity—for example, eating—break it into small, brief steps by giving only one instruction at a time.

    a. Remove covers from food plate and cups.

    b. Locate napkin and utensils.

    c. Add sugar and milk to coffee.

    d. Add condiments to food (sugar, salt, pepper).

    e. Cut foods.

    f. Proceed with eating.

6. Explain all activities.

    a. Offer simple explanations of tasks.

    b. Allow individuals to handle equipment related to each task.

    c. Allow individual to participate in task, such as washing his face.

    d. Acknowledge that you are leaving and say when you will return.

D. Increase person's self-esteem

1. Allow former habits (*e.g.*, reading in the bathroom).

2. Encourage the wearing of dentures.

3. Assist with removal of facial hair.

4. Ask family to provide spending money.

5. Ask person/significant others his usual grooming routine and encourage him to follow it.

6. Provide privacy at all times; when it is necessary to expose a body surface, take precautions to cover all other areas (*e.g.*, if washing a back, use towels or blankets to cover legs and front torso).

7. Provide for personal hygiene according to person's preferences (hair grooming, showers or bath, nail care, cosmetics, deodorants and fragrances).

E. Promote a well role

1. Discourage the use of nightclothes during the day; have person wear shoes, not slippers.

2. Encourage self-care and grooming activities.

3. Have person eat meals out of bed, unless contraindicated.

4. Promote socialization during meals (*e.g.*, set up lunch for four individuals in lounge).

5. Plan an activity each day to look forward to (*e.g.*, bingo, ice cream sundae gathering).

6. Encourage participation in decision making (*e.g.*, selecting what he or she wishes to wear).

F. Do not endorse confusion

1. Do not argue with person.
2. Never agree with confused statements.
3. Direct person back to reality; do not allow him to ramble.
4. Adhere to the schedule; if changes are necessary, advise person of them.
5. Avoid talking to coworkers about other topics in person's presence.
6. Provide simple explanations that cannot be misinterpreted.
7. Remember to acknowledge your entrance with a greeting and your exit with a closure. ("I will be back in 10 minutes.")
8. Avoid open-ended questions.
9. Replace five- to six-step tasks with two- to three-step tasks.

G. Prevent injury to the individual

1. Discourage the use of restraints; explore other alternatives.
   a. Put person in a room with others who can help watch him.
   b. Enlist aid of family or friends to watch person during confused periods.
   c. If person is pulling out tubes, use mitts instead of wrist restraints.
2. Refer to *Risk for Injury* for strategies for assessing and manipulating the environment for hazards.
3. Monitor medications and their reaction.
4. Register with an emergency medical system, including "wanderers list" with local police department.

Rationale

- It is important to differentiate acute (reversible) from chronic (irreversible) confusion (Stolley & Buckwalter, 1992).
- Unconditional positive regard communicates acceptance and affection to a person who has difficulty interpreting the environment (Stolley & Buckwalter, 1992).
- Careful listening is critical to evaluate responses to prevent escalation of anxiety and to detect physiologic discomforts (Miller, 1995).
- Memory loss and diminished intellectual functioning create a need for consistency (Stolley & Buckwalter, 1992).
- Sensory input is carefully planned to reduce excess stimuli, which increase confusion (Miller, 1995).
- Structured rest periods prevent fatigue and allow for lower-stress periods (Stolley & Buckwalter, 1992).
- Restraints are a violation of a person's rights and increase anxiety. All attempts to protect the person should be used before selecting restraints.
- "Functional or baseline behavior is likely to occur when the external demands (stressors) on the individual are adjusted to the level to which the person has adapted" (Hall, 1991).
- Four biologic mechanisms are required for coping: movement, energy production, sensing, and cerebral integrating. "As competence decreases, external environmental factors become increasingly important determinants of behavior and affect" (Hall, 1991).
- People with dementia can be assisted to maximize their function level by reducing or eliminating certain factors. These factors include (Hall & Buckwalter, 1987):
  - Fatigue
  - Change in routine, environment, or caregiver
  - High-stimulus activity (*e.g.*, crowds) or images (*e.g.*, frightening pictures or movies)
  - Frustration from trying to function beyond capabilities or from being restrained
  - Pain, discomforts, illness, or side effects from medications
  - Competing or misleading stimuli (*e.g.*, mirrors, television, costumes)
- Anxiety influences cognitive abilities through excessive self-focusing and worrying. Depression causes decreased concentration, attention deficits, and negative expectations (Miller, 1995).

Chronic Confusion

DEFINITION

Chronic Confusion: A state in which the individual experiences an irreversible, long-standing, and/or progressive deterioration of intellect and personality.

DEFINING CHARACTERISTICS
Major (Must Be Present)

Cognitive or intellectual losses
> Loss of memory   Inability to make choices, decisions
> Loss of time sense

Inability to problem-solve, reason
> Altered perceptions   Poor judgment
> Loss of language abilities

Affective or personality losses
> Loss of affect   Increasing self-preoccupations
> Diminished inhibition   Psychotic features
> Loss of tact, control of temper   Antisocial behavior
> Loss of recognition (others, environment, self)   Loss of energy reserve

Conative or planning losses
> Loss of general ability to plan   Impaired ability to set goals, plan

Progressive lowered stress threshold
> Purposeful wandering   Withdrawal or avoidance behavior
> Violent, agitated or anxious behavior   Compulsive repetitive behavior
> Purposeless behavior

RELATED FACTORS
Pathophysiologic (Hall, 1991)

Related to progressive degeneration of the cerebral cortex secondary to:
> Alzheimer's disease
> Multiinfarct disease (MID)
> Combination of senile dementia of the Alzheimer's type and MID

Related to disturbance in cerebral metabolism, structure, or integrity secondary to:
> Pick's disease
> Creutzfeldt-Jakob disease
> Toxic substance injection
> Degenerative neurologic disease
> Brain tumors
> Huntington's chorea
> End-stage diseases
>> AIDS   Cirrhosis
>> Cancer   Renal failure
>> Cardiac failure   Chronic obstructive pulmonary disease
> Psychiatric disorders

Author's Note
Refer to *Acute Confusion*

Errors in Diagnostic Considerations
Refer to *Acute Confusion*

Key Concepts
1. See *Acute Confusion*
2. Progressive dementing illnesses have four clusters of symptoms (Hall, 1988, 1994):
   a. Intellectual losses
      Loss of memory (recent initially)
      Loss of sense of time
      Inability to problem solve and reason
      Inability to make choices
      Altered ability to identify visual or auditory stimuli
      Loss of expressive and receptive language
   b. Affective personality losses
      Loss of affect   Emotional liability
      Decreased attention span   Loss of tact
      Decreased inhibitions   Increased self-preoccupation
   c. Cognitive or planning losses
      Loss of ability to plan   Loss of energy reserves
      Loss of instrumental functions (*e.g.*, money   Motor apraxia
         management, mail, shopping)   Frustration, refusal to
      Functional losses (*e.g.*, bathing, choosing   participate
         clothes)
   d. Progressively lowered stress threshold
      Confused or agitated night awakening   Violent, agitated, or anxious
      Purposeful wandering   behavior
                                              Compulsive repetitive behavior
3. Depression and dementia both cause cognitive impairments. It is critical to differentiate the underlying cause, because depression is treatable (Miller, 1995).

Focus Assessment Criteria

Refer to *Acute Confusion*

Outcome Criteria

The person will
- Participate to maximum level of independence in a therapeutic milieu
- Have decreased frustration when environmental stressors are reduced
- Have diminished episodes of combativeness
- Eliminate episodes of combative behavior
- Increase hours of sleep at night
- Stabilize or increase weight

Interventions
A. Refer to Interventions B through G under *Acute Confusion*

B. Assess who the person was before onset of dementia
   1. Educational level, career
   2. Hobbies, life-style
   3. Coping styles

C. Observe the person for 1 to 2 weeks to determine baseline behaviors (Hall, 1994)
    1. Client's best time of day
    2. Response time to a simple question
    3. Amount of distraction tolerable
    4. Judgment ability
    5. Insight into own disability
    6. Signs/symptoms of depression
    7. Usual routine

D. Promote communication that contributes to the person's sense of integrity (Miller, 1995)
    1. Adapt communication to the ability level of the person.
    2. Avoid "baby talk" and a condescending tone of voice.
    3. It may be necessary to use very simple sentences and to present one idea at a time.
    4. If person does not understand, repeat sentence using the same words.
    5. Use positive statements; avoid "don'ts."
    6. Unless a safety issue is involved, do not argue with the person.
    7. Avoid general questions, such as "What would you like to do?" Instead, ask "Do you want to go for a walk or work on your rug?"
    8. Be sensitive to the feelings the person is trying to express.
    9. Avoid questions you know he or she cannot answer.
    10. If possible, demonstrate to reinforce verbal communication.
    11. Use touch to gain attention or show concern unless a negative response is elicited.
    12. Maintain good eye contact and pleasant facial expressions.
    13. Determine which sense dominates the person's perception of the world (auditory, kinesthetic, olfactory, or gustatory). Communicate through the preferred sense (Feil, 1992).

E. Promote the client's safety
    1. Ensure that the person carries identification.
    2. Adapt the environment so that the person can pace or walk if desired.
    3. Keep the environment uncluttered.
    4. Keep medications, cleaning solutions, and other toxic chemicals in inaccessible places.
    5. If person cannot manipulate call button, use another method (*e.g.*, bell, an extension from bed call system).

F. Discourage use of restraints; explore other alternatives (Quinn, 1994)
    1. If person's behavior disrupts treatment (*e.g.*, nasogastric tube, urinary catheter, intravenous line) reevaluate whether treatment is appropriate.
        a. Intravenous therapy:
            Camouflage the tubing with loose gauze.
            Consider an intermittent access device instead of continuous IV therapy.
            If dehydration is a problem, institute a regular schedule for offering oral fluids.
            Use sites that are least restrictive.
        b. Urinary catheters:
            Evaluate causes of incontinence; institute specific treatment depending on type. Refer to *Altered Patterns of Urinary Elimination*.
            Place urinary collection bag at end of bed with catheter between legs rather than draped over legs. Velcro bands can hold catheter against leg.
        c. Gastrointestinal tubes:
            Check frequently for pressure against nares.
            Camouflage gastrostomy tube with a loosely applied abdominal binder.
            If person is pulling out tubes, use mitts instead of wrist restraints.
    2. Evaluate if restlessness is associated with pain. If analgesics are used, adjust dosage to reduce side effects.
    3. Put person in a room with others who can help watch him.
    4. Enlist aid of family or friends to watch person during confused periods.
    5. Give person something to hold (*e.g.*, stuffed animal).

G. Attempt to determine source of the fear and frustration that is associated with the person's combative episodes (Hall, 1994)
1. Fatigue
2. Change in routine, environment, or caregiver
3. Pressure from self or others to exceed functional capacity
4. Physical stressors, pain, infection, acute illness, discomfort
5. Misleading or inappropriate stimuli

H. If a dysfunctional episode or sudden functional loss has occurred
1. If a staff member is present, quickly substitute another staff person.
2. Address person by surname.
3. Assume a dependent position to the individual.
4. Distract with cues that require automatic social behavior (*e.g.*, "Mrs. Smith, would you like some juice now?").
5. After the episode has passed, discuss the episode with the individual.
6. Document antecedents, behavior observed, and consequences.

I. Ensure physical comfort and maintenance of basic health needs (*e.g.*, elimination, nutrition, bathing, toileting, hygiene, grooming). Refer to individual nursing diagnoses for individuals to assist a cognitively impaired person with self care.

J. Select modalities that provide favorable stimuli for the individual
1. Music therapy
   a. Provide soft, familiar music during meals.
   b. Arrange group song fests with consideration to cultural/ethical orientation.
   c. Play music during other therapies (physical, occupational, and speech).
   d. Have person exercise to music.
   e. Encourage construction of simple instruments and have individuals play them in a rhythm band.
   f. Organize guest entertainment.
   g. Use client-developed songbooks (large print and decorative covers).
   h. Play music to individuals that they preferred in their younger years.
2. Recreation therapy
   a. Encourage arts and crafts (knitting and crocheting).
   b. Suggest creative writing.
   c. Provide puzzles.
   d. Organize group games.
3. Remotivation therapy
   a. Organize group sessions into five steps (Dennis, 1984):
      Step 1: Climate of Acceptance (approx. 5 minutes)
         Relaxed atmosphere with introductions of leaders and participants
         Provide large-letter name tags and names on chairs
         Maintain assigned places for every session
      Step 2: Creating a Bridge to Reality (approx. 15 minutes)
         Use a prop (visual, audio, song, picture, object, poem) to introduce theme of session
      Step 3: Sharing the World We Live In (approx. 15 minutes)
         Group members discuss the topic
         Stimulation of senses should be promoted
      Step 4: Appreciation of the Work of the World (approx. 20 minutes)
         Discussion of how the topic relates to their past experiences (work, leisure)
      Step 5: Climate of Appreciation (approx. 5 minutes)
         Each member is thanked individually
         Announcement of the next session's topic and meeting date
   b. Use associations and analogies.
      "If ice is cold, then fire is . . . ?"
      "If day is light, then night is . . . ?"

    c. Topics for remotivation sessions are chosen based on suggestions from group leaders and the interest of the group. Examples are pets, bodies of water, canning fruits and vegetables, transportation, holidays (Janssen & Giberson, 1988).

4. Sensory training
    a. Stimulate vision (with brightly colored items of different shape, pictures, colored decorations, kaleidoscopes).
    b. Stimulate smell (with flowers, coffee, cologne).
    c. Stimulate hearing (ring a bell, play records).
    d. Stimulate touch (sandpaper, velvet, steel wool pads, silk, stuffed animals).
    e. Stimulate taste (spices, salt, sugar, sour substances).

5. Reminiscence therapy (Burnside & Haight, 1994; Smith, 1990).
    a. Consider instituting reminiscence therapy on a one-to-one or group basis. Discuss purpose and goals with client care team. Prepare oneself well before initiating. Refer to Burnside and Haight (1994) for specific protocols for one-to-one and group reminiscence.

K. Implement techniques to lower the stress threshold in individuals in middle or later stages of dementia (Hall & Buckwalter, 1987; Miller, 1995)

1. Reduce competing or excessive stimuli.
    a. Keep environment simple and uncluttered.
    b. Use simple written cues to clarify directions for use of radio and TV.
    c. Eliminate or minimize unnecessary noise.

2. Plan and maintain a consistent routine.
    a. Attempt to assign same caregivers.
    b. Elicit from family members specific methods that help or hinder care.
    c. Arrange personal care items in order of use (clothes, toothbrush, mouthwash, and so forth).
    d. Determine a daily routine with individual and family.
    e. Write down sequence for all caregivers
    f. Reduce the stress when change is anticipated
        Keep the change as simple as possible (*e.g.*, minimal holiday decorations).
        Ensure person is well rested.
        Institute change during person's best time of day if possible.

3. Focus on the person's ability level.
    a. Do not request performance of function beyond ability.
    b. Express unconditional positive regard for the person.
    c. Modify environment to compensate for ability (*e.g.*, use of Velcro fasteners, loose clothing, and elastic waistbands).
    d. Use simple sentences, demonstrate activity.
    e. Do not ask questions that the person cannot answer.
    f. Avoid open-ended questions (*e.g.*, "What do you want to eat?" or "When do you want to take a bath?").
    g. Avoid using pronouns; name objects.
    h. Offer simple choices (*e.g.*, "Do you want a cookie or crackers?").
    i. Use finger foods (*e.g.*, sandwiches) to encourage self-feeding.

4. Minimize fatigue (Hall, 1994)
    a. Provide rest periods twice daily.
    b. Determine with client a rest activity, such as reading or listening to music.
    c. Napping should be done in recliner chairs, not bed.
    d. Plan high-stress or fatiguing activities during best time for the individual.
    e. Allow the person to cease an activity at any time.
    f. Incorporate regular exercise in daily plan.
    g. Allow for wandering.
    h. Be alert to individual's expressions of fatigue and increasing anxiety and immediately reduce stimuli.

Rationale

- Assessing the individual's personal history can provide insight into current behavior patterns and communicates interest in the individual (Hall, 1994).

- Specific data about the person can increase individualization of the care (Hall, 1994).
- Baseline behavior is used to develop a plan for activities and daily care routines (Hall, 1994).
- Communication abilities (*i.e.*, receptive and expressive) are affected by Alzheimer's disease–related dementia (Hall, 1994).
- Individuals compensate for conative losses (ability to plan and sequence activities) by developing a daily routine.
- Dysfunctional episodes are transient changes characterized by cognitive and social inaccessibility (*e.g.*, inability to recognize familiar faces, withdrawn, belligerent, stubbornness) (Hall, 1994; Miller, 1995).
- Fatigue is the most frequent cause of dysfunctional episodes.
- Daytime rest periods help prevent night wakenings.
- Overstimulation, understimulation, or misleading stimuli can cause dysfunctional episodes because of impaired sensory interpretation (Hall, 1994).
- Attempting to perform functions that exceed cognitive capacity will result in fear, anger, and frustration (Hall, 1994).
- Physical stressors can precipitate a dysfunctional episode (*e.g.*, urinary tract infections, caffeine, constipation).
- Dysfunctional episodes are manifestations of fear; the goals of management are preventing injury, providing a sense of serenity, and promoting a sense of mastery in the person (Hall, 1994).

References/Bibliography

American Psychiatric Association (APA). (1994). *Diagnostic and statistical manual of mental disorders* (4th ed. revised). Washington, DC: American Psychiatric Press.

Alzheimer's disease and related disorders. (1988). In *Special care for Alzheimer's patients*. Chicago: Alzheimer's Disease and Related Disorders Association, Inc.

Blazer, D. G. (1986). Depression: Paradoxically a cause for hope. *Generations, 10*(3), 21–23.

Burnside, I., & Haight, B. (1994). Reminiscence and life review: Therapeutic interventions for older people. *Nurse Practitioner, 19*(4), 55–60.

Dennis, H. (1984). Remotivation therapy groups. In I. M. Burnside (Ed.). *Working with the elderly group: Process and techniques* (2nd ed.). Monterey, CA: Jones & Bartlett.

Feil, N. (1992). Validation therapy. *Geriatric Nursing, 13*(3), 129–133.

Hall, G. R. (1988). Care of the patient with Alzheimer's disease living at home. *Nursing Clinics of North America, 23*, 31–46.

Hall, G. R. (1991). Altered thought processes: Dementia. In M. Maas, K. Buckwalter, & M. Hardy (Eds.). *Nursing diagnoses and interventions for the elderly*. Menlo Park, CA: Addison-Wesley.

Hall, G. R. (1994). Caring for people with Alzheimer's disease using the conceptual model of progressively lowered stress threshold in the clinical setting. *Nursing Clinics of North America, 29*, 129–141.

Hall, G. R., & Buckwalter, K. C. (1987). Progressively lowered stress threshold: A conceptual model for care of adults with Alzheimer's disease. *Archives of Psychiatric Nursing, 1*, 399–406.

Janssen, J., & Giberson, D. (1988). Remotivation therapy. *Journal of Gerontological Nursing, 14*(6), 31–34.

Katzman, R. (1988). *Alzheimer's disease as an age dependent disorder, research and the aging population* (CIBA Foundation Symposium 1334). New York: John Wiley & Sons.

Miller, C. A. (1995). *Nursing care of older adults.* (2nd ed.). Glenview, IL: Scott, Foresman.

Parmelee, P. A., Katz, I. R., & Lawton, M. P. (1989). Depression among institutionalized aged: Assessment and prevalence estimation. *Journal of Gerontology: Medical Sciences, 44*, M22–M29.

Quinn, C. (1994). The four A's of restraint reduction: Attention, assessment, anticipation, avoidance. *Orthopaedic Nursing, 13*(2), 11–19.

Rasin, J. (1990). Confusion. *Nursing Clinics of North America, 25*, 909–918.

Smith, B. (1990). *Role of orientation therapy and reminiscence therapy: Alzheimer's disease*. St. Louis: C. V. Mosby.

Stolley, J., & Buckwalter, K. (1992). Confusion management. In G. Gulechek & J. McCloskey (Eds.). *Nursing interventions* (2nd ed.). Philadelphia: W. B. Saunders.

Wolanin, M., & Phillips, L. (1981). *Confusion: Prevention and care*. St. Louis: C. V. Mosby.

Resources for the Consumer

Literature

Hamby, R., Turnbull, J., Norman, L., & Lancaster M. (1990). *Alzheimers' disease: A handbook for caregivers*. St. Louis: C. V. Mosby.

Organizations

Alzheimer's Association (ADRDA), 919 North Michigan Avenue, Suite 100, Chicago, IL 60611; Tel. (800) 272-3900
- 24-hour hotline to provide information about Alzheimer's disease
- Free publications and newsletter
- Information about local chapters of the Alzheimer's Association

Alzheimer's Disease Education and Referral (ADEAR) Center, P.O. Box 8250, Silver Spring, MD 20907-8250; Tel. (301) 495-3311

Constipation

Colonic Constipation

Perceived Constipation

Constipation

DEFINITION

Constipation: The state in which an individual experiences or is at high risk of experiencing stasis of the large intestine resulting in infrequent elimination and/or hard, dry feces.

DEFINING CHARACTERISTICS

Major (Must Be Present)

Hard, formed stool and/or
Defecation occurs fewer than three times a week

Minor (May Be Present)

Decreased bowel sounds   Straining and pain on defecation
Reported feeling of rectal fullness   Palpable impaction
Reported feeling of pressure in rectum   Feeling of inadequate emptying

RELATED FACTORS

Pathophysiologic

Related to defective nerve stimulation, weak pelvic floor muscles, and immobility secondary to:

Spinal cord lesions   Cerebrovascular accident (CVA, stroke)
Spinal cord injury   Neurologic diseases (multiple sclerosis, Parkinson's)
Spina bifida   Dementia

Related to decreased metabolic rate secondary to:

Obesity   Hyperparathyroidism
Hypopituitarism   Pheochromocytoma
Uremia   Diabetic neuropathy
Hypothyroidism

Related to decreased response to urge to defecate secondary to:

Affective disorders

Related to pain (on defecation)

Hemorrhoids
Back injury

Related to decreased peristalsis secondary to hypoxia (cardiac, pulmonary)

Treatment-Related

Related to side effects of (specify):

Antacids (calcium, aluminum)	Calcium
Iron	Anticholinergics
Barium	Anesthetics
Aluminum	Narcotics (codeine, morphine)
Aspirin	Diuretics
Phenothiazines	Anti-Parkinson agents

Related to effects of anesthesia and surgical manipulation on peristalsis
Related to habitual laxative use
Related to mucositis secondary to radiation

Situational (Personal, Environmental)

Related to decreased peristalsis secondary to:

Immobility	Stress
Pregnancy	Lack of exercise

Related to irregular evacuation patterns
Related to cultural/health beliefs
Related to lack of privacy
Related to inadequate diet (lack of roughage, fiber, thiamine)
Related to inadequate fluid intake
Related to fear of rectal or cardiac pain
Related to faulty appraisal
Related to inability to perceive bowel cues

Author's Note

Two of the three constipation diagnoses contain their etiologic or contributing factors in the diagnostic labels *Colonic* and *Perceived*. Colonic constipation results from delayed passage of food residue in the bowel because of factors that the nurse can treat (*e.g.*, dehydration, insufficient dietary roughage, immobility). Perceived constipation refers to a faulty perception of constipation with self-prescribed overuse of laxatives, enemas, and/or suppositories.

When constipation results from factors other than those related to colonic or perceived constipation and are amenable to nursing interventions, the nursing diagnosis *Constipation* can apply.

Errors in Diagnostic Statements

Constipation related to reports of infrequent hard, dry feces

A report of infrequent hard, dry feces is a validation of constipation, not a contributing factor. If the nurse does not know the cause of constipation, the diagnosis can be written: *Constipation related to unknown etiology, as evidenced by reports of infrequent hard, dry feces.*

Key Concepts

1. Bowel elimination is controlled by the somatic and autonomic nervous system. Undigested food or feces passes through the large intestine propelled by involuntary muscles within the intestinal walls. At the same time, water that was needed for digestion is reabsorbed. The feces pass through the sigmoid colon, which empties into the rectum. At some point, the amount of stool in the rectum stimulates a defecation reflex, which causes the anal sphincter to relax and defecation to occur.
2. Bowel patterns are culturally or familially determined. The range of normal is wide, from three times a day to once every 3 days (McLane & McShane, 1991).
3. Table II-5 illustrates the components that are needed for normal bowel elimination and the conditions that impede these components.

Table II-5 **Components for Normal Bowel Elimination and Corresponding Barrier**

Components	Barriers
Daily diet of fiber (15–25 g)	Lack of access to fresh foods Financial constraints Insufficient knowledge*
6–8 glasses of water a day	Mobility problems Fear of incontinence Impaired thought process* Low motivation
Daily exercise	Minimal activity level Pain, fatigue Fear of falling
Cognitive appraisal	Impaired thought process Faulty appraisal
Toileting routine	Low motivation Change in routine Stress
Response to rectal cues	Mobility problems Decreased awareness Environmental constraints Self-care deficits

*These barriers can impede all the components.

4. Some medical conditions, such as brain disorders or spinal cord injuries, interfere with neurotransmission, whereas others, such as diabetes mellitus or rectal or anal trauma, cause rectal sphincter abnormalities. Inflammatory bowel disease, radiation proctitis, chronic constipation, and ileoanal surgery can decrease the fecal reservoir capacity and cause leaking (Maas & Specht, 1991).

5. Bulk and consistency of stool are influenced by dietary and fluid patterns. High-vegetable diet produces soft, bulky stools. High-meat diet produces small, dry, hard stools.

6. Diets high in unrefined fibrous food produce large, soft stools that decrease the colon's susceptibility to disease. Diets low in fiber and high in concentrated refined foods produce small, hard stools that increase the colon's susceptibility to disease.

7. Fiber that is not digested absorbs water, which adds bulk and softness to the stool, speeding up the passage through the intestines. Fiber without adequate fluid can aggravate, not facilitate, bowel function.

8. Laxatives and enemas are not components of a bowel management program, but are for emergency use only (McLane & McShane, 1991).

🌀 *Key Concepts—Child*

1. Constipation in children is not defined by frequency, as in adults, but by the character of the stool. The passage of firm or hard stool or hard masses with symptoms of difficulty in expulsion, blood-streaked bowel movements, and abdominal discomfort characterizes constipation in children (Jackson & Saunders, 1993).

2. As the infant ages, the stomach enlarges to hold a greater amount of food, and the rapid peristaltic activity of the gastrointestinal tract tract slows down. As a result, stools change in color, consistency, and frequency with maturation (Wong, 1993).

3. Voluntary withholding (functional constipation) is the most common cause of constipation beyond the neonatal period. Conflicts in toilet training or pain on defecation may lead to stool retention (Byrne, 1990).

4. Encopresis is fecal soiling or incontinence secondary to constipation. Previously toilet trained children with encopresis should be evaluated psychologically (Klish, 1994).

5. Children with functional constipation associate discomfort with defecation. When the sensation of relaxation of the internal anal sphincter occurs, the child contracts the external sphincter to prevent the expulsion of stools. Eventually the rectum dilates, resulting in more stool retention and diminished sensory response (Klish, 1994).

Key Concepts—Maternal

1. Constipation in pregnancy is caused by (May & Mahlmeister, 1994):
    a. Displacement of the intestines
    b. Increased water absorption from colon
    c. Hormonal influences
    d. Prolonged intestinal time
    e. Use of iron supplements
2. Postpartum causes of constipation are (May & Mahlmeister, 1994):
    a. Relaxed abdominal tone
    b. Decreased peristalsis
    c. Food and fluid restrictions during labor

Key Concepts—Older Adult

1. Older adults experience reduced mucus secretion in the large intestines and decreased elasticity of the rectal wall (Miller, 1995). However, no research validates that older adults are at higher risk for constipation because of age-related changes.
2. Some older adults are prone to constipation owing to such factors as decreased activity, insufficient dietary fiber and bulk, insufficient fluid intake, side effects of medications, laxative abuse, and inattention to defecation cues (Miller, 1995).

TRANSCULTURAL CONSIDERATIONS

1. Some cultures have folk medicine for elimination problems. For example, Mexican Americans differentiate diarrhea as a hot or cold condition. If the stool is green or yellow, it is hot and is treated with cold tea. If the stool is white, it is cold and is treated with hot tea (Giger & Davidhizar, 1991).

Focus Assessment Criteria

Subjective

A. Assess for defining characteristics
1. Elimination pattern
    Usual   Present
2. What frequency is considered normal?
3. Laxative/enema use
    Type   How often
4. Episodes of diarrhea
    How often?   Frequency?
    Duration?   Precipitated by what?
5. Associated symptoms/complaints of
    Headache   Thirst
    Weakness   Pain
    Lethargy   Cramping
    Anorexia   Weight loss/gain
6. Awareness of bowel cues

B. Assess for related factors
1. Life-style
    Activity level
    Occupation

Exercise (what? how often?)
Nutrition
24-Hour recall of foods and liquids taken
Usual 24-hour intake

Carbohydrates	Roughage
Fat	Liquids
Protein	

2. Current drug therapy

Antibiotics	Antacids
Iron	Central nervous system depressants
Steroids	

3. Medical–surgical history
Present conditions
Past conditions
Surgical history (colostomy? ileostomy?)
4. Awareness of bowel cues

Objective Data

A. Assess for defining characteristics
1. Stool

Color	Odor	Consistency
Brown	Normal	Soft, formed
Yellow	Foul	Soft, bulky
Yellow-green		Small, dry
Green		Pasty
Black		Diarrheal
Tan (clay-colored)		Hard
Red		

Size/Shape	Components
Narrow	Blood
Large caliber	Mucus
Small caliber	Pus
Round	Parasites
	Undigested food

2. Gastrointestinal motility (auscultation, light palpation)

Bowel Sounds	Abdominal Distention	Flatulence
High-pitched, gurgling (5/min)	None	None
	Slight	Occasionally
High-pitched, frequent, loud, pushing	Moderate	Frequent
	Severe	
Weak and infrequent		
Absent		

B. Assess for related factors
1. Nutrition

Food Intake	Fluid Intake
Type	Type
Amounts	Amounts

2. Perianal area/rectal examination

Hemorrhoids	Irritation
Fissures	Impaction
Control of rectal sphincter (presence of anal wink, bulbocavernosus reflex)	Presence/absence of stool in rectum

---

Outcome Criteria

The person will
- Describe therapeutic bowel regimen
- Relate or demonstrate improved bowel elimination
- Explain rationale for interventions

Interventions

A. Assess contributing factors
1. Irregular schedule
2. Inadequate exercise
3. Side effects of medical regimen
4. Imbalanced diet
5. Stress

B. Promote corrective measures
1. Regular time for elimination
   a. Identify normal defecation pattern before constipation began.
   b. Review daily routine.
   c. Advise that time for defecation be included as part of daily routine.
   d. Discuss suitable time (based on responsibilities, availability of facilities, and so forth).
   e. Provide stimulus to defecation (*e.g.*, coffee, prune juice).
   f. Advise that an attempt to defecate should be made about an hour or so after meal and that it may be necessary to remain in the bathroom a suitable length of time.
   g. Use bathroom instead of bedpan if possible.
   h. Offer bedpan or bedside commode if unable to use bathroom.
   i. Assist into position on bedpan or commode.
   j. Provide for privacy (close door, draw curtains around bed, play television or radio to mask sounds, have room deodorizer available).
   k. Provide for comfort (reading material as diversion) and safety (call bell available).
   l. Allow suitable position (sitting, if not contraindicated).
2. Adequate exercise
   a. Review current exercise pattern.
   b. Provide for moderate physical exercise on a frequent basis (if not contraindicated).
   c. Provide frequent ambulation of hospitalized patient when tolerable.
   d. Perform range-of-motion exercises for person who is bedridden.
   e. Teach exercises for increased abdominal muscle tone (unless contraindicated).
      Contract abdominal muscles several times frequently throughout day.
      Do sit-ups, keeping heels on floor with knees slightly flexed.
      While supine, raise lower limbs, keeping knees straight.
3. Balanced diet
   a. Review list of foods high in bulk:

Fresh fruits with skins	Whole-grain breads and cereals
Bran	Cooked fruits and vegetables
Nuts and seeds	Fruit juices

   b. Discuss dietary preferences.
   c. Take into account any food intolerances or allergies.
   d. Include approximately 800 g of fruits and vegetables (about four pieces of fresh fruit and large salad) for normal daily bowel movement.

e. Suggest use of bran in moderation at first (may irritate GI tract, produce flatulence, cause diarrhea or blockage).

f. Gradually increase amount of bran as tolerated (may add to cereals, baked goods, and the like). Explain the need for fluid intake with bran.

g. Consider financial limitations (encourage the use of fruits and vegetables in season).

4. Adequate fluid intake

a. Encourage intake of at least 2 L (8–10 glasses) unless contraindicated.

b. Discuss fluid preferences.

c. Set up regular schedule for fluid intake.

d. Recommend a glass of hot water to be taken one-half hour before breakfast, which may act as stimulus to bowel evacuation.

5. Optimal position

a. Assist to normal semisquatting position to allow optimum use of abdominal muscles and effect of force of gravity.

b. Assist onto bedpan if necessary and elevate head of bed to high Fowler's position or elevation permitted.

c. Use fracture bedpan for comfort, if preferred.

d. Stress the avoidance of straining.

e. Encourage exhaling during straining.

f. Place call bell within easy reach.

g. Maintain safety (side rails).

h. Provide privacy.

i. Chart results (color, consistency, amount).

C. Eliminate or reduce contributing factors

1. Untoward side effects of current medical regimen.

a. Administer mild laxative after oral administration of barium sulfate.*

b. Assess elimination status while on antacid therapy (may be necessary to alternate magnesium-type antacid with other types).*

c. Encourage increased intake of high-roughage foods and increased fluid intake as adjunct to iron therapy (*e.g.*, fresh fruits and vegetables with skins; bran, nuts, and seeds; whole wheat bread).

d. Encourage early ambulation, with assistance if necessary, to counter effects of anesthetic agents.

e. Assess elimination status while receiving certain narcotic analgesics (morphine, codeine) and alert physician if the patient is experiencing difficulty with defecation.

2. Laxative abuse

a. See *Perceived Constipation*.

3. Stress

a. See Appendix X for relaxation techniques for stress reduction.

4. Inadequate dietary and fluid intake: see *Altered Nutrition: Less Than Body Requirements*.

D. Conduct health teaching, as indicated

1. Explain to person and family the relationship of life-style changes to constipation.

2. Explain interventions that relieve symptoms.

3. Explain techniques to reduce the effects of stress and immobility.

Rationale

- A normal bowel elimination pattern is maintained by a daily diet of fiber, 6–8 glasses of water, and daily exercise. In addition, the person must be able to appraise the need to evacuate and establish a toileting routine (McLane & McShane, 1991).

* May require a primary care provider's order.

- Regular physical activity promotes muscle tonicity needed for fecal expulsion. It also increases circulation to the digestive system, which promotes peristalsis and easier feces evacuation (Maas & Specht, 1991).
- Sufficient fluid intake, at least 2 L daily, is necessary to maintain bowel patterns and promote proper stool consistency.
- A well-balanced diet high in fiber content stimulates peristalsis. Foods high in fiber should be avoided during episodes of diarrhea. These include:
  - Whole grains and nuts (bran, shredded wheat, brown rice, whole wheat bread)
  - Raw and coarse vegetables (broccoli, cauliflower, cucumbers, lettuce, cabbage, turnips, Brussels sprouts)
  - Fresh fruits, with skins
- The gastrocolic reflex and duodenocolic reflex stimulate mass peristalsis two or three times a day, most often after meals.
- Voluntary contraction of the muscles of the abdominal wall aids in the expulsion of feces.
- Frequency and consistency of stool are related to fluid and food intake. Fiber increases fecal bulk and enhances absorption of water into the stool. Adequate dietary fiber and fluid intake promote firm, but soft, well-formed stools and decrease the risk of hard, dry, constipated stools. Physical activity promotes peristalsis, aids digestion, and facilitates elimination.
- Laxatives upset a bowel program, because they cause much of the bowel to empty and can cause unscheduled bowel movements. With constant use, the colon loses tone and stool retention becomes difficult. Chronic use of bowel aids can lead to inconsistent stool consistency, which interferes with the scheduled bowel program and bowel management. Stool softeners may not be necessary if diet and fluid intake are adequate. Enemas lead to overstretching of the bowel and loss of bowel tone, contributing to further constipation (Toth, 1988).

Intervxentions—*Child Focus*

1. Discuss some causes of constipation in infants and children (*e.g.*, underfeeding, high protein-low carbohydrate diet, lack of roughage, dehydration).
2. If bowel movements are infrequent with hard stools
   a. With infants, add corn syrup to feeding or fruit to diet. Avoid apple juice or sauce.
   b. With children, add bran cereal, prune juice, and fruits and vegetables high in bulk.
3. Persistent constipation should be evaluated medically.
4. If child has functional constipation, consult with primary care provider for a laxative regimen.
5. Explain to adolescents the effects of fluids, fiber, and exercise on bowel function.

Rationale

- Several factors play a causative role in constipation:
  - Insufficient roughage or bulk
  - A bland diet, too high in dairy products, which results in reduced colonic motility
  - Insufficient oral intake of fluids, which allows the normal reabsorption of water from the colon to dehydrate the feces too much, or dehydration stemming from any activities that increase loss of fluids from sweating
  - Fecal retention by the child
  - Medications (*e.g.*, narcotics or anticonvulsants) that may have a side effect of promoting constipation
  - The child's emotional state (Christopherson, 1991)
- Children with long-standing functional constipation need a program of daily laxatives to allow the rectum to return to normal size (Klish, 1994).

⚙ **Interventions**—*Maternal Focus*

1. Explain the risks of constipation in pregnancy and postpartum:
   a. Decreased gastric motility
   b. Prolonged intestinal time
   c. Pressure of enlarging uterus
   d. Distended abdominal muscles (post)
   e. Relaxation of intestines (post)
2. Explain aggravating factors for hemorrhoid development (straining at defecation, constipation, prolonged standing, wearing constrictive clothing).
3. If woman has a history of constipation, discuss how to use bulk-producing laxatives to keep stool soft.
4. Postdelivery
   a. Assess abdomen (bowel sounds, distention, presence of flatus).
   b. Assess for hemorrhoids and perineal swelling.
   c. Provide relief of rectal and/or perineal pain.
   d. Instruct to take sitz baths and use cool, astringent compresses for hemorrhoids.

Rationale

- Explaining the causes of constipation during pregnancy and during the postpartum period can increase participation in behaviors that decrease or prevent constipation.

Colonic Constipation

DEFINITION
Colonic Constipation: The state in which an individual experiences or is at risk of experiencing a delay in passage of food residue, resulting in dry, hard stool.

DEFINING CHARACTERISTICS*
Major (80%–100%)
   Decreased frequency
   Hard, dry stool
   Straining at stool
   Painful defecation
   Abdominal distention

Minor (50%–79%)
   Rectal pressure
   Headache, appetite impairment
   Abdominal pain

---

* Adapted from McLane, A. M., & McShane, R. E. (1986). Empirical validation of defining characteristics of constipation: A study of bowel elimination practices of healthy adults. In M. E. Hurley (Ed.). *Classification of nursing diagnosis: Proceedings of the sixth conference*. St. Louis: C. V. Mosby.

RELATED FACTORS
Pathophysiologic

Related to defective innervation, weak pelvic floor muscles, and immobility secondary to:

Spinal cord lesions	Cerebrovascular accident (CVA, stroke)
Spinal cord injury	Neurologic diseases (multiple sclerosis, Parkinson's)
Spina bifida	Dementia

Related to decreased metabolic rate secondary to:
Obesity
Hypopituitarism
Hypothyroidism
Hyperparathyroidism
Affective disorder

Related to decreased peristalsis secondary to hypoxia (cardiac, pulmonary)

Treatment-Related

Related to side effects (specify):

Antacids	Anesthetics
Iron	Narcotics (codeine, morphine)
Barium	Aspirin
Aluminum	Phenothiazines
Calcium	Diuretics
Anticholinergics	Anti-Parkinson agents

Related to effects of anesthesia and surgical manipulation on peristalsis
Related to habitual laxative use

Situational (Personal, Environmental)

Related to decreased peristalsis secondary to:
Immobility
Stress
Lack of exercise
Related to irregular evacuation patterns
Related to lack of privacy
Related to inadequate diet (lack of roughage/thiamine)
Related to dehydration
Related to fear of pain
Related to inadequate fluid intake
Related to displacement of intestines, prolonged intestinal time, and iron supplements secondary to pregnancy
Related to relaxed abdominal tone, decreased peristalsis, and food/fluid restrictions secondary to labor and delivery.

Author's Note
Refer to Author's Note under *Constipation*

Errors in Diagnostic Statements
Refer to Errors in Diagnostic Statements under *Constipation*

Key Concepts
Refer to Key Concepts under *Constipation*

Focus Assessment Criteria

Refer to Focus Assessment Criteria under *Constipation*

Outcome Criteria

Refer to Outcome Criteria under *Constipation*

Interventions

Refer to Interventions under *Constipation*

■ Colonic Constipation
Related to Effects of Immobility on Peristalsis

Outcome Criteria

The person will
- Describe therapeutic bowel regimen
- Relate or demonstrate improved bowel elimination
- Explain rationale for interventions

Interventions

A. Assess causative factors of immobility

Musculoskeletal (*e.g.*, fractures, sprain, contractures, hip replacement)
Reliance on life-support systems
Chronic or acute illness
Trauma (*e.g.*, burns, head injury)
Physical handicap
Inappropriate coping mechanisms
Bed rest
Psychosomatic illness
Degenerative joint changes (arthritis)
Surgery
Minimal activity level

B. Eliminate or reduce contributing factors

1. Fecal impaction
   a. If fecal impaction is suspected, perform digital examination of rectum. Have client assume position lying on left side. Don glove, lubricate forefinger, and insert; attempt to break up any hardened fecal mass and remove pieces.
   b. If impaction is out of reach of gloved finger:
      Administer oil retention enema to aid in removal of mass.*
      Instruct person to retain enema at least 60 minutes or possibly overnight.
      Follow with cleansing enema* (both enemas may need to be repeated; may need to follow with repeated attempt to break up mass digitally).

* May require a primary care provider's order.

    c. Make client comfortable and allow to rest.

    d. Client may require temporary use of stool softener or mild cathartic.*

    e. Maintain accurate bowel elimination record.

2. Severe constipation

    a. First day, insert glycerin suppository and have client attempt bowel movement through intermittent straining efforts.

    b. If ineffective, on second day, insert glycerin suppository and follow same routine.

    c. If no results, on third day, request prescription for suppository, which if not effective should be followed by enema.*

    d. To aid in stimulation of reflex emptying, a suppository may be followed in 20–30 minutes by digital stimulation of anal sphincter.

    e. Return to first-day routine and follow until pattern is established (may be every 2–3 days).

C. Conduct health teaching, as indicated

1. Explain the interventions required to prevent constipation (*e.g.*, diet, exercise) versus those required to treat it.

Rationale

- Defecation involves the coordinated relaxation of the puborectalis and external anal sphincter muscles simultaneously with increased intraabdominal pressure forcing stool toward the rectum.
- Immobility can interfere with bowel elimination through loss of muscle tone, decreased gastrointestinal motility, and decreased gravity filling of lower rectum with a resulting diminished defecation reflex.

Perceived Constipation

DEFINITION

Perceived Constipation: The state in which an individual self-prescribes the daily use of laxatives, enemas, and/or suppositories to ensure a daily bowel movement.

DEFINING CHARACTERISTICS†

Major (80%–100%)

Expectation of a daily bowel movement with the resulting overuse of laxatives, enemas, and suppositories

Expected passage of stool at same time, every day

---

*May require a primary care provider's order.

† Adapted from McLane, A. M., & McShane, R. E. (1986). Empirical validation of defining characteristics of constipation: A study of bowel elimination practices of healthy adults. In M. E. Hurley (Ed.). *Classification of nursing diagnosis: Proceedings of the sixth conference.* St. Louis: C. V. Mosby.

RELATED FACTORS
Pathophysiologic

Related to faulty appraisal secondary to:

Obsessive–compulsive disorders   Depression
Central nervous system deterioration

Situational (Personal, Environmental)

Related to inaccurate information secondary to:

Cultural beliefs
Family beliefs

Author's Note

Refer to Author's Note under *Constipation*

Key Concepts

Refer to Key Concepts under *Constipation*

Focus Assessment Criteria

Refer to Focus Assessment Criteria under *Constipation*

Outcome Criteria

The person will
- Verbalize acceptance of bowel movement every 2–3 days
- Not use laxatives regularly
- Relate the causes of constipation
- Describe the hazards of laxative use
- Relate an intent to increase fiber, fluid, and exercise in daily life as instructed

---

Interventions

A. Assess causative or contributing factors

1. Cultural/familial belief
2. Faulty appraisal

B. Explain that bowel movements are needed every 2–3 days, not daily

1. Be sensitive to person's beliefs.
2. Be patient.

C. Explain the hazards of regular laxative use

1. Provide only temporary relief
2. Promote constipation by interfering with peristalsis
3. Can interfere with absorption of vitamins A, D, E, and K
4. Can cause diarrhea

D. If a laxative is necessary, teach how to use bulk-forming agents, such as psyllium seed or bran

1. Start slowly with one-half the recommended dose.
2. Increase dose gradually over weeks.

E. Refer to *Constipation* for interventions to promote optimal elimination

Rationale

- Stimulant laxatives purge the bowel of stool so effectively that a bowel movement may not occur normally for a few days. The person's response is to take the laxative again. This begins the cycle of laxative dependence (DiPiro, Talbert, Hayes, Yee, Matzke, & Posey, 1993).
- The chronic laxative user should be taught a combination of measures consisting of dietary modifications and use of bulk-forming laxatives, with the elimination of stimulant laxatives.

References/Bibliography

Byrne, W. J. (1990). The gastrointestinal tract. In R. E. Behrman & R. Kliegman (Eds.). *Nelson essentials of pediatrics*. Philadelphia: W. B. Saunders.

Christopherson, R. D. (1991). Toileting problems in children. *Pediatric Annual, 20*, 240–244.

DiPiro, J., Talbert, R., Hayes, P., Yee, G., Matzke, G., & Posey, L. M. (1993). *Pharmacotherapy* (2nd ed.). Norwalk, CT: Appleton & Lange.

Evans, K. (1990). Pediatric management problems: Chronic constipation. *Pediatric Nursing, 16*, 590–591.

Giger, J. N., & Davidhizar, R. E. (1991). *Transcultural nursing: Assessment and interventions*. St. Louis: Mosby Year Book.

Hardy, M. A. (1991). Normal changes with aging. In M. Maas, K. Buckwalter, & M. Hardy (Eds.). *Nursing diagnoses and interventions for the elderly*. Redwood City, CA: Addison-Wesley Nursing.

Jackson, D. B., & Saunders, R. B. (1993). *Child health nursing*. Philadelphia: J. B. Lippincott.

Klish, W. J. (1994). Functional constipation and encopresis. In F. A. Oski (Ed.). *Principles and practice of pediatrics*. Philadelphia: J. B. Lippincott.

Lara, L. L. (1990). The risk of urinary tract infection in bowel incontinent men. *Journal of Gerontological Nursing, 16*(5), 24–26, 40–41.

Maas, M., & Specht, J. (1991). Bowel incontinence. In M. Maas, K. Buckwalter, & M. Hardy (Eds.). *Nursing diagnoses and interventions for the elderly*. Redwood City, CA: Addison-Wesley Nursing.

Maresca, T. (1986). Assessment and management of acute diarrheal illness in adults. *Nurse Practitioner, 11*(11), 15–16.

May, K. A., & Mahlmeister, L. R. (1994). *Maternal and neonatal nursing: Family-centered care* (3rd ed.). Philadelphia: J. B. Lippincott.

McLane, A., & McShane, R. (1991). Constipation. In M. Maas, K. Buckwalter, & M. Hardy (Eds.). *Nursing diagnoses and interventions for the elderly*. Redwood City, CA: Addison-Wesley Nursing.

McShane, R., & McLane, A. (1988). Constipation: Impact of etiological factors. *Journal of Gerontological Nursing, 14*(4), 31–34.

Miller, C. A. (1995). *Nursing care of older adults* (2nd ed.). Glenview, IL: Scott, Foresman.

Murray, F. E., & Bliss, C. M. (1991). Geriatric constipation: Brief update on a common problem, *Geriatrics, 46*(3), 64–68.

Toth, L. (1988). Alterations in bowel elimination. In *Neuroscience nursing: Phenomena and practice*. Norwalk, CT: Appleton & Lange.

Wong, D. L. (1993). *Essentials of pediatric nursing* (4th ed.). St. Louis: C. V. Mosby.

Yakabowich, M. (1990). Prescribe with care: The role of laxatives in the treatment of constipation. *Journal of Gerontological Nursing, 16*(7), 4–11, 42–43.

Coping, Ineffective Individual

Defensive Coping

Ineffective Denial

Coping, Ineffective Individual

DEFINITION
Ineffective Individual Coping: A state in which the individual experiences, or is at risk to experience, an inability to manage internal or environmental stressors adequately due to inadequate resources (physical, psychological, behavioral, and/or cognitive).

DEFINING CHARACTERISTICS*
Major (One Must Be Present)
Verbalization of inability to cope or ask for help

or

Inappropriate use of defense mechanisms

or

Inability to meet role expectations

Minor (May Be Present)
Chronic worry, anxiety

Reported difficulty with life stressors

Alteration in social participation

Destructive behavior toward self or others

High incidence of accidents

Frequent illnesses

Verbal manipulation

Inability to meet basic needs

Nonassertive response patterns

Change in usual communication pattern

Substance abuse

RELATED FACTORS
Pathophysiologic
Related to chronicity of condition or complex self-care regimens

Related to changes in body integrity secondary to:

Loss of body part

Disfigurement secondary to trauma

Related to altered affect caused by changes secondary to:

Body chemistry   Intake of mood-altering substance

Tumor (brain)   Mental retardation

Treatment-Related
Related to separation from family and home (*e.g.*, hospitalization, confinement to a nursing home)

---

* Adapted from Vincent, K. G. (1985). The validation of a nursing diagnosis. *Nursing Clinics of North America, 20,* 631–639.

Related to disfigurement due to surgery

Related to altered appearance due to drugs, radiation, or other treatment

Situational (Personal, Environmental)

Related to increased food consumption in response to stressors

Related to changes in physical environment secondary to:

War	Poverty
Natural disaster	Homelessness
Relocation	Inadequate finances
Seasonal work (migrant worker)	

Related to disruption of emotional bonds secondary to:

Death	Institutionalization
Relocation	Desertion
Separation or divorce	Orphanage
Jail	Educational institution
Foster home	

Related to unsatisfactory support system

Related to sensory overload secondary to:

Factory environment

Urbanization: crowding, noise pollution, excessive activity

Related to inadequate psychological resources secondary to:

Poor self-esteem	Helplessness
Excessive negative beliefs about self	Lack of motivation to respond
Negative role modeling	

Related to culturally related conflicts with (specify)

Premarital sex

Abortion

Maturational

Child / adolescent

Related to:

Poor impulse control	Childhood trauma
Peer rejection	Parental substance abuse
Poor social skills	Parental rejection
Inconsistent methods of discipline	Repressed anxiety
Fear of failure	Panic level of anxiety

Adolescent

Related to inadequate psychological resources to adapt to:

Physical and emotional changes	Sexual awareness
Independence from family	Educational demands
Sexual relationships	Career choices

Young adult

Related to inadequate psychological resources to adapt to:

Career choices	Marriage
Educational demands	Parenthood
Leaving home	

Middle adult

Related to inadequate psychological resources to adapt to:

Physical signs of aging	Problems with relatives
Career pressures	Social status needs
Child-rearing problems	Aging parents

Older adult

Related to inadequate psychological resources to adapt to:

Physical changes	Retirement
Changes in financial status	Response of others to older people
Changes in residence	

Author's Note

Ineffective Individual Coping describes an individual experiencing difficulty in adapting to stressful event(s). Usual effective coping mechanisms may be inappropriate or ineffective for this event, or the person may have a poor history of coping with stressors.

If the event is recent, ineffective individual coping may be a premature judgment. For example, a person may respond to overwhelming stress with a grief response such as denial, anger, or sadness, making a *Grieving* diagnosis appropriate.

Impaired Adjustment may be more useful than *Ineffective Individual Coping* in the initial period after a stressful event. *Ineffective Individual Coping* and its related diagnoses may be more applicable to prolonged or chronic coping problems, such as *Defensive Coping* for a person with a long-standing pattern of ineffective coping.

Errors in Diagnostic Statements

Ineffective Individual Coping related to perceived effects of breast cancer on life goals, as evidenced by crying and refusal to talk

If this diagnosis was recent, the person's response of crying and refusal to talk would be normal grief responses. Thus, the proper diagnosis would be *Grieving related to perceived effects of breast cancer on life goals.* If this response was prolonged and evidence of "moving ahead" was not present (*e.g.,* initiation of social activities), *Ineffective Individual Coping* may be appropriate.

Ineffective Individual Coping related to reports of substance abuse

Substance abuse is a reportable or observable cue validating a diagnosis. If the person acknowledged the abuse and desires assistance, the diagnosis would be *Ineffective Individual Coping related to inability to manage stressors without drugs.* If the substance abuse was observed but the person denied that it existed or that it was a problem, the diagnosis would be *Ineffective Denial related to unknown etiology, as evidenced by lack of acknowledgment of drug dependency.*

Key Concepts

1. Lazarus (1985) defines coping as "constantly changing cognitive and behavioral efforts to manage specific external and/or internal demands that are taxing or exceeding the resources of the person."
2. Expectations of mastery encourage maturation and persistence. Expectations of failure induce avoidance behaviors (Potocki & Everly, 1989).
3. Coping behaviors fall into two broad categories (Lazarus & Folkman, 1984):
   a. Problem-focused: Efforts to improve the situation by changing things or taking some action
   b. Emotion-focused: Those thoughts or actions that relieve the emotional distress caused by the situation. Emotion-focused coping behaviors do not alter the situation, but do make the person feel better.
   Examples include:

Problem-Focused	Emotion-Focused
Making appointment with the boss to discuss pay raise	Playing basketball three times per week
Writing out time schedule for homework and adhering to it	Denying anything is wrong
Studying	Using food to relax
Seeking help	Joking

4. Emotion-focused behaviors include the following:
   a. *Minimization* occurs when the seriousness of a problem is minimized. This may be useful as a way to provide needed time for appraisal, but it may become dysfunctional when it precludes appraisal.

    b. *Projection, displacement*, and *suppression of anger* occur when anger is attributed to or expressed toward a less threatening person or thing, which may reduce the threat enough to allow an individual to deal with it. Distortion of reality and disturbance of relationships may result, which further compound the problem. Suppression of anger may result in stress-related physical symptoms.

    c. *Anticipatory preparation* is the mental rehearsal of possible consequences of behavior or outcomes of stressful situations, which provides the opportunity to develop perspective as well as to prepare for the worst. It becomes dysfunctional when the anticipation creates unmanageable stress, as, for example, in anticipatory mourning.

    d. *Attribution* is the finding of personal meaning in the problem situation, which may be religious faith or individual belief. Examples are fate, the will of the divine, and luck. Attribution may offer consolation but becomes maladaptive when all sense of self-responsibility is lost.

5. Addictive behavior is a habitual maladaptive way of coping with stress.

6. According to Miller (1995), individuals "who have a rigid set or narrow range of coping skills are at more risk for impaired coping because different types of coping strategies are effective in different situations."

7. Crisis is defined by Miller (1983) as "the experiencing of an acute situation where one's repertoire of coping responses is inadequate in effecting a resolution of the stress." For an individual, it usually represents a turning point in his or her life and a reorganization of some of the important aspects of his or her psychological structure.

8. An individual crisis can be described in four sequential stages: shock, defensive retreat, acknowledgment, and adaptation.

9. Stress may be defined as the nonspecific response of the body to any demand (Selye, 1974).

10. Stress and disease may be linked in three ways:

    a. Overstimulating a target organ through the neuroendocrine system

    b. Engaging in styles of living that are damaging, such as pressured life-style, poor diet, heavy use of tobacco or drugs

    c. Minimizing the significance of symptoms, leading to neglect or delay in seeking medical care (Monat & Lazarus, 1985)

11. Responses to stress vary among individuals due to personal perceptions of the event. Both positive and negative life events may initiate a stress response.

12. Personal and environmental factors influence how a person copes with a disability. Research findings have supported that motivation and morale are affected by social support, self-concept, locus of control, and hardiness (Evans & Halar, 1985; Sinyor, Amato, Kaloupek, Becker, Goldenberg, & Coopersmith, 1986).

13. Successful coping with physical injury or loss (Hamburg & Adams, 1953):

    a. Reduces stress to manageable limits

    b. Maintains feelings of personal worth

    c. Restores relationships with significant others

    d. Seeks recovery of physical functions

    e. Initiates a situation that is a positive contribution

    f. Initiates a situation (project, job, tasks) after maximum recovery that is viewed as socially acceptable and personally valued

    g. Gains pleasure from mastery

14. Responses to illness, disability, or treatments are influenced by:

    a. Attitude toward event (*e.g.*, punishment, weakness, challenge)

    b. Developmental level or age

    c. The extent of interference of the disability in goal-directed activity and the significance of the goal

15. Reactive depression occurs as a response to a situational stressor.

16. Endogenous depression, possibly somatic in origin, is a maladaptive response to often unidentifiable causes.

Reactive vs. Endogenous Depression

Element	Reactive Depression	Endogenous Depression
Precipitating event	Identifiable	Unclear
Family history	Unrelated	Familial tendency
Symptoms	Related to grief and anxiety; worse at night	Seemingly unrelated to events; worse in morning
Activity	Diminished motor and cognitive behavior	Agitated, restless
Emotion	Client feels sad	Alternates between sadness and manic gaiety
Cognitive abilities	May be slightly diminished	Retarded psychomotor performance
Orientation	Oriented and responsive to environment	May not be oriented or responsive
Treatment	Responds well to counseling and environmental change	May require somatic treatment in addition to counseling

17. Beck's cognitive theory of depression includes the tenets that depressed people process information in negative ways, even when there is evidence to the contrary. They filter information through a view of the world that is negatively toned, thus leading to distortions in thought (Calarco & Krone, 1991).
18. Depression can be conceptualized as a model with acute or chronic stressors interacting with the person's cognitive, interpersonal, and biologic factors (Calarco & Krone, 1991).

Key Concepts—Child

1. A child's ability to cope is affected by inborn traits, social support, and family coping (Wong, 1995).
2. Children who are more vulnerable to stress and demonstrate poorer coping skills include boys, those between 6 months and 4 years of age, those with a difficult temperament, and those with below-average intelligence (Wong, 1995).
3. As children mature, they develop and expand their coping strategies (Byrne & Hunsberger, 1989).
4. Three to 5% of children in the United States have attention deficit disorder (ADD), with boys outnumbering girls nine to one (American Psychiatric Association [APA], 1994).
5. ADD is a developmental disorder, with symptoms changing over time. The diagnosis is made when symptoms of inattention or hyperactivity–impulsivity persist for at least 6 months and are maladaptive and inconsistent with developmental level (APA, 1994).

Key Concepts—Older Adult

1. Miller (1995) identified six major psychosocial challenges of older adults: retirement, death of friends, chronic illness, relocation from family, disruption of household, and stereotypes associated with 65th birthday.
2. Folkman, Lazarus, Pimley, and Novacek (1987) reported that younger subjects reported more stressors related to finances and work, whereas older subjects reported stress related to concerns about health, home maintenance, and social and environmental issues.
3. Anticipation and perceived control over circumstances are predictors of the impact of stress for older adults (Willis, Thomas, Garry, & Goodwin, 1987).
4. In older adults, coping is facilitated in those with higher incomes, higher occupational status, and feelings of high self-efficacy. However, when significant life changes are necessary, higher occupational status and feelings of high self-efficacy are liabilities, because these individuals hold an unrealistic view of what is controllable (Simons & West, 1984).
5. No one life event has a consistently negative impact on an older adult; rather, a number of events in a short period of time represents the greatest challenge (Miller, 1995).

6. Older adults with feelings of high self-efficacy may suffer more when challenged by a disability (Simons & West, 1984).
7. Financial stability enhances coping in older adults (Simons & West, 1984).

TRANSCULTURAL CONSIDERATIONS

1. Three major components of cultural systems influence responses to illness or chronic disease and a person's ability to make healthful changes in lifestyle. These components are family support systems, coping behaviors, and health beliefs and practices (Boyle & Andrews, 1995).
2. In certain cultures, the family plays a critical role in all aspects of the client's life, including "rejection or reinforcement of healthy life style changes" (Boyle & Andrews, 1995, p. 232).
3. The Asian cultures emphasize maintaining harmony and respect. It is not unusual for an Asian client, who sees the nurse as an authority, to agree with all that is suggested. Agreeing does not mean intended compliance, but only good manners. This behavior is opposite to the assertive, questioning behavior emphasized in the dominant American culture (Boyle & Andrews, 1995).
4. Some cultures do not have a vocabulary for expressing emotional distress. There may be strong sanctions or taboos against complaining about one's fate (Mechanic, 1972).
5. Some symptoms that would be interpreted as mental illness by Western medicine are considered normal in some cultures. Visions, hexes, and hearing voices are acceptable in some subcultures in the United States: Appalachian, Asian, African-American, Hispanic, and Native American (Flaskerud, 1984).
6. East Indian Hindu Americans believe in internal and external forces of control. Psychological factors, such as anger, shame, and envy, that are not controlled make the person more susceptible to disease. Illness is also thought to be caused by an external event or misfortune, such as the wrath of a disease goddess, malevolent spirits of dead ancestors, sins committed in previous lives, or jealous living relatives. Hindus wear charms to ward off evil intentions of others (Henderson & Primeaux, 1981).
7. The Chinese culture views mental illness as shameful. Because of this social stigma, families wait until a family member's mental illness is unmanageable before seeking Western medicine (Liu, 1986).
8. Alcoholism is the number one health problem in the black community, reducing longevity with high incidences of acute and chronic alcohol-related diseases (Ronan, 1987). Unemployment has been identified as the primary factor. Treatment programs must be accessible within the community or by public transportation. Black churches serve a dual role as a site for therapy meetings and as a referral service (Giger & Davidhizar, 1991).
9. Among American ethnic groups, Irish Americans rank as the "highest or near highest in terms of heavy alcohol intake, loss of control and negative social consequences" (Giger & Davidhizar, 1991, p. 327). Their alcoholism is attributed to a need for reassurance, to escape psychological burdens, and to repress sexuality and aggression. Treatment includes teaching positive ways to alleviate stress and tension.
10. Alcohol consumption is a way of celebrating life for Mexican Americans. Alcohol contributes to the increased incidence of accidents and violence. Family pride protects the alcoholic male as long as he provides for the family (Arrendondo, Weddige, Justice, & Fitz, 1987).
11. Alcoholism is present in Native Americans in very high percentages. It is responsible for violence, suicides, and fetal alcohol syndrome. Studies have shown an increased sensitivity to alcohol in this group (Giger & Davidhizar, 1991).

Focus Assessment Criteria

Ineffective coping can be manifested in a variety of ways. A person or family may respond with an alteration in another functional pattern (*e.g.*, spiritual distress, altered parenting, violence). The nurse should be aware of this and use assessment data to ascertain the dimensions affected.

Subjective Data

A. Assess for defining characteristics
  1. Physiologic—stress-related symptoms
     a. Cardiovascular

Headache	Fainting (blackouts, spells)
Chest pain	Palpitations
Increased pulse	Increased blood pressure

     b. Respiratory

Shortness of breath	Increased rate and depth of breathing
Smoking history	Chest discomfort (pain, tightness, ache)

     c. Gastrointestinal

Nausea	Change in stool
Vomiting	Change in appetite
Abdominal pain (cramps, stomach ache)	Obesity/frequent weight changes

     d. Musculoskeletal
        Pain
        Weakness
        Fatigue
     e. Genitourinary
        Menstrual changes
        Urinary discomforts (pain, burning, urgency, hesitancy)
        Sexual difficulty (pain, impotence, altered libido, anorgasmia)
     f. Dermatologic

Itching	"Sweats"
Rash	Eczema

     g. Mental health

Phobias	"The blues"
Panic	"Bad nerves"
Insomnia	

  2. Perception of stressor
     a. How did you feel when this occurred? (Threatened or challenged?)
     b. How do you feel now?
     c. How have these stressors affected you?
     d. How are the problems working out?
  3. Obtain history of drinking pattern from client or significant others (Kappas-Larson & Lathrop, 1993).
     a. What was the day of last drink?
     b. How much was consumed on that day?
     c. On how many days out of the last 30 was alcohol consumed?
     d. What was the average intake?
     e. What was the most you drank?
  4. Determine attitude towards drinking by asking CAGE questions:
     a. Have you ever thought you should *C*ut down your drinking?
     b. Have you ever been *A*nnoyed by criticism of your drinking?
     c. Have you ever felt *G*uilty about your drinking?
     d. Do you drink in the morning (*i.e., E*yeopener) (Ewing, 1984)?
  5. Symptoms of depression (Depression Guideline Panel, 1993)*
     a. Depressed mood most of day, nearly every day
     b. Markedly diminished interest or pleasure in almost all activities most of the day, nearly every day
     c. Significant weight loss/gain
     d. Insomnia/hypersomnia
     e. Psychomotor agitation/retardation
     f. Fatigue (loss of energy)

* Diagnostic criteria for a major depressive disorder include that at least five of the eight symptoms and at least one of the first two symptoms must be present most of the day nearly daily for at least 2 weeks.

g. Impaired concentration (indecisiveness)

h. Recurrent thoughts of death or suicide

B. Assess for related factors

1. Current/recent stressors (number, type, duration)
2. Major life events and everyday stresses
3. Social—financial change, job pressure, marital/family conflicts, role changes, retirement, pregnancy, marriage, divorce, aging, school, death
4. Psychological—anxiety, depression, low self-esteem, lack of interpersonal skills, loneliness
5. Environmental—moving, hospitalization, loss of privacy, sensory deprivation/overload

Objective Data

A. Assess for defining characteristics

1. Appearance

Altered affect ("poker" face)	Poor grooming
Appropriate	Inappropriate dress

2. Behavior

Calm	Sudden mood swings
Hostile	Withdrawn
Tearful	

3. Cognitive function

Altered orientation to time, place, person	Impaired memory
Impaired concentration	Impaired judgment
Altered ability to solve problems	

4. Abusive behaviors

a. To self

Excessive smoking	Reckless driving
Excessive alcohol intake	Suicide attempts
Excessive food intake	Unsafe sexual practices
Drug abuse	

b. To others

Does not care

Neglects needs of dependent family members

Is unwilling to listen

Does not communicate

Imposes physical harm on family member (bruises, burns, broken bones)

Unsafe sexual practices

5. In children, attention difficulties (Johnson, 1995)

Difficulty listening	Speech problems
Easily distracted	Reading problems
Difficulty concentrating	Oppositional, stubborn
Impulsivity	Low frustration
Poor judgment	Labile mood
Motor hyperactivity	

Outcome Criteria

The person will

- Verbalize feelings related to his emotional state
- Identify his coping patterns and the consequences of the behavior that results
- Identify personal strengths and accept support through the nursing relationship
- Make decisions and follow through with appropriate actions to change provocative situations in personal environment

Interventions

A. Assess causative and contributing factors
   1. Negative self-concept
   2. Moral or ethical conflict (see *Spiritual Distress*)
   3. Disapproval by others
   4. Inadequate problem solving
   5. Loss-related grief (see *Grieving*)
   6. Sudden change in life pattern
   7. Recent change in health status of self or significant other
   8. Inadequate support system

B. Establish rapport
   1. Spend time with the individual. Provide supportive companionship.
   2. Avoid being overly cheerful. Avoid clichés such as "things will get better."
   3. Convey honesty and empathy.
   4. Offer support. Encourage expression of his feelings. Let him know that you understand his feelings. Don't argue with his expressions of worthlessness by saying things such as "How can you say that? Look at all you accomplished in life."
   5. Offer matter-of-fact appraisals. Be realistic.
   6. Allow extra time for the person to respond.

C. Assess individual's present coping status
   1. Determine onset of feelings and symptoms and their correlation with events and life changes.
   2. Assess ability to relate facts.
   3. Listen carefully as client speaks, to collect facts and observe facial expressions, gestures, eye contact, body positioning, and tone and intensity of voice.
   4. Determine risk of client's inflicting self-harm and intervene appropriately.
       a. Assess for signs of potential suicide.
          History of previous attempts or threats (overt and covert)
          Changes in personality, behavior, sexual life, appetite, sleep habits
          Preparations for death (putting things in order, making a will, giving away personal possessions, acquiring a weapon)
          A sudden elevation in mood
       b. See *Risk for Suicide* for additional information on suicide prevention.

D. Assess level of depression and intervene according to assessed level
   1. Severely depressed or suicidal individuals need environmental controls, usually hospitalization.
   2. Severely depressed people need assistance with decision making, grooming and hygiene, and nutrition.
   3. As depression lifts, individuals can solve problems and increase their coping behaviors.
   4. Involve them in activities. Do not allow social withdrawal.

E. Assist client to develop appropriate problem-solving strategies based on his personal strengths and previous experiences
   1. Have client describe previous encounters with conflict and how he managed to resolve them.
   2. Encourage to evaluate his own behavior.
       a. "Did that work for you?"
       b. "How did it help?"
       c. "What did you learn from that experience?"
   3. Discuss possible alternatives (*i.e.*, talk over the problem with those involved, try to change the situation, or do nothing and accept the consequences).

4. Assist to identify problems that he cannot control directly and help him to practice stress-reducing activities for control (*e.g.*, exercise program, yoga); see Appendix VII for problem-solving techniques.
5. Be supportive of functional coping behaviors.
    a. "Your way of handling this situation 2 years ago worked well for you then; can you do it now?"
    b. Give options; however, the decision making must be left to the client.
6. Mobilize into a gradual increase in activity.
    a. Identify activities that were previously gratifying but have been neglected: personal grooming or dress habits, shopping, hobbies, athletic endeavors, arts and crafts.
    b. Encourage to include these activities in daily routine for a set time span (*e.g.*, "I will play the piano for 30 minutes every afternoon.").
    c. Stress importance of activity in helping client to recover from depression; state that depression is immobilizing and that client must make a conscious effort to fight it to recover.
7. Find outlets that foster feelings of personal achievement and self-esteem.
    a. Make time for relaxing activities (*e.g.*, dancing, exercising, sewing, woodworking).
    b. Find a helper to take over responsibilities from time to time (*e.g.*, sitter).
    c. Learn to compartmentalize (do not carry problems around with you all the time; enjoy free time).
    d. Take longer vacations (not just a few days here and there).
    e. Provide opportunities to learn and use stress management techniques (*e.g.*, jogging, yoga; see also Appendix X).
8. Facilitate emotional support from others.
    a. Seek out people who share a common challenge: establish telephone contact, initiate friendships within the clinical setting, develop and institute educational and support groups.
    b. Establish a network of people who understand your situation.
    c. Decide who is best able to act as a support system (do not expect empathy from people who themselves are overwhelmed with their own problems).
    d. Make time to share personal feelings and concern with coworkers (encourage ventilation; frequently people who share the same circumstances are helpful to one another).
    e. Maintain a sense of humor.
    f. Allow tears.

F. **Initiate health teaching and referrals, as indicated**
    1. For depression-related problems beyond the scope of nurse generalists, refer to appropriate professional (marriage counselor, psychiatric nurse therapists, psychologist, psychiatrist).
    2. Instruct in relaxation techniques; emphasize the importance of setting 15–20 minutes aside each day to practice relaxation. Write down the following guidelines (see Appendix X for additional relaxation techniques).
        a. Find a comfortable position in chair or on floor.
        b. Close eyes.
        c. Keep noise to a minimum (only very soft music, if desired).
        d. Concentrate on breathing slowly and deeply.
        e. Feel the heaviness of all extremities.
        f. If muscles are tense, tighten, then relax, each one from toes to scalp.
    3. Teach assertiveness skills.
    4. Teach use of cognitive therapy techniques.

Rationale

- Effectiveness of coping is influenced by the number, duration, and intensity of the stressors; past experiences; support system; and personality of the individual (Fuller & Schaller-Ayers, 1990).

- Coping effectively requires successful management of many tasks: maintenance of self-concept, maintenance of satisfying relationships with others, maintenance of emotional balance, and management of stress.
- Individuals can be taught problem-solving techniques, such as:
  - *Goal-setting* is the conscious process of setting time limitations on behaviors, which is useful when goals are attainable and manageable. It may become stress inducing if unrealistic or short-sighted.
  - *Information-seeking* is the process of learning about all aspects of a problem, which provides perspective and, in some cases, reinforces self-control.
  - *Mastery* is the learning of new procedures or skills, which facilitates self-esteem and self-control: for example, self-care of colostomies, insulin injection, or catheter care.
  - *Help-seeking* is the reaching out to others for support. Sharing feelings with others provides an emotional release, reassurance, and comfort, as, for example, with weight loss and other self-help and support groups.
- Everyone has implicit or explicit goals. Through experience, patterns of successful behavior in achieving these individual goals are developed. The person then regularly uses this behavior to achieve goals.
- Goals are established to maintain:
  - Physical well-being
  - Self-esteem
  - Productive satisfying interactions with others
- The behavior of individuals is such that:
  - People act to meet needs and achieve goals.
  - Relatively stable patterns of behavior are developed.
  - Behavior is disrupted when both needs and goals are threatened.
- Cognitive adaptation to threatening events (*e.g.*, illness) focuses on searching for meaning, gaining control over the situation, and comparing one's situation with others (Taylor, 1983).
- To facilitate client coping, the nurse must focus on "the thoughts and actions individuals engage in to overcome threats to health, and deal with life crises encountered, in order to attain or retain optimal health and functioning" (Nyamathi, 1989).
- Individuals who work through the anticipated event (*e.g.*, retirement, surgery) are more likely to cope more effectively than those who avoid thinking about the upcoming event (Fiske, 1980).
- Optimal intervention can occur only when the defensive attempts have failed and the person has begun a self-examination of the current situation.
- Adaptation is the process whereby an individual strives to achieve comfortable and effective functioning in the environment. Adaptation is not static; it is an ongoing process.
- Cognitive interventions assist in helping the person to regain control over his life. Included is the identification of automatic thoughts and replacing them with positive thoughts about self.

🌀 Interventions—*Child Focus*

1. If attention disorders are present, explain their etiology and behavioral manifestations to child and caregivers.
2. Help child to understand he or she is not "bad" or "dumb."
3. Establish target behaviors with child and caregivers.
4. Work with parents and teachers to learn more effective behavioral strategies to support success.
   a. Establish eye contact before giving instructions.
   b. Set firm, responsible limits.
   c. Avoid lectures, simply state rules.
   d. Maintain routines as much as possible.
   e. Attempt to keep a calm and simple environment.
   f. Reinforce appropriate behavior with a positive reinforcer (*e.g.*, praise, hug).
5. Assist to improve play with peers (Johnson, 1995).
   a. Start with short play periods.
   b. Use simple, concrete games.

    c. Begin with sympathetic siblings or family members.
    d. Initially, select a quieter and less demanding peer as playmate.
    e. Provide immediate and instant feedback (*e.g.*, "I see you are being distracted"; "You are playing nicely").
6. Initiate health teaching and referrals as needed.
    a. Provide information about medication therapy if indicated.
    b. Consult with specialists as needed (*e.g.*, psychological, learning specialists).

Rationale (Johnson, 1995)

- Interventions focus on helping the child develop self-control and self-respect.
- Children with attention disorders are often very intelligent and do not need repetitive lectures on behavior.
- Routine helps to reduce stress for caregivers and child.
- Children with attention disorders are unable to filter out extraneous stimuli and therefore respond to all, thus losing focus.
- Success with peers in play is critical for positive reinforcement and self-esteem.

Interventions—*Older Adult*

1. Assess for risk factors for ineffective coping in older adults (Miller, 1995)
    a. Inadequate economic resources
    b. Immature developmental level
    c. Unanticipated stressful events
    d. Occurrence of several major events in short period of time
    e. Unrealistic goals

Rationale

- Miller (1995) has identified the following factors as risks for high levels of stress and poor coping in older adults: diminished economic resources, an immature developmental level, the occurrence of unanticipated events, the occurrence of several daily hassles at the same time, the occurrence of several major life events in a short period of time, high social status, and high feelings of self-efficacy in situations that cannot change.

Defensive Coping

DEFINITION

Defensive Coping: The state in which an individual repeatedly presents falsely positive self-evaluation as a defense against underlying perceived threats to positive self-regard.

DEFINING CHARACTERISTICS*
Major (80%–100%)

    Denial of obvious problems/weaknesses
    Projection of blame/responsibility

---

* Source: Norris, J., & Kunes-Connell, M. (1987). Self-esteem disturbance: A clinical validation study. In A. McLane (Ed.). *Classification of nursing diagnoses: Proceedings of the seventh conference.* St. Louis: C. V. Mosby.

Rationalization of failures
Hypersensitivity to slight criticism
Grandiosity

Minor (50%–79%)

Superior attitude toward others
Difficulty in establishing/maintaining relationships
Hostile laughter or ridicule of others
Difficulty in testing perceptions against reality
Lack of follow-through or participation in treatment or therapy

RELATED FACTORS

See *Chronic Low Self-Esteem, Powerlessness*, and *Impaired Social Interaction*

Author's Note

This diagnosis is intimately related to the diagnosis of *Ineffective Individual Coping*. It diverges insofar as it discriminates the exclusive manifestation of a specific, chronic pattern of ineffective coping.

In selecting this diagnosis, it is important to consider the potentially related diagnoses of *Chronic Low Self-Esteem, Powerlessness*, and *Impaired Social Interaction*, because these diagnoses may express how the individual established, or why he maintains, the defensive pattern.

This diagnosis is defined by the individual's dysfunction and inability to cope over time, and is reinforced if the nurse can establish a correlation between exacerbations in this pattern and identified stressors. If, at any point in time, a related, etiologic diagnosis appears applicable, the choice of the *Defensive Coping* diagnosis stems from a determination that the defensive pattern is a barrier to addressing the other diagnosis effectively (Harris, E., personal communication, February, 1996).

Key Concepts

1. Defensive functioning is the ability to use defense mechanisms to protect the ego from overwhelming anxiety. if defensive mechanism are overused, they become ineffective or ego defeating (Johnson, 1993).
2. See Key Concepts under *Ineffective Individual Coping*.

Focus Assessment Criteria

See *Ineffective Individual Coping*

Outcome Criteria

The person will
- Establish realistic goals in concert with caregivers
- Work effectively toward the achievement of these goals without progress being compromised by defensive dynamics

---

Interventions

A. Reduce demands on the individual as stress level or signs of defensive coping increase

1. Environmental—modify the level of, or remove the patient from, environmental stimuli (*e.g.*, noise, activity).

2. Interpersonal—decrease (or limit) contacts with others (*e.g.*, visitors, other patients, staff) as required.

3. Task—clearly articulate minimal expectations for activities. Decrease or increase expectations as tolerated.

4. Therapeutic—structure interactions with staff so that the client knows to whom he is to talk, when, for how long, and on what topics.

5. Strategic—identify stressors that are making demands on the client's coping resources, and develop plans to deal with them. The goal of these efforts is maximally to freeze, reduce, or eliminate stress in general; more specifically, it is to target and deal with those stressors that are exacerbating the defensive pattern most.

B. Establish a therapeutic stance that reduces defensive binds and increases effective actions

1. Maintain a neutral, matter-of-fact tone with a consistent positive regard. Ensure that all staff relate in a consistent fashion, with consistent expectations.

2. Focus on simple, here-and-now, goal-directed topics when encountering the client's defenses.

3. Encourage client to express goals, and then establish agreement with the client in at least one or two areas. (Note that "reflecting-in" statements, such as, "It sounds like you are saying 'x' " *can* produce declarative statements from the patient such as "No, I'm saying '-x'," which can then be agreed with.)

4. Do not react to, defend, or dwell on the client's negative projections or displacements. Try instead to shift the person to more neutral, positive, or goal-directed topics.

5. Disengage from disagreement or allow the patient to disengage.

6. Avoid directive statements. Encourage patient-initiated activities.

7. Avoid control issues, or attempt to present sets of positive options to the client, which allows him or her a measure of choice.

8. Do not challenge distortions or unrealistic/grandiose self-expressions. Try instead to redirect the conversation toward more neutral topics or more realistic topics when some agreement has already been established.

9. Avoid evaluative statements (whether negative *or* positive). Encourage the person to evaluate his or her own progress.

10. In an effort to limit maladaptive behaviors, identify for the client those actions that compromise the achievement of established goals.

11. To promote learning from the person's own actions (*i.e.*, "natural consequences"), identify for the person those actions that have interfered with the achievement of established goals.

12. Reinforce more adaptive coping patterns (*e.g.*, sublimation, formal problem solving, rationalization) that are assisting the person in achieving established goals.

13. Evaluate interactions, progress, and approach with other team members to ensure consistency within the treatment milieu.

C. Work to establish a therapeutic relationship with the client to decrease the need to defend and permit a more direct addressing of underlying, related factors (see *Chronic Low Self-Esteem*)

1. Validate the client's reluctance to trust in the beginning. Over time, reinforce the consistency of your statements, responses, and actions. Give special attention to your meeting of (reasonable) requests or your following through with plans and agreements.

2. Engage the client in diversional, non–goal-directed, noncompetitive activities (*e.g.*, relaxation therapy, games, outings).

3. Encourage self-expression of neutral themes, positive reminiscences, and so forth.

4. Encourage other means for self-expression (*e.g.*, writing, art) if verbal interaction is difficult or if this is an area of personal strength.

5. Listen passively to *some* grandiose or negative self-expression to reinforce your "positive regard." If this does not lead to more positive self-expression or activity, then such listening may prove counterproductive.

6. Establish an ego-support role for yourself by assisting the client to review and examine his or her interactive patterns with others. Note that this is a complex and latter-stage role that begins to address the roots of the defensive pattern itself. It requires significant trust and may not be achievable or recommended for many patients (for whom just becoming more functional at a given point in time may be a more realistic goal). If it is sought-after role, then its operation would incorporate the principles reflected in interventions B1, 9, 11, and 12.

Rationale

- Balance diversional, supportive interactions or activities with goal-directed/problem-focused interactions according to the client's tolerance.
- Increased levels of stress increase defensive coping (Johnson, 1993).
- Interventions attempt to put the person at ease and to focus the person on self-evaluation (Johnson, 1993).
- Interventions that increase trust may provide the person with the opportunity to use cognitive appraisal that could reduce the perceived threat (Nyamathi, 1989).
- If an ego-support role can be established, it is then possible for the client to begin to learn new, more effective coping strategies. Active stressors continue to elicit and reinforce the established defensive pattern, however, so this effort can be expected to be limited by the degree to which the client remains stressed or threatened.

Ineffective Denial

DEFINITION

Ineffective Denial: The state in which an individual minimizes or disavows symptoms or a situation to the detriment of his health.

DEFINING CHARACTERISTICS*
Major (Must Be Present)

Delays seeking or refuses health care attention to the detriment of health
Does not perceive personal relevance of symptoms or danger

Minor (May Be Present)

Uses home remedies (self-treatment) to relieve symptoms
Does not admit fear of death or invalidism
Minimizes symptoms
Displaces source of symptoms to other areas of the body
Unable to admit impact of disease on life pattern
Makes dismissive gestures or comments when speaking of distressing events
Displaces fear of impact of the condition
Displays inappropriate affect

---

* Source: Lynch, C. S., & Phillips, M. W. (1989). Nursing diagnosis: Ineffective denial. In R. M. Carroll-Johnson (Ed.). *Classification of nursing diagnosis: Proceedings of the eighth conference.* Philadelphia: J. B. Lippincott.

RELATED FACTORS
Pathophysiologic
Related to inability consciously to tolerate the consequences of any chronic or terminal illness

Treatment-Related
Related to prolonged treatment with no positive results

Situational/Psychological
Related to inability consciously to tolerate the consequences of:
    Loss of job
    Loss of spouse/significant other
    Financial crisis
    Feelings of negative self-concept, inadequacy, guilt, loneliness, despair, sense of failure
    Drug use
    Alcohol use
    Smoking
    Obesity
Related to feelings of increased anxiety/stress, need to escape personal problems, anger and frustration
Related to feelings of omnipotence
Related to culturally permissive attitudes toward alcohol/drug use

Biologic/Genetic
Related to family history of alcoholism

Author's Note
This type of denial differs from the denial in response to a loss. The denial in response to an illness or loss is necessary to maintain psychological equilibrium and is beneficial. Ineffective denial is not beneficial when the individual will not participate in regimens to improve health or the situation (*e.g.*, denial of substance abuse). If the cause of the ineffective denial is not known, *Ineffective Denial related to unknown etiology* can be used, such as *Ineffective Denial related to unknown etiology as evidenced by repetitive refusal to admit barbiturate use is a problem*.

Errors in Diagnostic Statements
See *Ineffective Individual Coping*

Key Concepts
1. Denial is a set of dynamic processes that protect the person from a threat to self-esteem.
2. The cost or benefits of denial must be evaluated in terms of the situation and resources available (Lazarus, 1985).
3. Denial is common in the grieving process.
4. When action is essential to change a threatening or damaging situation, denial is maladaptive; however, when no action is needed or when the outcome cannot be changed, denial can be positive and can help reduce stress (Lazarus, 1985).
5. A strong, intact denial system interferes with the person's realistic perceptions of the consequences of the situation (*e.g.*, loss, abuse, substance abuse) (Tweed, 1989).
6. Denial can take several forms:
    a. Denial of relevance to the person
    b. Denial of immediacy of the threat
    c. Denial of responsibility

    d. Denial that threat is anxiety provoking
    e. Denial of threatening information
    f. Denial of any information
7. Denial in alcoholism may include denial of loss of control, of family pain, or of the alcoholic's part in the family problem. Denial of alcohol/drug abuse may also be present among relatives and colleagues, because it is difficult to accept.
8. Alcoholics are those excessive drinkers whose dependence on alcohol has attained such a degree that they show a noticeable mental disturbance in or an interference with their bodily and mental health, their interpersonal relations, and their smooth social and economic functioning; or who show the prodromal signs of such developments (Expert Committee on Mental Health, 1951).

Focus Assessment Criteria

1. See *Ineffective Individual Coping* for general assessment
2. If substance abuse is suspected:

Assessment

Subjective Data

The person will
    Deny that alcohol/drug use is problematic
    Justify his use of alcohol/drugs
    Blame others for his use of alcohol/drugs
    Verbalize need of daily use
    Report unsuccessful attempts to reduce or stop use
    Express grandiosity, inflated self-esteem
    Express suspiciousness
    Report need for increased amount to achieve same effect (tolerance)
    Frequent complaints of illness or marital problems

Objective Data

The person will demonstrate inference in:
    Occupational functioning

Absenteeism	Daytime fatigue
Frequent unexplained brief absences	Failed assignments
Elaborate excuses	Loss of job

    Social functioning

Mood swings	Boisterousness/talkativeness
Isolation (avoidance of others)	Impulsiveness
Arguments with mate/friends	Poor judgment
Violence while intoxicated	Apathy
Traffic accidents/citations	Signs of intoxication, overdose
Legal difficulties	

    Physical complications
        Alcohol abuse

Blackout	Liver dysfunction
Memory impairment	Gout symptoms
Lower extremity paresthesias	Anemia
Malnutrition	Gastritis/gastric ulcers
Impatience	Pancreatitis
Unsteady gait	Cardiomyopathy

        Withdrawal symptoms (*e.g.*, tremors, nausea, vomiting, increased blood pressure, pulse, sleep disturbances, disorientation, hallucinations, agitation, seizures)
      Opiate abuse

Drowsiness	Impaired memory
Slurred speech	Slowed motor movements
Pupillary constriction	Malnutrition

Skin infections   Respiratory depression
Liver disease   Constipation
Low testosterone levels   Respiratory infections
Gastric ulcers   Decreased response to pain
Withdrawal symptoms (*e.g.*, tearing, runny nose, gooseflesh, yawning, dilated pupils, mild hypertension, tachycardia, nausea, vomiting, restlessness, abdominal cramps, joint pain)

Amphetamine and cocaine abuse

Hyperactivity   Tetanus
Increased alertness   Skin infections
Decreased appetite/weight loss   Cerebrovascular accident
Increased heart rate   Hallucinations
Dilated pupils   Cardiac dysrhythmias
Chills   Seizures
Nausea and vomiting   Respiratory depression
Hepatitis

Hallucinogen abuse

Increased heart rate   Tremors
Sweating   Incoordination
Palpitations   Hallucinations
Blurred vision   Flashbacks

Cannabis abuse

Dry mouth   Increased appetite
Increased heart rate   Impaired lung structure
Conjunctival infection   Sinusitis

Barbiturate/sedative/hypnotic abuse

Drowsiness   Endocarditis
Impaired memory   Pneumonia
Cellulitis   Respiratory depression
Hepatitis   Signs of intoxication and withdrawal

Outcome Criteria

The person will
• Acknowledge the source of anxiety or stress
• Use alternative coping mechanism instead of denial

Interventions

A. Initiate a therapeutic relationship

1. Assess effectiveness of denial
2. Avoid confronting that denial is being used.
3. Approach in direct, matter-of-fact, nonjudgmental manner.

B. Encourage sharing of their perceptions of the situation (*e.g.*, fears, anxieties)

1. Focus on the feelings shared.
2. Use reflection to encourage more sharing.

C. When appropriate, help with problem solving

Rationale

• Partial, tentative, or minimal denial allows the person to use problem-focused coping skills while reducing the distress (an emotion-focused coping skill) of the situation (Lazarus, 1985).

- Denial may be valuable in the early stages of coping when resources are not sufficient to manage more problem-focused approaches (Lazarus, 1985).
- As denial is reduced, interventions to focus on emerging strong feelings of anxiety and fear are needed.

■ Ineffective Denial
Related to Impaired Ability to Accept Consequences of His/Her Behavior as Evidenced by Lack of Acknowledgment of Substance Abuse/Dependency

Outcome Criteria

The person will
- Acknowledge an alcohol/drug abuse problem
- Explain the psychological and physiologic effects of alcohol or drug use
- Abstain from alcohol/drug use
- State recognition of the need for continued treatment
- Express a sense of hope
- Use alternative coping mechanisms to cope with stress
- Have a plan for high-risk situations for relapse

Interventions

A. Assist to improve self-esteem
   1. Be nonjudgmental.
   2. Assist person in gaining an intellectual understanding that this is an illness, not a moral problem.
   3. Provide opportunities to perform successfully; gradually increase responsibility.
   4. Provide educational information about the progressive nature of substance abuse and its effects on the body and interpersonal relationships.
   5. Refer to *Self-Esteem Disturbance* for further interventions.

B. Instill a sense of hope
   1. Maintain a positive attitude.
   2. Communicate the expectation that person can overcome problems.
   3. Promote setting of realistic, short-term goals.
   4. Facilitate interactions with people who have recovered or are recovering.
   5. Refer to *Hopelessness* for further interventions.

C. Assist in identifying and altering patterns of substance abuse
   1. Explore situations in which the person is expected to use alcohol/drugs (*e.g.*, at home with TV, after work with friends).
   2. Encourage avoidance of situations in which alcohol/drugs are being used.
   3. Assist person in replacing drinking/smoking buddies with nonusers. (Alcoholics Anonymous/Narcotics Anonymous are helpful alternatives here. Each

AA/NA group is unique; encourage person to find a group he or she is comfortable with.)

4. Assist in organizing and adhering to a daily routine.
5. Have person chart his alcohol/drug use (amount, time, situation); useful with early-stage substance abusers who are resistant to treatment (Metzger, 1988).

D. Assist in meeting physiologic and safety needs
1. Observe for signs of withdrawal. See collaborative problem, *Potential Complication: Alcohol withdrawal*
2. Provide supportive care through the detoxification period.
3. Prevent access to abused substances. Monitor visitors and belongings as appropriate.
4. Assess for presence of medical consequences of alcohol/drug use.
   a. Prostatitis
   b. Fetal alcohol syndrome (mental retardation, malformations, hyperactivity, growth deficiency, cardiac problems)
   c. White blood cell, red blood cell, platelet deficiencies
   d. Bleeding tendencies (decreased vitamin K production)
   e. Peripheral neuropathy, myopathy
   f. Hypertension
   g. Cardiac tissue damage, cardiomyopathy
   h. Gastritis, pancreatitis
   i. Hepatitis (alcoholic) cirrhosis
   j. Vitamin metabolism defects
   k. Esophageal varices, hemorrhoids, ascites
   l. HIV-positive or AIDS (high-risk sexual behavior or sharing of needles)
5. Assess potential for violence; refer to *Risk for Violence* for further interventions.
6. Assess for suicide potential; refer to *Risk for Self-Harm* for further interventions.
7. Teach side effects and appropriate interventions associated with medications (*e.g.*, disulfiram [Antabuse], methadone, antianxiety drugs [Librium]).

E. Assist person to identify effects of substance abuse on his life and significant others
1. Avoid labeling the client (*e.g.*, alcoholic, drug addict) or pressing diagnostic labels, which may evoke resistance to accept the substance abuse problems (Amodeo & Liftik, 1990; Miller, 1989).
2. Explore the client's own concerns about use of alcohol/drugs.
3. Assist the person to explore problems that have resulted from substance abuse (*e.g.*, marriage, relationships, health, finance, job, self-esteem).
4. Assist the person to discuss reasons for drug/alcohol use (*e.g.*, dealing with painful emotions, boredom, stress).
5. Assist the person to discuss what changes he wants to make (*e.g.*, What areas of life are important enough to change for—job, family, health? What are the gains or losses? What is his or her perception of life in a few years? Will substance abuse interfere?).

F. Discuss alternative coping strategies
1. Teach relaxation techniques and meditation. Encourage use when the client recognizes anxiety. Refer to Appendix X for stress management techniques.
2. Teach thought-stopping techniques to use when thoughts about drinking/substance use occur. Instruct him to say vocally or subvocally "STOP, STOP" and to replace that thought with a positive one. The technique must be prac-

ticed and the individual may need assistance in identifying replacement thoughts.

3. Assist in anticipating stressful events (*e.g.*, job, family, social situations) in which alcohol/drug use is expected; role-play alternative strategies.
   a. Teach assertiveness skills.
4. Teach how to handle anger constructively.

G. Assist person to achieve abstinence

1. Assist in setting short-term goals (*e.g.*, stopping one day at a time versus insisting never to drink/use again).
2. Assist in structured planning (Washton, 1989):
   a. Discard supplies.
   b. Break contact with dealers/users.
   c. Avoid high-risk places.
   d. Structure free time.
   e. Avoid large blocks of time without activities.
   f. Plan leisure activities that are not associated with alcohol/drug use.
3. Assist in recognizing stressors that lead to substance abuse (*e.g.*, boredom, the drug, interpersonal situations).
4. Assist person in evaluating the negative consequences of the behavior. Visualization may be helpful.
5. When person denies alcohol/drug use, look for nonverbal clues to substantiate facts (*e.g.*, is there verbal and nonverbal congruence, deteriorating appearance, job performance, or social skills?).
6. When on firm ground and a trusting relationship has been established, confront the client's denial.
7. Discourage person from attempting to correct other problems such as obesity and smoking during this time.
8. Do not attempt to probe past history in early abstinence.

H. Assist in resocialization

1. Involve in groups and in establishing an alcohol/drug-free network.
2. Establish a trusting relationship.
3. Involve the family in the treatment process.

I. Initiate health teaching and referral, as indicated

1. Refer to Alcoholics Anonymous, Alanon, AlaTeen.
2. Refer to treatment facility.
3. Teach side effects of drug use.
4. Provide nutritional counseling.

Rationale

- The client probably has been reprimanded by many and is distrustful. The nurse's personal experiences with alcohol may increase or decrease her empathy for the client.
- Historically, alcoholics have been viewed as immoral and degenerate. Acknowledgment of alcoholism as a disease can increase the client's sense of trust.
- Confrontation with family and peers may help to break down the client's denial.
- The client may try to focus on the reasons for using alcohol in an attempt to minimize the problem's significance.
- Participation in a structured treatment program greatly increases the chance of successful recovery from alcoholism.
- Recovering alcoholics provide honest, direct confrontation with the realities of alcoholism.
- A sense of hope can be promoted by affording the client direct contact with an expert who can help.

- The client's family needs assistance to identify enabling behavior and strategies for dealing with a recovering or existing alcoholic.
- Denial in alcoholism may include denial of loss of control, of family pain, or of the alcoholic's part in the family problem. Denial of alcohol/drug abuse may also be present among relatives and colleagues because it is difficult to accept.
- Alcohol and drug abuse is reinforced by the drug itself (*e.g.*, feelings of being high, increased congeniality, gaining attention) or avoiding unpleasant situations. Treatment approaches must be aimed at removing identified reinforcers (Washton, 1989).
- The purpose of the interventions is to assist the person to recognize and affirm the negative relationship between his denial and the resulting adverse consequences (health or social) (Tweed, 1989).
- "Sobriety in the alcoholic represents a major change and necessitates a redefinition of family member relationships if this change is to be maintained" (Captain, 1989, p. 57).
- Helping families work through manageable changes is critical (Captain, 1989).
- A substance-dependent person sees the substance as a solution to every problem. New problem-solving techniques are needed (Smith-DiJulio, 1994).

References/Bibliography

General

American Psychiatric Association. (1994). *Diagnostic and statistical manual of mental disorders* (4th ed.). Washington, DC: Author.

Arrendondo, R., Weddige, R., Justice, C., & Fitz, J. (1987). Alcoholism in Mexican-Americans: Intervention and treatment. *Hospital and Community Psychiatry, 38*, 180–183.

Bink, Y., Devins, G., & Orme, C. (1989). Psychological stress and coping in end-stage renal disease. In R. Neufeld (Ed.). *Advances in the investigation of psychological stress*. New York: John Wiley & Sons.

Boyle, J., & Andrews, M. (1995). *Transcultural concepts in nursing*. Glenview, IL: Scott, Foresman.

Byrne, C., & Hunsberger, M. (1989). Concepts of illness: Stress, crisis, and coping. In R. L. Foster, M. M. Hunsberger, & J. J. T. Anderson (Eds.). *Family-centered nursing care of children*. Philadelphia: W. B. Saunders.

Calarco, M., & Krone, K. (1991). An integrated nursing model of depressive behavior in adults. *Nursing Clinics of North America, 26*, 573–583.

Captain, C. (1989). Family recovery from alcoholism. *Nursing Clinics of North America, 24*, 55–67.

Depression Guideline Panel. (1993, April). *Depression in primary care: Detection, diagnosis and treatment quick reference guide for clinicians, no. 5*. AHCPR Pub. No. 93-0552. Rockville, MD: U.S. Department of Health Care Policy and Research.

Evans, R. L., & Halar, E. M. (1985). Cognitive therapy to achieve personal goals: Results of telephone group counseling with disabled adults. *Archives of Physical Medicine and Rehabilitation, 66*, 693–696.

Expert Committee on Mental Health. (1951). *First report of the alcoholism subcommittee*. WHO Technical Report Series, No. 42. Geneva: World Health Organization.

Fiske, M. (1980). Tasks and crises of the second half of life: The interrelationship of commitment, coping, and adaptation. In J. E. Birren & R. B. Sloan (Eds.). *Handbook of mental health and aging*. Englewood Cliffs, NJ: Prentice-Hall.

Flaskerud, J. H. (1984). A comparison of perceptions of problematic behavior by six minority groups and mental health professionals. *Nursing Research, 33*, 190–197.

Folkman, S., Lazarus, R., Pimley, S., & Novacek, J. (1987). Age differences in stress and coping processes. *Psychology and Aging, 2*, 171–184.

Fuller, J., & Schaller-Ayers, J. (1990). *Health assessment: A nursing approach*. Philadelphia: J. B. Lippincott.

Giger, J. N., & Davidhizar, R. E. (1991). *Transcultural nursing: Assessment and interventions*. St. Louis: Mosby Year Book.

Hamburg, D. A., & Adams, J. E. (1953). A perspective on coping behavior. *Archives of General Psychiatry, 17*, 1–20.

Henderson, G., & Primeaux, M. (1981). *Transcultural health care reading*. Boston: Addison-Wesley.

Johnson, B. S. (1993). *Psychiatric–mental health nursing: Adaptation and growth* (3rd ed.). Philadelphia: J. B. Lippincott.

Johnson, B. S. (1995). *Child, adolescent and family psychiatric nursing*. Philadelphia: J. B. Lippincott.

Johnson, J., & Morse, J. (1990). Regaining control: The process of adjustment after myocardial infarction. *Heart and Lung, 19*, 126–135.

Keller, C. (1990). Coping strategies of chronically ill adolescents and their parents. *Issues in Comprehensive Pediatric Nursing, 13*(2), 73–80.

Lazarus, R. (1985). The costs and benefits of denial. In A. Monat & R. Lazarus (Eds.). *Stress and coping: An anthology* (2nd ed.). New York: Columbia.

Lazarus, R., & Folkman, S. (1984). *Stress, appraisal and coping.* New York: Springer.

Liu, W. T. (1986). Health services for Asian elderly. *Research on Aging, 8*(1), 156–175.

Mechanic, D. (1972). Social psychological factors affecting the presentation of bodily complaints. *New England Journal of Medicine, 286,* 1132–1139.

Miller, C. A. (1995). *Nursing care of older adults* (2nd ed.). Glenview, IL: Scott, Foresman.

Miller, P. (1983). Family health and psychosocial response to cardiovascular diseases. *Health Values, 7*(6), 10–15.

Monat, A., & Lazarus, R. (Eds.). (1985). *Stress and coping: An anthology.* New York: Columbia.

Nyamathi, A. (1989). Comprehensive health seeking and coping paradigm. *Journal of Advanced Nursing, 14,* 281–290.

Potocki, E., & Everly, G. (1989). Control and the human stress response. In G. Everly (Ed.). *A clinical guide to treatment of human stress response.* New York: Plenum Press.

Ronan, L. (1987). Alcohol-related health risks among black Americans. *Alcohol Health and Research World, 12,* 36–39.

Selye, H. (1974). *Stress without distress.* Philadelphia: J. B. Lippincott.

Simons, R. L., & West, G. E. (1984). Life changes, coping resources and health among the elderly. *International Journal of Aging and Human Development, 20,* 173–189.

Sinyor, D., Amato, P., Kaloupek, D. G., Becker, R., Goldenberg, M., & Coopersmith, H. (1986). Poststroke depression: Relationship to functional impairment, coping strategies, and rehabilitation outcome. *Stroke, 17,* 1102–1107

Taylor, S. (1983). Adjustment to threatening events. *American Psychologist, 38,* 1161–1173.

Vincent, K. G. (1985). The validation of a nursing diagnosis. *Nursing Clinics of North America, 20,* 631–639.

Wong, D. L. (1993). *Essentials of pediatric nursing* (4th ed.). St. Louis: C. V. Mosby.

Willis, L., Thomas, P., Garry, P. J., & Goodwin, J. (1987). A prospective study of response to stressful life events in initially healthy elders. *Journal of Gerontology, 42,* 627–630.

Substance Abuse

Amodeo, M., & Liftik, J. (1990). Working through denial in alcoholism. *Families in Society: The Journal of Contemporary Human Services, 71,* 131–135.

Chychula, M. M. (1990). The cocaine epidemic: A comprehensive review of use, abuse and dependence. *Nurse Practitioner, 15*(7), 31–39.

Daley, D. C., & Raskin, M. S. (Eds.). (1991). *Treating the chemically dependent and their families.* Newbury Park, CA: Sage Publications.

Ewing, J. A. (1984). Detecting alcoholism: The CAGE questionnaire. *Journal of the American Medical Association, 252,* 1905–1907.

Kappas-Larson, P., & Lathrop, L. (1993). Early detection and intervention for hazardous ethanol use. *Nurse Practitioner, 18*(7), 50–55.

Lynch, C. S., & Phillips, M. W. (1989). Nursing diagnosis: Ineffective denial. In R. M. Carroll-Johnson (Ed.). *Classification of nursing diagnoses: Proceedings of the eighth conference.* Philadelphia: J. B. Lippincott.

Metzger, L. (1988). *From denial to recovery: Counseling problem drinkers, alcoholics, and their families.* San Francisco: Jossey-Bass.

Miller, W. R. (1989). Evaluation and motivation. In R. K. Hester & W. R. Miller (Eds.). *Handbook of alcoholism treatment approaches: Effective alternatives.* New York: Pergamon Press.

Smith-DiJulio, K. (1994). People who depend on alcohol. In E. M. Varcarolis (Ed.). *Foundations of psychiatric mental health nursing.* Philadelphia: W. B. Saunders.

Tweed, S. H. (1989). Identifying the alcoholic client. *Nursing Clinics of North America, 24,* 13–32.

Washton, A. M. (1989). *Cocaine addiction: Treatment, recovery, and relapse prevention.* New York: W. W. Norton.

Resources for the Consumer

Literature

Alcoholics Anonymous. (1976). *Alcoholics anonymous* (3rd ed.). New York: A.A. World Services.

Bradshaw, J. (1988). *Bradshaw on: The family, a revolutionary way of self-discovery.* Pompano Beach, FL: Health Communications.

Gorski, T. T., & Miller, M. (1986). *Staying sober: A guide for relapse prevention.* Independence, MO: Independence Press.

Narcotics Anonymous. (1988). *Narcotics anonymous* (5th ed.). Van Nuys, CA: Author.

Peluso, E., & Peluso, L. S. (1988). *Women and drugs: Getting hooked, getting clean.* Minneapolis: Compcare Publishers.

Wholey, D. (1988). *Becoming your own parent: The solution for adult children of alcoholic and other dysfunctional families.* Des Plaines, IL: Doubleday.

Yoder, B. (1990). *The recovery resource book.* New York: Simon & Schuster.

Organizations

Al-Anon Family Group Headquarters, Inc., PO Box 862, Midtown Station, New York, NY 10018-0862; (212) 302-7240.

Alcoholics Anonymous, Box 459, Grand Central Station, New York, NY 10017; (212) 686-1100.

Cocaine Anonymous, 6125 Washington Boulevard, Suite 202, Los Angeles, CA 90230; (213) 559-5833.

Families Anonymous, Inc., PO Box 528, Van Nuys, CA 91408; (818) 989-7841.

Narcotics Anonymous, PO Box 9999, Van Nuys, CA 91409; (818) 780-3951.

Coping, Ineffective Family: Disabling

DEFINITION

Ineffective Family Coping: Disabling: The state in which a family demonstrates, or is at risk to demonstrate, destructive behavior in response to an inability to manage internal or external stressors due to inadequate resources (physical, psychological, cognitive).

DEFINING CHARACTERISTICS

Major (One Must Be Present)

Abusive or neglectful care of individual(s)
Decisions/actions that are detrimental to family well-being
Abusive or neglectful relationships with other family members

Minor (May Be Present)

Distortion of reality regarding the person's health problem
Intolerance
Rejection
Abandonment
Agitation
Depression
Aggression
Hostility
Impaired restructuring of a meaningful life for self
Prolonged overconcern for client
Desertion
Psychosomaticism
Taking on illness signs of client

RELATED FACTORS

Biopathophysiologic

Related to impaired ability to fulfill role responsibilities secondary to:
Any acute or chronic illness

Situational (Personal, Environmental)

Related to impaired ability to constructively manage stressors secondary to:

Addiction	Low self-esteem
Alcoholism	History of ineffective relationship with own parents
Negative role modeling	History of abusive relationship with parents

Related to unrealistic expectations of child by parent
Related to unrealistic expectations of self by parent
Related to unrealistic expectations of parent by child
Related to unmet psychosocial needs of child by parent
Related to unmet psychosocial needs of parent by child

Author's Note

Ineffective Family Coping: Disabling describes a family with a history of overt or covert destructive behavior or response to a stressor. This diagnosis necessitates long-term care from a nurse therapist with advanced specialized education in family systems and abuse.

The use of this diagnosis in this book focuses on nursing interventions appropriate for a nurse generalist in a short-term relationship (*e.g.,* emergency unit, nonpsychiatric in-house unit) and for any nurse in the position to prevent *Ineffective Family Coping* through teaching, counseling, or referrals.

Errors in Diagnostic Statements

Ineffective Family Coping: Disabling related to reports of beatings by alcoholic husband

This diagnostic statement is incorrectly formulated and legally inadvisable for a nurse to write. Reported beating by an alcoholic husband is not the contributing factor to the diagnosis, but rather a diagnostic cue. This diagnosis should be written as *Ineffective Family Coping: Disabling related to unknown etiology, as evidenced by wife reporting "My husband is an alcoholic and beats me frequently."* The quoted statement represents the data as reported by the wife, rather than the nurse's judgment.

Key Concepts

1. See *Altered Family Processes* for key concepts of the family.
2. Patterns of maltreatment in families can take many forms, including physical abuse, endangerment, sexual abuse, emotional abuse, neglect (physical, emotional, educational), or economic abuse (Smith-DiJulio & Holzapfel, 1994).
3. Abuse is "willful infliction of physical injury or mental anguish and the deprivation by the caregiver of essential services" (Verwoerdt, 1976, as cited in Smith-DiJulio & Holzapfel, 1994) and nurturing.
4. Individuals involved in family violence have higher levels of depression, suicidal feelings, self-contempt, inability to trust, and inability to develop intimate relationships in later life (Smith-DiJulio & Holzapfel, 1994).
5. Children who witness abuse in their homes after the age of 5 or 6 years develop an identification with the aggressor and lose respect for the victim (Smith-DiJulio & Holzapfel, 1994).
6. Abusive families are characterized by:
   a. Poor differentiation of individuals within the family
   b. Lack of autonomy
   c. Insulation from the influence of others; social isolation
   d. Desperate competition for affection and nurturance among members
   e. Feelings of helplessness and hopelessness
   f. Abuse/violence learned as a way to reduce tension
   g. Low frustration tolerance; poor impulse control
   h. Closeness and caring confused with abuse/violence
   i. Communication patterns characterized by mixed and double messages
   j. High level of conflict surrounding family tasks
   k. Nonexistent parental coalition
7. The role of the victim is a critical factor in the occurrence of child and spouse abuse. The role is socially learned and characterized by helplessness. This occurs when victims learn over time that they cannot control their lives (Shapiro, 1984).
8. Guilt reactions are common among victims; they frequently feel responsible for the incident. This helps to protect them against feelings of powerlessness.

Spouse Abuse
1. "Domestic violence is a behavior that is chosen by a batterer in order to exercise power and control over another person. The batterer, and only the batterer, decides to use abusive and violent behavior. A battered partner cannot make the abuser stop being violent and/or abusive, as the batterer chooses to use this behavior as a form of control. A battered partner does not ask for, invite or provoke the abuser to be violent. The batterer does not become violent because of the use or abuse of alcohol and/or drugs." (AWARE, 1994, p. 1)

2. Spouse abuse in the form of beatings occurs in 1% of all families. Fifty percent of American families are disrupted by some form of violence. Fifteen percent of all homicides are spouse killings; 50% of the victims are women. Women usually kill their husbands with guns and knives, whereas husbands usually beat wives to death (Novello & Soto-Torres, 1992).
3. The battered wife syndrome has three major concepts—the cycle of violence (Fig. II-1), learned helplessness, and anticipatory fear (Blair, 1986).
4. Learned helplessness can be the result of childhood experiences, witnessing or receiving abuse, or the outcome of the battering relationship (Blair, 1986).

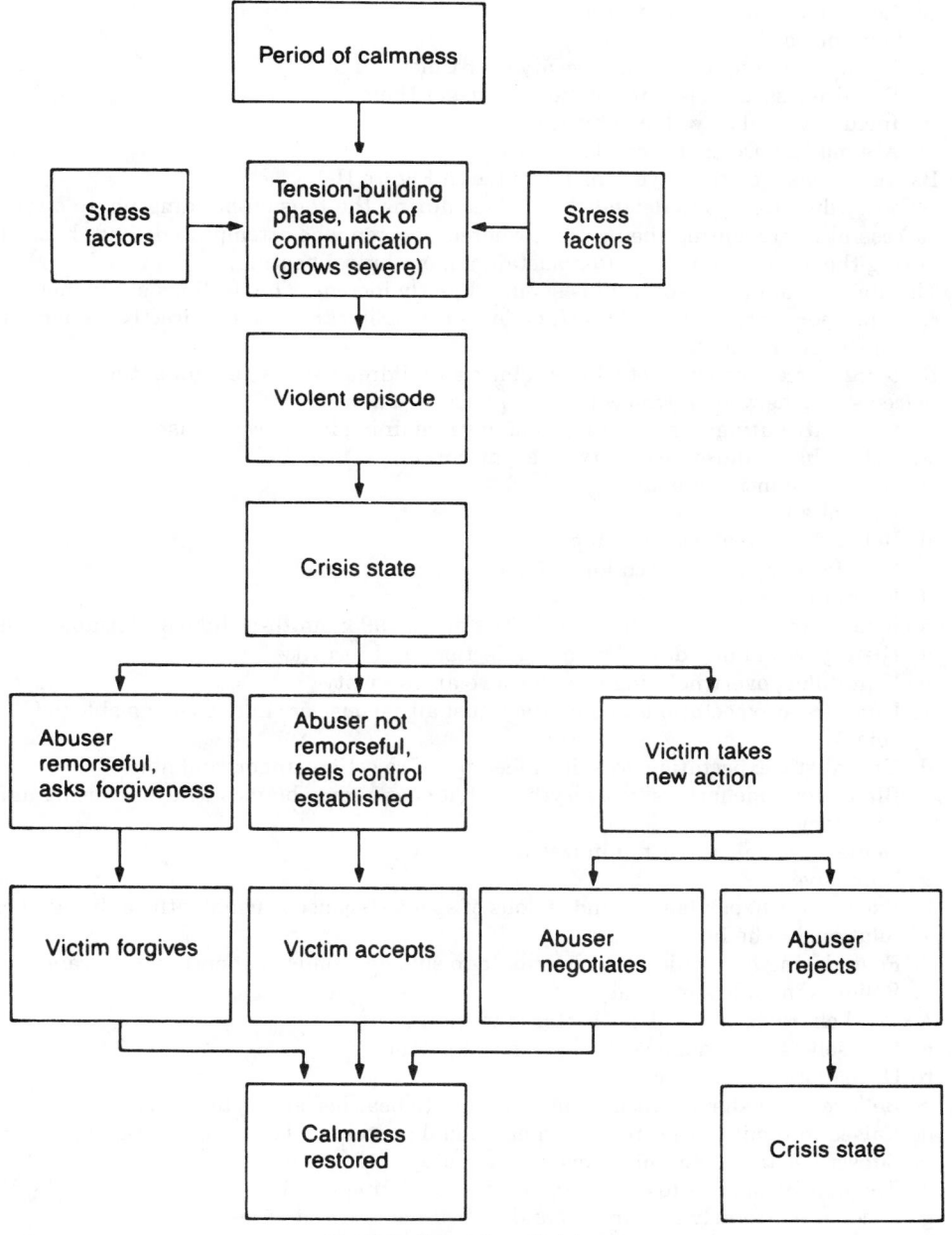

Fig. II-1 Escalation of violence.

5. Victims of abuse are "brainwashed by terror." The victim of abuse uses denial and rationalization when she remains in the battering relationship (Blair, 1986).
6. Battered women rarely report the incident to the health care provider, but instead seek assistance with psychosomatic conditions (chest pain, choking sensations, abdominal pain, fatigue, gastrointestinal disorders, and pelvic pain) or with injuries with inappropriate explanations for them (Greany, 1984).
7. The victims seldom report abuse because of (Blair, 1986):
    a. Feelings of guilt and shame
    b. Fear of social stigmatization
    c. Fear of the abuser
    d. View of violence as normal
    e. Lack of alternative resources
8. Violent episodes
    a. Escalate in frequency and severity over time
    b. Require less and less provocation to trigger them
    c. Include verbal as well as physical abuse
    d. Are made more brutal by alcohol use
9. Battering has a distinct cycle, as indicated in Figure II-1.
10. Women who attempt to defend themselves during the tension-building phase often are successful in preventing the beating, whereas women who attempt to defend themselves during the assaultive phase often sustain a more brutal beating.
11. The abuser's ability to control his spouse directly increases his feelings of autonomy and esteem. Therefore, the fear of loss (and loss of control) of his spouse directly influences his feelings about himself.
12. Battered women who did not witness abuse as children usually remain in the relationship twice as long as women who witnessed abuse as children.
13. Factors contributing to a battered woman's remaining in the relationship are
    a. Belief that children need a two-parent family
    b. Lack of financial support
    c. Lack of a place to go
    d. Belief that the abuse will stop
    e. Fear for her life or her children's lives
    f. Fear of unknown future
14. Personal characteristics of the abuser (Else et al., 1993; Smith-DiJulio & Holzapfel, 1994):
    a. History of a family devoid of love, affection, and security
    b. Unfulfilled, overwhelming need for love and security
    c. Unrealistic expectations about others (usually spouse or child) as being able to fill this void from childhood
    d. Unrealistic expectations result in feelings of rejection, anger, and abuse
    e. Blames outside factors for everything that goes wrong; blames wife for causing him to get angry
    f. Denies the violence or minimizes its severity
    g. Impulsive
    h. Excessively dependent on and jealous of spouse (spouse is usually the only significant relationship he has)
    i. Fears losing her, which can contribute to suicide, homicide, depression, or anger
    j. Believes in male supremacy
15. Personal characteristics of the battered woman:
    a. Low self-esteem, defines self in terms of partner
    b. Unrealistic hopes for change
    c. Believes that she has incited her husband to beat her and is to blame
    d. Raised in families that restricted emotional expression (e.g., anger, hugging)
    e. Subscribes to the feminine sex-role stereotype
    f. Frequently marries to escape restrictive, confining family
    g. Becomes extremely resourceful and self-sufficient to survive
    h. Usually was not abused as a child and did not witness abuse

i. Views herself as a victim with no option but to appease her spouse

j. Gradually increased social isolation

k. Believes partner "can't help it"

16. The likelihood of a woman seeking and using assistance for abuse is increased if (Sammons, 1981):

a. She has been in the relationship less than 5 years

b. She is employed

c. She has friends or relatives who live nearby (within a few miles)

d. She discussed the abuse with others

e. The abuse is frequent (daily, weekly), severe (required medical treatment/hospitalization), or increasing in frequency

🌀 Key Concepts—Child

1. About 2.7 million cases of suspected child abuse and neglect were reported in 1991. Of these cases, 33% were substantiated (National Center on Child Abuse and Neglect, 1993). A federally funded study conducted by Westat, Inc. in 1986 estimated that the professionals they surveyed failed to report almost 40% of the sexually abused children they saw, 30% of fatal or serious physical abuse cases, almost 50% of moderate physical abuse cases, and 70% of neglect cases. At the same time, an equally serious problem is a high number of "unfounded" (not indicated) reports of child maltreatment (Besharov, 1990).

2. The discrepancy between the reported cases of child abuse and neglect and the estimated number is related to differences in laws defining abuse/neglect, professionals' failure to recognize the signs, ignorance of the law, fear of court involvement, and lack of faith in child protective services (Thomas, 1989). Only about one third of cases recognized by professionals are reported (Wissow, 1994).

3. The nurse may come in contact with an abused child in an emergency room, school, or physician's office or in her personal life (Kauffman, Neill, & Thomas, 1986).

4. To minimize misdiagnosis of child abuse, health care professionals should be aware that (Hurwitz & Castells, 1987; Wong, 1987):

a. False allegations of abuse are common.

b. Child abuse may be mistaken for diseases such as hemophilia, erythema multiforme, or osteogenesis imperfecta, or accidental injuries such as car seat burns.

c. Child abuse may be used as a charge in custody battles.

d. Anatomically correct dolls and drawings are tools to help confirm abuse, but they are not confirmation in themselves.

e. Parents or accused people may not have been given adequate opportunity to present their account of the incident.

5. Child abuse is a symptom of a family in crisis or a family dysfunction. The crisis can be illness, financial difficulties, or any recent change in the family unit (*e.g.*, new members, loss of a member, relocation [Kauffman et al., 1986]).

6. Separation of the infant from its parents, as in the case of prematurity, can reduce the attachment and nurturing behaviors of the mother toward her child. A disproportionate number of abused children were premature or ill at birth (Kauffman et al., 1986).

7. Children are usually abused by someone they know: a parent, a babysitter, a relative, or a friend of the family. It must be remembered that most people who abuse a child are well intentioned adults who know the child and care about his or her welfare. The intent was to punish or teach the child a lesson. The abuser usually feels extremely guilty and is often relieved when help is offered. The child also may feel guilt, sensing that he is "bad" and therefore required the discipline (Wong, 1995).

8. Factors that contribute to child abuse include (Wong, 1995):

a. Lack of or unavailability of the extended family

b. Economic conditions (*e.g.*, inflation, unemployment)

c. Lack of role model as a child

d. High-risk children (*e.g.*, unwanted, of undesired sex or appearance, physically or mentally handicapped, hyperactive, terminally ill)

    e. High-risk parents (*e.g.*, single, adolescent, emotionally disturbed, alcoholic, drug addicted, physically ill)

9. Characteristic personal patterns of abusers include (Kauffman et al., 1986):
   a. No dominant ethnic or socioeconomic characteristics
   b. History of abuse by their parents and lack of warmth and affection from them
   c. Social isolation (few friends or outlets for tensions)
   d. Marked lack of self-esteem, with low tolerance for criticism
   e. Emotional immaturity and dependency
   f. Distrust of others
   g. Inability to admit the need for help
   h. Unrealistic expectations for/of child
   i. Desire for the child to give them pleasure

10. The nonabusing parent, who is usually passive and compliant in the abuse, must be included in the treatment plan (Kauffman et al., 1986).

11. The impact of abuse on the parent includes termination of parental rights, angry reactions from professionals, court proceedings and court-ordered treatment, reactions of family members and community, and financial obligations (due to medical and legal expenses) (Kauffman et al., 1986).

🖉 *Key Concepts—Maternal*

1. Studies have shown that 3.9%–8% of women are battered during pregnancy (Campbell, Poland, Waller, & Ager, 1992).
2. There is a correlation of low birth weight and trauma to the fetus and battering (Bullock & McFarlane, 1989).

🏛 *Key Concepts—Older Adult*

1. Older adults are increasingly vulnerable to abuse as they become economically, physically, socially, and emotionally more dependent and resources of the caretakers are limited.
2. Elder abuse is defined as maltreatment, intentional or unintentional, resulting from actions or inactions of others, usually caregivers. Types of elder abuse include physical and psychological mistreatment, misuse of property, and violation of personal rights (Miller, 1995).
3. An estimated 1.5 million elders are abused or mistreated each year (Fulmer, 1989).
4. Research on elder abuse has found origins in both the victim and the perpetrator and also in the relationship between the two (Miller, 1995).
5. Abusive caregivers have been associated with factors such as social isolation, recent decline in health, dependency, coresidency, and poor interpersonal relations with elder (Anetzberger, 1987).
6. According to Miller (1995), "Mandatory reporting laws do not require reporters to know that abuse or neglect has occurred, but merely to report it if they suspect its occurrence."

TRANSCULTURAL CONSIDERATIONS

1. Domestic violence is cross-cultural. It exists in every culture and is a sign of individual and family dysfunction.
2. Traditional Native American life did not include spouse or child abuse. Unfortunately, domestic violence has evolved and is frequently alcohol related (Spector, 1993).

Focus Assessment Criteria

Owing to the complexity and variability of this nursing diagnosis, the nurse must determine the type and extent of the assessment needed with each family.

A. Individual coping patterns of adult members: refer to assessment criteria for *Ineffective Individual Coping*

B. Family coping patterns: refer to assessment criteria for *Altered Family Processes*

C. Parenting patterns: refer to assessment criteria for *Altered Parenting*

D. Violence potential: refer to assessment criteria for *Risk for Violence*

E. Assess for defining characteristics
   1. Domestic abuse* (Subjective)
      a. Have you ever been emotionally or physically abused by your partner or someone important to you?
      b. In the last year, have you been hit, slapped, kicked, or otherwise physically hurt by someone?
      c. Are you or have you ever been pregnant? If yes, have you been hit, slapped, kicked, or otherwise physically hurt by someone? If yes, by whom? How many times?
      d. Within the last year, has anyone forced you to have sexual activities? If yes, who? Number of times?
      e. Are you afraid of your partner or anyone else you listed above?
      f. Has your partner (Campbell, 1989):

Tried to choke you?	Been violent to your children?
Threatened you with a weapon?	Been violent outside the home?
Threatened to try suicide?	Threatened to kill you?

      g. Does your partner (Campbell, 1989):
         Drink to excess?
         Use drugs?
         Try to control your daily activities?
         Try to control who you can be friends with?
         Have a gun?
         Exhibit violent jealousy?
   2. Child abuse suspicion (Subjective, Objective)
      a. Trauma (fractures, lacerations, bruises, welts, burns, dislocations)
         Unexplained injuries
         Nature and extent of injury not consistent with explanation
         Injuries in various stages of healing
         Injuries to face
         Abdominal injuries
      b. Physical indicators of sexual abuse

Vaginal or penile discharges	Venereal diseases
Genital or anal injuries or swelling	Pain or itching in genital area
Pain while urinating	Difficulty walking

      c. Behavioral indicators (Heindl, 1979)

Wary of adult contact	Afraid to go home
Fearful of parents	High pain threshold
Excessive effort to please	Excessive seeking of affection

      d. Indicators of neglect (subjective, objective) (Heindl et al., 1979)

Hunger	Poor growth patterns
Inappropriate dress for weather	Delinquency
Consistent lack of supervision	Assumes adult responsibilities
Unattended medical or dental needs	Constant fatigue or listlessness
Abandonment	

      e. How soon was medical care sought? Immediately after injury, day or more later?
      f. Is medical care sought at the same place or are different places used? Why?
      g. Caregiver–child interaction:
         Is child afraid of adult?   Are they interacting with each other?
         Is adult concerned?

* Source: Nursing Research Consortium on Violence and Abuse, 1989.

F. Assess for related factors
    1. Employment status
            Unemployed   Job satisfaction
    2. Housing
        Physical space: adequate, crowded
            Cleanliness   Privacy
    3. Transportation
            Car   Proximity to work/school/shopping
            Bus   Shared
            Dependency on other
    4. Financial
            Resources   Medical expenses
            Additional expenses
    5. Mental illness of caregiver
    6. Child/elder care provisions
            Who shares burden   Legal history
            Change in job/school status History of criminal/delinquent offenses

---

Outcome Criteria

The person will
• Appraise coping behaviors that are unhealthy for family members
• Relate expectations for self and for the family
• Relate community resources available

Interventions

A. Assist members to appraise family behaviors (usually before a crisis)

B. Discuss the impact of behaviors on individuals and family unit
    1. Emotions
    2. Roles
    3. Support
    4. Performance

C. Assist family to set goals
    1. Short-term
    2. Long-term

D. Promote family stabilization
    1. Identify stressors that can be reduced or eliminated.
        a. Ask each family member to identify one behavior that they could control in them-
           selves.
    2. Begin to help members to work through resentments of the past.

E. Explore with family how their functioning was negatively affected
   (Captain, 1989)
    1. Role-appropriate behaviors
    2. Importance of open communication
    3. Identifying and expressing feelings
    4. Problem-solving strategies
    5. Negotiating techniques

F. Determine family recreational activities that include all members and are enjoyable

G. Initiate referrals as needed
   1. Support groups
   2. Family therapy

Rationale

- Interventions focus on helping the family renegotiate roles and patterns of interacting and functioning (Captain, 1989).
- Each family member is provided an opportunity to share their feelings about the present and past (Smith-DiJulio & Holzapfel, 1994).
- Families with a dysfunctional member (*e.g.*, an alcoholic) are assisted to see that the entire family is dysfunctional, not just the individual (Captain, 1989).
- Short-term goals focus on stabilizing the family as much as possible. Long-term goals focus on changes needed in functioning and establishing patterns to foster lasting change (Captain, 1989).
- Dysfunctional families have a history of isolation. Interventions focus on increasing their socialization and use of community resources (Captain, 1989).
- Family recreational activities foster family cohesion with positive experiences (Captain, 1989).

■ Ineffective Family Coping: Disabling
Related to (Specify), as Evidenced by Domestic Abuse

Domestic abuse is defined as any action that is intended to harm another person (physical, emotional, financial, social, sexual).

Outcome Criteria

The person will
- Discuss the physical assaults
- Identify factors that contribute to violence
- Seek assistance for abusive behavior
- Relate community resources available when help is desired

Interventions

The interventions needed to address the complexity and the magnitude of the problems inherent in domestic violence are usually out of the scope of a nurse generalist. The interventions provided here are to assist the nurse who has a short-term interaction with the individual.

A. Develop rapport
   1. Interview in private. Be empathic.
   2. Don't assume you know what the person needs.
   3. Ask, "How can I help you?"

4. Avoid displaying shock or surprise at the details.

5. If contact is made by phone, find out how to get in touch with victim.

B. **Evaluate potential danger to victim and others**

1. Assess actual physical abuse.
   a. Current and past physical/sexual abuse
   b. When did it happen last?
   c. Are you hurt now?
   d. Are the children hurt?
   e. Assess danger to children.

2. Assess support system.
   a. Does she have a safe place to go?
   b. Does she want police called?
   c. Does she need an ambulance?

3. Assess drug and alcohol use.
   a. Is victim using drugs/alcohol?
   b. Is abuser using drugs/alcohol?

C. **Assess for the presence of factors that inhibit victims from seeking aid**

1. Personal beliefs
   a. Fear for safety of self or children
   b. Fear of embarrassment
   c. Low self-esteem
   d. Guilt (punishment justified)
   e. Myths ("It is normal" or "It will stop")

2. Lack of knowledge of
   a. The severity of the problem
   b. Community resources
   c. Legal rights

3. Lack of financial independence

4. Lack of support system

D. **Encourage decision-making**

1. Provide an opportunity to validate abuse and talk about feelings; if the acutely injured person is accompanied by spouse/caregiver who is persistent about staying, make an attempt to see the person alone (*e.g.*, tell her you need a urine specimen and accompany her to the bathroom).

2. Be direct and nonjudgmental (Blair, 1986).
   a. How do you handle stress?
   b. How does your partner or caregiver handle stress?
   c. How do you and your partner argue?
   d. Are you afraid of him?
   e. Have you ever been hit, pushed, or injured by your partner?

3. Provide options but allow them to make a decision at their own pace.

4. Encourage a realistic appraisal of the situation; dispel guilt and myths.
   a. Violence is not normal for most families.
   b. Violence may stop, but it usually becomes increasingly worse.
   c. The victim is not responsible for the violence.

5. Establish a safety plan (refer to abuse specialists).

E. **Provide referral information**

1. Discreetly inform of community agencies available to victim and abuser (emergency and long-term).
   a. Hotlines
   b. Legal services

c. Shelters
d. Counseling agencies
2. Discuss the availability of the social service department for assistance.
3. Consult with the legal resources in the community and familiarize the victim with the state laws regarding:
   a. Eviction of abuser
   b. Counseling
   c. Temporary support
   d. Protection orders
   e. Criminal law
   f. Types of police interventions
4. Refer for individual, group, or couples counseling.

F. Assist in developing support system
   1. Provide a safe environment, if consenting.
   2. Discuss the importance of regular social contacts to provide opportunities to share and to prevent isolation.
   3. Assist in arranging respite care and other home health services (hot meals, patient aides) for the elderly.

G. Document findings and dialogue for possible future court use (Blair, 1986)
   1. Occurrence, frequency
   2. Type of injury
   3. Record suspect injuries when "the pattern of injuries is inconsistent with the history."

H. Initiate health teaching if indicated
   1. Teach the community about the problem of spouse/elder abuse.
      a. Parent–school organizations
      b. Women's clubs
      c. Programs for schoolchildren
   2. Instruct caregivers in how properly to manage an elderly client at home (*e.g.,* transferring to chair, modified appliances, how to maintain orientation).
   3. Refer for financial assistance and transportation arrangements.
   4. Refer for assertiveness training (see Appendix X).
   5. Inform family of senior citizen centers or day care programs.
   6. Refer the abuser to the appropriate community service (only refer men who have asked for assistance or admitted their abuse, because revealing the wife's confidential disclosure may trigger more abuse).
   7. To secure additional information, contact National Clearinghouse on Domestic Violence, P.O. Box 2309, Rockville, MD 20852.

Rationale

- Nursing interventions should focus on safety and protection.
- Nurses must be cautious not to pressure the victim into a decision prematurely.
- Strategies to address domestic violence must be carefully planned with experts. Consequences of rash decisions can be fatal.
- Myths that offer explanations and tolerance for battering and give an illusion of control and rationality must be openly dispelled (Smith-DiJulio & Holzapfel, 1994).
- Information and referrals are provided to encourage decision making.
- A safety plan is a specific plan for a fast escape if the victim identifies "now is the time to leave" (*e.g.,* destination, money, articles of clothing, insurance information, essential items, medications) (AWARE, 1994).

■ Ineffective Family Coping: Disabling
Related to (Specify), as Evidenced by Child Abuse/Neglect

Child abuse is an action or inaction that brings injury to a child, including physical and psychological injury, neglect, and sexual abuse.

Outcome Criteria

The child will
- Seek comfort from the nurse
- Be free from injury or neglect

The parent will
- Seek assistance for the abusive behavior
- Demonstrate nurturing behavior toward the child

Interventions

A. Identify families at risk for child abuse
  1. Refer to Key Concepts.

B. Intervene before abuse with families at risk
  1. Establish a relationship with parents that encourages them to share difficulties ("Being a parent is sure hard [frustrating] work, isn't it?").
  2. Provide parents with access to information about parenting and child development (see *Altered Growth and Development*).
  3. Provide anticipatory guidance relative to growth and development (*e.g.,* the need to cry in early months; toilet training).
  4. Stress the importance of support systems (*e.g.,* encourage parents to exchange experiences with other parents).
  5. Encourage parents to allow time for their own needs (*e.g.,* attend an exercise class three times a week).
  6. Discuss with parents how they respond to parental frustrations (share feelings with other parents?) and instruct them not to discipline children when very angry.
  7. Explore other methods of discipline aside from physical punishment.
  8. Refer parents to expert help.
  9. Inform parents of community services (telephone hotlines, clergy).

C. Identify suspected cases of child abuse
  1. Assess for and evaluate
      a. Evidence of maltreatment (refer to Focus Assessment Criteria)
      b. History of incident or injury
          Conflicting stories
          Story improbable for age of child
          Story not consistent with injury
      c. Parental behaviors
          Care sought for a minor complaint (*e.g.,* cold) when other injuries are seen
          Exaggerated or absent emotional response to the injury

Unavailable for questioning

Fails to show empathy for child

Angry or critical of child for being injured

Demands to take child home if pressured for answers

   d. Child behaviors

Does not expect to be comforted

Adjusts inappropriately to hospitalization

Defends parents

Blames self for inciting parents to rage

D. **Report suspected cases of child abuse**

   1. Know your state's child abuse laws and procedures for reporting child abuse (*e.g.*, Bureau of Child Welfare, Department of Social Services, Child Protective Services).

   2. Maintain an objective record

     a. Description of injuries

     b. Conversations with parents and child in quotes

     c. Description of behaviors, not interpretation (*e.g.*, avoid "angry father," instead, "Father screamed at child, 'If you weren't so bad this wouldn't have happened.'")

     d. Description of parent–child interactions (*e.g.*, shies away from mother's touch)

     e. Nutritional status

     f. Growth and development compared to age-related norms

E. **Promote a therapeutic environment during hospitalization for child and parent**

   1. Provide the child with acceptance and affection.

     a. Show child attention without reinforcing inappropriate behavior.

     b. Use play therapy to allow child self-expression.

     c. Provide child with consistent caregivers and reasonable limits on behavior; avoid pity.

     d. Avoid asking too many questions and criticizing parent's actions.

     e. Ensure that play and educational needs are met.

     f. Explain in detail all routines and procedures in age-appropriate language.

   2. Assist child with grieving if foster home placement is necessary.

     a. Acknowledge that child will not want to leave parents despite how severe the abuse was.

     b. Allow opportunities for child to ventilate feelings.

     c. Explain the reasons for not allowing child to return home; dispel belief that this is a punishment.

     d. Encourage foster parents to visit child in hospital.

   3. Provide interventions that promote parent's self-esteem and sense of trust.

     a. Tell them it was good that they brought the child to the hospital.

     b. Welcome parents to the unit and orient them to activities.

     c. Promote their confidence by presenting a warm, helpful attitude and acknowledging any competent parenting activities.

     d. Provide opportunities for parents to participate in their child's care (*e.g.*, feeding, bathing).

F. **Promote comfort and reduce fear for child (Smith-DiJulio & Holzapfel, 1994)**

   1. Do not display anger, horror, or shock

   2. Do not blame abuser

   3. Reassure child that he or she was not "bad" or at fault
   4. Do not pressure child to give answers
   5. Do not force child to undress

G. Initiate health teaching and referrals, as indicated
   1. Provide anticipatory guidance for families at risk.
      a. Assist individuals to recognize stress and to practice techniques to manage stress (*e.g.*, planning for time alone away from child; see Appendix X).
      b. Discuss the need for realistic expectations of the child's capabilities.
      c. Teach about child development and constructive methods for handling developmental problems (enuresis, toilet training, temper tantrums); refer to literature in Bibliography.
      d. Discuss methods of discipline other than physical (*e.g.*, deprive the child of his favorite pastime: "May not ride your bike for a whole day"; "May not play your stereo").
      e. Emphasize rewarding positive behavior.
   2. Refer abusive parents to community agencies and professionals for counseling.
   3. Disseminate information to the community about the problem of child abuse (*e.g.*, parent–school organizations, radio, television, newspaper).
      a. Discuss with parents and parents-to-be the problems of parenting.
      b. Teach those who are at risk of being future abusers.
      c. Discuss constructive stress management.
      d. Teach the signs and symptoms of abuse and the method for reporting.
      e. Focus on abuse as a problem that results from child-rearing difficulties, not parental deficiencies.
      f. Relay your understanding of stresses but do not condone abuse.
      g. Focus on the parent's needs; avoid an authoritative approach.
      h. Take opportunities to demonstrate constructive methods for working with children (give the child choices; listen carefully to the child).
   4. Consider developing parenting classes for parents (preventive, corrective) to increase their skills as nurturers and teachers. Weekly topic examples:
      a. What is parenting?
      b. Child development and play
      c. Discipline and toilet training
      d. Play and nutrition
      e. Safety and health
      f. Discipline and common problems
      g. Parental needs
      h. Expectations versus realities (Seditus & Mock, 1988)

Rationale

- The identification of child abuse depends on the nurse recognizing the physical signs, specific parent behavior, specific child behavior, inconsistencies in the history of the injury, and contributing factors (*e.g.*, familial, environmental) (Kauffman et al., 1986).
- The nurse should consult the legislation mandating the reporting of child abuse for the specifics of legal definition, penalties for failure to report, reporting procedure, and legal immunity for reporting (Kauffman et al., 1986).
- The first priority of care for the abused child is preventing further injury (Wong, 1995).
- Successful interactions with abusing parents must be provided in the context of acceptance and approval to compensate for their low self-esteem and fear of rejection (Wissow, 1994).

- Strong negative feelings can interfere with the nurse's judgment and effectiveness (Smith-DiJulio & Holzapfel, 1994).
- Parents' involvement in the treatment plan may help in stopping abuse.
- Children, being egocentric, assume they are responsible for the maltreatment or neglect (Wong, 1995).
- Maltreatment of children can be reduced with programs that teach parents to interpret and understand their children's behaviors and appropriate responses (Wissow, 1994).

■ High Risk for Ineffective Family Coping: Disabling
Related to Multiple Stressors Associated With Elder Care

Outcome Criteria

The caregiver will
- Discuss the stressors of elder care
- Relate strategies to reduce stressors
- Identify community resources available

The older adult will
- Describe methods to increase socialization beyond caregiver
- Identify resources available for assistance

Interventions

A. Identify individuals (caregiver, older adult) at high risk for abuse

1. Caregiver
   a. Social isolation
   b. Dependency on elder (financial, emotional); coresidency
   c. Health problems (physical, mental)
   d. Substance abuse
   e. Poor relationship history with elder
   f. Financial problems
   g. Transgenerational violence
   h. Relationship problems

2. Older adult
   a. Dependent on others for activities of daily living
   b. Isolated
   c. Financially insecure
   d. Impaired cognitive functioning
   e. Depressive personality
   f. History of abuse to caregiver
   g. Incontinence

B. Assist caregivers to reduce stressors

1. Establish a relationship with caregivers that encourages them to share difficulties.
2. Encourage them to share experiences with others in same situation.
3. Evaluate caregiver's ability to provide long-term in-home care.
4. Explore sources of help (*e.g.*, housekeeping, home-delivered meals, day care, respite care, transportation assistance).
5. Encourage caregiver to discuss sharing responsibilities with other family members.
6. Discuss alternative sources of care (*e.g.*, nursing home, senior housing).
7. Discuss how caregiver can allow time for his or her own needs.
8. Discuss community resources available for help (*e.g.*, crisis hotline, social service, voluntary emergency caregivers).

C. Assist older adults to reduce risks of abuse by providing the following suggestions (American Association of Retired Persons, 1987)

1. Keep contact with old friends and neighbors if you relocate with relative.
2. Plan a weekly contact in person with friend, neighbor.
3. Participate in community activities as much as possible.
4. Take care of own personal needs.
5. Have your own telephone.
6. Acquire legal advice for possible future disability.
7. Do not accept personal care in exchange for transfer of assets or property without legal advice.
8. Do not live with someone who has a history of violence or substance abuse.

D. Identify suspected cases of elder abuse; observe for these signs

1. Failure to adhere to therapeutic regimens, which can pose threats to life (*e.g.*, insulin administration, ulcerated conditions)
2. Evidence of malnutrition, dehydration
3. Bruises, swelling, lacerations, burns, bites
4. Pressure ulcers
5. Caregiver not allowing nurse to be alone with elder
6. Consult with home health nurse to plan a home visit for assessment of signs of abuse or neglect (Smith-DiJulio & Holzapfel, 1994).
   a. House in poor repair
   b. Inadequate heat, lighting, furniture, or cooking utensils
   c. Unpleasant odors
   d. Inaccessible food
   e. Old food
   f. Older adult lying on soiled materials (*e.g.*, urine, food)
   g. Medication not being taken
   h. Presence of garbage

E. Report suspected cases (Anetzberger, 1987)

1. Consult with supervisor for procedures for reporting suspected cases of abuse.
2. Maintain an objective record, including:
   a. Description of injuries
   b. Conversations with elder and caregivers
   c. Description of behaviors
   d. Nutritional, hydration status

3. Consider the elder's right to choose to live at risk of harm providing he is capable of making that choice.
4. Do not initiate an action that could increase the elder's risk of harm or antagonize the abuser.
5. Respect the elder's right to secrecy and the right for self-determination.

F. Initiate health teaching and referrals, as indicated
1. Refer high-risk caregivers for counseling.
2. Refer elder for counseling to explore choices.
3. Explore support services (*e.g.*, respite, home health aide, homemaker services).
4. Disseminate information to community regarding prevention.
    a. Publicize support services.
    b. Seek to assist caregiving families (*e.g.*, companions, respite care, day care centers).
    c. Seek to establish weekly contact with dependent elderly.
    d. Attempt to reduce isolation of caregivers and elders.
    e. Develop procedures for investigation, public education.

Rationale

- Strategies for management of abuse include identification, access and assessment, intervention, follow-up, and prevention (O'Malley, Everitt, O'Malley, & Campion, 1983).
- Multiple, interrelated variables seem to be responsible for elder abuse. Invisibility of the problem and vulnerability of the older person are common to all elder abuse (Miller, 1995).
- Steinmetz (1988) reported that caregivers' perceptions of stress and feelings of burden are strong predictors of elder abuse.
- Abused elders usually do not report abuse because of fear of reprisal or abandonment. Rather, elder abuse must be detected.
- Interventions are focused on assisting caregivers to reduce stress and select constructive coping responses (Miller, 1995).
- Educational programs serve to advocate for elders and to raise the consciousness of the community.
- Each state has specific guidelines for reporting suspected cases of elder abuse.
- Caregivers should be given an opportunity to share their feelings of frustration and stress.

Compromised Family Coping

DEFINITION

Compromised Family Coping: That state in which a usually supportive primary person (family member or close friend) is providing insufficient, ineffective, or compromised support, comfort, assistance, or encouragement that may be needed by the client to manage or master adaptive tasks related to his or her health challenge.

DEFINING CHARACTERISTICS
Subjective Data

Client expresses or confirms a concern or complaint about significant other's response to his or her health problem.

Significant person describes preoccupation with personal reactions (*e.g.*, fear, anticipatory grief, guilt, anxiety) to client's illness, disability, or to other situational or developmental crises.

Significant person describes or confirms an inadequate understanding or knowledge base, which interferes with effective assistive or supportive behaviors.

Objective Data

Significant person attempts assistive or supportive behaviors with less than satisfactory results.

Significant person withdraws or enters into limited or temporary personal communication with the client at time of need.

Significant person displays protective behavior disproportionate (too little or too much) to the client's abilities or need for autonomy.

RELATED FACTORS

See *Altered Family Processes*

Author's Note

This nursing diagnosis describes situations that are similar to the diagnosis *Altered Family Processes*. Until clinical research differentiates this diagnosis from the aforementioned diagnosis, use *Altered Family Processes*.

Coping, Family: Potential for Growth

DEFINITION

Family Coping: Potential for Growth: Effective managing of adaptive tasks by family member involved with the client's health challenge, who now is exhibiting desire and readiness for enhanced health and growth in regard to self and in relation to the client.

DEFINING CHARACTERISTICS

Family member attempting to describe growth impact of crisis on his or her own values, priorities, goals, or relationships

Family member moving in direction of health-promoting and enriching life-style that supports and monitors maturational processes, audits and negotiates treatment programs, and generally chooses experiences that optimize wellness

Individual expressing interest in making contact on a one-to-one basis or on a mutual-aid group basis with another person who has experienced a similar situation

RELATED FACTORS

See *Health-Seeking Behaviors* and *Altered Family Processes*

Author's Note

This nursing diagnosis describes components that are found in *Altered Family Processes* and *Health-Seeking Behaviors*. Until clinical research differentiates the category from the aforementioned categories, use *Altered Family Processes* or *Health-Seeking Behaviors*, depending on the data presented.

References/Bibliography

Aiken, M. M. (1990). Documenting sexual abuses in prepubertal girls. *American Journal of Maternal–Child Nursing, 15*, 176–177.

AWARE. (1994). *Safety strategies for battered women & their children.* Mercer County, PA: AWARE.

Blair, K. (1986). The battered woman: Is she a silent partner? *Nurse Practitioner, 11*(6), 38.

Bullock, L. F., & McFarlane, J. (1989). Higher prevalence of low birthweight infants born to battered women. *American Journal of Nursing, 89*, 1153–1155.

Bullock, L. F., McFarlane, J., Bateman, L., & Miller, V. (1989). Characteristics of battered women in a primary care setting. *Nursing Practitioner, 14*, 47–55.

Campbell, J. C. (1989). A test of two explanatory models of women's responses to battering. *Nursing Research, 38*, 18–24.

Campbell, J., Poland, M., Waller, J., & Ager, J. (1992). Correlates of battering during pregnancy. *Research in Nursing and Health, 15*, 219–226.

Captain, C. (1989). Family recovery from alcoholism. *Nursing Clinics of North America, 24*, 55–67.

Else, L., et al. (1993). Personality characteristics of men who physically abuse women. *Hospital and Community Psychiatry, 44*(10), 54–62.

Greany, G. (1984). Is she a battered woman? A guide for emergency response. *American Journal of Nursing, 84*, 725–727.

Novello, A. C., & Soto-Torres, L. E. (1992). Women and the hidden epidemics: HIV/AIDS and domestic violence. *The Female Patient, 17*, 17.

O'Malley, T. A., Everitt, D. F., O'Malley, H., & Campion, E. (1983). Identifying and preventing family mediated abuse and neglect of elderly. *Annals of Internal Medicine, 93*, 998–1004.

Sammons, L. (1981). Battered and pregnant. *Maternal-Child Nursing Journal, 6*, 246–250.

Shapiro, R. (1984). Therapy with violent families. In S. Saunders, A. Anderson, C. Hart, C., et al. (Eds.). *Violent individuals and families: A handbook for practitioners.* Springfield, IL: Charles C Thomas.

Smith-DiJulio, K., & Holzapfel, S. K. (1994). Families in crises: Family violence. In E. M. Varcarolis (Ed.). *Foundations of psychiatric mental health nursing.* Philadelphia: W. B. Saunders.

Spector, R. (1993). Culture, ethnicity and nursing. In P. Potter & A. Perry (Eds.). *Fundamentals of nursing* (pp. 95–115). St. Louis: C. V. Mosby.

Child

Besharov, D. J. (1990, Spring). Gaining control over child abuse reports: Public agencies must address both under reporting and over reporting. *Public Welfare,* 34–40.

Heindl, C. (1979). The nurse's role in the prevention and treatment of child abuse and neglect. Publication No. 79-30202. Washington, DC: U.S. Department of Health, Education and Welfare.

Helfer, R. E., & Kempe, C. H. (1972). *Helping the battered child and his family.* Philadelphia: J. B. Lippincott.

Hurwitz, A., & Castells, S. (1987). Misdiagnosed child abuse and metabolic diseases. *Pediatric Nursing, 13*, 33–36.

Kauffman, C. K., Neill, M. K., & Thomas, J. N. (1986). The abusive parent. In S. H. Johnson (Ed.). *High-risk parenting: Assessment and nursing strategies for families at risk.* Philadelphia: J. B. Lippincott.

National Center on Child Abuse and Neglect. (1993). *A coordinated response to child abuse and neglect: A basic manual.* Washington, DC: NCCAN.

Seditus, C., & Mock, D. (1988). Interrupting the cycle of child abuse. *Maternal–Child Nursing Journal, 13*, 196–198.

Thomas, B. H. (1989). Nursing strategies: Child abuse and maltreatment. In R. L. Foster, M. M. Hunsberger, & J. J. T. Anderson (Eds.). *Family-centered nursing care of children.* Philadelphia: W. B. Saunders.

Wissow, L. (1994). Child maltreatment. In F. Oski (Ed.). *Principles and practice of pediatrics* (2nd ed.). Philadelphia: J. B. Lippincott.

Wong, D. L. (1987). False allegations of child abuse: The other side of the tragedy. *Pediatric Nursing, 13*, 329–333.

Wong, D. L. (1995). *Essentials of pediatric nursing* (3rd ed.). St. Louis: C. V. Mosby.

Elder Abuse

Anetzberger, G. J. (1987). *The etiology of elder abuse by adult offspring.* Springfield, IL: Charles C Thomas.

Fulmer, T. T. (1989). Mistreatment of elders. *Nursing Clinics of North America, 24,* 707–716.

Miller, C. A. (1995). *Nursing care of older adults* (2nd ed.). Glenview, IL: Scott, Foresman.

Steinmetz, S. K. (1988). *Duty bound: Elder abuse and family care.* Newberry Park, CA: Sage.

Resources for the Consumer

Literature

American Association of Retired Persons. (1987). *Domestic mistreatment of the elderly: Towards prevention—some do's and don't's* (pamphlet).

Child Care Manual, ROCOM Press, P.O. Box 1577, Newark, NJ 07101.

Christophersen, E. R. (1977). *Little people: Guidelines for common sense child rearing.* Lawrence, KS: H & H Enterprises.

Forward, S. (1986). *Men who hate women and the women who love them.* New York: Bantam Books.

Salk, L., & Kramer, R. (1973). *How to raise a human being.* New York: Warner Books.

Your child from 1 to 6. U.S. Department of Health, Education, and Welfare, Children's Bureau, Publication No. 30, Washington, DC, 20014.

Organizations

American Humane Association (AHA), Denver, CO.

LaLeche League International, 9616 Minneapolis Avenue, Franklin Park, IL 60131; also local chapters.

National Aging Resource Center on Elder Abuse, 810 First St. NE, Suite 500, Washington DC 20002-4205.

Parent Effectiveness Training, 531 Stevens Avenue, Solana Beach, CA 92075.

Parents Without Partners, 7910 Woodmount Avenue, #1000, Washington, DC 20014; also local chapters.

Local Counseling Services

Catholic Charities, Jewish Family Services, Christian Family Services, community agencies, and mental health centers.

Coping, Ineffective Community

DEFINITION
Ineffective Community Coping: The state in which a community's pattern of activities for adaptation and problem solving is unsatisfactory for meeting the demands or needs of the community.

DEFINING CHARACTERISTICS
Major (Must Be Present)
Community does not meet its own expectations
Unresolved community conflicts
Expressed difficulty in meeting demands for change
Expressed vulnerability

Minor (May Be Present)

Angry	Bitter
Indifferent	Apathetic
Helpless	Hopeless
Overwhelmed	

RISK FACTORS
Presence of risk factors (see Related Factors)

RELATED FACTORS
Situational
Related to lack of knowledge of resources
Related to inadequate communication patterns
Related to inadequate community cohesiveness
Related to inadequate problem solving
Related to inadequate community resources
Related to inadequate law-enforcement services
Related to overwhelming community destruction secondary to:

Flood	Hurricane
Earthquake	Epidemic
Avalanche	

Related to traumatic effects of:

Airplane crash	Industrial disaster
Large fire	Environmental accident

Related to threat to community safety (*e.g.*, murder, rape, kidnaping, robberies)
Related to sudden rise in community employment

Maturational
Related to inadequate resources for:

Children	Working parents
Adolescents	Older adult

Author's Note

This diagnosis is useful for nurses who practice with aggregates. An aggregate is a group of people "who have in common one or more personal or environmental characteristics" (Williams, 1977). Thus an aggregate can be the population of a small town, high-school girls, or Hispanic men with hypertension in Philadelphia.

This diagnosis may be more frequently used as a Risk diagnosis than an actual one. Nurses practicing with community aggregates would identify risk factors that could cause *Ineffective Community Coping*. The focus would be assisting the community to prevent the diagnosis.

Errors in Diagnostic Statements

Ineffective Community Coping related to unresolved community conflicts

Unresolved community conflicts are a sign of *Ineffective Community Coping*, not a contributing factor. The nurse needs to assess the community for causes of unresolved conflicts, such as lack of knowledge or insufficient resources.

Key Concepts

1. "In community settings, there is a generally broader focus on both physical and mental health than on the disease per se and on the variables that affect health directly or indirectly, such as life style, family interaction patterns and community resources (public transportation and adequate housing)" (Aroskar, 1979, p. 36).
2. The community is viewed as a system itself with a number of interacting subsystems, such as the health care system (Spradley, 1990).
3. "The values of the community are reflected in their identification of health needs and how they are met or not met based on some notion of rights to health and justice" (Aroskar, 1979, p. 36).
4. Community health care is different from home health care. The following illustrates the difference:

Community Health Care	Home Health Care
Continuous	Episodic
Targets populations	Targets individuals, families
Focuses on groups that do not seek care	Focuses on individuals who seek care
Emphasizes wellness and primary prevention	Emphasizes restoring health after an acute episode

5. Nurses who focus on populations or aggregates in the community must use epidemiologic approaches to establish an accurate data base. Epidemiology is the study of the distribution and determinants of health, disease, and injuries in populations. Sources of this data are vital statistics, census data, reportable diseases (state determined), registries (*e.g.*, cancer, tuberculosis), the Food and Drug Administration, the Consumer Product Safety Commission, the Environmental Protection Agency, and the National Center for Health Statistics Health Surveys. This information is available nationally, by states and counties, and through local health departments (Spradley, 1990).

6. The goal of epidemiology is to identify populations at risk so as to institute programs and services to prevent or halt the progression of disease (Clemen-Stone, Eigasti, & McGuire, 1992).

7. Community competence describes the collective functioning of the total community unit (Goeppinger, Lassiter, and Wilcox, 1982).

8. In 1976, Cottrell noted that a competent community has four important characteristics (Spradley, 1990).
   a. They can collaborate effectively in identifying community needs and problems.
   b. They can achieve a working consensus on goals and priorities.
   c. They can agree on ways and means to implement the agreed-on goals.
   d. They can collaborate effectively in the required actions.

9. Interventions with communities are categorized in the same way as interventions for individuals—primary prevention, secondary prevention, and tertiary prevention.
   a. Primary preventions are interventions that seek to strengthen the normal line of defense. Examples of primary prevention are immunization programs and classes for adults to prevent osteoporosis.
   b. Secondary preventions are interventions that seek to detect and treat existing health problems at the earliest stage possible. Examples of secondary prevention are hypertension screening programs and teaching self-breast or self-testicular exams to high-school students.
   c. Tertiary preventions are interventions that attempt to reduce the extent and severity of a health problem and to reestablish system equilibrium. Examples of tertiary prevention are posters to warn children playing in vacant lots about rats and Alcoholics Anonymous.

10. Community health nursing interventions can be grouped under the categories of educative, engineering, and enforcement. Educative interventions provide knowledge to foster preventive health behaviors. Engineering focuses on environmental modification to reduce or eliminate barriers to healthy living (*e.g.*, unsafe walkways). Enforcement involves using regulatory agencies to promote health and protect the community from harm (White, 1982).

Focus Assessment Criteria

A. Assess for defining characteristics
   1. Expressed vulnerability
   2. History of unresolved conflicts
   3. Response to present situation

Angry	Indifferent	Bitter	Apathetic
Helpless	Overwhelmed	Hopeless	

B. Assess for related factors
   1. Support available

Financial	Housing	Counseling	Food, clothing

   2. Problem-solving ability

Past	Present

3. Adequacy of community resources

    Emergency relief (funds, food, shelter)?   Counseling?

    Required health services?   Community meeting place?

    Law enforcement?

4. Community limitations

    Lack of cohesiveness   Inadequate communication system

    Isolating patterns   Inadequate information

5. Channels of communication

    Closed   Disregards subgroups

    Top-down style

Outcome Criteria

The community will
- Access information to improve coping
- Use communication channels to access assistance

Interventions

A. Assess for causative or contributing factors
1. Lack of knowledge of available resources
2. Inadequate problem solving
3. Inadequate communication links
4. Value conflicts
5. Threat to community safety

B. Provide opportunities for community members to meet and discuss the situation (*e.g.*, schools, churches, synagogues, town hall)
1. Demonstrate acceptance of their anger, withdrawal, or denial.
2. Correct misinformation as needed.
3. Discourage blaming.

C. Promote community competence in coping (Spradley, 1990)
1. Focus on community goals, not individuals.
2. Engage subgroups into group discussions and planning.
3. Ensure resource access for all members (*e.g.*, flexible hours for working members).
4. Devise a method for formal disagreements.
5. Evaluate each decision's impact on all community members.

D. Explore techniques that may improve coping; elicit suggestions from the group

E. Discuss resources that can be accessed; prepare the group to accept outside help
1. Emergency shelter, funds, food, clothes
2. Counseling
3. Transportation
4. Health care

F. Plan how to access isolated people in community

G. Establish a method to access information and support (*e.g.*, local health department, hospital, churches, synagogues, community center)

H. Initiate referrals as indicated
1. Counseling
2. Public assistance

Rationale

- Assessment of the community involves studying the interacting variables that influence a community's health (Spradley, 1990).
- Certain behaviors or beliefs can interfere with problem solving. These factors (*e.g.*, anxiety, fear, value conflicts) should be explored in discussions (Clemen-Stone et al., 1992).
- Community-oriented nursing addresses the health needs of population groups at risk, or aggregates, and ways of organizing the community to meet the identified needs.
- Spradley described essential conditions for community competence (1990, p. 385). A healthy community:
  - Has a high degree of awareness that "we are a community"
  - Uses its natural resources while taking steps to conserve them for future generations
  - Openly recognizes the existence of subgroups and welcomes their participation in community affairs
  - Is prepared to meet crises
  - Is a problem-solving community; it identifies, analyzes, and organizes to meet its own needs
  - Has open channels of communication that allow information to flow among all subgroups of citizens in all directions
  - Seeks to make each of its systems' resources available to all members of the community
  - Has legitimate and effective ways to settle disputes that arise within the community
  - Encourages maximum citizen participation in decision making
  - Promotes a high level of wellness among all its members
- The interventions for *Ineffective Community Coping* ideally would be secondary prevention rather than tertiary. Interventions to treat early community disequilibrium can prevent serious problems.

References/Bibliography

Aroskar, M. (1979). Ethical issues in community health nursing. *Nursing Clinics of North America, 14*, 35–44.

Clemen-Stone, E., Eigasti, D. G., & McGuire S. L. (1992). *Comprehensive family and community health nursing* (3rd ed.). St. Louis: Mosby Year Book.

Goeppinger, J., Lassiter, P., & Wilcox, B. (1982). Community health is community competence. *Nursing Outlook, 30*, 464–467.

Spradley, B. W. (1990). *Community health nursing* (3rd ed.). Glenview, IL: Scott, Foresman.

White, M. S. (1982). Construct for public health nursing. *Nursing Outlook, 30*, 527–530.

Williams C. (1977). Community health nursing—what is it? *Nursing Outlook, 25*, 250–254.

Coping, Potential for Enhanced Community

DEFINITION

Potential for Enhanced Community Coping: A state in which a community's pattern for adaptation and problem solving is satisfactory for meeting the demands or needs of the community, but the community desires to improve management of current and future problems/stressors.

DEFINING CHARACTERISTICS
Major (Must Be Present)
Successful coping with a previous crisis

Minor (May Be Present)
Active planning by community for predicted stressors
Active problem solving by community when faced with issues
Agreement that community is responsible for stress management
Positive communication among community members
Positive communication between community/aggregates and larger community
Programs available for recreation and relaxation
Resources sufficient for managing stressors

RISK FACTORS
Presence of risk factors (see Related Factors)

RELATED FACTORS
Situational
Related to availability of community programs to augment (specify)

Nutritional status	Exercise program
Weight control	Self-actualization
Stress management	Social support

Maturational
Related to availability of community programs to augment coping with life cycle events, such as

Aging	Parenting
Adolescence	Retirement
Pregnancy	"Empty nest"

Author's Note
This diagnosis can be used to describe a community that wishes to improve an already effective pattern of coping. For a community to be able to be assisted to a higher level of functioning, its basic needs for food, shelter, safety, a clean environment, and a supportive network must first be addressed. When these needs are met, programs can focus on higher functioning, such as wellness and self-actualization. Community programs can be designed after a community assessment and because of community requests. They can focus on enhancing health promotion with topics related to optimal nutrition, weight control, regular exercise programs, constructive stress management, social support, role responsibilities, and preparing for and coping with life cycle events such as retirement, parenting, and pregnancy.

Errors in Diagnostic Statements
Potential for Enhanced Coping related to present destructive response to the flood disaster
     When a community is assessed as having a destructive response to a disaster, *Potential for Enhanced Coping* is incorrect. The diagnosis should be *Ineffective Community Coping*. Interventions would focus on problem solving and accessing resources to promote effective coping.

Key Concepts
1. A community has four major elements: people, social interaction, area, and common ties (Clemen-Stone, Eigasti, & McGuire, 1992). Communities are a social unit "of people living in an environment that has the ability to meet their life goals and needs" (Clemen-Stone et al., 1992, p. 73).

2. Communities have six common components: people, goals, needs, environment, service systems, and boundaries (Clemen-Stone et al., 1992).
   a. *People:* the most important resource or core of the community. Functional, cohesive communities have shared values.
   b. *Goals/needs:* The goals and needs of individuals and groups in the community reflect the community goals and needs. As in Maslow's hierarchical order of needs, the community must have fulfilled needs in physiology, safety, and social affiliation before it can address meeting the higher needs of esteem and self-actualization.
   c. *Community environment:* The environment (climate, natural resources, buildings, food, water supply, flora, animals, insects, economics, health and welfare services, leadership, social networks, recreation, and religion) has a major impact on health.
   d. *Service systems:* A network of agencies and organizations in the community that help to meet the basic needs (social welfare, education, economic) and the health needs of the community.
   e. *Boundaries:* Communities are defined by boundaries. Some boundaries are concrete, such as geographic, political (*e.g.*, cities, states) or situational (*e.g.*, home, school, work). Conceptual boundaries are defined by interests, such as postmastectomy women.
3. Communities have functions to achieve life goals and needs of the population. These functions are:
   a. *Production/distribution/consumption:* Goods and services that are essential for community well-being and functioning are available. Tax funds are used to fund this system.
   b. *Socialization:* This is the process of relating in a social environment. Knowledge, values, beliefs, customs, and behaviors are transmitted to community members.
   c. *Social control:* Norms and rules of social control provide safety and order. Law agencies, courts, and government enforce social order.
   d. *Social participation:* Interactions with others meet basic needs for self-expression and self-fulfillment.
   e. *Mutual support:* Communities provide networks of people helping each other as individuals, religious groups, and official agencies.
4. There are differences between urban and rural communities. Rural communities have fewer than 2500 residents. Rural people are more self-reliant and reluctant to seek assistance from others (Bushy, 1990).
5. Researchers have found that rural people "define health as the ability to work and to do what needs to be done" (Bushy, 1990, p. 89). Comfort, cosmetic issues, and health promotion are not valued. Health care services are accessed when the person cannot work (Bushy, 1990).
6. Rural communities often are resistant to outsiders' ideas and prefer health care professionals who live in their community. However, because people all know one another, they are reluctant to ask for help or share problems for fear neighbors will find out (Bushy, 1990).
7. In population-based planning, the assessment phase involves conducting a needs assessment, analyzing the data, prioritizing the needs, and setting objectives (Clemen-Stone et al., 1992).

Focus Assessment Criteria

Community Screening Assessment (Clemen-Stone et al., 1992)

When assessing each area, consider the community's major strengths and needs.
1. Population
   a. Density
   b. Composition

Gender ratio	Ethnic origins
Age distribution	Race distribution

   c. Characteristics

Mobility	Educational level
Socioeconomic status	Marriage rate
Level of employment	Divorce rate

    d. Mortality rates

        Overall rate   Age-specific rates

        Infant mortality   Leading causes of death

        Maternal mortality

    e. Morbidity rates

        Specific diseases incidence rate

    f. Community norms

        Values, attitudes

    g. Family composition

        Head of household

        Number of members in household

        Number of children per family

2. Environmental
   a. Climate
   b. Types and frequency of natural disasters
   c. Housing types
   d. Air quality
   e. Water supply, quality
   f. Industrial pollutants, toxins
   g. Types of plants
   h. Types of animals, insects, reptiles

3. Health systems

        Emergency   Hospice, respite

        Hospitals   Home care

        Long-term care   School health services

        Preventive services Ambulatory services

4. Public assistance

        Type available   Housing

        Transportation   Special services

        Meals

5. Public safety

        Police

        Fire

        Ambulance

6. Education

        Public   Private

        Libraries   Special educational services (*e.g.*, health)

        Educational level of members

7. Economic

        Major industry   Major occupations

        Banks, credit unions Median income

        Sources of income   Percentage of population below poverty level

        Percentage of retired people

8. Government

        Official leadership

        Town, city offices

        Accessibility

9. Recreation

        Public   Leisure activities (frequently used)

        Private   Programs for special populations

        Recreational activities (frequently used)   (*e.g.*, elderly)

10. Religion

        Types   Community programs, services

11. Communication ability

        TV, radio   Community groups

        Local newspaper

■ Potential for Enhanced Community Coping
Related to Availability of Community Programs to Augment (Specify)

Outcome Criteria

The community will
- Access programs designed to improve overall community well-being

---

Interventions

A. Meet with influential members of target populations to determine health promotion needs (Archer, 1983)
  1. For what needs of members could the nursing agency develop services?
  2. How can the agency promote or market the services to motivate people to use them?
  3. Will enough members of the targeted population use the service?
  4. Based on past programming, what improvements can be made for the future?
  5. Are similar services provided by another agency or organization (hospital, religious)?

B. Plan the development of programs targeted for a specific population, such as
  1. Adolescents (13–18 years)
     a. Career planning
     b. Stress management
  2. Pregnant women
     a. Adolescent, adult
  3. Young adults (18–29 years)
     a. Career selection
     b. Constructive relationships
     c. Balancing one's life
     d. Parenting issues
  4. Middle age (30–50 years)
     a. Launching children
     b. Reciprocal relationships
     c. Aging parents
  5. Older adults (51–65 years)
     a. Aging parents
     b. Balancing one's life
     c. Retirement issues
     d. Facts and myths of aging
  6. All ages
     a. Civic planning
     b. Meeting the needs of all community members
     c. Crisis intervention
     d. Grieving

C. Define the target health promotion needs
  1. Analyze assessment of community (*e.g.*, risk groups, health problems).

    2. Prioritize the needs.
      a. Severity of the risk
      b. Probability of success
      c. Cost–benefit ratio (*e.g.*, resources available)
    3. Select a health promotion program.
    4. Identify target population (*e.g.*, entire community, older adults, adolescents).
    5. Delineate a timetable for the planning and implementation stages.

D. Develop detailed program objectives and the evaluation framework to be used
    1. Content
    2. Time needed
    3. Ideal teaching method for targeting group
    4. Teaching aids (*e.g.*, large-print materials)

E. Establish resources needed and sources
    1. Space
    2. Transportation facilities
    3. Optimal day of week
    4. Optimal time of year
    5. Supplies, audiovisual equipment
    6. Financial (budgeted, donations)

F. Market the program
    1. Media (*e.g.*, newspaper, TV, radio)
    2. Posters (food market, train station)
    3. Flyers (distribute via school to home)
    4. Word of mouth (religious organizations, community clubs, schools)
    5. Guest speaker (community clubs, schools)

G. Provide program and evaluate if desired results (objectives) were achieved
    1. Number of participants
    2. Actual expenditures versus budgeted
    3. Objectives achieved
      a. Participant evaluations
      b. Statistics (*e.g.*, bicycle accidents)
    4. Revisions for future planning
      a. Adequate planning
      b. Shared responsibility
      c. Negative feedback

Rationale

- For a community that has a history of effective coping with problems and stressors, the community nurse can offer programs and services to promote high-level wellness. These programs would focus on:
  - Optimal nutrition
  - Weight control
  - Stress management
  - Exercise programs
  - Self-actualization
  - Social support
  - Coping with life cycle events

- Life cycle events are predictable developmental tasks of young adults, middle-aged adults, and older adults. These events include (Clemen-Stone et al., 1992):
  - *Young Adult* (18–29 years)
    - Gaining autonomy from parents
    - Selecting and choosing a career
    - Developing an intimate relationship
    - Developing parenting skills
    - Developing personal life-style
    - Accepting one's citizen's role
  - *Middle-Aged Adult* (30–50 years)
    - Evaluating one's career
    - Helping children become autonomous
    - Sustaining a few deep friendships
    - Supporting aging parents
    - Participating in civic or social activities
    - Maintaining home property
    - Having satisfying leisure time
    - Adapting to changes associated with aging
  - *Older Adult* (51–65 years)
    - Being flexible in views
    - Seeking to update knowledge
    - Seeking to develop mutually supportive relationships with children and the younger generation
    - Nurturing partner relationships
    - Adjusting to personal losses
    - Helping aged parents
    - Using increased leisure time pleasurably
    - Preparing for retirement or another career
    - Adapting to losses associated with aging
- Involving community leaders in planning can increase community commitment and participation with their personal influence (Clemen-Stone et al., 1992).
- Effective community functioning can be promoted when service systems are functioning to reduce community member stressors (Clemen-Stone et al., 1992).
- Programs to reduce developmental-related stressors can reduce tension-producing stimuli that can disrupt a community (Clemen-Stone et al., 1992).
- Health care program planning provides an orderly structure for organizing large quantities of data to achieve community health goals successfully (Clemen-Stone et al., 1992).

References/Bibliography

Archer, S. E. (1983). Marketing public health nursing services. *Nursing Outlook, 31*, 49–53.

Bushy, A. (1990). Rural determinants in family health: Considerations for community nurse. *Family and Community Health, 12*(4), 89–94.

Clemen-Stone, S., Eigsti, D., & McGuire, S. (1992). *Comprehensive family and community health nursing* (3rd ed.). St. Louis: Mosby Year Book.

Decisional Conflict

DEFINITION

Decisional Conflict: The state in which an individual/group experiences uncertainty about a course of action when the choice involves risk, loss, or challenge.

DEFINING CHARACTERISTICS*

Major (80%–100%)

Verbalized uncertainty about choices
Verbalization of undesired consequences of alternative actions being considered
Vacillation between alternative choices
Delayed decision making

Minor (50%–79%)

Verbalized feeling of distress while attempting a decision
Self-focusing
Physical signs of distress or tension (*e.g.*, increased heart rate, increased muscle tension, restlessness) whenever the decision comes within focus of attention
Questioning personal values and beliefs while attempting to make a decision

RELATED FACTORS

Many situations can contribute to decisional conflict, particularly those that involve complex medical interventions of great risk. Any decisional situation can precipitate conflict for an individual; thus, the examples listed below are not exhaustive, but reflective of situations that may be problematic and possess factors that increase the difficulty.

Treatment-Related

Related to risks versus the benefits of (specify test, treatment):
(Surgery)

Tumor removal	Joint replacement
Cataract	Hysterectomy
Laminectomy	Transplant
Orchiectomy	Cesarean section
Cosmetic	

(Diagnostics)

Amniocentesis	X-rays
Ultrasound	

Chemotherapy
Radiation
Dialysis
Mechanical ventilation
Enteral feedings
Intravenous hydration
Use of preterm labor medications

---

* Supporting research from Hiltunen, E. (1989). Nursing diagnosis: Decisional conflict (specify). In R. M. Carroll-Johnson (Ed.). *Classification of nursing diagnoses: Proceedings of the eighth conference.* Philadelphia: J. B. Lippincott.

Situational

Related to risks versus the benefits of:
Personal

Marriage	Breast vs. bottle feeding
Separation	Institutionalization (child, parent)
Divorce	Abortion
Parenthood	Sterilization
Birth control	Nursing home placement
Artificial insemination	Transport from rural facilities
Adoption	Foster home placement
Circumcision	

Work/task

Career change	Business investments
Relocation	Professional ethics

Related to:

Lack of relevant information   Confusing information

Related to:

Disagreement within support systems
Inexperience with decision making
Unclear personal values/beliefs
Conflict with personal values/beliefs
Resignation
Family history of poor prognosis
Hospital environment—loss of control
Ethical dilemmas of:

Quality of life	Termination of pregnancy
Cessation of life-support systems	Organ transplant
"Do not resuscitate" orders	

Maturational

Related to risks versus benefits of:
(Adolescent)

Peer pressure	Use of birth control
Sexual activity	Whether to continue a relationship
Alcohol/drug use	College
Illegal/dangerous situations	Career choice

(Adult)

Career change	Relocation
Retirement	

(Older adult)

Retirement   Nursing home placement

Author's Note

The nurse has an important role in assisting clients and families with decision making. Because nurses usually do not benefit financially from decisions made regarding treatments and transfers, they are in an ideal position to assist with decisions. Although, according to Davis (1989), "nursing or medical expertise does not enable health care professionals to know the values of patients or what patients think is best for themselves," nursing expertise does enable nurses to facilitate systematic decision making that considers all possible alternatives and possible outcomes, and takes into account individual beliefs and values. The focus is on assisting with logical decision making, not on promoting a certain decision. "When people are making a treatment decision of considerable risk, they do not necessarily experience conflict. In situations where the treatment option is 'choosing life,' individual perception may be one of submitting to fate and be relatively unconflicted. Because of this, nurses must be cautious in labeling patients with the nursing diagnosis of 'Decisional Conflict' without sufficient validating cues" (Soholt, 1990).

Errors in Diagnostic Statements

Decisional Conflict related to failure of physician to gain permission for mechanical ventilation from family

If this situation did occur, this statement represents an unprofessional and legally problematic approach to the situation. Failure of the physician to gain permission for mechanical ventilation would be a practice dilemma necessitating formal reporting to the appropriate parties. Should the family have evidence that this treatment was not desired by the client (*i.e.*, a living will), this situation would not be described as *Decisional Conflict*, because there is no uncertainty about a course of action. The nurse should further assess the family for responses fitting other nursing diagnoses, such as *Grieving*.

Decisional Conflict related to uncertainty about choices

Uncertainty about choices validates *Decisional Conflict*; it is not a causative or contributing factor. If the person needed more information, the diagnosis would be *Decisional Conflict related to insufficient knowledge about choices and their effects*.

Key Concepts

1. An antecedent condition of decision making is a problem. Problems exist when goals are to be attained and there is uncertainty about an appropriate solution. A problem suggests more than one alternative solution.
2. Making a decision is a systematic process—a means, rather than an end (McDevitt-Graham, 1987). Decision making is a sequential process in which each step builds on the previous one (Lancaster & Lancaster, 1982). Optimal decision making is more likely to occur when done systematically, but it does not necessarily have to be a rigid, step-by-step process.
3. The logical steps of decision making are well identified in clinical practice (Bailey & Hendricks, 1987; Lancaster & Lancaster, 1982; Minogue & Reedy, 1988). They can be summarized in the following steps:
   a. Definition of the problem
   b. Listing of the possible alternatives or options
   c. Identification of the probable outcomes of the various alternatives
   d. Evaluation of the alternatives based on actual or potential threats to beliefs/values
   e. Making a decision
4. People usually are not taught a systematic method for making a decision, so frequently they rely on past experiences and intuition (Bailey & Hendricks, 1987). The intuitive mode of decision making is characterized by interaction and association among ideas that seem to coexist simultaneously (Nugent, 1982; Soholt, 1990).
5. Soholt (1990) identified that the following factors may influence a person when making a health care treatment decision:
   a. Reliance on the truth of medical advice
   b. Submission to fate when the treatment option is "choosing life"
   c. Consideration of values
   d. Regard for public opinion
6. The decision-making process is complicated when there is a need for a rapid decision (Minogue & Reedy, 1988). Making an intelligent decision during a period of acute stress is difficult, if not impossible. The stress can be enormous if the decision is compounded by a sense of urgency (Valanis & Rumpler, 1985).
7. Decisional conflict occurs when a person has simultaneous opposing tendencies to accept or reject a course of action (Janis & Mann, 1977).
8. Decisional conflict becomes more intense when it involves a threat to status and self-esteem (Zotti, 1987).
9. Decisional conflict is greater when none of the alternatives is good.
10. Jezewski (1993) reported that both intrapersonal and interpersonal conflict occurs when do-not-resuscitate decisions are being made. Intrapersonal conflict occurs because of discord with individual values and life events. The most common interpersonal conflict arises between staff and family members and among family members.

11. There are essentially three decision-making models in health care (Bille, 1987; Burke, 1980; Gauthier & Krasser-Maxwell, 1991; Valanis & Rumpler, 1985):
   a. Paternalism
      Health care providers make all of the decisions regarding patient care
      Based on a perceived need to protect the patient
      Locus of control is external to the patient and significant others
   b. Consumerism
      Health care providers only provide the patient and significant others with the information they request
      Based on the premise that the patient "knows best"
      Locus of control is internal for the patient and significant others
   c. Humanism/advocacy
      Health care providers collaborate with the patient and significant others to arrive at a decision
      Based on mutual respect for individual dignity and worth
      Locus of control is shared and all participants have an equal role in decision making
12. The most important right that a person possesses is the right of self-determination, the right to make the ultimate decision concerning what will or will not be done to his body (Marsh, 1986). Choice is facilitated when an individual is free to make it (Kohnke, 1980).
13. Value conflicts often lead to confusion, indecision, and inconsistency. Decision making is more complicated for a person when his goals conflict with those of his significant others. People may decide in contradiction to their values if the need to please others is greater than the need to please themselves (Kohnke, 1980).

🌹 *Key Concepts—Child*

1. In most cases, children do not make major decisions for themselves. A surrogate, usually a parent, must make the decision on behalf of the child (Brunnquell, 1990).
2. A child's ability to understand a situation and make a decision depends on age, developmental level, and past experience. However, understanding should not be confused with legal competence (Brunnquell, 1990).
3. As the adolescent matures, he gains the ability to analyze problems and make decisions (Scott, 1989).
4. Researchers working with children should seek assent from children with a mental age of 7 years or older. Parents must give written, informed consent for the child to participate in the study (Wong, 1995).

🏛 *Key Concepts—Older Adult*

1. Decisions are often made for, not with, older adults.
2. Barriers to decision making by older adults include dementia, depression, long-term passivity regarding decisions, and hearing or other communication problems (Miller, 1995).
3. Reasons why decision makers exclude elderly people from involvement in decisions that profoundly affect their lives include beliefs that the elderly are incompetent, not qualified, or not interested, and the desire to avoid discussion of sensitive topics (*e.g.*, finances, relocation) (Miller, 1995).
4. Family members making a decision to place an elderly family member in a long-term facility found information from health care professionals inadequate. Friends who validated the situation were most helpful (Dellasega & Mastrian, 1995).

TRANSCULTURAL CONSIDERATIONS

1. Fatalism is a belief that little can be done to change life events and the best response is submission and acceptance. Americans of Latin, Irish, Appalachian, Filipino, Puerto Rican, and Russian Orthodox origins frequently have this external focus of control (Giger & Davidhizar, 1991).
2. Northern European and African Americans have been found to have both internal and external foci of control (Giger & Davidhizar, 1991).

Focus Assessment Criteria

Decisional conflict is a subjective state that the nurse must validate with the individual. The nurse should assess each individual to determine the person's level of decision making within the present conflict situation. Some of the same cues may be seen in people with diagnoses of *Hopelessness*, *Powerlessness*, and *Spiritual Distress*.

Subjective Data

A. Assess for defining characteristics

    1. Decision-making patterns

        "Tell me about the decision you need to make."

        "How would you describe your usual method of making decisions?"

        Person may say:

            "I simply cannot decide."

            "What should I do?"

            "What would you do if you were me?"

            "Why don't you just tell me what I should do?"

    2. Perception of the conflict

        "How does it make you feel when you think about the decision you have to make?"

        "Has there been a change in your sleep patterns, appetite, activity level?"

        Person may state:

            "The risk is too great for me to decide."

            "This whole situation makes me very anxious."

            "I can't believe I got myself into this predicament."

            "I feel so uptight every time I think about the decision I have to make."

            "I feel like I have no control over the decision that needs to be made."

B. Assess for related factors

    1. "Why is this a stressful decision for you?"

    2. "What things make you uncomfortable about deciding?"

    3. "In the past, how did you arrive at decisions that had a positive outcome?"

    4. "What decisions have you made that you felt confident about?"

    5. "When you make a decision, do you do it alone or do you like to involve other people? If so, whom do you consult for advice?"

Objective Data

A. Assess for defining characteristics

    1. Body language

        Posture (rigid)

        Facial expression (annoyed, tense)

        Hands (rigid, wringing)

        Eye contact (darting)

    2. Motor activity

        Immobile   Pacing

        Increased   Agitation

    3. Affect

        Labile   Flat   Inappropriate

Outcome Criteria

The individual/group will

- Relate the advantages and disadvantages of choices
- Share their fears and concerns regarding choices and responses of others
- Make an informed choice

Interventions

A. Assess causative/contributing factors

   1. Lack of experience with or ineffective decision making
   2. Value conflict
   3. Fear of outcome/response of others
   4. Insufficient/inconsistent information
   5. Controversy with support system
   6. Unsatisfactory health care environment

B. Reduce or eliminate causative or contributing factors

   Internal
   1. Lack of experience with or ineffective decision making
       a. Review past decisions made by the person and what steps were taken to help him decide. Focus on major life events and what the final outcome was. Capitalize on past decisions that have served the person well.
       b. Facilitate a logical decision-making process.
           Assist the person in recognizing what the problem is and clearly identify the decision that needs to be made.
           Generate a list of all the possible alternatives or options.
           Help identify the probable outcomes of the various alternatives.
           Aid in evaluating the alternatives based on actual or potential threats to beliefs/values.
           Encourage the person to make a decision.
       c. Assess the person's usual locus of control (see *Powerlessness*) and support decision-making patterns.
       d. Encourage the person's significant others to be involved in the entire decision-making process.
       e. Suggest that the person use significant others as a sounding board when considering the decision alternatives.
       f. Regard the person as a competent decision maker—treat decisions and desires with respect.
       g. Be available to review the decision that needs to be made and the various alternatives.
       h. Teach and assist with relaxation techniques (see Appendix X) when the decision causes anxiety and stress.
       i. Facilitate refocusing on the decision that needs to be made when the person experiences fragmented thinking during periods of high anxiety.
       j. Encourage the person to take time in deciding.
       k. With adolescents, focus on the present—what will happen versus what will not. Help identify the important things in their life, because they do not have extensive past experiences on which to base decisions.
   2. Value conflict (also refer to *Spiritual Distress*)
       a. Explore the whys of how the person is feeling.
       b. Assist the individual in exploring personal values and relationships that may have an impact on the decision. Consider using a values history tool (Doukus & McCullough, 1991) to elicit the values of the patient and provide fuller understanding of his preferences and directions.
       c. Explore obtaining a referral with the person's spiritual leader.
       d. Use values clarification techniques to assist the person in reviewing the parts of his life that reflect what he believes in.
           Have the person identify the most prized and cherished activities in his life.
           Ask reflective statements that lead to further clarification.
           Review past decisions in which the person needed to make public affirmation of opinions and beliefs.

Evaluate stands the person has taken on controversial subjects. Does he view them in black-and-white terms, or various shades of gray?

Identify values the person is proud of. Rank them in order of importance.

e. Encourage the person to base decision on the most important values.

f. Support individual making the decision—even if decision conflicts with own values. Use health care team conferences to discuss any issues that would bias the person making the decision.

Consult own spiritual leader.

Change patient assignments so person can be cared for by nurse with compatible beliefs.

Arrange for discussions among health care team to share feelings.

3. Fear of outcome/response of others (also refer to *Fear*)

a. Provide clarification regarding potential outcomes and correct misconceptions.

b. Explore with the person what the risks of not deciding would be.

c. Encourage expression of feelings.

d. Promote self-worth.

e. Encourage the person to face fears.

f. Encourage the person to share what he fears with significant others.

g. Actively reassure the person that the decision is his to make and that he has the right to do so.

h. Assist the person in recognizing that it is his life; if he feels comfortable with the decision, others will respect the conviction.

i. Reassure the person that individuality is acceptable.

External

4. Insufficient or inconsistent information

a. Provide information in a comprehensive and sensitive manner.

b. Correct misinformation.

c. Give concise information that covers the major points when the decision must be made quickly.

d. Inform the person of his right to know.

e. Enable the person to determine the amount of information that he desires to obtain.

f. Encourage verbalization to determine the person's perception of choices.

g. Ensure that the person clearly understands what is involved concerning the decision and the various alternatives (*i.e.*, informed choice).

h. Encourage the person to seek second professional opinions regarding health.

i. Collaborate with other health care members/significant others to determine appropriate timing for truthfulness.

5. Controversy with support system

a. Ensure the person that he does not have to give in to pressure from others, whether they are family, friends, or health professionals.

b. Advocate for the person's wishes if others attempt to undermine his ability to make the decision personally.

c. Identify leaders within the support system and provide information.

d. Advocate for the deciding person if the family/significant others are excluding him from the decision making.

6. Unsatisfactory health care environment

a. Establish a trusting and meaningful relationship that promotes mutual understanding and caring.

b. Provide a quiet environment for thought; reduce sensory stimulation.

c. Allow uninterrupted periods with significant others.

d. Promote accepting, nonjudgmental attitudes.

e. Reduce the number of small decisions that the person needs to make to facilitate focusing on the decision in conflict.

f. Avoid using paternalistic/materialistic attitudes and actions. Foster acceptance of responsibility for the person's own decisions.

C. Initiate health teaching and referrals, when indicated
1. Explore with individual and family whether they have discussed and recorded their end-of-life decisions.
2. Describe the possible future dilemmas when these discussions are avoided.
3. Instruct the individual and family members to provide directives in the following areas:
    a. Person to contact in emergency
    b. Person individual most trusts with personal decisions
    c. Decision to be kept alive if individual will be mentally incompetent
    d. Preference to die at home, hospital, no preference
    e. Desire to sign a living will
    f. Decision regarding organ donation
    g. Funeral arrangements, burial, cremation
    h. Circumstances (if any) when information should be withheld from individual
4. Document these decisions and make two copies (retain one and give one to the person who is designated to be the decision maker in an emergency).
5. Discuss the purpose of a living will. Provide information when requested. To obtain a copy of your state's living will, write to the Society for the Right to Die, 250 West 57th Street, New York, NY 10107.

Rationale

*   When a person is experiencing physical and mental fatigue, the ability to concentrate or make a rational decision is limited (Pinch & Spielman, 1990).
*   Mastering content for effective decision making requires time. Time allows a person to choose the option that provides the most benefit with the least amount of risk.
*   Difficult decisions create stress and conflict. Conflict occurs when values and actions are not in congruence.
*   Conflict can create fears and anxieties that negatively affect the ability to make an effective decision. External resources become very important for the person in decisional conflict who has a low level of confidence in his ability to make an autonomous decision.
*   Sims, Boland, and O'Neill (1992) interviewed families involved in caregiving and concluded that the process by which a person "frames" a problem is key to understanding decision making. It was observed that values, feelings, and previous experiences significantly influenced caregivers' decision making. What information caregivers lack to make a decision is balanced by their intimate "person-specific" knowledge about the client.
*   Resolution of decisional conflict may not be possible in settings such as critical care (Hiltunen, 1994). Decision making may be delayed until physiologic stressors have lessened.
*   Roberts, Krouse, and Michaud (1995) involved students with upper respiratory symptoms in a study to determine differences in patient perceptions of two types of nurse–patient interactive styles. Results demonstrate that patients involved in an actively negotiated process of decision making have stronger feelings of decision-making control.
*   Individual values and the roles of values greatly influence the resolution of ethical decision-making dilemmas (Raines, 1993).
*   Value conflicts often lead to confusion, indecision, and inconsistency. Decision making is more complicated for a person when his goals conflict with those of his significant others. People may decide in contradiction to their values if the need to please others is greater than the need to please themselves (Kohnke, 1980; Taylor, 1993).
*   Health care providers' own values and attitudes shape their interaction with patients and families facing ethical decisions (Minogue & Reedy, 1988; Taylor, 1993).
*   Geary (1987) reported decision conflict for patients in critical care when faced with life-and-death decisions. The difficult decision making was precipitated by conflicts in patient and family religious beliefs and personal values. Taylor et al. (1993) also found conflict in discussions about death and related issues when the patient thought that his or her wishes were different from those of the family.
*   Every decision made and course of action taken is based on consciously or unconsciously held beliefs, attitudes, and values (Simon, Howe, & Kirschenbaum, 1978).

- People are the experts in their own life goals and values; therefore, health care professionals need to use a participatory decision-making model (Brady, 1990).
- Personal characteristics influence the desire to maintain control over the decision-making process. People who are strongly self-directed and have in the past taken responsibility for their own health practices are more likely to assume an active role in decision making.

References/Bibliography

Bailey, J. T., & Hendricks, D. E. (1987). Decisions made easy. *Nursing Life, 7*(4), 18–19.

Bille, D. A. (1987). Locus of decision making in patient and family education: Its effects on promoting wellness. *Nursing Administration Quarterly, 2*(3), 62–65.

Brady, T. J. (1990). Point: Patient control of treatment is essential. *Arthritis Care and Research, 3,* 163–166.

Brunnquell, D. (1990, May). *Difficult decisions: Overcoming factors which make discussion of ethical issues difficult.* Paper presented at the meeting of the Association for the Care of Children's Health, Washington, DC.

Burke, G. (1980). Ethics and medical decision-making. *Primary Care, 7,* 615–624.

Davis, A. J. (1989). Clinical nurses' ethical decision making in situations. *Advanced Nursing Science, 11*(3), 63–69.

Dellasega, C., & Mastrian, K. (1995) The process and consequences of institutionalizing an elder. *Western Journal of Nursing Research, 17,* 133–140.

Doukus, D. J., & McCullough, L. B. (1991) The values history: The evaluation of the patient's values and advance directives. *Journal of Family Practice, 32,* 145–153.

Gauthier, C. C., & Krasser-Maxwell, E. (1991). Time demands and medical ethics in women's health care. *Health Care for Women International, 12,* 153–165.

Geary, C. M. B. (1987). Nursing grand rounds: The patient with viral cardiomyopathy. *Journal of Cardiovascular Nursing, 2*(1), 48–52.

Giger, J. N., & Davidhizar, R.E. (1991) *Transcultural nursing: Assessment interventions.* St. Louis: Mosby Year Book

Hiltunen, E. (1987). Decisional conflict: A phenomenological description from the points of view of the nurse and the client. In A. M. McLane (Ed.). *Classification of nursing diagnosis: Proceedings of the seventh conference.* St. Louis: C. V. Mosby.

Hiltunen, E. (1989). Nursing diagnosis: Decisional conflict (specify). In R. M. Carroll-Johnson (Ed.). *Classification of nursing diagnosis: Proceedings of the eighth conference.* Philadelphia: J. B. Lippincott.

Hiltunen, E. (1994). Validation of decisional conflict by critical care nurses. In R. M. Carroll-Johnson & Paquette M. (Eds.). *Classification of nursing diagnoses: Proceedings of the tenth conference.* Philadelphia: J. B. Lippincott.

Janis, I. L., & Mann, L. (1977). *Decision making: A psychological analysis of conflict, choice, and commitment.* New York: The Free Press.

Jezewski, M. A. (1993). Consenting to DNR: Critical care nurses' interactions with patients and family members. *American Journal of Critical Care, 2,* 302–309.

Johnson, R. A., & Justin, R. (1988). Documenting patients' end of life decisions. *Nurse Practitioner, 13*(6), 41.

Kohnke, M. F. (1980). The nurse as advocate. *American Journal of Nursing, 80,* 2038–2040.

Lancaster, W., & Lancaster, J. (1982). Rational decision making: Managing uncertainty. *Journal of Nursing Administration, 12*(2), 23–28.

Marsh, F. L. (1986). Refusal of treatment. *Clinical Geriatric Medicine, 2,* 511–520.

McDevitt-Graham, S. M. (1987). Decision-making: The multi-attribute model. *Nursing Management, 18*(3), 18–19.

Miller, C. A. (1995). *Nursing care of older adults* (2nd ed.). Glenview, IL: Scott, Foresman.

Minogue, J. P., & Reedy, N. J. (1988). Companioning parents in perinatal decision making. *Journal of Perinatal and Neonatal Nursing, 1*(3), 25–35.

Myers, M. B. (1991). Conception of a nursing diagnosis-decision making family: Required. In R. M. Carrol-Johnson (Ed.). *Classification of nursing diagnoses: Proceedings of the ninth conference.* Philadelphia: J. B. Lippincott.

Nugent, P. S. (1982). Management and modes of thought. *Journal of Nursing Administration, 12*(2), 19–25.

O'Connor, A. M. (1995). Validation of a decisional conflict scale. *Medical Decision Making, 15*(1), 25–30.

Pinch, W. J., & Spielman, M. L. (1990). The parent's perspective: Ethical decision making in neonatal intensive care. *Journal of Advanced Nursing, 15,* 712–719.

Raines, D. A. (1993). Values: A guiding force. *AWHONNS Clinical Issues in Perinatal and Womens Health Nursing, 4,* 533–541.

Roberts, S. J., Krouse, H. J., & Michaud, P. (1995). Negotiated and nonnegotiated nurse–patient interactions: Enhancing perceptions of empowerment. *Clinical Nursing Research, 4*(1), 67–77.

Scott, P. N. (1989). Families with adolescents. In R. L. Foster, M. M. Hunsberger, & J. J. T. Anderson (Eds.). *Family-centered nursing care of children.* Philadelphia: W. B. Saunders.

Sims, S. L., Boland, D. L., & O'Neill, C. A. (1992). Decision making in home health care. *Western Journal of Nursing Research, 14,* 186–200.

Simon, S. B., Howe, L. W., & Kirschenbaum, H. (1978). *Values clarification: A handbook of practical strategies for teachers and students.* New York: A & W Publishers.

Soholt, D. (1990). *A life experience: Making a health care treatment decision.* Unpublished master's thesis, South Dakota State University, Brookings.

Taylor, E. J. (1993). Managing cancer pain at home: The decisions and ethical conflicts of patients, family caregivers, and homecare nurses. *Oncology Nursing Forum, 20*, 919–927.

Valanis, B. G., & Rumpler, C. H. (1985). Helping women to choose breast cancer treatment alternatives. *Cancer Nursing, 8*, 167–175.

Wong, D. L. (1995). *Essentials of pediatric nursing* (4th ed.). St. Louis: C. V. Mosby.

Zotti, M. E. (1987). Nursing intervention to assist patients' decision making with respect to family planning. *Public Health Nursing, 4*(3), 146–150.

Diarrhea

DEFINITION
Diarrhea: The state in which the individual experiences or is at risk of experiencing frequent passage of liquid stool or unformed stool.

DEFINING CHARACTERISTICS
Major (Must Be Present)
Loose, liquid stools and/or
Increased frequency (more than three times a day)

Minor (May Be Present)
Urgency
Cramping/abdominal pain
Increased frequency of bowel sounds
Increase in fluidity or volume of stools

RELATED FACTORS
Pathophysiologic
Related to malabsorption or inflammation secondary to:

Kwashiorkor	Crohn's disease
Gastritis	Colon cancer
Peptic ulcer	Spastic colon
Diverticulitis	Celiac disease (sprue)
Ulcerative colitis	Irritable bowel

Related to lactose deficiency
Related to increased peristalsis secondary to increased metabolic rate (hyperthyroidism)
Related to dumping syndrome
Related to infectious process secondary to:

Trichinosis	Shigellosis
Dysentery	Typhoid fever
Cholera	Infectious hepatitis
Malaria	

Related to excessive secretion of fats in stool secondary to liver dysfunction
Related to inflammation and ulceration of gastrointestinal mucosa secondary to high levels of nitrogenous wastes (renal failure)

Treatment-Related

Related to malabsorption or inflammation secondary to surgical intervention of the bowel

Related to side effects of (specify):

Thyroid agents	Chemotherapy
Antacids	Analgesics
Laxatives	Cimetidine
Stool softeners	Iron sulfate
Antibiotics	

Related to solute tube feedings

Situational (Personal, Environmental)

Related to stress or anxiety

Related to irritating foods (fruits, bran cereals)

Related to changes in water and food secondary to travel

Related to change in bacteria in water

Related to bacteria, virus, parasite to which no immunity is present

Related to hot weather

Related to increased caffeine consumption

Maturational

Infant: Related to breast milk

Author's Note

See *Constipation.*

Errors in Diagnostic Statements

Diarrhea related to opportunistic enteric pathogens secondary to AIDS

Diarrhea, sometimes chronic, occurs in 60%–90% of people with AIDS. Prolonged diarrhea represents a collaborative problem: *Potential Complication: Fluid/electrolyte/nutritional imbalances related to diarrhea.*

Besides cotreating this collaborative problem with a physician, the nurse treats other responses to chronic diarrhea such as *Risk for Impaired Skin Integrity* or *Risk for Social Isolation.*

Key Concepts

1. Diarrhea can be acute or chronic. Acute diarrhea can be caused by infection, drug reactions, heavy metal poisoning, fecal impaction, and dietary changes. Chronic diarrhea can be caused by irritable bowel syndrome, lactose deficiency, colon cancer, inflammatory bowel disease, malabsorption disorders, alcohol use, and laxative use (Wadle, 1991).

2. Drugs that can induce diarrhea are laxatives, antacids, certain antibiotics (*e.g.*, tetracyclines), certain hypertensives (*e.g.*, reserpine), cholinergics, and selected cardiac agents (*e.g.*, digoxin) (DiPiro, Talbert, Hayes, Yee, Matzke, & Posey, 1993).

3. Rapid transit of feces through the large intestine results in less water absorption and an unformed, liquid stool. Dehydration and electrolyte imbalance occur if diarrhea continues.

4. Hyperperistalsis is the motor response to intestinal irritants.

5. Diarrhea may be related to an inflammatory process in which the intestinal mucosal wall becomes irritated, resulting in increased moisture content in the fecal masses.

Key Concepts—Child

1. Acute gastroenteritis and its related diarrhea cause dehydration and are responsible for 300–500 deaths each year of children younger than 5 years of age in the United States (Goepp & Santosham, 1994).

2. Oral rehydration therapy is indicated for children with mild or moderate dehydration (Goepp & Santosham, 1994).
3. Signs of mild dehydration are slightly dry mucous membranes and increased thirst. Signs of moderate dehydration are sunken eyes, sunken fontanelle, loss of skin turgor, and dry mucous membranes. Signs of severe dehydration are those included in moderate plus one or more signs, such as rapid, thready pulse, cyanosis, rapid breathing, delayed capillary refill, lethargy, and coma (Goepp & Santosham, 1994).
4. Children who live in warm environments and in conditions of poor sanitation and refrigeration, and children who live in crowded and substandard environments are at risk for eating contaminated food.

 ### *Key Concepts—Older Adult*

1. Age-related loss of elasticity in abdominal muscles and loss of muscle tone in the perineal floor and anal sphincter can cause diarrhea in some older people (Hardy, 1991).
2. Refer to Key Concepts related to dehydration in older adults under *Fluid Volume Deficit*.

Focus Assessment Criteria

Refer to criteria for *Constipation*.

Outcome Criteria

The person will
- Describe contributing factors when known
- Explain rationale for interventions
- Report less diarrhea

Interventions

A. Assess causative contributing factors
   1. Tube feedings
   2. Dietary indiscretions/contaminated foods
   3. Dietetic foods
   4. Food allergies
   5. Foreign travel

B. Eliminate or reduce contributing factors
   1. Side effects of tube feeding
      a. Control infusion rate (depending on delivery set).
      b. Administer smaller, more frequent feedings.*
      c. Change to continuous-drip tube feedings.*
      d. Administer more slowly if signs of gastrointestinal intolerance occur.
      e. Control temperature.
      f. If refrigerated, warm in hot water to room temperature.
      g. Dilute strength of feeding temporarily.*
      h. Follow standard procedure for administration of tube feeding.
      i. Follow tube feeding with specified amount of water to ensure hydration.
      j. Be careful of contamination/spoilage (unused but opened formula should not be used after 24 hours; keep unused portion refrigerated).
   2. Contaminated foods (possible sources)
      a. Raw seafood

* May require a primary care professional's order.

   b. Shellfish
   c. Excess milk consumption
   d. Raw milk
   e. Restaurants
   f. Improperly cooked/stored food
3. Dietetic foods: eliminate foods containing large amounts of the hexitol, sorbitol, and mannitol used as sugar substitutes in dietetic foods, candy, and chewing gum.

C. Reduce diarrhea

1. Discontinue solids.
2. Avoid milk (lactose) products, fat, whole grains, and fresh fruits and vegetables.
3. Gradually add semisolids and solids (crackers, yogurt, rice, bananas, applesauce).
4. Avoid opiate-containing antidiarrheal drugs with acute infectious diarrhea (*e.g.*, Lomotil, Imodium).
5. For mild or moderate diarrhea, advise to use bismuth subsalicylate (Pepto-Bismol), 30 mL or 2 tablets every ½ hour–1 hour, up to 8 doses in 24 hours. Avoid in individuals with salicylate contraindications.
6. Instruct to seek medical care if blood in stool and fever greater than 101°F.

D. Replace fluids and electrolytes

1. Increase oral intake to maintain a normal urine specific gravity or to approximate volume of diarrhea losses.
2. Encourage liquids (water, apple juice, flat ginger ale).
3. When diarrhea is severe, use an oral rehydration solution (*e.g.*, over-the-counter packets or homemade (½ teaspoon salt, ½ teaspoon baking soda, 4 tablespoons sugar in 1 liter of water; discard in 24 hours).
4. Teach to monitor the color of urine to determine hydration needs.
5. Caution against use of very hot or cold liquids.
6. See *Fluid Volume Deficit* for additional interventions.

E. Conduct health teaching as indicated

1. Explain the interventions required to prevent future episodes.
2. Explain the effects of diarrhea on hydration.
3. Teach precautions to take when traveling to foreign lands.
   a. Avoid foods served cold, salads, milk, fresh cheese, cold cuts, and salsa.
   b. Drink carbonated or bottled beverages, avoid ice.
   c. Peel fresh fruits and vegetables.
   d. Avoid foods not stored at proper temperature.
4. Consult with primary health care provider for prophylactic use of bismuth subsalicylate (*e.g.*, Pepto-Bismol) 30–60 mL or 2 tablets qid during travel and 2 days after return; or antimicrobials, for prevention of traveler's diarrhea.
5. Explain how to prevent food-borne diseases at home.
   a. Refrigerate all perishable foods.
   b. Cook all food at high temperature (212°F) and boil for at least 15 minutes before serving.
   c. Avoid allowing food to stand at warm temperatures for several hours.
   d. Thoroughly clean kitchen equipment after contact with perishable foods (*e.g.*, meats, dairy, fish).
6. Explain that a diet primarily made up of dietetic foods containing sugar substitutes (hexitol, sorbitol, and mannitol) can cause diarrhea from slow absorption and rapid small bowel motility.

Rationale

- Most acute episodes of diarrhea are managed with symptomatic therapy with fluid and electrolyte replacement.
- Foods with complex carbon dehydrates (*e.g.*, rice, toast, cereal) facilitate fluid absorption into the intestinal mucosa (Bennett, 1995).

- Soft drinks (nondietetic or dietetic) and sport drinks are unsatisfactory for fluid replacement for moderate or severe fluid loss because of their sugar and salt content (Bennett, 1995).
- Opiate-containing antidiarrheals do not alter the natural cause of the disease and are harmful if invasive pathogens are the cause (Bennett, 1995).
- Bismuth subsalicylate (Pepto-Bismol) has been found to be safe in a variety of diarrheal illnesses and to have antibacterial activity as well. It is also effective in controlling symptoms of traveler's diarrhea (Bennett, 1995).
- Diarrheal stool can cause excoriation of the anal area because it is usually acidic and contains digestive enzymes.
- High-solute tube feedings may cause diarrhea if not followed by sufficient amounts of water.

🌀 Interventions—*Child Focus*

1. Monitor fluid and electrolyte losses
   a. Fluid volume lose
   b. Urine color and output
   c. Skin color
   d. Mucous membranes
   e. Capillary refill time
2. Consult with primary care provider if
   a. Diarrhea persists
   b. Blood or mucus in stools
   c. Signs of moderate dehydration
   d. Sudden increase in stools
   e. Vomiting
3. Reduce diarrhea
   a. Avoid milk (lactose) products, fat, whole grains, and fresh fruits and vegetables.
   b. Avoid high-carbohydrate fluids (*e.g.*, soft drinks) gelatin, fruit juices, caffeinated drinks, chicken or beef broths.
4. Provide oral rehydration (Goepp & Santosham, 1994).
   a. Use oral rehydration solutions (*e.g.*, Pedialyte, Lytren, Ricelyte, Resol).
   b. Provide 60–80 mL/kg over 2-hour period for mild to moderate diarrhea.
5. Reintroduce food
   a. Begin with bananas, rice, cereal, and crackers in small qualities.
   b. Gradually return to regular diet (except milk products) after 36–48 hours; after 3–5 days, gradually add milk products (half-strength skim milk to skim milk to half-strength whole milk to whole milk).
   c. Gradually introduce formula (half-strength formula to full-strength formula).
6. For breast-fed infants
   a. Continue breast-feeding
   b. Use oral rehydration therapy if needed
7. Protect skin from irritation.
8. Teach parents signs to report (refer to Key Concepts).

Rationale

- Children with signs of moderate or severe dehydration should be referred for possible parenteral therapy (Wong, 1995).
- Lactose-containing fluids or foods can worsen diarrhea in some children (Goepp & Santosham, 1995).
- Fluids high in carbohydrate content can exacerbate diarrhea because of their high osmolality. They are also low in electrolytes (Wong, 1995).
- Early reintroduction of normal nutrients has nutritional advantages and may reduce number of stools, weight loss, and the duration of the disease, and enhance intestinal mucosal healing (Brown, 1991).

- Breast-feeding should be continued with fluid replacement therapy. Reduced severity and duration of the illness is attributed to breast milk's low osmolality and its antimicrobial effects (Brown, 1991).

References/Bibliography

Bennett, R. (1995). Acute gastroenteritis and associated conditions. In L. R. Barker, J. Burton, & P. Zieve (Eds.). *Principles of ambulatory medicine*. Baltimore: Williams & Wilkins.

Brown, K. C. (1991). Dietary management of acute childhood diarrhea: Optimal timing of feeding and appropriate use of mil and mixed diets. *Journal of Pediatrics, 118*, S92–S98.

DiPiro, J., Talbert, R., Hayes, P., Yee, G., Matzke, G., & Posey, L. M. (1993). *Pharmacotherapy* (2nd ed.). Norwalk, CT: Appleton & Lange.

Goepp, J., & Santosham, M. (1994). Oral rehydration therapy. In F. Oski (Ed.). *Principles and practice of pediatrics*. Philadelphia: J. B. Lippincott.

Wadle, K. (1991). Diarrhea. In M. Maas, K. Buckwalter, & M. Hardy (Eds.). *Nursing diagnoses and interventions for the elderly*. Redwood City, CA: Addison-Wesley.

Wong, D. L. (1995). *Essentials of pediatric nursing* (4th ed). St. Louis: C. V. Mosby.

Disuse Syndrome

DEFINITION

Disuse Syndrome: The state in which an individual is experiencing or at risk for deterioration of body systems or altered functioning as the result of prescribed or unavoidable musculoskeletal inactivity.

DEFINING CHARACTERISTICS

Presence of a cluster of actual or risk nursing diagnoses related to inactivity

- *Risk for Impaired Skin Integrity*
- *Risk for Constipation*
- *Risk for Altered Respiratory Function*
- *Risk for Altered Peripheral Tissue Perfusion*
- *Risk for Infection*
- *Risk for Activity Intolerance*
- *Risk for Impaired Physical Mobility*
- *Risk for Injury*
- *Risk for Sensory—Perceptual Alterations*
- *Powerlessness*
- *Body Image Disturbance*

RELATED FACTORS

Some examples of inactivity or immobility are

Pathophysiologic

Related to: (optional)
Decreased sensorium
Unconsciousness

Neuromuscular impairment
    Multiple sclerosis   Muscular dystrophy
    Parkinsonism   Partial/total paralysis
    Guillain-Barré syndrome   Spinal cord injury
(Musculoskeletal)
    Fractures
    Rheumatic diseases
(End-stage disease)
    AIDS   Cardiac
    Renal   Cancer
(Psychiatric/mental health disorders)
    Major depression
    Catatonic state
    Severe phobias

Treatment-Related

Related to: (optional)
    Surgery (amputation, skeletal)   Mechanical ventilation
    Traction/casts/splints   Invasive vascular lines
    Prescribed immobility

Situational (Personal, Environmental)

Related to: (optional)
    Depression   Debilitated state
    Fatigue   Pain

Maturational

Related to: (optional)
    (Newborn/infant/child/adolescent)
        Down's syndrome   Risser-Turnbuckle jacket
        Legg-Calvé-Perthes disease   Juvenile arthritis
        Osteogenesis imperfecta   Autism
        Cerebral palsy   Mental/physical disability
        Spina bifida
    (Older Adult)
        Decreased motor agility
        Muscle weakness
        Presenile dementia

Author's Note

Disuse Syndrome describes a situation in which a person is experiencing or is at risk for the adverse effects of immobility. Syndrome nursing diagnoses should not be written as "Risk for" because clustered under them are risk and actual diagnoses. *Disuse Syndrome* identifies an individual as vulnerable to certain complications and also experiencing altered functioning in a health pattern. As a syndrome diagnosis, it contains its etiology in the diagnostic label (*Disuse*); a "related to" statement is not applicable. As discussed in Chapter 2, a syndrome diagnosis comprises a cluster of actual or risk nursing diagnoses predicted to be present because of the situation. Eleven risk or actual nursing diagnoses are clustered under *Disuse Syndrome* (see Defining Characteristics).

    The nurse no longer needs to use separate diagnoses, such as *Risk for Altered Respiratory Function* or *Risk for Impaired Skin Integrity*, because they are incorporated into this syndrome category. However, if an individual who is immobile manifests the signs or symptoms of impaired skin integrity or another diagnosis, the specific diagnosis should be used. The nurse should continue to use *Disuse Syndrome* so that deterioration of the other body systems does not occur.

Errors in Diagnostic Statements

Disuse Syndrome related to reddened sacral area (3 cm)

A reddened sacral area is evidence of the diagnosis *Impaired Skin Integrity*. Thus, the nurse should use two diagnoses for this person: *Impaired Skin Integrity related to effects of immobility, as evidenced by reddened sacral area (3 cm)* and *Disuse Syndrome*.

Key Concepts

1. "Immobility is inconsistent with human life." Mobility provides a person control over his environment; without mobility, a person is at the mercy of his environment (Christian, 1982).
2. Society values youthfulness, energy, and productivity. Immobility is contradictory to these values.
3. Immobility restricts the person's ability to seek out sensory stimulation. Conversely, immobile people may be unable to remove themselves from an environment that is too stressful or noisy (Christian, 1982).
4. Musculoskeletal inactivity or immobility has adverse effects on all the body systems. Table II-6 outlines the effects of immobility on body systems.
5. A muscle loses about 3% of its original strength each day it is immobilized.
6. Prolonged immobility has adverse effects on psychological health, learning, socialization, and ability to cope. Table II-7 illustrates these effects.

Key Concepts—Child

1. Mobility is essential for physical growth and development and mastery of developmental tasks (Wong, 1995). Restricted movement can thwart achievement of developmental tasks. Refer to Table II-11 in the diagnostic category *Altered Growth and Development*.
2. Physical activity serves as a vehicle for communication and expression for children.
3. The major psychological/emotional consequences of immobility include:
   a. Sensory deprivation, leading to altered self-perception and environmental awareness
   b. Isolation from peers
   c. Feelings of helplessness, frustration, anxiety, and boredom (Wong, 1995; Wright, 1989).
5. Children who are restrained by casts, splints, or straps during the first 3 years of life have more difficulty with language than children whose activities are unrestricted (Wong, 1995).
6. Children's responses to immobility may range from active protest to withdrawal or regression (Wong, 1995; Wright, 1989).

Key Concepts—Older Adult

1. Aging affects muscle functioning because of progressive loss of muscle mass and loss of strength and endurance.
2. Age-related changes in joint and connective tissue include impaired flexion and extension movements, decreased flexibility, and reduced cushioning protection for joints (Whitbourne, 1985).
3. After menopause, women experience an accelerated loss of trabecular and cortical bone: 9%–10% per decade (Miller, 1995).
4. Bed rest can cause an average vertical bone loss of 0.9% per week (Krolner & Toft, 1983).

Focus Assessment Criteria

Subjective Data

A. Assess for related factors

1. Neurologic
   Cerebrovascular accident, head trauma, increased intracranial pressure
   Multiple sclerosis, poliomyelitis, Guillain-Barré syndrome, myasthenia gravis
   Spinal cord injury, tumor, birth defect

Table II-6 **Adverse Effects of Immobility on Body Systems**

System	Effect
Cardiac	Decreased myocardial performance
	Decreased aerobic capacity
	Decreased heart rate and stroke volume
	Decreased oxygen uptake
Circulatory	Venous stasis
	Orthostatic intolerance
	Dependent edema
	Reduced venous return
	Increased intravascular pressure
Respiratory	Stasis of secretions
	Impaired cilia
	Drying of sections of mucous membranes
	Decreased chest expansion
	Slower, more shallow respirations
Musculoskeletal	Muscle atrophy
	Shortening of muscle fiber (contracture)
	Decreased strength/tone (*e.g.*, back)
	Osteoporosis
	Joint degeneration
	Fibrosis of collagen fibers (joints)
Metabolic/Hemopoietic	Decreased nitrogen excretion
	Impaired glucose tolerance
	Decreased red blood cells
	Decreased phagocytosis
	Hypercalcemia
	Anorexia
	Decreased metabolic rate
	Obesity
	Elevated creatine levels
Gastrointestinal	Constipation
Genitourinary	Urinary stasis
	Urinary calculi
	Urinary retention
	Inadequate gravitational force
Integumentary	Decreased capillary flow
	Tissue acidosis to necrosis
Neurosensory	Reduced innervation of nerves

(From Caswell [1993]; Porth [1994]; Tyler [1984]; and Wong [1993].)

2. Cardiovascular
   Myocardial infarction   Congestive heart failure
   Congenital heart anomaly
3. Musculoskeletal
   Osteoporosis   Arthritis
   Fractures
4. Respiratory
   Chronic obstructive pulmonary disease (COPD)   Pneumonia
   Orthopnea   Dyspnea on exertion
5. Debilitating diseases
   Cancer   Renal disease
   Endocrine disease

Table II-7 **Psychosocial Effects of Immobility**

	Effect
Psychological	Increased tension
	Negative change in self-concept
	Fear, anger
Learning	Decreased motivation
	Decreased ability to retain, transfer learning
	Decreased attention span
Socialization	Change in roles
	Social isolation
Growth and development	Dependency

(Zubek, J. P., & McNeil, M. [1967]. Perceptual deprivation phenomena: Role of the recumbent position. *Journal of Abnormal Psychology, 72,* 147.)

6. History of symptoms (complaints of)
   Pain
   Muscle weakness
   Fatigue
7. History of recent trauma or surgery
   Fractures
   Head injury
   Abdominal surgery or injury

Objective Data

A. Assess for defining characteristics
   1. Dominant hand
      Right
      Left
      Ambidextrous
   2. Motor function

Right	Strong	Weak	Absent	Spastic
Left arm	Strong	Weak	Absent	Spastic
Right leg	Strong	Weak	Absent	Spastic
Left leg	Strong	Weak	Absent	Spastic

   3. Mobility

Ability to turn self	Yes	No	Assistance needed (specify)
Ability to sit	Yes	No	Assistance needed (specify)
Ability to stand	Yes	No	Assistance needed (specify)
Ability to transfer	Yes	No	Assistance needed (specify)
Ability to ambulate	Yes	No	Assistance needed (specify)

      Weight-bearing (assess both right and left sides)
         Full
         Partial
         As tolerated
         Non–weight bearing
   4. Gait
      Stable
      Unstable
   5. Range of motion (shoulders, elbows, arms, hips, legs)
      Full
      Limited (specify)
      None

B. Assess for related factors
    1. Assistive devices

Crutches	Wheelchair
Cane	Prosthesis
Braces	Other
Walker	

    2. Restrictive devices

Cast or splint	Foley
Traction	Intravenous line
Braces	Monitor
Ventilator	Dialysis
Drain	

    3. Motivation (as perceived by nurse and/or reported by person)
        Excellent
        Satisfactory
        Poor

Outcome Criteria

The person will demonstrate continued
- Intact skin/tissue integrity
- Maximum pulmonary function
- Maximum peripheral blood flow
- Full range of motion
- Bowel, bladder, and renal functioning within normal limits
- Use of social contacts and activities when possible

The person will
- Explain rationale for treatments
- Make decisions regarding care when possible
- Share feelings regarding immobile state

Interventions

A. Identify causative and contributing factors
    1. Pain; refer also to *Altered Comfort*.
    2. Fatigue; refer also to *Fatigue*.
    3. Decreased motivation; refer also to *Activity Intolerance*.
    4. Depression; refer also to *Ineffective Individual Coping*.

B. Promote optimal respiratory function
    1. Vary the position of the bed, thus gradually changing the horizontal and vertical position of the thorax, unless contraindicated.
    2. Assist to reposition, turning frequently from side to side (hourly if possible).
    3. Encourage deep breathing and controlled coughing exercises five times every hour.
    4. Teach individual to use blow bottle or incentive spirometer every hour when awake (with severe neuromuscular impairment, the person may have to be awakened during the night as well).
    5. For child, use colored water in blow bottle; have him blow up balloons, blow soap bubbles, blow cotton balls with straw.
    6. Auscultate lung fields every 8 hours; increase frequency if altered breath sounds are present.
    7. Encourage small, frequent feedings to prevent abdominal distention.

C. Maintain usual pattern of bowel elimination; refer to *Constipation* for specific interventions

D. Prevent pressure ulcers (Maklebust & Sieggreen, 1996)
  1. Use repositioning schedule that relieves vulnerable area most often (*e.g.*, if vulnerable area is the back, turning schedule would be left side to back, back to right side, right side to left side, and left side to back); post "turn clock" at bedside.
  2. Turn person or instruct him to turn or shift weight every 30 minutes to 2 hours, depending on other causative factors present and the ability of the skin to recover from pressure.
  3. Frequency of turning schedule should be increased if any reddened areas that appear do not disappear within 1 hour after turning.
  4. Position person in normal or neutral position with body weight evenly distributed.
  5. Keep bed as flat as possible to reduce shearing forces; limit Fowler's position to only 30 minutes at a time.
  6. Use foam blocks or pillows to provide a bridging effect to support the body above and below the high-risk or ulcerated area so that affected area does not touch bed surface; do not use foam donuts or inflatable rings because they increase the area of pressure.
  7. Alternate or reduce the pressure on the skin surface with:
      a. Foam mattresses
      b. Air mattresses
      c. Air-fluidized beds
      d. Vascular boots to suspend heels
  8. Use enough personnel to lift person up in bed or chair rather than pull or slide skin surfaces; use protectors to reduce friction on elbows and heels.
  9. To reduce shearing forces, support feet with footboard to prevent sliding.
  10. Promote optimum circulation when person is sitting.
      a. Limit sitting time for person at high risk for ulcer development.
      b. Instruct person to lift self using chair arms every 10 minutes if possible, or assist person in rising up off the chair every 10–20 minutes, depending on risk factors present.
  11. Inspect areas at risk of developing ulcers with each position change.
      a. Ears
      b. Occiput
      c. Heels
      d. Sacrum
      e. Scrotum
      f. Elbows
      g. Trochanter
      h. Ischia
      i. Scapula
  12. Observe for erythema and blanching and palpate for warmth and tissue sponginess with each position change.
  13. Massage nonreddened, vulnerable areas gently with each position change.
  14. Refer to *Impaired Skin Integrity* for additional interventions.

E. Promote factors that improve venous blood flow
  1. Elevate extremity above the level of the heart (may be contraindicated if severe cardiac or respiratory disease is present).
  2. Avoid standing or sitting with legs dependent for long periods of time.
  3. Consider the use of below-knee elastic stocking to prevent venous stasis.
  4. Reduce or remove external venous compression, which impedes venous flow.
      a. Avoid pillows behind the knees or get bed that is elevated at the knees.
      b. Avoid leg crossing.
      c. Change positions, move extremities, or wiggle fingers and toes every hour.
      d. Avoid garters and tight elastic stockings above the knees.
  5. Measure baseline circumference of calves and thighs daily if individual is at risk for deep venous thrombosis, or if it is suspected.

F. Maintain limb mobility and prevent contractures
  1. Increase limb mobility.
    a. Perform range of motion exercises (frequency to be determined by condition of the individual).
    b. Support extremity with pillows to prevent or reduce swelling.
    c. Encourage the person to perform exercise regimens for specific joints as prescribed by physician or physical therapist.
  2. Position the person in alignment to prevent complications.
    a. Avoid placing pillows under knee; support calf instead.
    b. Point toes and knees toward ceiling when the client is in a supine position.
    c. Use footboard to prevent footdrop.
    d. Avoid prolonged periods of hip flexion (*i.e.*, sitting position).
    e. To position hips, place rolled towel lateral to hip to prevent external rotation.
    f. Keep arms abducted from the body with pillows.
    g. Keep elbows in slight flexion.
    h. Keep wrist in a neutral position, with fingers slightly flexed and thumb abducted and slightly flexed.
    i. Change position of shoulder joints during the day (*e.g.*, abduction, adduction, range of circular motion).

G. Prevent urinary stasis and calculi formation
  1. Provide a daily intake of fluid of 2000 mL or greater (unless contraindicated); refer to *Fluid Volume Deficit* for specific interventions.
  2. Maintain urine pH below 6.0 (acidic) to reduce the formation of calcium calculi with acid ash foods (cereals, meats, poultry, fish, cranberry juice, apple juice).
  3. Teach to avoid foods high in calcium and oxalate (*very high), such as:
    a. Milk, milk products, cheese
    b. Bran cereals
    c. *Spinach, cranberries, plums, raspberries, gooseberries
    d. Sardines, shrimp, oysters
    e. Legumes, whole-grain rice
    f. *Chocolate
    g. Asparagus, rhubarb, kale, Swiss chard, turnip greens, mustard greens, broccoli, beet greens
    h. Peanut butter, ripe olives

H. Reduce and monitor bone demineralization
  1. Monitor for hypercalcemia.
    a. Serum levels
    b. Nausea/vomiting, polydipsia, polyuria, lethargy
  2. Provide weight-bearing when possible.
    a. Tilt-table
  3. Maintain vigorous hydration.
    a. Adults: 2000 mL/day
    b. Adolescents: 3000–4000 mL/day

I. Promote sharing and a sense of well-being
  1. Encourage to share feelings and fears regarding restricted movement.
  2. Encourage client to wear own clothes rather than pajamas.
    a. Encourage the wearing of unique adornments as an expression of individuality (*e.g.*, baseball caps, colorful socks).

J. Reduce the monotony of immobility
  1. Vary daily routine when possible (*e.g.*, give bath in the afternoon, so that the person can watch a special show or talk with a visitor who drops in to see him).

2. Include the individual in planning schedule for daily routine.
   a. Allow the person to make as many decisions as possible.
   b. Make daily routine as normal as possible (*e.g.*, have the person wear street clothes during the day if feasible).
3. Plan time for visitors.
   a. Encourage person to make a schedule for visitors so everyone does not come at once or at an inconvenient time.
   b. Spend quality time with the person (*i.e.*, not time that is task oriented; rather, sit down and talk).
4. Be creative; vary the physical environment and daily routine when possible.
   a. Update bulletin boards, change the pictures on the walls, move the furniture within the room.
   b. Maintain a pleasant, cheerful environment (*e.g.*, plenty of light, flowers, conversation pieces).
   c. Place the person near a window if possible.
   d. Provide reading material, radio, television, "books on tape" (if person is visually impaired).
   e. Plan an activity daily to give person something to look forward to; always keep your promises.
   f. Discourage the use of television as the primary source of recreation unless it is highly desired.
   g. Consider using a volunteer to spend time reading to the person or helping with an activity.
   h. Encourage suggestions and new ideas (*e.g.*, "Can you think of things you might like to do?").

K. Provide opportunities for individual to control decisions
   1. Allow person to manipulate surroundings, such as deciding what is to be kept where (shoes under bed, picture on window).
   2. Keep needed items within reach (call bell, urinal, tissues).
   3. Discuss daily plan of activities and allow person to make as many decisions as possible about it.
   4. Increase decision-making opportunities as person progresses.
   5. Respect and follow individual's decision if you have given him options.
   6. Record person's specific choices on care plan to ensure that others on staff acknowledge preferences ("Dislikes orange juice," "Takes shower," "Plan dressing change at 7:30 before shower").
   7. Keep promises.
   8. Provide opportunity for person and family to express feelings.
   9. Provide opportunities for person and family to participate in care.
   10. Plan a care conference to allow staff to discuss methods of individualizing care; encourage each nurse to share at least one action that she discovered a particular individual liked.
   11. Shift emphasis from what one cannot do to what one can do.
   12. Set goals that are short-term, practical, and realistic.

Rationale

- See Tables II-6 and II-7 for effects of immobility prevented by specific interventions.
- Activity, mobility, and flexibility are integral to a person's life-style. Immobility has a serious impact on self-concept and life-style (Christian, 1982).
- The more portions of the body immobilized and the longer the immobilization, the greater the adverse effects.
- Joints without range of motion develop contractures in 3–7 days because flexor muscles are stronger then extensor muscles.
- Increased serum calcium resulting from bone destruction caused by lack of motion and weight bearing increases the coagulability of the blood. This, in addition to circulatory stasis, makes the person vulnerable to thrombosis formation.

- The peristaltic contractions of the ureters are insufficient when in a reclining position; thus, there is stasis of urine in the renal pelvis.
- Compression of nerves by casts, restraints, or improper positions can result in ischemia and nerve degeneration. Compression of the peroneal nerve results in footdrop; compression of the radial nerve results in wristdrop.
- Interventions to maintain hydration prevent hypercoagulability and clot formation and urine concentration of stone-forming elements (Porth, 1994).

✤ Interventions—*Child Focus*

1. Plan appropriate activities for children.
   a. Provide an environment with accessible playthings that suit the child's developmental age, and ensure that they are well within reach.
   b. Encourage family to bring in child's favorite playthings, including items from nature that will keep the "real world" alive (*e.g.*, goldfish, leaves in fall).
2. Use play therapy (Appendix IX) to encourage child to share feelings (*e.g.*, put cast on doll).
3. Transport outside the room as much as possible
4. Engage in participation in self-care.
   a. Plan daily routine.
   b. Select diet, snacks.
   c. Select clothes (*e.g.*, baseball cap).
5. Allow to wear street clothes as soon as possible.

Rationale

- Play therapy decreases the monotony of immobilization and decreases tension and frustration (Wong, 1995).
- Changes in environment provide varied stimuli and increased social contact (Wong, 1995).
- Increasing self-care activities and decision making allows expressions of autonomy and individualization (Wong, 1995).

References/Bibliography

Caswell, D. (1993). Thromboembolic phenomena. *Critical Care Nursing Clinics of North America, 5,* 489–497.

Christian, B. J. (1982). Immobilization: Psychosocial aspects. In C. Norris (Ed.). *Concept clarification in nursing.* Rockville, MD: Aspen Publications.

Houk, N. G. (1980). The disabled adolescent: Promoting a positive self-concept by achievement of developmental tasks. In P. L. Chinn & K. B. Leonard (Eds.). *Current practice in pediatric nursing.* St. Louis: C. V. Mosby.

Krolner, B., & Toft, B. (1983). Vertical bone loss: An unheeded side effect of therapeutic bedrest. *Clinical Science, 64,* 537–540.

Maklebust, J., & Sieggreen, M. (1996). *Pressure ulcers: Guidelines for prevention and nursing management* (2nd ed.). Springhouse, PA: Springhouse.

Miller, C. A. (1995). *Nursing care of older adults: Theory and practice* (2nd ed.). Glenview, IL: Scott, Foresman.

Porth, C. M. (1994) *Pathophysiology: Concepts of altered health states.* Philadelphia: J. B. Lippincott.

Tyler, M. (1984). The respiratory effects of body positioning and immobilization. *Respiratory Care, 29,* 472–481.

Whitbourne, S. K. (1985). Appearance and movement. In S. K. Whitbourne (Ed.). *The aging body.* New York: Springer-Verlag.

Wong, D. L. (1995). *Essentials of pediatric nursing* (4th ed.). St. Louis: C. V. Mosby.

Wright, S. (1989). Nursing strategies: Altered musculoskeletal function. In R. L. Foster, M. M. Hunsberger, & J. J. T. Anderson (Eds.). *Family-centered nursing care of children.* Philadelphia: W. B. Saunders.

Diversional Activity Deficit

DEFINITION

Diversional Activity Deficit: The state in which the individual or group experiences or is at risk of experiencing decreased stimulation from, or interest in, leisure activities.

DEFINING CHARACTERISTICS

Major (Must Be Present)

Observed and/or statements of boredom/depression due to inactivity

Minor (May Be Present)

Constant expression of unpleasant thoughts or feelings
Yawning or inattentiveness
Flat facial expression
Body language (shifting of body away from speaker)
Restlessness/fidgeting
Weight loss or gain
Hostility

RELATED FACTORS

Pathophysiologic

Related to difficulty accessing or participating in usual activities secondary to:
Communicable disease
Pain

Treatment-Related

Related to difficulty accessing or participating in usual activities secondary to isolation or immobility

Situational (Personal, Environmental)

Related to unsatisfactory social behaviors
Related to no peers or friends
Related to monotonous environment
Related to long-term hospitalization or confinement
Related to lack of motivation
Related to difficulty accessing or participating in usual activities secondary to:
Excessively long hours of stressful work
No time for leisure activities
Career changes (*e.g.*, teacher to homemaker, retirement)
Children leaving home ("empty nest")
Immobility
Decreased sensory perception (*e.g.*, blindness, hearing loss)
Multiple role responsibilities

Maturational

(Infant/child)
Related to lack of appropriate stimulation toys/peers
(Older adult)
Related to difficulty accessing or participating in usual activities secondary to:

Sensory/motor deficits	Lack of peer group
Lack of transportation	Limited finances
Fear of crime	Confusion

Author's Note

A deficit in diversional activities is expressed by the person, who alone can determine whether types and amounts of activity are problematic. Miller (1995) writes that a person's self-concept is affirmed through activities associated with various role supports.

To validate a nursing diagnosis of *Diversional Activity Deficit*, the nurse needs to explore the etiology of factors that are amenable to nursing interventions, with the main focus on increasing or improving the quality of leisure activities. For a person with personality problems that hinder relationships and result in decreased social activities with others, the diagnosis *Impaired Social Interactions* would be more valid. The nurse would focus on helping the person identify the behavior as a barrier to socialization.

Errors in Diagnostic Statements

Diversional Activity Deficit related to boredom and reports of no leisure activities

This diagnosis does not reflect the required treatment. Boredom and reports of no leisure activities represent manifestations of the diagnosis, not contributing factors. Thus, the diagnosis should be written as: *Diversional Activity Deficit related to unknown etiology, as evidenced by reports of boredom and no leisure activities.*

Diversional Activity Deficit related to inability to sustain meaningful relationships, as evidenced by "no one calls me to go out"

This diagnosis would focus nursing interventions on enhancing the person's diversional activities. In this situation, the nurse should delay making a formal diagnosis and should collect more data to explore more specifically the meaning of "no one calls me to go out." Other diagnoses may be more applicable, such as *Impaired Social Interactions, Self-Concept Disturbance*, and *Ineffective Coping.*

Key Concepts

1. All human beings need stimulation. In the adult, lack of stimulation results in boredom and depression. In the infant or child, it causes "failure to thrive" and may stunt growth severely.
2. A significant relationship exists between informal activity and life satisfaction. The quality or type of interaction is more important than the quantity of activity (Rantz, 1991).
3. Boredom paralyzes an individual's productivity and causes a feeling of stagnation. It is often a major contributing factor to substance abuse (overeating, drug abuse, alcoholism, and smoking).
4. The bored person has introspective feelings of being oppressed and trapped, which give rise to conscious or unconscious anger or hostility.

Key Concepts—Child

1. Children at special risk for diversional activity deficit include:
   a. Those who are bored
   b. Those who are immobilized
   c. Those who are hospitalized for long periods of time
   d. Those who are isolated to protect themselves or others
   e. Those who have diminished contact with family and/or friends
2. Age-appropriate activities should be provided to promote mental health and human development (Scipien, Chard, Howe, & Barnard, 1990). Refer to Table II-11 in the diagnosis *Altered Growth and Development.*
3. Children who are bored may be at greater risk for injury. Refer to the diagnosis *Risk for Injury related to maturational age of the hospitalized child* for more information.
4. See also Key Concepts—Child for *Anxiety* and *Altered Growth and Development.*

Key Concepts—Older Adult

1. The older individual's cultural background strongly influences his use of diversional activities because of the value placed on work versus leisure activities (Matteson & McConnell, 1988).

2. Older, less educated, rural people tend to place less value on leisure activities (Matteson & McConnell, 1988).
3. In our society, retirement usually occurs from age 62–70 years. About 80% of men and 90% of women older than 65 years of age are identified as being retired. The lost work role for the man can result in a void and subsequent depression, particularly if there has been no preretirement planning (Matteson & McConnell, 1988; McPherson & Guppy, 1979).
4. The aging process is enhanced when the person has cultivated varied interests and activities throughout life (Ebersole & Hess, 1990; Matteson & McConnell, 1988; McPherson & Guppy, 1979).
5. A change in living arrangements or environment might subject the elderly to a diversional activity deficit. For example, an organic gardener in his own private yard moves to a senior high-rise apartment where no land is available for a garden, or an older man who plays the drums moves in with his adult children who have neither the space for his drum set nor the inclination to listen to his drum solos (Matteson & McConnell, 1988).
6. Social isolation resulting from death of a spouse, lack of transportation, hearing impairment, limited finances, fear of crime, or other physical or psychological disabilities places the older individual at risk for diversional activity deficit (Hogstel, 1990; Rantz, 1991).
7. Cognitive impairments, musculoskeletal impairment, pain, metabolic abnormality, or sensory deficit may force an elderly person to consider modification of long-time leisure activities or development of new activities. For example, a person who likes to cook but has poor eyesight might obtain large-print cookbooks, have a friend write favorite recipes in bold print, or tape-record recipes (Rantz, 1991)
8. Volunteer activities provide diversion for 21% of individuals aged 55–64 years and 14% of those aged 65 years and older. Those aged 65 and older volunteered an average of 8 hours per week. Reasons cited for not volunteering included transportation difficulties, financial concerns, and age discrimination by some community organizations (Ebersole & Hess, 1990; Hogstel, 1990; Matteson & McConnell, 1988).

Focus Assessment Criteria

Subjective Data

A. Assess for defining characteristics

    1. Perception of person's current activity level

        Too busy (not enough time for relaxing activities)

        Busy but able to find time to do relaxing activities

        Bored, trapped, wishes there was more recreational activity

    2. Past activity patterns (type, frequency)

        Work

        Leisure

    3. Activities the person desires

Objective Data

A. Assess for related factors

    1. Motivation

        Interested   Withdrawn

        Disinterested   Hostile

    2. Presence of barriers to recreational activities

    3. Physical status

        Immobility   Pain

        Altered level of consciousness   Sensory deficits (visual, auditory)

        Fatigue   Equipment (traction, IV lines)

        Altered hand mobility   Communicable disease/isolation

    4. Psychological/cognitive status

        Lack of motivation   Depression

        Lack of knowledge   Embarrassment

        Fear

5. Socioeconomic status
    Lack of support system   Financial limitations
    Previous patterns of inactivity   Transportation difficulties
    Language barrier

Outcome Criteria

The person will
- Relate feelings of boredom and discuss methods of finding diversional activities
- Relate methods of coping with feelings of anger or depression caused by boredom
- Report an increase in enjoyable activities

Interventions

A. Assess causative factors

1. Monotony
2. Inability to make decisions concerning his own plan of care (see *Powerlessness*)
3. Diminished socialization (see *Social Isolation*)
4. Lack of motivation/depression

B. Reduce or eliminate causative factors

1. Monotony
    a. Vary daily routine when possible (*e.g.*, give bath in the afternoon, so that the person can watch a special show or talk with a visitor who drops in to see him).
    b. Include the individual in planning schedule for daily routine.
        Allow the person to make as many decisions as possible.
        Make daily routine as normal as possible (*e.g.*, have the person wear street clothes during the day, if feasible).
    c. Plan time for visitors.
        Encourage person to make a schedule for visitors so everyone does not come at once or at an inconvenient time.
        Spend quality time with the person (*i.e.*, not time that is task oriented; rather, sit down and talk).
    d. Be creative, vary the physical environment and daily routine when possible.
        Update bulletin boards, change the pictures on the walls, move the furniture within the room.
        Maintain a pleasant, cheerful environment (*e.g.*, plenty of light, flowers, conversation pieces).
        Place the person near a window if possible.
        Provide reading material, radio, television, "books on tape" (if person is visually impaired).
        Plan an activity daily to give person something to look forward to, and always keep your promises.
        Discourage the use of television as the primary source of recreation unless it is highly desired.
        Consider using a volunteer to spend time reading to the person or helping with an activity.
        Encourage suggestions and new ideas (*e.g.*, "Can you think of things you might like to do?").
        Recognize that computers and telephones can help the confined become involved.
    e. Provide opportunities for reminiscence individually or in groups (*e.g.*, past trips, hobbies, special interest).
    f. Provide music therapy with audio cassette players with lightweight headphones.

g. For group music therapy (Rantz, 1991):

Introduce a topic.   Play related music.

Develop the topic with discussion.   Discuss responses.

h. Consider pet therapy (Rantz, 1991):

Animals must be well groomed, healthy, and clean.

Animals should be relaxed with strangers.

Animals should eliminate before entering the facility.

Sponsors should always ask the individual if that type of animal is liked before approaching the person.

2. Lack of motivation

a. Stimulate motivation by showing interest and encouraging sharing of feelings and experiences.

Explore fears and concerns about participating in activities.

Discuss the person's likes and dislikes.

Encourage sharing of feelings of present and past experiences.

Spend time with the person purposefully talking about other topics (*e.g.*, "I just got back from the shore. Have you ever gone there?").

Point out the need to "get oneself going" and try something new.

b. Help the person to work through feelings of anger and grief.

Allow him to ventilate.

Take the time to be a good listener.

See *Anxiety* for additional interventions.

c. Encourage the person to join a group that might be of interest or help (may have to participate via intercom or special arrangement).

d. Consider the use of music therapy (Buckwalter, Hartsock, & Gaffney, 1985) or reminiscence therapy (Halmilton, 1985).

C. Identify factors that promote activity and socialization

1. Encourage socialization with peers and all age groups (frequently the very young and the very old mutually benefit from interaction with each other).

2. Acquire assistance to increase the person's ability to travel.

a. Arrange transportation to activities if necessary.

b. Acquire aids for safety (*e.g.*, wheelchair for going to shopping center, a walker for ambulating in hallways).

3. Increase the person's feelings of productivity and self-worth.

a. Encourage person to use his strengths to help others and himself (*e.g.*, give him tasks to perform in a general project).

b. Acknowledge efforts made by the person (*e.g.*, "You look nice tonight" or "Thank you for helping Mr. Jones with his dinner").

c. Encourage open communication; value the person's opinion ("Mr. Jones, what do you think about . . . ?").

d. Encourage the person to challenge himself with learning a new skill or pursuing a new interest.

e. Refer to *Social Isolation* for additional interventions.

Rationale

- Informal activities promote well-being more than formally structured activities. Solitary activities have little effect on life satisfaction (Longino & Kart, 1982).
- Being aware that one is bored allows one to redirect activities to increase stimulation.
- Music therapy can be a valuable intervention in relieving boredom, sparking interest, and assisting individuals in coping with social problems (Rantz, 1991).
- Membership in a group or a support group can boost self-esteem and self-worth, provide a sense of belonging, and encourage activities that the person otherwise may have shied away from. Support groups can often assist individuals with stressful, costly, or time-consuming problems.
- Reminiscing, or spending time focusing on recalling significant memories, can be a satisfying and stimulating pastime for the bored, ill, confined, or elderly individual (Rantz, 1991).

🌀 Interventions—*Child Focus*

1. Provide an environment with accessible playthings that suit the child's developmental age, and ensure that they are well within reach.
2. Keep toys in all waiting areas.
3. Encourage family to bring in child's favorite playthings, including items from nature that will help to keep the "real world" alive (*e.g.*, goldfish, leaves in fall).

Rationale

- Play is essential to a child's mental, emotional, and social well-being (Wong, 1993).
- Play provides diversion and increased feelings of security (Wong, 1993).
- Provides an expressive outlet for feelings.
- Provides opportunities for choices and to be in control (Wong, 1993).

🏛 Interventions—*Older Adult*

1. Explore interests and the feasibility of trying a new activity (*e.g.*, mobility, vision).
2. Arrange for someone to accompany or orient during initial encounters.
3. Explore possible volunteer opportunities (*e.g.*, Red Cross, hospitals, schools).
4. Initiate referrals, if indicated.
   a. Suggest joining AARP (American Association of Retired Persons).
   b. Write local health and welfare council or agencies.
   c. Provide a list of associations with senior citizen activities:

YMCA	Sixty Plus Club
Churches	XYZ Group (Extra Years of Zest)
Golden Age Club	Young at Heart Club
Encore Club	SOS (Senior Outreach Services)
MORA (Men of Retirement Age)	Leisure Hour Group
Gray Panthers	

Rationale

- The older individual's cultural background strongly influences his use of diversional activities because of the value placed on work versus leisure activities (Matteson & McConnell, 1988).
- Cognitive impairments, musculoskeletal impairment, pain, metabolic abnormality, or sensory deficit may force an elderly person to consider modification of long-time leisure activities or development of new activities. For example, a person who likes to cook but has poor eyesight might obtain large-print cookbooks, have a friend write favorite recipes in bold print, or tape-record recipes (Rantz, 1991)
- Change, although a welcome relief from boredom, does increase anxiety initially.

References/Bibliography

Buckwalter, K., Hartsock, J., & Gaffney, J. (1985). Music therapy. In G. Bulechek & J. McCloskey (Eds.). *Nursing interventions: Treatments for nursing diagnoses*. Philadelphia: W. B. Saunders.

Ebersole, P., & Hess, P. (1990). *Toward healthy aging: Human needs and nursing response* (3rd ed.). St. Louis: C. V. Mosby.

Halmilton, D. (1985). Reminiscence therapy. In G. Bulechek & J. McCloskey (Eds.). *Nursing interventions: Treatments for nursing diagnoses*. Philadelphia: W. B. Saunders.

Hogstel, M. O. (1990). *Geropsychiatric nursing*. St. Louis: C. V. Mosby.

Longino, C. F., & Kart, C. S. (1982). Explicating activity theory: A formal replication. *Journal of Gerontology, 37,* 713–722.

Matteson, A. M., & McConnell, E. S. (1988). *Gerontological nursing: Concepts and practice*. Philadelphia: W. B. Saunders.

McPherson, B., & Guppy, N. (1979). Preretirement lifestyle and the degree of planning for retirement. *Journal of Gerontology, 34,* 254–263.

Miller, C. A. (1995). *Nursing care of the older adult* (2nd ed.). Glenview, IL: Scott, Foresman.

Rantz, M. (1991). Diversional activity deficit. In M. Maas, K. Buckwalter, & M. Hardy (Eds.). *Nursing diagnoses and interventions for the elderly*. Redwood City, CA: Addison-Wesley Nursing.

Scipien, G. M., Chard, M. A., Howe, J., & Barnard, M. U. (1990). *Pediatric nursing care*. St. Louis: C. V. Mosby.

Wong, D. L. (1993). *Essentials of pediatric nursing* (4th ed.). St. Louis: C. V. Mosby.

Dysreflexia

DEFINITION
Dysreflexia: The state in which an individual with a spinal cord injury at T7 or above experiences or is at risk to experience a potential life-threatening uninhibited sympathetic response of the nervous system to a noxious stimulus.

DEFINING CHARACTERISTICS
Major (Must Be Present)
Individual with spinal cord injury (T7 or above) with:
>Paroxysmal hypertension (sudden periodic elevated blood pressure in which systolic pressure is above 140 mm Hg and diastolic is above 90 mm Hg)
>Bradycardia or tachycardia (pulse rate of less than 60 or over 100 beats/min)
>Diaphoresis (above the injury)
>Red splotches on skin (above the injury)
>Pallor (below the injury)
>Headache (a diffuse pain in different portions of the head and not confined to any nerve distribution area)
>Apprehension

Minor (May Be Present)
>Chilling
>Conjunctival congestion
>Horner's syndrome (contraction of the pupil, partial ptosis of the eyelid, enophthalmos, and, sometimes, loss of sweating over the affected side of the face)
>Paresthesia
>Pilomotor reflex
>Blurred vision
>Chest pain
>Metallic taste in mouth
>Nasal congestion

RELATED FACTORS
Pathophysiologic
>Related to visceral stretching and irritation secondary to:
>(Bowel)
>>Constipation
>>Fecal impaction
>>Acute abdominal condition
>(Bladder)
>>Distended bladder
>>Urinary calculi
>>Infection
>Related to stimulation of skin (abdominal, thigh)
>Related to spastic sphincter

Treatment-Related
>Related to removal of fecal impaction
>Related to clogged or nonpatent catheter
>Related to visceral stretching and irritation secondary to surgical incision

Situational (Personal, Environmental)

Related to lack of knowledge of prevention or treatment
Related to sexual activity
Related to menstruation

Author's Note

Dysreflexia represents a life-threatening situation that nurses can prevent or treat through nurse-prescribed interventions. Prevention involves teaching the client to reduce sympathetic nervous system stimulation and avoiding nursing interventions that can cause sympathetic stimulation. When dysreflexia occurs, nursing interventions focus on reducing or eliminating the noxious stimulus (*e.g.*, fecal impaction, urinary retention). If nursing actions do not eliminate the stimuli and resolve symptoms, initiation of medical intervention is critical. When a client requires medical treatment for all or most episodes of dysreflexia, the situation would be labeled as a collaborative problem: *Potential Complication: Dysreflexia*.

Errors in Diagnostic Statements

Dysreflexia related to paroxysmal hypertension

Paroxysmal hypertension is a sign of dysreflexia, not a causative or contributing stimulus. The diagnosis should be restated as *Risk for Dysreflexia related to possible reflex stimulation by visceral or cutaneous irritation, as evidenced by (specify)*.

Clinically, *Risk for Dysreflexia* is a more descriptive diagnosis than *Dysreflexia*. The client is in a potential state most of the time, with associated nursing responsibilities of prevention, teaching, and early removal of stimulus.

Key Concepts

1. The autonomic nervous system, sympathetic and parasympathetic, is located in the cerebrum, hypothalamus, medulla, brain stem, and spinal cord. With spinal cord injury, the cord activity below the injury is deprived of the controlling effects from the higher centers, which results in poorly controlled responses (Zejdlik, 1992).
2. When sensory receptors are stimulated below a spinal lesion, sympathetic discharge, mediated by the spinothalamic tract and posterior columns, results. This reflex stimulation of the sympathetic nervous system causes spasms of the pelvic viscera and the arterioles. These spasms cause vasoconstriction below the level of the injury. Baroreceptors in the aortic arch and carotid sinus respond to the hypertensive state with superficial vasodilatation, flushing, diaphoresis, and piloerection (gooseflesh) above the level of the spinal lesion. Vagal stimulation slows the heart rate, but because the cord is severed, vagal impulses to dilate vessels are prohibited (Zejdlik, 1992).
3. Failure to reverse dysreflexia can result in status epilepticus, stroke, and death. Uncontrolled hypertension can cause systolic blood pressure to rise as high as 240–300 mm Hg (Zejdlik, 1992).
4. Three types of stimuli can initiate a dysreflexia response: visceral distention (*e.g.*, full bladder or rectum), stimulation of pain receptors (*e.g.*, diagnostic procedure, pressure), and visceral contractions (*e.g.*, ejaculation, bladder spasms, or uterine contractions) (Porth, 1994).

Focus Assessment Criteria

Subjective Data

A. Assess for defining characteristics

    1. Initial symptoms

        Headache

        Sweating, where?

Chills
Metallic taste in mouth
Nasal congestion
Blurred vision
Numbness
Other _____
  Medications used? What? Any recent changes?
  Bladder program (type, problems, any recent changes?)
  Bowel program (type, problems, any recent changes?)

B. Assess for related factors
  1. History of dysreflexia
     Triggered by
     Bladder distention   Sexual activity
     Bowel distention   Menstruation
     Tactile stimulation   Diagnostic study
     Skin lesion   Pressure
  2. Knowledge of dysreflexia
     Cause   Medical treatment
     Self-treatment   Prevention

Outcome Criteria

The individual/family will
- State factors that cause dysreflexia
- Describe the treatment for dysreflexia
- Relate when emergency treatment is indicated

Interventions
A. Assess for the presence of causative or contributing factors
  1. See Related Factors

B. If signs of dysreflexia occur, stand person up or raise the head of the bed and remove the noxious stimuli
  1. Bladder distention
     a. Check for distended bladder
     b. If catheterized
        Check catheter for kinks or compression.
        Irrigate with only 30 mL of saline, very slowly.
        Replace catheter if it will not drain.
     c. If not catheterized, insert catheter using dibucaine hydrochloride ointment (Nupercainal) and remove 500 mL, then clamp for 15 minutes; repeat cycle until bladder is drained.
  2. Fecal impaction
     a. First apply Nupercainal to the anus and into the rectum for 1 inch (2.54 cm).
     b. Gently check rectum with a well lubricated glove using index finger.
     c. Insert rectal suppository or gently remove impaction.
  3. Skin irritation
     a. Spray skin lesion that is triggering dysreflexia with a topical anesthetic agent.

C. Remove support hose

D. Continue to monitor blood pressure every 3–5 minutes

   E. Immediately consult physician for pharmacologic treatment if hypertension or noxious stimuli are not eliminated

   F. Initiate health teaching and referrals as indicated
     1. Teach signs and symptoms and treatment of dysreflexia to person and family.
     2. Teach when immediate medical intervention is warranted.
     3. Explain what situations can trigger dysreflexia (menstrual cycle, sexual activity, bladder or bowel routines).
     4. Teach to watch for early signs and to intervene immediately.
     5. Teach to observe for early signs of bladder infections and skin lesions (pressure ulcers, ingrown toenails).
     6. Advise consultation with physician for long-term pharmacologic management if individual is very vulnerable.

Rationale

- An upright position and removal of hose increase venous pooling, reduce venous return, and decrease blood pressure (Porth, 1994).
- Failure to reverse severe hypertension can result in status epilepticus, cerebrovascular accident, and death (Zejdlik, 1992).
- Intravenous pharmacologic intervention may be warranted if the noxious stimuli cannot be removed or hypertension reduced. Medications used may include diazoxide (Hyperstat), hydralazine (Apresoline), sodium nitroprusside (Nipride), and ganglionic blocking agents such as phenoxybenzamine (Dibenzyline) and guanethidine sulfate (Ismelin). Nifedipine capsule (10 mg) administered sublingually has been used to relieve hypertension in dysreflexia (Zejdlik, 1992).
- Good teaching can help the client and family successfully prevent or treat dysreflexia at home.

References/Bibliography

Hickey, J. (1992). *Neurological and neurosurgical nursing* (3rd ed.). Philadelphia: J. B. Lippincott.

Johnson, K. M. S. (1991). Growing up with a spinal cord injury. *SCI Nursing, 8*(1), 11–19.

Niederpruem, M. S. (1984) Autonomic dysreflexia. *Rehabilitation Nursing, 9,* 29–31.

Porth, C. M. (1994) *Pathophysiology: Concepts of altered health states.* Philadelphia: J. B. Lippincott.

Zejdlik, C. P. (1992). *Management of spinal cord injury* (2nd ed.). Boston: Jones & Bartlett.

Energy Field Disturbance

DEFINITION

Energy Field Disturbance: The state in which a disruption of the flow of energy surrounding a person's being results in a disharmony of the body, mind, and/or spirit.

DEFINING CHARACTERISTICS

Perception of changes in patterns of the energy flow, such as:
   Temperature change
     Warmth   Coolness

Visual changes
        Image   Color
Disruption of the field
        Vacant   Hole
        Spike   Bulge
Movement
        Wave   Spike
        Tingling   Dense
        Flowing
Sounds
        Tone   Word

RELATED FACTORS
Pathophysiologic

Related to slowing or blocking of energy flows secondary to:
        Illness (specify)
        Pregnancy
        Injury

Treatment-Related

Related to slowing or blocking of energy flows secondary to:
        Immobility
        Perioperative experience
        Labor and delivery

Situational (Personal, Environmental)

Related to the slowing or blocking of energy flows secondary to:
        Pain   Fear
        Anxiety   Grieving

Maturational

Related to age-related developmental difficulties or crises (specify)

Author's Note

This diagnosis is unique for two reasons. It represents a specific theory—human energy field theory—and the interventions used require specialized instruction and supervised practice. Meehan (1991) recommends preparation by:

- At least 6 months' experience in professional practice in an acute care setting
- Guided learning by a nurse with at least 2 years' experience
- Conformance with practice guidelines
- Thirty hours of instruction in the theory and practice
- Thirty hours of supervised practice with relatively healthy individuals
- Successful completion of written and practice evaluations

This diagnosis may be considered unconventional by some. Perhaps each nurse needs to be reminded that there are many theories, philosophies, and frameworks of nursing practice, just as there are many definitions of clients and practice settings. Some nurses practice on street corners with homeless people, whereas others practice in an office attached to their home. Nursing diagnosis should not represent only the practices of nurses in the mainstream practice setting (acute care, long-term care, home health). Rather than criticize a diagnosis as having little applicability to one's own practice, perhaps instead we should celebrate the diversity among us. Fundamentally, nurses are all connected as each of us and all of us seek to improve the condition of clients, families, groups, and communities.

Key Concepts

1. Therapeutic touch is rooted in Eastern philosophy. Because of our Western culture orientation, we search for research to explain its effects. To the Eastern mind, if it works, research is not necessary to prove how it works. The Eastern mind does not care how it works, only that it does (Carpenito, R., 1994, personal communication).
2. Therapeutic touch is derived from the basic premise that all living organisms are sustained by universal life energy. Health is defined as the state in which all an individual's energies are in harmony or dynamic balance. Health is compromised when there is disequilibrium, blockage, and/or deficit in the flow of energy (Macrae, 1988).
3. In nursing, the Rogerian conceptual system has provided the foundation for therapeutic touch. This model affirms that energy fields are fundamental units of human beings and their environment (Meehan, 1991).
4. "Therapeutic touch is a knowledgeable and purposive patterning of the patient–environmental energy field process" (Meehan, 1991, p. 201). It requires specialized instruction and supervised practice. Refer to Author's Note for this diagnosis for recommended preparation.
5. Life-giving, healing energy flows within the universal flow of energy. This life-giving, healing energy is present in all living systems. It is composed of intelligence, order, and compassion (Bradley, 1987).
6. Rogers states that therapeutic touch is an example of how a nurse "seeks to strengthen the coherence and integrity of human and environmental fields and to knowingly participate in the patterning of human and environmental fields for the realization of optimum well-being" (Meehan, 1991).
7. In a pilot study, Quinn and Strelkauskas (1993) found that all the recipients of therapeutic touch had a dramatic increase in all dimensions of positive affect (joy, vigor, contentment, and affection) and a dramatic decrease in all of the dimensions of negative affect (anxiety, guilt, hostility, and depression). They also identified a shift in consciousness during therapeutic touch, which was measured by perception of time. The same time distortions were reported by the practitioner and the recipients, indicating a shift in consciousness.

Focus Assessment Criteria

Because the assessment of the energy field is quickly followed by the intervention and reassessment continues throughout the intervention, refer to Interventions for assessment.

Outcome Criteria

The person will
- Report relief of symptoms after therapeutic touch
- Report increase sense of relaxation
- Report a decrease in pain using a scale of 0–10 before and after therapies

---

Interventions

Note: The following phases of therapeutic touch are learned separately but are rendered concurrently. The presentation of these interventions is for the purpose of describing the process for nurses who do not practice therapeutic touch. This discussion may help nurses to support colleagues who practice therapeutic touch and also to initiate referrals. As discussed previously, to prepare oneself for therapeutic touch requires specialized instruction, which is beyond the scope of this book.

A. Prepare the client and environment for therapeutic touch
   1. Provide as much privacy as possible.
   2. Explain therapeutic touch and obtain verbal permission.
   3. Give person permission to stop the therapy at any time.
   4. Allow person to assume a comfortable position (*e.g.*, lying or sitting on a bed or couch).

B. Shift from a direct focus on one's environment to an inner focus, which is perceived as the center of life within the nurse (centering)

C. Assess by scanning the person's energy field for openness and symmetry (Krieger, 1979)
   1. Move hands, palms toward person, at a distance of 2–4 inches over the person's body from head to feet in a smooth, light movement.
   2. Sense the cues to energy imbalance (*e.g.*, warmth, coolness, tightness, heaviness, tingling, emptiness).

D. Facilitate a rhythmic flow of energy by moving hands more vigorously from head to toe (unruffling/clearing)

E. Focus one's intent on the specific repatterning of areas of imbalance and impeded flow. Using one's hands as focal points, move the hands in gentle, sweeping movements from head to feet one time
   1. Note energy flow over lower legs and feet.
   2. If energy flow is not open in this area, continue to move hands or hold feet physically to facilitate energy flow.
   3. Briefly shake hands to dispel congestion from field if needed.
   4. When therapeutic touch is complete, place hands over the solar plexus area (just above the waist) and focus on facilitating the flow of healing energy to the person.
   5. Provide the person with an opportunity to rest.

F. Encourage the person to provide feedback
   1. Assess if the person exhibits a relaxation response:
      a. Drops of several decibels in voice volume
      b. Slower, deeper respirations
      c. Audible sign of relaxation (*e.g.*, sigh)
      d. Peripheral flush perceived on face

G. Document both the procedure and the feedback

Rationale

- Early beliefs regarding therapeutic touch attributed its effects to an energy transfer and exchange between the practitioner and recipient (Quinn, 1989). It is now believed that the practitioner shifts "consciousness into a state that may be thought of as a 'healing meditation,' facilitates repatterning of the recipient's energy field through the process of resonance, rather than 'energy exchange or transfer'" (Quinn & Strelkauskas, 1993, p. 14).
- The practitioner using therapeutic touch facilitates the flow of healing energy.
- "At the core of the therapeutic touch process is the intent of the practitioner to help the recipient" (Quinn & Strelkauskas, 1993, p. 14). The practitioner focuses completely on the recipient in an act of unconditional love and compassion. The healer has intentionality and motivation to help the healed, who has a willingness to accept the change.

References/Bibliography

Bradley, D. B. (1987). Energy fields: Implications for nurses. *Journal of Holistic Nursing, 5*(1), 32–35.

Dossey, B. M., Keegan, L., Guzzetta, C. E., & Kolmeier, L. G. (1995). *Holistic nursing: A handbook for practice* (2nd ed.). Rockville, MD: Aspen Publishers.

Krieger, D. (1975). Therapeutic touch: The imprimatur of nursing. *American Journal of Nursing, 75*, 784–787.

Krieger, D. (1979). *The therapeutic touch: How to use your hands to help or to heal*. Englewood Cliffs, NJ: Prentice-Hall.

Krieger, D. (1981). *Foundations of holistic health nursing practices: The Renaissance nurse*. Philadelphia: J. B. Lippincott.

Krieger, D. (1987). *Living the therapeutic touch: Healing as a lifestyle*. New York: Dodd, Mead.

Lionberger, H. J. (1986). Therapeutic touch: A healing modality or a caring strategy. In P. Chinn (Ed.). *Nursing research methodology: Issues and implementation*. Rockville, MD: Aspen Publishers.

Macrae, J. (1988). *Therapeutic touch: A practical guide*. New York: Knopf.

Meehan, T. C. (1991). Therapeutic touch. In G. Bulechek & J. McCloskey (Eds.). *Nursing interventions: Essential nursing treatments*. Philadelphia: W. B. Saunders.

Quinn, J. F. (1989). Therapeutic touch as energy exchange: Replication and extension. *Nursing Science Quarterly, 2*(2), 79–87.

Quinn, J., & Strelkauskas, A. (1993). Psychoimmunologic effects of therapeutic touch on practitioners and recently bereaved recipients: A pilot study. *Advances in Nursing Science, 15*(4), 13–26.

Environmental Interpretation Syndrome, Impaired

DEFINITION

Impaired Environmental Interpretation Syndrome: Consistent lack of orientation to person, place, time, or circumstances over more than 3 to 6 months, necessitating a protective environment.

DEFINING CHARACTERISTICS

Major

Consistent disorientation in known and unknown environments
Chronic confusional states

Minor

Loss of occupation or social functioning from memory decline
Inability to follow simple directions, instructions

Inability to reason
Inability to concentrate
Slow in responding to questions

RELATED FACTORS

Dementia (Alzheimer's disease, multiinfarct dementia, Pick's disease, AIDS dementia)
Parkinson's disease

Huntington's disease
Depression
Alcoholism

Author's Note

Impaired Environmental Interpretation Syndrome describes an individual who needs a protective environment because of consistent lack of orientation to person, place, time, or circumstances. This diagnosis is already described under *Chronic Confusion* and *Risk for Injury*. Interventions would focus on maintaining the maximum level of independence and preventing injury.

Until clinical research differentiates this diagnosis from the aforementioned diagnoses, use *Chronic Confusion* and/or *Risk for Injury*, depending on the data presented.

Family Processes, Altered

Family Processes, Altered: Alcoholism

Family Processes, Altered

DEFINITION
Altered Family Processes: The state in which a usually supportive family experiences, or is at risk to experience, a stressor that challenges its previously effective functioning.

DEFINING CHARACTERISTICS
Major (Must Be Present)
Family system cannot or does not:
>Adapt constructively to crisis
>Communicate openly and effectively between family members

Minor (May Be Present)
Family system cannot or does not:
>Meet physical needs of all its members
>Meet emotional needs of all its members
>Meet spiritual needs of all its members
>Express or accept a wide range of feelings
>Seek or accept help appropriately

RELATED FACTORS
Any factor can contribute to *Altered Family Processes*. Some common factors are listed below.

Pathophysiologic
>Related to impact of illness (specify)
>Related to change in the family member's ability to function

Treatment-Related
Related to:
>Disruption of family routines due to time-consuming treatments (*e.g.*, home dialysis)
>Physical changes due to treatments of ill family member
>Emotional changes in all family members due to treatments of ill family member
>Financial burden of treatments for ill family member
>Hospitalization of ill family member

Situational (Personal, Environmental)
Related to loss of family member

Death	Incarceration
Going away to school	Desertion
Separation	Hospitalization
Divorce	

Related to gain of new family member
    Birth   Marriage
    Adoption   Elderly relative
Related to losses associated with:
    Poverty
    Disaster
    Relocation
    Economic crisis
    Change in family roles
        Working mother
        Retirement
    Birth of child with defect
Related to conflict (moral, goal, cultural)
Related to breach of trust between members
Related to social deviance by family member (*e.g.*, crime)

Author's Note

Altered Family Processes describes a family that reports usual constructive function but a current challenge from a stressor has altered the family's functioning. The family is viewed as a system, with interdependence between members. Thus, life challenges for individual family members also challenge the family system. Certain situations have the potential negatively to influence family functioning; examples include illness, elderly relative moving in, relocation, separation, or divorce. The diagnosis *Risk for Altered Family Process* can represent such a situation.

Altered Family Processes is different from *Caregiver Role Strain*. Certain situations require a family member or members to assume a caregiver role for a family member. Caregiver role responsibilities can vary from ensuring an elderly parent has three balanced meals daily to providing for all the hygiene and self-care activities for an adult or child.

Caregiver Role Strain describes the burden that the caregiver role places on individuals, mentally and physically. All the caregiver's concurrent relationships and role responsibilities are influenced. *Caregiver Role Strain* focuses specifically on the individual or individuals who have multiple direct caregiver responsibilities.

Errors in Diagnostic Statements

Altered Family Process related to family not discussing the situation

A family's failure to discuss a situation does not represent a related factor, but rather a possible validation of the problem. If this situation is usual for the family, the diagnosis *Ineffective Family Coping: Disabling* should be investigated. If a failure to support each other represents a response to a stressor affecting the family system, the diagnosis *Altered Family Processes related to (specify stressor), as evidenced by report of family not discussing the situation* may be appropriate.

Key Concepts

1. Each family has a personality to which each member contributes.
2. The family unit may be viewed as a system with
   a. Interdependence between members
   b. Interactional patterns that provide structure and support for members
   c. Boundaries between the family and the environment and between members with varying degrees of permeability
3. Families change with time. They must accomplish specific tasks that originate from the needs of their members. Table II-8 illustrates the tasks of the family.
4. Each family responds to life challenges in ways that reflect experiences in the past and goals for the future.

Table II-8 **Stage-Critical Family Developmental Tasks Through the Family Life Cycle**

Stage of the Family Life Cycle	Positions in the Family	Stage-Critical Family Developmental Tasks
1. Married couple	Wife Husband	Establishing a mutually satisfying marriage Adjusting to pregnancy and the promise of parenthood Fitting into the kin network
2. Childbearing	Wife–mother Husband–father Infant daughter or son or both	Having, adjusting to, and encouraging the development of infants Establishing a satisfying home for both parents and infant(s)
3. Preschool-age	Wife–mother Husband–father Daughter–sister Son–brother	Adapting to the critical needs and interests of preschool children in stimulating, growth-promoting ways Coping with energy depletion and lack of privacy as parents
4. School-age	Wife–mother Husband–father Daughter–sister Son–brother	Fitting into the community of school-age families in constructive ways Encouraging children's educational achievement
5. Teenage	Wife–mother Husband–father Daughter–sister Son–brother	Balancing freedom with responsibility as teenagers mature and emancipate themselves Establishing postparental interests and careers as growing parents
6. Launching center	Wife–mother–grandmother Husband–father–grandfather Daughter–sister–aunt Son–brother–uncle	Releasing young adults into work, military service, college, marriage, etc., with appropriate rituals and assistance Maintaining a supportive home base
7. Middle-aged parents	Wife–mother–grandmother Husband–father–grandfather	Rebuilding the marriage relationship Maintaining kin ties with older and younger generations
8. Aging family members	Widow–widower Wife–mother–grandmother Husband–father–grandfather	Coping with bereavement and living alone Closing the family home or adapting it to aging Adjusting to retirement

(Duvall, E.M. [1977]. *Marriage and family development* [5th ed.]. Philadelphia: J. B. Lippincott, reproduced with permission)

5. Within a family, members interact in a variety of roles, which result from individual and group needs: parent, spouse, child, sibling, friend, teacher, and so on. Illness of a family member may cause great changes, putting the family at high risk for maladaptation (Fife, 1985).

6. Each family member influences the family unit. Thus, the health of an individual influences the health of the family. Family equilibrium depends on a balance of roles in the family and reciprocation (Duvall, 1977; Freidman, 1981).

7. *Stress* is defined as the body's response to any demand made on it. Stress has the potential for becoming a crisis when the person or family cannot cope constructively. A *crisis* is an event that occurs when the person's usual problem-solving methods are inadequate to resolve the situation.

8. The family in response to crisis does one of the following: returns to precrisis functioning, develops a more optimal level of functioning (adaptation), or develops a destructive form of functioning (maladaptation).

9. Constructive or functional coping mechanisms of families faced with a stress crisis are (Friedman, 1981).
   a. Greater reliance on each other
   b. Maintenance of a sense of humor
   c. Increased sharing of feeling and thoughts
   d. Promotion of each member's individuality
   e. Accurate appraisal of the meaning of the problem
   f. Search for knowledge and resources about the problem
   g. Use of support systems
10. Destructive or dysfunctional coping mechanisms of families faced with a stress or crisis are (Friedman, 1981):
    a. Denial of the problem
    b. Exploitation of one or more of the family members (threats, violence, neglect, scapegoating)
    c. Separation (hospitalization, institutionalization, divorce, abandonment)
          Authoritarianism (no negotiation)
          Preoccupation of family or members (who lack affection) with appearing close
11. Parenthood is a crisis. Some common problems are
    a. Increase in mate arguments
    b. Fatigue resulting from schedule
    c. Disrupted social life
    d. Disrupted sex life
    e. Multiple losses—actual or perceived (*e.g.*, independence, career, appearance, attention)
12. Characteristics of families prone to crisis include (Fife, 1985):
    a. Apathy (resigned to state in life)
    b. Poor self-concept
    c. Low income
    d. Inability to manage money
    e. Unrealistic preferences (materialistic)
    f. Lack of skills and education
    g. Unstable work history
    h. Frequent relocations
    i. History of repeated inadequate problem solving
    j. Lack of adequate role models
    k. Lack of participation in religious or community activities
    l. Environmental isolation (no telephone, inadequate public transportation)
13. There exists a time lag between identification of symptoms and help-seeking behavior, which may vary between families, depending on previous experience with the health care system, cultural interpretations of health and illness, and financial concerns.
14. Successful outcomes of family efforts to achieve a new level of adaptation after a crisis depend on (Nugent, Hughes, Ball, & Davis, 1992):
    a. Cohesiveness in response to past stressors
    b. Interacting with others in support group
    c. Belief that family can handle the crisis

☺ *Key Concepts—Child*

1. Two of the most significant stresses a child and family may experience are illness and hospitalization. The stresses of separation from parents, loss of control in a strange environment, and fear of bodily injury and pain make children particularly vulnerable (Wong, 1995).
2. Parents share many of the same stresses as hospitalized children. In addition, they may experience stress if their roles as primary caretakers are taken over by hospital staff. Parents are responsible as well for the care of siblings, who are affected by the crisis of illness and hospitalization (Craft & Craft, 1989).
3. Parents of hospitalized children often are not aware of the number of changes that siblings experience (Craft & Craft, 1989).
4. Keeping the "family secrets" consumes the child's attention and energy (Johnson, 1995a).

TRANSCULTURAL CONSIDERATIONS

1. The dominant American culture values two goals for families: the encouragement and nurturance of each individual and the cultivation of healthy, autonomous children. Marital partners are expected to be supportive and share a sense of meaning. Each partner has the freedom for personality development. Children are encouraged to develop their own identity and life directions (Giger & Davidhizar, 1995).

2. The family was found to be the principal source of support during illness in seven minority groups (Orque, Bloch, & Monroy, 1983).

3. In Latin families, the needs of the family are more important than those of the individual. The father is the provider, head of household, and decision maker (Boyle & Andrews, 1989).

4. For Arab Americans, families are supposed to be supportive. A family is often criticized as a failure if a member is sent to the hospital for psychiatric care. Arab-American families may appear overindulgent and interfering to compensate for criticism (Giger & Davidhizar, 1995)

5. Japanese Americans identify themselves by the generation in which they are born. First- and second-generation Japanese Americans see the family as one of the most important factors in their lives. The father and other male members are in the top position. Problems are managed within the family structure. Achievement or failure of an individual member is a reflection on the entire family. Caring for elderly parents is expected, usually by the oldest son or unmarried child. Adult children freely provide their parents with goods, money, and assistance (Hashizume & Takano, 1983).

6. The nuclear family and the greater Jewish community is the center of the Jewish culture. Their families are closely knit and child oriented. The commandments dictate the expected behavior toward parents and within the community (Giger & Davidhizar, 1995).

7. The family has been the chief source of cohesion and continuity for hundreds of years for the Vietnamese people. The immediate family includes the parents, unmarried children, and sometimes the husband's parents and sons with their wives and children. Behavior and misbehavior reflect on the whole family. A member is expected to give up personal wishes or ambitions if they disrupt family harmony. Family loyalty is "filial piety," which commands children to obey and honor their parents even after death (Giger & Davidhizar, 1995).

Focus Assessment Criteria

Subjective/Objective

A. General
1. Family composition (who resides in home, who does not)
2. Family strengths
3. Rules/discipline
4. Financial status
5. Participation in community activities
6. Family Process (Clemen-Stone, Eigasti, & McGuire, 1991)
    How does the family
        Integrate its roles, relationships?
        Use information from outside the family?
        Adapt to changes?
        Make and implement decisions?
        Respond to conflict or disagreements?
        Preserve family integrity as well as family members' autonomy?

B. Assess for defining characteristics
1. Communication patterns
    Straight messages
    No manipulation
    Express positive and negative feelings openly

2. Emotional/supportive pattern
   a. Constructive

Rely on each other	Appraise problem accurately
Seek knowledge and resources	Optimistic
Share feelings, thoughts	Deal with problems
Use support systems	

   b. Destructive
      Denial of problems
      Abandonment
      Authoritarianism
      Exploitation of members (threats, violence, neglect, scapegoating)
      Apathy
3. Socialization function
   Family members developing in a healthy pattern
   Roles and responsibilities are negotiated
4. Parenting and marriage roles
   Satisfying
   Mutual agreement
5. Child behavior
   Home
   School

C. Assess for related factors
1. Gain of new family member

Birth	Adoption
Marriage	Elderly relative

2. Loss of family member

Relocation	Illness
Death	

3. Change in family roles
4. Financial crisis
5. Disaster
6. Conflicts
7. Family member with a coping problem
8. Relocation history

Outcome Criteria

The family members will
- Frequently verbalize feelings to professional nurse and each other
- Maintain functional system of mutual support for each member
- Identify appropriate external resources available

Interventions

A. Assess causative and contributing factors
1. Illness-related factors
   a. Sudden, unexpected nature of illness
   b. Burdensome problems of a chronic nature
   c. Potentially disabling nature of illness
   d. Symptoms creating disfiguring change in physical appearance
   e. Social stigma associated with illness
   f. Financial burden

2. Factors related to behavior of ill family member
   a. Refuses to cooperate with necessary interventions
   b. Engages in socially deviant behavior associated with illness: suicide attempts, violence, substance abuse
   c. Isolates self from family
   d. Acts out or is verbally abusive to health professionals and family members
3. Factors related to the family as a whole
   a. Presence of unresolved guilt, blame, hostility, jealousy
   b. Inability to problem-solve adequately
   c. Ineffective patterns of communication among members
   d. Changes in role expectations and resulting tension
4. Factors related to illness in family (refer also to *Caregiver Role Strain*)
   a. Lack of family members available for support
   b. Inadequate finances
   c. Lack of knowledge of caregiver
   d. History of poor relationship between caregiver and ill member
   e. Overburdened caregiver
5. Factors related to health care environment
   a. Intervening professionals lack expertise in crisis intervention, counseling, or basic communication skills.
   b. Not enough health professionals can spend time with the family.
   c. Lack of continuity of care
   d. Lack of physical facilities in institution to ensure privacy or individualized care
6. Factors related to the community
   a. Lack of support from spiritual resources (philosophical and/or religious)
   b. Lack of relevant health education resources
   c. Lack of supportive friends
   d. Lack of adequate community health care resources (*e.g.*, long-term follow-up care, hospice, respite agency)

B. Acknowledge your feelings about the family and their situation
   1. Attempt to resolve these feelings.
      a. Pity
      b. Identifying with own family
      c. Blaming ill person or family for circumstances
      d. Judgmental attitude toward family
      e. Practicing punishing behavior (*e.g.*, ignoring people involved)
   2. Gain experience in crisis intervention and communication skills.

C. Provide ongoing information
   1. Approach the family with warmth, respect, and support.
   2. Avoid vague and confusing advice and clichés, such as "Take it easy, everything will be OK."
   3. Reflect family emotions to confirm these feelings ("This is very painful for you"; "You are very frightened").
   4. Keep family members abreast of changes in ill member's condition when appropriate.
   5. Avoid discussions of what caused the problem, or blaming.

D. Promote cohesiveness
   1. Facilitate communication.
   2. Encourage verbalization of guilt, anger, blame, and hostility and subsequent recognition of own feelings in family members.
   3. Enlist help of other professionals when indicated (*e.g.*, social worker, clinical psychologist, nurse therapist, clinical specialist, psychiatrist, child care specialist, school nurse).

E. Assist family with appraisal of the situation
   1. What is at stake? Encourage family to have a realistic perspective by providing accurate information and answers to questions.
   2. What are the choices? Assist family to reorganize roles at home and set priorities to maintain family integrity and reduce stress.
   3. Initiate discussions regarding stressors of home care (physical, emotional, environmental, financial).

F. Initiate health teaching and referrals, as necessary
   1. Include family members in group education sessions.
   2. Refer families to lay support and self-help groups.

Al-Anon	Arthritis Foundation
Syn-Anon	National Multiple Sclerosis Society
Alcoholics Anonymous	American Cancer Society
Sharing and Caring (American	American Heart Association
Hospital Association)	American Diabetes Association
Ostomy Association	American Lung Association
Reach for Recovery	Alzheimer's Disease and Related Disorders
Lupus Foundation of America	Association

   3. Facilitate family involvement with social supports.
      a. Assist family members to identify reliable friends (*e.g.*, clergy, significant others) and encourage seeking help (emotional, technical) when appropriate.

Rationale

- The goal of crisis management is to assist the family to return to its precrisis functioning. If the precrisis functioning was destructive (*e.g.*, alcoholism), the goal would be to develop a more optimal level of functioning. (See Appendix VII for guidelines for crisis management.)
- Common sources of family stress are (Miller & Winstead-Fry, 1982; Minuchin, 1974):
  - External sources of stress that one member is experiencing (*e.g.*, job or school related)
  - External sources of stress that influence the family unit (*e.g.*, finances, relocation)
  - Developmental stressors (*e.g.*, child-bearing, new baby, child-rearing, adolescence, new member or members—arrival of older grandparent, marriage of single parents— or loss of spouse)
  - Situational stressors (*e.g.*, illness, hospitalization, separation)

■ Altered Family Processes
Related to Impact (Specify) of Ill Member on Family System

Outcome Criteria

See Outcome Criteria for *Family Processes, Altered*
The family members will
- Participate in care of ill family member
- Facilitate return of ill family member from sick role to well role

Interventions

A. Create a private and supportive hospital environment for family

1. Keep client's door closed if possible.
2. Provide family members with a meeting place alternative to client's room.
3. Make sure family members are oriented to visiting hours, bathrooms, vending machines, cafeteria, and so forth.
4. If possible, provide pillows/blankets for family members spending the night.
5. Promote positive family visits (Harkulich & Calamita, 1986).
   a. Relate a positive experience that you have observed that represents a strength or individuality of the person.
   b. Encourage the person to be well dressed and groomed for visits.
   c. Encourage activities that the person enjoys (*e.g.*, walking, crafts, card games).
   d. If appropriate, share the weekly schedule of activities.
   e. Elicit suggestions from family for unmet needs.

B. Facilitate family strengths

1. Acknowledge these strengths to family when appropriate.
   a. "I can tell you are a very close family."
   b. "You know just how to get your mother to eat."
   c. "Your brother means a great deal to you."
2. Involve family members in care of ill member when possible (feeding, bathing, dressing, ambulating).
3. Involve family members in client care conferences, when appropriate.
4. Encourage family to acquire substitutes to care for the ill person, to provide the family with time away.
5. Promote self-esteem of individual family members ("Your daughter may respond to your drawings if we place them in her crib") (see *Self-Concept Disturbance*).
6. If appropriate, help ill member identify how to give support to caregiver (*e.g.*, praise, listening).
7. Mobilize ill individual to accept responsibility for some activities that contribute to family functioning (*e.g.*, shopping list, phone inquiries, peel vegetables).

C. Facilitate understanding, in other family members, of how ill member feels

1. Discuss stresses of hospitalization.
2. Describe implications of "sick role" and how it will return to "well role."
3. Aid family members to change their expectations of the ill member in a realistic manner.

D. Assist family with appraisal of the situation

1. Emphasize the importance of respites to prevent isolating behaviors that foster depression.
2. Discuss with the nonprimary caregivers their responsibilities in caring for the primary caregiver.

E. Provide the family with anticipatory guidance as illness continues

1. Inform parents of the effects of prolonged hospitalization on children (appropriate to developmental age).
2. Prepare family members for signs of depression, anxiety, and dependency, which are a natural part of the illness experience.

3. If the ill family member is an elderly parent undergoing surgery, inform the children that the patient may be confused or disoriented for a limited period of time after surgery.

4. Refer to *Caregiver Role Strain* if indicated.

F. Discuss the implications of caring for ill family member with all household members; cover:

1. Available resources (finances, environmental)
2. 24-Hour responsibility
3. Effects on other household members
4. Likelihood of progressive deterioration
5. Sharing of responsibilities (with other household members, siblings, neighbors)
6. Likelihood of exacerbation of long-standing conflicts
7. Impact on life-style
8. Alternative or assistive options (*e.g.*, community-based health care providers, life care centers, group living, nursing home)

Rationale

- Successful coping with illness requires the family to complete the following tasks: acknowledge the problem and seek help, accept the problem and its implications, and adjust as the member begins reconstruction (Clark & Gwin, 1993).
- The family acknowledges the problem by identifying the symptoms as serious enough to warrant investigation, and gaining knowledge of accessible resources (Clark & Gwin, 1993).
- The family must face the diagnosis and its implications. This task is multidimensional, including (Tilden & Weinert, 1987):
  - Experiencing the initial shock
  - Engaging in open communication between members
  - Minimizing anxiety and its disabling consequences
  - Preventing prolonged despair, guilt, blame, hostility
  - Accepting a valid diagnosis
- Studies have shown that family members of people with cancer "have perceived needs for information, communication skills, coping strategies and support services" (Clark & Gwin, 1993, p. 470).
- The family must adjust, as the member begins to recover, by
  - Adapting to new ways of living and making appropriate changes as recovery ensues
  - Fostering independence of recovering member
  - Accepting residual disability and making any necessary accommodations
  - Recognizing depression and anxiety in family member during change from "sick role" to "well role"
- The family must return to normality by returning to previous activities as much as possible and incorporating the recovered member back into the flow of family activities and responsibilities.

Family Processes, Altered: Alcoholism

DEFINITION

Altered Family Processes: Alcoholism: The state in which the psychosocial, spiritual, economic, and physiologic functions of the family members and system are chronically disorganized because of the effects of alcohol abuse.

DEFINING CHARACTERISTICS (LINDEMAN, HOKANSON, & BARTEK, 1994)

Major (80%–100%)

Behaviors

Loss of control of drinking
Denial of problems
Alcohol abuse
Impaired communication
Rationalization
Broken promises
Inability to meet emotional needs of members
Manipulation

Inappropriate expression of anger
Dependency
Refusal to get help
Blaming
Enabling behaviors
Ineffective problem-solving skills
Inadequate understanding or knowledge of alcoholism
Criticizing

Roles and Relationships

Deterioration in family relationships
Disturbed family dynamics
Marital problems
Ineffective spouse communication
Disruption of family roles

Inconsistent parenting
Family denial
Intimacy dysfunction
Closed communication systems

Feelings

Decreased self-esteem
Anger
Frustration
Powerlessness
Tension
Insecurity
Suppressed rage
Anxiety
Repressed emotions
Responsibility for alcoholic's behavior
Lingering resentment
Embarrassment

Hurt
Unhappiness
Guilt
Distress
Emotional isolation
Vulnerability
Worthlessness
Shame
Loneliness
Mistrust
Hopelessness
Rejection

Minor (70%–79%)

Behaviors: Minor

Inability to express or accept wide range of feelings
Orientation toward tension relief rather than achievement of goals
Family's special occasions are alcohol centered
Escalating conflict
Lying
Failure to send clear messages
Immaturity

Inability to get help or receive help appropriately
Ineffective decision making
Contradictory, paradoxical communication
Failure to deal with conflict
Harsh self-judgment
Isolation
Nicotine addiction
Difficulty having fun

Control of communication
Inability to adapt to change
Immaturity
Power struggles
Stress-related physical illnesses
Inability to deal with traumatic
experiences constructively
Seeking approval and affirmation
Lack of reliability
Disturbances in academic
performance in children

Disturbances in concentration
Chaos
Substance abuse other than alcohol
Difficulty with life cycle transitions
Verbal abuse of spouse or parent
Failure to accomplish current or
past developmental tasks
Agitation
Diminished physical contact

Feelings
Being different from other people
Depression
Hostility
Fear
Emotional control by others
Confusion
Dissatisfaction
Self-blaming
Unresolved grief

Loss
Feelings misunderstood
Abandonment
Confused love and pity
Moodiness
Failure
Being unloved
Lack of identity

Roles and Relationships
Triangulating family relationship
Inability to meet spiritual needs of its members
Reduced ability of family members to relate to each other for mutual growth and
maturation
Lack of skills necessary for relationships
Lack of cohesiveness
Disrupted family rituals
Family unable to meet security needs of members
Family does not demonstrate respect for autonomy and individuality of its members
Decreased sexual communication
Low perception of parental support
Pattern of rejection
Economic problems
Neglected obligations

RELATED FACTORS

Because the cause of this diagnosis is alcohol abuse by a family member, no related factors
are needed.

Author's Note

Alcoholism is a family disease. This nursing diagnosis represents the consequences of the
disturbed family dynamics related to alcohol abuse by a family member. The NANDA definition of *Altered Family Processes* is "the state in which a family that normally functions
effectively experiences a dysfunction" (NANDA, 1992, p. 41). The alcoholic family does not
have a history of effective functioning. The diagnosis *Ineffective Family Coping: Disabling*
would be more descriptive of the alcoholic family. The diagnosis could be stated as *Ineffective Family Coping: Alcoholism*. Further assessment will determine the effects of alcoholism on physical, psychological, spiritual, financial, and developmental aspects of the
family unit. If clinical research validates that alcoholism affects all these dimensions in all
or most families, the diagnosis *Alcoholic Family Process Syndrome* may prove very useful.

Errors in Diagnostic Considerations

Altered Family Processes: Alcoholism related to effects of alcohol on family

The "related to" for this diagnosis is a duplicate of the diagnostic statement. The inclusion of the term *alcoholism* in the diagnostic statement eliminates the need for related factors. Thus, the diagnosis can be stated as *Altered Family Processes: Alcoholism as evidenced by denial of severity of the problem, guilt, and repressed emotions.*

Key Concepts

1. Alcoholism is a family disease. There are approximately 10 million alcoholics in the United States and at least 4 million others intimately affected (Captain, 1989).
2. Alcoholic family members "lack trust in each other, lack nurturing closeness and solve problems in a piecemeal fashion" (Smith-DiJulio, 1994, p. 651).
3. Alcoholic families are dominated by the presence of alcoholism and its denial. Developmental tasks are thwarted or ignored when alcohol is the center of the family. "To keep the family unit intact, each member must change his or her cognitive perceptions to fit into the family's scheme of enabling the drinking to continue, while at the same time denying that it is a problem" (Starling & Martin, 1990, p. 16).
4. Alcoholic people initially use denial with regard to the use of alcohol to relieve stress. After dependence sets in, denial is used to conceal from the self and others how important alcohol is to functioning (Grisham & Estes, 1982).
5. As destructive interactions continue, family members and the alcoholic person move away from each other. The alcoholic person turns to liquor, while the family finds other means to escape (Collins, Leonard, & Searles, 1990).
6. "Meaningful sobriety is characterized by more than just the abstinence of the alcoholic person. It necessitates an ongoing growth process for all family members to work together toward the goal of a well-functioning family" (Grisham & Estes, 1982, p. 257).
7. Wegscheider (1981) described six roles typical in families affected by alcoholism:
   a. Alcoholic
   b. Chief enabler—often the spouse; super-responsible, takes on duties vacated by the alcoholic
   c. Family hero—high achiever to provide family with some pride to cover up family's failures
   d. Scapegoat—defiant, angry, diverts family focus from alcoholism
   e. Lost child—helpless, powerless
   f. Mascot—clowning, joking; a form of tension relief to mask underlying terror
8. Wing (1991) describes a four-stage theory of alcoholism, recovery, and goal setting:
   a. Stage I: Denial—alcoholics are coerced into treatment; their goals are to avoid punishment; no sincere desire to stop drinking.
   b. Stage II: Dependence—alcoholics admit that they have a drinking problem, seek treatment to maintain job or a relationship.
   c. Stage III: Behavior change—alcoholic attempts to replace unhealthy behaviors with healthy behaviors.
   d. Stage IV: Life planning—alcoholic integrates family, career, and educational goals with sobriety.
9. A genogram is a three-generation map of the family structure and relationships. It can assist the nurse and family in understanding that their present structure, roles, values, and entire system evolved from the past (Johnson, 1995b) (see Fig. II-2).

Key Concepts—Child

1. Children learn definitions of love, intimacy, and trust in their families of origin. The environment in the alcoholic family is one of chaos and unpredictability. Roles are unclear. Sometimes the children become the parents and the alcoholic member an outsider in the family (Collins et al., 1990).
2. Children report being most disturbed by parents arguing rather than one parent's drinking. Children can respond in varied ways (*e.g.*, peacemaker, aggression at school).

3. Behavioral problems in children need to be assessed in the context of what purpose they serve for the family (Johnson, 1995a).
4. Children of alcoholics are accustomed to extra and inappropriate responsibilities (Smith-DiJulio, 1994).

Focus Assessment Criteria

This assessment focuses on the individual family members and the family unit. For an assessment of the alcoholic family member, refer to a specific assessment tool (*e.g.*, Michigan Alcoholism Screening Test [MAST] or CAGE Screening Test [see p. 264]). For a general family assessment, refer to *Altered Family Processes*.

Subjective Data

A. General

1. Family composition
2. Family roles
    Breadwinner
    Decision-maker(s)
3. Family strengths
4. Rules/discipline
5. Financial status
6. Participation in community activities

B. Assess for defining characteristics

1. Denial of the problem
2. Responses of family members

Afraid	Alcohol use influences what you do or don't do
Worried	Overall feelings
Embarrassed	Effects on each family member
Attempts to hide	Behavioral problems (children)
Guilt feelings	

3. Characteristics of alcoholic person

Friends drink heavily	Justifies his or her alcohol use
Promises to quit or reduce intake	Drives under influence
Fails to remember events when drinking	Verbally or physically abusive
Avoids conversations about alcohol use	Periods of remorse

4. Family/social functions
    Unsatisfactory, tense
    Always include alcohol
    Negative comments of others on drinking behavior
    Financial, legal problems

Objective Data

A. Prepare a three-generation genogram (Fig. II-2) (Johnson, 1995b)

1. Use symbols □ (male) and ○ (female).
2. Give name, age, birth date, death date, highest level of education, occupation, significant health problems, and date of diagnosis for parents, siblings, children of person, and spouse.
3. Link symbols with lines that indicate:
    Marriage
    Separation
    Divorce
    Living together
4. Indicate death with × in symbol
    or miscarriage with △
    or abortion with ×

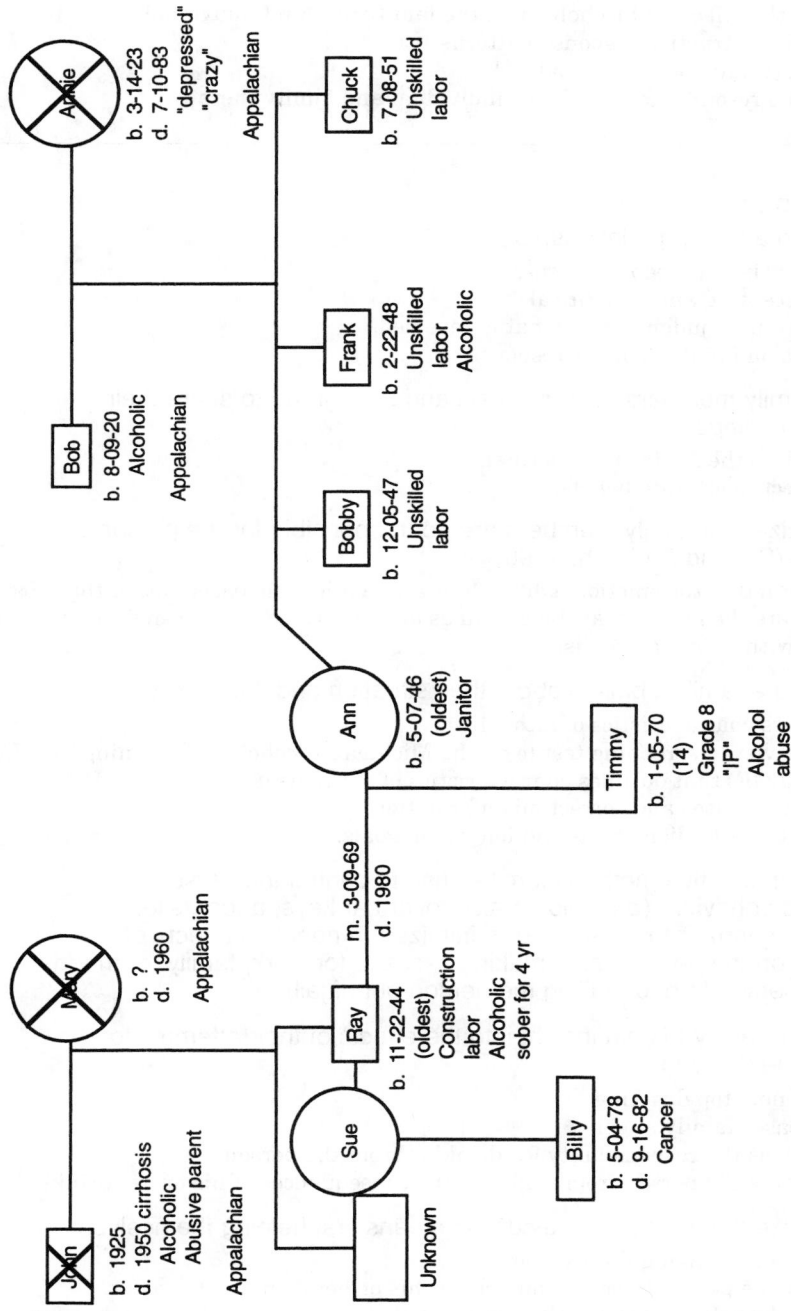

Fig. II-2 Genogram for the M. family. (Redrawn from Johnson, B. S. [1995]. *Psychiatric mental health nursing: Adaptation and growth* [3rd ed.]. Philadelphia: J. B. Lippincott.)

Outcome Criteria

The family will
• Acknowledge the alcoholism in the family
• Relate the effects of alcoholism on the family unit and individuals
• Identify destructive response patterns
• Set short- and long-term goals
• Describe resources available for individual and family therapy

Interventions

A. Establish a trusting relationship
1. Be consistent, keep promises.
2. Be accepting and noncritical.
3. Do not pass judgment on what is revealed.
4. Focus on family member responses.

B. Allow family members as individuals and as a group to share their pent-up feelings
1. Validate the feelings are normal.
2. Correct inaccurate beliefs.

C. Emphasize that family members are not responsible for the person's drinking (Starling & Martin, 1990)
1. Explain that the emotional difficulties are relationship based rather than "psychiatric."
2. Educate the family that their feelings and experiences are seen frequently in association with family alcoholism.

D. Explore the family's beliefs about their situation and their goals
1. Discuss characteristics of alcoholism.
   a. Review a screening test (e.g., the Michigan Alcoholism Screening Test [MAST] or CAGE) that outlines characteristics of alcoholism.
2. Discuss causes and correct misinformation.
3. Assist to establish short- and long-term goals.

E. Discuss ineffective methods families use to control the person's alcoholic behaviors (e.g., hiding alcohol or car keys, anger, silence, threats, crying) or to cover up or minimize the negative effects of drinking on the person (e.g., making excuses for work, family, or friends, putting person to bed, bailing the person out of jail)

F. Assist the family to gain insight into the effects of their attempts to control the drinking
1. Does not stop drinking
2. Increases family anger
3. Removes the responsibility for drinking from the person
4. Prevents the person from suffering the consequences of his or her drinking behavior

G. Emphasize that helping the alcoholic means first helping themselves
1. Focus on changing their response.
2. Allow the person to be responsible for his or her drinking behavior.
3. Describe activities that will improve their life, as individuals and as a family.
4. Initiate one stress management technique (e.g., aerobic exercises, assertiveness course, walking, meditation, relaxation breathing; refer to Appendix X, Stress Management).
5. Plan time as a family together outside the home (e.g., museum, zoos, picnic). If the alcoholic person is included, the person must contract not to drink during the activity and agree on a consequence if he or she does.

H. Discuss with the family that during recovery, their usual family dynamics will be dramatically changed
   1. The alcoholic is removed from the center of attention.
   2. All family roles will be challenged.
   3. Family members will have to focus on themselves instead of the alcoholic person.
   4. Family members will have to assume responsibility for their behavior, rather than blaming someone else.
   5. Behavioral problems of children serve a purpose for the family.

I. Discuss the possibility of relapse and the contributing factors (refer to Key Concepts, No. 8)

J. If additional family or individual nursing diagnoses exist, refer to specific diagnosis (*e.g.*, Child abuse, Domestic violence)

K. Initiate health teaching regarding community resources and referrals as indicated
   1. AL-ANON
   2. Alcoholics Anonymous
   3. Family therapy
   4. Individual therapy
   5. Self-help groups (*e.g.*, Adult Children of Alcoholics)

Rationale

- Cessation of the drinking behavior is a threat to the family because equilibrium is centered around the alcoholism (Smith-DiJulio, 1994).
- Interventions are focused on assisting the family to change their ineffective communication and response patterns (Smith-DiJulio, 1994).
- Denial is used by family members to avoid the shame of admitting the problem, to avoid having to deal with their contribution to the problem, and in the hope that it will disappear if it is not disclosed (Collins et al., 1990).
- Communication in the family is disturbed. Sharing feelings is uncommon because of a history of disappointment. Diminished sharing of thoughts and feelings and silence can maintain disturbed families for long periods. Communication is mainly focused on family members trying to control the other person's drinking behavior (Grisham & Estes, 1982).
- "The potential value of reaching the alcoholic person by first assisting family members should not be underestimated" (Grisham & Estes, 1982, p. 257). It is important that the family and the health care professional accept that no certain outcome can be promised for the alcoholic person even when the family receives help.
- Wing (1994) proposes that relapses occur for different reasons in each stage. In Stage I, relapse occurs when the threat of punishment is removed. Relapse in Stage II occurs when the object of dependence (*e.g.*, marriage, job) is secured or lost. Relapses in Stage III and IV occur less frequently. They are triggered by unexpected, stressful events. Nursing interactions for people in Stages I and II would focus on confronting the denial and helping them to become more internally focused. People recovering in Stages III and IV need to be assisted to learn how to cope with unexpected, stressful events without alcohol (Wing, 1994).
- Common issues that families face when in therapy are (Vanicelli, 1987):
   a. Coping with sudden disequilibrium
   b. Feelings that they are strangers
   c. Attributing all family problems to the alcohol problem
   d. Loss of fantasy that everything will be fine when drinking ceases
   e. Learning appropriate ways to express anger
- Self-help and support groups promote acceptance of the disease concept of alcoholism and can reduce burdens of guilt, shame, and hostility (Smith-DiJulio, 1994).

References/Bibliography

Boyle, J., & Andrews, M. (1995). *Transcultural concepts in nursing* (2nd ed.). Philadelphia: J. B. Lippincott.

Clemen-Stone, S., Eigasti, D. G., & McGuire, S. L. (1991). *Comprehensive family and community health nursing* (3rd ed.). St. Louis: Mosby-Year Book.

Clark, J., & Gwin, R. (1993). Psychological responses of the family. In S. Groenwald, M. Frogge, M. Goodman, & C. Yarbo (Eds.). *Cancer nursing: Principles and practice*. Boston: Jones and Bartlett.

Craft, M. J., & Craft, J. L. (1989). Perceived changes in siblings of hospitalized children: A comparison of sibling and hospitalized and parent reports. *Children's Health Care, 18*(1), 42–48.

Duvall, E. M. (1977). *Marriage and family development* (5th ed.). Philadelphia: J. B. Lippincott.

Fife, B. L. (1985). A model for predicting the adaptation of families to medical crisis: An analysis of role integration. *Image: Journal of Nursing Scholarship, 18*(4), 108–112.

Friedman, M. (1981). *Family nursing: Theory and assessment.* New York: Appleton-Century-Crofts.

Giger, J. N., & Davidhizar, R. E. (1995). *Transcultural nursing: Assessment and interventions* (2nd ed.). St. Louis: Mosby-Year Book.

Harkulich, J., & Calamita, B. (1986). *A manual for caregivers of Alzheimer's disease clients in long-term care* (2nd ed.). Beachwood, OH: Nursing Home Training Center, Menorah Park Center for the Aged.

Hashizume, S., & Takano, J. (1983). Nursing care of Japanese American patients. In M. S. Orque, B. Bloch, & L. S. A. Monroy (Eds.). *Ethnic nursing care: A multicultural approach.* St. Louis: C. V. Mosby.

Miller, S., & Winstead-Fry, P. (1982). *Family systems theory in nursing practice.* Norwalk, CT: Reston Publishing.

Minuchin, A. (1974). *Families and family therapy.* Cambridge, MA: Harvard University Press.

Nugent, K., Hughes, R., Ball, B., & Davis, K., (1992). A practice model for pediatric support groups. *Pediatric Nursing, 18*(1), 11–16.

Orque, M. S., Bloch, B., & Monroy, L. S. A. (Eds.). (1983). *Ethnic nursing care: A multicultural approach.* St. Louis: C. V. Mosby.

Tilden, V. P., & Weinert, C. (1987). Social support and the chronically ill individual. *Nursing Clinics of North America, 22,* 613–620.

Wong, D. L. (1993). *Essentials of pediatric nursing* (4th ed.). St. Louis: C. V. Mosby.

Alcoholism

Captain, C. (1989). Family recovery from alcoholism. *Nursing Clinics of North America, 24,* 55–67.

Collins, R. L., Leonard, K., & Searles, J. (1990). *Alcohol and the family: Research and clinical perspectives.* New York: Guilford Press.

Grisham, K., & Estes, N. (1982). Dynamics of alcoholic families. In N. Estes & M. E. Heinemann (Eds.). *Alcoholism: Development, consequences and interventions.* St. Louis: Mosby-Year Book.

Johnson, B. S. (1995a). *Child, adolescent and family psychiatric nursing.* Philadelphia: J. B. Lippincott.

Johnson, B. S. (1995b). *Psychiatric mental health nursing: Adaptation and growth* (3rd ed.). Philadelphia: J. B. Lippincott.

Lindeman, M., Hokanson, J., & Bartek, J. (1994). The alcoholic family. *Nursing Diagnoses, 5*(2), 65–73.

North American Nursing Diagnosis Association. (1992). *NANDA nursing diagnosis: Definitions and classifications.* Philadelphia: Author.

Smith-DiJulio, K. (1994). People who depend on alcohol. In E. M. Varcarolis (Ed.). *Foundations of psychiatric mental health nursing.* Philadelphia: W. B. Saunders.

Vanicelli, M. (1987). Treatment of alcoholic couples in outpatient group therapy. *Group 11, 4,* 247–257.

Wegscheider, S. (1981). *Another chance.* Palo Alto, CA: Science and Behavior Books.

Wing, D. M. (1991). Goal setting and recovery from alcoholism. *Archives of Psychiatry in Nursing, 5,* 178–184.

Wing, D. M. (1994). Understanding alcoholism relapse. *Nurse Practitioner, 19*(4), 67–69.

Resources for the Consumer

Beattie, M. (1992). *Codependent no more—how to stop controlling others and start caring for yourself.* Center City: Hazelden.

Peele, S., & Brodsky, A. (1992). *The truth about addiction and recovery.* New York: Simon & Schuster.

Woititz, J. G. (1990). *Adult children of alcoholics.* Deerfield Beach: Health Communications, Inc.

Fatigue

DEFINITION

Fatigue: The self-recognized state in which an individual experiences an overwhelming, sustained sense of exhaustion and decreased capacity for physical and mental work that is not relieved by rest.

DEFINING CHARACTERISTICS*

Major (80%–100%)

Verbalization of an unremitting and overwhelming lack of energy
Inability to maintain usual routines

Minor (50%–79%)

Perceived need for additional energy to accomplish routine tasks
Increase in physical complaints
Emotionally labile or irritable
Impaired ability to concentrate
Decreased performance
Lethargic or listless
Lack of interest in surroundings/introspection
Decreased libido
Accident prone

RELATED FACTORS

Many factors can cause fatigue; it may be useful to combine related factors, such as Related to muscle weakness, build-up of waste products, inflammatory process, and infections secondary to hepatitis.

Pathophysiologic

Related to hypermetabolic state secondary to:
Viruses
Fever
Endocarditis
Related to inadequate tissue oxygenation secondary to:

Congestive heart failure	Anemia
Chronic obstructive lung disease	Peripheral vascular disease

Related to biochemical changes secondary to:
(Endocrine/metabolic disorders)

Diabetes mellitus	Pituitary disorders
Hypothyroidism	Addison's disease

Chronic diseases (*e.g.*, renal failure, cirrhosis, Lyme disease)
Related to muscular weakness secondary to:

Myasthenia gravis	Parkinson's disease
Multiple sclerosis	AIDS
Amyotrophic lateral sclerosis	

Related to hypermetabolic state, competition between body and tumor for nutrients, anemia, and stressors associated with cancer

* Voith, A. M., Frank, A. M., & Pigg, J. S. (1987). Validations of fatigue as a nursing diagnosis. In A. M. McLane (Ed.). *Classification of nursing diagnosis: Proceedings of the seventh conference.* St. Louis: C. V. Mosby.

Related to nutritional deficits or changes in nutrient metabolism secondary to:

Nausea	Side effects of medications
Vomiting	Gastric surgery
Diarrhea	Diabetes mellitus

Related to chronic inflammatory process secondary to:

AIDS	Cirrhosis
Arthritis	Inflammatory bowel disease
Lupus erythematosus	Renal failure
Hepatitis	

Treatment-Related

Related to chemotherapy
Related to radiation therapy
Related to side effects of (specify):
Related to surgical damage to tissue and anesthesia
Related to increased energy expenditure secondary to:
  Amputation
  Gait disorder
  Use of walker, crutches

Situational

Related to prolonged decreased activity and deconditioning secondary to:

Anxiety	Social isolation
Fever	Nausea/vomiting
Diarrhea	Depression
Pain	

Related to excessive role demands
Related to overwhelming emotional demands
Related to extreme stress
Related to sleep disturbance

Maturational

Child/Adolescent
Related to hypermetabolic state secondary to:
  Mononucleosis   Fever
Related to insufficient nutrients secondary to:
  Obesity   Excessive dieting
  Eating disorders
Adult/adolescent
(Pregnancy, postpartum)
Related to effects of newborn care on sleep patterns and need for continuous attention
Related to changes in metabolic, respiratory, circulatory, gastrointestinal, renal, and
  endocrine function during first trimester

Author's Note

Fatigue is different from tiredness. Tiredness is a transient, temporary state (Rhoten, 1982) caused by lack of sleep, improper nutrition, increased stress, sedentary life-style, or a temporary increase in work or social responsibilities. Fatigue is a pervasive, subjective, drained feeling that cannot be eliminated, but the individual can be assisted to adapt to fatigue. Activity intolerance is different from fatigue in that the person with activity intolerance will be assisted in increasing endurance to progress and will increase his activity.

The person with fatigue is not focused on increasing endurance. If the cause of fatigue resolves or abates (*e.g.*, acute infection, chemotherapy, radiation), the *Fatigue* diagnosis is discontinued and the diagnosis *Activity Intolerance* can be initiated to focus on improving the deconditioned state.

Errors in Diagnostic Statements

Fatigue related to feelings of lack of energy for routine tasks

When a person reports insufficient energy for routine tasks, the nurse performs a focus assessment and collects additional data to determine whether *Fatigue* is the appropriate diagnosis or whether fatigue is actually a symptom of another diagnosis, such as *Activity Intolerance, Ineffective Coping, Altered Family Processes, Anxiety*, or *Altered Health Maintenance*. When fatigue is caused by acute or chronic disorders or therapies, the nurse needs to determine whether the person increases endurance (which would call for the diagnosis *Activity Intolerance*) or whether energy conservation techniques will be needed to help the person accomplish desired activities.

When fatigue results from ineffective stress management or poor daily health habits, the diagnosis of *Fatigue* or *Activity Intolerance* is not indicated. During data collection to determine contributing factors, the nurse can record the diagnosis as: *Possible Fatigue related to reports of lack of energy*. Labeling the diagnosis as "possible" indicates the need for additional data collection to rule out or confirm.

Key Concepts

1. Fatigue can be a simple or complex problem. It is a subjective experience with physiologic, situational, and psychological components.
2. Normal fatigue or tiredness is an expected response to physical exertion, change in daily activities, additional stress, or inadequate sleep (Kellum, 1985).
3. American society values energy and productivity. Those without energy are viewed as sluggish or lazy. Energy and vitality are valued positively, whereas fatigue and tiredness are viewed negatively (Rhoten, 1982).
4. Fatigue can result from pathophysiology such as:
   a. Decreased cardiac output
   b. Prolonged circulatory time
   c. Accumulation of metabolic wastes
   d. Decreased oxygen transport
5. Fatigue can be manifested in areas of cortical inhibition such as (Jiricka, 1994; Rhoten, 1982):
   a. Decreased attention
   b. Slowed and impaired perception
   c. Impaired thinking
   d. Decreased motivation
   e. Decreased performance in physical and mental activities
   f. Loss of fine coordination
   g. Poor judgment
   h. Indifference to surroundings
6. Hargreaves (1977) described a high incidence of "fatigue syndrome" in young married women moving to a new town. Factors that contributed to the fatigue were increased physical work, changes in support systems, and other stresses in relocation.
7. People with rheumatoid arthritis reported that their fatigue was related to joint pain. In addition, clients with flare were observed to awaken more often and take longer to walk and perform activities than nonflare clients and the control group (Crosby, 1991).
8. Prolonged stress may be the main cause of chronic fatigue in people with cancer (Aistars, 1987).
9. The stressors (pathophysiologic, situational, treatment-related) contributing to fatigue in cancer clients are illustrated in Table II-9.
10. Women receiving localized radiation to the breast reported fatigue decreased the second week but increased and plateaued after week 4 until 3 weeks after the treatment ceased. Fatigue levels did not change significantly on the weekends between treatments (Greenberg, Sawicka, Eisenthal, & Ross, 1992).
11. When fatigue is a side effect of treatment, it does not resolve when the treatment is finished, but gradually lessens over a period of months (Nail & Winningham, 1993).

Table II-9 **Fatigue-Contributing Factors in Cancer Clients**

Pathophysiologic*
Hypermetabolic state associated with active tumor growth
Competition between the body and the tumor for nutrients
Chronic pain
Organ dysfunction (*e.g.*, hepatic, respiratory, gastrointestinal)

Treatment-Related*
Accumulation of toxic waste products secondary to radiation, chemotherapy
Inadequate nutritional intake secondary to nausea, vomiting
Anemia
Analgesics, antiemetics
Diagnostic tests
Surgery

Situational (Personal, Environmental)
Uncertainty about future
Fear of death, disfigurement
Social isolation
Losses (role responsibilities, occupational, body parts, function, appearance, economic)
Separation for treatments

*Aistars, J. (1987). Fatigue in the cancer patient: A conceptual approach to a clinical problem. *Oncology Nursing Forum, 14*(6d), 25–30.

12. Depression slows one's thought processes and produces a decrease in physical activities. Work output decreases, and endurance is reduced. The effort to continue activity produces fatigue.
13. Anxiety can interfere with thought processes, increase movements, and disturb gastrointestinal function, thus causing fatigue.

🐣 *Key Concepts—Child*

1. Infants and small children are unable to express fatigue. This information can be elicited by the nurse from interviewing the parents and carefully assessing key functional health patterns (*e.g.*, sleep–rest, activity–exercise [which may reveal respiratory difficulties or activity intolerance], and nutrition–metabolic [which may reveal feeding difficulties]).
2. Children at risk for fatigue include those with acute or chronic illness, congenital heart disease, exposure to toxins, prolonged stress, and anemia (Oski, 1994).
3. Children depend on parents/caregivers to modify their environment to mitigate the effects of fatigue.

🐚 *Key Concepts—Maternal*

1. Gardner (1992) reported that levels of fatigue in postpartum women increased at 2 weeks postpartum but decreased by 6 weeks.
2. Factors associated with high levels of postpartum fatigue were sleep alterations, additional children, child care problems, less household help, less education, low family income, and young age of mother (Gardner & Campbell, 1991).

🏛 *Key Concepts—Older Adult*

1. The normal effects of aging do not in themselves increase the risk of or cause fatigue.
2. Fatigue in older adults has basically the same etiologies as in younger adults. The difference lies in the fact that older adults tend to experience more chronic diseases than younger adults. Thus, fatigue in older adults is not the result of age-related factors, but rather to such risk factors as chronic diseases, medications, and others.
3. Depression is the most common psychosocial impairment in older adults. Depression-related affective disturbances affect 27% of adults in a community-living setting (Miller, 1995).

4. Chronic fatigue and diminished energy are functional consequences of late-life depression (Miller, 1995).

5. According to Miller (1995), "the activity theory proposed that older adults would remain psychologically and socially fit if they remained active." A person's self-concept is affirmed through participation in activities.

6. Chronic fatigue, reported by approximately 70% of the elderly, can result in diminished motor activity and muscle tone. Note that anemia, very common in the elderly, is another possible contributor to chronic fatigue complaints (Matteson & McConnell, 1988; Mitchell, 1986).

Focus Assessment Criteria

Subjective Data

A. Assess for defining characteristics

    1. Description of fatigue

Onset?	Pattern: morning, evening, transient, unfading
Precipitated by what?	Relieved by rest?

    2. Effects of fatigue on:

Activities of daily living	Libido
Concentration	Mood
Leisure activities	Motivation

B. Assess for related factors

    1. Medical condition (acute, chronic)

    2. Nutritional imbalances

    3. Treatments

Chemotherapy	Medication side effects
Radiation therapy	

    4. Stressors

Excessive role demands	Financial
Depression	Career
Family	

Outcome Criteria

The person will
- Discuss the causes of fatigue
- Share feelings regarding the effects of fatigue on his or her life
- Establish priorities for daily and weekly activities
- Participate in activities that stimulate and balance physical, cognitive, affective, and social domains

---

Interventions

The nursing interventions for this diagnosis are interventions for individuals with fatigue with etiologies that cannot be eliminated. The focus of nursing care is to assist the individual and family to adapt to the fatigue state.

A. Assess causative or contributing factors

    1. Lack of sleep; refer to *Sleep Pattern Disturbance*

    2. Poor nutrition; refer to *Altered Nutrition*

    3. Sedentary life-style; refer to *Health-Seeking Behaviors*

4. Inadequate stress management; refer to *Health-Seeking Behaviors*
5. Physiologic impairment
6. Treatment (chemotherapy, radiation, medications)
7. Chronic excessive role or social demands
8. The quality or type of activity reportedly is more important than the quantity (Lemon, Bengston, & Peterson, 1972). Informal activities promoted well-being the most, followed by formal structured activities, and last by solitary activities, which were found to have little or no effect on life satisfaction (Longino & Kart, 1982).

B. Explain the causes of fatigue (see Key Concepts)

C. Allow expression of feelings regarding the effects of fatigue on life
1. Identify those activities that are difficult.
2. Verbalize how fatigue interferes with role responsibilities.
3. Convey how fatigue causes frustration.

D. Assist the individual to identify strengths, abilities, interests
1. Identify client's values and interests.
2. Identify client's areas of success and usefulness; emphasize his past accomplishments.
3. Use this information to develop goals with the client.
4. Assist to identify sources of hope (*e.g.* relationships, faith, things to accomplish).
5. Assist to develop realistic short- and long-term goals (progress from simple to more complex; may use a "goals poster" to indicate type and time for achieving specific goals).

E. Assist individual to identify energy patterns and the need to schedule activities
1. Instruct to record fatigue levels every hour during a 24-hour period, select a usual day (Aistars, 1987).
   a. Ask to rate his fatigue 0–10 using the Rhoten fatigue scale (0 = not tired, peppy; 10 = total exhaustion).
   b. Record the activities at the time of each rating.
2. Analyze together the 24-hour fatigue levels.
   a. Times of peak energy
   b. Times of exhaustion
   c. Activities associated with increasing fatigue

F. Assist individual to identify what tasks can be delegated
1. Explore what activities are viewed as important for the individual to maintain self-esteem.
2. Attempt to divide the vital activities or tasks into components; delegate parts of the task but retain certain components (*e.g.*, meal preparation, shopping, storing, preparing food for cooking, cooking, serving, cleaning up).
3. Plan the important tasks during periods of high energy (*e.g.*, prepare all the day's meals in the morning).

G. Explain the purpose of pacing and prioritization
1. Assist individual to identify priorities and to eliminate nonessential activities.
2. Plan each day to avoid energy- and time-consuming nonessential decision making.
3. Organize work with work items within easy reach.
4. Distribute difficult tasks throughout the week.
5. Rest before difficult tasks and stop before fatigue ensues.

H. Teach energy conservation techniques
1. Modify the environment.
   a. Replace steps with ramps.
   b. Install grab rails.

    c. Elevate chairs 3–4 inches.

    d. Organize kitchen or work areas.

    e. Reduce trips up and down stairs (*e.g.*, put a commode on first floor).

  2. Plan small, frequent meals to decrease energy required for digestion.

  3. Use taxi instead of driving self.

  4. Delegate housework (*e.g.*, employ a high school student for a few hours after school).

I. **Explain the effects of conflict and stress on energy levels and assist to learn effective coping skills**

  1. Teach the importance of mutuality in sharing concerns.

  2. Explain the benefits of distraction from negative events.

  3. Teach the value of confronting issues.

  4. Teach and assist with relaxation techniques (see Appendix X) before anticipated stressful events. Encourage mental imagery to promote positive thought processes (see Appendix X).

  5. Allow the client time to reminisce to gain insight into past experiences.

  6. Teach to maximize aesthetic experiences (*e.g.*, smell of coffee, back rub, or feeling the warmth of the sun or a breeze).

  7. Teach to anticipate experiences the client takes delight in each day (*e.g.*, walking, reading favorite book, writing letter).

J. **Explain the psychological and physiologic benefits of exercise and discuss what is realistic**

  1. Refer to *Health-Seeking Behaviors* for specific information.

K. **Provide significant others opportunities to discuss their feelings in private regarding**

  1. Changes in the person with fatigue

  2. Their care-taking responsibilities

  3. Financial issues

  4. Changes in life-style, role responsibilities, relationships

  5. Refer to *Caregiver Role Strain* for additional strategies for caregivers.

L. **Initiate health teaching and referrals, as indicated**

  1. Counseling

  2. Community services (Meals-On-Wheels, housekeeper)

  3. Financial assistance

Rationale

- In many chronic diseases, fatigue is the most common, disruptive, and distressing symptom experienced because it interferes with self-care activities (Hart, Freel, & Milde, 1990). Exploring with the client the effects of fatigue helps both the nurse and client plan interventions.

- Identifying times of peak energy and exhaustion can aid in planning activities to maximize energy conservation and productivity.

- Focusing the client on strengths and abilities may provide him with insight into positive events and lessen the tendency to overgeneralize the severity of disease, which can lead to depression (Beck, 1984).

- The client requires rest periods before or after some activities. Planning can provide for adequate rest and reduce unnecessary energy expenditure. Such strategies can enable continuation of activities, contributing to positive self-esteem.

- There are many stressors related to chronic illness (*e.g.*, pain, threats to independence, self-concept, future plans, and fulfillment of roles). Clients who learn self-help responses face definable, manageable adversities by maintaining control of everyday problems (Braden, 1990).

- Reciprocity or returning support to one's support system is vital for balanced and healthy relationships (Tilden & Weinert, 1987). Individuals who are fatigued have difficulty with reciprocity.

- Winningham (1992) found the following in cancer clients:
  - Too much as well as too little rest contributes to feelings of fatigue.
  - Too little as well as too much activity contributes to feelings of fatigue.
  - A balance between activity and rest promotes restoration; an imbalance promotes fatigue and deterioration.
  - Any symptom that contributes to decreased activity leads to increased fatigue and decreased functional status.
- Preparatory information is used to clarify the person's expectations about chemotherapy or radiation therapy. Such information regarding fatigue, with suggestions about planning for rest periods, has had positive effects on clients' abilities to maintain usual activities (Nail & Winningham, 1993).

Interventions—*Maternal Focus*

1. Explain the reason for fatigue in first and third trimesters.
   a. Increased basal metabolic rate
   b. Changes in hormonal levels
   c. Anemia
   d. Increased cardiac output (third trimester)
2. Emphasize the need for naps and 8 hours of sleep.
3. Discuss the importance of exercise (*e.g.*, walking).
4. Advise to avoid overexertion.
5. For postpartum women, discuss factors that increase fatigue (Gardner & Campbell, 1991).
   a. Labor more than 30 hours, difficult labor or reports of high labor pain
   b. Hemoglobin >10 g/dL or postpartum hemorrhage
   c. Preexisting chronic disease
   d. Episiotomy, tear, or cesarean section
   e. Sleeping difficulties
   f. Ill neonate or a congenital anomaly
   g. Nonsupportive partner
   h. Dependent children at home
   i. Child care problems
   j. Unrealistic expectations

Rationale

- Explaining the reasons for fatigue can allay fears.

Interventions—*Older Adult Focus*

1. Consider if chronic fatigue is the consequence of late life depression.
2. Refer individual suspected of depression for evaluation.

Rationale

- Late-life depression causes chronic fatigue and diminished energy (Miller, 1995).

References/Bibliography

Aistars, J. (1987). Fatigue in the cancer patient: A conceptual approach to a clinical problem. *Oncology Nursing Forum, 14*(6d), 25–30.

Beck, A. T. (1984). Cognitive approaches to stress. In R. F. Woolfolk & P. M. Lehrer (Eds.). *Principles and practice of stress management.* New York: Guilford Press.

Braden, C. J. (1990). A test of the self-help model: Learned response to chronic illness experience. *Nursing Research, 39*(1), 42–47.

Crosby, L. (1991). Factors which contribute to fatigue associated with rheumatoid arthritis. *Journal of Advanced Nursing, 16,* 974–981.

Gardner, D. L. (1992). Fatigue in postpartum women. *Applied Nursing Research, 4*(5), 57–62.

Gardner, D. L., & Campbell, B. (1991). Assessing postpartum fatigue. *Maternal–Child Nursing Journal, 16,* 264–266.

Greenberg, D., Sawicka, J., Eisenthal, S., & Ross, D. (1992). Fatigue syndrome due to localized radiation. *Journal of Pain and Symptom Management, 7*(1), 38–45.

Hargreaves, M. (1977). The fatigue syndrome. *Practitioner, 218,* 841–843.

Hart, L., Freel, M., & Milde, F. (1990). Fatigue. *Nursing Clinics of North America, 25,* 967–976.

Jiricka, M. K. (1994). Alterations in activity tolerance. In C. M. Porth (Ed.). *Pathophysiology: Concepts of altered health states.* Philadelphia: J. B. Lippincott.

Kellum, M. D. (1985). Fatigue. In M. M. Jacobs & W. Geels (Eds.). *Signs and symptoms in nursing.* Philadelphia: J. B. Lippincott.

Lemon, B. W., Bengston, V. L., & Peterson, J. A. (1972). An exploration of activity theory of aging. *Journal of Gerontology, 27,* 511–523.

Longino, C. F., & Kart, C. S. (1982). Explicating activity theory: A formal replication. *Journal of Gerontology, 37,* 713–722.

Matteson, M. A., & McConnell, E. S. (1988). *Gerontological nursing: Concepts and practices.* Philadelphia: W. B. Saunders.

Miller, C. A. (1995). *Nursing care of older adults* (2nd ed.). Glenview, IL: Scott, Foresman.

Mitchell, C. A. (1986). Generalized chronic fatigue in the elderly: Assessment and intervention. *Journal of Gerontological Nursing, 12*(4), 19–23.

Morris, M. (1982). Tiredness and fatigue. In C. Norris (Ed.). *Concept clarification in nursing.* Rockville, MD: Aspen Systems.

Nail, L., & Winningham, M. (1993). Fatigue. In S. Groenwald, M. Frogge, M. Goodman, & C. Yarbo (Eds.). *Cancer nursing: Principles and practice.* Boston: Jones and Bartlett.

Oski, F. (Ed.). (1994). *Principles and practice of pediatrics* (2nd ed.). Philadelphia: J. B. Lippincott.

Rhoten, D. (1982). Fatigue and the postsurgical patient. In C. Norris (Ed.). *Concept clarification in nursing.* Rockville, MD: Aspen Systems.

Tilden, V. P., & Weinert, C. (1987). Social support and the chronically ill individual. *Nursing Clinics of North America, 22,* 613–620.

Winningham, M. L. (1992). How exercise mitigates fatigue: Implications for people receiving cancer therapy. In R. M. Johnson (Ed.). *The biotherapy of cancer: V.* Pittsburgh: Oncology Nursing Press.

Fear

DEFINITION

Fear: A state in which an individual or group experiences a feeling of physiologic or emotional disruption related to an identifiable source that is perceived as dangerous.

DEFINING CHARACTERISTICS
Major (Must Be Present)

Feeling of dread, fright, apprehension and/or
Behaviors of
Avoidance
Narrowing of focus on danger
Deficits in attention, performance, and control

Minor (May Be Present)

Verbal reports of panic, obsessions
Behavioral acts of

Crying	Dysfunctional immobility
Aggression	Compulsive mannerisms
Escape	Increased questioning/verbalization
Hypervigilance	

Visceral–somatic activity

Musculoskeletal
Trembling
Muscle tightness
Fatigue/weakness of the limbs

Genitourinary
Urinary frequency/urgency

Cardiovascular
Palpitations
Rapid pulse
Increased blood pressure

Skin
Flush/pallor
Sweating
Paresthesia

Respiratory
Shortness of breath
Increased rate

CNS/Perceptual
Syncope
Insomnia
Lack of concentration
Irritability
Absentmindedness
Nightmares
Pupil dilation

Gastrointestinal
Anorexia
Nausea/vomiting
Diarrhea/urge to defecate
Dry mouth/throat

RELATED FACTORS

Fear can occur as a response to a variety of health problems, situations, or conflicts. Some common sources are indicated in the following.

Pathophysiologic

Related to perceived immediate and long-term effects of:

Loss of body part
Loss of body function
Disabling illness
Cognitive impairment

Long-term disability
Terminal disease
Sensory impairment

Treatment-Related

Related to loss of control and unpredictable outcome secondary to:

Hospitalization
Surgery and its outcome
Anesthesia

Invasive procedures
Radiation

Situational (Personal, Environmental)

Related to loss of control and unpredictable outcome secondary to:

Pain
New environment
New people
Lack of knowledge

Change or loss of significant other
Divorce
Success
Failure

Related to potential loss of income

Maturational

(Preschool, school-age)
Related to separation from parents, peers

Not being liked
Being alone
Strangers

Animals
Bodily harm
Age-related fears (dark, strangers, ghosts, monsters)

(Adolescent)
Related to uncertainty of:
    Appearance   Scholastic success
    Peer support
(Adult)
Related to uncertainty of:
    Marriage   Job security
    Pregnancy   Effects of aging
    Parenthood
(Older adult)
Related to anticipated dependence
    Prolonged suffering   Financial insecurity
    Vulnerability to crime   Abandonment

Author's Note

See *Anxiety*

Key Concepts

1. Psychological defense mechanisms are distinctly individual and can be adaptive or maladaptive.
2. Fear differs from anxiety in that fear is a feeling aroused by an identified threat (specific object); anxiety is a feeling aroused by a threat that cannot be easily identified (nonspecific or unknown).
3. Both fear and anxiety lead to disequilibrium.
4. Anger may be an adaptive response to certain fears.
5. A sense of adequacy in confronting danger reduces fear. Fear disguises itself. The expressed fear may be a substitute for other fears that are not socially acceptable. Awareness of factors that cause intensification of fears enhances controls and prevents heightened feelings. Fear is reduced when the safe reality of a situation is confronted.
6. Fear can become anxiety (*i.e.*, fear becomes internalized and serves to disorganize instead of becoming adaptive).
7. Chronic physical reactions to stressors lead to susceptibility and chronic disease.
8. Physiologic responses are manifested throughout the body primarily from the hypothalamus's stimulation of the autonomic and endocrine systems.
9. Individuals interpret the degree of danger from a threatening stimulus. The physiologic and psychological systems react with equal intensity to the perceived threat ($\uparrow$ blood pressure, $\uparrow$ heart rate, $\uparrow$ respiratory rate).
10. Fear is adaptive and is a healthy response to danger.
11. Fear is different from phobia. Phobia is defined as an irrational, persistent fear of a circumscribed stimulus (object or situation) other than fear of having a panic attack (panic disorder) or of humiliation or embarrassment in certain social situations (social phobia) (American Psychiatric Association, 1991).

🌀 Key Concepts—*Child*

1. Infants and small children experience fear but are unable verbally to identify the threat. Verbal (crying, protesting, *e.g.*, "NO") and nonverbal responses (kicking, biting, holding back) are important indicators of children's fear (Broome, Bates, Lillis, & McGahee, 1990; Hunsberger, 1989).
2. Fear behaviors are *consistent* and *immediate* on exposure or mention of a specific stressor; if the response is erratic, the diagnosis might more accurately be anxiety (Hunsberger, 1989). Refer to Table II-11 in the diagnosis *Altered Growth and Development* or to Key Concepts—Child for the diagnosis *Anxiety*.
3. Fears throughout childhood follow a developmental sequence and are influenced by culture, environment, and parental fears (Wong, 1995).

4. Main fears of different age groups include (Anderson, 1989; Hunsberger, 1989; Wong, 1995):
   a. *Infants and toddlers (birth to 2 years):* Fears evolve from physical stimuli (*e.g.*, loud noises, separation from parents/caregivers, strangers, sudden movements, animals, certain situations [doctor's office]).
   b. *Preschoolers (3–5 years):* Fears evolve from real or imagined situations (*e.g.*, injury or mutilation, ghosts, devils, monsters, the dark, bathtub and toilet drains, being alone, dreams, robbers).
   c. *School-age (6–12 years):* Fears are numerous and include large machines, bodily injury, loss of self-control, not being liked, separation from parents and peers, failure, unattractive physical appearance, supernatural beings, dark, storms.
   d. *Adolescents:* Fears can be verbalized and include loss of self-control, disturbance to body image, death, separation from peers, inept social performance, sexuality gossip.
5. "Fear is a momentary reaction to danger based on a low estimate of one's own power" (Wong, 1995, p. 147).

Key Concepts—*Older Adult*

1. Cesarone (1991) clustered the sources of fear in the elderly into five categories:
   a. Fear of disease, suffering
   b. Fear of dependence, abandonment
   c. Fear of dying
   d. Fear of illness or death of loved ones
   e. Miscellaneous reasons (crime, financial insecurity, diagnostic tests)

Focus Assessment Criteria

Subjective/Objective Data

A. Assess for defining characteristics
   1. Onset
      Have the person tell you his "story" about his fearfulness.
   2. Manner of communication
      Verbal reports of distress?
      Fear-related behavioral acts?
      Visceral or somatic activity?
   3. Thought process and content
      How does person organize his thoughts?
      Are thoughts clear, coherent, logical, confused, or forgetful?
      Can he concentrate or is he preoccupied?
      Do misperceptions interfere with reality testing?
   4. Emotional state
      Is emotional feeling tone appropriate or inappropriate to the situation?
      Do facial expressions, voice tone, and body posture correspond to the intensity of the person's verbal expression of fear?
   5. Perception and judgment
      Is fear still present after stressor is eliminated?
      Do only major events lead to fearfulness, or do minor events trigger fears?
      Can the person comprehend the present and focus on his actions or is he overwhelmed by future anticipations?
      Is the fear a response to a present stimulus or is it distorted by influences in the past?
   6. Assess for the presence of visceral–somatic activity

Musculoskeletal	Genitourinary
Trembling	Urinary frequency/urgency
Muscle tightness	
Fatigue/weakness of the limbs	

Cardiovascular
Palpitations
Rapid pulse
Increased blood pressure

Respiratory
Shortness of breath
Increased rate

Gastrointestinal
Anorexia
Nausea/vomiting
Diarrhea/urge to defecate
Dry mouth/throat

Skin
Flush/pallor
Sweating
Paresthesia

CNS/Perceptual
Syncope
Insomnia
Lack of concentration
Irritability
Absentmindedness
Nightmares
Pupil dilation

Outcome Criteria

The adult will
• Relate increase in psychological and physiologic comfort
• Differentiate real from imagined situations
• Describe effective and ineffective coping patterns
• Identify his own coping responses

The child will
• Discuss his fears
• Exhibit or relate an increase in psychological comfort

Interventions

The nursing interventions for the diagnosis *Fear* represent interventions for any individual with fear regardless of the etiologic or contributing factors.

A. Assess possible contributing factors
1. Perception of threatening stimulus (realistic)
a. Unfamiliar environment (new home, hospital admission, new people)
b. Intrusion on personal space
c. Life-style change (promotion, marriage/divorce, retirement)
d. Biologic and physiologic change (dysfunction, disability, pain)
e. Self-esteem threat (abandonment, rejection)
2. Distorted perceptions of dangerous stimulus

B. Reduce or eliminate contributing factors
1. Unfamiliar environment
a. Orient to environment using simple explanations.
b. Speak slowly and calmly.
c. Avoid surprises and painful stimuli.
d. Use soft lights and music.
e. Remove threatening stimulus.
f. Plan one-day-at-a-time, familiar routine.
g. Encourage gradual mastery of a situation.

      h. Provide transitional object with symbolic safeness (security blanket, religious medals).
   2. Intrusion on personal space
      a. Allow personal space.
      b. Move person away from stimulus.
      c. Remain with person until fear subsides (listen, use silence).
      d. Later, establish frequent and consistent contacts; use family members and significant others to stay with person.
      e. Use touch as tolerated (sometimes holding person firmly helps him maintain control).
   3. Threat to self-esteem
      a. Support preferred coping style when adaptive mechanisms are used.
      b. Initially, decrease the person's number of choices.
      c. Use simple, direct statements (avoid detail).
      d. Give direct suggestion to manage everyday events (some prefer details; others, general explanations).
      e. Encourage expression of feelings (helplessness, anger).
      f. Give feedback about expressed feelings (support realistic assessments).
      g. Refocus interaction on areas of capability rather than dysfunction.
      h. Encourage normal coping mechanisms.
      i. Encourage sharing common problems with others.
      j. Give feedback of effect person's behavior has on others.
      k. Encourage person to face the fear.
   4. Distorted perceptions
      a. Encourage responses that reflect reality.
      b. Ask straightforward questions (*e.g.,* "Do you feel pain?" "Does my asking you about your feelings make you uncomfortable?").
      c. Provide information to reduce distortions (*e.g.,* "No, I will not harm you." "That was only a shadow and not a monster.").
      d. Encourage specifics and discourage generalizations; have person give details, not vague general assumptions (*e.g.,* "Who are you referring to when you say 'they' are trying to kill you?").
      e. Explore superficial interactions.
         Examine the person's reason for avoiding feelings.
         Allow individual to know that it is okay to feel.
         Share your reaction to the event (*e.g.,* "I can see why you're upset; if that happened to me I would have felt like screaming.").
      f. Provide an emotionally nonthreatening atmosphere.
         Provide situations that are predictable.
         Allow for consistency in personnel to enhance comfort and familiarity.
         Announce changes in the environment.

C. When intensity of feelings has decreased, assist with insight and controlling response
   1. Bring behavioral cues into the person's awareness.
      a. Teach signs that indicate increased fear (*e.g.,* "Your face flushes and you clench your fists when we discuss your discharge.").
      b. Indicate adaptiveness of behavior.
   2. Explain how expressed fear of one thing may be hidden fear of something else.
   3. Teach how to problem-solve.
      a. What is the problem?
      b. Who or what is responsible for the problem?
      c. What are the options?
      d. What are advantages and disadvantages of each option?
   4. Teach ways for enhancing control.
      a. Include the person in the treatment process (*e.g.,* "Please raise your hand if the procedure causes pain.").

  b. Share test results when appropriate.
  c. Inform ahead of time about tests (time interval depends on ability to cope).
  d. Identify activities that rechannel emotional energy to diffuse intensity.
  e. Use night light or flashlight to diffuse fear (child with fear of dark can be given a flashlight to use when needed).
  f. Before tests or surgery, prepare patient as to what to expect, especially sensations, and define this role and how to participate in the role (*e.g.*, postoperative breathing exercises may take mind off of fears and dissipate physical reaction).

D. Initiate health teaching and referrals as indicated
  1. Recommend or instruct concerning methods that increase comfort or relaxation (see Appendix X).
    a. Progressive relaxation technique
    b. Reading, music, breathing exercises
    c. Desensitization, self-coaching
    d. Thought stopping, guided fantasy
    e. Yoga, hypnosis, assertiveness training
  2. Participate in community functions to teach parents age-related fears and constructive interventions (*e.g.*, parent–school organizations, newsletters, civic groups).

Rationale

- Safety feelings increase when a person identifies with another person who has successfully dealt with a similar fearful situation.
- Open, honest dialogue may help initiate constructive problem solving and can instill hope.
- Support people and coping mechanisms are important tools in anxiety reduction.
- Minimizing environmental stimuli can help reduce escalation of fear (Varcarolis, 1994).
- Physical activity helps redirect and dissipate tension (Varcarolis, 1994).
- Severe fear or panic can interfere with concentrating and information processing (Varcarolis, 1994).
- A quiet, calm professional can communicate calm to the person (Varcarolis, 1994).

Interventions—*Child*

1. Provide child with opportunities to express his fears and to learn healthy outlets for anger or sadness, such as play therapy (see Appendix IX).
2. Acknowledge illness, death, and pain as real and refrain from protecting children from the reality of their existence; encourage open, honest sharing.
3. Accept the child's fear and provide him with an explanation, if possible, or some form of control; share with child that these fears are okay.
  a. Fear of imaginary animals, intruders (*e.g.*, "I don't see a lion in your room, but I will leave the light on for you, and if you need me again, please call.")
  b. Fear of parent being late (establish a contingency plan, *e.g.*, "If you come home from school and Mommy is not here, go to Mrs. S. next door.")
  c. Fear of vanishing down a toilet or bathtub drain
      Wait until child is out of tub before releasing drain.
      Wait until child is off the toilet before flushing.
      Leave toys in bathtub and demonstrate how they do not go down the drain.
  d. Fear of dogs, cats
      Allow child to watch a child and a dog playing from a distance.
      Do not force child to touch the animal.
  e. Fear of death
      See Key Concepts for *Grieving*
  f. Fear of pain
      See *Pain* under Interventions—Child Focus.
  g. Refusal to go to sleep (Wong, 1995)
      Establish a realistic hour for retiring
      Contract for a reward if child is successful
      Do not sleep with child or take child to parent's room

4. Discuss with parents the normality of fears in children; explain the necessity of acceptance and the negative outcomes of punishment, shaming, or of forcing the child to overcome the fear.
5. Provide child with opportunity to observe other children cope successfully with feared object.
6. Demonstrate strength and self-confidence.
   a. Take child's hand and gently guide into shallow water.
   b. Allow child to watch you pet a dog.

Rationale

- Children's fears can be reduced by the presence of an adult who is seen as a protector (Wong, 1995).
- "Desensitization by gradually facing a fearsome object or situation is effective with most children" (Wong, 1995, p. 148).
- Providing the child with some control (*e.g.*, flashlight can help to reduce fear of the dark).

References/Bibliography

American Psychiatric Association. (1991). *Diagnostic and statistical manual of mental disorders IV*. Washington, DC: Author.

Anderson, J. J. (1989). Families with school-age children. In R. L. Foster, M. M. Hunsberger, & J. J. T. Anderson (Eds.). *Family-centered nursing care of children*. Philadelphia: W. B. Saunders.

Broome, M. E., Bates, T. A., Lillis, P. P., & McGahee, T. W. (1990). Children's medical fears, coping behaviors, and pain perceptions during a lumbar puncture. *Oncology Nursing Forum, 17*, 361–367.

Cesarone, D. (1991). Fear. In M. Maas, K. Buckwalter, & M. Hardy (Eds.). *Nursing diagnoses and interventions for the elderly*. Redwood City, CA: Addison-Wesley Nursing.

Hunsberger, M. (1989). Principles and skills adapted to the care of children. In R. L. Foster, M. M. Hunsberger, & J. J. T. Anderson (Eds.). *Family-centered nursing care of children*. Philadelphia: W. B. Saunders.

Taylor-Loughran, A. E., O'Brien, M. E., LaChapelle, R., & Rangel, S. (1989). Defining characteristics of the nursing diagnoses fear and anxiety: A validation study. *Applied Nursing Research, 2*, 178–186.

Varcarolis, E. (1994). *Foundations of psychiatric health nursing*. Philadelphia: W. B. Saunders.

Vaughn, V. C., & Litt, I. F. (1990). Fears. In *Child and adolescent development: Clinical implications*. Philadelphia: W. B. Saunders.

Wong, D. (1995). *Nursing care of infants and children* (5th ed.). St. Louis: C. V. Mosby.

Yocum, C. (1984). The differentiation of fear and anxiety. In M. Kim, G. McFarland, & A. McLane (Eds.). *Classification of nursing diagnoses: Proceeding of fifth national conference*. St. Louis: C. V. Mosby.

Fluid Volume Deficit

DEFINITION

Fluid Volume Deficit: The state in which an individual who is able to take fluids (not NPO) experiences or is at risk of experiencing vascular, interstitial, or intracellular dehydration.

DEFINING CHARACTERISTICS
Major (Must Be Present)

Insufficient oral fluid intake

Negative balance of intake and output

Dry skin/mucous membranes

Weight loss

Minor (May Be Present)

Increased serum sodium
Decreased urine output or excessive urine output
Concentrated urine or urinary frequency
Decreased skin turgor
Thirst/nausea/anorexia

RELATED FACTORS
Pathophysiologic

Related to excessive urinary output
    Uncontrolled diabetes
    Diabetes insipidus (inadequate antidiuretic hormone)
Related to increased capillary permeability and evaporative loss from burn wound (nonacute)
Related to losses secondary to:
    Fever or increased metabolic rate
    Abnormal drainage
        Wound
        Excessive menses
        Other
    Peritonitis
    Diarrhea

Situational (Personal, Environmental)

Related to vomiting/nausea
Related to decreased motivation to drink liquids secondary to:
    Depression   Fatigue
Related to fad diets/fasting
Related to high-solute tube feedings
Related to difficulty swallowing or feeding self secondary to:
    Oral pain   Fatigue
Related to extreme heat/sun/dryness
Related to excessive loss through:
    Indwelling catheters   Drains
Related to insufficient fluids for exercise effort or weather conditions
Related to excessive use of:
    Laxatives or enemas   Diuretics or alcohol

Maturational

Infant/child
    Related to increased vulnerability secondary to:
        Decreased fluid reserve and decreased ability to concentrate urine
    Older Adult
    Related to increased vulnerability secondary to:
        Decreased fluid reserve and decreased sensation of thirst

Author's Note

Fluid Volume Deficit frequently is used to describe people who are NPO, in hypovolemic shock, or experiencing bleeding, as well as people with insufficient oral fluid intake. The current NANDA-approved defining characteristics contribute to its clinical misuse in cases of hemoconcentration, change in serum sodium, or hypotension. Related factors are listed as active fluid volume loss and failure of regulatory mechanisms.

A validation study of *Fluid Volume Deficit* yielded additional critical indicators: thready pulse, decreased venous filling, and decreased cardiac output; according to the authors, "pinpointing which indicators are most relevant can help the practitioner collect and interpret data when researching and assessing fluid volume status" (Gershan et al., 1990). Should the nursing diagnosis *Fluid Volume Deficit* be used to represent such clinical situations as shock, renal failure, or thermal injury? Most nurses would agree that these are all problems that should be reported to the physician for collaborative management.

Errors in Diagnostic Statements

Risk for Fluid Volume Deficit related to increased capillary permeability, protein shifts, inflammatory process, and evaporation secondary to burn injuries

This diagnosis does not represent a situation for which nurses could prescribe interventions for outcome achievement (*e.g.*, "The client will have stable vital signs and adequate urine output (0.5–1.0 mL/kg)." Because both nurse- and physician-prescribed interventions are needed to accomplish this outcome, this situation is actually the collaborative problem *Potential Complication: Fluid/Electrolyte Imbalance* with the nursing goal of "The nurse will monitor to detect fluid and electrolyte imbalances."

Fluid Volume Deficit related to effects of NPO status

Managing fluid balance in an NPO client is a nursing responsibility involving both nurse- and physician-prescribed interventions. Thus, this situation is best described with the collaborative problem *Potential Complication: Fluid/Electrolyte Imbalance*. If the nurse wants to specify etiology, the diagnosis can be written: *Potential Complication: Fluid/Electrolyte Imbalance related to NPO state*. This usually is not necessary, however.

When a person can drink but is not drinking sufficient amounts, the nursing diagnosis *Fluid Volume Deficit related to decreased desire to drink fluids secondary to fatigue and pain* may apply.

Key Concepts

1. Table II-10 shows the average intake and output for an adult in a 24-hour period.
2. To maintain homeostasis, body fluid shifts between two major compartments:
   a. The intracellular compartment, the fluid inside the cells, which makes up two thirds of body fluids and is found primarily in skeletal muscles
   b. The extracellular compartment, the fluid outside the cells, which makes up one third of body fluids and is found in the intravascular space (in blood vessels), in the interstitial space (in fluid surrounding the cell), and in the transcellular space (in sweat, digestive secretions, and cerebrospinal, pericardial, synovial, intraocular, and pleural fluids)
   c. Abnormal shifts between compartments may cause fluid excess or deficit. Dehydration may occur within the vascular tree, while fluid within the interstitial space may be excessive (edema).

Table II-10 **Average Intake and Output in an Adult for a 24-Hour Period**

Intake		Output	
Oral liquids	1300 mL	Urine	1500 mL
Water in food	1000 mL	Stool	200 mL
Water produced by metabolism	300 mL	Insensible Lungs	300 mL
Total	2600 mL	Skin	600 mL
		Total	2600 mL

(Metheny N. [1992]. *Fluid and electrolyte balance: Nursing considerations.* Philadelphia: J. B. Lippincott.)

3. There are two main causes of fluid volume deficit; inadequate intake or increased losses (*e.g.*, gastrointestinal, urinary, skin, third-space [edema]) (Porth, 1994).
4. Vomiting or gastric suctioning results in fluid and potassium and hydrogen loss.
5. Fluid intake is primarily regulated by the sensation of thirst. Fluid output is primarily regulated by the kidneys' ability to concentrate urine.
6. The specific gravity of urine reflects the kidneys' ability to concentrate urine; the range of urine specific gravity varies with the state of hydration and the solids to be excreted. (Specific gravity is elevated when dehydration is present, signifying concentrated urine.) Values are

> Normal: 1.010–1.025   Diluted: <1.010
> Concentrated: >1.025

7. People at high risk for fluid imbalance include:
   a. People on medication for fluid retention, high blood pressure, seizures, or "anxiety" (tranquilizers)
   b. People who suffer from diabetes, cardiac disease, excessive alcohol intake, malnourishment, obesity, or gastrointestinal distress
   c. Adults older than 60, and children younger than 6 years of age
   d. People who are confused, depressed, comatose, or lethargic (no sensation of thirst)
8. Blood is the cooling fluid of the body. Dehydration (and resulting decrease in blood volume) causes an increased body temperature, pulse, and respirations.
9. Excessive fluid loss can be expected during

> Fever or increased metabolic rate   Excessive vomiting or diarrhea
> Extreme exercise or diaphoresis   Burns, tissue insult, fistulas
> Climate extremes (heat/dryness)

🍩 *Key Concepts—Child*

1. In determining the 24-hour intake requirement for an infant or child, both caloric and fluid intake should be measured. The following calculations can be used:

   Calorie Intake
   For a child up to 10 kg of body weight: 100 cal/kg
   For a child between 11 and 20 kg: 1000 cal plus 50 cal/kg for each kg above 20

   Fluid Intake for Maintenance
   Approximately 120 mL/100 cal of metabolism
   Abnormal fluid loss must be replaced in addition to the above.
2. Infants are vulnerable to fluid loss due to the following factors:
   a. More water can be lost rapidly because their bodies have a higher proportionate water content. A greater proportion of fluid is in the extracellular space, from which it is lost more easily.
   b. Infants have a greater metabolic turnover of water.
   c. Homeostatic regulation (*i.e.*, renal function) is immature.
   d. Infants have a greater surface area relative to body mass (Rimar, 1989; Wong, 1995).

🏛 *Key Concepts—Older Adult*

1. A general decrease in thirst with aging puts an elderly person at risk for not drinking sufficient fluids to maintain adequate hydration.
2. The older adult is more susceptible to fluid loss and dehydration because of (Miller, 1995):
   a. Decreased renal blood flow
   b. Decreased glomerular filtration
   c. Impaired ability to regulate temperature
   d. Decreased ability to concentrate urine
   e. Increase in physical disabilities decreases access to fluids
   f. Self-limiting of fluids for fear of incontinence
3. About 75% of the fluid intake in elderly people typically occurs between 6 A.M. and 6 P.M. (Miller, 1995).
4. Cognitive impairments can interfere with recognition of cues of thirst.

Focus Assessment Criteria

Subjective Data

A. Assess for defining characteristics
  1. Fluid intake (amounts, type)
  2. Skin (dry, turgor)
  3. Thirst
  4. Weight loss (amount, duration)
  5. Urine output (decreased, increased)

B. Assess for related factors
  1. History of contributing and causative factors
      Diabetes mellitus (diagnosed, family history)/diabetes insipidus
      Cardiac disease
      Renal disease
      Gastrointestinal disorders or surgery
      Alcohol use
      Medications
          Laxatives/enemas   Side effects that are gastrointestinal irritants (anti-
          Diuretics   biotics, chemotherapy)
      Allergies (food, milk)
      Extreme heat/humidity
      Extreme exercise effort accompanied by sweating
      Depression
      Pain
  2. Current antihypertensive or diuretic therapy
      Type, dosage
      Frequency (last dose taken when?)

Objective Data

A. Assess for defining characteristics
  1. Present weight/usual weight
  2. Intake (last 24–48 hours)
  3. Output (last 24–48 hours)
  4. Signs of dehydration
      a. Skin
          Mucosa (lips, gums) (dry)   Moisture (dry or diaphoretic)
          Tongue (furrowed/dry)   Fontanelles of infants (depressed)
          Turgor (decreased)   Eyeballs (sunken)
          Color (pale or flushed)
      b. Urine output
          Amount (varied; very large or minimal amount)
          Color (amber; very dark or very light)
          Specific gravity (increased or decreased)
      c. Blood
          Increased sodium level   Decreased hematocytes

B. Assess for related factors
  1. Abnormal or excessive fluid loss
      Liquid stools
      Vomiting or gastric suction (*e.g.*, fistulas, drains)
      Diuresis or polyuria
      Diaphoresis
      Abnormal or excessive drainage
      Loss of skin surfaces (*e.g.*, healing burns)
      Fever

2. Decreased fluid intake related to
>   Fatigue
>   Decreased level of consciousness
>   Depression/disorientation
>   Nausea or anorexia
>   Physical limitations (*e.g.*, unable to hold glass)

Outcome Criteria

The person will
- Increase intake of fluids to a specified amount according to age and metabolic needs
- Relate the need for increased fluid intake during stress or heat
- Maintain a urine specific gravity within a normal range
- Demonstrate no signs and symptoms of dehydration

Interventions

A. Assess causative factors
1. Inability to feed self
2. Dislike of available liquids
3. Sore throat/mouth
4. Extreme fatigue or weakness
5. Lack of knowledge (of the need for increased fluid intake)
6. Difficulty swallowing (see *Impaired Swallowing*)

B. Reduce or eliminate causative factors
1. Inability to feed self (see *Self-Care Deficit*)
2. Dislike of available liquids
   a. Assess likes and dislikes; provide favorite fluids within dietary restrictions.
   b. Plan an intake goal for each shift (*e.g.*, 1000 mL during day; 800 mL during evening; 300 mL at night).
   c. Make a set schedule for supplementary liquids.
3. Sore throat/mouth
   a. Offer warm or cold fluids; consider frozen ices.
   b. Consider warm saline gargle or anesthetic lozenges before fluids.
4. Extreme fatigue or weakness
   a. Give smaller amounts more frequently.
   b. Provide for periods of rest before meals.
5. Lack of knowledge
   a. Assess the person's understanding of the reasons for maintaining adequate hydration and methods for reaching goal of fluid intake.
   b. Include significant others.
   c. Proceed with teaching.
   d. See Key Concepts under *Health-Seeking Behaviors*.

C. Have person maintain a written record (log) of fluid intake and urinary output and daily weight (if necessary)

D. Prevent dehydration in high-risk individuals (see Key Concepts for Children and Older Adults)
1. Monitor intake; ensure at least 2000 mL of oral fluids every 24 hours.
2. Monitor output; ensure at least 1000–1500 mL every 24 hours.
3. Offer fluids in large glasses, 120 or 240 mL.

4. Weigh daily in same clothes, at same time. A 2%–4% weight loss indicates mild dehydration; 5%–9% weight loss indicates moderate dehydration.
5. Monitor urine and serum electrolytes, blood urea nitrogen, and osmolality, creatinine, hematocrit, and hemoglobin.
6. For people scheduled for fasting before diagnostic studies, increase their fluid intake 8 hours before fasting.
7. Review client's medications. Do they contribute to dehydration (*e.g.*, diuretics)? Do they require increased fluid intake (*e.g.*, lithium)?
8. Teach that coffee, tea, and grapefruit juice are diuretics and can contribute to fluid loss.
9. Consider the additional fluid losses associated with vomiting, diarrhea, fever.

E. Initiate health teaching, as indicated
1. Give verbal and written directions for desired fluids and amounts.
2. Include the person/family in keeping a written record of fluid intake, output, daily weights.
3. Provide a list of alternative fluids (*e.g.*, ice cream, pudding).
4. Explain the need to increase fluids during exercise, fever, infection, and hot weather.
5. Teach how to observe for dehydration (especially in infants) and to intervene by increasing fluid intake (see Objective and Subjective Data for signs of dehydration).
6. Seek medical consultation for continued dehydration.

Rationale

- Output may exceed intake, which already may be inadequate to compensate for insensible losses. Dehydration may increase the glomerular filtration rate, making output inadequate to clear wastes properly and leading to elevated blood urea nitrogen and electrolyte levels.
- Accurate daily weights can detect fluid loss.
- To monitor weight effectively, weights should be done at the same time on the same scale wearing the same clothes. A 2%–4% weight loss indicates mild dehydration; a 5%–9% weight loss indicates moderate dehydration.
- Large amounts of sugar, alcohol, and caffeine act as diuretics that increase urine production and may cause dehydration.
- People receiving tube feedings are at high risk for dehydration, because the high solute concentration of the tube feeding may cause diarrhea and diuresis. *Tube feedings must be supplemented with specific amounts of water to maintain adequate hydration.*
- Adequate protein intake is necessary to maintain normal osmotic pressures. Foods that have a high protein content are meats, fish, fowl, soybeans, eggs, legumes, and cheese.

Interventions—*Child Focus*

1. To increase fluid intake
   a. Offer:
      Appealing forms of fluids (popsicles, frozen juice bars, snow cones, water, milk, Jell-O with vegetable coloring added; let child help make it)
      Unusual containers (colorful cups, straws)
      A game or activity
   b. Read a book to child and have him drink a sip when a page is turned, or have a tea party.
   c. Have child take a drink when it is his turn in a game.
   d. Make a set schedule for supplementary liquids to promote the habit of in-between-meal fluids (*e.g.*, juice or Kool-Aid at 10 A.M. and 2 P.M. each day).
   e. Decorate straws.
   f. Let child fill small cups with a syringe.
   g. Make a progress poster, use stickers or stars to indicate fluid goals met.
2. For fever in children younger than 5 years of age:

a. Work to attain a temperature less than 101°F (38.4°C) with medication* (acetaminophen or ibuprofen) only.
b. Use tepid water (85°–90°F/29.4°–37.7°C) for sponging or bathing the child.
c. Caution parents not to cover the child with blankets and to be aware of the increased risk of febrile seizures.
d. Give the child small amounts of *clear liquids only* (15 mL) frequently.
e. Teach the parents how to protect the child should a seizure occur, and *instruct them to seek immediate medical consultation.*

3. For fluid replacement, refer to Interventions—Child Focus under *Diarrhea.*

Rationale

- Older children usually respond to the challenge of meeting a specific goal for intake (Wong, 1995).
- Rewards and contracts are also effective (*e.g.*, sticker for drinking a certain amount).
- Young children usually respond to games that integrate drinking fluids.

■ Fluid Volume Deficit
Related to Abnormal Fluid Loss

Abnormal fluid loss describes fluid loss by vomiting, diarrhea, excessive diaphoresis, or drains, not by hemorrhage or acute burns.

Outcome Criteria

The person will
- Maintain adequate intake of fluid and electrolytes, as evidenced by (specify)
- Identify abnormal fluid loss, relate methods of decreasing this loss (if possible) and replace fluids as needed
- Maintain a urine specific gravity within normal range

Interventions

A. Assess causative factors
1. Vomiting
2. Fever
3. Gastric suction
4. Diarrhea/loose stools
5. Impaired swallowing (see *Impaired Swallowing*)

B. Remove or reduce causative factors
1. Vomiting
   a. Encourage small, frequent amounts of ice chips or clear liquids such as weak tea or apple juice (adults 30 mL, children 15 mL; see *Diarrhea* for replacement therapy.

* May require a primary care professional's order. Do not give aspirin or products containing aspirin to children younger than 18 years of age with flu symptoms because of risk of potentially fatal Reye's syndrome.

  2. Fever (see also *Hyperthermia*)
     a. Maintain temperature lower than 101°F (38.4°C) with medication (*e.g.,* ibuprofen or acetaminophen).*
        Eliminate excessive clothing and bed covers.
        Keep the room temperature cool.
        Encourage cool, clear liquids when medication is at peak effectiveness and temperature is lowest.
        Substitute frozen ices or popsicles if necessary (be resourceful).
        If the temperature is extremely high, above 103°F (39.5°C), use tepid water for sponging.*
  3. Gastric suction (nasogastric or other)
     a. Use only normal saline for irrigation of gastric tubes to minimize electrolyte imbalance.
     b. Do not allow swallowing of water or ice chips; a "few small sips" can readily add up over a period of time.
     c. For the thirsty individual with gastric suction, *unless contraindicated by surgery or renal failure,* consult with the physician concerning ingestion of measured sips of Gatorade (1 oz/hour).
     d. Always subtract all fluid ingested (by either tube or mouth) from any total gastric drainage to attain net drainage.
     e. Keep a careful, clear record of intake and output: amount, character, color.
     f. Offer frequent mouth care.
  4. Diarrhea/loose stools (see *Diarrhea*)
  5. Wound drainage
     a. Keep careful records of the amount and type of drainage.
     b. Weigh dressings, if necessary, to estimate fluid loss (weigh the wet dressing; weigh a dry dressing of the same type; compare the difference).
     c. Weigh the person daily if the drainage is excessive and difficult to measure (*e.g.,* soaked sheets).
     d. Replace fluid loss (may be contraindicated in cardiac failure, renal failure, or head trauma).

C. Initiate health teaching, as indicated
  1. Assess the person's understanding of the type of fluid loss he is experiencing (what electrolytes are lost) and the fluids that provide replacement (see Key Concepts).
  2. Give verbal and written instructions for fluid replacement (*e.g.,* "Drink at least 3 quarts of liquid a day, including 1 quart of Gatorade.").
  3. Teach the person to
     a. Avoid sudden exposure and overexposure to heat, sun, and exercise.
     b. Gradually increase exposure and activity in hot weather.
     c. Eat three balanced meals a day.
     d. Increase fluid intake during hot days.
     e. Decrease activity during extreme weather.

Rationale

- The focus of treatment is replacing both water and electrolytes lost (Porth, 1994).
- Fluids high in sugar (*e.g.,* soda, Jell-O) can cause osmotic diarrhea (Porth, 1994).
- Refer to Rationale in *Diarrhea*.
- For child, refer to Rationale under Interventions—Child Focus in *Diarrhea*.

* May require a primary care professional's order. Do not give aspirin or products containing aspirin to children younger than 18 years of age with flu symptoms because of risk of potentially fatal Reye's syndrome.
* May require a primary care professional's order.

References/Bibliography

See *Fluid Volume Excess*

Fluid Volume Excess

DEFINITION

Fluid Volume Excess: The state in which an individual experiences or is at risk of experiencing intracellular or interstitial fluid overload.

DEFINING CHARACTERISTICS
Major (Must Be Present)

Edema (peripheral, sacral)
Taut, shiny skin

Minor (May Be Present)

Intake greater than output
Shortness of breath
Weight gain

RELATED FACTORS
Pathophysiologic

Related to compromised regulatory mechanisms secondary to:
Renal failure, acute or chronic
Related to increased preload, decreased contractility, and decreased cardiac output secondary to:
Myocardial infarction
Congestive heart failure
Left ventricular failure
Valvular disease
Tachycardia/arrhythmias
Related to portal hypertension, lower plasma colloidal osmotic pressure, and sodium retention secondary to:
Liver disease
Cirrhosis
Ascites
Cancer
Related to impaired venous return secondary to:

Varicose veins	Chronic phlebitis
Peripheral vascular disease	Immobility
Thrombus	

Treatment-Related

Related to sodium and water retention secondary to:
Corticosteroid therapy

Situational (Personal, Environmental)

Related to excessive sodium intake/fluid intake
Related to low protein intake
  Fad diets
  Malnutrition
Related to dependent venous pooling/venostasis secondary to:
  Immobility
  Tight cast or bandage
  Standing or sitting for long periods of time
Related to venous compression by pregnant uterus
Related to inadequate lymphatic drainage secondary to:
  Mastectomy

Maturational

Older Adult
  Related to impaired venous return secondary to increased peripheral resistance and
    decreased efficiency of valves

Author's Note

Fluid Volume Excess frequently is used to describe pulmonary edema, ascites, and renal failure.

Pulmonary edema, ascites, and renal failure are all collaborative problems that should not be renamed as *Fluid Volume Excess*. This diagnosis represents a situation for which nurses can prescribe if the focus is on peripheral edema. Nursing interventions would center on teaching the client or family how to minimize edema and on protecting tissue.

Errors in Diagnostic Statements

Risk for Fluid Volume Excess related to left-sided mastectomy

For this diagnosis, the nurse would institute strategies to reduce edema and teach the client how to manage the edema. Thus, the diagnosis should be written as: *Risk for Fluid Volume Excess related to lack of knowledge of techniques to reduce edema secondary to compromised lymphatic function.*

If edema were present, the nurse might use *Risk for Impaired Physical Mobility related to effects of lymphedema on motion.*

Fluid Volume Excess related to portal hypertension and decreased colloid osmotic pressure secondary to cirrhosis

This diagnosis requires frequent monitoring, electrolyte replacement, diuretic therapy, dietary restrictions, and plasma expander therapy. These interventions call for three collaborative problems to describe this situation:

  Potential Complication: Ascites
  Potential Complication: Negative nitrogen balance
  Potential Complication: Hypokalemia

Because edema predisposes skin to injury and breakdown, the nurse also could use the diagnosis: *Risk for Impaired Skin Integrity related to vulnerability of skin secondary to edema.*

Key Concepts

1. See *Fluid Volume Deficit.*
2. Fluid volume excess can result from inadequate sodium and water excretion, excessive sodium intake, venous or lymphatic insufficiency, trauma, or cardiac failure (Porth, 1994).
3. People with cardiac pump failure are at high risk for both vascular and tissue fluid excess (*i.e.*, pulmonary and peripheral edema). Pulmonary edema should be considered a medical emergency.
4. The most frequent vascular cause of tissue edema is increased venous pressure, which causes increased capillary blood pressure.

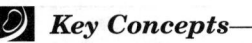 ***Key Concepts**—Maternal*

1. Increased estrogen levels during pregnancy cause water retention of 6–8 L to supply tissue needs for water and electrolytes (May & Mahlmeister, 1994).

***Key Concepts**—Older Adult*

1. The older adult is prone to stasis edema of the feet and ankles as a result of (Miller, 1995):
   a. Increased vein tortuosity
   b. Increased vein dilatation
   c. Decreased valve efficiency

Focus Assessment Criteria

Subjective Data

A. Assess for defining characteristics
   1. History of symptoms
      Complaints of
         Shortness of breath   Weakness/fatigue
         Weight gain   Edema
      Onset/duration
      Location
      Description

B. Assess for related factors
   1. History of contributing and causative factors
      Family or personal history of diabetes   Steroid therapy
      Pregnancy   Malnutrition
      Premenses   Excessive salt intake
      Cardiac or renal disease   Excessive use of tap-water enemas
      Liver disease   Lymphatic obstruction (*e.g.*, after
      Alcoholism   lymph node dissection)
      Hyperthyroidism or hypothyroidism   Excessive parenteral fluid
      Hypertension   replacement
   2. Dietary intake
      Estimated protein intake (adequate/inadequate)
      Estimated caloric intake (adequate/inadequate/excess)
      Estimated fluid intake (adequate/inadequate/excess)
      Daily alcohol consumption
         Type
         Amount
      24- to 72-hour intake and output

Objective Data

A. Assess for defining characteristics
   1. Signs of fluid overload
      Pulse (bounding or dysrhythmic)
      Respirations
         Rate (tachypnea)   Lung sounds (rales or rhonchi)
         Quality (labored or shallow)
      Blood pressure (elevated)
   2. Edema
      Press thumb for at least 5 seconds into the skin and note any remaining indentations.
      Note degree and location (feet, ankles, legs, arms, sacral, generalized).
   3. Weight gain (weigh daily on the same scale, at the same time)
   4. Neck vein distention (distended neck veins at 45° elevation of the head may indicate fluid overload or decreased cardiac output)

> **Outcome Criteria**
>
> The person will
> - Relate causative factors and methods of preventing edema
> - Exhibit decreased peripheral and sacral edema

Interventions

A. Identify contributing and causative factors
1. Improper diet (excessive sodium intake, inadequate protein intake)
2. Dependent venous pooling/venostasis
3. Venous pressure point (*e.g.*, tight cast or bandage)
4. Inadequate lymphatic drainage
5. Immobility/neurologic deficit
6. Lack of knowledge of or compliance with medical regimen

B. Reduce or eliminate causative and contributing factors
1. Improper diet
   a. Assess dietary intake and habits that may contribute to fluid retention.
      Be specific; record daily and weekly intake of food and fluids.
      Assess weekly diet for adequate protein or excessive sodium intake.
         Discuss likes and dislikes of foods that provide protein.
         Teach to plan weekly menu that provides protein at a price that is affordable.
   b. Encourage to decrease salt intake.
      Teach to
         Read labels for sodium content.
         Avoid convenience foods, canned foods, and frozen foods.
         Cook without salt and use spices to add flavor (lemon, basil, tarragon, mint).
         Use vinegar in place of salt to flavor soups, stews, etc. (*e.g.*, 2–3 teaspoons of vinegar to 4–6 quarts, according to taste).
      Ascertain with physician whether salt substitute may be used (caution individual that he must use exactly the substitute prescribed).
2. Dependent venous pooling
   a. Assess for evidence of dependent venous pooling or venostasis.
   b. Encourage alternating periods of horizontal rest (legs elevated) with vertical activity (standing); this may be contraindicated in congestive heart failure.
   c. Keep edematous extremity elevated above the level of the heart whenever possible (unless contraindicated by heart failure).
      Keep edematous arms elevated on two pillows or with IV pole sling.
      Elevate legs whenever possible, using pillows under legs (avoid pressure points, especially behind knees).
      Discourage leg and ankle crossing.
   d. Reduce constriction of vessels.
      Assess wearing apparel for proper fit and constrictive areas.
      Instruct person to avoid panty girdles/garters, knee-highs, and leg crossing and to practice keeping legs elevated when possible.
   e. Consider using antiembolism stockings or Ace bandages; measure legs carefully for stockings/support hose.*
      Measure from back of heel to back of knee, or top of thigh, depending on desired stocking length.
      Measure circumference of calf and thigh.

* May require a primary care professional's order.

Consider both measurements in choosing a stocking, matching measurements with size requirement chart that accompanies the stockings.

Apply stockings while lying down (*e.g.*, in the morning before arising).

Check extremities frequently for adequate circulation and evidence of constrictive areas.

3. Venous pressure points
   a. Assess for venous pressure points associated with casts, bandages, tight stockings.

   Observe circulation at edges of casts, bandages, stockings.

   For casts, insert soft material to cushion pressure points at edges.

   Check circulation frequently.
   b. Shift body weight in cast to redistribute weight within the cast (unless contraindicated).

   Encourage person to do this himself every 15–30 minutes during waking hours to prevent venostasis.

   Encourage wiggling of fingers or toes and isometric exercise of unaffected muscles within the cast.*

   If the person is unable to do this himself, assist him at least hourly to shift body weight.

   See *Impaired Physical Mobility*.

4. Inadequate lymphatic drainage
   a. Keep extremity elevated on pillows.

   If edema is marked, the arm should be elevated, *but not in adduction* (this position may constrict the axilla).

   The elbow should be higher than the shoulder.

   The hand should be higher than the elbow.
   b. Take blood pressures in unaffected arm.
   c. Do not give injections or start intravenous fluids in affected arm.
   d. Protect the affected limb from injury.

   Teach the person to avoid strong detergents, carrying heavy bags, holding a cigarette, injuring cuticles or hangnails, reaching into a hot oven, wearing jewelry or a wristwatch, or using Ace bandages.

   Advise the person to apply lanolin or similar cream several times a day to prevent dry, flaky skin.

   Encourage the person to wear a "Medic Alert" tag engraved with *Caution: lymphedema arm—no tests—no needle injections*.

   Caution the person to see a physician if the arm becomes red, swollen, or unusually hard.
   e. After a mastectomy, encourage range-of-motion exercises and use of affected arm to facilitate development of a collateral lymphatic drainage system (explain to the person that lymphedema is often decreased within a month, but that she should continue massaging, exercising, and elevating the arm for 3 or 4 months after surgery).

5. Immobility/neurologic deficit
   a. Plan passive or active range-of-motion exercises for all extremities every 4 hours, including dorsiflexion of the foot to massage veins.
   b. Change the individual's position at least every 2 hours, using the four positions (left side, right side, back, abdomen), if not contraindicated (see *Impaired Skin Integrity*).
   c. If the person must be maintained in high Fowler's position, assess for edema of the buttocks and sacral area and help the person to shift body weight every 2 hours to prevent pressure on edematous tissue.

6. Lack of knowledge
   a. Assess the person's knowledge of

   Medical diagnosis (*e.g.*, congestive heart failure, renal failure)

   Diet

---

* May require a primary care professional's order.

Medications (*e.g.*, diuretics, cardiotonics)
Activity
Use of Ace bandages, antiembolus stockings
   b. Proceed with health teaching, as indicated.

C. Protect edematous skin from injury
1. Inspect skin for redness and blanching.
2. Reduce pressure on skin areas; pad chairs and footstools.
3. Prevent dry skin.
   a. Use soap sparingly.
   b. Rinse off soap completely.
   c. Use a lotion to moisten skin.
4. See *Impaired Skin Integrity* for additional information on preventing injury

D. Initiate health teaching and referrals, as indicated
1. Give clear instructions verbally and in writing for all medications: what, when, how often, why, side effects; pay special attention to drugs directly influencing fluid balance (*e.g.*, diuretics, steroids).
2. Write down instructions for diet, activity, use of Ace bandages, stockings, and so forth.
3. Have the person demonstrate the instructions.
4. Have the person keep a written record of intake/output.
5. With severe fluctuations in edema, have the person weigh himself every morning and before bedtime daily; instruct the person to keep a written record of weights.
6. For less severe illness, the person may need to weigh himself daily only and record.
7. Caution to call physician for excessive edema/weight gain (>2 lb/day) or increased shortness of breath at night or on exertion.
8. Explain that no. 7 may be indicative of early heart problems and may require medication to prevent them from getting worse.
9. Consider home care or visiting nurses referral to follow at home.
10. Provide literature concerning low-salt diets; consult with dietitian if necessary.

Rationale

- Edema inhibits blood flow to the tissue, resulting in poor cellular nutrition and increased susceptibility to injury.
- A high intake of sodium causes increased retention of water. Foods with high sodium content include salted snacks, bacon, cheddar cheese, pickles, soy sauce, processed luncheon meats, MSG (monosodium glutamate), canned vegetables, catsup, and mustard. Some over-the-counter drugs, such as antacids, also are high in sodium.
- Corticosteroids contain both glucocorticoid and mineralocorticoid elements. The mineralocorticoid element promotes sodium reabsorption and potassium excretion from distal renal tubules. Resultant sodium retention expands extracellular fluid volume by preventing water excretion (Truhan & Ahmeh, 1989).
- Edema develops as increased extracellular fluid enters interstitial spaces and the blood, increasing interstitial fluid and blood volume.
- Lymph flow is propelled by contracting skeletal muscles. Exercise increases muscle efficiency (Sieggreen, 1989).
- Besides the increased risk of skin injury due to edema, the loss of perivascular collagen in the small vessels of the skin makes them more susceptible to damage.

Interventions—*Maternal Focus*

1. Explain the cause of edema of ankles and fingers.
2. Explain not to limit salt intake severely unless advised.
3. Instruct to lie on left side for short periods several times a day (*e.g.*, in bath).

Rationale

- Limiting salt can decrease circulating volume to a point so low that kidney function is decreased (May & Mahlmeister, 1994).

- Lying on the left side removes weight of gravid uterus from vessels, increases venous return to heart, and improves renal function (May & Mahlmeister, 1994).
- Research has suggested that edema during pregnancy may be better reduced by rest periods in water (*i.e.*, taking a bath) than by bed rest (Staff, 1990).

References/Bibliography

Books

Bulechek, G., & McCloskey, J. (1989). *Nursing interventions* (2nd ed.). Philadelphia: W. B. Saunders.

May, K., & Mahlmeister, L. (1994). *Maternal and neonatal nursing: Family-centered care* (3rd ed.). Philadelphia: J. B. Lippincott.

Metheny, N. (1992). *Fluid and electrolyte balance: Nursing considerations.* Philadelphia: J. B. Lippincott.

Miller, C. A. (1995). *Nursing care of older adults* (2nd ed.). Glenview, IL: Scott, Foresman.

Porth, C. (1994) *Pathophysiology: Concepts of altered health status* (4th ed.). Philadelphia: J. B. Lippincott.

Rimar, J. M. (1989). Principles of fluid and electrolyte maintenance. In R. L. Foster, M. M. Hunsberger, & J. J. T. Anderson (Eds.). *Family-centered nursing care of children.* Philadelphia: W. B. Saunders.

Sergent, E., Strauss, C., Jaffe, M., Majewsky, E., & Mitchell, C. (1991). Diagnostic content validity of fluid volume excess: A construct replication. In R. Carroll-Johnson (Ed.). *Classification of nursing diagnoses: Proceedings of the ninth conference.* Philadelphia: J. B. Lippincott.

Sieggreen M. (1989). Nursing management of adults with venous and lymphatic disorders. In P. Beare & J. Myers (Eds.). *Principles and practice of adult health nursing.* St. Louis: C. V. Mosby.

Smeltzer, S., & Beare, P. (Eds). (1996). *Brunner and Sudarth's textbook of medical–surgical nursing* (8th ed.). Philadelphia: Lippincott–Raven Publishers.

Webber, J. (1993). *Nurses' handbook of health assessment* (2nd ed.). Philadelphia: J. B. Lippincott.

Wong, D. L. (1995). *Nursing care of infants and children* (5th ed.). St. Louis: C. V. Mosby.

Articles

Ellison, D. (1994). Diuretic prescriptions and the treatment of edema: From clinic to bench and back again. *American Journal of Kidney Disease, 23,* 623–643.

Gershan, J. (1990). Fluid volume deficit: Validating indicators. *Heart and Lung, 19,* 152–156.

Porth, C. (1992). Physiology of thirst and drinking: Implications for nursing practice. *Heart and Lung, 21,* 273–284.

Staff. (1990). Clinical news: Watering down edema. *American Journal of Nursing, 90*(7), 18.

Truhan, A. P., & Ahmeh, A. R. (1989). Corticosteroids: A review with emphasis on complications of prolonged systemic therapy. *Annals of Allergy, 62,* 375–391.

Grieving

Grieving, Anticipatory

Grieving, Dysfunctional

Grieving*

DEFINITION

Grieving: A state in which an individual or family experiences a natural human response involving psychosocial and physiologic reactions to an actual or perceived loss (person, object, function, status, relationship).

DEFINING CHARACTERISTICS
Major (Must Be Present)

The person

Reports an actual or perceived loss (person, object, function, status, relationship)

Minor (May Be Present)

Denial

Guilt

Anger

Despair

Inability to concentrate

Visual, auditory, and tactile hallucinations about the object or person

Feelings of worthlessness

Suicidal thoughts

Crying

Sorrow

Longing/searching behaviors

Delusions

Phobias

Anergia

RELATED FACTORS

Many situations can contribute to feelings of loss. Some common situations are:

Pathophysiologic

Related to loss of function or independence secondary to:

Neurologic

Cardiovascular

Sensory

Musculoskeletal

Digestive

Respiratory

Renal

Trauma

Treatment-Related

Related to losses associated with:

Long-term dialysis

Surgery (mastectomy, colostomy, hysterectomy)

* This diagnosis is not currently on the NANDA list but has been included for clarity or usefulness.

Situational (Personal, Environmental)

Related to the negative effects and losses secondary to:
Chronic pain
Terminal illness
Death
Related to losses in life-style associated with
Childbirth   Child leaving home (*e.g.*, college or marriage)
Marriage   Divorce
Separation
Related to loss of normalcy secondary to:
Handicap
Scars
Illness

Maturational

Related to changes attributed to aging:
Friends   Function
Occupation   Home
Related to loss of hope, dreams

Author's Note

Grieving, Anticipatory Grieving, and *Dysfunctional Grieving* represent three types of responses of individuals or families experiencing a loss. *Grieving* describes normal grieving after a loss and participation in grief work. *Anticipatory Grieving* describes someone engaged in grief work before an expected loss. *Dysfunctional Grieving* represents a maladaptive process occurring when grief work is suppressed or absent or when a person exhibits prolonged exaggerated responses. For all three diagnoses, the goal of nursing is to promote grief work. In addition, for *Dysfunctional Grieving*, the nurse directs interventions to reduce excessive, prolonged, problematic responses.

In many clinical situations, the nurse expects a grief response (*e.g.*, loss of body part, death of significant other). Other situations that evoke strong grief responses are sometimes ignored or minimized (*e.g.*, abortion, newborn death, death of one twin or triplet, death of illicit lover, suicide, loss of children to foster homes, adoption) (Lazare, 1979).

Errors in Diagnostic Statements

Dysfunctional Grieving related to excessive emotional reactions (crying, anger) to recent death of son

People respond to losses in highly individualized ways. Regardless of its severity, no response to acute loss should be labeled as "dysfunctional." *Dysfunctional Grieving* is characterized by a sustained or prolonged detrimental response; validation of this diagnosis cannot be done until several months to a year after the loss. This diagnosis should be reworded as *Grieving related to recent death of son, as evidenced by emotional responses of anger and profound sadness.*

Anticipatory Grieving related to perceived effects of spinal cord injury on life goals

Using *Anticipatory Grieving* in this situation places the focus on anticipated losses rather than current, actual losses. Because this individual is grieving over both actual and anticipated losses, the diagnosis should be rewritten as *Grieving related to actual or anticipated losses associated with recent spinal cord injury.*

Key Concepts

1. American culture is devoted to youth and life. Even though death surrounds each person, it is viewed as pertaining to someone else, not oneself. Society today has been called "death defying," failing to recognize and confront the realities of death and grief (Rando, 1984).

2. Caregivers need to recognize that their own attitudes and beliefs about death, dying, and grief have a significant impact on their care of individuals experiencing loss (Hare, 1989; Rando, 1984).
3. Loss can occur without death; when a person experiences any loss (object, relationship), grief and mourning ensue.
4. Grief is the emotional response to loss; grief work, the adaptive process of mourning. Grief work involves:
   a. Accepting the reality of the loss
   b. Experiencing the pain of grief
   c. Adjusting to an environment from which the lost person or object is missing
   d. Reinvesting in another relationship (Worden, 1982)
5. An individual's grief is affected by many factors, such as personality, previous losses, intimacy of relationship, and personal resources.
6. Staging (of grieving process) can create problems if the nurse applies the stages universally to all people, disregarding individual differences. Staging also may encourage the nurse to focus on the symptoms as opposed to the strength of the person/family.
7. The following stages (Engle, 1964) are specific enough to assist the nurse to intervene and broad enough to prevent labeling.

I. Shock and disbelief
   Initial denial   Decreased activity
   Numbed feelings   Sporadic periods of despair
II. Developing awareness of loss
   Sadness   Guilt
   Anger   Crying
III. Restitution (usually requires at least a year)
   The work of mourning   Preoccupation with thoughts of loss
   Painful void in life
IV. In the months to follow
   Beginning to put the lost relationship in perspective (its positive and negative qualities)

---

8. "The notion that grief is a neat, orderly, linear process completed at some arbitrary point in time" has been refuted (Haylor, 1987).
9. Terminal illness with its concurrent treatments and its progression produces a multitude of losses:
   a. Loss of function (all systems/roles)
   b. Loss of financial independence
   c. Change in appearance
   d. Loss of friends
   e. Loss of self-esteem
   f. Loss of self
10. Divorce presents many losses for the partners, children, grandparents, and so forth. The losses are roles, relationships, homes, possessions, finances, control, routines, and patterns.

🌰 *Key Concepts—Child*

1. The child responds to death depending on his developmental age and the response of significant others:
   a. Age under 3 years: Cannot comprehend death, fears separation
   b. Age 3–5 years: Views illness as a punishment for real or imagined wrongdoing
      Has little concept of death as final because of immature concept of time
      May view death as a kind of sleep

May feel he caused the event to happen (magical thinking) (*e.g.*, by bad thoughts about person)

c. Age 6–10 years: Begins to fear death

Attempts to put meaning to the event (*e.g.*, devil, ghost, God)

Associates death with mutilation and punishment

Can feel responsibility for the event

d. Age 10–12 years: Usually has an adult concept of death (inevitable, irreversible, universal)

Attitudes greatly influenced by reactions of parent and others

Very interested in postdeath services and rituals

e. Adolescence: Has a mature understanding of death

May suffer from guilt and shame

Least likely to accept death, particularly if it is their own (Wong, 1995)

2. Children may learn early that discussions about death are taboo (Homedes & Ahmed, 1987).

3. Children may use symbolic or nonverbal language to communicate their awareness of death and dying (McCowan, 1989).

Key Concepts—Maternal

1. The death of a fetus or infant presents multiple stresses for the family.

2. The birth of a child with congenital anomalies creates emotional difficulties for the parents, their relationship with the child, and family functioning (Reeder, Martin, & Koniak, 1992).

Key Concepts—Older Adult

1. Grief in elderly people often can be related to losses within self, such as role changes, body image changes, or decreased body function. These losses sometimes are less easily accepted than the loss of a significant other (Matteson & McConnell, 1988).

2. In many cultures, the death of a mate is documented as the most stressful life event. Increasing longevity brings increased potential for 50-plus years of marriage to the same spouse, with a concomitantly greater impact of the loss of that spouse. The spouse possibly could be the older person's only close family member and social contact (Gallagher, Breckenridge, Thompson, & Peterson, 1983).

3. One study of people older than 50 years of age looked at the following factors over a period of 2 years after the loss of spouse: emotional shock, helplessness/avoidance, psychological strength/coping, anger/guilt/confusion, and grief resolution behaviors. Statistically significant changes were seen in all areas except psychological strength/coping. There also was no significant change in life satisfaction scores in this study (Caserta, Lund, & Dimond, 1985).

4. There seems to be some support for extending traditional bereavement periods to an expected point of at least 24 months for older individuals who have lost a spouse. Of greater impact than the loss of significant other is the loss of a crucial relationship that provides meaning to the person's life. Even in young widows, the estimate of adjustment period has been extended, based on research showing movement at the 24-month mark from high distress to low distress (as measured on the Goldberg General Health Questionnaire) (Caserta, Lund, & Dimond, 1985; Ebersole & Hess, 1990; Oberfield, 1984; Vachon, Lyall, Rogers, Freedman-Letofsky, & Freeman, 1980).

5. Bereavement is a risk factor for suicide. About 25% of all suicides are committed by older adults. Suicide attempts are less frequent in the elderly; however, the rate of attempted suicide to successful suicide increases to 4:1 after age 60 years, compared with 20:1 in the 40-year-old and younger group. Men aged 65 years and older have the highest incidence of suicide: men aged 65–74 years have 30.4 suicides per 100,000: men aged 75–84 years have 42.3 suicides per 100,000; and men aged 85+ years have 50.6 suicides per 100,000 (Abrams & Berkow, 1990; Hogstel, 1990).

6. The death of a pet can be a significant loss for an isolated older person and result in a grieving process (Hungelman, Kenkel-Rossi, Klassen, & Stollenwerk, 1985).

7. Reminiscence therapy or life review can help integrate losses. Frequently, the older person uses reminiscence to move through Erikson's eighth developmental stage of Ego Integrity versus Despair (Matteson & McConnell, 1988).

8. Social supports, strong religious beliefs, good prior mental health, and a greater number of resources are related to less psychosocial or physical dysfunction (Matteson & McConnell, 1988).

TRANSCULTURAL CONSIDERATIONS

1. Mourning is a behavioral response to death or loss and is culturally determined (Andrews & Hansen, 1989).
2. "Even if bereavement is regarded as a universal stressor, the magnitude of the stress and its meaning to the individual varies significantly cross-culturally" (Andrews & Hansen, 1989, p. 376). In the dominant American culture, it is assumed that the death of a child is more stressful than that of an older relative.
3. Puerto Ricans believe that a person's spirit is not free to enter the next life if that person has left something unsaid before death. Heightened grieving may occur if closure has not been properly completed, such as through sudden death (Andrews & Hansen, 1989).
4. Hispanics sometimes express grief with seizure-like behavior, hyperkinetic episodes, aggression, or stupor. This syndrome is called *elliptic* (Andrews & Hansen, 1989).
5. The degree of mourning in the Chinese culture depends on the mourner's closeness to and the importance of the deceased person (Andrews & Hansen, 1989).

Focus Assessment Criteria

Subjective Data

A. Assess for defining characteristics
   1. Present interactions between or among family members
      Adults
      Children
         Maturational level
         Understanding of crisis
         Degree of participation
      Knowledge of expected grief reactions
      Relationship to ill or deceased person
   2. Expressions of
      Ambivalence   Anger
      Denial   Depression
      Fear   Guilt
      Concerns
   3. Report of
      Gastrointestinal disturbances
         Indigestion   Weight gain or loss
         Nausea or vomiting   Constipation or diarrhea
         Anorexia
      Insomnia
      Preoccupation with sleep
      Fatigue (decreased or increased activity level)
      Inability to carry out self-care, social, and work responsibilities

B. Assess for related factors
   1. Family
      Previous coping patterns for crisis
      Quality of the relationship of the ill or deceased person with each family member
      Position or role responsibilities of the ill or deceased person
      Sociocultural expectations for bereavement
      Religious expectations for bereavement

2. Individual family members

Previous experiences with loss or death (as child, adolescent, or adult)

Did family talk out their grief?

Did they practice any particular religious rituals associated with bereavement?

Objective Data

A. Assess for defining characteristics

1. Normative

Shock

Disbelief, denial	Withdrawal
Anger	Preoccupation with lost object
Crying	Hopelessness
Sorrow	

2. Pathologic pattern (profound; increases in intensity; continuous over 12 months)

Anger	Stoic
Depression	Denial
Isolation	Regression
Despair	Obsession
Worthlessness	Hallucinations
Guilt	Delusions
Suicidal thoughts	Phobias

Outcome Criteria

The individual will
- Express his grief
- Describe the meaning of the death or loss to him
- Share his grief with significant others (children, spouses)

Interventions

A. Assess for causative and contributing factors that may delay the grief work

Unavailable or lack of support system

Dependency

Multiple losses

Uncertainty of loss (*e.g.*, MIA, missing children)

Failure to grieve prior losses

Inability to grieve (cultural, social, age related)

History of previous emotional illness

Personality structure

Early object loss

Nature of the relationship with the lost person or object

B. Reduce or eliminate causative or contributing factors, if possible

1. Promote a trust relationship.
   a. Promote feelings of self-worth through one-on-one or group sessions.
   b. Allow for established time to meet and discuss feelings.
   c. Communicate clearly, simply, and to the point.
   d. Never try to lessen the loss (*e.g.*, "She didn't suffer long"; "You can have another baby").
   e. Assess what the person and the family are learning by the use of feedback.

    f. Offer support and reassurance.

    g. Create a therapeutic milieu.

    h. Establish a safe, secure, and private environment.

    i. Demonstrate respect for the person's culture, religion, race, and values.

    j. Provide privacy but be careful not to isolate the person or family inadvertently.

    k. Provide a presence of simply "being" with the bereaved.

2. Support the person's and the family's grief reactions.

    a. Explain grief reactions:

        Shock and disbelief

        Developing awareness

        Restitution

    b. Describe varied acceptable expressions:

        Elated or manic behavior as a defense against depression

        Elation and hyperactivity as a reaction of love and protection from depression

        Various states of depression

        Various somatic manifestations (weight loss or gain, indigestion, dizziness)

    c. Assess for past experiences with loss:

        Loss of significant other in childhood

        Losses in later life

3. Promote family cohesiveness.

    a. Support the family at its level of functioning.

    b. Encourage self-exploration of feelings with family members.

    c. Explain the need to discuss behaviors that interfere with relationships.

    d. Recognize and reinforce the strengths of each family member.

    e. Encourage the family to evaluate their feelings and support one another.

4. Promote grief work with each response.

    a. Denial

        Recognize that this is a useful and necessary response.

        Explain the use of denial by one family member to the other members.

        Do not push client to move past denial without emotional readiness.

    b. Isolation

        Convey a feeling of acceptance by allowing grief.

        Create open, honest communications to promote sharing.

        Reinforce the person's self-worth by allowing privacy.

        Encourage client/family gradually to increase social activities (*e.g.*, support groups, church groups).

        Prepare client/family that they may experience avoidance from some friends and family who may not be comfortable with their situation of loss or their grief responses.

        Encourage client/family to let significant others know what their needs are (*e.g.* need for support, privacy, or permission to share their experience).

    c. Depression

        Reinforce the person's self-esteem.

        Identify the level of depression and develop the approach accordingly.

        Use empathetic sharing; acknowledge grief ("It must be very difficult").

        Identify any indications of suicidal behavior (frequent statements of intent, revealed plan).

        See *Risk for Self-Harm* for additional information.

    d. Anger

        Understand that this feeling usually replaces denial.

        Explain to family that anger serves to try to control one's environment more closely because of inability to control loss.

        Stress that the illness or death did not result from being bad or because the well child wished it.

6. Identify people who are at high risk for dysfunctional grieving reactions.

    a. Absence of any emotion

    b. Previous conflict with deceased person

    c. History of ineffective coping patterns

7. Teach individual/family signs of pathologic grieving, especially people who are at risk:

    a. Prolonged hallucinations

    b. Continued searching for the deceased (frequent moves/relocations)

    c. Delusions

    d. Isolation

    e. Egocentricity

    f. Overt hostility (usually toward a family member)

8. Promote physical well-being: nutrition, rest, exercise.

9. For survivors of suicide (Johnson, 1993)

    a. Encourage survivors to access their primary care professional for care.

    b. Elicit their interpretation of the event. Clarify distortions.

    c. Discuss plans for funeral, notification of friends and relatives.

    d. Discuss the hazards of secrecy.

    e. Allow for ventilation of guilt, rage and blaming (*e.g.*, of professionals).

    f. Follow up with telephone contacts to family.

    g. Refer all survivors to counseling, especially high-risk survivors (surviving children, those with inadequate support, those who respond with blaming, scapegoating, or secrecy).

C. Provide health teaching and referrals, as indicated

1. Teach the person and the family signs of resolution.

    a. Griever no longer lives in the past but is future oriented and establishing new goals.

    b. Griever redefines relationship with the lost object/person.

    c. Griever begins to resocialize.

2. Identify agencies that may be helpful.

    a. Community agencies

    b. Religious groups

Rationale

- Grief work cannot begin until the loss is acknowledged. Nurses can encourage this acknowledgment by open, honest dialogue, by providing the family with an opportunity to view the dead person, and by recognizing and validating the experience of grief for the individual.
- Life review is a process whereby a dying person reminisces about the past, especially unresolved conflicts, in an attempt to resolve them. Life review also provides the person with an opportunity to evaluate his successes and failures.
- Anger is often perceived as negative. Anger, however, can energize behavior, facilitate expression of negative feelings, and function to help the client defend against a threat (Taylor, Baird, Malone, & McCorkle, 1993).
- Sudden death or suicide is a catastrophic event. Interventions would focus on helping survivors with valid perceptions of the event, and, in the case of suicide, the shame and embarrassment (Johnson, 1993).
- Interventions must begin immediately after a completed suicide, since those left behind experience guilt, rejection, and disillusionment. The death of a child can put an extreme strain on a marital relationship (Pallikkathayil & Flood, 1991).
- Mourners who were very busy with the practical and necessary caregiving tasks of the dying person do not address the impending loss and therefore are at risk for delayed grieving response (Stuart & Sundeen, 1995).
- The purpose of mourning and mourning rituals is to achieve acknowledgment of the loss, providing for a return of energy for reinvestment in daily life and for coping with the changes required (Kahn, 1995).
- Acceptance of crying can be conveyed by silent presence and use of touch (Kahn, 1995).
- Acknowledging that grief responses are expected and normal can support anxious grievers (Kahn, 1995).

- Helping the person identify perceptions of dying and death can provide opportunities to examine their accuracy (Kahn, 1995).
- Secrecy related to suicide impedes grief work because open discussion is thwarted (Wilson & Kneisel, 1992).

✿ Interventions—*Child Focus*

1. Explain what caused the death.
   a. Clarify child's perceptions.
   b. Openly clarify that the child did not cause the death.
2. Openly discuss possible responses.
   a. "Sometimes when someone dies we feel bad if we said or did something bad to them."
   b. "Sometimes we feel glad we didn't die and then feel bad because _____ did."
   c. "When someone dies, we can become afraid that we may die also."
   d. "I remember when _____ said or did _____. What do you remember?"
3. Explain rituals.
4. Allow to grieve at own pace.
5. Consider a sibling support group if indicated.

Rationale

- Children can be encouraged to communicate symbolically through writing or telling stories or by drawing pictures (see Appendix IX for play therapy guidelines) (McCowan, 1989).
- Children need to feel the joys and sorrows of life to begin to incorporate both in their lives appropriately (Kübler-Ross, 1983).
- Children can feel rejected or unloved if parents or significant other are unable to offer emotional support and nurturing because of their own grief (Bourne & Meier, 1988; McCowan, 1989).
- Children of parents who commit suicide have a higher risk for future psychopathology and depression (Wilson & Kneissel, 1992).
- Siblings of deceased children may have feelings of guilt, anger, jealousy, and fear (Wong, 1995).

◑ Interventions—*Maternal Focus*

1. Assist parents of a deceased infant (newborn, stillbirth, miscarriage) with grief work (Mina, 1985; Reeder, Martin, & Koniak, 1992):
2. Promote grieving.
   a. Use baby's name when discussing loss.
   b. Allow parents to share the hopes and dreams they had for the child.
   c. Provide parents with access to hospital chaplain or own religious leader.
   d. Encourage parents to see and hold their infant to validate the reality of the loss.
   e. Design a method to communicate to auxiliary departments that the parents are in mourning (*e.g.*, rose sticker on door, chart).
   f. Prepare a memory packet (wrapped in clean baby blanket) (photograph [Polaroid], ID bracelet, footprints with birth certificate, lock of hair, crib card, fetal monitor strip, infant's blanket).
   g. Encourage parents to take memory packet home. If they prefer not to, keep the packet on file in case parents change their minds later.
   h. Encourage parents to share the experience with siblings at home (refer to pertinent literature for consumers).
   i. Provide for follow-up support and referral services after discharge (*e.g.*, social service, support group).
3. Assist others to comfort grieving parents.
   a. Stress the importance of openly acknowledging the death.
   b. If the baby or fetus was named, use the name in discussions.
   c. Never try to lessen the loss with discussions of future pregnancies or other healthy siblings.
   d. Send sympathy cards.

e. Be sensitive of the gravity of loss for both the mother and father.

f. Create a remembrance for the infant (*e.g.*, plant a tree).

Rationale

- Researchers have found 100% of parents who held their deceased babies reported positive experiences. Parents who did not hold their infants reported problems with resolution of grief process (Ransohoff-Adler & Berger, 1989).
- In a study, 80% of the parents who did not hold their deceased infants reported it was the decision of a health care professional (Ransohoff-Adler & Berger, 1989).

Grieving, Anticipatory

DEFINITION

Anticipatory Grieving: The state in which an individual/group experiences reactions in response to an expected significant loss.

DEFINING CHARACTERISTICS

Major (Must Be Present)

Expressed distress at potential loss

Minor (May Be Present)

Denial

Guilt

Anger

Sorrow

Change in eating habits

Change in sleep patterns

Change in social patterns

Change in communication patterns

Decreased libido

RELATED FACTORS

See *Grieving*

Key Concepts

See *Grieving*

Focus Assessment Criteria

See *Grieving*

Outcome Criteria

The person will

- Express his grief
- Participate in decision making for the future
- Share his concerns with significant others

Interventions

A. Assess for causative and contributing factors of anticipated or potential loss

Terminal illness

Separation (divorce, hospitalization, marriage, relocation, job)

Socioeconomic status

Body image changes

Self-esteem changes

Aging

B. Assess individual response

Denial

Rejection

Bargaining

Isolation

Helplessness/hopelessness

Shock

Anger

Depression

Guilt

Fear

1. Encourage the person to share concerns.
   a. Use communication techniques of open-ended questions and reflection ("What are your thoughts today?"; "Are you sad?").
   b. Acknowledge the value of the person and his grief by using touch and by sitting with him and verbalizing your concern ("This must be a very difficult time for you," "What is most important to you now?").
   c. Recognize that some individuals may choose not to share their concerns, but convey that you are available if they desire to do so later ("What do you hope for?").
2. Assist the person and the family to identify strengths.
   a. "What do you do well?"
   b. "What are you willing to do to improve your life?"
   c. "Is religion a source of strength for you?"
   d. "Do you have close friends?"
   e. "Who do you turn to in times of need?"
   f. "What does this person do for you?"
3. Promote the integrity of the person and the family by acknowledging strengths.
   a. "Your brother looks forward to your visit."
   b. "Your family is so concerned for you."
4. Support person and family with grief reactions.
   a. Prepare person and family for grief reactions.
   b. Explain grief reactions to person and family.
   c. Focus on the present life situation until the person or family indicates the desire to discuss future.
5. Promote family cohesiveness.
   a. Identify availability of a support system.
      Meet consistently with family members.
      Identify family member roles, strengths, weaknesses.
   b. Assess communication patterns.
      Listen and clarify the messages being sent.
      Identify the patterns of communication within the family unit by assessing positive and negative feedback, verbal and nonverbal communications, and body language.
   c. Provide for the concept of hope by
      Supplying accurate information
      Resisting the temptation to give false hope
      Discussing concerns willingly
   d. Promote group decision making to enhance group autonomy.
      Establish consistent times to meet with person and family.
      Encourage members to talk directly with each other and to listen to each other.
6. Promote grief work with each response.
   a. Denial
      Initially support and then strive to increase the development of awareness (when individual indicates readiness for awareness).

   b. Isolation

   Listen and spend designated time consistently with person and family.

   Offer the person and the family opportunity to explore their emotions.

   Reflect on past losses and acknowledge loss behavior (past and present).

   c. Depression

   Begin with simple problem solving and move toward acceptance.

   Enhance self-worth through positive reinforcement.

   Identify the level of depression and indications of suicidal behavior or ideas.

   Be consistent and establish times daily to speak with person and family.

   d. Anger

   Allow for crying to release this energy.

   Listen to and communicate concern.

   Encourage concerned support from significant others as well as professional support.

   e. Guilt

   Listen and communicate concern.   Promote more direct expression of

   Allow for crying.   feelings.

   Explore methods to resolve guilt.

   f. Fear

   Help person and family recognize the feeling.

   Explain that this will help cope with life.

   Explore person's and family's attitudes about loss, death, and the like.

   Explore person's and family's methods of coping.

   g. Rejection

   Allow for verbal expression of this feeling state to diminish the emotional strain.

   Recognize that expression of anger may cause rejection by significant others.

7. Provide for expression of grief.

   a. Encourage emotional expressions of grieving.

   b. Caution about the use of sedatives and tranquilizers, which may prevent or delay emotional expressions of loss.

   c. Encourage verbalization on the part of clients and families of all age groups.

   Support family cohesiveness.

   Promote and verbalize strengths of the family group.

   d. Encourage person and family to engage in life review.

   Focus and support the social network relationships.

   Reevaluate past life experiences and integrate them into a new meaning.

   Convey empathetic understanding.

   Explore unfinished business.

8. Identify potential pathologic grieving reactions.

Delusions	Suicidal indications
Hallucinations	Difficulty crying or controlling crying
Phobias	Loss of control of environment leading to
Obsessions	hopelessness, helplessness
Isolations	Intense reactions lasting longer than 6 months
Conversion hysteria	with few signs of relief
Agitated depression	Restrictions of pleasure
Delay in grief work	

9. Refer individual with potential for pathologic grieving responses for counseling (psychiatrist, nurse therapist, counselor, psychologist).

C. Provide health teaching and referrals, as indicated

1. Explain what to expect

Sadness	Rejection
Feelings of aloneness	Anger
Guilt	Emotions will be very labile initially and become more
Fear	stable as grief work is accomplished

2. Teach person and family signs of resolution.
   a. Griever no longer lives in past but is future oriented, establishing new goals.
   b. Griever redefines relationship with the lost object/person.
   c. Griever begins to resocialize.
3. Teach signs of pathologic responses and referrals needed.
   a. Defenses used in uncomplicated grief work that become exaggerated or maladaptive responses
   b. Persistent absence of any emotion
   c. Prolonged intense reactions of anxiety, anger, fear, guilt, helplessness
4. Identify agencies that may enhance grief work.
   a. Self-help groups
   b. Widow-to-widow groups
   c. Parents of deceased children
   d. Single parent groups
   e. Bereavement groups

Rationale

- The knowledge that no further treatment is warranted and that death is imminent may give rise to feelings of powerlessness, anger, profound sadness, and other grief responses. Open, honest discussions can help the client and family members accept and cope with the situation and their response to it (Hull, 1992).
- Research validates that "professional interventions and professionally supported voluntary and self-help services are capable of reducing risk of psychiatric and psychoanalytic disorders resulting from bereavement" (Martinez & Wagner, 1993).

Grieving, Dysfunctional

DEFINITION

Dysfunctional Grieving: The state in which an individual or group experiences prolonged unresolved grief and engages in detrimental activities.

DEFINING CHARACTERISTICS
Major (Must Be Present)

Unsuccessful adaptation to loss
Prolonged denial, depression
Delayed emotional reaction
Unable to assume normal patterns of living

Minor (May Be Present)

Social isolation or withdrawal
Failure to develop new relationships/interests
Failure to restructure life after loss

RELATED FACTORS

See *Grieving*

Key Concepts

1. Unresolved grief may be difficult to determine because there is no clearly defined end point to the grief experience, and nor is there a "right way" to grieve (Raphael, 1983). Some individuals do experience factors that interfere with the natural progress of grief work and therefore the resolution of grief. Rando (1984) outlines seven variations of unresolved grief:
   a. *Absent grief:* as if the death never occurred
   b. *Inhibited grief:* able to mourn only certain aspects of the loss
   c. *Delayed grief:* unable to experience grief at the time of loss (*i.e.*, the mourner feels grief cannot be dealt with at the time of loss: "I must be strong for my children right now.")
   d. *Conflicted grief:* often associated with a previous dependent or ambivalent relationship
   e. *Chronic grief:* ongoing experience of intense grief reaction, sometimes serves to keep the deceased "alive" through grief
   f. *Unanticipated grief:* unable to grasp the full implications of loss; extreme bewilderment, anxiety, self-reproach, and depression
   g. *Abbreviated grief:* often confused with unresolved grief, this is a shortened but normal form of grief; might occur when a significant amount of grief work has been done before the loss
2. Unresolved grief is a pathologic response or prolonged denial of the loss or a profound psychotic response. Examples of such responses are
   a. Refusal to remove possessions of the deceased after a reasonable length of time
   b. Lasting loss of normal patterns of social behavior
   c. Progressively deeper regression, depression
   d. Progressively deeper isolation
   e. Somatic manifestations (prolonged)
   f. Obsessions, phobias
   g. Delusions, hallucinations
   h. Attempted suicide
3. Factors that contribute to unresolved grief are
   a. Quality of the individual's attachment to the loved object
   b. Presence of lowered self-esteem
   c. Guilt, multiple loss, victims of violence
   d. Perception of fairness
4. Lazare (1979) describes the social factors that can contribute to unresolved grief as social negation of the loss (*e.g.*, abortion, newborn, death of twin, death of frail elderly parent) and socially defined as inappropriate to discuss (*e.g.*, death of lover, suicide).

Focus Assessment Criteria

See *Grieving*

Outcome Criteria

The individual/group will
- Acknowledge the loss
- Describe feelings expected with loss
- Verbalize an intent to seek professional assistance

Interventions

A. Assess for causative and contributing factors that may contribute to dysfunctional grieving
   1. Unavailable (or lack of) support system
   2. Was very dependent on deceased

3. History of a difficult relationship with the lost person or object
4. Multiple past losses
5. Ineffective coping strategies
6. Unexpected death
7. Expectations to "be strong"

B. Promote a trust relationship
   1. Promote feelings of self-worth through one-on-one or group sessions.
   2. Allow for established time to meet and discuss feelings.
   3. Communicate clearly, simply, and to the point.
   4. Assess what the person and the family are learning by the use of feedback.
   5. Offer support and reassurance.
   6. Create a therapeutic milieu.
   7. Establish a safe, secure, and private environment.
   8. Demonstrate respect for the person's culture, religion, race, and values.

C. Support the person and the family's grief reactions
   1. Explain grief reactions.
      a. Shock and disbelief
      b. Developing awareness
      c. Restitution
   2. Describe varied acceptable expressions.
      a. Elated or manic behavior as a defense against depression
      b. Elation and hyperactivity as a reaction of love and protection from depression
      c. Various states of depression
      d. Various somatic manifestations (weight loss or gain, indigestion, dizziness)
   3. Assess for past experiences with loss.
      a. Loss of significant other in childhood
      b. Losses in later life
   4. Promote family cohesiveness.
      a. Support the family at its level of functioning.
      b. Encourage self-exploration of feelings with family members.
      c. Slowly and carefully identify the reality of the situation (*e.g.*, "After your husband died, who helped you most?").
      d. Explain the need to discuss behaviors that interfere with relationships.
      e. Recognize and reinforce the strengths of each family member.
      f. Encourage the family to evaluate their feelings and support one another.

D. Promote grief work with each response
   1. Denial
      a. Explain the use of denial by one family member to the other members.
      b. Do not force client to move past denial without emotional readiness.
   2. Isolation
      a. Convey a feeling of acceptance by allowing grief.
      b. Create open, honest communications to promote sharing.
      c. Reinforce the person's self-worth by allowing privacy.
      d. Encourage client/family gradually to increase social activities (*e.g.*, support groups, church groups).
   3. Depression
      a. Reinforce the person's self-esteem.
      b. Identify the level of depression and develop the approach accordingly.
      c. Use empathetic sharing; acknowledge grief ("It must be very difficult").
      d. Identify any indications of suicidal behavior (frequent statements of intent, revealed plan).
      e. See *Risk for Self-Harm* for additional information.
   4. Anger
      a. Understand that this feeling usually replaces denial.

    b. Explain to family that anger serves to try to control one's environment more closely because of inability to control loss.

    c. Encourage verbalization of the anger.

    d. See *Anxiety* for additional information for anger.

  5. Guilt/ambivalence

    a. Acknowledge the person's expressed self-view.

    b. Role play to allow person to "express" to the dead person what he wants to say or how he feels.

    c. Encourage client to identify positive contributions/aspects of the relationship.

    d. Avoid arguing and participating in the person's system of shoulds and should nots.

    e. Discuss the person's preoccupation with him and attempt to move verbally beyond the present.

  6. Fear

    a. Focus on the present and maintain a safe and secure environment.

    b. Help the person to explore reasons for a meaning of the behavior.

    c. Consider alternative ways of expressing his feelings.

E. **Provide health teaching and referrals, as indicated**

  1. Teach the person and the family signs of resolution.

    a. Griever no longer lives in past but is future oriented and establishing new goals.

    b. Griever redefines relationship with the lost object/person.

    c. Griever begins to resocialize, seeks new relationships, experiences.

  2. Teach individual/family signs of pathologic grieving, especially people who are at risk, and to seek professional counseling.

    a. Prolonged depression

    b. Denial

    c. Lives in past

    d. Prolonged hallucinations

    e. Continued searching for the deceased (frequent moves/relocations)

    f. Delusions

    g. Isolation

    h. Egocentricity

    i. Over-hostility (usually toward a family member)

  3. Identify agencies that may be helpful.

    a. Community agencies' support groups, mental health agencies

    b. Religious groups

    c. Psychotherapists, grief specialists

Rationale

- Risk of death is greater in men than in women during the first 6 months of conjugal bereavement. Changes in health behavior patterns, such as nutrition, alcohol use, smoking, and decreased physical activity levels, may contribute to this increased mortality rate (Kaprio & Koskenvuo, 1987).
- The more dependent the person was on the deceased person, the more difficult the resolution (Varcarolis, 1995).
- Unresolved conflicts disrupt successful grief work (Varcarolis, 1995).
- Individuals with few supportive relationships have a more difficult grieving (Varcarolis, 1995).

References/Bibliography

Books

Abrams, S., & Berkow, R. (Eds.). (1990). *The Merck manual of geriatrics.* Rahway, NJ: Merck & Co.

Andrews, M., & Hanson, P. (1989). Religious beliefs: Implications for nursing practice. In J. Boyle & M. Andrews (Eds.). *Transcultural concepts in nursing.* Glenview, IL: Scott, Foresman.

Ebersole, P., & Hess, P. (1990). *Toward healthy aging: Human needs and nursing response* (3rd ed.). St. Louis: C. V. Mosby.

Hogstel, M. O. (1990). *Geropsychiatric nursing.* St. Louis: C. V. Mosby.

Johnson, B. S. (1993). *Psychiatric–mental health nursing* (3rd ed.). Philadelphia: J. B. Lippincott.

Kahn, A. M. (1995) Coping with fear and grieving. In J. M. Lubkin (Ed.). *Chronic illness: Impact and interventions* (3rd ed.). Boston: Jones & Bartlett.

Kübler-Ross, E. (1975). *Death: The final stage of growth.* Englewood Cliffs, NJ: Prentice-Hall.

Kübler-Ross, E. (1983). *On children and death.* New York: Macmillan.

Lazare, A. (1979). Unresolved grief. In A. Lazare (Ed.). *Outpatient psychiatry: Diagnosis and treatment.* Baltimore: Williams & Wilkins.

Martinez, J., & Wagner, S. (1993). Hospice care. In S. L. Greenwald, M. Goodman, M. H. Frogge, & C. Yarbo (Eds.). *Cancer nursing: Principles and practice* (3rd ed.). Boston: Jones & Bartlett.

Matteson, M. A., & McConnell, E. S. (1988). *Gerontological nursing: Concepts and practice.* Philadelphia: W. B. Saunders.

McCowan, D. (1989). Impact of death and dying. In R. L. Foster, M. M. Hunsberger, & J. J. T. Anderson (Eds.). *Family-centered nursing care of children.* Philadelphia: W. B. Saunders.

Rando, T. A. (1984). *Grief, dying, and death: Clinical interventions for caregivers.* Champaign, IL: Research Press.

Raphael, B. (1983). *The anatomy of bereavement.* New York: Basic Books.

Reeder, S., Martin, L., & Koniak, D. (1992). *Maternity nursing* (17th ed.). Philadelphia: J. B. Lippincott.

Stuart, G. W., & Sundeen, S. (1995). *Principles and practice of psychiatric nursing* (5th ed.). St. Louis: Mosby Yearbook

Varcarolis, E. M. (1995) Alterations in mood: Grief and depression. In E. M. Varcarolis (Ed.). *Foundations of psychiatric mental health nursing* (2nd ed.). Philadelphia: W. B. Saunders.

Wilson, H. S., & Kneisel, C. R. (1992) *Psychiatric nursing* (4th ed.) Redwood, CA: Addison-Wesley Nursing.

Wong, D. L. (1995). *Essentials of pediatric nursing* (5th ed.). St. Louis: C. V. Mosby.

Worden, J. (1982). *Grief counseling and grief therapy: A handbook for the mental health practitioner.* New York: Springer Publishing.

Journals

Antonacci, M. (1990). Sudden death: Helping bereaved parents in the PICU. *Critical Care Nurse, 10*(4), 65–70.

Bourne, V., & Meier, J. (1988). What happens now? A book to be read to children who have lost a loved one. *Oncology Nursing Forum, 15*(1), 81–85.

Caserta, M. S., Lund, D. A., & Dimond, M. F. (1985). Assessing interviewer effects in a longitudinal study of bereaved elderly adults. *Journal of Gerontology, 40,* 637–640.

Engle, G. (1964) Grief and grieving. *American Journal of Nursing, 64,* 93–97.

Gallagher, D. E., Breckenridge, J. N., Thompson, L. W., & Peterson, J. A. (1983). Effects of bereavement on indicators of mental health in elderly widows and widowers. *Journal of Gerontology, 38,* 565–571.

Grogan, L. B. (1990). Grief of an adolescent when a sibling dies. *American Journal of Maternal Child Nursing, 15*(1), 21–24.

Gyulag, J. (Ed.) (1989). The death of a child. *Issues in Comprehensive Pediatric Nursing, 12*(4), 1–137.

Hare, J. (1989). Nurses' fear of death and comfort with dying patients. *Death Studies, 13,* 349–360.

Haylor, M. (1987). Human response to loss. *Nurse Practitioner, 12*(5), 63.

Homedes, N., & Ahmed, S. M. (1987). In my opinion . . . death education for children. *Children's Health Care, 16*(10), 34–36.

Hull, M. M. (1992). Coping strategies of family caregivers in hospice home care. *Oncology Nursing Forum, 19,* 1179–1187.

Hungelman, J., Kenkel-Rossi, B., Klassen, L., & Stollenwerk, R. M. (1985). Spiritual well-being in older adults: Harmonious interconnections. *Journal of Religion and Health, 24,* 147–153.

Kaprio, J., & Koskenvuo, R. H. (1987). Mortality after bereavement: A prospective study of 95,647 widowed persons. *American Journal of Public Health, 77,* 283–287.

Miles, A. (1990). Caring for families when a child dies. *Pediatric Nursing, 16,* 346–347.

Mina, C. (1985) A program for helping grieving parents. *Maternal–Child Nursing Journal, 10,* 118–121.

Parkman, S. E. (1992). Helping families say goodbye. *American Journal of Maternal–Child Nursing, 17,* 14–17.

Oberfield, R. A. (1984). Terminal illness: Death and bereavement: Toward an understanding of its nature. *Perspectives in Biology and Medicine,* 287–301.

Oehler, J. (1981). The frog family books: Color pictures sad or glad. *Maternal–Child Nursing Journal, 6,* 281.

Page-Liegerman, J., & Hughes, C. (1990). How fathers perceive perinatal death. *Journal of Maternal–Child Nursing, 15,* 320–322.

Pallikkathayil, L., & Flood, M. (1991). Adolescent suicide. *Nursing Clinics of North America, 26*(3), 623–630.

Ransohoff-Adler, M., & Berger, C. S. (1989). When newborns die: Do we practice what we preach. *Journal of Perinatal, 9,* 311–316.

Taylor, E. J., Baird, S., Malone, D., & McCorkle, R. (1993). Factors associated with anger in cancer patients and their caregivers. *Cancer Practice, 1,* 101–109.

Vachon, M. L., Lyall, W. A., Rogers, J., Freedman-Letofsky, B., & Freeman, S. J. (1980). A controlled self-help intervention for widows. *American Journal of Psychiatry, 137,* 1380–1384.

Wheeler, S. R., & Limbo, R. K. (1990). Blueprint for a perinatal bereavement support group. *Pediatric Nursing, 16,* 341–344, 377.

Resources for the Consumer

For Children

A Cradle Song. (1988). Produced by Dennis Spalsbury. Distributed by Fanlight Productions, 47 Halifax Street, Boston, MA 02130; 617-524-0980. Videotape, 29 minutes. Purchase $295; rental $100/week, $50/day.

Buscaglia, L. D. (1982). *The fall of Freddie the leaf.* New York: Charles B. Slack.

Rofes, E. (Ed.) (1986). *The kids' book about death and dying.* New York: Little, Brown. (Researched and written by 11-to-14-year-old students who also recommend other books about death and dying; covers topics such as euthanasia, organ donation, autopsy, emotions, and how children feel about the death of a friend, pet, parent, or their own life-threatening illness. However, section on brain death needs updating.)

What happens now? (single copy): St. Luke's Hospital, 2900 West Oklahoma Avenue, Milwaukee, WI 53215.

Growth and Development, Altered

DEFINITION

Altered Growth and Development: The state in which an individual has, or is at risk for, impaired ability to perform tasks of his or her age group or impaired growth.

DEFINING CHARACTERISTICS
Major (Must Be Present)

Inability or difficulty performing skills or behaviors typical of his or her age group (*e.g.*, motor, personal/social, language/cognition) (Table II-11) and/or

Altered physical growth: weight lagging behind height by 2 standard deviations; pattern of height and weight percentiles indicate a drop in pattern

Minor (May Be Present)

Inability to perform self-care or self-control activities appropriate for age (see Table II-11)

Flat affect, listlessness, decreased responses, slow in social responses, shows limited signs of satisfaction to caregiver, shows limited eye contact, difficulty feeding, decreased appetite, lethargic, irritable, negative mood, regression in self-toileting, regression in self-feeding (see Focus Assessment Criteria)

Infants: watchfulness, interrupted sleep pattern

RELATED FACTORS
Pathophysiologic

Related to compromised physical ability and dependence secondary to:
(Circulatory impairment)
    Congenital heart defects, congestive heart failure
(Neurologic impairment)
    Cerebral damage, congenital defects, cerebral palsy, microencephaly
(Gastrointestinal impairment)
    Malabsorption syndrome, gastroesophageal reflux, cystic fibrosis
(Endocrine or renal impairment)
    Hormonal disturbance
(Musculoskeletal impairment)

Congenital anomalies of extremities	Repeated acute illness, chronic illness
Acute illness	Inadequate caloric, nutritional intake
Prolonged pain	Muscular dystrophy

Table II-11 **Age-Related Developmental Tasks**

Developmental Tasks/Needs	Parental Guidance	Implications for Nursing
Birth to 1 Year		
PERSONAL/SOCIAL	Encourage parent to respond to cry, meet infant's need *consistently*	Encourage parent to participate in care:
Learns to trust and anticipate satisfaction	Teach parent not to be afraid they will "spoil" infant with too much attention	Bathing
Sends cues to mother/caretaker	Talk and sing to child; hold and cuddle often	Feeding
Begins understanding self as separate from others (body image)	Provide variety of stimulation	Holding
MOTOR	Allow infant to feed self (cereal, etc.)	Teach parent guidance information
Responds to sound	Do not prop bottle	Provide ongoing stimulation while confined through use of toys, mirrors, mobiles, music
Social smile	TOYS	Hold, speak to infant, maintain eye contact
Reaches for objects	Brightly colored crib toys, mobiles	Investigate crying
Begins to sit, creep, pull up, and stand with support	Stuffed toys: of varied textures	Do not restrain
Attempting to walk	Music boxes	
LANGUAGE/COGNITION	SAFETY	
Learns to signal wants/needs with sounds, crying	Be aware of rapidly changing locomotive ability (*i.e.*, childproof kitchen, stairways; small objects within reach; tub safety)	
Begins to vocalize with meaning (two syllable words: Dada, Mama)		
Comprehends some verbal/nonverbal messages (no, yes, bye-bye)		
Learns about words through senses		
FEARS		
Loud noises		
Falling		
1–3½ Years		
PERSONAL/SOCIAL	Provide child with peer companionship	Allow child to take liquids from a cup (including medicines)
Establishes self-control, decision making, self-independence (autonomy)	Allow for brief periods of separation under familiar surroundings	Allow child to perform some self-care tasks:
Extremely curious, prefers to do things himself	Practice safety measures that guard against child's increased motor ability and curiosity (poisoning, falls)	Wash face and arms
Demonstrates independence through negativism	Tell the truth	Brush teeth
Very egocentric: believes he controls the world		
Learns about words through senses		

MOTOR

Begins to walk and run well

Drinks from cup, feeds self

Develops fine motor control

Climbs

Begins self-toileting

LANGUAGE/COGNITION

Has poor time sense

Increasingly verbal (4–5 word sentences by age 3½)

Talks to self/others

Misconceptions about cause/effect

FEARS

Loss/separation from parents

Darkness

Machines/equipment

Intrusive procedures

Disciplining child for violation of safety rules:
Running in street
Touching electricial wires

Allow child some control over fears:
Favorite toy
Night light

Allow exploration within safe limits

Explain as simply as possible why things happen

Allow child to explain why he thinks things are happening

Correct misconceptions

Include child in domestic activities when possible:
Dusting
Cleaning spoons

Discuss differences in opinions (between parents) in front of child

Do not threaten child with what will happen if he does not behave

Always follow through with punishment

TOYS

Manipulative toys

Puzzles

Bright-colored, simple books

Large-muscle devices (gym sets, etc.)

Music (songs, records)

Expect resistant behavior to treatments; reinforce treatments, not punishments

Use firm, direct approach and provide child with choices only when possible

Restrain child when needed

Explain to parents methods for disciplining child:
Slap hand once (for dangerous touching, *e.g.*, stove)
Sit in chair for 2 minutes (if child gets up, put him back and reset timer)

Explain the need for consistency

Allow expression of fear, pain, displeasure

Assign consistent caregiver

Let child play with simple equipment (stethoscope)

Provide materials for play (favorite toy, night light, etc.)

Be honest about procedure

Praise child for helping you:
Holding still
Holding the Band-Aid

Give child choices whenever possible

Tell child he can cry or squeeze your hand, but you expect him to hold still

Have parents present for procedures when at all possible

Explore with child his fantasies of the situation:
Use play therapy

Explain the procedure immediately beforehand if short (*i.e.*, injection) and when appropriate if longer or intrusive (*e.g.*, x-ray, IV insertion)

Follow home routines when possible

3½–5 Years

PERSONAL/SOCIAL

Attempts to establish self as like his parents, but independent

Explores environment on his own initiative

Teach parents to listen to child's fears, feelings

Encourage hugs, touch as expressions of acceptance

Provide explanations—simply

Encourage expressing of fears

Reinforce reality of body image

Encourage self-care, decision making when possible

(continued)

Table II-11 **Age-Related Developmental Tasks** (continued)

Developmental Tasks/Needs	Parental Guidance	Implications for Nursing
Boasts, brags, has feelings of indestructibility	Limit stimulation from television to avoid intense material	Involve parents in teaching
Family is primary group	Focus on positive behaviors	Provide peer stimulation
Peers increasingly important	Allow child to help as much as possible	Limit physical restraint
Assumes sex roles	Provide child with regular contact with other children (e.g., nursery school)	Provide play opportunities for acting out fantasy, story-telling
Aggressive	Explain that television, movies are make-believe	Explain to child how he can cooperate (e.g., hold still), and expect that he will
MOTOR	Practice definite limit-setting behavior	Use play therapy to allow child free expression
Locomotion skills increase, and coordinates easier	Offer child choices	Explain all procedures:
Rides tricycle/bicycle	Allow child to express anger verbally but limit motor aggression ("You may slam a door but you may not throw a toy")	Use equipment if possible; allow therapeutic play
Throws ball, but has difficulty catching	Discipline (examples):	Encourage child to ask questions
LANGUAGE/COGNITION	Sit in chair 5 minutes	Tell child the exact body parts that will be affected
Egocentric	Forbid a favorite pastime (no bicycle riding for 2 hours)	Use models, pictures
Language skills flourish	Be consistent and firm	Explain when procedure will occur in relation to daily schedule (e.g., after lunch, after bath)
Generates many questions: how, why, what?	Teach safety precautions about strangers	
Simple problem solving; uses fantasy to understand, problem-solve	TOYS AND GAMES	
FEARS	Enjoys "make-believe" play (play house, toy models, etc.)	
Mutilation	Simple games with others, books, puzzles, coloring	
Castration		
Dark		
Unknown		
Inanimate, unfamiliar objects		

5–11 Years

PERSONAL/SOCIAL

Learns to include values and skills of school, neighborhood, peers

Peer relationships important

Focuses more on reality, less on fantasy

Family is main base of security and identity

Sensitive to reactions of others

Seeks approval, recognition

Enthusiastic, noisy, imaginative, desires to explore

Likes to complete a task

Enjoys helping

MOTOR

Moves constantly

Physical play prevalent (sports, swimming, skating, etc.)

LANGUAGE/COGNITION

Organized, stable thought

Concepts more complicated

Focuses on concrete understanding

FEARS

Rejections, failures

Immobility

Mutilation

Death

Teach appropriate foods needed each day, provide choices

Encourage interaction outside home

Include cooking and cleaning in home activities

Teach safety (bicycle, street, playground equipment, fire, water, strangers)

Maintain limit-setting and discipline

Prepare child for bodily changes of pubescence and provide with concrete sex education information (late childhood)

Expect fluctuations between immature and mature behavior

Respect peer relationships but do not compromise your values (e.g., "But, Mom, all the other girls are wearing makeup!")

Promote responsibility, contribution to family (i.e., duties for helping, etc.)

Promote exploration and development of skills (i.e., joining clubs, sports, hobbies, etc.)

TOYS AND GAMES

Group games, board games, art activities, crafts, video games, reading

---

Promote family and peer interactions (e.g., visiting, telephone)

Explain all procedures and impact on body

Encourage questioning, active participation in care

Be direct about explanation of procedures (i.e., body part involved, use anatomic names, pictures, etc.); explain step by step

Be honest

Reassure child that he is liked

Provide privacy

Involve parents but make direction of care the child's decision

Reason and explain

Encourage continuance of school work, activities if condition permits (i.e., homework, contact with classmates)

Encourage continuance of hobbies, interests

(continued)

Table II-11 **Age-Related Developmental Tasks** (continued)

Developmental Tasks/Needs	Parental Guidance	Implications for Nursing
11–15 Years		
PERSONAL/SOCIAL	Encourage independent problem solving, decision making within established values	Respect privacy
Family values continue to be significant influence	Be available	Accept expression of feelings
Peer group values have increasing significance	Compliment child's achievements	Direct discussions of care and condition to child
Early adolescence: outgoing and enthusiastic	Listen to interests, likes, dislikes without passing judgment	Ask for opinions, allow input into decisions
Emotions are extreme, mood swings, introspection	Respect privacy	Be flexible with routines, explain all procedures/treatments
Sexual identity fully mature	Allow independence while maintaining safety limits	Encourage continuance of peer relationships
Wants privacy/independence	Provide concrete information about sexuality, function, bodily changes	Listen actively
Develops interests not shared with family	Teach about:	Identify impact of illness on body image, future functioning
Concern with physical self	Auto safety	Correct misconceptions
Explores adult roles	Drug abuse	Encourage continuance of school work, hobbies, interests
MOTOR	Alcohol hazards	
Well developed	Tobacco hazards	
Rapid physical growth	Mechanical safety	
Secondary sex characteristics	Sexuality relations	
	Dating	
LANGUAGE/COGNITION	GAMES/INTERESTS	
Plans for future career	Intellectual games	
Able to abstract solutions and problem-solve in future tense	Reading	
	Arts, crafts, hobbies	
FEARS	Video games	
Mutilation	Problem-solving games	
Disruption in body image	Computers	
Rejection from peers		

420

Treatment-Related

Related to separation from significant others or school, or inadequate sensory stimulation secondary to:

Prolonged, painful treatment

Traction or casts

Isolation due to disease processes

Repeated or prolonged hospitalization

Prolonged bed rest

Confinement for ongoing treatment

Situational (Personal and Environmental)

Related to:

Parental knowledge deficit

Stress (acute, transient, or chronic)

Change in usual environment

Separation from significant others (parents, primary caretaker)

Inadequate, inappropriate parental support (neglect, abuse)

Inadequate sensory stimulation (neglect, isolation)

Parent–child conflict

School-related stressors

Maternal or parental anxiety

Loss of significant other

Loss of control over environment (established rituals, activities, established hours of contact with family)

Maturational

Infant–Toddler
(birth to 3 years)

Related to limited opportunities to meet social, play, or educational needs secondary to:

Separation from parents/significant others

Restriction of activity secondary to (specify)

Inadequate parental support

Inability to trust significant other

Inability to communicate (deafness)

Multiple caregivers

Preschool Age
(4–6 years)

Related to limited opportunities to meet social, play, or educational needs secondary to:

Loss of ability to communicate

Lack of stimulation

Lack of significant other

Related to loss of significant other (death, divorce)

Related to loss of peer group

Related to removal from home environment

School Age
(6–11 years)

Related to loss of significant others

Related to loss of peer group

Related to strange environment

Adolescent
(12–18 years)

Related to loss of independence and autonomy secondary to: (specify)

Related to disruption of peer relationships

Related to disruption of body image

Related to loss of significant others

Author's Note

Specific developmental tasks are associated with various age groups (*e.g.*, age 18–30 years, to establish lasting relationships; age 1–3 years, to gain autonomy and self-control [*e.g.*, toileting]). An adult's failure to accomplish a developmental task may cause or contribute to altered functioning in a functional health pattern—for example, *Impaired Social Interactions, Powerlessness*. Because nursing interventions focus on the altered functioning rather than on achievement of past developmental tasks, the diagnosis *Altered Growth and Development* has limited uses for adults. It is most useful for a child or adolescent experiencing difficulty achieving a developmental task.

Errors in Diagnostic Statements

Altered Growth and Development related to inability to perform toileting self-control appropriate for age (4 years)

Inability to perform toileting self-control is not a contributing factor, but rather a diagnostic cue. The diagnosis should be rewritten as *Altered Growth and Development related to unknown etiology, as evidenced by inability to perform toileting self-control appropriate for age (4 years)*. The use of "unknown etiology" directs nurses to collect more data on reasons for the problem.

Altered Growth and Development related to mental retardation secondary to Down syndrome

When *Altered Growth and Development* is used to describe an individual with mental or physical impairment, what is the nursing focus? What client goals would nursing interventions achieve? If physical impairments represent barriers to achieving developmental tasks, the diagnosis can be written as *Risk for Altered Growth and Development related to impaired ability to achieve developmental tasks (specify—e.g., socialization) secondary to disability*.

For a mentally impaired child, the nurse should determine what functional health patterns are altered or at high risk for alteration and amenable to nursing interventions, and address the specific problem (*e.g., Toileting Self-Care Deficit*).

Key Concepts

1. Development can be defined as the patterned, orderly, lifelong changes in structure, thought, or behavior that evolve as a result of maturation of physical and mental capacity, experiences, and learning. Development results in the person achieving a new level of maturity and integration. Growth refers to increase in body size, function, and complexity of body cell content (Wong, 1995). For the purpose of this diagnosis, growth and development are synonymous, because any disruption that does not affect development most likely results in a diagnosis of *Altered Nutrition*.
2. The following assumptions concerning development are relevant (Santrock, 1989; Wong 1995):
   a. The most rapid growth and development occurs in the early stages of life.
   b. Childhood is the foundation period of life and establishes the basis for successful or unsuccessful development throughout life.
   c. Growth and development are continuous and occur in spurts, rather than in a straight, upward direction.
   d. Development follows a definable, predictable, and sequential pattern.
   e. Critical periods exist when development is occurring rapidly and the individual's ability to respond to stressors is limited.
   f. Growth proceeds in a cephalocaudal, proximodistal direction.
   g. Development proceeds from simple to complex.
   h. Development occurs in all components of a person (*i.e.*, motor, intellectual, personal, social, language).
   i. Development results from biologic, maturational, and individual learning.

3. Often development is defined in terms of stages or levels, as illustrated in Erikson's stages of man and Piaget's stages of cognition. In addition, development may be defined in terms of tasks that must be accomplished. A developmental task is a growth responsibility that occurs at a particular time in the life of a person. Successful achievement of the task leads to success with later tasks. Development is affected through either an acceleration of the process or a slowing down of the process by a variety of influences. Physiologic disruptions, through either genetic malfunction or insult from illness, may potentially alter development, temporarily or permanently. Psychological and social influences may also alter development positively or negatively. The alteration of development in a child is particularly critical because the alteration may establish a basic foundation that then remains faulty for the life of the child. Because of the rapid acceleration of development in childhood, several critical periods exist when influences can easily modify development (Wong, 1995).

Focus Assessment Criteria

See Table II-11 for descriptions of appropriate developmental milestones/behaviors for each age group, as well as information for nursing intervention and parental guidance.

Subjective Data

(Data should be verified with primary caregiver.)

A. Assess for defining characteristics
  1. Developmental level: Behaviors listed under Developmental Tasks (see Table II-11) may be assessed through direct observation or report of parent/primary caregiver. The Denver Developmental Screening Tool may be used for children younger than 6 years of age.

B. Assess for related factors
  1. Current nutritional patterns
      Diet recall for past 24 hours (from parent or child, type of food, amounts)
      Diet history
      Height/weight at birth
      Intake pattern
      Child's reaction to eating, feeding
      Parental/child knowledge of nutrition
  2. Physiologic alterations
      Presence of nausea, vomiting, diarrhea
      Allergies
      Food intolerances
      Dysphagia
      Fatigue
      Report of other physical symptoms (*e.g.*, rash, upper respiratory infection)
  3. Parental attitudes
      What are the parents' expectations for the child?
      What are the parents' feelings about being parents?
      Did the parents experience poor parenting themselves?
      Parenting approach to care and discipline of child?
      How do the parents feel about home situation?
      How do the parents feel about child's illness, treatments/hospitalization?
      Assess family functioning with appropriate assessment tool.
  4. Stressors in environment
      Illness in family
      Conflict in family
      History of illness or hospitalization of child
      Child's behavior/success in school
      Child's peer/sibling relationships

Objective Data

A. Assess for defining characteristics

    1. General appearance

        Cleanliness, grooming   Response to stimulation

        Eye contact   Mood (*e.g.*, crying, elated)

        Facial responses

    2. Response/interaction with parent

        Spontaneous, happy when comforted by parent

        Reaction when separated

        Response to procedures, strangers

    3. Nutritional status

        Height/weight (compare to norms)

        Frontal/occipital circumference (also see Focus Assessment Criteria under *Nutrition, Altered: Less Than Body Requirements*)

    4. Bowel and bladder control

    5. Personal/social

        Language/cognition

        Motor activity: Assess for achievement of developmental skills in appropriate age group (see Table II-11)

    6. Developmental level (see behaviors described under Developmental Tasks, Table II-11)

Outcome Criteria

The child will

- Demonstrate an increase in behaviors in personal/social, language, cognition, motor activities appropriate to age group (specify the behaviors)

Interventions

A. Assess causative or contributing factors

    1. Lack of knowledge—parental (caregiver)

    2. Acute or chronic illness

    3. Stress

    4. Inadequate stimulation

    5. Parent–child conflict

    6. Change in environment

B. Teach parents the age-related developmental tasks and parental guidance information (see Table II-11)

C. Carefully assess child's level of development in all areas of functioning by using specific assessment tools (*e.g.*, Brazelton Assessment Table, Denver Developmental Screening Tool)

D. Provide opportunities for an ill child to meet age-related developmental tasks (see Implications for Nursing in Table II-11 to assist with designing interventions)

Birth to 1 Year

    1. Provide increased stimulation using variety of colored toys in crib (*e.g.*, mobiles, musical toys, stuffed toys of varied textures, frequent periods of holding and speaking to infant).

    2. Hold while feeding; feed slowly and in relaxed environment.

3. Provide periods of rest before feeding.
4. Observe mother and child during interaction, especially during feeding.
5. Investigate crying promptly and consistently.
6. Assign consistent caregiver.
7. Encourage parental visits/calls and involvement in care, if possible.
8. Provide buccal experience if infant desires (*i.e.*, thumb, pacifier).
9. Allow hands and feet to be free, if possible.

1–3½ Years

1. Assign consistent caregiver.
2. Encourage self-care activities (*e.g.*, self-feeding, self-dressing, bathing).
3. Reinforce word development by repeating words child uses, naming objects by saying words, and speaking to child often.
4. Provide frequent periods of play with peers and with a variety of toys (puzzles, books with pictures, manipulative toys, trucks, cars, blocks, bright colors).
5. Demonstrate all procedures on a doll before you do them.
6. Provide safe area where the child can locomote.
7. Encourage parental visits/calls and involvement in care, if possible.
8. Provide comfort measures after painful procedures.

3½–5 Years

1. Encourage self-care: self-grooming, self-dressing, mouth care, hair care.
2. Provide frequent play time with others and with variety of toys (*e.g.*, models, musical toys, dolls, puppets, books, mini-slide, wagon, tricycle).
3. Read stories aloud.
4. Ask for verbal responses and requests.
5. Say words for equipment, objects, and people and ask the child to repeat.
6. Allow time for individual play and exploration of play environment.
7. Encourage parental visits/calls and involvement in care, if possible.
8. Monitor television and use television as means to help child understand time ("After *Sesame Street*, your mother will come.").

5–11 Years

1. Talk with child about care provided.
2. Request input from child (*e.g.*, diet, clothes, routine).
3. Allow child to dress in clothes instead of pajamas.
4. Provide periods of interaction with other children on unit.
5. Provide craft project that can be completed each day or week.
6. Continue school work at intervals each day.
7. Praise positive behaviors.
8. Read stories, and provide variety of independent games, puzzles, books, video games, painting.
9. Introduce child by name to people on unit.
10. Encourage visits with or telephone calls from parents, siblings, and peers.

11–15 Years

1. Speak frequently with child about feelings, ideas, concerns over condition or care.
2. Provide opportunity for interaction with others of the same age on unit.
3. Identify interest or hobby that can be supported on unit in some manner, and support it daily.
4. Allow hospital routine to be altered to suit child's schedule.
5. Dress in his own clothes if possible.
6. Involve in decisions about his care.
7. Provide opportunity for involvement in variety of activities (*i.e.*, reading, video games, movies, board games, art, trips outside or to other areas).
8. Encourage visits or telephone calls from parents, siblings, and peers.

E. Initiate health teaching and referrals, when indicated

1. Provide anticipatory guidance for parents regarding constructive handling of developmental problems and support of developmental process (see Table II-11 and *Altered Parenting*).
2. Refer to appropriate agency for counseling or follow-up treatment of abuse, parent–child conflict, chemical dependency, and the like (see *Ineffective Family Coping*).
3. Refer to appropriate agency for structured, ongoing stimulation program when functioning is likely to be impaired permanently (*e.g.*, schooling).
4. Refer to community programs specific to contributing factors (*e.g.*, WIC, social services, family services, counseling).
5. Provide list of parent support groups (*e.g.*, ARC, Down Syndrome Awareness, Muscular Dystrophy Association, National Epilepsy).

Rationale

- All dimensions of growth and development have a predictable, definite sequence. New behaviors or biologic parts come from previously established ones. Each stage is affected by those before and affects those that follow (Wong, 1995).
- Of the range of possible physiologic, psychological, and social influences that may affect development, many exist within the context of illness and wellness care and are often encountered by nurses as they provide care to children. As a result, nursing interventions should be designed with particular developmental tasks and developmental information as a basis for intervention. As part of the care of the child, the nurse must also consider the impact of the primary caregiver or parent figure on the development of the child. The parent essentially controls most of the psychological and social influences present in the early years of childhood. By virtue of the child's dependence on the parent, these influences can modify development (Hunsberger, 1989; Wong 1995).
- Illness, hospitalization, separation from parents, conflict, or inadequate support from parents, as well as specific pathophysiologic processes that interfere with growth, may ultimately affect development in a child. The nurse must support the family as well as the child in ensuring continuance of the child's developmental processes throughout the course of his illness if optimal recovery is to be achieved. In addition, the nurse must seek to stimulate as well as maintain the child's unique developmental level to promote optimal recovery. Stimulation of the developmental process may occur through parental support, parental teaching, referral, or direct intervention (see also *Altered Parenting*) (Farkas, 1983).

References/Bibliography

Abbott, K. (1990). The therapeutic use of play in the psychological preparation of preschool children undergoing cardiac surgery. *Issues in Comprehensive Pediatric Nursing, 13,* 265–277.

Blackman, J. A. (1992). The validity of continuing developmental follow-up of high-risk infants to age five years. *American Journal of Diseases of Children, 146,* 70–75.

Farkas, S. C. (1983). *Hospitalized children: The family's role in care and treatment.* Washington, DC: The Catholic University of America.

Gorski, P. A. (1991). Promoting infant development during neonatal hospitalization: Critiquing the state of the science. *Children's Health Care, 20,* 250–257.

Hunsberger, M. (1989). Nursing care during hospitalization. In R. L. Foster, M. M. Hunsberger, & J. J. T. Anderson (Eds.). *Family-centered nursing care of children.* Philadelphia: W. B. Saunders.

King, E. H. (1992). Risk factors for developmental delay among infants and toddlers. *Children's Health Care, 21,* 39–52.

Krietemeyer, B. C., & Heiney, S. P. (1992). Storytelling as a therapeutic technique in a group for school-aged oncology patients. *Children's Health Care, 21,* 14–20.

Santrock, J. W. (1989). *Lifespan development.* Dubuque, IA: William C. Brown.

Wong, D. L. (1995). *Nursing care of infants and children* (5th ed.). St. Louis: C. V. Mosby.

Health Maintenance, Altered

DEFINITION

Altered Health Maintenance: The state in which an individual or group experiences or is at risk of experiencing a disruption in health because of an unhealthy life-style or lack of knowledge to manage a condition.

DEFINING CHARACTERISTICS (IN THE ABSENCE OF DISEASE)
Major (Must Be Present)

Reports or demonstrates an unhealthy practice or life-style, such as:

Reckless driving of vehicle	Overeating
Substance abuse	High-fat diet

Minor (May Be Present)

Reports or demonstrates:

Skin and nails
    Malodorous   Sunburn
    Unusual color, pallor   Unexplained scars
    Skin lesions (pustules, rashes, dry or scaly skin)
Respiratory system
    Frequent infections
    Dyspnea with exertion
    Chronic cough
Oral cavity
    Frequent sores (on tongue, buccal mucosa)
    Loss of teeth at early age
    Lesions associated with lack of oral care or substance abuse (leukoplakia, fistulas)
Gastrointestinal system and nutrition
    Obesity   Chronic bowel irregularity
    Chronic anemia   Chronic dyspepsia
    Anorexia   Cachexia
Musculoskeletal system
    Frequent muscle strain, backaches, neck pain
    Diminished flexibility and muscle strength
Genitourinary system
    Frequent venereal lesions and infections
    Frequent use of potentially unhealthful over-the-counter products (*e.g.*, chemical douches, perfumed vaginal products)
Constitutional
    Chronic fatigue, malaise, apathy
Neurosensory
    Presence of facial tics (nonconvulsant)
    Headaches
Psychoemotional
    Emotional fragility
    Behavior disorders (compulsiveness, belligerence)
    Frequent feelings of being overwhelmed

RELATED FACTORS

A variety of factors can produce *Altered Health Maintenance*. Some common causes are listed.

Situational (Personal, Environmental)

Related to:

Information misinterpretation   Lack of access to adequate health care services
Lack of motivation   Inadequate health teaching
Lack of education or readiness   Impaired ability to understand secondary to:
          (specify)

Maturational

Related to lack of education of age-related factors. Examples include:

Child

Sexuality and sexual development   Substance abuse
Safety hazards   Nutrition

Adolescent

Same as children   Substance abuse (alcohol, other drugs,
Cycle, automobile safety practices   tobacco)

Adult

Parenthood   Safety practices
Sexual function

Older Adult

Effects of aging
Sensory deficits

See Table II-12 for age-related conditions.

Author's Note

The nursing diagnosis *Altered Health Maintenance* is applicable to both well and ill populations. Health is a dynamic, ever-changing state defined by the individual based on the perception of his or her highest level of functioning (*e.g.*, a marathon runner's definition of health will differ from a paraplegic person's). Because individuals are responsible for their own health, *Altered Health Maintenance* represents a diagnosis that the individual is motivated to treat. An important nursing responsibility associated with health maintenance involves raising the person's consciousness that better health is possible.

This diagnosis is appropriate for a person expressing a desire to change an unhealthy life-style. Examples of an unhealthy life-style are excessive dissatisfaction with occupation; lack of exercise; failure to be refreshed after rest; diet high in fat, salt, simple carbohydrates; tobacco use; obesity; excessive alcohol use; and insufficient social support.

The nursing diagnosis *Risk for Altered Health Maintenance* is useful to describe an individual who needs teaching or referrals before discharge from an acute care center to prevent problems with health maintenance after discharge.

Health-Seeking Behaviors is used to describe an individual or a group desiring health teaching related to the promotion and maintenance of high-level wellness (*e.g.*, preventive behavior, age-related screening, optimal nutrition) or, according to the NANDA definition, "seeking ways to alter personal health habits in order to move to a higher level of health." In most cases, this diagnosis describes an asymptomatic person. However, it also can be used for a person with a chronic disease to help that person attain a higher level of wellness in a particular area. Different from good health, high-level wellness can be defined as an integrated method of functioning oriented toward maximizing the potential of which the individual is capable (Dunn, 1959). For example, a woman with multiple sclerosis with many physical problems could be taught breast self-examination or relaxation exercises using the diagnosis *Health-Seeking Behaviors: Breast self-exam.*

Health Seeking-Behaviors is best written as a one-part diagnostic statement with the sought-after health practice specified (*e.g., Health-Seeking Behaviors: Breast self-exam*). Using "related to" for *Health-Seeking Behaviors* is unnecessary; it is understood that all people with the diagnosis are motivated to achieve a higher level of health. Related factors could not represent causative or contributing factors, unless the nurse wants to repeat the

Table II-12 **Primary and Secondary Prevention for Age-Related Conditions**

Developmental Level	Primary Prevention	Secondary Prevention

Infancy (0–1 year)	Parent education
	  Infant safety
	  Nutrition
	  Breast feeding
	Sensory stimulation
	  Infant massage and touch
	  Visual stimulation
	    Activity
	    Colors
	  Auditory stimulation
	    Verbal
	    Music
	Immunizations
	  DPT or DTaP
	  TOPV or IPV, Hib } at 2, 4, and 6 months
	  Hepatitis B
	  Influenza (for high risk > 6 months)
	Oral hygiene
	  Teething biscuits
	  Fluoride (if needed > 6 months)
	  Avoid sugared food and drink
		Complete physical exam every 2–3 months
		Screening at birth
		  Congenital hip
		  PKU
		  G-6-PD deficiency in blacks, Mediterranean, and Far Eastern origin children
		  Sickle cell
		  Hemoglobin or hematocrit (for anemia)
		  Cystic fibrosis
		  Vision (startle reflex)
		  Hearing (response to and localization of sounds)
		  TB test at 12 months
		  Developmental assessments
		Screen and intervene for high risk
		  Low birth weight
		  Maternal substance abuse during pregnancy
		    Alcohol: fetal alcohol syndrome
		    Cigarettes: SIDS
		    Drugs: addicted neonate, AIDS
		  Maternal infections during pregnancy

Preschool (1–5 years)	Parent education
	  Teething
	  Discipline
	  Nutrition
	  Accident prevention
	  Normal growth and development
	Child education
	  Dental self-care
	  Dressing
	  Bathing with assistance
	  Feeding self-care
	Immunizations
	  DTaP
	  TOPV } at 18 months
	  MMR at 12–15 months
	  HIB at 24 months
	  Influenza (for high risk)
	Dental/oral hygiene
	  Fluoride treatments
	  Fluoridated water
		Complete physical exam between 2 and 3 years and preschool (UA, CBC)
		TB test at 3 years
		Development assessments (annual)
		  Speech development
		  Hearing
		  Vision
		Screen and intervene
		  Lead poisoning
		  Developmental lag
		  Neglect or abuse
		  Strong family history of arteriosclerotic diseases (e.g., MI, CVA, peripheral vascular disease), diabetes, hypertension, gout, or hyperlipidemia—fasting serum cholesterol at age 2 years, then every 3–5 years if normal
		  Strabismus
		  Hearing deficit
		  Vision deficit

School age (6–11 years)	Health education of child
	  "Basic 4" nutrition
	  Accident prevention
	  Outdoor safety
	  Substance abuse counsel
	  Anticipatory guidance for physical changes at puberty
		Complete physical exam
		TB test every 3 years (at ages 6 and 9)
		Developmental assessments
		  Language
		  Vision: Snellen charts at school
		    6–8 years, use "E" chart
		    Over 8 years, use alphabet chart
		  Hearing: audiogram

(continued)

Table II-12 **Primary and Secondary Prevention for Age-Related Conditions** (continued)

Developmental Level	Primary Prevention	Secondary Prevention

	Immunizations
	  Tetanus age 10
	  MMR
	  DTaP } boosters between
	  TOPV } 4 and 6 years
	Dental hygiene every 6–12 months
	  Continue fluoridation
	Complete physical exam
		Cholesterol profile, if high risk, every 3–5 years
		Serum cholesterol one time (not high risk)

Adolescence
(12–19 years)
	Health education
	  Proper nutrition and healthful diets
	  Sex education
	    Choices
	    Risks
	    Precautions
	  Sexually transmitted diseases
	Safe driving skills
	Adult challenges
	  Seeking employment and career choices
	  Dating and marriage
	  Confrontation with substance abuse
	Safety in athletics, water
	Skin care
	Dental hygiene every 6–12 months
	Immunizations
	  Hepatitis B series if needed
	  TOPV booster at 12–14 years
		Complete physical exam (prepuberty or age 13)
		  Blood pressure
		  Cholesterol profile
		  TB test at 12 years
		  VDRL, CBC, U/A
		  Female: breast self-exam (BSE)
		  Male: testicular self-exam (TSE)
		  Female, if sexually active: Pap and pelvic exam twice, 1 year apart (cervical gonorrhea culture with pelvic); then every 3 years if both are negative
		Screening and interventions if high risk
		  Depression
		  Suicide
		  Substance abuse
		  Pregnancy
		Family history of alcoholism or domestic violence

Young adult
(20–39 years)
	Health education
	  Weight management with good nutrition as BMR changes
	  Low cholesterol diet
	Life-style counseling
	  Stress management skills
	  Safe driving
	  Family planning
	  Divorce
	  Parenting
	  Sexual practices
	  Parenting skills
	  Regular exercise
	  Environmental health choices
	  Alcohol, drug use
	Dental hygiene every 6–12 months
	Immunizations
	  Tetanus at 20 years and every 10 years
	  Female: rubella, if serum negative for antibodies
	  Hepatitis-B for high-risk people
		Complete physical exam at about 20 years, then every 5–6 years
		Cancer checkup every 3 years
		Female: BSE monthly
		Male: TSE monthly
		All females: baseline mammography between ages 35 and 40
		Parents-to-be: high-risk screening for Down syndrome, Tay-Sachs
		Female pregnant: screen for VD, rubella titer, Rh factor, amniocentesis for women 35 years or older (if desired)
		Screening and interventions if high risk
		  Female with previous breast cancer: annual mammography at 35 years and after
		  Female with mother or sister who has had breast cancer, same as above
		  Family history colorectal cancer or high risk: annual stool guaiac, digital rectal, and sigmoidoscopy
		PPD if exposed to TB
		Glaucoma screening at 35 years and along with routine physical exams
		Cholesterol profile every 5 years, if normal
		Cholesterol profile every 1–2 years if borderline

Table II-12 **Primary and Secondary Prevention for Age-Related Conditions** (continued)

Developmental Level	Primary Prevention	Secondary Prevention

Middle-aged adult (40–59 years)	Health education: continue with young adult
	Midlife changes, male and female counseling
	  "Empty nest syndrome"
	  Anticipatory guidance for retirement
	  Grandparenting
	Dental hygiene every 6–12 months
	Immunizations
	  Tetanus every 10 years
	  Influenza—annual if high risk (i.e., major chronic disease [COPD, CAD])
	  Pneumococcal—single dose
		Complete physical exam every 5–6 years with complete laboratory evaluation (serum/urine tests, x-ray, ECG)
		Cancer checkup every year
		Female: BSE monthly
		Male: TSE monthly
		All females: mammogram every 1–2 years (40–49 years) then annual mammography 50 years and over
		Schiotz's tonometry (glaucoma) every 3–5 years
		Sigmoidoscopy at 50 and 51, then every 4 years if negative
		Stool guaiac annually at 50 and thereafter
		Screening and intervention if high risk
		  Endometrial cancer: have endometrial sampling at menopause
		  Oral cancer: screen more often if substance abuser

Older adult (60–74 years)	Health education: continue with previous counseling
	  Home safety
	  Retirement
	  Loss of spouse, relatives, friends
	  Special health needs
	    Nutritional changes
	    Changes in hearing or vision
	Dental/oral hygiene every 6–12 months
	Immunizations
	  Tetanus every 10 years
	  Influenza—annual if high risk
	  Pneumococcal—(one time only)
		Complete physical exam every 2 years with laboratory assessments
		Annual cancer checkup
		Blood pressure annually
		Female: BSE monthly
		Male: TSE monthly
		Female: annual mammogram
		Annual stool guaiac
		Sigmoidoscopy every 4 years
		Schiotz's tonometry every 3–5 years
		Podiatric evaluation with foot care PRN
		Screen for high risk
		  Depression
		  Suicide
		  Alcohol/drug abuse
		  "Elder abuse"

Old-age adult (75 years and over)	Health education: continue counsel
	Anticipatory guidance
	  Dying and death
	  Loss of spouse, relatives, friends
	  Increasing dependency on others
	Dental/oral hygiene every 6–12 months
	Immunizations
	  Tetanus every 10 years
	  Influenza—annual
	  Pneumococcal—if not already received
		Complete physical exam annually
		  Laboratory assessments
		  Cancer checkup
		  Blood pressure
		  Stool guaiac
		Female: annual mammogram, sigmoidoscopy every 4 years
		Schiotz's tonometry every 3–5 years
		Podiatrist PRN

same factors for each client (*e.g., Health-Seeking Behaviors: Breast self-exam related to desire to maximize health*).

As focus shifts from an illness/treatment-oriented health care system to a health-oriented one, *Altered Health Maintenance* and *Health-Seeking Behaviors* are becoming increasingly significant nursing diagnoses. The increasingly high acuity and shortened lengths of stay in hospitals require that nurses be creative in addressing health promotion—for example, by using printed materials, TV instruction, and community-based programs.

Errors in Diagnostic Statements

Altered Health Maintenance related to refusal to quit smoking

Refusal to quit smoking represents significant data that require further clarification—for example, is the person making an informed decision? Does the person know the effects of smoking on respiratory and cardiovascular functioning? Does the person know where assistance can be acquired to stop smoking? If the answers to these questions are "yes," then the diagnosis *Altered Health Maintenance* is incorrect. On the other hand, if the person is not fully aware of the deleterious effects of smoking or the availability of self-help resources, the diagnosis *Altered Health Maintenance related to insufficient knowledge of effects of tobacco use and self-help resources available* may be appropriate.

Note: The nurse should be cautioned about timing attempts to encourage a person to quit smoking or control eating after an acute episode, such as myocardial infarction. In such a situation, denying the person his or her usual coping mechanism, no matter how unhealthy it is, may be more problematic to the person's overall health. The nurse should emphasize teaching so the person can make informed choices, not merely prohibit certain choices.

Health-Seeking Behaviors related to increased alcohol and tobacco use in response to marital break-up and heavy family demands

This represents an inappropriate diagnosis for this person, who wants to alter personal habits but is not in good or excellent health. A more appropriate focus would be to promote constructive stress management without tobacco or alcohol, through the nursing diagnosis *Ineffective Individual Coping related to inability to constructively manage the stressors associated with marital break-up and family demands*.

Key Concepts

1. Many members of the population view health as absence of disease. Rather, health can be viewed as a return (or recovery) to a previous state or to a heightened awareness of the individual's full potential and life meaning (Flynn, 1980).
2. The control of major health problems in the United States depends directly on modification of individual behavior and habits of living (Flynn, 1980).
3. Belloc and Breslow (1972) correlated well-being and increased life span to the following seven practices:
   a. Sleeping 7–8 hours nightly
   b. Eating three meals at regular times
   c. Eating breakfast daily
   d. Maintaining desirable body weight
   e. Avoiding excessive alcohol consumption
   f. Participating in regular exercise
   g. Abstaining from smoking
4. In addition to addressing life-styles to promote wellness, total health depends on (Flynn, 1980):
   a. Eradication of poverty and ignorance
   b. Availability of jobs
   c. Adequate housing, transportation, and recreation
   d. Public safety
   e. Esthetically pleasing and beneficial environment

5. The goals of prevention are
    a. Avoidance of disease by choosing a healthy life-style
    b. Decrease in mortality due to disease by early detection and intervention
    c. Improvement of quality of life
6. The three levels of prevention are primary, secondary, and tertiary.
7. The primary level of prevention involves actions that prevent disease and accidents and promote well-being. Key concepts are as follows:

Concept	Examples
Wellness	Diet low in salt, sugar, and fat
A life-style that incorporates the principles of health promotion and is directed by self-responsibility	Regular exercise and stress management
	Elimination of smoking
	Minimal alcohol intake
Self-help	
Mutual sharing with others who have similar needs	LaLeche League
	Childbirth education
	Assertiveness training
	Specific written resources (books, pamphlets, magazines)
	Public media (radio, television)
Safety	Adherence to speed limits
	Use of seat belts and car seats
	Proper storage of household poisons
Immunizations	Children: Varicella
	Nonpregnant women of childbearing age: Rubella vaccine if antibody titer is negative
	Elderly: influenza, pneumonia

8. The secondary level of prevention concerns actions that promote early detection of disease and subsequent intervention, both routine physical examination by a health professional at regular intervals and self-examination.
9. The tasks of screening are to
    a. Identify major disabling conditions.
    b. Investigate the personal and social benefits of early detection and intervention for asymptomatic persons with the condition (*e.g.*, facilitate family coping, minimize disability and cost, prevent premature death, improve productivity of affected persons, decrease overall morbidity and mortality).
    c. Identify people at high risk for specific conditions through *personal health history* (*e.g.*, concurrent disease such as diabetes mellitus involves greater risk for hypertension), *family health history* (*e.g.*, breast cancer, diabetes, hypertension), and *social history* (*e.g.*, substance abuse—cancer, heart disease; sexual patterns—venereal disease; domestic violence—person abuse).
    d. Identify tests and procedures that accurately detect the condition (who will do them? how often are they done? who bears the cost?).
    e. Plan a strategy for disseminating screening information to health care professionals and the public.
    f. Plan evaluation of screening effectiveness.
10. Types of screening measures include
    a. Physical findings (periodic examinations by health care professionals and self-exams of breast, testicles, and skin)
    b. Survey of risk factors (smoking, alcohol abuse)
    c. Laboratory tests (serum—*e.g.*, sickle-cell in blacks, phenylketonuria in newborns; urine—*e.g.*, renal disease in the elderly; x-ray—*e.g.*, dental caries, chest tuberculosis)
11. The tertiary level of prevention involves actions that restore and rehabilitate in the presence of illness. For example, for a person with coronary artery disease, these would be
    a. Restorative (surgery, such as coronary artery bypass, angioplasty, and medications)

    b. Rehabilitative (stress management, exercise program, stop smoking, "zipper club" [self-help group])

12. Potential barriers to prevention are found both in the health care system and in the individual.

    a. The system may be

        Disease-oriented rather than health-oriented

        Composed of health care professionals who are taught to focus on fragment systems of the human body rather than to take a holistic approach

        Functioning on a financial system that rewards treatment of illness, not prevention

        Difficult to reach or may have previously proved unsatisfactory

    b. The client may

        Believe that the health/illness state is determined by forces (fate, luck) outside himself (external locus of control)

        Perceive the behavior needed as unacceptable or uncomfortable

        Practice sociocultural behaviors that are not healthful (*e.g.*, obesity is considered desirable, salt is prevalent in diet)

        Experience psychological disturbances that impede incentive to practice healthy behaviors

        Lack financial resources

Nutrition

See Key Concepts for *Altered Nutrition*.

Exercise

1. Regular exercise can provide the person with increased

    Cardiovascular–respiratory endurance   Ability to deliver nutrients to tissue

    Muscle strength   Ability to tolerate psychological stress

    Muscle endurance   Ability to reduce body fat content

    Flexibility

2. An exercise program should include

    A warm-up session (10 minutes of   Endurance exercises

      a slower pace)   A cool-down session (slower pace and stretching, 5–10 minutes)

Weight Reduction

1. Overeating is a complex, multidimensional problem with physical, social, and psychological components.

2. Overweight people are usually nutritionally deprived.

3. Internal motivation is essential for a successful weight loss program.

4. An individual's body image and coping patterns influence the weight loss program's success or failure.

5. The body uses a higher percentage of energy (calories) to convert carbohydrates to body fat than it does to convert fat to body fat. The body only needs 135–225 fatty calories to supply daily essential fatty acids.

6. Fluctuations in body weight are common, especially in women. Daily weights can be misleading and disheartening. Body measurements are a better measurement of losses. Regular exercise causes lean muscle mass to increase. Because muscle weighs more than fat, this may be reflected on the scale as a weight gain.

Smoking

1. Smoking has immediate and long-term effects on the respiratory system.

2. Immediate effects are paralysis of the ciliary cleansing mechanism of the lungs (which should keep breathing passages free of inhaled irritants and bacteria); irritation of the lining of the lungs, causing an inflammatory response; increased production of mucous; and decreased oxygenation.

3. Long-term effects are *permanent* disabling of the ciliary cleansing mechanism; reduction of the number of macrophages in the airways; a *permanent* decrease in the lung's ability

to fight infection; increased production of mucous cells; a significant increase in the risk for development of pulmonary disease (a history of 15–20 "pack years" indicates a high risk); possible enlargement of the distal air passages; and chronic CO_2 retention, which results in hypoxia becoming the drive to breathe, rather than hypercarbia (increased CO_2).

4. Smoking has immediate and long-term effects on the cardiovascular system. Immediate effects are vasoconstriction and decreased oxygenation of the blood, elevated blood pressure, increased heart rate and possible dysrhythmias, and an increase in the work of the heart. Long-term effects include an increased risk for coronary artery disease, stroke, increased lipidemia, and myocardial infarction. Smoking also contributes to hypertension, peripheral vascular disease (*e.g.*, leg ulcers), and chronically abnormal arterial blood gases (low oxygen, or PO_2, and high carbon dioxide, or PCO_2).

5. The use of smokeless tobacco (snuff, chewing tobacco) is associated with oral leukoplakia (premalignant lesions), oral cancer, and nicotine addiction. At least 12 million Americans are at risk, mostly male teens and male adults (Young, Koch, & Mauger, 1988).

6. Tobacco use is a significant risk factor for the following cancer sites: tongue and oral mucosa, larynx, lungs, bladder, and cervix. Combined with other carcinogens (*e.g.*, alcohol, asbestos, coal dust, radon), the health risk intensifies. The rate of cancer recurrence increases in clients who continue tobacco use during and after treatment.

7. Nicotine is the primary addicting substance in tobacco smoke and juice. Tobacco use is an addiction; these clients need special assistance with short-term withdrawal and long-term maintenance of a tobacco-free life.

8. Passive smoking, the inhalation of tobacco smoke by nonsmokers, has been shown to have negative health effects.
   a. People with angina experience more discomfort in a smoke-filled room.
   b. Bronchospasm is increased when an asthmatic is exposed to tobacco smoke.
   c. Children living with smoking parents have more upper respiratory infections than those living with nonsmokers.
   d. Passive smoking causes lung cancer in nonsmokers (U.S. Department of Health and Human Services, 1986).

9. In the last 25 years, most health professions have seen a significant decline in the smoking behavior of its members—*but not nursing*. Estimates show that 25%–29% of nurses still smoke. Studies of nurses link occupational stress and social influences with tobacco use (Cinelli & Glover, 1988). A nurse who smokes sends the wrong signals to clients. According to Ash (1987), "a role model does not smoke, thus exemplifying behavior which is desired, and behaves in a way that provides guidance and that others will want to imitate."

Osteoporosis

1. Age-related changes beginning around 40 years of age decrease cortical bone by 3%/decade for men and women (Riggs & Melton, 1986).

2. After menopause, women experience an increase in cortical bone loss to 9%–10%/decade (Riggs & Melton, 1986).

3. Loss of trabecular bone begins in the fourth decade and progresses at a rate of 6%–8%/decade. The rate is accelerated in women after menopause (Riggs & Melton, 1986).

4. Osteoporosis is classified as primary (associated with age and menopause-related changes) or secondary (caused by medications or diseases) (Miller, 1995).

5. Factors that contribute to a woman's risk of osteoporosis include loss of female hormones after menopause, low calcium intake, insufficient exercise, small stature, fair skin, family history, cigarette smoking, excessive alcohol consumption, excessive caffeine intake and excessive protein consumption, excessive use of aluminum-type antacids, and long-term use of corticosteroids (Chestnut, 1984).

🕮 *Key Concepts—Child*

1. Anticipatory health promotion, or anticipatory guidance, is an essential component of comprehensive health care and varies in content with the age of the child. It involves teaching parents and older children what is likely to occur in the child's development in the upcoming weeks or months (Scipien, Chard, Howe & Barnard, 1990).

2. Health maintenance begins with the prenatal visit and continues with comprehensive health supervision during the child's developmental years (Wong, 1995).

3. The child depends on a parent/adult caregiver to provide a safe environment and promote health (*e.g.*, immunizations, well-child check-ups, and chronic disease management) (Wong, 1995).

4. The risk of altered health maintenance varies with the child's age and health status. For example, the toddler is at risk for accidental poisoning, whereas the adolescent is more likely to engage in high-risk behavior (Wong, 1995).

5. Malnutrition, lack of immunizations, or an unsafe environment may be related to parental knowledge deficit, alteration in parenting, or barriers to health care (Wong, 1995).

6. Many factors can influence a child's nutritional needs, including periods of rapid growth, stress, illness, metabolic errors, some medications, and socioeconomic factors such as inadequate income, poor housing, and lack of food (Scipien et al., 1990).

7. An increase in the use and abuse of drugs (including alcohol and tobacco) has been reported among school-age children and adolescents (Scipien et al., 1990; Wong, 1995).

8. By conservative estimates, more than one million youth run away from home each year (Farrow, 1991, p. 491). Alienated youth are frequently outside the health care system and tend to remain there unless efforts are made to identify them and develop health services that are acceptable to them. The adoption of destructive life-styles by many of these youth contributes heavily to physical and psychological morbidity and to an alarmingly high mortality rate (Farrow, 1991).

9. The most frequent complication of adolescent obesity is its persistence into adulthood, with high resistance to treatment (Wong, 1995).

10. The most destructive complications of adolescent obesity are psychosocial, resulting from ridicule and rejection by peers and family (Wong, 1995).

11. Good weight management for children and adolescents focuses on weight maintenance or slow loss, meeting nutrient and energy needs, avoiding hunger, preservation of lean body mass, and increasing physical activity and growth (Wong, 1995).

12. Current trends in the care of chronically ill or disabled children focus on the developmental versus chronologic age of the child, and on normalization (Wong, 1995). Children with chronic illness or disability can achieve wellness when they function at their optimal level (Hunsberger, 1989).

Key Concepts—Maternal

1. Smoking during pregnancy has been associated with small-for-gestational-age (SGA) newborns, miscarriage, stillbirths, and sudden infant death syndrome (Institute of Medicine, 1985). Pregnant women who quit smoking before the second trimester eliminate the (smoking-related) risk of having an SGA newborn (Novella, 1990).

Key Concepts—Older Adult

1. According to Miller (1995), health is "the ability of older adults to function at their highest capacity, despite the presence of age-related changes and risk factors."

2. Miller (1995) also states, "Of all the age-related changes . . . osteoporosis is the one that is most likely to cause serious negative functional consequences, even in the absence of additional risk factors."

3. About 70% of people older than 65 years of age rate their health as excellent (U.S. Department of Health and Human Services, 1987).

4. It is important to differentiate between age-related changes and risk factors that affect functioning of older people. Such risk factors as inadequate nutrition, fluid intake, exercise, and socialization can have a greater effect on functioning than can most age-related changes.

5. The mortality rate from pneumonia or influenza for people older than 65 years is 9/100,000. For people who smoke, have kyphosis, or have chronic diseases, this rate increases to 979/100,000. Older adults should be immunized yearly against influenza in late fall (Miller, 1995).

6. Oxygen consumption at anaerobic threshold varies inversely with age. Therefore, in the older individual there is a lower anaerobic threshold, with earlier rise in lactic acid accumulation and earlier onset of muscle fatigue (Posner, Gorman, Klein, & Woldow, 1986).

7. Maximal aerobic capacity and maximal heart rate decline with age. For aerobic conditioning, an older individual must exercise to reach target heart rate for at least 20–30 minutes three times a week. The following formula will obtain target heart rate: 220 − Individual's age × 60%–70% = Target Training Heart Rate. Older adults must be taught to monitor carotid pulse for rate and rhythm. There is a greater time threshold for older individuals to return to baseline heart rates, blood pressure, and respiratory rate after exercise (Harris, 1982).

8. Elderly people have decreased thermoregulation with diminished ability to cool the body by perspiration after physical exertion, affecting their tolerance of physical activity (Matteson & McConnell, 1988).

9. There is an age-related increase in systolic blood pressure at rest and at submaximal workloads. The cardiovascular system has a diminished sensitivity to the chronotropic, inotropic, and vasodilatory effects of catecholamines. Studies have shown that catecholamines or β-adrenergic stimulation, when administered during exercise, had greater effects on young individuals as opposed to those of advanced age (Abrams & Berkow, 1990; Fleg, 1986).

10. Because the current generation of elderly people has not typically been involved in structured exercise programs and fitness clubs, many individuals have not developed endurance for sustained physical activity. In their culture, exercise and perspiration resulted in a completed task such as a plowed field or a painted house.

11. A regular exercise program has been shown to correlate positively with increased self-esteem. Adult learning principles support encouraging an exercise program or regular activity that has meaning to the older individual if compliance is expected. When exercising, the older individual should be encouraged to exercise to the point of mild symptoms of intolerance and then cut back by 25% (Matteson & McConnell, 1988).

TRANSCULTURAL CONSIDERATIONS

1. Health and illness are culturally prescribed. An obese person may be viewed as "strong and healthy in one culture and as weak and unhealthy in another" (Boyle & Andrews, 1994, p. 26).

2. "Nurses must keep in mind that a treatment strategy that is consistent with the person's belief may have a better chance of being successful" (Boyle & Andrews, 1994, p. 103).

3. A future orientation to illness, disease, and health care is necessary for prevention. The dominant American culture is oriented to the future over the present. Some cultures have a present-oriented perception (*e.g.*, African-Americans, Hispanic, Southern Appalachian, and traditional Chinese Americans). Some members of these cultures have acquired the dominant culture's values and have become future oriented (Tripp-Reimer & Lively, 1988).

4. Some cultures believe that the fate of the world and humans is dependent on the actions of God or other supernatural forces. Humans are at the mercy of these forces despite their behavior. "Health is seen as a gift or reward given as a sign of God's blessing or good will" (Boyle & Andrews, 1994, p. 27).

5. Some Asian cultures believe in the concept of balance and harmony for health. Moderation is emphasized; excesses are avoided. In the yin/yang theory, the yin force in the universe represents the female aspect of nature—cold and darkness. The yang force represents the male aspect of nature—fullness, light, and warmth. An imbalance of yin and yang creates illness (Capra, 1982).

6. In Hispanic and black cultures, health is maintained by the hot/cold humoral theory. This ancient Greek concept describes four body humors: yellow bile, black bile, phlegm, and blood. When these humors are balanced, health is present. The treatment of illness consists of restoring the body's humoral balance through the addition or deletion of substances. Substances—foods, beverages, herbs, and drugs—are either hot or cold. For example, an earache is classified as cold, thus needing hot substances for treatment (Boyle & Andrews, 1994).

7. Because the family is usually the client's most important social unit, the nurse can use the family to support life-style changes and promote health (Boyle & Andrews, 1994).
8. Blacks, Hispanics, and Asians in the United States smoke more than whites and have higher death rates from cancer. More emphasis on creating culturally based cessation programs and materials is needed (Koepke, Flay, & Johnson, 1990).

Focus Assessment Criteria

Subjective Data

A. Assess for defining characteristics
   1. Health status
      a. Client's description of health
      b. Immediate health concerns
      c. Frequency of
         Bowel irregularity
         Respiratory infections
         Influenza
         Urinary tract infections
         Headaches
         Fatigue
         Mouth lesions
         Skin rashes
         Feelings of being overwhelmed

B. Assess for related factors
   1. Influencing factors: health management and adherence behavior
      What factors make it difficult to follow health advice?
      What daily health management activities are practiced?
   2. Risk factors
      Family incidence of:
      Cardiovascular disease   Abuse or violence
      Hypertension   Drug or alcohol abuse
      Cancer   Genetic disorders
      Diabetes mellitus   Other (specify)
      Psychiatric illness
      Health habits
      Do you smoke? How much?
      Alcohol use (frequency, amount, type)
      Drug use (prescribed, over-the-counter)
      Dietary consumption of fat/salt/sugar
      Exercise program
   3. Environmental risk factors
      Do you use seat belts or child restraints?
      Is home child-proofed? (If appropriate, determine measures taken)
      Any factors in the home or at work that could cause falls or accidents?
      Are there any other factors you can identify that could potentially threaten your health or cause injury?
   4. Preventive health screening activities
      Self-examinations (breast, testicles, blood pressure): Indicate frequency and perceived problems
      Last professional examination (dental, pelvic, rectal, vision, hearing, complete physical)
      Last laboratory or other diagnostic testing (electrocardiogram, complete blood count, cholesterol, occult blood, Pap, chest x-ray)

Objective Data

A. Assess for defining characteristics

1. General appearance
2. Weight, height

Outcome Criteria

The individual or caregiver will:
- Identify barriers to health maintenance
- Verbalize an intent or engage in health maintenance behaviors

---

Interventions

A. Assess for barriers to health maintenance

1. Lack of knowledge
2. Lack of access or finances
3. Low priority
4. Family life-style patterns

B. Explain the primary and secondary preventions for age (see Table II-12)

C. Identify strategies to improve access (*e.g.*, community centers, school-based clinics)

D. Assist the individual or family to identify health behaviors that are compatible with their life-style

Rationale

- "Many of the most serious disorders can be prevented or postponed by immunizations, chemoprophylaxis and healthy life-styles or detected early with screening and treated effectively" (U. S. Department of Health and Human Services, 1994, p. xvii).
- The focus of low-income families is usually directed toward meeting basic needs; providing for food, shelter, and safety and seeking help with curing an illness, not prevention (Hanson & Boyd, 1996).
- Life-style patterns are passed on from one generation to another. When one family member initiates a change (*e.g.*, diet, smoking cessation), other family members are affected (Hanson & Boyd, 1996).
- Providing information and resources can help to increase the sense that change is possible.

■ Altered Health Maintenance
Related to Insufficient Knowledge of Effects of Tobacco Use and Self-Help Resources Available*

Outcome Criteria

The individual will
- Identify short-term and long-term health effects of tobacco use
- Identify benefits of abstinence from tobacco use
- Verbalize commitment to personal health and desire to eliminate tobacco use†
- Devise strategies to assist in smoking/chewing cessation†
- Significantly decrease amount of tobacco used or stop altogether†

Interventions

A. Define tobacco use behavior
　　1. Type and quantity
　　　　Cigarettes
　　　　　　Filter/nonfilter
　　　　　　Regular/reduced tar and nicotine
　　　　　　Pack years
　　　　Cigars
　　　　　　Inhaled/not inhaled
　　　　　　Number/day, number of years
　　　　Pipe
　　　　　　Inhaled/not inhaled
　　　　　　Number of bowls/day
　　　　Smokeless tobacco (chewing)
　　　　　　Number of minutes/day
　　　　　　Number of years
　　2. Associated activities
　　　　Job: Works in a smoke-filled room (note exposure to carcinogens in workplace, *e.g.*, asbestos, arsenic, coal-tar fumes)
　　　　Home: Presence of radon greatly increases lung cancer risk
　　　　Relaxation
　　　　Stressful events
　　　　Recreation
　　　　Use of alcohol/drugs
　　3. Previous attempts to abstain from tobacco use
　　　　What strategies were used?
　　　　Why were they not successful?
　　　　What was helpful during previous abstentions from tobacco?
　　　　What trigger factors precipitated relapse?

---

* This nursing diagnosis can be used in two different situations—for the individual who does not know the hazards of tobacco use and for the individual who desires to quit.

† These outcome criteria are established only *if* the client desires to quit tobacco use. For the client who does not wish to change tobacco use behaviors, provide information regarding health risks and benefits so that an *informed* choice is made. Avoid being judgmental. Always "keep the door open" should the client later change his mind.

B. Promote understanding of personal tobacco use behavior
　1. Identify negative aspects of tobacco use with client.
　　　Physical: exercise intolerance, cough, sputum, frequent respiratory infections, dental disease, increased risk of diseases, premature facial wrinkling, bad breath
　　　Environmental: burned clothing/furniture, discolored interiors of home/workplace, malodorous clothing/furniture, dirty ashtrays, house and occupational fires
　　　Social: inability to smoke in public places; offensive nature of tobacco use behaviors to family members, friends, coworkers
　　　Financial: calculate monetary cost of client's habit with client
　　　Psychological: unpleasant withdrawal symptoms that occur when tobacco is not available (*e.g.*, midnight "nicotine fits"), decreased self-esteem due to dependency
　2. Identify positive aspects of tobacco use with client (use client's own words).

C. Provide information
　1. Health risks of tobacco use to self
　　　Cancer (oral, lung, bladder)
　　　Chronic obstructive pulmonary disease (COPD) and respiratory infections
　　　Arteriosclerosis (coronary and peripheral)
　　　Hypertension and cerebrovascular accident
　　　Periodontal disease
　2. Health risks of tobacco use to others
　　　Unborn child　　People with angina
　　　Infants　　　　People with allergies
　　　Asthmatics　　People sharing living/working space
　3. Benefits of quitting
　　　Decreased pulse and blood pressure
　　　Decreased sputum production
　　　Pulmonary mucosa regenerates
　　　Decreased risk of cancer, stroke, myocardial infarction, COPD
　　　Improved dental hygiene
　　　Improved senses of taste/smell
　　　Increased social acceptance
　4. Strategies available
　　　Individual methods: self-help books and tapes, "cold turkey"
　　　Group methods: contact local chapters of American Cancer Society, American Lung Association, and private businesses
　　　Hypnosis
　　　Acupuncture
　　　Over-the-counter products: filters, tablet regimens, nontobacco cigarettes, nicotine-containing chewing gum
　　　Transdermal nicotine patch: stress the hazards of smoking with patch
　5. Discuss strategies to minimize weight gain and increase exercise.
　6. Discuss symptoms of nicotine withdrawal and assist client to prepare for them (McAndrew, 1994).
　　　Craving for tobacco
　　　Irritability
　　　Anxiety
　　　Difficulty concentrating
　　　Restlessness
　　　Headache

Drowsiness

Gastrointestinal upsets: diarrhea, cramps

If client has experienced these symptoms before, suggest he choose a time to quit in which he is experiencing relatively low stress.

D. Provide support and encouragement to promote success

1. Identify with client significant others who will provide ongoing support of client's abstinence from tobacco use.
2. Identify with client people who may sabotage efforts and devise strategies to minimize their impact.
3. Reinforce with client his personal reasons for tobacco use cessation; encourage client to make visible reminders.

Rationale

- Benefits of cessation extend to people of all ages. Life expectancy and quality of life are enhanced after quitting, even in people older than 60 years of age. It is never too late to quit (Novella, 1990).
- To assist an individual to initiate a health behavior change, the nurse would provide interventions to increase the person's perception of the seriousness of the behavior and his susceptibility to disease if behavior continues (Edelman & Mandel, 1990).
- Providing information on the benefits of smoking cessation can help to motivate (Edelman & Mandel, 1990).
- Information that increases the person's confidence in a success may precipitate a decision to cease smoking (Edelman & Mandel, 1990).

Interventions—*Child Focus*

1. Assess if adolescent knows someone who smokes (peers, relatives).
   a. Use an open-ended, nonjudgmental approach (*e.g.*, "What do you think about smoking?").
2. Relate the short-term rather then long-term consequences of smoking (*e.g.*, early wrinkling of skin, yellow stains on teeth, fingers, tobacco odor on breath and clothing).
3. Emphasize the ostracization of smokers in society (*e.g.*, standing outside a building in the cold to smoke).
4. Direct to adults who smoke if they would like to quit.
5. Role play with a nonsmoker how to deal with peer pressure.
6. Discuss the hazards of smokeless tobacco (cancer of the mouth, tongue, tooth erosion and loss, foul breath).

Rationale

- Helping the adolescent appreciate that most smokers would like to quit may deter starting (Wong, 1995).
- Programs that focus on negative long-term effects of smoking are not effective with teenagers (Winklesteen, 1991).
- Teenagers are very preoccupied with appearance and peer acceptance (Wong, 1995).
- Smokeless tobacco is seen as less of a health hazard by children. The incidence of use has increased in school-age children (U.S. Department of Health and Human Services, 1994).

Interventions—*Maternal Focus*

1. Explain the adverse effects of smoking (Reeder, Martin, & Koniak, 1992).
   a. During pregnancy

   Crosses the placenta

   Reduces oxygen to the fetus

   Reduces transport of nutrients, calcium, glucose, hormones

Causes low birth weight
Causes stillbirths
Congenital deformities
  b. Infants, children
Allergies, otitis media
Bronchitis, asthma
Sudden infant death syndrome
2. If desired, establish a plan to decrease number of cigarettes smoked per day and, if possible, set a date for total cessation.
3. Approach relapses as temporary setbacks (O'Connor et al., 1992).
  a. Identify situations that lead to smoking.

Rationale

- Adverse effects of smoking are proportional to daily cigarettes smoked; therefore, any decrease is beneficial.

■ Altered Health Maintenance
Related to Increased Food Consumption in Response to Stressors and Insufficient Energy Expenditure for Intake

Outcome Criteria

The individual will
- Identify patterns of eating associated with consumption/energy expenditure imbalance
- Identify stressors and effective response patterns
- Describe the relationship among metabolism, intake, and exercise
- Commit to exercise program (specify type, amount)
- Commit to reduced caloric intake program (adults only)
- Commit to eating a balanced diet

Interventions

A. Assess for causative and contributing factors
  1. Lack of knowledge
    a. Balanced nutritional intake
    b. Exercise requirements
  2. Inappropriate response to external stressors
  3. Lack of initiative, motivation
  4. Imbalance in composition of foods (*e.g.*, excess fat or simple carbohydrate intake)
  5. Cultural, familial, genetic factors
  6. Poor eating habits (*e.g.*, eating out, eating on the run, skipping meals)
  7. Sedentary life-style or occupation, recent smoking cessation
  8. Sabotage by family or significant others

B. Increase awareness of components of intake/activity balance

1. Multiply female weight by 11 and male weight by 12 to determine calorie intake/day needed to maintain current weight.
2. One pound of fat is roughly equivalent to 3500 cal. To lose 2 lb/week, a person must cut 7000 cal from weekly intake or increase exercise caloric expenditure.
3. Exercise caloric expenditure charts may be used to determine amount of calories burned per duration increment of activity.
4. Weight-loss goals may be achieved through a combination of caloric intake reduction and energy expenditure (through exercise).
5. Successful weight reduction/maintenance is contingent on a balance of reduced caloric intake and caloric expenditure through exercise.

C. Assist client to identify realistic weight-loss program to fit his or her needs

1. Decide on amount of loss desired
2. Time and duration of program
3. Cost of various programs
4. Nutritional soundness of program
5. Compatibility with life-style

D. Assist client to anticipate environmental considerations

1. Friends, family, coworkers—what are their habits? Would they be supportive?
2. What types of foods are found in the home? At parties? At work? In the lunch room?
3. What types of leisure/recreational activities are engaged in? Is person sedentary?
4. What routes are taken to work? Does client pass by fast-food establishments?
5. Who does the housework? Gardening? Yard? Errands?
6. How much television is watched? Do commercials trigger eating?
7. Has person responded to gimmick advertisements for rapid weight loss (*e.g.*, "sleep away," belts, garments, wraps, lotions)?

E. Assist to self-assess present eating/exercise habits by keeping a diary for a week, including usual

1. Food intake/exercise
2. Location/time of meals
3. Emotions around meal time
4. People client eats with
5. Skipped meals
6. Snacks

F. Familiarize with cues that often trigger eating

1. Eating while doing another activity (*e.g.*, watching TV)
2. Eating standing up (*e.g.*, can give illusion of not eating)
3. Eating out of boredom or stress
4. Eating because everyone else is eating

G. Teach basics of balanced nutritional intake, including supportive measures

1. Choose a diet plan that encourages high intake of complex carbohydrates and limited fat intake.
2. Know what you are eating. The "basic four" label is misleading (*e.g.*, a chicken-fried steak is a protein converted to high fat content through its preparation [frying]).

3. Attempt to obtain more calories from fruits and vegetables instead of meat and dairy products.
4. Eat more chicken and fish because they contain less fat and fewer total calories than beef. Remove fat and skin.
5. Be aware of salad toppings and especially dressings with mayonnaise (216–308 calories per 2-oz serving).
6. Completely avoid fast foods, because they have high fat and total caloric content.
7. Dine in or make special requests in restaurants for food selection/preparations (*e.g.*, salad dressing on side, omit sauce from entree).
8. Plan meals in advance.
9. If attending a party or restaurant, decide what you will eat ahead of time and stick to it.
10. Adhere to grocery list.
11. Involve family in meal planning for better nutrition.
12. Buy the highest-quality beef. Ground round = 10% fat; hamburger = 25% fat.
13. Choose a variety of foods.
14. Avoid serving family-style.
15. Drink 8–10 8-oz glasses of water daily.
16. Measure foods and count calories; keep records.
17. Read labels on foods and note food composition and calories per serving.
18. Eat slowly.
19. Experiment with spices, substitutes, and low-calorie recipes.

H. Discuss benefits of exercise
   1. Reduces caloric absorption
   2. Is an appetite suppressant
   3. Increases metabolic rate
   4. Preserves lean muscle mass
   5. Increases oxygen uptake
   6. Improves self-esteem
   7. Decreases depression, anxiety, and stress
   8. Increases caloric expenditure
   9. Increases the odds for weight-loss maintenance
   10. Increases restful sleep
   11. Improves body posture
   12. Provides fun, recreation, and diversion
   13. Increases resistance to degenerative diseases of middle/later years (*e.g.*, heart, blood vessels)

I. Assist client to identify realistic exercise program to fit his or her needs, considering
   1. Personality, life-style
   2. Time factor, time of day
   3. Season—anticipate and plan
   4. Sedentary/active occupation
   5. Safety (*e.g.*, sports injuries, environmental hazards)
   6. Costs—club membership, equipment
   7. Age, physical size, physical condition

J. Monitor or discuss getting started on the exercise program
   1. Start slow and easy. Obtain clearance from physician.
   2. Choose activities using many parts of the body.
   3. Choose an activity that is vigorous enough to cause "healthful fatigue."
   4. Read, consult experts, talk with friends/coworkers who exercise.

5. Plan a daily walking program and gradually increase rate and length of walk.
   a. Start out at 5–10 blocks for 0.5–1.0 mile/day; increase 1 block or 0.1 mile/week.
   b. Remember, progress slowly.
   c. Avoid straining or pushing too hard and becoming overly fatigued.
   d. Stop immediately if any of the following signs occur:

Lightness or pain in chest	Dizziness
Severe breathlessness	Loss of muscle control
Lightheadedness	Nausea

   e. If pulse is 120 beats/minute (bpm) 5 minutes after stopping exercise, 100 bpm 10 minutes after stopping exercise, or if short of breath 10 minutes after exercise, slow down either the rate of walking or the distance.
   f. If unable to walk 5 blocks or 0.5 mile without signs of overexertion appearing, decrease length of walking for 1 week to point before signs appear and then start to add 1 block/0.1 mile each week.
   g. Walk at same rate; time self with stopwatch or second hand on watch; after reaching 10 blocks (1 mile), try to increase speed.
   h. Remember, increase only the rate or the length of walk at one time.
   i. Establish a regular time of day to exercise, with the goal of three to five times/week for a duration of 15–45 minutes and with a heart rate of 80% of stress test or gross calculation (170 bpm for 20–29-year-old age group; decrease 10 bpm for each additional decade of life, *e.g.*, 160 bpm for ages 30–39 years, 150 bpm for ages 40–49 years).
6. Encourage significant others also to engage in walking program.
7. Add supplemental activity (*e.g.*, park far away, work on garden, walk up stairs, spend weekends at leisure activities, such as festivals or art fairs, that require walking).
8. Work up to 1 hour of exercise per day at least 4 days per week.
9. Avoid lapses of more than 2 days between exercise days.

K. Teach about the risks of obesity
   1. Vascular insufficiency
   2. Arteriosclerosis, heart disease, hypertension
   3. Left ventricular hypertrophy
   4. Diabetes mellitus, gallbladder disease
   5. Increased risk of complications of surgery
   6. Respiratory disease
   7. Joint degeneration
   8. Increased risk of cancer (*e.g.*, breast)
   9. Increased risk of accident/injury

L. Assist to increase interest and motivation in weight reduction/exercise program
   1. Develop contract listing realistic short- and long-term goals.
   2. Keep intake/activity records.
   3. Hang an admired photograph on the refrigerator.
   4. Get family involved in project.
   5. Record body measurements and limit weighing to once per week.
   6. Increase knowledge by reading and talking with health-conscious friends and coworkers.
   7. Make new friends who are health conscious.
   8. Get a friend to go on program too or be a central support.
   9. Avoid people who may sabotage attempts.
   10. Reward self on a regular basis.
   11. Remind self that self-image and behavior are learned and can be unlearned.

12. Build a support system of people who value growth and value you as an individual.
13. Be aware of rationalization (*e.g.*, a lack of time may be a lack of prioritization).
14. Keep a list of positive outcomes.

M. Reduce inappropriate responses to stressors
   1. Teach to distinguish between urge and hunger.
   2. Use distraction, relaxation, imagery.
   3. Use alternative response training.
      a. Make a list of external cues/situations that lead to off-target behavior.
      b. List what you can do constructively instead of indulging in off-target behavior when this occurs (*e.g.*, take a walk).
      c. Post the list of alternate behaviors on the refrigerator.
      d. Reevaluate whether plan is realistic and effective every 1–2 weeks.

N. Assist to plan for life-long weight maintenance
   1. Understand issues of dependency, control, and esteem.
   2. Decide on *your* plan for *your* control.
   3. Set realistic short- and long-term goals: revise as necessary.
   4. Think positively, start slowly.
   5. Give self credit for each achievement; avoid perfectionism.
   6. Build healthy support system.

O. Initiate health teaching and referrals, as indicated
   1. Refer to support groups (*e.g.*, Weight Watchers, Overeaters Anonymous, TOPS, trim clubs, The Diet Workshop, Inc.).
   2. Consult dietitian for meal planning.
   3. Consult physician for morbid obesity and evaluation of other health problems.

Rationale

- Intake must be reduced to 500 cal/day less than requirement to obtain a 1 lb/week weight loss. The desirable weight loss rate is 1–2 lb/week.
- An American's diet currently consists of 42% fat, 12% protein, 22% complex carbohydrates, and 24% simple carbohydrates. Recommended U.S. dietary goals are 30% fat, 12% protein, 48% complex carbohydrates, and 10% simple carbohydrates (*Healthy People 2000*).
- Any increase in activity increases energy output and increases caloric deficits of a person following a dietary regimen.
- Often, obesity is facilitated/aggravated by inappropriate response to external cues, including, most often, stressors. This response sets off an ineffective pattern whereby the individual eats in response to stress cues rather than physiologic hunger.
- The safest activities for the unconditioned obese person are walking, water aerobics, swimming, and cycling.
- A regular exercise program should
  - Be enjoyable
  - Use a minimum of 400 calories in each session
  - Sustain a heart rate of approximately 120–150 beats/minute
  - Involve rhythmic, alternating contracting and relaxing of muscles
  - Be integrated into the person's life-style 4–5 days/week (at least 30–60 minutes)
- Before beginning an exercise program, the person must consider
  - Physical limitations (consult nurse or physician)

- Personal preferences
- Life-style
- Community resources
- What clothing is needed (shoes)
- How to monitor pulse before, during, and after exercise

- The person is taught to monitor his pulse before, during, and after exercise to assist him to achieve his target heart rate and not to exceed his maximum advisable heart rate for his age.

Age	Maximum Heart Rate	Target Heart Rate
30	190	133–162
40	180	126–153
50	170	119–145
60	160	112–136

Interventions—*Child Focus*

1. Assist the child and family to realize the shared responsibility of weight control.
2. Assist the child to identify habits or behaviors that contribute to overeating.
3. Elicit how weight has been a problem for the child.
   a. Sports
   b. Peers
4. Advise to avoid calories restriction diets.
5. Teach how to adjust eating by (Copeland & Baucon-Copeland, 1981):
   a. Reducing the quantity of eating
   b. Improve the quality (*e.g.*, substitute a low-calorie food like pretzels for high-calorie foods like chips).
   c. Reduce associations between eating and other stimuli, such as eating while watching TV.
6. Emphasize that regular physical exercise is necessary for successful long-term weight loss.
7. Encourage the entire family to eat the healthy foods, with emphasis on reduced portions for those needing weight reduction.
8. Initiate referrals as indicated.
   a. If desired, enlist the help of the school nurse (*e.g.*, weigh-ins, support).
   b. Consider summer camps for overweight teens.
   c. Make use of community resources (*e.g.*, adolescent support groups).

Rationale

- Sharp reductions in calories, which can result in large losses of lean body mass in children, should be avoided (Wong, 1995).
- Substituting high-fat and high-calorie foods with healthy, low-fat and low-calorie choices while the child grows into his or her weight prevents an increase in body fat (Copeland & Baucon-Copeland, 1981).
- "The most successful diets are those that use ordinary foods in controlled portions rather than diets that require the avoidance of any specific foods" (Wong, 1995, p. 900).

References/Bibliography

Belloc, N., & Breslow, L. (1972). The relation of physical health status and health practice. *Preventive Medicine, 1,* 409–421.

Boyle, J., & Andrews, M. (1994). *Transcultural concepts in nursing* (2nd ed.). Glenview, IL: Scott, Foresman.

Capra, F. (1982). *The turning point.* New York: Bantam Books.

Dunn, H. L. (1959). What high-level wellness means. *Canadian Journal of Public Health, 50,* 447–457.

Edelman, C. L., & Mandle, C. L. (1990). *Health promotion throughout the lifespan.* St. Louis: Mosby-Year Book.

Flynn, P. A. (1980). *Holistic health: The art and science of care.* Bowie, MD: Robert J. Brady.

Hanson, S. M., & Boyd, S. T. (1996). *Family health care nursing: Theory, practice and research*. Philadelphia: W. B. Saunders.

Tripp-Reimer, T., & Lively, S. (1988). Cultural considerations in therapy. In C. K. Beck, R. P. Rawlins, & S. Williams (Eds.). *Mental health–psychiatric nursing*. St. Louis: C. V. Mosby.

U. S. Department of Health and Human Services, Public Health Service. *Healthy people 2000*. Washington, DC: U.S. Government Printing Office.

U. S. Department of Health and Human Services. (1994). *Clinician's handbook of preventive services*. Washington, DC: U.S. Government Printing Office.

Gerontologic

Abrams, W. B., & Berkow, R. (Eds.). (1990). *The Merck manual of geriatrics*. Rahway, NJ: Merck & Co.

Fleg, J. L. (1986). Alterations in cardiovascular structure and function with advancing age. *American Journal of Cardiology, 57*, 33C–44C.

Matteson, M. A., & McConnell, E. S. (1988). *Gerontological nursing: Concepts and practices*. Philadelphia: W. B. Saunders.

Miller, C. A. (1995). *Nursing care of older adults* (2nd ed.). Glenview, IL: Scott, Foresman.

Posner, J. D., Gorman, K. M., Klein, H. S., & Woldow, A. (1986). *American Journal of Cardiology, 57*, 52C–58C.

Schneider, E. L. (1983). Infectious diseases in the elderly. *Annals of Internal Medicine, 98*, 395–400.

U.S. Department of Health and Human Services. (1987). *Current estimates for the national health interview survey*. Hyattsville, MD: Author.

Tobacco Use

Ash, C. R. (1987). Smoking and lung cancer. *Cancer Nursing, 10*(4), 171.

Cinelli, B., & Glover, E. (1988). Nurses' smoking in the work-place: Causes and solutions. *Journal of Community Health Nursing, 5*, 255–261.

Institute of Medicine. (1985). *Preventing low birthweight*. Committee to Study the Prevention of Low Birthweight, Division of Health Promotion and Disease Prevention. Washington, DC: National Academy Press.

Koepke, D., Flay, B., & Johnson, C. A. (1990). Health behaviors in minority families: The case of cigarette smoking. *Family and Community Health, 13*, 35–43.

McAndrew, M. (1994). People who depend on substances other than alcohol. In E. M. Varcarolis (Ed.). *Foundations of psychiatric–mental health nursing*. Philadelphia: W. B. Saunders.

Novella, A. C. (1990). Surgeon General's report on the health benefits of smoking cessation. *Public Health Reports, 105*, 545–548.

O'Connor, A., Davies, B., Dulberg, C., Buhler, P., Nadon, C., McBride, B., & Benzie, R. (1992). Effectiveness of a pregnancy smoking cessation program. *Journal of Obstetric, Gynecologic, and Neonatal Nursing, 21*, 385–392.

U.S. Department of Health and Human Services. (1986). *The health consequences of involuntary smoking: A report of the Surgeon General*. DHHS (CDC) Publication No. 87-8398. Washington, DC: U.S. Government Printing Office.

U.S. Department of Health and Human Services. (1994). *Preventing tobacco use among young people: A report of the surgeon general*. Washington, DC: U.S. Government Printing Office.

Winklesteen, M. (1991). Adolescent smoking: Influential factors, past preventive efforts and future nursing interventions. *Pediatric Nursing, 7*, 120–127.

Young, E. W., Koch, P. B., & Mauger, J. L. (1988). Smokeless tobacco: Substituting the spittoon for the ashtray. *Journal of Community Health Nursing, 5*, 167–176.

Obesity

See *Altered Nutrition: Less Than Body Requirements* for additional sources of information.

Bal, D. G., & Foester, S. B. (1991). Changing the American diet: Impact on cancer prevention policy recommendations and program implications for the American Cancer Society. *Cancer, 67*, 2671–2680.

Copeland, E. T., & Baucon-Copeland, S. (1981). Childhood obesity: A family system views. *American Family Physician, 24*, 153–155.

Fleury, J. D. (1991). Empowering potential: A theory of wellness motivation. *Nursing Research, 40*, 286–291.

Jeffery, R. W. (1991). Population perspectives on the prevention and treatment of obesity in minority populations. *American Journal of Clinical Nutrition, 53*(6 Suppl), 1621S–1624S.

Pencak, M. (1991). Workplace health promotion programs: An overview. *Nursing Clinics of North America, 26*, 233–240.

Reeder, S., Martin, L., & Koniak, D. (1992). *Maternity nursing: Family, newborn, and women's health care* (17th ed.). Philadelphia: J. B. Lippincott.

Osteoporosis

Bellantoni, M. F., & Blackman, M. R. (1988). Osteoporosis: Diagnostic screening and its place in current care. *Geriatrics, 43*(2), 63–70.

Chestnut, C. H. (1984). Treatment of postmenopausal osteoporosis. *Comprehensive Therapy, 10*(7), 41–47.

Lindsay, R. (1989). Osteoporosis: An updated approach to prevention and management. *Geriatrics, 44*(1), 45–54.

Miller, C. A. (1995). *Nursing care of older adults* (2nd ed.). Glenview IL: Scott, Foresman.

Riggs, L. B., & Melton, L. J. (1986). Involutional osteoporosis. *New England Journal of Medicine, 314*, 1676–1685.

Pediatric

Farrow, J. A. (1991). Youth alienation as an emerging pediatric health care issue. *American Journal of Diseases of Children, 145*, 491–492.

Hunsberger, M. (1989). Impact of acute illness. In R. L. Foster, M. M. Hunsberger, & J. J. T. Anderson (Eds.). *Family-centered nursing care of children*. Philadelphia: W. B. Saunders.

Scipien, G. M., Chard, M. A., Howe, J., & Barnard, M. U. (1990). *Pediatric nursing care*. St. Louis: C. V. Mosby.

Wong, D. L. (1995). *Nursing care of infants and children* (5th ed.). St. Louis: Mosby-Yearbook.

Resources for the Consumer

Billigmeier, S. B. (1991). *Inner eating: How to free yourself forever from the tyranny of food*. Nashville: Thomas Nelson Publishers.

Hirshmann, J. R., & Munter, C. H. (1989). *Overcoming overeating*. New York: Addison-Wesley.

Organizations

American Cancer Society, American Dental Association, American Heart Association, American Lung Association

---

Health-Seeking Behaviors

DEFINITION

Health-Seeking Behaviors: The state in which an individual in stable health actively seeks ways to alter personal health habits and/or the environment in order to move toward a higher level of wellness.*

DEFINING CHARACTERISTICS
Major (Must Be Present)

Expressed or observed desire to seek information for health promotion

Minor (May Be Present)

Expressed or observed desire for increased control of health
Expression of concern about current environmental conditions on health status
Stated or observed unfamiliarity with wellness community resources
Demonstrated or observed lack of knowledge in health-promotion behaviors

RELATED FACTORS
Situational (Personal, Environmental)

Related to anticipated role changes (specify)
    Marriage   "Empty-nest" syndrome
    Parenthood   Retirement
Related to lack of knowledge of:
    Preventive behavior (disease)   Regular exercise program
    Screening practices for age and risk   Constructive stress management
    Optimal nutrition and weight control   Supportive social networks

Maturational

See Table II-12 for age-related situations.

Author's Note

See *Altered Health Maintenance*

---

* Stable health status is defined as age-appropriate illness prevention measures are achieved, client reports good or excellent health, and signs and symptoms of disease, if present, are controlled.

Key Concepts

1. A major focus of nursing care is to promote effective health-seeking behaviors in clients. Nursing activities that promote health-seeking behaviors include nurturing, encouraging, teaching, communicating, and providing (Nyamathi, 1989).

2. According to Nyamathi (1989), "The health goals of the client and desired goals of the nurse are mutually concerned with enhancing the individual's motivation to attain and maintain health and function, to avoid disease and disability, and to attain or retain the highest possible level of health, function or productivity."

3. Adequate dietary intake of complex carbohydrates, found in grains, fruits, legumes, and vegetables, improves human health in many ways (*e.g.*, decreasing the incidence of obesity, cardiovascular disease, cancer, malnutrition, diabetes, and dental caries). Current recommendations advise an increase in total dietary carbohydrates to 55% of daily calories and a reduction of total simple sugars (concentrated nonnutritive sweets) to only 10% of daily calories.

4. Recent studies prove that the risk of heart disease can be reduced by decreasing serum cholesterol through diet and drugs, if necessary (American Heart Association, 1989).

   a. Recommended dietary changes (to reduce serum cholesterol) include:

   A decrease in total fats, saturated fats, and cholesterol

   In overweight people, reduced daily caloric intake to attain desired body weight (Ernst & Cleeman, 1989)

   Increased intake of nutrients that may help decrease the risk of cardiovascular disease (*e.g.*, oat bran and other water-soluble fibers, fruit gums, vegetables, garlic, polyunsaturated fats, olive oil, legumes, and fatty fish)

   b. Many people find it difficult to maintain health-seeking diets even when they have been successful. Examples of helpful approaches include behavioral contracts (Neale, Singleton, Dupius, & Hess, 1989), positive self-talk (Kayman, 1989), and strengthening family supports (Torisky, Hertzler, Johnson, Keller, Hodges, & Mifflin, 1989).

   c. Risk factors for cardiovascular disease include (Ernst & Cleeman, 1989):

   Male gender

   Family history of myocardial infarction or sudden death in parent or sibling younger than then 55 years of age

   Smokes more than 10 cigarettes/day

   Hypertension

   High-density lipoprotein cholesterol level less than 35 mg/dL

   History of definite occlusive vascular disease (peripheral or cerebral)

   Morbid obesity (greater than 30% overweight).

   d. Guidelines for cholesterol screening are (Ernst & Cleeman, 1989):

   Less than 200 mg/dL: Desirable

   200–239 mg/dL: Borderline high

   240 mg/dL and over: High blood cholesterol

   For all readings over 200 mg/dL, the test should be repeated within 8 weeks, along with lipoprotein analysis and medical follow-up.

   e. Dietary recommendations for children older than age 2 years include (American Heart Association, 1990):

   Provide a variety of foods daily

   Maintain desirable body weight

   Limit total dietary fat to 30% of calories

   Limit total daily cholesterol to 100 mg/1000 calories and not more than 300 mg/day

   Limit daily protein intake to 15% of calories

   Limit daily carbohydrate intake to 55% of calories

   Limit sodium intake by reducing processed foods and keeping salt shaker off the table

5. There has been much research on both animals and human beings that suggests a link between nutrition and cancer; some nutrients act as promoters of carcinogens, others are protectors against cancer (Whitney, Cataldo, & Rolfes, 1987).

a. Dietary behaviors associated with cancer include high consumption of fats (all types), vitamin A deficiency, excessive use of nitrite-containing foods, consumption of cancer-producing chemicals through food chain (*e.g.*, pesticides, herbicides, radiation, toxic waste in water source), high intake of alcohol.

b. Dietary nutrients that protect against cancer include vegetable and grain fibers, vitamins A and C, cruciferous vegetables, and vegetables and fruits rich in carotene.

6. The exact relationship between dietary sodium and essential hypertension has yet to be unequivocally described. Studies show, however, that blood pressure in many (not all) clients with hypertension decreases when dietary sodium is restricted. All hypertensive people should be given a trial of a reduced sodium diet (2 g sodium/day.) If successful, continued dietary support is needed.

Key Concepts—*Child*

1. Children who are intrinsically motivated in health behavior reinforce their own sense of competency and self-determinism through the process of choosing and accomplishing positive health behaviors (Cox, 1990).

2. Children who are extrinsically motivated need interventions that are based on a program of external rewards for positive health behaviors (Cox, 1990).

Focus Assessment Criteria

Subjective Data

A. Assess for defining characteristics
1. Does the individual/family report good or excellent health?
2. Does the person/family desire to adopt a behavior to maximize health?

Outcome Criteria

The person will
• Describe screening that is appropriate for age and risk factors
• Perform self-screening for cancer
• Participate in a regular physical exercise program
• State an intent to use positive coping mechanisms and constructive stress management
• Agree with self-responsibility for wellness (physical, dental, safety, nutritional, family)

Interventions

A. Assess for factors that contribute to the promotion and the maintenance of health
1. Knowledge of disease and preventive behavior
2. Appropriate screening practices for age and risk
3. Good nutrition and weight control
4. Regular exercise program
5. Constructive stress management
6. Supportive social networks

B. Promote health behaviors in the person and the family
1. Determine the person's or family's knowledge or perception of
   a. Specific diseases (*e.g.*, heart disease, cancer, respiratory disease, childhood diseases, infections, dental disease)
   b. Susceptibility (*e.g.*, presence of risk factors, family history)

    c. Seriousness

    d. Value of early detection

2. Determine the person's or family's past patterns of health care.

    a. Expectations

    b. Interactions with health care system or providers

    c. Influences of family, cultural group, peer group, mass media

3. Provide specific information concerning screening for age-related conditions (see Table II-12).

4. Discuss the role of nutrition in health maintenance and the prevention of illness (see Key Concepts for *Altered Nutrition* for specific explanations).

    a. Basic four food groups

    b. Nutrient needs related to age, level of physical activity, pregnancy, and lactation

    c. The prudent use of

        Salt (see *Fluid Volume Excess* for foods high in sodium)

        Canned vegetables

        Fried foods

        Red meats

        Fats (butter, margarines)

        High-calorie desserts

        Snack foods (potato chips, candy, soda)

        Refined sugar

        Foods containing nitrosamines (smoked meats, preservatives)

    d. The generous use of health-promoting foods

        Cruciferous vegetables (broccoli, cabbage, cauliflower, Brussels sprouts)—protect against colorectal cancer

        High-fiber foods—protect against colorectal cancer

        Calcium-containing foods (*e.g.*, dairy, dark leafy vegetables)—protect against osteoporosis

    e. See *Altered Health Maintenance* for specific information concerning weight control.

5. Discuss the benefits of a regular exercise program.

    a. See Key Concepts for *Altered Health Maintenance* for the positive effects of a regular exercise program.

    b. Determine the optimal exercise for the individual, considering physical limitations, preferences, and life-style.

Walking briskly	Aerobic dancing
Jogging	Swimming
Running	Bicycling
Aerobic exercises	Skipping rope

    c. Stress the importance of beginning any physical activity slowly.

6. Discuss the elements of constructive stress management.

    a. Assertiveness training

    b. Problem solving

    c. Relaxation techniques

    d. See Appendix X for relaxation techniques and Appendix VII for guidelines for problem solving.

7. Discuss strategies for developing positive social networks.

    a. Relate the functions of a support system:

        Provide love and affection

        Share common social concerns

        Serve as buffers against life's stressors

        Prevent isolation

        Respect mutual pursuits of members

        Cooperate for the common purpose

        Provide dependable assistance (emotional and economic, if appropriate)

    b. Suggest methods for strengthening this system:

        Be supportive of others.

Practice active listening by allowing yourself to listen attentively to the other person, such as:

Don't interrupt the person.

Allow a few seconds to lapse between dialogue to provide time to gather thoughts and to reduce the "rush to speak."

c. Provide others with opportunities to share their concerns without judgment. Refrain from giving solutions to problems of others; rather, a discussion of options may be indicated (*e.g.*, "You have several options: You can quit your job, request a transfer, discuss the problem with your boss, or do nothing").

d. When confronted with a relationship problem, review the situation.

What is the problem?

Who/what is responsible for the problem?

What are the options?

What are the advantages and disadvantages of each option? (See Appendix VII for guidelines for problem-solving.)

e. Show love and mutual respect to significant others.

Show unconditional love to own children.

Provide encouragement to significant others facing a challenge.

Avoid criticism, punishment, excessive praise, or pampering.

Demonstrate genuine warmth and affection.

f. Practice mutual goal setting to direct common efforts, and reevaluate them periodically.

g. Offer sincere assistance to individuals to promote trust.

h. Build relationships with individuals and families who share common interests and values.

i. Recognize when additional assistance is needed.

Marital counseling	Health professional
Self-help groups	Religious affiliation

j. Allow oneself and each member of the family—children, spouse, parents—to enhance personal identity by pursuing individual interests (refer to *Altered Growth and Development* for age-related needs of children).

C. Initiate health teaching and referrals, as indicated

1. Review the daily health practices of the individual (adults, children).

   a. Dental care

   b. Food intake

   c. Fluid intake

   d. Exercise regimen

   e. Leisure activities

   f. Responsibilities in the family

   g. Use of

Tobacco	Alcohol
Salt, sugar, fat products	Drugs (over-the-counter, prescribed)

   h. Knowledge of safety practices

   Fire prevention

   Water safety

   Automobile (maintenance, seat belts, car seats, air bags)

   Bicycle

   Poison control

2. Suggest selective disease-preventing behaviors when appropriate.

   a. Skin cancers

   Avoid frequent sun exposure.

   Avoid tanning salons.

   Wear effective sunscreens and protective clothing.

   Plan outdoors activities for before 10 A.M. and after 2 P.M. During these hours, wear a hat and sunscreen.

b. Sexually transmitted diseases

Use barrier contraceptive methods.

Avoid casual sex.

Avoid high-risk partners (*e.g.*, history of multiple partners, does not use condoms).

c. AIDS

Use condoms.   Avoid use of contaminated needles.

Avoid high-risk sexual practices.

d. Hepatitis B

Hepatitis vaccine   Use of condoms

e. Hearing loss

Use ear protection routinely (*e.g.*, mowing lawn, around machinery).

Avoid loud music (*e.g.*, headphones).

Avoid prolonged exposure to loud noises.

Treat infections promptly.

f. Congenital deformities

Avoid the use of alcohol and drugs during pregnancy.

g. Oral cancers

Avoid tobacco chewing.

Avoid concurrent heavy use of alcohol and tobacco.

h. Lung cancers, chronic obstructive pulmonary disease

Avoid tobacco smoking.

Avoid chronic exposure to known inhalable carcinogens (*e.g.*, asbestos).

Include carotene-rich foods in diet (*e.g.*, yellow vegetables and fruits).

Avoid smoke-filled rooms; discourage smoking in your living and work spaces.

Routinely test home for radon.

i. Coronary artery disease

Avoid obesity.

Avoid tobacco use.

Practice stress management.

Exercise regularly.

Avoid dietary cholesterol and saturated fats, and reduce total dietary fats.

Maintain normal blood pressure.

Increase daily intake of water-soluble fibers in diet (*e.g.*, oat bran, fruit pectins, psyllium).

j. Stroke

Avoid tobacco use, especially if taking oral contraceptives.

Maintain normal blood pressure.

Avoid dietary cholesterol and saturated fats, and reduce total dietary fats.

k. Reye syndrome

Avoid aspirin products in children with viral infections.

l. Osteoarthritis

Avoid obesity.

Avoid repeated trauma to joints.

m. Osteoporosis for high-risk women (refer to *Altered Health Maintenance*)

Take vitamin D and calcium supplements.

Use hormone replacement therapy when advisable.

Exercise regularly.

Reduce intake of or abstain from caffeine, alcohol.

n. Colorectal cancer

Avoid chronic constipation.

Avoid foods containing nitrites (cured and smoked meats) and consume orange juice or other vitamin C-rich product with same meal when nitrites are included in diet.

Include generous amounts of cruciferous vegetables (*e.g.*, cabbage, broccoli, Brussels sprouts, cauliflower) and other sources of fiber in diet.

   o. Breast cancer
      Avoid high-fat diet.
   p. Gastroenteritis due to contaminated food
      Avoid foods prepared with raw egg.
      Avoid raw or incompletely cooked seafood, poultry, or meats.
      Avoid shellfish from polluted waters.
   q. Hematologic cancers
      Avoid consumption of fish from dangerously polluted waters (mercury, PCBs).
   r. Lyme disease
      Avoid tick-infested wooded or grassy areas during peak seasons (usually late
         spring, summer, early fall).
      If entering hazardous areas, wear long sleeves, hat, long pants with socks
         pulled over cuffs of pants. Light colors make ticks more visible.
      Use effective insect repellent on adults only.
      Search clothes, body, and pets for ticks after hiking in hazardous areas.
      Because deer ticks are the size of a dot, inspect all skin areas for reddened dots
         or rash. Have a physician or nurse evaluate the bite or rash.
3. Refer to selected nursing diagnoses for additional information on and assessment of
   a. Safety needs: see *Risk for Injury*
   b. Activity needs: see *Diversional Activity Deficit*
   c. Affiliative needs: see *Social Isolation*
   d. Parenting needs: see *Altered Parenting*
   e. Family needs: see *Altered Family Processes*
   f. Spiritual needs: see *Spiritual Distress*
   g. Sexual needs: see *Altered Sexuality Patterns*
   h. Self-care needs: see *Impaired Home Maintenance Management*
   i. Emotional needs: see *Ineffective Individual Coping; Anxiety; Fear; Grieving; Self-Concept Disturbance;* and *Powerlessness*

Rationale

- Health-seeking and coping behaviors are closely intertwined; nurses assist clients to maximize their abilities to handle stress throughout life (Nyamathi, 1989).
- The process of seeking and attaining positive life-style change is known as "empowering potential" (Fleury, 1991). Empowering potential occurs in three stages: appraising readiness, changing, and integrating change. As an individual strives to improve his health, he moves through a process of introspection, planning new, healthier activities, coping with barriers and setbacks, and ultimately absorbing these new behaviors into everyday life.
- The individual is responsible for choosing a healthy pattern of living. The nurse is responsible for explaining the choices (Edelman & Mandel, 1990).
- Healthy eating can prevent disease and decrease the complications of disease that cannot be prevented (Edelman & Mandel, 1990). A regular exercise program improves cardiovascular endurance, increases muscle strength and endurance, and lowers low-density lipoprotein cholesterol, triglyceride levels, blood pressure, and body fat (Edelman & Mandel, 1990).
- Social support is needed to maintain health and prevent disequilibrium (Edelman & Mandel, 1990).

References/Bibliography

General

See also References/Bibliography for *Altered Health Maintenance*

American Heart Association. (1989). *Cholesterol and your heart*. Dallas: National Center.

American Heart Association. (1990). *Help your heart: Children and cholesterol*. Philadelphia: American Heart Association.

Edelman, C. L., & Mandel, C. L. (1990). *Health promotion throughout the lifespan*. St. Louis: Mosby-Year Book.

Ernst, N., & Cleeman, J. (1989). Reducing high blood cholesterol levels: Recommendations from the National Cholesterol Education Program. *Journal of Nutrition Education, 20,* 23–29.

Fleury, J. D. (1991). Empowering potential: A theory of wellness motivation. *Nursing Research, 40*, 286–291.

Kayman, S. (1989). Applying theory from social psychology and cognitive behavioral psychology to dietary behavior change and assessment. *Journal of the American Dietetic Association, 89*, 191–193.

Neale, A., Singleton, S., Dupius, M., & Hess, J. Correlates of adherence to behavioral contracts for cholesterol reduction. *Journal of Nutrition Education, 21*, 221–225.

Nyamathi, A. (1989). Comprehensive health seeking and coping paradigm. *Journal of Advanced Nursing, 14*, 281–290.

Torisky, C., Hertzler, A., Johnson, J., Keller, J., Hodges, P., & Mifflin, B. (1990). Virginia EFNEP homemakers' dietary improvement and relation to selected family factors. *Journal of Nutrition Education, 21*, 249–257.

Whitney, E., Cataldo, C., & Rolfes, S. (1987). *Understanding normal and clinical nutrition.* St. Paul: West Publishing.

Pediatric

Cox, C. L. (1990). The health self-determinism index for children. *Research in Nursing and Health, 13*, 237–246.

Wong, D. (1995). *Nursing care of infants and children* (5th ed.). St. Louis: Mosby-Yearbook.

Home Maintenance Management, Impaired

DEFINITION

Impaired Home Maintenance Management: The state in which an individual or family experiences or is at risk to experience a difficulty in maintaining a safe, hygienic, growth-producing home environment.

DEFINING CHARACTERISTICS
Major (Must Be Present)

Expressions or observations of
Difficulty in maintaining home hygiene
Difficulty in maintaining a safe home
Inability to keep home up
Lack of sufficient finances

Minor (May Be Present)

Repeated infections
Infestations
Accumulated wastes
Unwashed cooking and eating equipment
Offensive odors
Overcrowding

RELATED FACTORS
Pathophysiologic

Related to compromised functional ability secondary to:
Chronic debilitating disease
Diabetes mellitus
Chronic obstructive pulmonary disease
Congestive heart failure
Cerebral vascular accident
Cancer
Arthritis
Multiple sclerosis
Muscular dystrophy
Parkinson's disease

Situational (Personal, Environmental)

Related to change in functional ability of (specify family member) secondary to:
  Injury (fractured limb, spinal cord injury)
  Surgery (amputation, ostomy)
  Impaired mental status (memory lapses, depression, anxiety–severe panic)
  Substance abuse (alcohol, drugs)
Related to unavailable support system
Related to loss of family member
Related to lack of knowledge
Related to insufficient finances

Maturational

(Infant)
Related to multiple care requirements secondary to:
  High-risk newborn
(Older Adult)
Related to multiple care requirements secondary to:
  Family member with deficits (cognitive, motor, sensory)

Author's Note

With the rising life expectancy and declining mortality rate, an increasing number of older adults are living in their homes. Eighty percent of people aged 65 years or older report one or more chronic diseases. Of adults aged between 65 and 74 years, only 20% report that they have activity limitations, and 15% are unable to perform at least one activity of daily living independently (U.S. Department of Health and Human Services, 1987).

The shift from health care primarily in the hospital to reduced lengths of stay has resulted in the discharge of many functionally compromised individuals to their homes. Often a false assumption is made that someone will assume the management of the household responsibilities until the individual has recovered.

Impaired Home Maintenance Management describes situations in which a person or family needs teaching, supervision, or assistance to manage care of the household. For the most part, assessment of the home environment and the person's functioning at home is best accomplished by a community health nurse. The nurse in the acute setting can make a referral for a home visit for assessment.

A nurse who diagnoses the need for teaching to prevent household problems may use the diagnosis *Risk for Impaired Home Maintenance Management related to insufficient knowledge of (specify)* to describe this situation.

Errors in Diagnostic Statements

Impaired Home Maintenance Management related to caregiver burnout

Caregiver burnout is not a sign or related factor for *Impaired Home Maintenance Management*. Caregiver burnout is associated with the diagnosis *Caregiver Role Strain*. *Impaired Home Maintenance Management* may also be present if the caregiver is overwhelmed with multiple responsibilities. In this situation, both diagnoses are needed because the interventions are different.

Key Concepts

1. Home care by professionals should be preventive, supportive, and therapeutic.
    a. *Preventive* measures include health education, home safety, and stress management.
    b. *Supportive* care can be legal, financial, nutritional, social, religious, and homemaking.
    c. *Therapeutic* care involves nursing, therapies (occupational, speech), dental, and medical.

🌀 *Key Concepts—Child*

1. Children are dependent on family members for managing home care (Foster, 1989).
2. Trends in the treatment of children with chronic illness or disability include home care, early discharge, focus on the developmental age of the child, and assessment of the strengths and uniqueness of the child (Wong, 1995).
3. Interventions are geared toward the family as a whole rather than merely toward the ill child (Foster, 1989).
4. High-risk graduates of neonatal intensive care units require technically complex home care. Discharge is planned as early as possible for cost containment and to help reduce the adverse effects of hospitalization on the infant and the family system (Baker, Kuhlmann, & Magliaro, 1989).

🏛 *Key Concepts—Older Adult*

1. Older people have a greater incidence of chronic disease, impaired function, and diminished economic resources, and a smaller social network than do younger people (Arling, 1987; Matteson & McConnell, 1988).
2. After age 75 years, most elderly people living in the community live alone. Of older people living alone, 60% own a home (Matteson & McConnell, 1988).
3. Functional ability includes activities of daily living (ADLs) and also instrumental activities of daily living (IADLs)—those skills needed to live independently (*e.g.*, procuring food, cooking, using the telephone, housekeeping, and handling finances). IADLs are integrally connected to physical and cognitive abilities (Kane & Kane, 1981; Kane, Orslander, & Abrass, 1984; Matteson & McConnell, 1988). The elderly person who lives alone is at great risk of being institutionalized if he cannot perform IADLs. There is a great possibility that there is no social network to meet these deficits (Hogstel, 1990).
4. Approximately 9 of 10 older people have one or more chronic health problems with differing effects on function (Hogstel, 1990).
5. Chronic conditions cause approximately 6 of 10 people older than age 75 years to limit their ADLs (Hogstel, 1990).
6. Along with diminished cognitive or physical ability, the older individual frequently has diminished financial resources, sporadic kin, or neighborhood social supports. The person also may live in substandard housing or housing that does not allow simple adaptation to meet individual physical or cognitive deficits (Matteson & McConnell, 1988; Schank & Lough, 1990).
7. In some cultures and some family structures, older adults can seek assistance in some areas of home management and still retain a feeling of independence. These individuals have determined that by choosing selective resources to meet their needs, they will be able to maintain independent living for a longer period of time (Arling, 1987; Schank & Lough, 1990).

Focus Assessment Criteria

Subjective Data

A. Assess for defining characteristics
    1. Assessment of individual function
       a. Housekeeping activities: ability to

Clean	Shop
Launder clothes	Prepare food

B. Assess for related factors
    1. Assessment of individual function
       a. Vision
           Adequate
           Corrected (date of last prescription)
           Complaints of

Blurriness	Difficulty in focusing
Loss of side vision	Inability to adjust to darkness

    b. Hearing
        Adequate
        Use of hearing aid (condition, batteries)
        Need to lip-read
    c. Thermal/tactile
        Adequate
        Altered sense of cold/hot
    d. Mental status
        Alert
        Drowsy
        Confused
        Oriented to time, place, events
        Complaints of
            Vertigo
            Altered sense of balance
            Orthostatic hypotension
    e. Mobility
        Ability to ambulate
            Around room   Around house
            Up and down stairs   Outside house
        Ability to travel
            Drive car (date of last reevaluation)   Get in and out of vehicles
            Use public transportation
        Devices
            Cane   Prosthesis
            Wheelchair   Condition of devices
            Walker   Competence in their use
        Shoes/slippers
            Proper fit   Nonskid soles
            Condition
    f. Self-care activities: ability to
        Dress and undress   Use the toilet
        Groom self   Eat
        Bathe
    g. Miscellaneous
        Drug therapy
            Type, dosage   Storage
            Labeling   Ability to self-medicate safely
        Communication: ability to
            Write   Contact emergency assistance
            Use phone
    h. Support system
        Help available from relatives, friends, neighbors
        Club or religious contacts
        Emergency help available

Objective Data

A. Assess for defining characteristics
    1. Assessment of housing
        a. Type (rent, own)
            Apartment   Single family house
            Duplex
        b. Appearance: presence of
            Insects (flies, roaches)   Unwashed cooking equipment
            Rodents/vermin   Accumulation of dirt, food wastes, or hygiene
            Offensive odors   wastes

  c. Physical facilities

Number of rooms for family members	Lighting
Toilet facilities (accessibility)	Water supply
Heating	Sewage disposal
Ventilation	Garbage disposal
Handrails (stairs)	Screens

  d. Safety

    Are there any adaptations that need to be made in the home for the individual?

      Better communication (telephone)

      Access (in and out of home, to rooms)

      Bathroom (*e.g.*, grab bar, bath bench, nonskid floors)

Refer to Focus Assessment Criteria for *Risk for Injury* for an assessment of hazards in the home.

  2. Assessment of home environment of children

    a. Provisions for play

      Appropriate play materials

      Safe play area (indoors, outdoors)

      Special place designated for child's possessions

    b. Stimulating environment

      Selected use of television (amount, type)

      Activities for age-related development (see *Altered Growth and Development*)

      Family time (meal, joint activities)

      Family outings

    c. Affectionate environment

Touching, holding	Conversations convey positive feelings
Speaks with pride about child	

Outcome Criteria

The person or caretaker will
- Identify factors that restrict self-care and home management
- Demonstrate the ability to perform skills necessary for the care of the home
- Express satisfaction with home situation

Interventions

The following interventions apply to many individuals with impaired home management, regardless of etiology.

A. Assess for causative or contributing factors

  1. Lack of knowledge

  2. Insufficient funds

  3. Lack of necessary equipment or aids

  4. Inability to perform household activities (illness, sensory deficits, motor deficits)

  5. Impaired cognitive functioning

  6. Impaired emotional functioning

B. Reduce or eliminate causative or contributing factors, if possible

  1. Lack of knowledge for home care

  a. Determine with the person and family the information needed to be taught and learned.

    Monitoring skills needed (pulse, circulation, urine)

    Medication administration (procedure, side effects, precautions)

Treatment/procedures

Equipment use/maintenance

Safety issues (*e.g.*, environmental)

Community resources

Follow-up care

Anticipatory guidance (*e.g.*, emotional and social needs of family, alternatives to home care)

   b. Initiate the teaching and give detailed written instruction.

   c. Refer to a community nursing agency for follow-up.

2. Lack of necessary equipment or aids

   a. Determine the type of equipment needed, considering availability, cost, and durability.

   b. Seek assistance from agencies that rent or loan supplies.

Teach the care and maintenance of supplies that increase length of use.

Consider adapting equipment to reduce cost.

3. Insufficient funds

   a. Consult with social service department for assistance.

   b. Consult with service organizations for assistance.

American Heart Association

The Lung Association

American Cancer Society

4. Inability to perform household activities

   a. Determine the type of assistance needed (*e.g.*, meals, housework, transportation) and assist the individual to obtain them.

Meals

Discuss with relatives the possibility of freezing complete meals that require only heating (*e.g.*, small containers of soup, stew, casseroles).

Determine the availability of meal services for ill people (Meals on Wheels, church groups).

Teach people about foods that are easily prepared and nutritious (*e.g.*, hard-boiled eggs).

Housework

Contract with an adolescent for light housekeeping.

Refer to community agency for assistance.

Transportation

Determine the availability of transportation for shopping and health care.

Request rides with neighbors to places they drive routinely.

5. Impaired mental processes

   a. Assess the ability of the individual safely to maintain a household.

   b. Refer to *Risk for Injury* related to lack of awareness of hazards.

   c. Initiate appropriate referrals.

6. Impaired emotional functioning

   a. Assess the severity of the dysfunction.

   b. Refer to *Ineffective Individual Coping* for additional assessment and interventions.

C. Initiate health teaching and referrals, as indicated

1. Refer to support groups (*e.g.*, stroke club, local Alzheimer's Association, American Cancer Society).

2. Refer to community nursing agency.

3. Refer to community agencies (*e.g.*, volunteer visitors, meal programs, homemakers, adult day care).

Rationale

- Discharge planning begins at admission, with the nurse determining the anticipated needs of the person and family after discharge: the individual's self-care ability, the availability of support, homemaker services, equipment needs, community nursing services, and therapy (physical, speech, occupational).

- The home environment must be assessed for safety before discharge: location of bathroom, access to water, cooking facilities, and environmental barriers (stairs, narrow doorways).
- In determining an individual's ability to care for himself at home, assess his ability to function and protect self. Consider such things as motor deficits, sensory deficits, and mental status.

References/Bibliography

Arling, G. (1987). Strain, social support and distress in old age. *Journal of Gerontology, 42,* 107–113.

Baker, K., Kuhlmann, T., & Magliaro, B. (1989). Homebound. *Nursing Clinics of North America, 24,* 655–664.

Foster, R. L. (1989). Principles and strategies of home care. In R. L. Foster, M. M. Hunsberger, & J. J. T. Anderson (Eds.). *Family-centered nursing care of children.* Philadelphia: W. B. Saunders.

Hogstel, M. O. (1990). *Geropsychiatric nursing.* St. Louis: C. V. Mosby.

Kane, R. A., & Kane, R. L. (1981). *Assessing the elderly: A practical guide to measurement.* Lexington, MA: Lexington Books.

Kane, R. L., Orslander, J. G., & Abrass, I. B. (1984). *Essentials of clinical geriatrics.* New York: McGraw-Hill.

Matteson, M. A., & McConnell, E. S. (1988). *Gerontological nursing.* Philadelphia: W. B. Saunders.

Schank, M. J., & Lough, M. A. (1990). Profile: Frail elderly women, maintaining independence. *Journal of Advanced Nursing, 15,* 674–682.

U.S. Department of Health and Human Services. (1987). *Current estimates for the national health interview survey.* Hyattsville, MD: Author.

Wong, D. L. (1991). Transition from hospital to home for children with complex medical care. *Journal of Pediatric Oncology Nursing, 8*(1), 3–9.

Wong, D. L. (1995). *Nursing care of infants and children* (5th ed.). St. Louis: Mosby-Yearbook.

Organizations

Alzheimer's Disease and Related Disorders Association, 70 East Lake Street, Chicago, IL 60601-5997.

American Cancer Society, 90 Park Avenue, New York, NY 10016.

American Parkinson Disease Association, 116 John Street, New York, NY 10038.

National Multiple Sclerosis Society, 205 East 42nd Street, New York, NY 10017.

National Parkinson Foundation, 1591 N.A. Ninth Avenue, Miami, FL 31316.

National Spinal Cord Injury Association, 369 Elliot Street, Newton Upper Falls, MA 02164.

Hopelessness

DEFINITION

Hopelessness: A sustained subjective emotional state in which an individual sees no alternatives or personal choices available to solve problems or to achieve what is desired and cannot mobilize energy on own behalf to establish goals.

DEFINING CHARACTERISTICS
Major (Must Be Present)

Expresses profound, overwhelming, sustained apathy in response to a situation perceived as impossible with no solutions (overt or covert).

Examples of expressions are:

"I might as well give up because I can't make things better."
"My future seems awful to me."
"I can't imagine what my life will be like in 10 years."
"I've never been given a break, so why should I in the future?"
"Life looks unpleasant when I think ahead."
"I know I'll never get what I really want."
"Things never work out how I want them to."
"It's foolish to want or get anything because I never do."
"It's unlikely I'll get satisfaction in the future."
"The future seems vague and uncertain."

Physiologic
   Slowed responses to stimuli
   Lack of energy
   Increased sleep

Emotional
   The hopeless person often has difficulty experiencing feelings, but may feel:
      Unable to seek good fortune, luck, or God's favor
      A lack of meaning or purpose in life
      "Empty or drained"
      A sense of loss and deprivation
      Helpless
      Incompetent
      Entrapped

Person exhibits
   Passiveness and a lack of involvement in care
   Decreased verbalization
   Decreased affect
   Lack of ambition, initiative, and interest
   "Giving up–given up complex"
   Inability to accomplish anything
   Pessimism
   Impaired interpersonal relationship
   Slowed thought processes
   Does not take responsibility for own decisions and life

Cognitive
   Decreased problem-solving and decision-making capabilities
   Deals with past and future, not here and now
   Decreased flexibility in thought processes
   Rigid (*e.g.*, all-or-none thinking)
   Lacks imagination and wishing capabilities
   Unable to identify or accomplish desired objectives and goals
   Unable to plan, organize, or make decisions
   Unable to recognize sources of hope
   Suicidal thoughts

Minor (May Be Present)

Physiologic
   Anorexia
   Weight loss

Emotional
   Person feels:

"A lump in his throat"	Overwhelmed (feels he just "can't . . .")
Discouraged with self and others	Loss of gratification from roles and
"At the end of his rope"	relationships
Tense	Vulnerable

Person exhibits
Poor eye contact; turns away from speaker; shrugs in response to speaker
Decreased motivation
Despondency
Sighing
Social withdrawal
Lack of initiative
Lack of involvement in self-care (may be cooperative in nursing care but offers little help to self)
Anorexia
Regression
Resignation
Depression
Cognitive
Decreased ability to integrate information received
Loss of time perception for past, present, and future
Decreased ability to recall from the past
Confusion
Inability to communicate effectively
Distorted thought perceptions and associations
Unreasonable judgment

RELATED FACTORS
Pathophysiologic

Any chronic or terminal illness can cause or contribute to hopelessness (*e.g.*, heart disease, kidney disease, cancer, AIDS).
Related to:
Failing or deteriorating physiologic condition
New and unexpected signs or symptoms of previous disease process
Prolonged pain, discomfort, weakness
Impaired functional abilities (walking, elimination, eating)

Treatment-Related
Related to:
Prolonged treatments (*e.g.*, chemotherapy, radiation) that cause discomfort
Prolonged treatments with no positive results
Treatments that alter body image (*e.g.*, surgery, chemotherapy)
Prolonged diagnostic studies that yield no significant results
Prolonged dependence on equipment for life support (*e.g.*, dialysis, respirator)
Prolonged dependence on equipment for monitoring bodily functions (*e.g.*, telemetry)

Situational (Personal, Environmental)
Related to:
Prolonged activity restriction (*e.g.*, fractures, spinal cord injury)
Prolonged isolation due to disease processes (*e.g.*, infectious diseases, reverse isolation for suppressed immune system)
Abandonment of or separation from significant others (parents, spouse, children, others), or isolation
Inability to achieve goals in life that one values (marriage, education, children)
Inability to participate in activities one desires (walking, sports, work)
Loss of something or someone valued (spouse, children, friend, financial resources)
Prolonged caretaking responsibilities (spouse, child, parent)
Exposure to long-term physiologic or psychological stress
Loss of belief in transcendent values/God
Stressful stimuli, major decisions

Maturational

Related to:
(Child)
>   Loss of caregiver
>   Loss of trust in significant other (parents, sibling)
>   Abandonment by caregivers
>   Loss of autonomy related to illness (*e.g.*, fracture)
>   Loss of bodily functions
>   Inability to achieve developmental tasks (trust, autonomy, initiative, industry)

(Adolescent)
>   Loss of significant other (peer, family)
>   Loss of bodily functions
>   Change in body image
>   Inability to achieve developmental task (role identity)

(Adult)
>   Impaired bodily functions, loss of body part
>   Impaired relationships (separation, divorce)
>   Loss of job, career
>   Loss of significant others (death of children, spouse)
>   Inability to achieve developmental tasks (intimacy, commitment, productiveness)

(Older Adult)
>   Sensory deficits
>   Motor deficits
>   Loss of independence
>   Loss of significant others, things
>   Inability to achieve developmental tasks (integrity)

Author's Note

Hopelessness describes a person who sees no possibility that his or her life will improve and maintains that no one can do anything to help. *Hopelessness* differs from *Powerlessness*, in that a hopeless person sees no solution to his problem or no way to achieve what is desired, even if he feels in control of his life. In contrast, a powerless person may see an alternative or answer to the problem, yet be unable to do anything about it because of lack of control or resources. Sustained feelings of powerlessness may lead to hopelessness. Hopelessness is commonly related to grief, depression, and suicide. For a person at risk for suicide, the nurse also should use the diagnosis *Risk for Suicide*.

Errors in Diagnostic Statements

Hopelessness related to AIDS

This diagnostic statement does not describe a situation that the nurse can treat. The statement should include specific factors that the person has identified as overwhelming, as in the following diagnostic statement: *Hopelessness related to recent diagnosis of AIDS and rejection by parents*.

Key Concepts
Hope

1. Hope is a multidimensional, dynamic human attribute (Notwotny, 1989).
2. Hope is an unconscious cognitive behavior that energizes and allows a person to act, achieve, and use crisis as an opportunity for growth. It activates the motivation system and defends against despair (Korner, 1970).
3. Hope is described as desires, wishes, and waiting for "the not yet hour" (Fromm, 1968).
4. Hope has been defined as any expectation greater than zero for achieving a given goal (Stotland, 1969).

5. Hope is a "common human experience in that it is a way of propelling self towards envisioned possibilities in everyday encounters with the world" (Parse, 1990).

6. Hope is future- and reality-oriented. A hopeful person wants a desired change in his current life. He feels that change is possible and that there is a way out of his difficulties.

7. Early childhood experiences influence a person's ability to hope. A person learns to hope if a trusting environment is promoted.

8. Hope is related to faith because many people experience hope by recognizing their reliance on higher powers to restore meaning and purpose in their lives.

9. Plummer (1988) found high indices of hope to be in individuals who have a relationship with a higher being, participate in religious services, and are able to control their immediate environment. Spiritual practices provide a source of hope (Herth, 1990).

10. Watson (1979) has identified hope as both a curative and a "carative" factor in nursing. Hope, along with faith and trust, provides psychic energy to draw on to aid in the curative process.

11. It has been observed that hope prolongs life in critical survival conditions, whereas a loss of hope often results in death (Korner, 1970).

12. A hoping person feels autonomous in making decisions about choices open to him.

13. Kübler-Ross (1975) observed that those who expressed hope coped more effectively during their difficult dying periods. She also noted that death occurred soon after these individuals stopped expressing hope.

14. A person's level of hope is directly related to his level of coping and vice versa (Herth, 1989; Davies, 1993). Christman (1990) found uncertainty and less hope to be associated with adjustment problems during radiation therapy.

15. Hope directly influences survival, response to therapy, and the quality of life (Engel, 1989).

16. According to Hickey (1986), "hope enables the living to continue on and the dying to die better." Gottschalk (1974) found high hope scores in clients to be correlated with survival and going home, versus hospitalization.

17. Notwotny (1989) identified six dimensions of hope: confidence in outcome, possibility of a future, relating to others, spiritual beliefs, emergence from within, and active involvement.

18. Owen (1989) found hopeful cancer patients able to set goals, be optimistic, redefine the future, find meaning in life, feel peaceful, and give out or use energy.

19. Miller (1989) studied 60 critically ill clients to determine hope-inspiring strategies; findings included:
    a. Thinking to buffer threatening perceptions
    b. Positive thinking
    c. Feelings that life has meaning and growth results from crises
    d. Beliefs and practices enabling transcendence of suffering
    e. Receiving from caregivers a constructive view of patient, expectations of patient's ability to manage difficulty, and confidence in therapy
    f. Sustaining relationships with loved ones
    g. Perception that one's knowledge and actions can affect an outcome
    h. Having desired activities and outcomes to attain
    i. Other specific coping behaviors that thwarted feelings of despair, including distraction and humor

20. Meaning and purpose in one's life gives one a sense of control (O'Connor, Wicher, & Germino, 1990).

21. Significant correlations have been found between one's perceived level of control and hope and information seeking.

22. Coward (1991) found self-transcendence to directly affect emotional well-being and emotional well-being to have a negative effect on illness distress in a study of 107 women with breast cancer.

23. It has been postulated that hope is a powerful resource that can promote wound healing through the electrochemical reaction that affects the autonomic, endocrine, and immune systems (Jackson, 1993).

Hopelessness

1. Hopelessness is an emotional state in which a person feels that life is too much to handle—that it is impossible. A person who lacks hope sees no possibility that his life will improve and no solution to problems. He believes that neither he nor others can do anything to help.

2. Hopelessness is related to despair, helplessness, doubt, grief, apathy, sadness, depression, and suicide; hopelessness is present- and past-oriented. It is a deenergizing state.

3. It has been observed that hope reflected in clients' drawings has a direct relationship to the clients' improvement, whereas a lack of hope is related to recurrence of disease. Therefore, a nurse can be helpful to clients in finding their resources of hope.

4. The presence of cancer has been significantly predicted in individuals on the basis of identifying the presence of hopelessness in the person's life before the diagnosis of cancer. Therefore, terminal illness may result in hopelessness, and a life state of hopelessness may result in terminal illness (Schmale & Iher, 1966).

5. Hopelessness results in three basic categories of feelings:
   a. Sense of the impossible; what the person feels he must do, he cannot; he feels trapped
   b. Overwhelmed; tasks and others are perceived as too big and difficult to handle and the self is perceived as small
   c. Apathy; the person has no goals; no sense of purpose

6. Hopeless people lack internal resources or strengths (*e.g.*, autonomy, self-esteem, integrity) to draw on. Regardless of age, they reach outside themselves for help because their internal resources may be depleted.

7. Some degree of hopelessness is involved in everyone's life. It occurs in various forms and is a more common and usual feeling than reported (*e.g.*, we all must die; it is hopeless to hope for anything else).

8. Hopelessness is most often observed in those who are rigid and inflexible in their thoughts, feelings, and actions.

9. Often people have ideals that are hopeless in reality (*e.g.*, not to die, we can trust everyone, all people should always act appropriately).

10. Engel (1989) identified the "giving up–given up" complex as having five characteristics:
    a. Feeling of giving up experienced as helplessness or hopelessness
    b. Depreciated image of the self
    c. Sense of loss of gratification from relationships or roles
    d. Feeling of disruption
    e. Reactivation of memories of earlier periods of giving up
    Engel proposed that this state of coping activates neurally regulated biologic emergency patterns, which may decrease one's capacity to fight off pathogenic processes. Therefore, the "giving up–given up" complex is a contributing factor for development of disease.

11. Often when a person's internal and external resources are exhausted, he relies on his relationship with God for hope. He may feel more secure in placing hope in God than in other people or himself. Hoping in God may not mean an abrupt end to crisis, but gives the person a sense of God's control of circumstances and ability to support a person during this time. Meaning and purpose for life and suffering may be found in a client's relationship with God and the knowledge of His control. Hope for a client's future may depend on his perception of a promise of eternal fellowship with God that continues after this present life on earth ends. With this eternal relationship with God comes the belief in God's promise to end all suffering and restore harmonious relationships—man with God, himself, and others.

12. Hope and hopelessness are not mutually exclusive. Hope is not the complete absence of hopelessness (LeGresley, 1991).

🌹 *Key Concepts—Child*

1. Hope may be fostered in children by consistent nurturing, trustworthiness, and achievement of hoped-for things and events (Drew, 1990).

2. Families of children with life-threatening diseases may feel hopeless and become dysfunctional. The nurse may need to identify dysfunctional family interactions, use strategies from family therapy, or make appropriate referrals.

3. Hinds (1984) introduced a definition of hope for adolescents through the use of grounded theory methodology. Hope was defined as the degree to which an adolescent believes that a personal tomorrow exists.

4. To achieve adulthood, an adolescent must first achieve hopefulness. Hinds and Martin (1988) found that adolescents with cancer progress through four sequential, self-sustaining phases to cope and achieve hopefulness:
   a. Cognitive discomfort
   b. Distraction
   c. Cognitive comfort
   d. Personal competence
   These phases have implications for nurses in planning appropriate strategies to assist the adolescent achieve hopefulness.

5. Hinds (1988) identified that adolescent hopefulness differs from adult hopefulness in that adolescents experience a wider range or greater intensity of hopefulness. In addition, adolescents usually focus on hope for others and believe in the value of forced effort—that is, identifying an area of hope and fostering it.

6. Nursing interventions that have been found to influence hopefulness in adolescents include truthful explanations, doing something with them, nursing knowledge of survivors, caring behaviors, focusing on future, competency, and conversing about less sensitive areas. In addition, humor has been identified as promoting cognitive distraction and facilitating hope. Nursing interventions that inhibit cognitive distraction, such as focusing on nursing tasks and on negative adolescent behaviors, promote hopelessness (Hinds, Martin, & Vogel, 1987).

🏛 *Key Concepts—Older Adult*

1. The older adult is at risk for hopelessness because of the numerous psychosocial and physiologic changes that are part of the normal aging process (McGill, 1992). These changes often are perceived as losses. The older adult also has decreased energy, which is necessary for hopefulness.

2. Healthy coping in the older adult is related to the acquisition of developmental resources in later adulthood. The older adult must learn to give up less useful operations and acquire more effective resources to deal with life changes, which is part of the aging process (Reed, 1986).

3. Stressors for the older adult are unique and differ from those of other age groups. These include changes in personal care, longing for missing children or grandchildren, fear of being a victim of crime, and fear of being taken advantage of by the "system." The nurse may be able to assist the elderly client with identifying these stressors and locating resources to assist the client with preventing hopelessness.

TRANSCULTURAL CONSIDERATIONS

1. Cultural differences concerning values, expectations, and locus of control may be misinterpreted by the nurse who subscribes to the dominant American culture. A nurse who misdiagnoses the client as hopeless may not actively intervene—"Why even try?" (Leininger, 1978).

2. The concept of hopelessness may not be relevant to some cultures that are not future oriented. Hopelessness focuses on an inability to achieve goals, which is more future oriented.

Focus Assessment Criteria

Hopelessness is a subjective emotional state that the nurse must validate with the individual. Emotional and cognitive areas must be assessed carefully by the nurse to make the inference that the person is experiencing hopelessness. Some of these same cues may be seen in people with diagnoses of *Social Isolation, Powerlessness, Self-Concept Disturbance, Spiritual Distress*, or *Ineffective Coping*. The Herth Hope Scale is a tool that can be used to determine the level of hope in adult clients of varied ages and with different levels of illness (Herth, 1992).

Subjective Data

A. Assess for defining characteristics
　　1. Activities of daily living
　　　　a. Exercise: amount, type
　　　　b. Sleep: time, amount, quality
　　　　c. Hobbies: self-interest activities
　　　　d. Self-care participation: grooming habits
　　　　e. Appetite: eating habits
　　2. Energy and motivation
　　　　a. Does the person feel exhausted, tired?
　　　　b. Does the person have any goals or desires?
　　　　c. What are these goals and desires? Are they realistic?
　　　　d. Does this person feel he can achieve them?
　　　　e. Does this person feel overwhelmed?
　　　　f. What does he feel he can achieve?
　　　　g. Does he express an interest in self-care?
　　　　h. Does he express an interest in social activities?
　　　　i. Does he express an interest in any activities?
　　3. Meaning and purpose in life
　　　　a. What does this person value most in life? Why?
　　　　b. Is he able to achieve this value?
　　　　c. What does this person describe as his purpose or role in life?
　　　　d. Is this purpose/role fulfilled?
　　　　e. What in life has the most meaning to this person?
　　　　f. Is this available to this person at this time?
　　　　g. Are his perceptions of his meaning and purpose realistic or achievable?
　　　　h. What kind of relationship does he have with God or a higher being?
　　　　i. Does this relationship give meaning or purpose to his life?
　　　　j. What does this illness mean to the person?
　　　　k. What has changed most in his life since he has had this illness?
　　4. Choice or control in situations
　　　　a. What does he perceive as his most difficult problem? Why?
　　　　b. What does he feel the solution to the problem is? Is this solution realistic?
　　　　c. What kind of problem-solving or decision-making skills does this person have? Planning skills? Organizing skills?
　　　　d. Is his perception of the problem distorted? If so, how?
　　　　e. Have other alternatives to his problem been considered or tried?
　　　　f. Does this person feel he has any controlling influence in the situation?
　　　　g. How flexible or rigid are this person's thought processes?
　　5. Future options
　　　　a. What does the person believe the future will bring? Negative or positive things?
　　　　b. Does this person look forward to the future? What does he say about his past?
　　　　c. What does he see as worth living for?
　　　　d. How does the future look to this person?
　　　　e. How does this person perceive his present illness? Its effect on his life? Its effect on his relationships?
　　　　f. How does this person perceive his current treatments for his illness? Promising, or stressful and useless?
　　　　g. Does this person recognize any sources of hope?
　　　　h. Does this person have any wishes or dreams?
　　　　i. What does he want most in life?
　　　　j. Does this person have suicidal thoughts? If so, explore why.

B. Assess for related factors
　　1. Presence of illness or treatment
　　　　a. Chronic, prolonged, deteriorating, exhausting

2. Significant relationships
    a. Who does this person perceive as the most significant other in his life?
    b. What is this person's current relationship with this significant other?
    c. What are this person's feelings toward this significant other now?
    d. Is this relationship currently pleasing or helpful to this person?
    e. Does this person have contact with this significant other now?
    f. Has divorce or death of spouse, or death of child, sibling, friend, pet, occurred recently?
    g. Has this person moved away from significant others recently?

Objective Data

A. Assess for defining characteristics
    1. General appearance
        Grooming   Eye contact
        Posture   Speed of activities

Outcome Criteria

Short-Term
The person will
- Share suffering openly and constructively with others
- Reminisce and review his life positively
- Consider his values and the meaning of life
- Express feelings of optimism about the present
- Express confidence in a desired outcome and goals
- Express confidence in self and others
- Practice energy conservation

Long-Term
- The person will demonstrate an increase in energy level, as evidenced by activities (*i.e.*, self-care, exercise, hobbies, and the like)
- Express positive expectations about the future
- Demonstrate initiative, self-direction, and autonomy in decision making and problem solving
- Make statements similar to the following:
  - "I am looking forward to . . ."
  - "When things are not so good, it helps me to think of . . ."
  - "I have enough time to do what I want."
  - "There are more good times ahead."
  - "I expect to succeed in . . ."
  - "I expect to get more out of the good things in life."
  - "My past experiences have helped me be prepared for my future."
  - "In the future, I'll be happier."
  - "I have faith in the future."
- Develop, improve, and maintain positive relationships with others
- Participate in a significant role
- Express spiritual beliefs
- Redefine the future and set realistic goals
- Exhibit peace and comfort with situation

Interventions

A. Assist to identify and express feelings
    1. Listen actively and treat the person as an individual (Miller & Wake, 1994).

2. Convey empathy to promote verbalization of doubts, fears, and concerns (Miller & Wake, 1994).
3. Validate and reflect impressions with the person. It is important to realize that cancer patients often have their own reality, which may differ from the nurse's own view of reality (Yates, 1993).
4. Accept the person's feelings (*i.e.*, trust his will to live if it exists, accept his anger).
5. Encourage to verbalize why and how hope is significant in his life.
6. Encourage expressions of how hope is uncertain in his life and areas in which hope has failed him.
7. Assist to recognize that hopelessness is a part of everyone's life that demands recognition. It can be used as a source of energy, imagination, and freedom that encourages a person to consider alternate choices. It leads to self-discovery.
8. Assist to understand that he can deal with the hopeless aspects of his life by separating them from the hopeful aspects. Help the person identify areas of hopelessness in his life and acknowledge them. Help him to distinguish between the possible and the impossible. The nurse mobilizes a client's internal and external resources to promote hope. Assist clients to identify their own personal reasons for living that provide meaning and purpose to their lives.

B. **Assess and mobilize the person's internal resources (autonomy, independence, rationality, cognitive thinking, flexibility, spirituality)**

1. Emphasize strengths, not weaknesses.
2. Compliment on appearance or efforts when appropriate.
3. Promote motivation by:
   a. Identifying reasons for living (Poncar, 1994)
   b. Identifying areas of success and usefulness; emphasize his past accomplishments. Use this information to develop goals with the client
   c. Assist clients to identify things they have fun doing and things they perceive as humorous. This can serve as a distraction to discomfort and allow the client to move on to cognitive comfort (Hinds & Martin, 1988).
   d. Assist to identify sources of hope (*i.e.*, relationships, faith, things to accomplish) (Poncar, 1994).
   e. Assist to adjust and develop realistic short- and long-term goals (progress from simple to more complex; may use a "goals poster" to indicate type and time for achieving specific goals). Attainable expectations promote hope (Herth, 1993).
   f. Teach to monitor specific signs of progress to use as self-reinforcement.
   g. Encourage "means–end" thinking in positive terms (*i.e.*, If I do this and . . . , then I'll be able to . . .).
   h. Foster lightheartedness and the sharing of uplifting memories (Herth, 1990).
4. Assist with problem solving and decision making (see Appendix VII).
   a. Respect the client as a competent decision maker; treat his decisions and desires with respect.
   b. Encourage verbalization to determine the client's perception of choices.
   c. Clarify the client's values to determine what is important (Poncar, 1994).
   d. Correct misinformation.
   e. Assist to identify those problems he cannot resolve to advance to problems he can resolve. In other words, assist the client to move away from dwelling on the impossible and hopeless and to begin to deal with matters that are realistic and hopeful.
   f. Assess the client's perceptions of self and others in relation to size. (This person often perceives others in the world as large and difficult to deal with and perceives himself as small.) If his perceptions are unrealistic, assist him to reassess them to restore proper scale to his world.
   g. Promote flexibility. Encourage the client to try alternatives and take risks.
   h. Teach and support to use rational inquiry (to seek more information).
5. Assist to learn effective coping skills.
   a. Assist with setting realistic, attainable short- and long-term goals.

b. Teach the importance of mutuality in sharing concerns.

c. Explain the benefits of distraction from negative events.

d. Teach the value of confronting issues.

e. Teach and assist with relaxation techniques (see Appendix X) before anticipated stressful events.

f. Encourage mental imagery to promote positive thought processes (see Appendix X).

g. Allow the client time to reminisce to gain insight into past experiences.

h. Teach the client to "hope to be" the best person possible today and to appreciate the fullness of each moment.

i. Teach to maximize esthetic experiences (*e.g.*, smell of coffee, back rub, or feeling the warmth of the sun or a breeze), which can inspire hope (Poncar, 1994).

j. Teach to anticipate experiences he takes delight in each day (*e.g.*, walking, reading favorite book, writing letter).

k. Assist in expressing spiritual beliefs.

l. Teach ways to conserve and generate energy. Moderate physical exercise and rest can enhance hope (Owen, 1989).

C. **Assess and mobilize person's external resources (significant others, health care team, support groups, God or higher powers)**

1. Family or significant others

a. Involve family or significant others in plan of care.

b. Foster and encourage the client to spend increased time or thoughts with loved ones in healthy relationships.

c. Teach the family their role in sustaining hope through a supportive, positive relationship (Herth, 1993; Poncar, 1994).

d. Convey hope, information, and confidence to family because their feelings will be conveyed to the client.

e. Discuss the client's attainable goals with family.

f. Use touch and closeness with the client to demonstrate to the family that this is acceptable (provide privacy).

g. Help the client to recognize that he is loved, cared about, and important to the lives of others regardless of his failing health.

h. The following strategies were found by Herth (1993) to foster hope in caregivers of terminally ill people:

Cognitive reframing through positive self-talk, praying/meditating, and envisioning hopeful images. This may involve letting go of expectations for things to be another way.

Time refocusing by focusing less on the future and more on living one day at a time

Belief in a power greater than self to empower the caregiver's hope

Balancing available energy through listening to music or other favorite activities to empower the caregiver's hope through uplifting energy

2. Health care team

a. Develop positive, trusting nurse–client relationship by:

Answering questions	Touching
Respecting client's feelings	Providing comfort
Providing consistent care	Being honest
Following-through on requests	Conveying positive attitude

b. Convey attitude of "We care too much about you to let you just give up," or "I can help you."

c. Hold conferences and share client's goals with staff.

d. Provide staff support groups, use team care conferences.

e. Encourage the client to use and work with the health care team to cope with problems.

f. Share advances in technology and research for treatment of diseases.

g. Have available a list of laughter resources (*i.e.*, books, films).

3. Support groups
   a. Encourage person to share concerns with others who have had similar problem or disease and have had positive experiences from coping effectively with it.
   b. Provide information on self-help groups (*i.e.*, "Make today count"—40 chapters in United States and Canada; "I can cope"—series for cancer clients; "We Can Weekend"—for families of cancer patients).
   c. Initiate referrals when indicated.
4. God or higher powers
   a. Assess belief support system (value, past experiences with, religious activities, relationship with God, meaning and purpose of prayer; refer to *Spiritual Distress*).
   b. Create environment in which client feels free to express self spiritually.
   c. Acknowledge the client's belief system.
   d. Allow the client time and opportunities to reflect on the meaning of suffering, death, and dying.
   e. Accept, respect, and support the patient's hope in God.

D. Identify the individual at risk for self-harm (refer to *Risk for Suicide*)

E. Initiate referrals, as indicated
   1. Counseling
      a. Spiritual
      b. Family
   2. Crisis hotline

Rationale

- Hope is related to help from others, in that a person feels his external resources may be supportive when his internal resources and strengths seem insufficient to cope with a situation (*e.g.*, a family or significant other is often a source of hope).
- Hope has been found to be directly related to the quality of the person's relationships with others (Gottschalk, 1974; Herth, 1990).
- Hope has been claimed to be capable of influencing a person's physical, psychological, and spiritual health (Cousins, 1989; Ingelfinger, 1980; Miller, 1985; Watson, 1979).
- Maintaining family role responsibilities is essential for hope and coping (Herth, 1989). In addition, the hope concept is essential for families of the critically ill to facilitate coping and adjustment (Coulter, 1989).
- Moderate physical exercise and adequate rest can enhance hope, because hope takes energy and gives energy (Owen, 1989).
- "Lightheartedness," humor, and uplifting memories were found to foster hope in terminally ill people (Herth, 1990).
- Hope maintained by family members has a contagious effect on clients (Miller, 1991).
- Isolation, concurrent losses, and poorly controlled symptom management hinder hope (Herth, 1993).
- A person experiencing hopelessness cannot imagine anything that can be done or is worth doing, nor can he imagine beyond what is currently occurring.
- If hopelessness is recognized and dealt with imaginatively, it can result in movement, growth, and resourcefulness. Rigidity never overcomes hopelessness.
- A person can cope with a part of his life he views as hopeless if he is able to realize that there are other factors in his life that are hopeful. For example, a person may realize he may never walk again, yet he will be able to go home and be in the company of his grandchildren and move around. Therefore, hopelessness can lead to the discovery of alternatives that provide meaning and purpose in life. It is essential to keep hopelessness out of the way of hope.
- Motivation is essential in the recovery process from hopelessness. The client must determine a goal even if he has low expectations of achieving it. The nurse is the catalyst to encourage the client to take the first step to identify a goal. After this is accomplished, another goal must be created.

- The health care team must be hopeful if the client is to be hopeful; otherwise, the client views efforts of the team as a waste of time.
- The more the client believes he can attain a goal, the more important that goal becomes in providing hope for the client.
- The nurse mobilizes the client's internal and external resources to strengthen his hope, motivation, and will to live.

References/Bibliography

Christman, N. J. (1990). Uncertainty and adjustment during radiotherapy. *Nursing Research, 39*(1), 17–20, 47.

Coulter, M. A. (1989). The needs of family members of patients in intensive care units. *Intensive Care Nursing, 5,* 4–10.

Cousins, N. (1989). *Head first: The biology of hope and the healing powers of the human spirit.* Harmondsworth, England: Penguin Books.

Coward, D. S. (1991). Self-transcendence and emotional well-being in women with advanced breast cancer. *Oncology Nursing Forum, 18,* 857–863.

Davies, H. N. (1993). Hope as a coping strategy for the spinal cord injured individual. *Axone, 15*(2), 40–45.

Drew, B. L. (1990). Differentiation of hopelessness, helplessness and powerlessness using Erikson's "Roots of Virtue." *Archives of Psychiatric Nursing, 14,* 332–337.

Engel, G. (1989). A life setting conducive to illness: The giving up–given up complex. *Annals of Internal Medicine, 69,* 293–300.

Fromm, E. (1968). *The evolution of hope.* New York: Harper.

Gottschalk, L. A. (1974). A hope scale applicable to verbal samples. *Archives of General Psychiatry, 30,* 779–787.

Herth, K. A. (1989). The relationship between level of hope and level of coping response and other variables in patients with cancer. *Oncology Nursing Forum, 16,* 67–72.

Herth, K. (1990). Fostering hope in terminally ill people. *Journal of Advanced Nursing, 15,* 1250–1259.

Herth, K. (1992). Abbreviated instrument to measure hope: Development and psychometric evaluation. *Journal of Advanced Nursing, 17,* 1251–1259.

Herth, K. (1993). Hope in the family caregiver of terminally ill people. *Journal of Advanced Nursing, 18,* 538–547.

Hickey, S. S. (1986). Enabling hope. *Cancer Nursing, 9,* 133–137.

Hinds, P. (1988). Adolescent hopefulness in illness and health. *Advances in Nursing Science, 10*(3), 79–88.

Hinds, P., Martin, J., & Vogel, R. (1987). Nursing strategies to influence adolescent hopefulness during oncologic illness. *Journal of the Association of Pediatric Oncology Nurses, 4*(1/2), 14–23.

Hinds, P. S. (1984). Inducing a definition of "hope" through the use of grounded theory methodology. *Journal of Advanced Nursing, 9,* 357–362.

Hinds, P. S., & Martin, J. (1988). Hopefulness and the self-sustaining process in adolescents with cancer. *Nursing Research, 37,* 336–340.

Ingelfinger, F. J. (1980). Arrogance. *New England Journal of Medicine, 30,* 1507–1511.

Jackson, B. S. (1993). Hope and wound healing. *Journal of Enterostomal Therapy in Nursing, 20*(2), 73–77.

Korner, I. N. (1970). Hope as a method of coping. *Journal of Consultation and Clinical Psychology 34,* 134–139.

Kübler-Ross, E. (1975). *Death: The final stage of growth.* Englewood Cliffs, NJ: Prentice-Hall.

LeGresley, A. (1991). Validation of hopelessness: Perceptions of the critically ill. In R. M. Carroll-Johnson (Ed.). *Classification of nursing diagnoses: Proceedings of the ninth conference.* Philadelphia: J. B. Lippincott.

Leininger, M. (1978). *Transcultural nursing: Concepts, theories, and practices.* New York: John Wiley & Sons.

McGill, J. S. (1992). Functional status as it relates to hope in elders. *Kentucky Nurse, 40*(4), 6.

Miller, J. F. (1985). Inspiring hope. *American Journal of Nursing, 85,* 22–25.

Miller, J. F. (1989). Hope inspiring strategies of the critically ill. *Applied Nursing Research, 2*(1), 23–29.

Miller, J. F. (1991). Developing and maintaining hope in the families of the critically ill. *Critical Care Nursing, 2,* 307–314.

Miller, J. F., & Powers, M. J. (1988). Development of an instrument to measure hope. *Nursing Research, 37*(1), 6–9.

Miller, J. F., & Wake, M. M. (1994). Multinational perspectives on nursing interventions for hopelessness. In R. M. Carroll-Johnson & M. Paquette (Eds.). *Classification of nursing diagnoses: Proceedings of the tenth conference.* Philadelphia: J. B. Lippincott.

Notwotny, M. L. (1989). Assessment of hope in patients with cancer: Development of an instrument. *Oncology Nursing Forum, 16,* 57–61.

O'Connor, A. P., Wicher, C. A., & Germino, B. B. (1990). Understanding the cancer patient's search for meaning. *Cancer Nursing, 13*(3), 167–175.

Owen, D. C. (1989). Nurses' perspectives on the meaning of hope in patients with cancer: A qualitative study. *Oncology Nursing Forum, 16,* 75–79.

Parse, R. R. (1990). Parse's research methodology within an illustration of the lived experience of hope. *Nursing Science Quarterly, 3*(3), 9–17.

Plummer, E. M. (1988). Measurement of hope in the elderly hospitalized institutionalized person. *New York State Nurses' Association, 19*(3), 8–11.

Poncar, P. J. (1994). Inspiring hope in the oncology patient. *Journal of Psychosocial Nursing, 32*(1), 33–38.

Reed, P. G. (1986). Developmental resources and depression in the elderly. *Nursing Research, 35*, 368–373.

Schmale, A. H., & Iher, H. P. (1966). The affect of hopelessness and the development of cancer. *Psychosomatic Medicine, 28*, 714–721.

Stotland, E. (1969). *The psychology of hope.* San Francisco: Jossey-Bass.

Wake, M. M., Fehring, R. J., & Fadden, T. C. (1994). Multinational diagnostic content vali-

dation of anxiety, hopelessness, and ineffective airway clearance. In R. M. Carroll-Johnson & M. Paquette (Eds.). *Classification of nursing diagnoses: Proceedings of the tenth conference.* Philadelphia: J. B. Lippincott.

Watson, J. (1979). *Nursing: The philosophy and science of caring.* Boston: Little, Brown.

Yates, P. (1993). Towards a reconceptualization of hope for patients with a diagnosis of cancer. *Journal of Advanced Nursing, 18*, 701–706.

Infant Behavior, Disorganized

DEFINITION

Disorganized Infant Behavior: The degree to which an infant has reached his organizational threshold and no longer is maintaining himself, as reflected in his use of varying physiologic, postural, or state strategies, and as reflected across all subsystems of behavioral adaptation (*i.e.*, autonomic, motor, state, and attention–interaction systems).

DEFINING CHARACTERISTICS (VANDENBERG, 1990)

Autonomic system
- Cardiac
  - Increased rate
- Respiration
  - Pauses, tachypnea, gasping
- Color changes
  - Paling around nostrils, perioral duskiness, mottled, cyanotic, gray, flushed, ruddy
- Visceral
  - Hiccups, gagging, grunting, spitting up
  - Straining as if actually producing a bowel movement
- Motor

Seizures	Sneezing
Tremoring/startling	Yawning
Twitching	Sighing
Coughing	

Motor system
- Fluctuating tone
- Flaccidity of

Trunk	Face
Extremities	

- Hypertonicity

Leg extensions	Arching
Salutes	Finger splays
Airplaning	Tongue extensions
Sitting on air	Fisting

Hyperflexions
Trunk   Fetal tuck
Extremities
Frantic diffuse activity
State system (range)
Diffuse states
Sleep
Twitches   Whimpers
Sound   Grimacing
Jerky moves   Fussy in sleep
Irregular respirations
Awake
Eye floating   Panicked, worried, or dull look
Glassy eyed   Weak cry
Strained, fussy   Irritability
Staring   Abrupt state changes
Gaze aversion
Attention–interaction system
Imbalance of withdrawal versus engaging behaviors
Impaired ability to orient, attend, engage in reciprocal social interactions
Difficult to console

RELATED FACTORS
Pathophysiologic

Related to immature or altered central nervous system secondary to:
Prematurity   Infection
Prenatal exposure to drugs   Hyperbilirubinemia
Congenital anomalies   Decreased oxygen saturation
Hypoglycemia   Perinatal factors
Related to nutritional deficits secondary to:
Reflux emesis   Swallowing problems
Colic   Feeding intolerances
Related to excess stimulation secondary to:
Pain
Hunger
Oral hypersensitivity
Temperature variation

Treatment-Related

Related to excess stimulation secondary to:
Invasive procedures   Medication administration
Chest physical therapy   Movement
Restraints   Feeding
Lights   Noise (*e.g.*, prolonged alarms, voices, environmental)
Tubes, tape
Related to inability to see caregivers secondary to eye patches

Situational (Personal, Environmental)

Related to unpredictable interactions secondary to multiple caregivers
Related to imbalance of task touch and consoling touch
Related to decreased ability to self-regulate secondary to:
Sudden movement
Noise
Fatigue
Disrupted sleep–wake cycles

Author's Note

This diagnosis describes an infant who has difficulty regulating and adapting to external stimuli. This difficulty is due to immature neurobehavioral development and increased environmental stimuli associated with neonatal units. When an infant is overstimulated or stressed, she or he uses energy to adapt, which depletes the supply of energy needed for physiologic growth. The goal of nursing care is to assist the infant with energy conservation by reducing environmental stimuli, by allowing the infant sufficient time to adapt to handling, and by providing sensory input appropriate to the infant's physiologic and neurobehavioral status.

Key Concepts

1. Als (1986) explained that an infant's primary route of communication of competency and efforts at self-regulation is through his behavioral indices.
2. The behavior of infants is a continual interaction with their environment by means of fine subsystems (Blackburn, 1993; Yecco, 1993):
   a. Autonomic/physiologic—regulation of respirations, color, and visceral functions (*e.g.*, gastrointestinal, swallowing)
   b. Motor—regulation of tone, posture, level of activity, specific movement patterns of the extremities, head, trunk, and face
   c. State/organizational—involves the range of states of consciousness, transition between states, and the quality of the states (*e.g.*, sleep to arousal, awake to alert, crying)
   d. Attention–interactive—ability to orient and focus on sensory stimuli (*e.g.*, faces, sounds, objects) and to take in cognitive, social, and emotional information
   e. Self-regulatory—maintains the integrity and balance of the other subsystems, a smooth transition between states, and relaxation between subsystems
3. These systems are synchronized and function smoothly in the full-term infant. The infant can regulate these five systems with ease. Less mature or ill infants are able to tolerate only one activity at a time. Loss of control results in instability or disorganization in one or more subsystems (Blackburn, 1993). The defining characteristics represent signs of the instability.
4. Blackburn and Barnard (1985) emphasized that immature infants are born early and thus must adapt to the extrauterine environment with underdeveloped body systems, usually in a neonatal intensive care unit (NICU) environment.
5. Although mortality and morbidity rates have been greatly reduced in high-risk infants, they experience a variety of neurobehavioral problems. These problems have been labeled as "the new morbidities of low birth weight infants," which include hyperexcitability, language problems, attention-deficit disorders, higher-order cognitive problems, and schooling problems (Blackburn, 1993).
6. There are six stages in central nervous system development: dorsal induction, ventral induction, proliferation and neurogenesis, neuron migration, organization, and myelinization. The first three occur completely before the fourth month of gestation. The last three stages continue to complete development. The migration stage involves the movement of millions of cells from their point of origin in the periventricular region to their terminal location within the cerebral cortex and cerebellum. The organization stage occurs at a peak time of 6 months' gestation to 1 year after birth. The myelinization stage peaks from 8 months' gestation to 1 year after birth. Myelinization insulates individual nerve fibers to facilitate specificity of connections, increases the number of alternative pathways, and increases the speed of transmission (Blackburn, 1993).
7. The neurologic dysfunctions resulting from neurologic underdevelopment include (Blackburn, 1993):
   a. Sparse myelin
   b. Long refractory period
   c. Weak transmission
   d. Decreased inhibitory potential

  e. Decreased ability to use various systems
  f. Slow nerve conduction
  g. Slow synaptic conduction
  h. Unable to sustain high firing rates
  i. Incomplete cell differentiation
  j. Decreased ability to process impulses for cell-to-cell communication
8. These limitations in neurologic function result in the behavior characteristics of immature infants (Blackburn, 1993):
  a. Irregular state of regulation
  b. Increased and decreased tone
  c. Deficits in primitive reflexes
  d. Easily exhausted
  e. Irritable, difficult to soothe
  f. Inability to inhibit
  g. Jerky movements
  h. Low arousal
  i. Difficulty to sustain an alert state
  j. Poor coordination
  k. Altered autonomic regulation
  l. Asymmetric, uncoordinated posture and movement
9. For too long it was believed that neonates could not perceive, respond to, or remember
  pain. Research has validated that neonates do feel and express pain. Williamson and
  Williamson (1983) found that infants who received local anesthesia for a circumcision
  cried less and had decreased variation in heart rate and higher oxygen saturation compared with infants who did not have a local anesthetic.
10. Loudness of sound is measured in decibels (db). Adult speech is recorded at about 45–50
  db. Sound levels in infant incubators have been reported to be from 50–80 db. Hearing
  loss in adults has been associated with levels above 80–85 db (Blackburn, 1993).
11. The incidence of sensorineural hearing impairment is 4% in low–birth-weight infants and
  13% in very–low-birth-weight infants (Thomas, 1989).

Focus Assessment Criteria

Note: Experts recommend two assessment tools for assessing neurobehavioral function; the
Brazelton Neonatal Behavioral Assessment Scale (NBAS) for healthy, full-term neonates,
Assessment of Preterm Infant Behavior (APIB) for preterm neonates, and NIDCAP (Newborn
Individualized Developmental Care and Assessment Program). All tools require training in
their use. Refer to References/Bibliography for information on training centers.

Objective
A. Assess for defining characteristics
  1. Autonomic system
    a. Respirations
        Pauses   Gasping   Deep, rapid
    b. Color changes
        Paling around nostrils   Gray
        Mottled   Flushed
        Cyanotic   Ruddy
    c. Visceral
        Gagging   Spitting up
        Grunting   Straining (as if having a bowel movement)
        Hiccoughs
    d. Motor
        Tremors   Coughing
        Startling   Sneezing
        Seizures   Yawning
        Twitching   Sighing

2. Motor system (fluctuating tone)
   a. Flaccid trunk, extremities, face
   b. Hypertonic

Arching	Toe, finger splays
Leg extensions	Tongue extensions
Fisting	Sitting on air
Salutes	

   c. Hyperflexions

Trunk	Fetal tuck
Extremities	

   d. Frantic, diffuse activity
3. State system (range)
   a. When sleeping

Twitches	Jerky movements
Grimaces	Whimpers
Fussy	

   b. When awake

Uncoordinated	Glassy eyes
Unfocused eyes	Staring
Panicked look	Weak cry
Irritable	

   c. Abrupt state charges
4. Attention–interaction system
   a. Imbalance of withdrawal versus engaging behaviors
   b. Impaired ability to

Orient	Engage in reciprocal social interactions
Attend	

   c. Difficult to console

Outcome Criteria (Blackburn, 1993, p. 1001)

The infant will
- Experience minimal fluctuation of tone and muscle extensions
- Demonstrate organized sleep states and calm, quiet alerting
- Demonstrate improvement of respiratory regularity and color during handling

The parent(s)/caregiver(s) will
- Describe techniques to reduce environmental stress in agency and/or at home

---

Interventions

A. Assess for causative/contributing factors
   1. Pain
   2. Fatigue
   3. Disorganized sleep–wake pattern
   4. Feeding problems

B. Reduce or eliminate contributing factors, if possible
   1. Pain
      a. Determine the baseline behavioral manifestations of the infant and document.
      b. Observe for responses different from baseline that have been associated with neonatal pain responses (Bozzette, 1993; Grunau & Craig, 1987):
         Facial responses (open mouth, brow bulge, grimace, chin quiver, nasolabial furrow, taut tongue)
         Motor responses (flinch, muscle rigidity, clenched hands, withdrawal)

    c. If unsure whether behavior indicates pain, but pain is suspected, consult with physician for an analgesic trial. Evaluate the infant's response.

    d. Aggressively manage obvious pain stimuli (*e.g.*, postsurgical, lack of feeding, painful procedures, hyperglycemia) (Acute Pain Management Guideline Panel, 1982a).

        Consult with physician for an analgesic.

        Provide an analgesic before painful procedures.

        Consider topical analgesia for frequent painful procedures (*e.g.*, heelstick, venipuncture).

    e. When administering analgesics (Acute Pain Management Guideline Panel, 1982b):

        Reduce initial dose and monitor respiratory response cautiously.

        Determine optimal dose and interval:

            Monitor when pain breaks through.

            Determine if infant appears comfortable after the dose.

        When indicated, wean infant slowly over a period of days from the drug. Assess response to withdrawal. Consult with physician to manage withdrawal symptoms if indicated.

    f. When painful or stressful procedures must be administered, consider facilitations to prepare the infant's state and calmness, including:

        Supporting the flexed position with another caregiver

        Providing opportunities to suck while shielding the infant from other stresses

    g. Consider the efficient execution of necessary manipulations while supporting the infant's behavioral organization during the manipulation.

    h. Consider *unhurried* reorganization and stabilization of the infant's regulation (*i.e.*, position in prone, opportunities to hold onto caregiver's finger and suck, encasement of trunk and back of head in caregiver's hand, inhibition provided to soles of feet) (Als, 1993).

    i. Consider spending 15–20 minutes after manipulation; over time, the infant's self-regulatory abilities will improve, making the caregiver's facilitation increasingly less necessary.

    j. Consider calming initiated on the caregiver's body and then transfer to the crib as necessary. For other infants, this may be too arousing, and transition is more easily accomplished in the isolette with the provision of steady boundaries and encasing without any stimulation.

2. Disrupted 24-hour diurnal cycles

    a. Evaluate the need and, if needed, the frequency of each intervention.

    b. Consider 24-hour caregiving assignment, and primary caregiving, to provide consistent caregiving throughout the day and night for the infant from the onset of admission. This is important in terms of responding to increasingly more mature sleep cycles, feeding ability, and especially emotional development.

    c. Consider supporting the infant's transition to sleep and supporting the maintenance of sleep by avoiding peaks of frenzy and overexhaustion, by continuously maintaining a calm, regular environment and schedule, and by establishing a reliable, repeatable pattern of gradual transition into sleep in prone and side-lying in the isolette or crib.

3. Facilitate a supportive, self-regulatory feeding experience.

    a. Observe and record infant's readiness for participation with feeding:

        Hunger cues

            Transitioning to drowsy or alert state

            Mouthing, rooting, or sucking

            Brings hands to mouth

            Cries and unconsoled with pacifier or nonnutritive sucking alone

        Physiologic stability

            Regulated breathing patterns

            Stable color

            Stable digestion

    b. Facilitate nurturing environment in support of coregulatory feeding experience:
        Decrease environmental stimulation.
        Provide comfortable seating (be especially sensitive to the needs of postpartum
            mothers, *e.g.*, soft cushions, small stool to elevate legs, supportive pillows
            for nursing).
        Encourage softly swaddling infant to facilitate flexion and balanced tone during feeding.
    c. Explore feeding methods that meet the needs of the infant as well as family goals (*i.e.*, breast feeding, bottle feeding, gavage).

C. Support the infant's own self-regulatory efforts

    1. When painful or stressful procedures must be administered, consider facilitations to prepare the infant's state and enhance calmness.
        a. Supporting the flexed position with another caregiver
        b. Providing opportunities to suck while shielding the infant from other stresses
    2. Consider the efficient execution of necessary manipulations while supporting the infant's behavioral organization during the manipulation.
    3. Consider *unhurried* reorganization and stabilization of the infant's regulation (*i.e.*, position in prone, opportunities to hold onto caregiver's finger and suck, encasement of trunk and back of head in caregiver's hand, inhibition provided to soles of feet).
    4. Consider removing extraneous stimulation (*e.g.*, stroking, talking, position shifts) to institute restabilization. Consider spending 15–20 minutes after manipulation; over time, the infant's self-regulatory abilities will improve, making the caregiver's facilitation increasingly less necessary.
    5. Consider supporting the infant's transition to sleep and supporting the maintenance of sleep by avoiding peaks of frenzy and overexhaustion, by continuously maintaining a calm, regular environment and schedule, and by establishing a reliable, repeatable pattern of gradual transition into sleep in prone and side-lying in the isolette or crib.
    6. Consider calming initiated on the caregiver's body and then transfer to the crib as necessary. For other infants, this may be too arousing, and transition is more easily accomplished in the isolette with the provision of steady boundaries and encasing without any stimulation.
    7. Critical review of the use of the automatic swing for the irritable infant may be indicated. For some infants, it appears to lead to momentary quieting, but not necessarily to increased internal regulatory control over time.
    8. Soothing, gentle instrumental music or the parent's voice may be comforting for some infants during transition to sleep.
    9. A nonstimulating sleep space with a lack of exciting visual targets, social inputs, and the like, may need to be made available in preparation to relaxing into sleep. A regularly implemented sleep routine may be helpful for many infants.

D. Reduce environmental stimuli

    1. Noise (Thomas, 1989)
        a. Do not tap on incubator.
        b. Place a folded blanket on top of the incubator if it is the only work surface available.
        c. Slowly open and close porthole.
        d. Pad incubator doors to reduce banging.
        e. Use plastic instead of metal waste cans.
        f. Remove water from ventilator tubing.
        g. Speak softly at the bedside and only when necessary.
        h. Slowly drop the head of the mattress.
        i. Eliminate radios.
        j. Close doors slowly.
        k. Position the infant's bed away from sources of noise (*e.g.*, telephone, intercom, unit equipment).

      l. Consider the following methods in reducing unnecessary noise in the NICU:
         Consider performing rounds away from the bedsides.
         Consider adaptations to large equipment to eliminate noise and clutter.
      m. Alert staff when the decibel level in unit exceeds 60 db (*e.g.*, by a light attached to a sound meter). Institute quiet time for 10 minutes to lower noise.
      n. Move more vulnerable infants out of unit traffic patterns.
  2. Lights
      a. Use full-spectrum light instead of white light at bedside.
      b. Cover cribs, incubators, and radiant warmers completely during sleep periods, partially during awake times.
      c. Install dimmer switches, shades, and curtains.
      d. Shade infants' eyes with a blanket tent or cutout box.

E. Position in postures that permit flexion and minimize flailing, arching, and squirming

  1. Consider gentle, *unhurried* reorganization and stabilization of the infant's regulation by supporting the infant in softly tucked prone positioning, with opportunities to hold onto caregiver's finger and suck, encasement of trunk and back of head in caregiver's hand, and inhibition provided to soles of feet.
  2. Position prone/side-lying.
  3. Avoid supine position.
  4. Swaddle if possible to maintain flexion.
  5. Create a nest using soft bedding (*e.g.*, natural sheepskin, soft cotton, flannel).

F. Reduce the stress associated with handling

  1. When moving or lifting an infant, contain the infant with hands by wrapping or placing rolled blankets around his or her body.
  2. Maintain containment during procedures and caregiving activities.
  3. Handle slowly and gently.
  4. Initiate all interactions and treatments with one sense stimulus at a time (*e.g.*, touch), then slowly progress to visual, auditory, and movement.
  5. Assess for cues for readiness, impending disorganization, or stability; respond to cues.
  6. Support minimal disruption of the infant's own evolving 24-hour sleep–wake cycles.
  7. Use PRN suctioning or postural drainage instead of routine.
  8. Use minimal amount of adhesive tape. Remove carefully.

G. Reduce disorganized behavior during active interventions (weighing, transfers out of incubator, and supportive positioning during interventions such as x-rays) and transport

  1. Have a plan for transport with assigned roles for each team member.
  2. Establish behavior cues of stress of this infant with the primary nurse before transport.
  3. Minimize sensory input:
      a. Use calm, quiet voices.
      b. Shade the infant's eyes from light.
      c. Protect the infant from unnecessary touch.
  4. Support the infant's softly tucked postures with your hands and offer something to grasp (your finger or corner of a soft blanket or cloth).
  5. Swaddle the infant or place in a nest made of blankets.
  6. Ensure that the transport equipment (*e.g.*, ventilator) is ready. Warm mattress or use sheepskin.
  7. Carefully and smoothly move the infant. Avoid talking if possible.
  8. Consider conducting caregiving routines while infant is held supportively by parent(s) or designated caregiver in their absence whenever possible.

H. Enhance parents' and infant's evolving competencies and expectations in their own developmental progression
   1. Encourage parents to share their feelings, fears, and expectations.
   2. Consider involving the parents in developing the infant and family's developmental plan (Cole & Frappier, 1985)

   My strengths are:
   These things stress me:
   Time-out signals:
   How you can help me:

I. Initiate health teaching and referrals as indicated
   1. Review the following information relating to the growth and development of the infant and family in anticipatory guidance for home.
      a. Health concerns

Feeding, hygiene	Illness, infection
Safety, temperature	Growth and development

      b. State modulation
         Appropriate stimulation
         Sleep–wake patterns
      c. Parent–infant interaction
         Behavior cues
         Signs of stress
      d. Infant's environment
         Animate, inanimate stimulation   Playing with infant
         Role of father and siblings
      e. Parental coping and support
         Support network   Challenges
         Problem solving
   2. Discuss transition to community supports with the family (nursing respite, social and civic groups, religious affiliations).
   3. Refer for follow-up home visits.

Rationale

- When a premature neonate is ill, the combination of immature cerebral nervous system, exposure to inappropriate and unexpected patterned sensory input, and multiple caregivers leads to disorganization and imbalance of the behavioral indices to regulation.
- Preterm infants may have difficulties or demonstrate disorganization in progression in feeding behaviors (*e.g.*, feeding readiness, availability of hunger cues) and gastrointestinal motility issues related to prematurity (*i.e.*, esophageal motility, intestinal motility, and gastric emptying time).
- "If care providers are unsure whether a behavior indicates pain, and if there is a reason to suspect pain, an analgesic trial can be diagnostic as well as therapeutic" (Acute Pain Management Guideline Panel, 1992a, p. 12).
- Pharmacologic treatments may not be the first line of intervention with all infants. Utilize nonpharmacologic methods, if appropriate (*e.g.,* rocking).
- Noise levels in NICUs are hazardous because of potential damage to the cochlea with subsequent hearing loss, and because of arousal effects on infants who are unable to inhibit their responses. Noise interferes with sleep, increases heart rate, and leads to vasoconstriction (Blackburn, 1993). Energy that the infant needs for growth and to supply his or her brain with glucose and oxygen is expended on arousal caused by noise (Thomas, 1989).
- Thomas (1989) found that there is a loud, continuous pattern of background noise in NICUs. In addition, peak noises over the continuous noise level can raise the decibel level 10-fold. Examples of peak noises are monitor alarms (67 db), NICU radios (62 db), opening the plastic sleeve (67 db), tapping the hood (70 db), and turning a sink on and off (66 db).

References/Bibliography

Acute Pain Management Guideline Panel (1992a). *Acute pain management in infants, children, and adolescents: Operative and medical procedures.* Quick Reference Guide for Clinicians, AHCRP Pub. No. 92-0020. Rockville, MD: Agency for Health Care Policy and Research, Public Health Service, U.S. Department of Health and Human Services.

Acute Pain Management Guideline Panel (1992b). *Acute pain management: Operative or medical procedures and trauma.* Clinical Practice Guideline, AHCPR Pub. No. 92-0032. Rockville, MD: Agency for Health Care Policy and Research, Public Health Service, U.S. Department of Health and Human Services.

Als, H. (1986). A synactive model of neonatal behavioral organization: Framework for the assessment of neurobehavioral development in the premature infant and for the support of infants and parents in the neonatal intensive care environment. *Physical and Occupational Therapy in Pediatrics, 6,* 3–53.

Bill, S. G. (1994). The national pain management guideline: Implications for neonatal intensive care. *Neonatal Network, 13*(3), 9–17.

Blackburn, S. (1993). Assessment and management of neurologic dysfunction. In C. Kenner, A. Brueggemeyer, & L. Gunderson (Eds.). *Comprehensive neonatal nursing.* Philadelphia: W. B. Saunders.

Blackburn, S., & Barnard, K. E. (1985). Analysis of caregiving events in preterm infants in the special care unit. In A. Gottfried & J. Gaiter (Eds.). *Infants under stress: Environmental neonatology.* Baltimore: University Park Press.

Blackburn, S., & Vandenberg, K. (1993). Assessment and management of neonatal neurobehavioral development. In C. Kenner, A. Brueggemeyer, & L. Gunderson (Eds.). *Comprehensive neonatal nursing.* Philadelphia: W. B. Saunders.

Bozzette, M. (1993). Observations of pain behavior in the NICU: An exploratory study. *Journal of Perinatal and Neonatal Nursing, 7*(1), 76–87.

Broome, M. E., & Tanzillo, H. (1990). Differentiating between pain and agitation in premature neonates. *Journal of Perinatal and Neonatal Nursing, 4*(1), 33–62.

Cole, J., & Frappier, P. (1985). Infant stimulation reassessed. *Journal of Obstetrical, Gynecological, and Neonatal Nursing, 14,* 471–477.

Collins, S. K., & Kuck, K. (1991). Music therapy in the neonatal intensive care unit. *Neonatal Network, 9*(6), 23–26.

Flandermyer, A. A. (1993). The drug exposed neonate. In C. Kenner, A. Brueggemeyer, & L. Gunderson (Eds.). *Comprehensive neonatal nursing.* Philadelphia: W. B. Saunders.

Grunau, R., & Craig, K. (1987). Pain expression in neonates: Facial action and cry. *Pain, 28,* 395–410.

Hill, A., & Rath, L. (1993). The care and feeding of low birth weight infant. *Journal of Perinatal and Neonatal Nursing, 6*(4), 56–68.

Johnson-Crowley, N. (1993). Systematic assessment and home follow-up. In C. Kenner, A. Brueggemeyer, & L. Gunderson (Eds.). *Comprehensive neonatal nursing.* Philadelphia: W. B. Saunders.

Korner, A. F. (1986). The use of waterbeds in the care of preterm infants. *Journal of Perinatology, 6,* 142–147.

Reeder, S., Martin, L., & Koniak, D. (1992). *Maternity nursing: Family, newborn and women's health care* (17th ed.). Philadelphia: J. B. Lippincott.

Thomas, K. A. (1989). How the NICU environment sounds to a preterm infant. *MCN: American Journal of Maternal–Child Nursing, 14,* 249–251.

Vandenberg, K. (1990). The management of oral nippling in the sick neonate, the disorganized feeder. *Neonatal Network, 9*(1), 9–16.

Williamson, P. S., & Williamson, M. L. (1983). Physiologic stress reduction by local anesthetic during newborn circumcision. *Pediatrics, 7,* 36–40.

Yecco, G. J. (1993). Neurobehavioral development and developmental support of premature infants. *Journal of Perinatal and Neonatal Nursing, 7*(1), 56–65.

Resources for the Consumer

Center for Parent Education, 55 Chapel Street, Newton, MA 02150; (617) 964-2442.

Parent Care, Inc., 9041 Colgate Street, Indianapolis, IN 46268; (317) 872-9913.

Association for the Care of Children's Health (ACCH), 7910 Woodmont Avenue, Suite 300, Bethesda, MD 20814; (301) 655-6549.

Infant Behavior, Risk for Disorganized

DEFINITION
Risk for Disorganized Infant Behavior: The state in which the neonate is at risk for an alteration in integration and modulation of the physiologic and behavioral systems of adaptation (autonomic, motor, state, organizational, self-regulatory, and attentional–interactional).

RISK FACTORS
Refer to Related Factors.

RELATED FACTORS
Refer to *Disorganized Infant Behavior.*

Focus Assessment Criteria

Refer to *Disorganized Infant Behavior.*

Interventions

Refer to *Disorganized Infant Behavior.*

Infant Behavior, Potential for Enhanced Organized

DEFINITION
Potential for Enhanced Organized Infant Behavior: A pattern of modulation of the physiologic and behavioral systems of functioning of an infant (*i.e.,* autonomic, motor, state, organizational, self-regulatory, and attentional–interactional) that is satisfactory but that can be improved, resulting in higher levels of integration in response to environmental stimuli.

DEFINING CHARACTERISTICS (BLACKBURN & VANDENBERG, 1993)
Autonomic system
    Able to regulate color and respiration
    Reduction of tremors, twitches
    Reduction of visceral signals (*e.g.,* smooth)
    Digestive functioning, feeding tolerance
Motor system
    Smooth, well-modulated posture and tone

Synchronous smooth movements with:

Hand/foot clasping	Suck/suck searching
Grasping	Hand holding
Hand-to-mouth activity	Tucking

State system
 Well differentiated range of states
 Clear, robust sleep states
 Active self-quieting/consoling
 Focused, shiny-eyed alertness with intent or animated facial expressions
 "Ooh" face
 Cooing
 Attentional smiling

RELATED FACTORS

Because this is a diagnosis of effective functioning, the use of related factors is not warranted.

Author's Note

This diagnosis describes an infant who is responding to the environment with stable and predictable autonomic, motoric, and state cues. The focus of interventions is to promote continued stable development and to reduce excess environmental stimuli that may stress the infant.

Because this is a wellness diagnosis, the use of related factors is not needed. The diagnostic statement can be written as *Potential for Enhanced Organized Infant Behavior as evidenced by ability to regulate autonomic, motor, and state systems to environmental stimuli.*

Key Concepts

See *Disorganized Infant Behavior*.

Focus Assessment Criteria

Objective

A. Assess for defining characteristics
 1. Ability to regulate:

Respiratory rate	Color
Cardiac rate	

 2. Autonomic/visceral stability
  Smooth digestive functioning
  Reduction in twitches, tremors
 3. Posture/tone

Smooth	Well modulated
Balance of flexion/extension	Midline oriented

 4. Presence of synchronous, smooth movements

Hand/foot clasping	Grasping
Hand-to-mouth activity	Suck/suck searching
Hand holding	Tucking
Symmetric movements	

 5. Sleep–wake states

Well-differentiated range of states	Organized alertness
Clear states from deep sleep	Robust cry

 6. Self-regulatory ability
  Displays balance of engaging and withdrawal behavior
  Ability to orient and arouse to visual or auditory stimuli

7. Reciprocal interactions

Displays eye contact	Exploratory behavior
Mutual gazing	Easily consoled
Reaching toward	Attends to social stimuli

Outcome Criteria

The infant will
- Continue age-appropriate growth and development
- Not experience excessive environmental stimuli

The parent(s) will
- Demonstrate handling that promotes stability
- Describe developmental needs of infant
- Describe signs of stress or exhaustion
- Demonstrate (Reeder, Martin, & Koniak, 1992):
  - Gentle, soothing touch
  - Melodic tone of voice, coos
  - Mutual gazing
  - Rhythmic movements
  - Acknowledgment of all baby's vocalizations
  - Recognition of soothing qualities of actions

Interventions

A. Explain developmental needs of infants
1. Stimulation (visual, auditory, vestibular, tactile, olfactory, gustatory)
2. Periods of alertness
3. Sleep requirements

B. Explain to the parents the effects of excess environmental stress on the infant
1. Provide a list of signs of stress for their infant.
2. Teach to terminate stimulation if infant shows signs of stress.
3. When providing developmental intervention(s):
   a. Offer only when the infant is alert.
   b. If possible, show parents examples of their infant alert and not alert.
   c. Begin with one stimulus at a time (touch, voice).
   d. Provide intervention for a short time.
   e. Increase interventions according to infant's cues.
   f. Provide frequent, short-duration interventions instead of infrequent, long-term ones.

C. Explain, role-model, and observe parent engaging in developmental interventions
1. Visual (Reeder et al., 1992):
   a. Eye-to-eye contact
   b. Face-to-face experiences
   c. Provide with high-contrast colors, geometric shapes (*e.g.*, black and white shapes on paper mobile). For newborn up to 4 weeks, provide a simple mobile of four dessert-size paper plates with drawings of stripes, four-square checkerboard, a black dot, a simple bull's eye, hung with plates down 10–13 inches from baby's eyes.

    2. Auditory:
        a. Use high-pitched vocalization.
        b. Play classical music softly.
        c. Use a variety of voice inflections.
        d. Avoid loud talking.
        e. Call the infant by name.
        f. Avoid monotone speech patterns.
    3. Tactile:
        a. Use firm, gentle touch as initial approach.
        b. Use skin-to-skin contact in a warm room.
        c. For a massage, stroke skin very slowly and gently in a head-to-toe direction. Begin at trunk.
        d. Provide alternative textures (*e.g.,* sheepskin, velvet, satin).
    4. Vestibular (movement):
        a. Rock in chair.
        b. Place in sling and rock.
        c. Close infant's fist around a soft toy.
        d. Slowly change position during handling.
        e. Provide head support.
    5. Olfactory:
        a. Wear a light perfume.
    6. Gustatory:
        a. Allow nonnutritive sucking (*e.g.,* pacifier, hand in mouth).

D. Promote adjustment and stability to caregiving activities (Blackburn & Vandenberg, 1993)
    1. Waking:
        a. Enter room slowly.
        b. Turn on light, open curtains slowly.
        c. Avoid waking if asleep.
    2. Changing:
        a. Keep room warm.
        b. Gently change position: contain limbs during movement.
        c. Stop changing if infant is irritable.
    3. Feeding:
        a. Time feedings with alert states.
        b. Eliminate unnecessary noise.
        c. Hold infant close and, if needed, swaddle in blanket.
    4. Bathing:
        a. Ventral openness may be stressful.
        b. Cover body parts not being bathed.
        c. Proceed slowly; allow for rest.
        d. Offer a pacifier or hand to suck.
        e. Eliminate unnecessary noise.
        f. Use a soft, soothing voice.

E. Explain the need to reduce environmental stimuli when taking infant outside the home
        a. Shelter eyes from light.
        b. Swaddle the infant so his or her hands can reach the mouth.
        c. Protect from loud noises.

F. Praise parent(s) on their interaction patterns; point out infant's engaging responses

G. Initiate health teaching and referrals if needed
   1. Explain that developmental interventions will change as child develops. Refer to *Altered Growth and Development* for specific age-related developmental needs.
   2. Provide parent(s) with resources for assistance at home (*e.g.*, community resources).

Rationale

Refer to Rationale under *Disorganized Infant Behavior*.

References/Bibliography

Blackburn, S., & Vandenberg, K. (1993). Assessment and management of neonatal neurobehavioral development. In C. Kenner, A. Brueggemeyer, & A. Gunderson (Eds.). *Comprehensive neonatal nursing.* Philadelphia: W. B. Saunders.

Reeder, S., Martin, L., & Koniak, D. (1992). *Maternity nursing: Family, newborn and women's health care* (17th ed.). Philadelphia: J. B. Lippincott.

Infection, Risk for

DEFINITION

Risk for Infection: The state in which an individual is at risk to be invaded by an opportunistic or pathogenic agent (virus, fungus, bacteria, protozoa, or other parasite) from endogenous or exogenous sources.

RISK FACTORS

See Related Factors

RELATED FACTORS

A variety of health problems and situations can create favorable conditions that would encourage the development of infections.* Some common factors are:

Pathophysiologic

Related to compromised host defenses secondary to:
   Chronic diseases

Cancer	Hepatic disorders
Renal failure	Respiratory disorders
Arthritis	Collagen disorder
Hematologic disorders	Heritable disorders
Diabetes mellitus	AIDS

   Alcoholism
   Immunosuppression
   Immunodeficiency
   Altered or insufficient leukocytes
   Blood dyscrasias
   Altered integumentary system
   Periodontal disease

* See Key Concepts

Related to compromised circulation secondary to:
   Lymphedema
   Obesity
   Peripheral vascular disease

Treatment-Related

Related to a site for organism invasion secondary to:

Surgery	Presence of invasive lines
Dialysis	Intubation
Total parenteral nutrition	Enteral feedings

Related to compromised host defenses secondary to:
   Radiation therapy
   Organ transplant
   Medication therapy (specify; *e.g.*, chemotherapy, immunosuppressants)

Situational (Personal, Environmental)

Related to compromised host defenses secondary to:

History of infections	Malnutrition
Prolonged immobility	Stress
Increased length of hospital stay	Smoking

Related to a site for organism invasion secondary to:
   Trauma (accidental, intentional)
   Postpartum period
   Bites (animal, insect, human)
   Thermal injuries
   Warm, moist, dark environment (skin folds, casts)
Related to contact with contagious agents (nosocomial or community acquired)

Maturational

(Newborns)
   Related to increased vulnerability of infant secondary to:
      Lack of maternal antibodies (dependent on maternal exposures)
      Lack of normal flora
      Open wounds (umbilical, circumcision)
      Immature immune system
(Infant/childhood)
   Related to increased vulnerability secondary to:
      Lack of immunization
(Older adult)
   Related to increased vulnerability secondary to:
      Debilitated condition
      Diminished immune response
      Chronic diseases

Author's Note

All individuals are at risk for infection; secretion control, environmental control, and hand-washing before and after client care reduce the risk of transmission of organisms. Included in the population at risk for infection is a smaller group at high risk for infection. *Risk for Infection* describes an individual whose host defenses are compromised, thus increasing susceptibility to environmental pathogens or their own endogenous flora (*e.g.*, a person with chronic liver dysfunction or with an invasive line). Nursing interventions for such a person focus on minimizing introduction of organisms and on increasing resistance to infection (*e.g.*, by improving nutritional status). For an individual with an infection, the situation is best described by the collaborative problem *Potential Complication: Sepsis*.

Risk for Infection Transmission describes an individual at high risk for transferring an infectious agent to others. Some people are at high risk both for acquiring opportunistic agents and for transmitting infecting organisms, warranting the use of both *Risk for Infection* and *Risk for Infection Transmission.*

Errors in Diagnostic Statements

Risk for Infection related to progression of sepsis secondary to failure to treat infection

Sepsis is a collaborative problem, not a nursing diagnosis. This person is not at risk for infection but rather requires medical and nursing interventions to treat the sepsis and prevent septic shock.

Risk for Infection related to direct access to bladder mucosa secondary to Foley catheter and lack of staff knowledge of aseptic technique

If the staff's lack of knowledge of aseptic technique is valid, the nurse should proceed with reporting the situation to nursing management in an incident report. Adding this to a nursing diagnosis statement would be legally and professionally inadvisable. Nursing diagnostic statements should never be used to criticize a client, group, or a member of the health team or to expose unsafe or unprofessional practices or behavior. Other organizational channels of communication must be used for these purposes.

Key Concepts

1. There are two parameters that can assist in identifying individuals at risk for infection—predictive factors and confounding factors (Owen & Grier, 1987).
2. Confounding factors are
   a. Age
   b. Anatomic determinants
   c. Metabolic determinants
   d. Decreased numbers of neutrophils
   e. Diminished or defective immunoglobulin synthesis or rapid loss of immunoglobulin
   f. Defective cell-mediated immune mechanisms
   g. Antimicrobial therapy
3. Resistance to infection depends on the host's immune response (susceptibility), the dose of the infecting agent, and the virulence of the organism. Factors influencing the host's immune response include:
   a. Anatomic barriers—each system has specific lines of defenses.
   b. Therapies—pose a threat to normal lines of defense by either invasiveness or alteration of body function.
   c. Developmental and heritable factors—factors that have negative impact on the individual's immune system function (*e.g.*, newborn status; agammaglobulinemia).
   d. Hormonal factors—the male is more vulnerable to infection than the female; pregnancy increases the female's vulnerability; steroid therapy increases vulnerability in both sexes.
   e. Age—includes both extremes of age (immaturity or degeneration of the immune system).
   f. Nutrition influences protein synthesis and phagocytosis, decreasing the body's vulnerability to infection.
   g. Fever—hyperthermia may inhibit the growth of organisms; hypothermia may decrease the effects of the fever.
   h. Secretions such as mucus, saliva, and skin secretions contain substances that are bactericidal, decreasing the risk of infection and colonization.
   i. Endotoxins, a product of some gram-negative bacteria, have a limited ability to kill other bacteria or increase an individual's resistance to some infections.
   j. Interference—the interaction between two distinct organisms that are parasitizing the host leads to interference, in which one remains dominant and the other is suppressed.

k. The inflammatory response consists of the following: (1) activation of leukocytes, (2) plasma proteins, which localize and phagocytize the infectious process, and (3) increased blood and lymph flow that dilutes and flushes out toxic materials; this process causes a local increase in temperature.

l. Phagocytosis is the process by which parasites are removed by means of engulfment and digestion.

Host Defenses

Specific host defenses of each system that influence the immune response include:

Central Nervous System

Because the most common route for both bacterial and viral infections of the central nervous system is the hematogenous route, blood host defenses play an important primary role.

Cutaneous

1. Skin provides a first line of defense against organisms, both anatomically and chemically.
2. Sweat glands and sebaceous glands do not allow overgrowth of bacteria.
3. The acid pH of the skin does not allow pathogenic organisms to grow or survive on the skin for any length of time.
4. Eye infections are controlled by the flushing and lysozyme action of tears. Organisms are flushed through the lacrimal duct and deposited in the nasopharynx.

Blood

1. The circulating blood is the major vehicle for transporting internal defense mechanisms.
2. The febrile response is associated with the circulation of pyrogens to the hypothalamus.

Genitourinary Tract

1. Anatomic structure eliminates easy ascent of perineal microorganisms into the bladder.
2. Mucous layer allows entrapment of organisms and engulfment by bladder cells.
3. The pH and osmolality of urine prevent bacterial multiplication.
4. The ability to empty the bladder completely eliminates stasis of invading organisms and allows for continual flushing.

Respiratory Tract

1. The nares entrap most foreign matter on the mucous membranes as a result of turbulence caused by the turbinates and hairs.
2. The mucociliary transport system consists of cilia and mucus, which remove additional matter passing to the upper and lower bronchi.
3. Lysozymes and immunoglobulin A (IgA), a secretion of phagocytes, are found in nasal secretions and assist in the prevention of colonization.
4. Particles reaching as far as the alveoli can be removed through the expulsive action of sneezing and coughing, and the gag reflex.
5. Phagocytosis occurs in the alveoli, with the macrophages used as a major defense mechanism.

Gastrointestinal Tract

1. A mucous layer traps ingested microbes in the epithelium of the GI tract.
2. Gastric acids kill most organisms.
3. Peristalsis aids in the removal of organisms.
4. Intestinal secretions contain antibody (IgA), bile salts, lysozyme, glycolipids, and glycoproteins that prevent proliferation and adherence.
5. Normal gut flora interact to restrict over proliferation.

Wounds

1. Skin provides a first line of defense; the opening of the skin, either surgically or traumatically, potentiates infection.

2. A wound essentially closes within 24 hours, eliminating the risk of direct inoculations of organisms.
3. Wound infections rely on the capabilities of other host defenses to assist in the healing process.
4. Risk factors associated with wound infections depend on (1) endogenous factors such as presence of confounding factors, skin preparation, and the use of prophylactic antibiotics; and (2) exogenous factors such as the preoperative scrub, barrier techniques, airborne contamination, environmental disinfection, wound care, and the condition of the wound at the time of closure (Bennett & Brachman, 1992).
5. Wounds are at risk for infection owing to the following factors:
    a. Sutures and staples, unlike tape, create their own wounds, act like drains, and cause their own inflammatory response (Bennett & Brachman, 1992).
    b. Drains provide a site for microorganism entry (Bennett & Brachman, 1992).
    c. The incidence of infection in clients who are not shaved or clipped is 0.9%. It increases to 1.4% with electric shaving, 1.7% with clipping, and 2.5% with razor shaving (Kovach, 1990).

🕭 Key Concepts—Child

1. Congenital infections, those acquired in utero, usually result from exposure to such viruses as cytomegalovirus, rubella, hepatitis B, herpes simplex, herpes zoster, varicella, and Epstein-Barr. Some infections, such as toxoplasmosis, syphilis, tuberculosis, try-panosomiasis, and malaria, also may be caused by nonviral agents (Kenner, 1992, p. 16).
2. Congenital bacterial infections may arise from bacterial organisms that travel to the fetus through the placenta. The fetus may also become infected by organisms that reach the amniotic cavity through the mother's cervix (Kenner, 1992, p. 17).
3. Fetal skin and mucous membranes, intervillous placenta spaces, the umbilical cord, and respiratory airways (through aspiration) provide other avenues of infection (Kenner, 1992).
4. Approximately 80% of all childhood illnesses are due to infections, with respiratory infections occurring two to three times as often as other illnesses combined (Wong, 1995).
5. In general, acute illness is less frequent in children younger than age 6 months, increases from then on until age 3 or 4 years, and then gradually decreases throughout middle and older childhood (Wong, 1995).
6. According to Kliegman (1990), "the neonate is at higher risk for infections." By the time a child is a toddler, the production of antibodies is well established. Phagocytosis is much more efficient in toddlers than in infants (Wong, 1995).
7. Children who attend day care centers are at increased risk for infections caused by such organisms as *Shigella*, rotavirus, *Hemophilus influenzae* type b, and hepatitis A (Wong, 1995).
8. Good hygiene, optimal nutrition, immunizations, and strict sanitary practices can reduce the incidence of infectious disease during childhood.

🏛 Key Concepts—Older Adult

1. A slower rate of epidermal proliferation causes injured skin to take twice as long to heal in older adults.
2. Older adults also have compromised dermal immunologic responses because of a reduced number of Langerhans cells and reduced microcirculation (Miller, 1995).
3. In older adults, the lung's alveolar surface and elastic recoil are slightly decreased, and gas exchange in lower lung regions is decreased (Sparrow & Weiss, 1988).
4. Age-related changes in respiratory function do not significantly increase elderly people's risk for infection. Rather, the presence of non–age-related risk factors, such as smoking and exposure to occupational toxins, increases risk.
5. It is reported that 5%–20% of residents in long-term care facilities have infections. The most frequent infections are those of the urinary tract, respiratory system, and skin and soft tissues (usually a pressure ulcer) (Titler & Knipper, 1991).
6. The increased susceptibility of the elderly to infections is multifactorial (either host factors or environmental) (Titler & Knipper, 1991).

7. Host factors include underlying diseases, invasive treatment modalities, indiscriminate use of antibiotics, malnutrition, dehydration, impaired mobility, and incontinence (Titler & Knipper, 1991).
8. Environmental factors present in institutions include limited surveillance for infection, crowded areas, cross-contamination, and delay in early detection (Crossley, 1985).
9. Skin and urinary tract colonization is a greater problem in the elderly than in younger clients. Changes in immune competence with aging increase their susceptibility to fungal, viral, and mycobacterial pathogens (Stengle & Dries, 1994).
10. The elderly do not exhibit the usual signs of infection (fever, chills, tachypnea, tachycardia, leukocytosis), but instead present with anorexia, weakness, change in mental status, normothermia, or hypothermia (Stengle & Dries, 1994).

Focus Assessment Criteria

Subjective Data

A. Assess for related factors
  1. Does the person complain of:
     a. Previous infections

Urinary tract	Bone and joint
Pneumonia	Cardiovascular system
Surgical wound	Central nervous system
Skin and soft tissue	Eye, ear, nose, throat, mouth
Reproductive tract	Systemic
Lower respiratory tract	GI system
Blood	

     b. Pain or swelling
        Generalized   Localized
     c. Hemoptysis
     d. Productive, prolonged cough
     e. Chest pain associated with other criteria
     f. Systemic symptoms

Fever, continuous or intermittent	Easy fatigability
Chills	Loss of appetite
Night sweats	Weight loss

  2. History of recent travel
     a. Within United States
     b. Outside United States
  3. History of exposure to infectious diseases
     a. Airborne (most childhood infections result from communicable diseases, *e.g.*, chickenpox, tuberculosis)
     b. Vector-borne and other vector-associated infections (malaria, plague)
     c. Vehicle-borne and other food- and water-borne infections (hepatitis A, salmonellas)
     d. Contact spread (most common type of exposure)
        Direct (person to person)
        Indirect (instruments, clothing, and the like, to person)
        Contact droplet (*e.g.*, pneumonias, colds)
  4. History of risk factors associated with infections (see Related Factors)

Objective Data

A. Assess for related factors
  1. Presence of wounds
     a. Surgical
     b. Burns
     c. Invasive devices (tracheostomy, IV, drains)
     d. Self-induced
  2. Temperature, abnormal
  3. Nutritional status

Outcome Criteria

The person will:
- Demonstrate meticulous handwashing technique by the time of discharge
- Demonstrate knowledge of risk factors associated with potential for infection and will practice appropriate precautions to prevent infection

Interventions

A. Identify individuals at high risk for nosocomial infections (Owen & Grier, 1987)

1. Assess for predictors.
   a. Remote site of infection
   b. Abdominal or thoracic surgery
   c. Surgery longer than 2 hours
   d. Genitourinary procedure
   e. Instrumentation (ventilator, suction, catheters, nebulizers, tracheostomy, invasive monitoring)
   f. Anesthesia
2. Assess for confounding factors.
   a. Age younger than 1 year or older than 65 years
   b. Obesity
   c. Underlying disease conditions (chronic obstructive pulmonary disease, diabetes, cardiovascular, blood dyscrasias)
   d. Substance abuse
   e. Medications (steroids, chemotherapy, antibiotic therapy) that modify immune response
   f. Nutritional status (intake less than minimum daily requirements)
   g. Smoker
3. Consider a person who has one or more confounding factors and one or more predictors to be at *Risk for Infection.*
4. The following factors put people at risk for delayed wound healing (Kovach, 1990).
   a. Malnourishment
   b. Smoking
   c. Obesity
   d. Anemia
   e. Diabetes, cancer
   f. Corticosteroid therapy
   g. Renal insufficiency
   h. Hypovolemia
   i. Hypoxia
   j. Zinc, copper, magnesium deficiency
   k. Surgery >3 hours
   l. Night or emergency surgery
   m. Immune system compromise

B. Reduce the entry of organisms into individuals (Owen & Grier, 1987)

Surgical Wound

1. Before surgery, assess client for risk of remote site of infection.
2. If abdominal surgery, teach client (preop) importance of and technique for correct coughing, turning, and deep breathing.
3. If surgery is longer than 2 hours, assess client every shift for signs/symptoms of infection at surgical site.

4. Monitor temperature every 4 hours; notify physician if greater than 100.8°F.
5. Assess nutritional status to provide adequate protein and calorie intake for healing.
6. Assess wound site every 24 hours and during dressing changes, documenting any abnormal findings.
7. Evaluate all abnormal lab findings, especially culture/sensitivities, complete blood count (CBC).
8. Notify epidemiologist of any abnormal findings related to the development of infection.
9. Administer all prophylactic antibiotics within 15 minutes of scheduled administration time to ensure adequate therapeutic levels at surgery.
10. Instruct client and family on appropriate aseptic practice.
11. Use aseptic technique during dressing changes.
12. Use universal precautions with all body fluids from client.

Urinary Tract

1. Evaluate all abnormal lab findings, especially cultures/sensitivities, CBC.
2. Assess client for abnormal signs/symptoms after any urologic procedure, including frequency, urgency, burning, abnormal color, odor.
3. Monitor client temperature at least every 24 hours for elevation and notify physician if greater than 100.8°F.
4. Encourage fluids when appropriate.
5. Notify epidemiologist of any abnormal findings related to the development of infection.
6. Assess other wounds and systems to evaluate client's increased risk for development of infections at other sites.
7. Instruct client and family as to risk for development of urinary tract infections.
8. Use universal precautions with all fluids from client.
9. Use aseptic technique when emptying any urinary drainage device; keep bag off the floor, but below bladder or clamped during transport.
10. Administer all antibiotics within 15 minutes of scheduled administration time to ensure adequate therapeutic levels are maintained.
11. Reassess need for indwelling urinary catheter daily.

Circulatory

1. Assess all invasive lines every 24 hours for signs of redness, inflammation, drainage, tenderness.
2. Monitor client temperature at least every 24 hours and notify physician if greater than 100.8°F.
3. Maintain aseptic technique for all invasive devices, changing sites, dressings, tubing, and solutions per policy schedule.
4. Evaluate all abnormal lab findings, especially cultures/sensitivities, CBC.
5. Notify epidemiologist of any abnormal findings related to the development of infection.
6. Administer all antibiotics within 15 minutes of scheduled administration time.
7. Instruct client and family on appropriate aseptic practices to prevent infection.
8. Use universal precautions with all body fluids from client.
9. Assess nutritional status of client to provide adequate protein and calorie intake for healing.
10. Evaluate client for secondary sites of infection, either to bloodstream from another site or from bloodstream to other risk sites on patient.

Respiratory Tract

1. Evaluate client risk for infection after any instrumentation of the respiratory tract for at least 48 hours after procedure.
2. Notify epidemiologist of any abnormal findings related to the development of infection.
    a. Monitor temperature at least every 8 hours and notify physician if greater than 100.8°F.

    b. Evaluate sputum characteristics for frequency, purulence, blood, odor.

    c. Evaluate sputum and blood cultures, if done, for significant findings.

    d. Evaluate CBC for significant shift in white blood cell counts.

    e. Assessment of lung sounds every 8 hours or PRN.

  3. If client has abdominal/thoracic surgery, instruct before surgery on importance of coughing, turning, and deep breathing.

  4. If client has had anesthesia, monitor for appropriate clearing of secretions in lung fields.

  5. Administer cardiopulmonary treatments as ordered, with assessment of response to treatment documented.

  6. Evaluate need for suctioning if patient is unable adequately to clear secretions.

  7. Use universal precautions with all body fluids from client.

  8. Use aseptic technique with all invasive procedures of the respiratory tract.

  9. Assess for risk of aspiration, keeping head of bed elevated 30° unless otherwise contraindicated.

  10. Assess nutritional status of patient to provide adequate protein and calorie intake for healing.

  11. If oral feedings not tolerated without aspiration, contact physician for further action.

  12. Instruct on principles of cough and deep breathing and prevention of infection.

C. Protect the immune-deficient individual from infection

  1. Place in private room.

  2. Instruct client to ask all visitors and personnel to wash their hands before approaching.

  3. Limit visitors when appropriate.

  4. Screen all visitors for known infections or exposure to infections.

  5. Limit invasive devices to those that are absolutely necessary.

  6. Teach client and family members signs and symptoms of infection.

  7. Evaluate client's personal hygiene habits.

  8. Provide immune globulin to those exposed to specific diseases that might be life threatening (*e.g.*, chickenpox, hepatitis, measles).

D. Reduce client's susceptibility to infection

  1. Encourage and maintain caloric and protein intake in diet (see *Altered Nutrition*).

  2. Assess the client for adequate immunizations against childhood diseases, bacterial infections (*e.g.*, pneumococcal and *Hemophilus influenzae* vaccines), and other viral infections (flu virus vaccines).

  3. Monitor use or overuse of antimicrobial therapy.

  4. Administer prescribed antimicrobial therapy within 15 minutes of scheduled time.

  5. Observe for clinical manifestations of infection in individuals at high risk.

  6. Minimize length of stay in hospital to prevent colonization with nosocomial organisms.

  7. Observe for superinfection development in clients currently receiving antimicrobial therapy.

E. Initiate health teaching and referrals, as indicated

  1. Instruct client and family regarding the causes, risks, and communicability of the infection.

  2. Report communicable diseases as appropriate to public health department.

  3. Collaborate with nurse epidemiologist on needs of client and family.

Rationale

- Predictors are controllable factors that have been identified as increasing the risk of infection by interfering with or compromising the host defenses. Intervention can be implemented to control or influence the degree of risk associated with these factors (Owen & Grier, 1987).

- Confounding factors augment the risk of infection. They are not singularly controllable during hospitalization but can enhance a person's predictive risk for infection significantly (Owen & Grier, 1987).
- Nurses must use precautions with blood and body fluids from all clients to protect themselves from exposure to all potentially infectious organisms (Centers for Disease Control and Prevention, 1989).
  - Wash hands before and after all client or specimen contact.
  - Handle the blood of all clients as potentially infectious.
  - Wear gloves for potential contact with blood and body fluids.
  - Place used syringes immediately in nearby impermeable container; avoid recapping or manipulating needle! Recapping or needle removal must be accomplished through the use of a mechanical device or a one-handed technique (U.S. Department of Health and Human Services [DHHS], 1991, p. 64176).
  - Wear protective eyewear and mask if splatter with blood or body fluids is possible (*e.g.*, bronchoscopy, oral surgery).
  - Wear gowns when splash with blood or body fluids is anticipated.
  - Handle all linen soiled with blood or body secretions as potentially infectious.
  - Process all laboratory specimens as potentially infectious.
  - Wear mask for tuberculosis and other respiratory organisms (HIV is not airborne).
  - Place resuscitation equipment where respiratory arrest is predictable (U.S. DHHS, 1991).
  - Wear shoe covers or surgical caps or hoods in instances where gross contamination can reasonably be anticipated (*e.g.*, autopsy, orthopedic surgery, obstetrics).
- Antibiotics administered at the proper timing interval ensure adequate maintenance of therapeutic levels.
- Handwashing reduces the risk of cross-contamination.
- Subtle changes in vital signs may be early signs of sepsis, particularly fever.
- A wound healing by primary intention requires a dressing to protect it from contamination until the edges seal (usually 24 hours). A wound healing by secondary intention requires a dressing to maintain adequate hydration; the dressing is not needed after wound edges seal.
- To repair tissue, the body needs increased protein and carbohydrate intake and adequate hydration for vascular transport of oxygen and wastes.

References/Bibliography

Bennett, J. V., & Brachman, P. S. (Eds.). (1992). *Hospital infections* (2nd ed.). Boston: Little, Brown.

Centers for Disease Control and Prevention. (1989, June 23). Guidelines for prevention of transmission of human immunodeficiency virus and hepatitis B virus to health-care and public safety workers. *MMWR, 38*, 5–15.

Centers for Disease Control and Prevention. (1995). Guidelines for handwashing and hand antisepsis in health care settings. *MMWR, 44*, 1–17.

Crossley, K. B. (1985). Infection control practices in Minnesota nursing homes. *Journal of the American Medical Association, 254*, 2918–2921.

Goldschmidt, R. H., & Dong, B. J. (1995) Current report—HIV: Treatment of AIDS and HIV-related conditions. *Journal of the American Board of Family Practice, 8*, 139–162.

Kenner, C. A. (1992). Biological characteristics of adaptation. In *Nurses' clinical guide: Neonatal care*. Springhouse, PA: Springhouse Corp.

Kliegman, R. M. (1990). Fetal and neonatal medicine. In R. E. Behrman & R. Kliegman (Eds.). *Nelson essentials of pediatrics*. Philadelphia: W. B. Saunders.

Kovach, T. (1990) Nip it in the bud: Controlling wound infection with preoperative shaving. *Today's O.R. Nurse, 9*, 23–26.

Mandell, A., Bennett, G. H., & Dolin, L. (1990). *Principles and practices of infectious diseases* (4th ed). Los Angeles: Churchill Livingstone.

Miller, C. A. (1995). *Nursing care of older adults* (2nd ed.). Glenview, IL: Scott, Foresman.

Nyhus, L., & Baker, R. J. (1992) *Mastery of surgery* (2nd ed. Vol. 1). Boston: Little, Brown.

Owen, M., & Grier, M. (1987). *Infection risk assessment guide*. Orange, CA: CalOptima.

Sparrow, D., & Weiss, S. T. (1988). Pulmonary systems. In J. W. Rowe & C. Besdive (Eds.). *Geriatric medicine*. Boston: Little, Brown.

Stamm, W. E. (1991). Catheter-associated urinary tract infections: Epidemiology, pathogenesis, and prevention. *American Journal of Medicine, 91*, 65S–71S.

Stengle, J., & Dries, D. (1994). Sepsis in the elderly. *Critical Care Nursing Clinics of North America, 6,* 421–427.

Titler, M., & Knipper, J. (1991). Potential for infection. In M. Maas, K. Buckwalter, & M. Hardy. (Eds.). *Nursing diagnoses and interventions for the elderly.* Redwood City, CA: Addison-Wesley Nursing.

U.S. Department of Health and Human Services. (1991). Rules and regulations. *Federal Register, 56*(235), 47632–47649.

U.S. Department of Health and Human Services. (1994). Draft guidelines for isolation precautions in hospitals. *Federal Register, 59*(214), 55552–55570.

U.S. Department of Health and Human Services and Centers for Disease Control and Prevention. (1994). *Core curriculum on tuberculosis: What the clinician should know* (3rd ed.). Washington, DC: Public Health Service.

Weinstein, R. A. (1991). Epidemiology and control of nosocomial infections in adult intensive care units. *American Journal of Medicine, 91,* 179S–184S.

Wong, D. L. (1995). *Nursing care of infants and children* (5th ed.). St. Louis: Mosby-Yearbook.

Infection Transmission, Risk for*

DEFINITION
Risk for Infection Transmission: The state in which an individual is at risk for transferring an opportunistic or pathogenic agent to others.

RISK FACTORS
Presence of risk factors (see Related Factors)

RELATED FACTORS
Pathophysiologic
Related to:

    Colonization with highly antibiotic-resistant organism
    Airborne transmission exposure
    Contact transmission exposure (direct, indirect, contact droplet)
    Vehicle transmission exposure
    Vector-borne transmission exposure

Treatment-Related
Related to contaminated wound
Related to devices with contaminated drainage:

    Urinary, chest tubes
    Suction equipment
    Endotracheal tubes

Situational (Personal, Environmental)
Related to:

    Unsanitary living conditions (sewage, personal hygiene)
    Areas considered high risk for vector-borne diseases (malaria, rabies, bubonic plague)

* This diagnosis is not currently on the NANDA list but has been included for clarity or usefulness.

Areas considered high risk for vehicle-borne disease (hepatitis A, *Shigella, Salmonella*)
Lack of knowledge of sources or prevention of infection
Intravenous drug use
Multiple sex partners
Natural disaster (*e.g.*, flood, hurricane)
Disaster with hazardous infectious material

Maturational

(Newborn)

Related to birth outside hospital setting in uncontrolled environment
Related to exposure during prenatal or perinatal period to communicable disease through mother

Key Concepts

1. To spread an infection, three elements are required (refer to Figure II-3):
   a. A source of infecting organisms
   b. A susceptible host
   c. A means of transmission for the organism
2. Sources of infecting organisms include:
   a. Clients, personnel, and visitors with acute disease, incubating infection, or colonized organisms without apparent disease

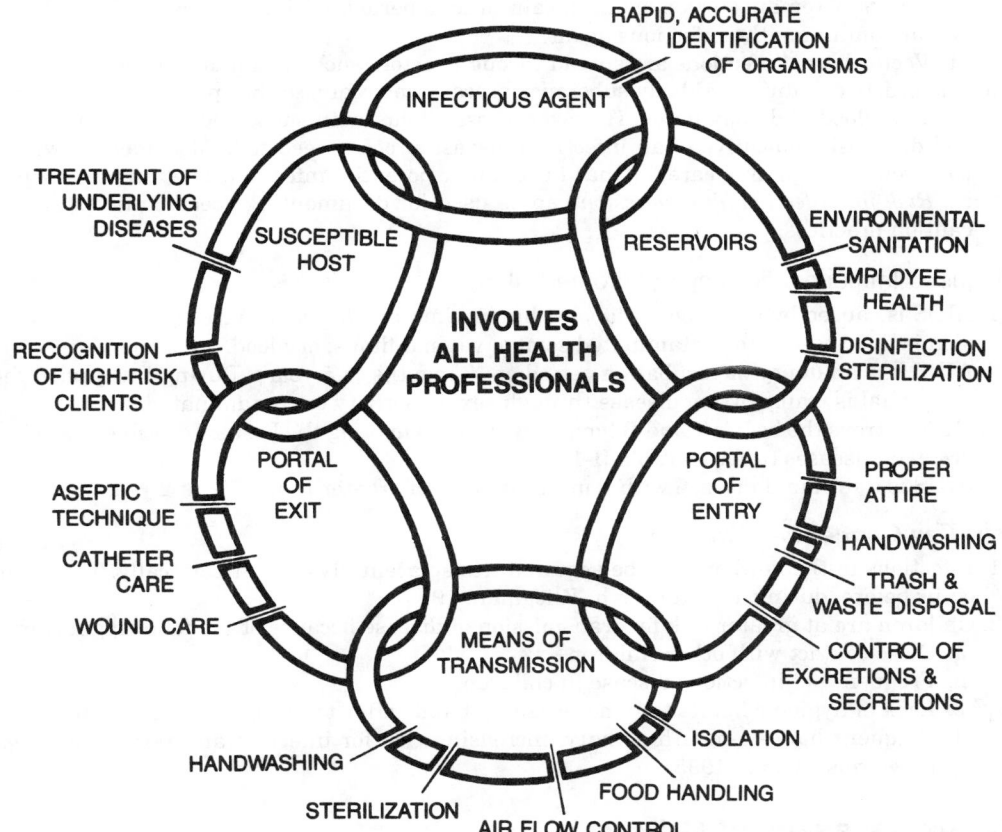

Fig. II-3 Breaking the chain of infection. (Adapted from the APIC Starter Kit with permission from the Association for Professionals in Infection Control and Epidemiology. Washington, DC, copyright APIC, 1978.)

    b. Person's own endogenous flora (autogenous infection)

    c. Inanimate environment, including equipment and medications

3. Susceptibility of the host varies according to

    a. Immune status of the host

    b. Ability to develop a commensal relationship with the infecting organism and become an asymptomatic carrier

    c. Preexisting diseases affecting the client

4. Means of transmission for the organism include one or more of the following:

    a. Contact transmission, the most frequent method of transferring organisms. It can be divided into three subgroups:

        Direct contact—involves direct physical transfer between a susceptible host and an infected or colonized person

        Indirect contact—involves the exchange of organisms between a host and contaminated objects, usually inanimate

        Droplet contact—involves the transfer of organisms from coughing, sneezing, or talking by an infected person into the conjunctivae, nose, or mouth of a susceptible host. Droplets travel no more than 3 feet.

    b. Vehicle route transmission infections are spread through a means such as:

        Food (*e.g.*, hepatitis A, *Salmonella*)

        Water (*e.g.*, *Legionella*)

        Drugs (*e.g.*, IV-contaminated products)

        Blood (*e.g.*, hepatitis B, HIV)

    c. Airborne infections are disseminated by droplet nuclei (residue of evaporated droplets that may remain suspended in the air for long periods of time) or dust particles in the air containing the infectious agent.

    d. Vector-borne infections are spread through vectors such as animals or insects.

5. The practice of universal body substance precautions requires that precautions be taken with all blood and body fluids. However, those clients with suspected or confirmed medical diagnosis indicative of an infectious disease process need to be documented with a comprehensive plan of care for that infection or potential infection. The nursing diagnosis *Risk for Infection Transmission* can be used for documenting specific universal precaution practices.

Acquired Immunodeficiency Syndrome (AIDS)

1. AIDS is caused by a retrovirus labeled human immunodeficiency virus (HIV). Transmission is by exposure to contaminated semen, vaginal fluids, or blood.

2. AIDS has a latency or incubation period of 18 months to 5 years. During this period the individual is transmitting disease through sexual activity or contaminated blood.

3. HIV destroys the body's T and B lymphocytes, thus making the host susceptible to a select group of diseases (refer to Table II-13).

4. AIDS is a terminal disease with a mortality rate of greater than 95% at 2 years.

✷ *Key Concepts—Child*

1. Infections in the newborn can be acquired transplacentally or transcervically. These can occur before, during, or after birth (Kliegman, 1990).

2. Children are at greater risk for transmission of disease because of the following factors:

    a. Close contact with other children

    b. Frequency of infectious disease in children

    c. Lack of hygienic habits (*e.g.*, not washing hands after toileting or before eating)

    d. Frequent hand-to-mouth activity, increasing risk for infection and reinfection (*e.g.*, pinworms) (Wong, 1995)

Focus Assessment Criteria

Refer to *Risk for Infection*

Table II-13   **List of Most Frequent Infections and Neoplasms in Acquired Immunodeficiency Syndrome (AIDS)**

Problem	Site
AIDS-Related Complex	
Candida albicans	Mouth (thrush)
Herpes simplex	Mucocutaneous; may be severe
Herpes zoster	Disseminated; may be severe
Lymphadenopathy	Generalized (always more than one lymph node)
Fevers	Usually greater than 100°F; persistent over months
Diarrhea	No organisms recovered, or conventional organisms recovered
Weight loss	Progressive and sustained
Night sweats	Characteristically severe and drenching; persistent and sustained over months
Thrombocytopenia	Often accompanied by petechia; may be severe and life threatening
Human immunodeficiency virus (HIV) encephalopathy	Clinical findings of disabling cognitive or motor dysfunction in absence of concurrent illness or condition other than HIV infection
HIV wasting syndrome	Profound, in the absence of concurrent illness or condition other than HIV infection
Infections	
Candida albicans	Mouth (thrush); throat
Cryptococcus neoformans	Central nervous system (CNS); pulmonary; disseminated
Pneumocystis carinii	Pneumonia
Toxoplasma gondii	CNS
Histoplasma gondii	CNS
Cryptosporidium	Intestine; diarrhea
Cytomegalovirus	Retinas; intestine; pulmonary; disseminated
Herpes simplex	Mucocutaneous; severe
Herpes zoster	Disseminated; severe
HIV	CNS, disseminated
Progressive multifocal leukoencephalopathy	CNS
Mycobacterium avium-intracellulare	Disseminated
Mycobacterium tuberculosis	Pulmonary (TB)
Neoplasms	
Kaposi's sarcoma	Skin; disseminated
Burkitt's lymphoma	Lymphatic system
Non-Hodgkin's lymphoma	Lymphatic system
Mycosis fungoides	Skin (dermal lymphoma)

(Adapted from Keating, S. B., & Kelman, G. B. [1988]. *Home health care nursing concepts and practice* [p 251]. Philadelphia: J. B. Lippincott.)

Outcome Criteria

The person will
- Relate the need to be isolated until noninfectious
- Describe the mode of transmission of disease by the time of discharge
- Demonstrate meticulous handwashing during hospitalization

Interventions

A. Identify susceptible host individuals based on focus assessment for risk for infection and history of exposure

B. Identify the mode of transmission based on infecting agent
  1. Airborne
  2. Contact
     a. Direct
     b. Indirect
     c. Contact droplet
  3. Vehicle-borne
  4. Vector-borne

C. Reduce the transfer of pathogens
  1. Isolate clients with airborne communicable infections (Table II-14).
  2. Secure appropriate room assignment depending on the type of infection and hygienic practices of the infected person.
  3. Use universal precautions to prevent transmission to self or other susceptible host.

D. Discuss the mode of transmission of infection with client, family and other significant individuals

Table II-14 **Airborne Communicable Diseases**

Disease	Apply Airborne Precautions for How Long	Comments
Anthrax, inhalation	Duration of illness	Promptly report to infection control office
Chickenpox (varicella)	Until all lesions are crusted	Immune person does not need to wear a mask. Exposed susceptible clients should be placed in a private special airflow room on STOP SIGN alert status beginning 10 days after initial exposure until 21 days after last exposure. Report to epidemiology.
Diphtheria, pharyngeal	Until 2 cultures from both nose and throat taken at least 24 hr after cessation of antimicrobial therapy are negative for *Corynebacterium diphtheriae*	Promptly report to epidemiology
Epiglottis, due to *Hemophilus influenzae*	For 24 hr after cessation of antimicrobial therapy	Report to epidemiology
Erythema infectiosum	For 7 days after onset	Report to epidemiology
Hemorrhagic fevers	Duration of illness	Call epidemiology office immediately. Physician may call the State Health Department and Centers for Disease Control and Prevention for advice about management of a suspected case.
Herpes zoster (varicella zoster), disseminated	Duration of illness	Localized does not require STOP SIGN
Lassa fever Marburg virus disease	Duration of illness	Call epidemiology office immediately. Physician may call the State Health Department and Centers for Disease Control and Prevention for advice about management of a suspected case.

Table II-14 **Airborne Communicable Diseases** *(continued)*

Disease	Apply Airborne Precautions for How Long	Comments
Measles (rubeola)	For 4 days after start of rash, except in immunocompromised patients with whom precautions should be maintained for duration of illness	Immune people do not need to wear a mask. Exposed susceptible clients should be placed in a private special air flow room on STOP SIGN alert status beginning the 5th day after exposure until 21 days after last exposure.
Meningitis *Hemophilus influenzae* known or suspected	For 24 hr after start of effective antibiotic therapy	Call epidemiology to report
Neisseria meningitidis (meningococci) known or suspected	For 24 hr after start of effective antibiotic therapy	Promptly report to epidemiology
Meningococcal pneumonia	For 24 hr after start of effective antibiotic therapy	Promptly report to epidemiology
Meningococcemia	For 24 hr after start of effective antibiotic therapy	Consult with epidemiology
Multiply resistant organisms	Until culture negative or as determined by epidemiology	Consult with epidemiology
Mumps (infectious parotitis)	For 9 days after onset of swelling	People with history do not need to wear a mask. Call epidemiology office to report.
Pertussis (whooping cough)	For 7 days after start of effective therapy	Call epidemiology to report
Plague, pneumonic	For 3 days after start of effective therapy	Promptly report to epidemiology
Pneumonia, *hemophilus* in infants and children any age	For 24 hr after start of effective therapy	Call epidemiology
Pneumonia, meningococcal	For 24 after start of effective antibiotic therapy	Promptly report to epidemiology
Rubella (German measles)	For 7 days after onset of rash	Immune people do not need to wear a mask. Promptly report to epidemiology.
Tuberculosis, bronchial, laryngeal, pulmonary, confirmed or suspect	Clients are not considered infectious if they meet all these criteria: Adequate therapy received for 2–3 weeks Favorable clinical response to therapy Three consecutive negative sputum smear results from sputum collected on different days	Call epidemiology to report; prompt use of effective antituberculosis drugs is the most effective means of limiting transmission.
Varicella (chickenpox)	Until all lesions crusted over	See chickenpox

(Centers for Disease Control and Prevention. [1996]. Isolation guidelines.)

E. Evaluate client for secondary sites of infection related to the spread of infection from primary site

F. Initiate health education and referrals as indicated

Rationale

- Nurses must use precautions with blood and body fluids from all clients to protect themselves from exposure to HIV and hepatitis B virus.
- To prevent transmission of infection the mode of transmission must be known (*i.e.*, airborne, contact, vehicle-borne or vector-borne) (Hoeprich, Jordon, & Ronald, 1994).

■ Risk for Infection Transmission

Related to Lack of Knowledge of Reducing the Risk of Transmitting the AIDS Virus

Outcome Criteria

The person will
- Describe the causes of AIDS and situations/factors contributing to its transmission
- Relate practices that reduce the transmission of the AIDS virus sexually
- Describe how to disinfect equipment

Interventions

A. Identify susceptible host individual
   1. Homosexual practices
   2. Bisexual practices
   3. Intravenous drug users
   4. Multiple blood transfusions (before March, 1985)
   5. Human immunodeficiency virus (HIV)-positive people
   6. Multiple sexual partners
   7. High-risk behaviors
   8. Presence of sexually transmitted diseases

B. Counsel susceptible host individuals to be tested for AIDS

C. Discuss the mode of transmission of the virus in semen or vaginal fluids and blood (Source: *Understanding AIDS*)
   1. Vaginal, anal, or oral sex with susceptible hosts
   2. Unprotected sex with infected person
   3. Sharing intravenous needles and syringes
   4. Contact of infected fluids with broken skin or mucous membrane

D. Prevent the transfer of virus and infection
   1. Teach to
      a. Abstain from sexual activity.
      b. Engage in sexual activity with one, mutually faithful, uninfected partner.
      c. Avoid intravenous (street) drug use.
   2. Use appropriate universal body substance precautions for all body fluids:
      a. Wash hands before and after all patient or specimen contact.
      b. Handle the blood of all patients as potentially infectious.
      c. Wear gloves for potential contact with blood and body fluids.
      d. Place used syringes immediately in nearby impermeable container; do not recap or manipulate needle in any way!
      e. Wear protective eyewear and mask if splatter with blood or body fluids is possible (*e.g.*, bronchoscopy, oral surgery).
      f. Wear gowns when splash with blood or body fluids is anticipated.
      g. Handle all linen soiled with blood or body secretions as potentially infectious.
      h. Process all laboratory specimens as potentially infectious.
      i. Wear mask for tuberculosis and other respiratory organisms (HIV is not airborne).
      j. Place resuscitation equipment where respiratory arrest is predictable.

3. Administer all antibiotics within 15 minutes of scheduled administration time to ensure adequate maintenance of therapeutic levels.
4. Monitor temperature at least every 4 hours during infectious process.
5. Evaluate all abnormal lab findings and report to physician, including culture with sensitivities to antibiotic administration.
6. Evaluate client for secondary sites of infection related to the spread of infection from a primary site.

E. Reduce the risk of transmission of AIDS with susceptible host people
1. Explain low-risk sexual behaviors.
   a. Mutual masturbation
   b. Massage
   c. Vaginal intercourse with condom
2. Explain the risk of ejaculate contact with broken skin or mucous membranes (oral, anal).
3. Teach to use condoms of latex rubber, not "natural membrane" condoms; teach appropriate storage to preserve latex.
4. Explain the need to use water-based lubricants to reduce prophylactic breaks. Avoid petroleum-based lubricants, which dissolve latex.
5. Explain that a condom with a spermicide may provide additional protection by decreasing the number of viable HIV particles.

F. Teach how to disinfect equipment possibly contaminated with the AIDS virus at home (needles, syringes, sex aids)
1. Wash under running water.
2. Fill or wash with household bleach.
3. Rinse well with water.

G. Provide facts to dispel the myths regarding AIDS transmission
1. The AIDS virus is not transmitted by mosquitoes, swimming pools, clothes, eating utensils, telephones, toilet seats, or close contact (*e.g.*, at work, school).
2. Saliva, sweat, tears, urine, and feces do not transmit the AIDS virus.
3. AIDS cannot be contracted during blood donations.
4. Blood for transfusions is tested to reduce substantially the risk of contracting the AIDS virus.

H. Initiate health teaching and referrals as indicated
1. Provide with AIDS hotline (1-800-342-AIDS) for more information.
2. Emphasize the need to be careful about the person the client becomes sexually involved with (past sexual partners, experimented with drugs).
3. Provide the community and schools with the facts regarding the transmission of AIDS, and dispel myths.
4. Refer to infection control practitioner for follow-up with the Health Department regarding family exposure and cause of exposure and to assist in appropriate plan of care for client
5. Client education regarding handwashing is the single most important measure to prevent the spread of infection.
6. Educate client regarding the chain of infection and client's responsibility in both the hospital and at home.

Rationale

- Handwashing is one of the most important means of preventing the spread of infection.
- Masks prevent transmission by aerosolization of infectious agents if oral mucosal lesions are present; gowns prevent soiling of clothes if contact with secretions/excretions is likely.

- Gloves provide a barrier from contact with infectious secretions and excretions.
- Eye coverings protect the eyes from accidental exposure to infectious secretions.
- Although to date no evidence of viral transmission to anyone other than sexual partners has been identified, still it is advisable that family members and others caring for or coming in contact with the client take simple precautions.
- Testing can predict onset of infection, enabling the person to receive medications prophylactically to slow disease progression.
- HIV is transmitted by sexual contact, by contact with infected blood and blood products, and perinatally (from mother to fetus).
- These measures aim to prevent contact of body fluids with mucous membranes.
- HIV is rapidly inactivated by exposure to disinfecting agents. Household bleach solution (dilute 1:10 with water) is an inexpensive choice.
- Dispelling myths and correcting misinformation can reduce anxiety and allow others to interact more normally with the client.

References/Bibliography

American Academy of Pediatrics Task Force on Pediatric AIDS. (1989, June). *Pediatric guidelines for HIV infection control*. San Francisco: AAP.

American Thoracic Society. (1994). Treatment of tuberculosis and tuberculosis infection in adults and children. *American Journal of Respiratory Critical Care Medicine, 149,* 1359–1374.

Becker, C. E., Cone, J. E., & Gerberding, J. (1989). Occupational infection with human immunodeficiency virus: Risks and risk reduction. *Annals of Internal Medicine, 110,* 653–656.

Bell, D. M. (1991). Human immunodeficiency virus transmission in healthcare settings: Risk and risk reduction. *American Journal of Medicine, 91,* 294S–300S.

Bennett, J. V., & Brachman, P. S. (Eds.). (1986). *Hospital infections* (2nd ed.). Boston: Little, Brown.

Centers for Disease Control and Prevention. (1991, July 12). Recommendations for preventing transmission of human immunodeficiency virus and hepatitis B virus to patients during exposure-prone invasive procedures. *MMWR, 40,* 1–9.

Centers for Disease Control and Prevention. (1992, December 18). 1993 Revised classification system for HIV infection and expanded surveillance case definition for AIDS among adolescents and adults. *MMWR, 41,* 1–19.

Garner, J. S., & Hughes, J. M. (1987). Options for isolation precautions [editorial]. *Annals of Internal Medicine, 107,* 248–250.

Hoeprich, P., Jordan, C., & Ronald, A. (1994). *Infectious diseases* (5th ed.). Philadelphia: J. B. Lippincott.

Jackson, M. M., Lynch, P., & McPerson, D. (1987). Why not treat all body substances as infectious? *American Journal of Nursing, 87,* 1137–1139.

Kliegman, R. M. (1990). Fetal and neonatal medicine. In R. E. Behrman & R. Kliegman (Eds.). *Nelson essentials of pediatrics*. Philadelphia: W. B. Saunders.

Lynch, P., Jackson, M. M., Cummings, M. F., & Stamm, W. E. (1987). Rethinking the role of isolation precautions in the prevention of nosocomial infections. *Annals of Internal Medicine, 107,* 243–246.

Miller, C. A. (1995). *Nursing care of older adults* (2nd ed.). Glenview, IL: Scott, Foresman.

U.S. Department of Health and Human Services. (1994). Draft guidelines for isolation precautions in hospitals. *Federal Register, 59*(214), 55552–55570.

U.S. Department of Health and Human Services. (1994). Guidelines for preventing the transmission of *Mycobacterium* tuberculosis in health-care facilities: Notice. *Federal Register, 59*(208), 54242–54303.

Wong, D. L. (1995). *Nursing care of infants and children* (5th ed.). St. Louis: Mosby-Year Book.

Resources for the Consumer

Literature

Available through state and county health departments (all major communicable diseases)

Understanding AIDS. DHHS Publication No. (CDC) HHS-88-8404. Washington, DC: Public Health Service.

Organizations

American Lung Association

Association for Professionals in Infection Control and Epidemiology (APIC, Washington, DC)

American Cancer Association

Public Health Service, AIDS Hotline USA, 1-800-342-2437

Injury, Risk for

Risk for Aspiration

Risk for Poisoning

Risk for Suffocation

Risk for Trauma

Injury, Risk for

DEFINITION

Risk for Injury: The state in which an individual is at risk for harm because of a perceptual or physiologic deficit, a lack of awareness of hazards, or maturational age.

RISK FACTORS

Presence of risk factor (see Related Factors)

RELATED FACTORS
Pathophysiologic

Related to altered cerebral function secondary to:

Tissue hypoxia	Syncope	Vertigo

Related to altered mobility secondary to:

Unsteady gait	Loss of limb
Amputation	Cerebrovascular accident
Arthritis	Parkinsonism

Related to impaired sensory function (specify)

Vision	Thermal/touch
Hearing	Smell

Related to fatigue
Related to orthostatic hypotension
Related to vertebrobasilar insufficiency
Related to vestibular disorders
Related to lack of awareness of environmental hazards secondary to:

Confusion	Depression
Hypoglycemia	Electrolyte imbalance

Related to tonic–clonic movements secondary to:
Seizures
Related to carotid sinus syncope

Treatment-Related

Related to effects of (specify) in mobility or sensorium:
Medications

Sedatives	Diuretics

> Vasodilators   Phenothiazine
> Antihypertensives   Psychotropics
> Hypoglycemics
>
> Related to casts/crutches, canes, walkers

Situational (Personal, Environmental)

Related to decrease in or loss of short-term memory
Related to faulty judgment secondary to:
  Dehydration (*e.g.*, in summer)
  Stress
  Alcohol, drugs
Related to prolonged bed rest
Related to vasovagal reflex
Related to household hazards (specify)

Unsafe walkways	Stairs
Unsafe toys	Slippery floors
Inadequate lighting	Faulty electric wires
Bathrooms (tubs, low toilets)	Improperly stored poisons

Related to automotive hazards
  Lack of use of seat belts or child seats
  Mechanically unsafe vehicle
Related to fire hazards
Related to unfamiliar setting (hospital, nursing home)
Related to improper footwear
Related to inattentive caretaker
Related to improper use of aids (crutches, canes, walkers, wheelchairs)
Related to history of accidents

Maturational

Infant/child
  Related to lack of awareness of hazards
Older Adult
  Related to faulty judgments secondary to motor and sensory deficits, medication (accidental overdose), cognitive deficits

Author's Note

This diagnosis has four subcategories: *Risk for Aspiration, Poisoning, Suffocation*, and *Trauma*. The interventions to prevent poisoning, suffocation, and trauma are included under the general category *Risk for Injury*. Should the nurse choose to isolate interventions only for prevention of poisoning, suffocation, or trauma, then the diagnosis *Risk for Poisoning, Risk for Suffocation*, or *Risk for Trauma* would be useful.

   Nursing interventions related to *Risk for Injury* focus on protecting a person from injury and teaching precautions to reduce the risk of injury. When the nurse is teaching a client or family safety measures to prevent injury, but is not providing on-site protection (as in the community or outpatient department, or for discharge planning), the diagnosis *Risk for Injury related to insufficient knowledge of safety precautions* may be more appropriate.

Errors in Diagnostic Statements

Risk for Injury: Hemorrhage related to abnormal blood profile secondary to cirrhosis
   This diagnosis does not represent a situation that a nurse can prevent, but rather one that the nurse monitors and comanages as the collaborative problem *Potential Complication: Hemorrhage related to altered clotting factors.*

Key Concepts

1. Injury is the fourth leading cause of death in the general population (40.1 deaths per 100,000), and the leading cause of death for children and young adults (National Center for Health Statistics, 1993).
2. The rate of accidents can be reduced with health education activities that focus on fire safety, home safety, water safety, seat belt use, motor vehicle safety, cardiopulmonary resuscitation (CPR) training, poison control, and first aid (Clemen-Stone, Eigasti, & McGuire, 1991).
3. Table II-15 lists common sources of poisoning in the home.

Postural Hypotension

1. Postural hypotension refers to a sudden drop in blood pressure of 20 mm Hg or greater for at least 1 minute when standing.
2. Studies have shown that postprandial hypotension occurs in about one third of healthy adults 1 hour after eating breakfast and lunch (Lipsitz & Fullerton, 1986).
3. Postural hypotension can seriously affect a person's quality of life if it contributes to falls or fear of falling.
4. Postural hypotension also can precipitate stroke and myocardial infarctions (Cunha, 1987).

🐢 Key Concepts—Child

1. Injuries rank as the number 1 cause of death in people between 1 and 19 years of age (Wong, 1995).
2. Five leading injuries include traffic accidents, drowning, burns and scalds, choking, poisoning, and falls (Children's National Medical Center, 1989).
3. Each year, car crashes injure and kill more children than any disease. Used properly, child safety seats and safety belts protect children in a crash and help save lives (Children's National Medical Center, 1989).

Table II-15 **Poisonous Substances Around the House**

Drugs

Aspirin	Cough medicines	Laxatives
Tranquilizers	Vitamins	Oral contraceptives
Barbiturates	Acetaminophen	

Petroleum Products

Cleaning Agents

Soaps and polishes	Disinfectants	Drain cleaners

Poisonous Plants

Amaryllis	Iris	Philodendron
Azalea	Jack-in-the-pulpit	Poinsettia
Baneberry	Jerusalem cherry	Poison hemlock
Bellodonna	Jimsonweed	Poison ivy
Bittersweet	Lily of the valley	Pokeweed
Bloodroot	Marijuana	Potato leaves
Castor-bean plant	Mistletoe	Rhododendron
Climbing nightshade	Morning glory	Rhubarb leaves
Daffodil	Mountain laurel	Schefflera
Devil's ivy	Mushrooms	Tomato leaves
Dieffenbachia	Oleander	Wisteria
Foxglove	Peacelily	Yew
Holly		

Miscellaneous

Baby powder	Cosmetics	Lead paint

4. Injury accounts for 78% of the total fatalities among late adolescents (age 15–19 years), the pediatric age group at highest risk for injury mortality (Guyer & Ellers, 1990).
5. Between 70% to 80% of infants will use a walker, usually between 5 and 12 months of age. Of those infants who use walkers, 30%–40% will have an accident (American Medical Association [AMA] Board of Trustees, 1991).
6. Most walker accidents are minor; however, serious trauma from head injuries, lacerations, and burns does occur occasionally. Parents should be counseled on the risk of injury from the use of infant walkers (AMA Board of Trustees, 1991).
7. School-age children are at greatest risk for bicycle accidents. Every day, more than 1000 children are injured, and 1 dies, in bicycle accidents. One third of children treated in emergency rooms for bicycle accidents have head injuries. The use of bicycle helmets could reduce the incidence of these injuries.
8. Drowning is the second leading cause of death from injury during childhood. Children younger than 4 years of age are at especially high risk (Children's National Medical Center, 1989).
9. Children should be taught early (when 2 years old) and constantly reminded about rules concerning streets, playground equipment, fires, water (pools, bathtubs), animals, strangers.
10. In 1982 in the United States, 738 children drowned and 3000 children experienced near-drowning, with one third left with neurologic deficits; 68,000 people had nonsubmersion accidents in and around swimming pools (Baxter, 1987).
11. Sixty-eight percent of the near-drowning accidents take place while a parent is supervising the child, resulting from a momentary lapse of attention (Baxter, 1987).
12. Effective swimming depends on intellectual as well as physical maturity. Organized swimming lessons may give parents a false sense of security that their child "can swim" (Baxter, 1987).
13. Swimming programs that use total submersion put an infant at risk for water intoxication, hypothermia, and bacterial infections. In addition, infants may learn to fear the water (Brill, 1987).
14. Children age 1–3 years are at greatest risk for scalds. More than one third of children age 3–8 years are burned while playing with matches. When a fire strikes, young children need help to escape (Children's National Medical Center, 1989).
15. For children younger than age 3 years, choking is the fourth leading cause of accidental death (Children's National Medical Center, 1989).
16. Toddlers are at highest risk for poisoning. Children are poisoned by medications as well as by common household items (*e.g.*, plants, make-up, and cleaning products) (Children's National Medical Center, 1989).
17. For children aged 1–4 years, the leading cause of accidental death and serious injury is falls in the home (Children's National Medical Center, 1989).

Key Concepts—Older Adult

1. Falls occur with greater frequency in the elderly, and the mortality, dysfunction, disability, and need for medical services that result are greater than in younger age groups. Unintentional injury, a category including falls, motor vehicle accidents, and burns, is the seventh leading cause of death in the elderly, and the incidence of falls represents over 60% of that category.
2. Approximately 25% of hospital admissions for older adults are directly related to falling; 47% of these people are admitted to long-term care facilities (Tideiksaar, 1989).
3. "Fallaphobia" refers to fears related to a person's loss of confidence to perform activities without falling. These fears actually increase the risk for falling, and the person eventually becomes house-bound (Tideiksaar, 1989).
4. A fall-free existence is not always possible for some individuals. Increased independence and mobility may be an important and valuable trade-off for an increased risk of falling. Collaboration among the client, family, and team members helps arrive at the decision of a less restricted environment.

5. The following factors increase the risk for falls in older adults (Berryman, Gaskin, Jones, Tolley, & MacMullen, 1989; Moss, 1992):
   a. History of falls
   b. Sensory–motor deficits (*e.g.*, vision, hearing, hemianopia, paresis, aphasia)
   c. Gait instability
   d. Improper footwear or foot problems (corns, bunions, calluses)
   e. Postural hypotension, especially with complaints of dizziness
   f. Confusion (persistent or acute)
   g. Incontinence, urinary urgency
   h. Cardiovascular disease affecting cerebral perfusion and oxygenation: dysrhythmias, syncopal episodes, congestive heart failure, fibrillation
   i. Neurologic disease affecting movement or judgment: cerebrovascular accident with impulsivity; parkinsonism; moderate Alzheimer's disease; seizure disorder, vertigo
   j. Orthopedic disorders or devices affecting movement or balance: casts, splints, slings, prostheses, recent surgery, severe arthritis
   k. Medications affecting blood pressure or level of consciousness: psychotropics, sedatives, analgesics, diuretics, antihypertensives, medication change, more than five drugs
   l. Agitation, increased anxiety, emotional lability
   m. Willfulness, uncooperativeness
   n. Situational factors: new admission, room change, roommate change

Focus Assessment Criteria

This entire assessment is indicated only when the client is at high risk for injury because of personal deficits, alterations (*e.g.*, mobility problems), or maturational age. In households without such a family member, the functional assessment of the individual can be deleted.

Subjective Data

These consist of the person's physical capabilities (as reported by person or caretaker).

A. Assess for related or risk factors
   1. Vision
      Adequate
      Corrected (date of last prescription)
      Complaints of
         Blurriness   Difficulty in focusing
         Loss of side vision   Inability to adjust to darkness
   2. Hearing
      Adequate   Need to read lips
      Use of hearing aid (condition, batteries)   Inadequate
   3. Thermal/tactile
      Adequate   Altered sense of hot/cold
   4. Mental status
      Alert
      Drowsy
      Confused
      Oriented to time, place, events
      Complaints of
         Vertigo   Orthostatic hypotension
         Altered sense of balance
      Cognitive stage (immature reasoning/judgment)
   5. Mobility
      Reports of
         Feeling lightheaded, dizzy   Losing balance
         Difficulty standing, sitting   Wandering
         Falling or almost falling

Ability to ambulate

    Around room   Around house

    Up and down stairs   Outside house

Ability to travel

    Drive car (date of last reevaluation)

    Use public transportation

Devices

    Cane   Walker   Condition of devices

    Wheelchair   Prosthesis   Competence in their use

Shoes/slippers

    Condition   Nonskid soles   Fit

Abilities related to developmental milestones

    Turning over   Climbing

    Sitting   Crawling

    Standing   Walking

6. Miscellaneous

Drug therapy

    Type, dosage   Storage

    Labeling   Ability to self-medicate safely

Communication

    Write   Contact emergency assistance

    Use phone   Make needs known

Support system/primary caregiver

Help available from relatives, friends, neighbors

    Club and church contacts

History of "blackouts"

Urinary frequency or incontinence

Objective Data

A. Assess for related factors

   1. Blood pressure (left, right, sitting/lying more than 5 minutes, 1 minute after standing)

   2. Gait/mobility

      Steady   Requires aids   Unsteady

   3. Cognitive processes

      Ability to communicate needs

      Ability to interact

      History of wandering (witnessed and reported by others)

      Ability to understand cause and effect

   4. Presence of

      Anger   Withdrawal

      Depression   Faulty judgment

   5. Ability for self-care activities

      Dress and undress   Bathe

      Groom self   Feed self

      Reach toilet

B. Assess for related factors in the home

   1. Safety

      Toilet facilities   Water supply

      Heating   Sewage

      Ventilation   Garbage disposal

   2. Safety of walkways (inside and outside)

      Sidewalks (uneven, broken)

      Stairs (inside and outside)

         Broken steps   Lighting

         No hand rails   Protection for children

Halls
  Cluttered
  Poor lighting
3. Electrical hazards
  Absence of outlet covers
  Cords frayed and unanchored
  Outlets overloaded; accessible to children; near water
  Switches too far from bedside
4. Inadequate lighting
  At night; and outdoors
  To bathroom at night
5. Unsafe floors
  Even or uneven
  Highly polished
  Rugs not anchored
6. Kitchen hazards
  Pot handles not turned inward
  Stove (grease or flammable objects on stove)
  Refrigerator (improperly stored food; inadequate temperatures)
7. Toxic substances
  Stored in food containers, not properly labeled and accessible to children
  Medications kept beyond date of expiration
  Poisonous household plants
8. Fire hazards
  Matches/lighters accessible to children
  No fire extinguishers
  Improper storage of corrosives, combustibles
  Lack of furnace maintenance
  No fire escape plan, no fire extinguishers
  Emergency telephone numbers not accessible (firehouse, police)
9. Hazards for children in nursery
  Cribs near drapery cords
  Cribs with wide slat openings
  Plastic bags
  Pillows in crib
  Space between mattress and crib rails
  Unattended without crib rails up
  Unattended on changing table
  Pacifier hung around infant's neck
  A propped bottle placed in infant's crib
  Toys with pointed edges, removable parts
10. Hazards for children in household
  Accessible purses with medications, lighters, matches
  Objects with lead paint
  Poisonous plants (see Table II-15 for specific plants)
  Open windows without screens or loose screens
  Plastic bags
  Furniture with glass or sharp corners
  Open doorways, stairways
11. Outdoor hazards for children
  Porches without rails
  Play area without fence
  Backyard pools
  Domestic/wild animals
  Poisonous plants

Outcome Criteria

The person will
- Identify factors that increase the risk for injury
- Relate an intent to use safety measures to prevent injury (*e.g.*, remove throw rugs or anchor them)
- Relate an intent to practice selected prevention measures (*e.g.*, wear sunglasses to reduce glare)
- Increase his daily activity, if feasible

Interventions

A. Assess for the presence of causative or contributing factors
   1. Unfamiliar surroundings
   2. Impaired vision
      a. Altered spatial judgment
      b. Blurred vision
      c. Diplopia
      d. Blind spots
      e. Cataracts
      f. Altered peripheral vision
      g. Hemianopia (loss of half the visual field)
      h. Increased susceptibility to visual glare
      i. Decreased ability to distinguish object from background
   3. Decreased hearing acuity
   4. Decreased tactile sensitivity (touch)
   5. Orthostatic hypotension
   6. Hypoglycemia
   7. Unstable gait
   8. Pain
   9. Fatigue
   10. Improper shoes or slippers
   11. Improper use of crutches, canes, walkers
   12. Joint immobility
   13. Side effects of medication (*e.g.*, tranquilizers, diuretics)
   14. Hazardous environmental factors

B. Reduce or eliminate causative or contributing factors, if possible
   1. Unfamiliar surroundings
      a. Orient each new admission to surroundings, explain the call system, and assess the person's ability to use it.
      b. Closely supervise the person during the first few nights to assess safety.
      c. Use night-light.
      d. Encourage to request assistance during the night.
      e. Teach about side effects of certain drugs (*e.g.*, dizziness, fatigue).
      f. Keep bed at lowest level during the night.
      g. Consider use of a movement detection monitor, if needed.
   2. Impaired vision
      a. Provide safe illumination and teach person to
         Provide adequate lighting in all rooms, with soft light at night.
         Have light switch easily accessible, next to bed.
         Provide background light that is soft.
      b. Teach how to reduce glare.
         Avoid all glossy surfaces (*e.g.*, glass, highly polished floors).
         Use diffuse light rather than direct light; use shades that darken the room.

Turn head away when switching on a bright light.

Wear sunglasses or hats with brims, or carry umbrellas, to reduce glare outside.

Avoid looking directly at bright lights (*e.g.*, headlights).

c. Teach person or family to provide sufficient color contrast for visual discrimination and to avoid green and blue.

Color-code edges of steps (*e.g.*, with colored tape).

Avoid white walls, dishes, counters.

Avoid clear glasses (*i.e.*, use smoked glass).

Choose objects colored black on white (*e.g.*, black phone).

Avoid colors that merge (*e.g.*, beige switches on beige walls).

Paint doorknobs bright colors.

3. Decreased tactile sensitivity

a. Teach preventive measures.

Assess temperature of bath water and heating pads before use.

Use bath thermometers.

Assess extremities daily for undetected injuries.

Keep feet warm and dry and skin softened with emollient lotion (lanolin, mineral oil).

b. See *Altered Tissue Perfusion: Peripheral* for additional interventions.

4. Decreased hearing acuity

a. Determine if the person has had his hearing evaluated professionally.

b. Assist him in making a decision concerning the use or type of hearing aid if indicated.

c. Teach, when driving, to leave car window partially open to allow warning signals to be heard (*e.g.*, sirens) and set air conditioner, heater, or radio low so that outside noises can be heard.

5. Orthostatic hypotension

a. See *Risk for Injury Related to Vertigo Secondary to Orthostatic Hypotension* for additional interventions.

6. Unstable gait

a. Crutches

Teach exercises to strengthen arm and shoulder muscles to facilitate use of crutches; use weights and parallel bars.

Measure and fit crutches to each person (2–3 inches between top of crutch and armpit); improper length of crutches may cause nerve damage or falls.

Instruct to wear shoes that fit properly and have nonskid soles.

Assess ability to walk and climb up and down stairs.

Consult with physical therapist for proper gait training.

b. Canes

Teach person to hold cane in hand opposite affected leg and move cane and impaired limb together.

Cane should be proper length to allow person to extend elbow and bear weight on hand.

Cane should be fitted with rubber tip.

Consult with physical therapist for proper gait training.

c. Walkers

Teach person exercises to strengthen triceps muscles used in proper crutch walking.

See that floors are clean and dry and free of obstacles and that rugs are anchored.

Instruct to wear properly fitted shoes with nonslip soles.

Consult with physical therapist for proper gait training.

d. Prosthesis

Teach to bathe and inspect stump daily.

Instruct to put on prosthesis soon after rising to minimize stump swelling.

Prepare person for crutch walking with triceps exercises using weights and
parallel bars.

Consult with physical therapist for proper gait training.

7. Side effects of medications
   a. Assess for the presence of side effects of drugs that may cause vertigo.

   Hypotension   Vasodilation

   Sedation   Vasoconstriction

   Hypokalemia

8. Hazardous environmental factors
   a. Teach to

   Eliminate throw rugs, litter, and highly polished floors.

   Provide nonslip surfaces in bathtub or shower by applying commercially available traction tapes.

   Provide hand grips in bathroom.

   Provide railings in hallways and on stairs.

   Remove protruding objects (*e.g.*, coat hooks, shelves, light fixtures) from stair-
   way walls.

   b. Instruct staff to

   Keep siderails on bed in place and bed at the lowest position when person is
   left unattended.

   Keep bed at lowest position with wheels locked when stationary.

   Teach person in wheelchair to lock and unlock wheels.

   Ensure that person's shoes or slippers have nonskid soles.

C. Describe and document falls

1. Document and describe injuries, previous falls, medications, and measures taken

D. Initiate health teaching and referrals, as indicated

1. Teach measures to prevent auto accidents.
   a. Frequently reevaluate ability to drive vehicles.
   b. Wear good-quality sunglasses (gray or green) to reduce glare.
   c. Keep windshields clean and wipers in good condition.
   d. Place mirrors on both sides of car.
   e. Stop periodically to stretch and rest eyes.
   f. Know the effects of medications on driving ability.
   g. Do not smoke while driving or drive after drinking.

2. Teach measures to prevent pedestrian accidents.
   a. Allow enough time to cross streets.
   b. Wear garments that reflect light (beige, white) at night.
   c. Wait to cross on the sidewalk, not the street.
   d. Look both ways.
   e. Do not rely solely on green traffic lights to provide safe crossing (right turn on red
   light may be legal, or driver may disobey traffic regulations).

3. Teach measures to prevent burns.
   a. Equip home with smoke alarm system and check its function each month.
   b. Have a hand fire extinguisher.
   c. Set thermostats for water heater to provide warm, but not scalding, water.
   d. Use baking soda or a lid cover to smother a kitchen grease fire.
   e. Do not wear loose-fitting clothing (*e.g.*, robes, nightgowns) when cooking.
   f. Do not smoke when sleepy.
   g. Ensure that portable heaters are safely used.
   h. See *Risk for Injury Related to Lack of Awareness of Environmental Hazards* for
   additional safety measures.

4. Refer individuals with motor or sensory deficits for assistance in identifying environmental hazards.
   a. Local fire company
   b. Community nursing agency
   c. Accident-prevention information (see References/Bibliography)

5. Discuss the benefits of a walking program to increase circulation if permissible; instruct to
   a. Rest 10–15 minutes before walking.
   b. Start slowly (10 minutes).
   c. Increase time gradually.
   d. Refrain from drinking caffeine products (coffee, tea, chocolate, cola) 2–3 hours before walking.
   e. Wait 2 hours after meals to walk.
   f. Expect some muscle soreness; reduce activity if pain or breathlessness occur.
6. Assist person and family to evaluate environmental hazards and the effects of restrictions on quality of life.
7. Refer to public health or visiting nurse for home visit.
8. Refer to physical therapist for evaluation of gait.

Rationale

- An unfamiliar environment and problems with vision, orientation, mobility, and fatigue can increase a client's risk of falling.
- Identifying the types of visual disturbances and options available allows the client to take the necessary precautions.
- A client with mobility problems needs such safety devices installed and hazards eliminated to aid in activities of daily living.
- Goals for prevention and management of falls focus on reducing the likelihood of falls by reducing environmental hazards, strengthening individual competence to resist falls and fall-related injury, and providing postfall injury care.
- Visual difficulty because of glare is often responsible for falls in the aged, who have an increased susceptibility to glare. Incandescent (nonfluorescent) lighting produces less glare and, therefore, provides better illumination for the aged.
- An unfamiliar environment coupled with vision and mobility difficulties can increase a client's risk of injury (*e.g.*, falls, burns).

■ Risk for Injury
Related to Lack of Awareness of Environmental Hazards

Outcome Criteria

The person or family will
- Identify potentially hazardous factors in the environment
- Report safe practices in the home
- Teach children safety habits

Interventions

A. Identify situations that contribute to accidents

       Unfamiliar setting (homes of others, hotels)
       Peak activity periods (during meal preparation, holidays)
       New equipment (bicycle, chain saw, lawn mower, snow blower)
       Lack of awareness of or disregard for environmental hazards

B. Reduce or eliminate hazardous situations
  1. New equipment
     a. Teach to read directions completely before using a new appliance or a piece of equipment.
     b. Determine the limitations of the equipment.
     c. Unplug and turn off any appliance that is not functioning before examining (*e.g.*, lawn mower, snow blower, electric mixer).
  2. Unsafe practices
     a. Automobiles
        Driving a mechanically unsafe vehicle
        Not using or misusing seat restraints
        Driving after partaking of alcohol or drugs
        Driving with unrestrained babies and children in the car
        Driving at excessive speeds
        Driving without necessary visual aids
        Driving with unsafe road or road crossing conditions
        Nonuse or misuse of necessary headgear for motorcyclist
        Children riding in front seat of car
        Backing up without checking location of small children
        Warming a car in a closed garage
     b. Flammables
        Igniting gas leaks
        Delayed lighting of gas burner or oven
        Experimenting with chemicals or gasoline
        Unscreened fires, fireplaces, heaters
        Inadequately stored combustibles, matches, or oily rags
        Smoking in bed or near oxygen
        Highly flammable children's toys or clothing
        Playing with fireworks or gunpowder
        Playing with matches, candles, cigarettes, lighters
        Wearing of plastic aprons or flowing clothing around open flame
     c. Household
        Kitchen
           Grease waste collected on stoves
           Wearing of plastic aprons or flowing clothing around open flame
           Use of cracked glasses or dishware
           Use of improper canning, freezing, or preserving methods
           Knives stored in an uncovered fashion
           Pot handles facing front of stove
           Use of thin or worn potholders or oven mitts
           Stove controls on front
           Lead in dishes
        Bathroom
           Unlocked medicine cabinet
           Lack of grab rails in bathtub
           Lack of nonskid mats or emery strips in bathtub
           Poor lighting in bathroom and hallways
           Improper placement of electrical outlets
        Chemicals and irritants
           Improperly labeled medication containers
           Medications kept in containers other than original ones
           Poor illumination at the medicine cabinet
           Improperly labeled containers of poisons and corrosive substances
           Expired medications that dangerously decompose
           Toxic substances stored in accessible areas (*e.g.*, under sink)

Inadequately stored corrosives (*e.g.*, lye)
Contact with intense cold
Overexposure to sun, sunlamps, heating pads
Lighting and electrical
Uncovered outlets
Unanchored electrical wires
Overloaded electrical outlets
Overloaded fuse boxes
Faulty electrical plugs, frayed wires, or defective electrical appliances
Inadequate lighting over landings and stairs
Inaccessible light switches (*e.g.*, bedside)
Use of machinery or appliances without prior instruction

Rationale

- The differentiation between accidents and injuries is a useful distinction for nurses to understand. The term *accident* implies lack of control of external forces. Nursing focuses on identifying variables (host, agent, environment) that can be controlled to prevent injuries (Green, 1989).
- The nurse can reduce host variables that increase risk for injury, such as lack of knowledge; agent variables, such as shear forces in bed; and environmental variables, such as spills and other hazards.
- Accidents occur more frequently
  - During the initial period of hospitalization and between the hours of 6 and 9 P.M.
  - During peak activity periods (mealtime, playtime)
  - In unfamiliar surroundings
  - With inadequate lighting
  - At holidays
  - On vacations
  - During home repairs
- Color contrast between the object and the background increases visualization (*e.g.*, white against black).

Interventions—*Child Focus*

A. Teach parents basic safety measures and assessments
1. Teach parents to expect frequent changes in infants' and children's abilities and to take precautions (*e.g.*, infant who suddenly rolls over for the first time might be on a changing table unattended).
2. Discuss with parents the necessity of constant monitoring of small children.
3. Provide parents with information to assist them in selecting a babysitter.
   a. Determine previous experiences and knowledge of emergency measures.
   b. Observe the interaction of the sitter with the child (*e.g.*, pick up the sitter one-half hour before you are ready to leave).
4. Teach parents to expect children to mimic them and to teach children what they can do with or without supervision.
   a. Tell the child to ask you before attempting a new task.
   b. Do not take pills in front of children.
5. Explain and expect compliance with certain rules (depending on age) concerning

Streets	Fire
Playground equipment	Animals
Water (pools, bathtubs)	Strangers
Bicycles	

6. Role-play with children to assess understanding of the problem

"You are walking home from school and a strange man pulls up in a car near you. What do you do?"

"While walking past a barbecue, your dress catches on fire. What do you do?"

B. Identify situations that contribute to accidents
1. Bicycles, wagons, skateboards, and skates
   a. No reflectors or lights
   b. Not in single file
   c. Riding a too-large bicycle
   d. Lack of knowledge of rules of the road
   e. Use of skateboards or skates in heavily traveled areas
   f. Lack of helmet, protective pads
2. Water and pools
   a. Discourage use of flotation or swim aids (water wings, tubs) with children who cannot swim.
   b. Teach safe water behavior:
      No running, pushing
      No jumping on others
      No swimming alone
      No playful screaming for help
      No diving in water less than 8 feet deep
      No swimming after meals
      No swimming during electrical storms
      Avoid excessive alcohol use
   c. Enclose pool:
      Use a 5–5½ foot fence.
      Use a fence that children cannot climb.
      Use self-locking gates.
   d. Remove pool cover completely.
   e. Avoid free-floating pool covers.
   f. Teach safe diving and sliding techniques.
      Allow diving only from diving boards.
      Discourage running dives.
      Teach to steer upward with hands and head.
      Descend pool slide sitting with feet first.
   g. Have lifesaving equipment at poolside (life preserver, rope, or hook).
   h. Learn CPR and how to respond to accidental submersion.
      Remove from water.
      If spinal injury is suspected, immobilize on a board and apply a cervical collar.
      Clear airway of debris.
      If person is unresponsive, place on side if vomiting occurs.
      Remove wet clothes, dry, and cover with blankets (including head)
      Begin CPR and continue until help arrives.
3. Miscellaneous
   a. Unsupervised contact with animals and poisons in environment (plants, pool chemicals, pills)
   b. Obstructed passageways
   c. Unsafe window protection in home with young children
   d. Guns or ammunition stored in unlocked fashion
   e. Large icicles hanging from roof
   f. Icy walkways
   g. Glass sliding doors that look open when closed

h. Low-strung clothesline

i. Discarded or unused refrigerators or freezers without removed doors

4. For infants and toddlers

a. Household

Pillows in crib

Staircases without stair gates

Crib mattresses that do not fit snugly

Cribs with slat opening to allow child's body to fall through, catching the head

Glass or sharp-edged tables

Porches and decks without railings

Poisonous plants (see Table II-15)

Furniture painted with lead paint

Unsupervised bathing

Open windows

Propped bottle in crib

b. Toys

Sharp edges	Balloons
Easily breakable parts	Lollipops
Removable small pieces	Pacifier around neck

c. Miscellaneous

Unattended in shopping cart

Unattended in car

Cribs, walkers, high chairs with movable parts that trap child (*e.g.*, springs)

Put in car safety seat in back seat only

C. Assist parents to analyze an accident

1. What happened?

2. How did it happen?

3. Where, when?

4. Why did the accident happen?

D. Teach how to prevent poisoning

1. Instruct how to "child-proof" the home.

2. Instruct to keep poisons and corrosive substances in tightly closed, carefully marked containers in locked closets.

3. Parents should discard unused supplies of medications and keep needed medications in locked, inaccessible medicine closet.

4. Parents should be taught how to administer antidotes for specific toxic substances, if advised by Poison Control Center.

5. Parents should also have the phone number of the Poison Control Center in a convenient place.

6. Refer individuals to local poison control center for "Mr. Yuk" poison warning stickers and advice on emergency procedures; teach the child what a Mr. Yuk sticker means.

7. Instruct parents on the use of ipecac and its availability.

E. Initiate health teaching and referrals, as indicated

1. Assist family to evaluate environmental hazards in home and when visiting others.

2. Install specially designed locks to prevent children from opening closets where combustible, corrosive, or flammable materials or medications are stored.

3. Instruct to use socket covers to prevent accidental electrical shocks to children.
4. Teach about hazards of lead paint ingestion and how to identify "pica" in a child.
5. Refer parents to public health department if lead paint screening is necessary.
6. Encourage use of childproof caps.
7. Advise to avoid storing dangerous substances in containers ordinarily used for foods.

Rationale

- The nurse should assess each child's unique risk of potential for injury. This includes the child with sensory or motor deficits and developmental delay. Environmental changes, such as hospitalization, visiting relatives' homes, and celebrating holidays pose special hazards for children.
- All environmental hazards cannot be removed. Strategies that include supervision and education of parents can reduce accidents (Clemen-Stone et al., 1991).
- Analysis of an accident may prevent recurrence.
- Injury prevention requires anticipation and recognition of where safety measures are applicable. Passive strategies provide automatic protection without choice (*e.g.*, air bags, product design). Active strategies require persuasion through teaching or legislation to practice safety measures (Wong, 1995).
- Prevention strategies to decrease serious injuries resulting from skateboarding include warnings against skateboard use by children younger than 5 years of age, prohibition of skateboards on streets and highways, and the promotion of use of helmets and other protective gear (Retsky, 1991).

■ Risk for Injury
Related to Lack of Awareness of Environmental Hazards Secondary to Maturational Age of Hospitalized Child

Outcome Criteria

The child/adolescent will be
- Free from injury from potentially hazardous factors that are identified in the hospital environment

The family will
- Reinforce and demonstrate safe practices in the hospital

Interventions

A. Protect the infant/child from injury in the hospital by controlling hazards that are age-related

Infant (1–12 Months)
Ensure that the infant can be identified by an identification band and a tag on his crib.

Do not shake powder directly on infant; rather, place powder in hand and then on infant's skin. Keep powder out of infant's reach.

Keep unsafe toys out of reach (*e.g.*, buttons, beads, balloons, broken toys, sharp-edged toys, other small toys).

Use mitts to prevent infant from removing catheters, eye patches, IV infusions, dressings, and feeding tubes, as needed.

Keep siderails up in locked position when child is in crib.

Pad siderails if infant is able to move out of bed or is at risk for seizures.

Do not use foam cushions for holding/feeding infant. (This type of pillow is filled with foam pellets.)

Use a cool-mist vaporizer.

Do not use an infant walker.

Ascertain identity of all visitors.

Use a firm mattress that fits crib snugly.

Do not feed honey to infants younger than 12 months of age owing to danger of botulism.

Fasten safety straps on infant seats, swings, highchairs, and strollers.

Do not allow bottles to be propped. The infant should be held with his head in an upright position.

Do not place pillows in crib.

Place one hand over the child while weighing, changing diapers, and so forth, to keep infant safe.

Do not allow infant to wear pacifier on a string around the neck.

Check bath water to make sure that the temperature is appropriate. Never leave infant alone while bathing! Support the small infant's head out of the water.

Check the temperature of formula, especially if it is heated in the microwave.

Position crib away from bedside stand, infusion pumps, and the like, to prevent child from reaching unsafe objects (*e.g.*, dials on infusion pump, suction machine, electrical outlets, flowers).

Do not allow parents to smoke or drink hot beverages in infant's room.

Foods that must be chewed or are small enough to occlude the airway should not be offered (*i.e.*, nuts, popcorn, hard candy, whole hot dogs). Forks and knives are not appropriate utensils for infants.

Discard syringes, needles, med packets, plastic bags safely.

Protect the feet of the infant who is able to walk with shoes or slippers.

Transport the infant safely to other areas of the hospital (*i.e.*, x-ray, laboratory).

Remind parents to have approved car seat in their automobile to transport the child home.

Assess each unique situation for risk for injury to the infant. Inform parents of the infant's risk for injury.

Early Childhood (13 Months–5 Years)

Ensure that the young child is identifiable by name band and name tag on crib.

Keep siderails up in locked position when child is in crib—top and bottom compartments; use siderails on youth beds.

Monitor child at all times when eating, bathing, playing, and toileting.

Keep cleaning agents, sharp items, and plastic bags out of reach.

Secure thermometer while taking temperature (use rectal or axillary method with toddler, oral method when child is old enough not to bite down on thermometer) or use infrared instant thermometer in the ear canal.

Assess for loose teeth, and document on records.

Check the temperature of bath water before immersing child.

Use electric beds with extreme caution. For example, children may get their fingers caught or get under the bed and be at risk for a crushing injury.

Position crib/bed away from bedside stand, infusion pumps, flowers, and the like, to prevent child from reaching unsafe objects.

Keep child safe when mobile:
> Protect child's feet with shoes or slippers when ambulating.
> Keep bathroom and closet doors firmly shut.
> Check any tubing attached to child to prevent kinking or dislodgment.
> Apply safety straps when child is in highchair, stroller, or on a cart.
> Transport safely to other areas of the hospital (*e.g.*, x-ray).
> Use mitts to prevent child from removing catheters, eye patches, IV infusion, dressings, and feeding tubes, as needed.
> Place one hand over child when weighing, changing diapers, and the like, to prevent falls.

Do not call medications "candy."

Do not permit the child to chew gum, eat hard candy, nuts, whole hot dogs, or fish with bones.

Set limits. Enforce and repeat to child what he can do in the hospital and to which areas he may go.

Provide with age-appropriate, safe toys (see manufacturer's guidelines).

Do not allow parents to smoke or drink hot beverages in the child's room.

Feed the child in a quiet environment; ensure that the child is seated while eating, to prevent choking.

Remind parents to have approved car seat in automobile to transport child home.

Ascertain identity of all visitors.

Assess each unique situation for risk for injury to the young child. Inform parents of the young child's risk for injury.

School-ager/Adolescent (6–12 Years/13–18 Years)

Ensure that the school-ager/adolescent can be identified by a name band and a tag on his bed. School-agers may claim to be someone else to joke with the nurse, not realizing the danger of this.

Assess for loose teeth and document on records.

Assess for self-care deficits and activity intolerance because the school-ager/adolescent may not ask for help when ambulating, bathing, toileting, and so forth.

Apply safety straps when transporting by cart or wheelchair.

Set limits. Enforce and reiterate to the child what he can do and to what areas he may go in the hospital.

Provide with age-appropriate activities. Supervise therapeutic play closely and do not allow child to use syringes as squirt guns.

Do not allow parents to smoke or drink hot beverages in the child's room.

Encourage child/adolescent to wear Medic Alert necklace or bracelet, if appropriate. Encourage to carry I.D. in wallet/purse.

Remind to wear seat belt in auto when discharged.

Discourage smoking and use of illicit drugs, including alcohol.

Assess each unique situation for risk for injury to the school-ager/adolescent. Inform parents of child's/adolescent's risk for injury.

Rationale

• To protect children from injury, caretakers must be aware of the age-related behavioral characteristics that increase the child's vulnerability to injury (Wong, 1995).

■ Risk for Injury
Related to Vertigo Secondary to Orthostatic Hypotension

Outcome Criteria

The individual will
- Identify situations that cause vertigo
- Relate methods of preventing sudden decreases in cerebral blood flow due to orthostatism
- Demonstrate maneuvers to change position and avoid sudden drop in cerebral pressure
- Relate fewer episodes of dizziness or vertigo

Interventions

A. Identify contributing factors, which may include
   1. Cardiovascular disorders (hypertension, cerebral infarct, anemia, dysrhythmias)
   2. Fluid or electrolyte imbalances
   3. Peripheral neuropathy, Parkinson's disease
   4. Diabetes
   5. Certain medications (antihypertensives, anticholinergics, barbiturates, vasodilators, tricyclic antidepressants, levodopa, nitrates, monoamine oxidase inhibitors, phenothiazine)
   6. Alcohol
   7. Age 75 years or older
   8. Prolonged bed rest
   9. Surgical sympathectomy
   10. Valsalva maneuver during voiding (Miller, 1995)
   11. Arthritis (spurs on vertebrae)

B. Assess for orthostatic hypotension
   1. Take bilateral brachial pressures with the person supine.
   2. If the brachial pressures are different, use the arm with the higher reading and take the blood pressure immediately after the client stands up quickly; report differences to the physician.
   3. Ask the client to describe sensations.

C. Discuss physiology of orthostatic hypotension with client
   1. Age-related changes in vessel
   2. Volume of blood in lower extremities
   3. Sympathetic nervous system response
   4. Effects of prolonged bed rest
   5. Postprandial effects

D. Teach techniques to reduce orthostatic hypotension
   1. Change positions slowly.
   2. Move from lying to an upright position in stages.
      a. Sit up in bed.
         Dangle first one leg, then the other over the side of the bed.

    b. Allow a few minutes before going on to each step.

    c. Gradually pull oneself from a sitting to a standing position.

    d. Place a chair, walker, cane, or other assistive device nearby to use to steady oneself when getting out of bed.

3. During day, rest in a recliner, rather than in bed.

4. Avoid prolonged standing.

5. Avoid stooping to pick something from the floor; use an assistive device available from an orthotics department or a self-help store to pick up items from the floor.

6. Evaluate the possible effectiveness of waist-high stockings.

    a. Put stockings on in morning before getting out of bed.

    b. Avoid sitting for long periods.

    c. Remove stockings when supine.

E. Encourage person to increase daily activity if permissible

1. Discuss the value of daily exercise (increases circulation, decreases the process of osteoporosis, increases energy levels, reduces stress, and contributes to an overall state of well-being).

2. Establish an exercise program.

F. Teach to avoid dehydration and vasodilation

1. Replace fluids during periods of excess fluid loss (*e.g.*, in hot weather).

2. Avoid diuretic fluids (*e.g.*, coffee, tea, cola).

3. Avoid alcohol consumption.

4. Avoid sources of intense heat, *e.g.*, direct sun, hot showers, baths, electric blankets.

5. Avoid taking nitroglycerin while standing.

G. Teach to reduce postprandial hypotension (Miller, 1995)

1. Take antihypertensive medications after meals, rather than before.

2. Eat small, frequent meals.

3. Remain seated or lie down after meals.

H. Institute environmental safety measures (Refer to *Risk for Injury Related to Lack of Awareness of Environmental Hazards*)

Rationale

- Older adults cannot compensate for hypertensive or hypotensive stimuli as efficiently as younger adults and are thus more sensitive to these states (see also Postural Hypotension under Key Concepts).
- The client's understanding of orthostatic hypotension may help him modify behavior to reduce the frequency and severity of episodes (Cunha, 1987).
- Use of the arm with the higher pressure gives a more accurate assessment of the mean blood pressure.
- Prolonged bed rest increases venous pooling. Gradual position change allows the body to compensate for venous pooling (Cunha, 1987).
- Adequate hydration is necessary to prevent decreased circulating volume.
- Certain medications (*e.g.*, vasodilators, antihistamines) can precipitate orthostatic hypotension.
- Studies have shown a blood pressure reduction of 20 mm Hg within 1 hour of eating the morning or noon meal in healthy older adults. This is thought to be due to impaired baroreflex compensatory response to splanchnic blood pooling during digestion (Miller, 1995).
- External heat may dilate the superficial vessels sufficiently to shunt blood from the brain, causing neurologic symptoms.

Risk for Aspiration

DEFINITION

Risk for Aspiration: The state in which a person is at risk for entry of secretions, solids, or fluids into the tracheobronchial passages.

RISK FACTORS

Presence of favorable conditions for aspiration (see Related Factors)

RELATED FACTORS

Pathophysiologic

Related to reduced level of consciousness secondary to:

Presenile dementia　　　　　Parkinson's disease
Seizures　　　　　　　　　　Head injury
Alcohol/drug-induced　　　　Anesthesia
Cerebral vascular accident　　Coma

Related to depressed cough/gag reflexes

Related to delayed gastric emptying secondary to:

Intestinal obstruction　　　Gastric outlet syndrome
Ileus

Related to increased intragastric pressure secondary to:

Lithotomy position　　　Obesity
Enlarged uterus　　　　Ascites

Related to impaired swallowing or decreased laryngeal and glottic reflexes secondary to:

Achalasia　　　　　　　　　Muscular dystrophy
Scleroderma　　　　　　　　Cerebrovascular accident
Esophageal strictures　　　　Parkinson's disease
Myasthenia gravis　　　　　Debilitating conditions
Guillain-Barré syndrome　　Catatonia
Multiple sclerosis

Related to tracheoesophageal fistula

Related to impaired protective reflexes secondary to:

Facial/oral/neck surgery or trauma　　Paraplegia or hemiplegia

Treatment-Related

Related to depressed laryngeal and glottic reflexes secondary to:

Presence of tracheostomy/endotracheal tube
Sedation
Tube feedings

Related to impaired ability to cough secondary to:

Wired jaw
Imposed prone position

Situational (Personal, Environmental)

Related to inability/impaired ability to elevate upper body
Related to eating when intoxicated

Maturational

Premature
Related to impaired sucking/swallowing reflexes

Neonate
    Related to decreased muscle tone of inferior esophageal sphincter
Older Adult
    Related to poor dentition

Author's Note

Risk for Aspiration is a clinically useful diagnosis for people at high risk for aspiration because of reduced level of consciousness, structural deficits, mechanical devices, and neurologic and gastrointestinal disorders. People with swallowing difficulties often are at risk for aspiration; the nursing diagnosis *Impaired Swallowing* should be used to describe a client who has difficulty swallowing who also is at risk for aspiration. *Risk for Aspiration* should be used to describe people who require nursing interventions to prevent aspiration, but not to improve swallowing for nutritional purposes.

Errors in Diagnostic Statements

Risk for Aspiration related to bronchopneumonia
    This diagnostic statement does not direct the nurse to the risk factors that could be reduced. If the nurse were monitoring and comanaging bronchopneumonia, the correct statement would be the collaborative problem *Potential Complication: Bronchopneumonia.*
    Risk for Aspiration related to difficulty swallowing
    Difficulty Swallowing is validation for *Impaired Swallowing*; thus, *Impaired Swallowing* would be correct. Nursing measures would also include prevention of aspiration.

Key Concepts

1. Swallowing is a complicated mechanism with three stages: voluntary, pharyngeal, and esophageal.
2. The voluntary stage is the moving of the food from the palate to the pharynx.
3. The pharyngeal stage is automatic.
    a. Soft palate is pulled up to close the posterior nares.
    b. Palatopharyngeal folds on the sides of the pharynx constrict to permit passage of properly masticated food.
    c. Epiglottis swings backward over larynx opening to prevent aspiration into the trachea.
    d. Relaxation of hypopharyngeal sphincter stretches the opening of the esophagus.
    e. Rapid peristaltic wave forces food into the upper esophagus.
4. The esophageal stage moves the food from the pharynx to the stomach by peristaltic movements controlled by vagal reflexes.
5. Central nervous system depression interferes with the protective mechanism of the sphincters.
6. Nasogastric and endotracheal tubes cause incomplete closure of the esophageal sphincters and depress gag and cough reflex.
7. Clients with debilitating conditions who aspirate are at high risk for aspiration pneumonia.
8. The volume and characteristics of the aspirated contents influence morbidity and mortality. Food particles can cause mechanical blockage. Gastric juice erodes alveoli and capillaries and causes chemical pneumonitis.

Key Concepts—Child

1. A proportionately oversized airway diameter in infants and small children increases the risk of aspiration of foreign objects (Hunsberger, 1989).
2. Common household objects and food items that are aspirated include:
    a. Baby powder
    b. Hot dogs, candy, nuts, grapes

    c. Balloons; toy rubber balloons are the leading cause of choking deaths from children's products (Ryan, 1990)

    d. Small batteries (Wong, 1995)

3. Children with certain congenital anomalies (*e.g.*, tracheoesophageal fistula, cleft palate, and gastroesophageal reflux) are at greater risk for aspiration.

Focus Assessment Criteria

Subjective Data

A. Assess for related factors

    1. History of a problem with swallowing or aspiration

    2. Presence or history of: (see Pathophysiologic Related Factors)

Objective Data

A. Assess for related factors

    1. Height and weight

    2. Ability to swallow, chew, feed self

    3. Neuromuscular impairment

        Decreased/absent gag reflex

        Decreased strength on excursion of muscles involved in mastication

        Perceptual impairment

        Facial paralysis

    4. Mechanical obstruction

        Edema

        Tracheostomy tube

        Tumor

    5. Perceptual patterns/awareness

    6. Level of consciousness

    7. Condition of oropharyngeal cavity

    8. Nasal regurgitation

    9. Hoarseness

    10. Aspiration

    11. Coughing a second or two after swallowing

    12. Dehydration

    13. Apraxia

Outcome Criteria

The person will

- Not experience aspiration
- Relate measures to prevent aspiration

Interventions

A. Assess causative or contributing factors

    1. Susceptible individual

        a. Reduced level of consciousness

        b. Autonomic disorders

        c. Debilitated

        d. Newborn

    2. Tracheostomy/endotracheal tubes

    3. Gastrointestinal tubes/feedings

B. Reduce the risk of aspiration in
1. Individuals with decreased strength, decreased sensorium, or autonomic disorders:
   a. Maintain a side-lying position if not contraindicated by injury.
   b. If the person cannot be positioned on his side, open oropharyngeal airway by lifting the mandible up and forward, with the head tilted backward (for a small infant, hyperextension of the neck may not be effective).
   c. Assess for position of the tongue, ensuring that it has not dropped backward, occluding the airway.
   d. Keep the head of the bed elevated, if not contraindicated by hypertension or injury.
   e. Maintain good oral hygiene: Clean teeth and use mouthwash on cotton swab; apply petroleum jelly to lips, removing incrustations gently.
   f. Clear secretions from mouth and throat with a tissue or gentle suction.
   g. Reassess frequently for presence of obstructive material in mouth and throat.
   h. Reevaluate frequently for good anatomic positioning.
   i. Maintain side-lying position after feedings.
2. Tracheostomies or endotracheal tubes:
   a. Inflate cuff:
      During continuous mechanical ventilation
      During and after eating
      During and 1 hour after tube feedings
      During intermittent positive-pressure breathing treatments
   b. Suction every 1–2 hours and PRN
3. Gastrointestinal tubes and feedings:
   a. Confirm that the placement of the tube has been verified by radiography or aspiration of greenish fluid.
   b. Confirm that tube position has not changed since it was inserted and verified.
   c. Elevate head of bed 30–45 minutes during feeding periods, and 1 hour after to prevent reflux by use of reverse gravity.
   d. Aspirate for residual contents before each feeding for tubes positioned gastrically.
   e. Administer feeding if residual contents are less than 150 mL (intermittent) or administer feeding if residual is no greater than 150 mL at 10%–20% of hourly rate (continuous).
   f. Regulate gastric feedings using an intermittent schedule allowing periods for stomach emptying between feeding intervals.
4. For an older adult with difficulties chewing and swallowing, see *Impaired Swallowing*.

C. Initiate health teaching and referrals, as indicated
1. Instruct person and/or family on causes and prevention of aspiration.
2. Have family demonstrate tube feeding technique.
3. Refer to community nursing agency for assistance at home.
4. Teach about the danger of eating when under the influence of alcohol.
5. Teach the Heimlich or abdominal thrust maneuver to remove aspirated foreign bodies.

Rationale

- Regurgitation is often silent in people with decreased sensorium or depressed mental states.
- Increased intragastric pressure can contribute to regurgitation and aspiration. Situations that increase intragastric pressure are bolus tube feedings, obstructions, obesity, pregnancy, and autonomic dysfunction.
- Verifying correct placement of feeding tubes is done most reliably by radiography. Aspiration of green-colored fluid or gastric aspirant with a pH of 6.5 or lower is also reliable. Verifying placement by instilling air and simultaneously auscultating or by aspirating nongreen fluid has proved inaccurate.
- After radiographic verification of correct feeding tube placement and knowledge that the position of the tube has not changed, routine testing of placement before feeding is not needed.

- Tracheostomy tubes interfere with the synchrony of the glottic closure. Inadequate cuff inflation provides a path for aspirate.
- Such regulation is necessary to prevent overfeeding and increased risk of reflux and aspiration. Gastric feedings should be administered intermittently when the potential for aspiration is high. Continuous feedings increase the risk of aspiration because the stomach contains a constant supply of formula.

❧ Interventions—*Child Focus*

1. For newborns with cleft lip and/or palate:
   a. Position infant's head in an upright position.
   b. Use a large, soft nipple with large hole or Lamb's nipple (long, soft).
   c. The nipple hole should be large enough for the feeding to be under 30 minutes.
   d. Do not position the nipple through the cleft.
   e. Apply gentle counterpressure on the base of the bottle to assist the infant with tongue and palate control of the milk flow.
   f. Burp frequently because of excessive air swallowing.
   g. If nipple feeding is unsuccessful, use a rubber-tipped syringe to deposit the formula on the back of the tongue.

Rationale

- All newborns have poor muscle tone of the cardiac sphincter of the esophagus, thus causing regurgitation easily (Wong, 1995).
- These infants cannot apply enough suction to use normal nipples.
- Sucking is important for muscle development for later speech development (Wong, 1995).
- Excessive air swallowing necessitates frequent burping.
- Gentle pressure at the base of bottle assists the infant with tongue and palate control.

Risk for Poisoning

DEFINITION

Risk for Poisoning: The state in which an individual is at risk of accidental exposure to or ingestion of drugs or dangerous substances.

RISK FACTORS

Presence of risk factors (see Related Factors for *Risk for Injury*)

Risk for Suffocation

DEFINITION

Risk for Suffocation: The state in which an individual is at risk for smothering and asphyxiation.

RISK FACTORS

Presence of risk factors (see Related Factors for *Risk for Injury*)

Risk for Trauma

DEFINITION

Risk for Trauma: The state in which an individual is at risk of accidental tissue injury (*e.g.*, wound, burns, fracture).

RISK FACTORS

Presence of risk factors (see Related Factors for *Risk for Injury*)

Injury, Risk for Perioperative Positioning

DEFINITION

Risk for Perioperative Positioning Injury: The state in which an individual is at risk for harm as a result of positioning requirements for surgery and loss of usual protective responses secondary to anesthesia.

RISK FACTORS

Presence of risk factors (see Related Factors)

RELATED FACTORS
Pathophysiologic

Related to increased vulnerability secondary to:

Chronic disease	Radiation therapy
Renal, hepatic dysfunction	Cancer
Osteoporosis	Infection
Compromised immune system	Thin body frame

Related to compromised tissue perfusion secondary to:

Diabetes mellitus	Cardiovascular disease
Peripheral vascular disease	Anemia
Hypothermia	History of thrombosis
Ascites	Dehydration
Edema	

Related to vulnerability of stoma during positioning

Related to preexisting contractures or physical impairments secondary to:

Rheumatoid arthritis

Polio

Treatment-Related

Related to position requirements and loss of usual sensory protective responses secondary to anesthesia*

Related to surgical procedures of 2 hours or longer

Related to vulnerability of implants or prostheses (*e.g.*, pacemakers) during positioning

Situational (Personal, Environmental)

Related to compromised circulation secondary to:

Obesity	Pregnancy
Cool operating suite	Tobacco use

Maturational

Related to increased vulnerability to tissue injury secondary to:

Infant status

Elder status

Author's Note

This diagnosis focuses on identifying the vulnerability for tissue, nerve, and joint injury resulting from required positions for surgery. The addition of the terms *perioperative positioning* to the *Risk for Injury* diagnoses adds etiology to the label.

If a client has no preexisting risk factors that make him or her more vulnerable to injury, this diagnosis could be used with no related factors because they are evident. If related factors are desired, the statement could read *Risk for Perioperative Positioning Injury related to position requirements for surgery and loss of usual sensory protective measures secondary to anesthesia.*

When a client has preexisting risk factors, the statement should include these—for example, *Risk for Perioperative Positioning Injuries related to compromised tissue perfusion secondary to peripheral arterial disease.*

Errors in Diagnostic Statements

Risk for Perioperative Positioning Injury related to inadequate protective measures

These related factors are legally problematic. Even if inadequate protective measures are a problem, they must not be included in the diagnostic statement. Instead, this problem should be referred to nursing management.

---

* This risk factor is always present and may be deleted from the diagnostic statement.

Key Concepts

1. The physiologic effects of positioning for surgical procedures vary with the specific position. Overall positioning affects the cardiovascular, respiratory, neurologic, and integumentary systems.
2. The pulmonary capillary blood flow volume is diminished with prolonged immobility. Lung expansion is limited owing to positional pressure on ribs or on the diaphragm's ability to force abdominal contents downward.
3. Anesthesia causes peripheral blood vessels to dilate, resulting in hypotension, and decreases blood return to heart and lungs. Prolonged immobility causes pooling in vascular beds.
4. Obese people are at higher risk for injury from surgical positions owing to the following factors (Fuller, 1994):
    a. Difficulty is experienced in lifting them into position.
    b. Massive tissue and pressure areas need extra padding.
    c. Length of surgery may be prolonged owing to the mechanics of manipulation of adipose tissue.
    d. Recovery period may be prolonged because adipose tissue retains fat-soluble agents and slows elimination of agents.
    e. Venous stasis decreases circulation, and adipose tissue has a poor blood supply.

 ### Key Concepts—Older Adult

1. Osteoarthritis, loss of subcutaneous fat, decreased peripheral circulation and wasted flaccid muscles can contribute to injury or trauma to bones, joints, nerves, and skin when on the operating table (Stanley & Beare, 1995).

Focus Assessment Criteria

Subjective Data

A. Assess for preexisting risk factors
    1. Medical conditions
        Cardiovascular disease   Cancer
        Renal, hepatic disorders   History of thrombosis
        Osteoporosis   Diabetes mellitus
        Anemia   History of cerebral vascular accident
        Peripheral vascular disease
    2. Compromised immune system
        Chemotherapy   AIDS
        Radiation therapy   Cancer
    3. Compromised tissue perfusion
        Pregnancy   Obesity
        Ascites   Edema
        Dehydration   Tobacco use
        Hypothermia
    4. Compromised mobility
        Rheumatoid arthritis   Polio
    5. Other
        Very young   Very old age
        Implants (e.g., pacemaker)   Prosthesis
        Stoma   Thin body frame

Objective Data

A. Assess for presurgical risk factors
    1. Skin
        Temperature (cool, warm)
        Color (pale, dependent rubor, flushed, cyanotic, brown discolorations)
        Ulcerations (size, location, description of surrounding tissue)

2. Bilateral pulses (radial, posterior tibial, dorsalis pedis)
Rate, rhythm
Volume
+0 = Absent, nonpalpable
+1 = Thready, weak, fades in and out
+2 = Present but diminished
+3 = Normal, easily palpable
+4 = Aneurysmal
3. Paresthesia (numbness, tingling, burning)
4. Edema (location, pitting)
5. Capillary refill (normal less than 3 seconds)
6. Range of motion (normal, compromised)

Outcome Criteria

The person will
• Have no evidence of neuromuscular damage or injury related to the surgical position

---

Interventions

A. Determine whether the client has preexisting risk factors (refer to Risk Factors), communicate findings to the surgical team

B. Before positioning, assess and document
1. Range-of-motion ability
2. Physical abnormalities
3. External/internal prostheses or implants
4. Neurovascular status
5. Circulatory status

C. Move the person from the transport stretcher to the OR bed
1. Have a minimum of two people with their hands free (*e.g.*, not holding an IV bag).
2. Explain the transfer to the client. Lock all wheels on the stretcher and bed.
3. Ask the person to move slowly to the OR bed. Assist during the move. Do not pull or drag person.
4. When on the OR bed, attach a safety belt a few inches above the knees with a space of three fingerbreadths.
5. Check that legs are not crossed and that feet are slightly separated and not over the edge.
6. Ensure that the person is not touching any metal of table or equipment.
7. Do not leave the person unattended.

D. Discuss with the surgeon the surgical position desired. Advise if any preexisting factors exist. Determine if the position will be arranged before or after anesthesia.

E. Always ask the anesthesiologist or nurse anesthetist for permission before moving or repositioning an anesthetized person

F. Reduce vulnerability to injury (soft tissue, joint, nerves, blood vessels)
1. Align the neck and spine at all times.
2. Gently manipulate joints. Do not abduct more than 90 degrees.
3. Do not let limbs extend off the OR bed. Reposition slowly and gently.
4. Use a draw-sheet above the elbows to tuck in arms at side or abduct arm on an arm board with padding.

G. Protect eyes and ears from injury
   1. Use padding or a special headrest to protect ears, superficial nerves, and blood vessels of face if the head is on its side.
   2. Ensure that the ear is not bent when positioned.
   3. If needed, protect eyes from abrasions with an eye patch or shield.

H. Depending on the surgical position used, protect vulnerable areas; document position and protection measures used
   1. Supine
      a. Pad the calcaneus, sacrum, coccyx, olecranon process, scapula, ischial tuberosity and occiput.
      b. Keep arms at side, palms down or abducted on arm board.
      c. Protect the head and ears if the head is turned to the side.
   2. Trendelenburg
      a. Use a well padded shoulder brace over the acromion process, not over soft tissue, and away from neck.
   3. Reverse Trendelenburg
      a. Use a padded foot board.
   4. Jack-knife (modified prone) at correct heights.
      a. Use padded arm boards at correct heights to allow elbows to bend comfortably.
      b. Place a soft pillow under the down ear.
      c. Cushion hips and thighs with large pillows.
      d. Cushion breasts.
      e. Cushion male genitalia in natural position.
      f. Use a large pillow under the lower legs and ankles to raise the toes off the bed.
      g. Use additional padding on the shoulder girdle, olecranon, anterosuperior iliac spine, patella, and dorsum of the foot.
      h. Apply a safety strap across the thighs.
   5. Prone
      a. Position two large body rolls longitudinally from the acromioclavicular joint to the iliac crest.
      b. Refer to Jack-knife for additional information.
   6. Laminectomy
      a. After induction of anesthesia, at least six people help roll the person from the stretcher to the OR bed onto laminectomy brace.
      b. Keep body aligned.
      c. Protect limbs from torsion.
      d. Place rolled towels in axillary regions.
      e. Follow precautions for jack-knife.
   7. Lithotomy
      a. Prepare stirrups with padding.
      b. Have two people simultaneously, slowly raise legs with slight rotation of the hips. Gently position the knees slightly flexed.
      c. Position buttocks about 1 inch over the end of the table.
      d. Use a small lumbar pad and extra padding in sacral area.
      e. Cover legs with cotton boots.
      f. Position arms on arm boards or loosely over abdomen, supported with a sheet.
   8. Fowler
      a. Position the neck in straight alignment.
      b. Use a padded foot board.
      c. Support the knees with a pillow.
      d. Cross arms loosely over the abdomen and tape on pillow.
   9. Sims (lateral)
      a. Position on the side with arms extended on double arm boards.
      b. Flex the lower leg.
      c. Use a small pillow under the head.

    d. Use a rolled towel in the axillary area of the downside arm.

    e. Elevate and pad the flank.

    f. Flex the lower leg and place a long pillow the length of the leg to the groin.

    g. Use a 4-inch strip of adhesive tape attached to one side of the table, over iliac crest and to other side.

    h. Protect ankles and feet from pressure.

    i. Protect male genitalia, female breasts, and ear as for jack-knife position.

I. If feasible, ask client if he or she feels pain, burning, pressure, or any discomfort after positioning

J. Continually assess that team members are not leaning on the client, especially limbs

K. Ensure that the head is lifted slightly every 30 minutes

L. When repositioning or returning person to supine position after certain surgical positions (*e.g.*, Trendelenburg, lithotomy, reverse Trendelenburg, jack-knife, lateral), slowly change position to prevent severe hypotension

M. Assess skin condition when surgery is completed and document findings. Inform postanesthesia nurses if preexisting risk factors are present that increase vulnerability postoperatively.

N. Continue to assess and relieve pressure to vulnerable areas during the postoperative period

Rationale

- Prolonged positioning can cause mechanical pressure on peripheral and superficial nerves. Hyperextension (>90-degree angle) of a limb of an anesthetized person can cause nerve injuries (Fairchild, 1993).
  - The brachial plexus (in the arm) can be injured by hyperextension of the arm on an arm board. Improper positioning of the brace can also injure the brachial plexus.
  - Ulnar nerve injuries occur when an elbow slips off the mattress and is compressed between the table and the medial epicondyle.
  - Radial nerve injuries occur when the nerve is compressed between the client and the table surface or from striking the table.
  - Saphenous and peroneal nerve damage occurs with the use of stirrups with lithotomy—compression of the peroneal nerve against the stirrups or of the saphenous nerve between the metal popliteal knee support stirrup and the medial tibial condyle.
- Tissue and skin can be injured by excessive pressure or bruised by hitting a hard surface. People more vulnerable to pressure injuries are the very young, elderly, dehydrated, very thin or obese, and those undergoing more than 2 hours of immobility.
- Anesthetic agents interfere with normal vasodilation and constriction, thus reducing perfusion to bony prominences, compressed, or dependent limbs (Fairchild, 1993).
- Injury to the face and eyes can be caused by excessive pressure of position, equipment, or the surgical team. Excessive pressure to the eyes can cause thrombosis of the central renal artery. Eyes should be kept closed and lubricated to prevent drying and scratching (Fairchild, 1993).
- If repositioning is necessary after induction, lifting the person, rather than rolling or pulling, avoids shearing forces and friction. Shearing occurs when the dermal layers stay in a fixed position because of the friction between linen and skin, and tissues attached to bony structures move with the weight of the torso (Fairchild, 1993). Tissue layers slide on each other, resulting in the kinking or stretching of subcutaneous blood vessels, thus obstructing blood flow to and from areas (Atkinson & Kohn, 1986).

- Prolonged immobilization of and pressure on the head can cause alopecia. Postoperatively, it first appears as edema and painful seroma leading to ulceration and localized hair loss (transient or permanent) (Atkinson & Kohn, 1986).
- Most surgical positions, except supine and prone, cause massive circulatory pooling. If the surgical position is reversed too quickly, severe hypotension can occur. Gradual and slow changes in position allow the person's cardiovascular system to adjust to the change (Atkinson & Kohn, 1986).

References/Bibliography

Berryman, E., Gaskin, D., Jones, A., Tolley, F., & MacMullen, J. (1989). Point by point: Predicting elders' falls. *Geriatric Nursing, 10,* 199–201.

Clemen-Stone, S., Eigasti, D. G., & McGuire, S. (1991). *Comprehensive family and community health nursing.* St. Louis: Mosby-Yearbook.

Green, P. M. (1989). Potential for injury. In G. McFarland & E. McFarlane (Eds.). *Nursing diagnosis and interventions.* St. Louis: C. V. Mosby.

Lipsitz, L. A., & Fullerton, K. J. (1986). Postprandial blood pressure reduction in health elderly. *Journal of the American Geriatrics Society, 34,* 267–270.

Miller, C. A. (1995). *Nursing care of older adults* (2nd ed.). Glenview, IL: Scott, Foresman.

Moss, A. B. (1992). Are the elderly safe at home? *Journal of Community Health Nursing, 9*(1), 13–19.

National Center for Health Statistics. (1993). *Monthly vital statistics report, 1991.* Hyattsville, MD: U.S. Public Health Service Publications.

Tideiksaar, R. (Ed.). (1989). *Falling in old age: Its prevention and treatment.* New York: Springer Publishing.

Child Safety

American Medical Association Board of Trustees. (1991). Use of infant walkers. *American Journal of Diseases of Children, 145,* 933–934.

Baxter, L. (1987, May). *Report on 1986–1987 CPSC study on immersion accidents.* Presented at Conference on Childhood Drowning: Current Issues and Strategies on Prevention, Newport Beach, CA.

Brill, J. (1987). Dispelling the myth of the drown proof child. *Contemporary Pediatrics, 4*(6), 30.

Children's National Medical Center (1989). *Safe kids are no accident.* Washington, DC: Author.

Guyer, B., & Ellers, B. (1990). Childhood injuries in the United States. *American Journal of Diseases of Children, 144,* 649–652.

Hunsberger, M. (1989). Nursing strategies: Altered respiratory function. In R. L. Foster, M. M. Hunsberger, & J. J. T. Anderson (Eds.). *Family-centered nursing care of children.* Philadelphia: W. B. Saunders.

Retsky, J. (1991). Skateboarding injuries in children: A second wave. *American Journal of Diseases of Children, 145,* 188–193.

Ryan, C. A. (1990). Childhood deaths from toy balloons. *American Journal of Diseases of Children, 144,* 1221–1224.

Weiss, B. D. (1992). Trends in bicycle helmet use by children: 1985 to 1990. *Pediatrics, 89,* 78–80.

Wong, D. L. (1995). *Nursing care of infants and children* (5th ed.). St. Louis: Mosby-Yearbook.

Orthostatic Hypotension

Cunha, U. V. (1987). Management of orthostatic hypotension in the elderly. *Geriatrics, 42*(9), 61–68.

Perioperative

Atkinson, L., & Kohn, M. (1986). *Berry and Kohn's introduction to operating room nursing.* New York: McGraw-Hill.

Fairchild, S. (1993). *Perioperative nursing: Principles and practice.* Boston: Jones and Bartlett.

Fuller, J. (1994). *Surgical technology: Principles and practice.* Philadelphia: W. B. Saunders.

Murphy, E. (1987). Cases involving ulnar nerve injuries demonstrate precautions nurses can and should take. *AORN Journal, 46,* 762–763, 768.

Rothrock, J. (1990). *Perioperative nursing care planning.* St. Louis: Mosby-Yearbook.

Smith, K. (1990). Positioning principles. *AORN Journal, 52,* 1196–1198, 1200–1202.

Stanley, M., & Beare, P.G. (1995). *Gerontological nursing.* Philadelphia: F. A. Davis.

Resources for the Consumer

Literature

Poison Prevention Packaging available free from the Consumer Product Safety Commission, Washington, DC 20207.

Kids aren't drownproof, The kids aren't drownproof coloring book, Is your pool safe? and *What every parent should know about water safety.* The Community Association for the Retarded, 3864 Middlefield Road, Palo Alto, CA 94303.

Never leave a child alone. Accident Prevention Committee, American Academy of Pediatrics, PO Box 2134, Inglewood, CA 90305.

Safe swimming for your boy or girl. The Injury Prevention Program (TIPP), American Academy of Pediatrics, Publications Department, 141 Northwest Point, PO Box 927, Elk Grove Village, IL 60007.

Booklets available on safety tips for children who ride school buses: National School Bus Safety Week, P.O. Box 2639, Springfield, VA 22152.

Buyers guide—*The safe nursery, and which toy for which child—Ages birth through five and ages six through twelve.* Order the catalogue from the U.S. Consumer Product Safety Commission, Washington, DC 20207.

Knowledge Deficit

DEFINITION

Knowledge Deficit: The state in which an individual or group experiences a deficiency in cognitive knowledge or psychomotor skills concerning the condition or treatment plan.

DEFINING CHARACTERISTICS

Major (Must Be Present)

Verbalizes a deficiency in knowledge or skill/request for information
Expresses "inaccurate" perception of health status
Does not correctly perform a desired or prescribed health behavior

Minor (May Be Present)

Lack of integration of treatment plan into daily activities
Exhibits or expresses psychological alteration (*e.g.*, anxiety, depression) resulting from misinformation or lack of information

---

Author's Note

Knowledge deficit does not represent a human response, alteration, or a pattern of dysfunction, but rather a related factor.* All of us have knowledge deficits. It is when this lack of knowledge causes or could cause a problem that the nurse acts on a nursing diagnosis. Lack of knowledge can contribute to a variety of responses (*e.g.*, anxiety, self-care deficits, noncompliance). All nursing diagnoses have related client/family teaching as a part of nursing interventions (*e.g., Altered Bowel Elimination, Impaired Verbal Communication*). When the teaching directly relates to a specific nursing diagnosis, incorporate the teaching in the plan. When lack of or insufficient knowledge is the primary cause of a diagnosis or a risk factor for a potential diagnosis, list lack of knowledge as a "Related to." For example, when specific teaching is indicated before a procedure, *Anxiety related to unfamiliar environment and procedures* can be used. When information giving is directed to assist a person or family with a decision, *Decisional Conflict* may be indicated. Other examples of diagnostic statements with lack of knowledge as the "Related to" are *Risk for Ineffective Management of Therapeutic Regimen related to lack of knowledge of diabetes mellitus, management, and signs/symptoms of complications; Risk for Impaired Home Maintenance Management related to lack of knowledge of home care and community resources*; and *Risk for Injury related to lack of knowledge of bicycle safety*.

---

* Jenny, J. (1987). Knowledge deficit: Not a nursing diagnosis. *Image, 19*(4), 184–185.

Loneliness, Risk for

DEFINITION
Risk for Loneliness: The state in which an individual is at risk for experiencing discomfort associated with a desire or need for contact with others.

RISK FACTORS
See Related Factors.

RELATED FACTORS
Pathophysiologic
Related to fear of rejection secondary to:
    Obesity
    Cancer (disfiguring surgery of head or neck, superstitions of others)
    Physical handicaps (paraplegia, amputation, arthritis, hemiplegia)
    Emotional handicaps (extreme anxiety, depression, paranoia, phobias)
    Incontinence (embarrassment, odor)
    Communicable diseases (acquired immunodeficiency syndrome [AIDS], hepatitis)
    Psychiatric illness (schizophrenia, bipolar affective disorder, personality disorders)
Related to difficulty accessing social events secondary to:
    Debilitating diseases
    Physical disabilities

Treatment-Related
Related to therapeutic isolation

Situational (Personal, Environmental)
Related to insufficient planning for retirement
Related to death of a significant other
Related to divorce
Related to disfiguring appearance
Related to fear of rejection secondary to:
    Obesity   Hospitalization or terminal illness (dying process)
    Extreme poverty   Unemployment
Related to moving to another culture (*e.g.*, unfamiliar language)
Related to history of unsatisfactory social experiences secondary to:
    Drug abuse   Unacceptable social behavior
    Alcohol abuse   Delusional thinking
    Immature behavior
Related to loss of usual means of transportation
Related to change in usual residence secondary to:
    Long-term care   Relocation

Maturational
Child
    Related to protective isolation or a communicable disease
Older Adult
    Related to loss of usual social contacts secondary to:
        Retirement   Death of (specify)
        Relocation   Loss of driving ability

Author's Note

Risk for Loneliness was added to the NANDA list in 1994. Currently, *Social Isolation* is also on the NANDA list. *Social Isolation* is a conceptually incorrect diagnosis because it does not represent a response but instead is the cause. *Loneliness* and *Risk for Loneliness* better describe the negative state of aloneness.

Loneliness is a subjective state that exists whenever a person says it does and is perceived as imposed by others. Social isolation is *not* the voluntary solitude that is necessary for personal renewal, nor is it the creative aloneness of the artist or the aloneness—and possible suffering—a person may experience as a result of seeking individualism and independence (*e.g.*, moving to a new city, going away to college).

Errors in Diagnostic Statements

Loneliness related to inability to engage in satisfying personal relationships since death of wife 1 year ago

When a person fails to resume activities or to renew or initiate social relationships after the death of a spouse, the nurse should suspect *Dysfunctional Grieving*. Prolonged social isolation after a death is a cue for unresolved grief. The nurse should conduct a focus assessment to identify other cues, such as prolonged denial, depression, or other evidence of unsuccessful adaptation to the loss of his wife. Until additional data are confirmed, the diagnosis *Possible Dysfunctional Grieving related to failure to resume or initiate relationships after wife's death 1 year ago* would be appropriate in this situation.

Loneliness related to multiple sclerosis

Using multiple sclerosis as a related factor clusters all people with multiple sclerosis as socially isolated and for the same reasons. This not only violates the uniqueness of each individual but does not specify how a nurse can intervene. If mobility and incontinence problems are present, but no data support social isolation, the nurse can record the diagnosis as *Risk for Loneliness related to mobility and incontinence problems secondary to multiple sclerosis*.

Key Concepts

1. Loneliness is an affective statement involving an awareness of being apart from others with an accompanying vague need for other people (Leiderman, 1969).
2. Loneliness differs from aloneness, solitude, and grief. Aloneness refers to being without company, not necessarily a negative state. Solitude involves being alone with a positive affective state. Grief is a response to the experience of a traumatic loss (Hillestad, 1984).
3. Social isolation can result in intense feelings of loneliness and suffering. The suffering associated with social isolation is not always visible. To diagnose this state, nurses must first be able to identify those people at risk.
4. The lonely or isolated person often aggravates his condition by suffering alone. The lonely tend to shun one another. The isolated person may resign himself to his situation and never seek companionship or help. He may deny his own feelings.
5. Illness, whether physical or psychiatric, may be the only legitimate way a socially isolated individual can get attention.
6. Lonely people are preoccupied with self, are hypervigilant to threats, and tend to interpret social cues as being hostile (Weiss, 1973).
7. Loneliness may become part of a person's self-image. Although ego dystonic, he may find the state familiar so that his discomfort level is outweighed by his fear of the social risks that would be required to overcome it.
8. The lonely often see the rest of the world (including health care providers) as a socially interactive milieu. They are not usually exposed to other individuals who suffer from loneliness and so believe that their pain is unique. As a result, there is a tendency to resent the nurse because she enjoys what the individual sees as unobtainable.
9. An individual cannot focus on meeting social needs until more basic ones (shelter, food, safety) are met (Maslow, 1968).

🔄 *Key Concepts—Child*

1. Children at high risk for social isolation include the chronically ill or disabled, terminally ill, and disfigured (Davis, 1990) and their siblings (Bender, 1990).
2. A child in protective isolation or with a communicable disease may not understand the rationale for separation from others (Hunsberger, 1989).
3. Gay or lesbian teenagers often suffer emotional isolation and lack access to information specific to their needs (*e.g.*, they are at increased medical risk for sexually transmitted diseases, substance use, and violence) (Bidwell & Deisher, 1991).

🏛 *Key Concepts—Older Adult*

1. "Resources valued by this society include knowledge, skills, power, and position, and the elderly may be ignored because they no longer have these in their control. This lack of control is noted in at least two contrasting views of the elderly. Some view the elderly as free to relax and enjoy freedom from worries and responsibilities. Others see the elderly as being slow and worthless, having nothing to contribute to society. In neither of these views is the older person seen as a contributing member of society" (Elsen & Blegen, 1991, p. 519).
2. Older adults are at high risk for loneliness because there often are fewer natural opportunities for being among people. Retirement from work, difficulty securing transportation, health problems that restrict visiting, sensory deficits making communication laborious or frustrating, or isolation from the mainstream in institutions (hospitals or nursing homes) each can significantly limit the natural encounters an older adult would have with people.
3. Family roles become altered and stressed when parents become dependent on their children, and children begin to assume traditional parental tasks or decision making. To help older adults meet their affiliative needs and increase satisfaction with social encounters, it is suggested that small groups be formed to promote interaction (rather than large, noisy crowds) and that one or two meaningful relationships (confidante) be encouraged.
4. Factors increasing social isolation in elderly people include hearing impairment, limited mobility, fatigue, caregiving responsibilities, inability to drive, mental or psychosocial impairments, and separation from spouse, friends, and/or relatives by death, illness, or physical distance (Miller, 1995).
5. Impaired ability to drive due to impaired vision, financial hardship, musculoskeletal functioning, and/or central nervous system functioning can increase an older adult's social isolation and dependency on others (Miller, 1995).
6. Sensory deficits rate highest on the list of problems in the older adult that have the potential for causing social isolation (Bernardini, 1985).

Focus Assessment Criteria

Subjective Data

A. Assess for related factors
  1. Social resources (support)
     "Who lives with you?"
     "About how many times did you talk to someone—friends, relatives or others—on the telephone in the past week (either you called them or they called you)?" If subject has no phone, question in the following manner.
     "How many times during the past week did you spend some time with someone who does not live with you; that is, you went to see them, or they came to visit you, or you went out to do things together?"
     "How often do you talk with the people/person with whom you live and about what kinds of things?"
     To whom does the person turn in time of need?
     Are there friends or neighbors on whom he relies for such things as meals and transportation?

"Do you see your relatives and friends as often as you want to, or are you somewhat unhappy about how little you see them?"

If institutionalized: "In the past year, about how often did you leave here to visit
your family or friends for weekends or holidays, or to go on shopping trips or
outings or are most of your friends here in the institution with you?"

2. Desire for more human contact

What kind of relationships would he like? (Same sex or opposite sex? Same age?
Someone with same situational or maturational problem?)

Is he able to make the effort to meet new people and go to new places?

What kind of group activities does he most enjoy? (Travel? A religious service or
activity?)

Has divorce or death (of spouse, child, sibling, friend, pet) occurred recently?

3. Barriers to social contacts

Does the person lack knowledge of resources available, where to meet others, how
to initiate conversation with strangers?

Is he housebound? (Illness or incapacity—lack of mobility on steps or curbs—and
weather hazards can physically isolate the elderly, as does loss of usual transportation, living in dangerous area, and lack of access to public transportation.)

Are there changes in the person's sensory ability (tactile sense, hearing, visual
acuity, ability to write letters)?

4. Change in living arrangement

Has the person moved recently (to nursing home or child's home, to an apartment,
to a strange location)?

Objective Data

A. Assess for related factors

1. Esthetic problems

Mutilating surgery	Extreme obesity
Odor (*e.g.*, ulcerating tumor)	Incontinence

2. Personality problems

"Does this individual lack certain social skills or have features in his personality
that may discourage others from befriending him" (*e.g.*, aggressive, egocentric,
racist, sexist, complaining, critical, problem drinker)?

Outcome Criteria

The person will
- Identify the reasons for his feelings of isolation
- Discuss ways of increasing meaningful relationships

Interventions

The nursing interventions for a variety of contributing factors that might be associated with
a diagnosis of *Risk for Loneliness* are very similar.

A. Identify causative and contributing factors (see Focus Assessment
Criteria)

B. Reduce or eliminate causative and contributing factors

1. Promote social interaction.

a. Support the individual who has experienced a loss as he works through his grief
(see *Grieving*).

b. Validate the normality of grieving.

   c. Encourage person to talk about his feelings of loneliness and the reasons why they exist.

   d. Encourage the development of or mobilize person's preexisting support system of family, friends, and neighbors.

   e. Discuss the importance of high-quality socialization, rather than a great number of interactions.

   f. Refer to social skills teaching (see *Social Interaction, Impaired*).

   g. Offer feedback on how the person presents himself to others (see *Social Interactions, Impaired*).

2. Decrease barriers to social contact.

   a. Assist with identification of transportation options.

   b. Determine available transportation in the community (public, church-related, volunteer).

   c. Determine if person must be taught how to use alternative transportation (*e.g.*, drive a car). Help densensitize to fear/stigma of using public transportation.

   d. Assist with the development of alternative means of communication for people with compromised sensory ability (*e.g.*, amplifier on phone, taped instead of written letters; see *Impaired Communication*).

   e. Assist with the management of esthetic problems (*e.g.*, consult enterostomal therapist if ostomy odor is a problem; teach those with cancer to control odor of tumors by packing area with yogurt or pouring in buttermilk, then rinsing well with saline solution).

   f. Assist person in locating stores that sell clothing specially made for those who have had disfiguring surgery (*e.g.*, mastectomy).

   g. Refer to *Altered Patterns of Urinary Elimination* for specific interventions to control incontinence.

3. Identify strategies to expand the world of the isolated.

   a. Senior centers and church groups

   b. Foster grandparent program

   c. Day care centers for the elderly

   d. Retirement communities

   e. House sharing, group homes, community kitchens

   f. Adult education classes, special interest courses

   g. Pets

   h. Regular contact so that the need to obtain attention by precipitating a crisis (*e.g.*, suicidal gesture) is diminished

   i. Psychiatric day hospital or activity program

4. For individuals with poor or offensive social skills:

   a. Engage in one-to-one social dialogue. Explain the difference between casual and meaningful conversation.

   b. Discuss the characteristics of meaningful conversation (Durham, 1983):

        Initiating interactions

        Being spontaneous

        Being alert

        Showing interest

        Giving and receiving compliments

        Showing interest in others, in activities

        Requesting help when needed

        Using increased eye contact

        Using appropriate speech tone and nonverbal behavior

   c. Allow the person opportunities to observe others engaged in meaningful conversation.

   d. Observe the person socializing, and discuss the interactions afterward. Offer praise. Gently discuss alternative approaches. Role-play skills.

5. Discuss the anticipatory effects of retirement on his or her life. Assist with preplanning (Stanley & Beare, 1994).

a. Plan to ensure adequate income.

b. Decrease time at work the last 2 to 3 years (*e.g.*, shorter days, longer vacations).

c. Cultivate friends outside of work.

d. Develop routines at home to replace work structure.

e. Rely on others rather than spouse for leisure activities.

f. Cultivate leisure activities that are realistic (energy, cost).

g. Prepare self for ambivalent feelings and short-term negative impact on self-esteem.

C. Initiate referrals, as indicated

1. Community-based groups that contact the socially isolated
2. Self-help groups for clients isolated because of specific medical problems (Reach to Recovery, United Ostomy Association)
3. Wheelchair groups
4. Psychiatric consumer rights associations

Rationale

- A socially isolated person usually is not able to initiate or coordinate various isolation-reduction activities on his or her own behalf.
- The functional ability of a person's senses has a strong influence on his or her perception of the world, his behavior, and the behavior of others toward him or her (Yurick, Spier, Robb, & Ebert, 1984). A person with visible deficits may be shunned.
- Chronic illness can contribute to social isolation because of lack of energy, decreased mobility, discomforts, fear of exposure to pathogens, and distancing by previous friends who are uncomfortable with the ill person's disabilities or the stigma associated with psychiatric problems (Miller, 1995).
- "Retirement is a significant life event that requires pre-planning and realistic expectations of life changes" (Stanley & Beare, 1994, p. 365).
- Longino and Karl (1982) reported that the type and quality of social interactions are more important than the quantity. Informal activities promote well-being to a greater degree than formal, structured activities.

References/Bibliography

Bender, S. J. (1990). Anxiety and isolation in siblings of pediatric cancer patients: The need for prevention. *Social Work in Health Care, 14*(3), 17–35.

Bernardini, L. (1985). Effective communication as an intervention for sensory deprivation in the elderly client. *Topics in Clinical Nursing, 1*(4), 72–81.

Bidwell, R. J., & Deisher, R. W. (1991). Adolescent sexuality: Current issues. *Pediatric Annals, 20*, 293–302.

Davis, B. (1990). Loneliness in children and adolescents. *Issues in Comprehensive Pediatric Nursing, 13*(1), 59–69.

Drew, N. (1991). Combating the social isolation of chronic mental illness. *Journal of Psychosocial Nursing and Mental Health Services, 29*(6), 14–17.

Durham, R. (1983). Long-stay psychiatric patients in hospital. In S. Spence & G. Shepherd (Eds.). *Development in social skills training.* New York: Academic Press.

Elsen, J., & Blegen, M. (1991). Social isolation. In M. Maas, K. Buckwalter, & M. Hardy (Eds.). *Nursing diagnoses and interventions for the elderly.* Redwood City, CA: Addison-Wesley Nursing.

Folden, S. L. (1990). On the inside looking out: Perceptions of the homebound. *Journal of Gerontological Nursing, 16*(1), 9–15.

Hillestad, E. A. (1984). Toward understanding of loneliness. In *Proceedings of conference on spirituality.* Milwaukee, WI: Marquette University.

Hunsberger, M. (1989). Principles and skills adapted to the care of children. In R. L. Foster, M. M. Hunsberger, & J. J. T. Anderson (Eds.). *Family-centered nursing care of children.* Philadelphia: W. B. Saunders.

Kelly, J. H., & Cavan Frisch, N. (1994). A transcultural concept analysis of social isolation. In R. Carrol-Johnson & Paquette, M. (Eds.). *Classification of nursing diagnosis: Proceedings of the tenth conference.* Philadelphia: J. B. Lippincott.

Leiderman, P. H. (1969). Loneliness: A psychodynamic interpretation. In E. S. Scheidman & M. J. Ortega (Eds.). *Aspects of depression: International psychiatric clinics.* Boston: Little, Brown.

Lien-Gieschen, T. (1993). Validation of social isolation related to maturational age: Elderly. *Nursing Diagnosis, 4*(1), 37–44.

Longino, C. F., & Karl, C. S. (1982). Explicating activity theory: A formal replication. *Journal of Gerontology, 37*, 713–722.

Lynch, J. J. (1979). *The broken heart: The medical consequences of loneliness.* New York: Basic Books.

Maslow, A. H. (1968). *Towards a psychology of being* (2nd ed.). New York: Van Nostrand.

Miller, C. A. (1995). *Nursing care of older adults* (2nd ed.). Glenview, IL: Scott, Foresman.

Stanley, M., & Beare, P. G. (1994). *Gerontological nursing.* Philadelphia: W. B. Saunders.

Warren, B. J. (1993). Explaining social isolation through concept analysis. *Archives of Psychiatric Nursing, 7*(5), 270–276.

Weiss, R. S. (1973). *Loneliness: The experience of emotional and social isolation.* Cambridge, MA: MIT Press.

Wong, D. (1995). *Nursing care of infants and children* (5th ed.). St. Louis: Mosby-Yearbook.

Yurick, A., Spier, B., Robb, S., & Ebert, N. (1989). *The aged person and the nursing process* (3rd ed.). Norwalk, CT: Appleton-Century-Crofts.

Management of Therapeutic Regimen, Effective: Individual

DEFINITION

Effective Management of Therapeutic Regimen: Individual: A pattern in which the individual integrates into daily living a program for treatment of illness and its sequelae that is satisfactory for meeting health goals.

DEFINING CHARACTERISTICS

Appropriate choices of daily activities for meeting the goals of a treatment or prevention program

Illness symptoms within a normal range of expectation

Verbalized desire to manage the treatment of illness and prevention of sequelae

Verbalized intent to reduce risk factors for progression or illness and sequelae

RELATED FACTORS

Refer to Author's Note for an explanation.

Author's Note

Effective Management of Therapeutic Regimen describes an individual who is successful in managing an illness or condition. The concept of "enhanced" is appropriate: the nurse can assist the person to enhance his or her management. The focus would be one of anticipatory guidance (*e.g.,* teaching the person what events could negatively affect his or her management and how to reduce the negative impact).

Errors in Diagnostic Statements

Effective Management of Therapeutic Regimen related to internal locus of control

This diagnosis does not need related factors. Writing related factors would only serve to repeat the characteristics of people who manage their conditions well (*e.g.,* motivated, knowledgeable).

Key Concepts

See *Ineffective Management of Therapeutic Regimen*

Focus Assessment Criteria

A. Assess for defining characteristics

    1. Knowledgeable about

        a. Illness/condition

            Severity

            Susceptibility to complications

            Prognosis

            Ability to cure it or control its progression

        b. Treatment/diagnostic studies

        c. Preventive measures

    2. Has a pattern of adherence to recommended health behaviors or regimen

    3. Expresses a desire to increase ability to manage condition (progression, sequelae)

    4. Reports that symptoms of condition are stable or diminished

---

Outcome Criteria

The person will
- Describe strategies to address progression or complications of his or her condition if they should arise
- Discuss situations that can challenge his or her continued successful management

---

Interventions

A. Discuss possible changes in client's condition that may affect illness and usual management

    1. Exacerbation

    2. Complications

    3. Side effects of medication

B. Advise early contact with care provider to discuss possible changes in management regimen

C. Discuss how increased levels of stress can negatively affect previous successful management and possibly decrease resistance to colds or influenza

D. Explore with the person his or her evaluation of the level of stress that he or she usually lives with

    1. Usual level of stress

    2. Signs of overload

E. Discuss to anticipate that stress comes with favorable and unfavorable life events (*e.g.*, marriage, divorce, birth, death, vacations, work)

F. When faced with upcoming additional stresses, plan to:

    1. Reduce stress in other aspects of life, if possible.

    2. Increase adherence to healthy habits.

        a. Sleep 7–8 hours.

        b. Eat breakfast.

        c. Exercise daily (at least a 30-minute brisk walk).

        d. Eliminate or minimize alcohol intake.

        e. Increase intake of complex carbohydrates.

        f. Decrease intake of fat.

        g. Decrease caffeine intake.

3. Increase spiritually related activities.
   a. Meditation
   b. Listening to relaxing music
   c. Nature walking (*e.g.*, woods, near water, mountains)
   d. Reading poetry

G. Initiate health teaching and referrals regarding stress reduction techniques (Refer to Appendix X)

Rationale

- The dynamic nature of chronic conditions necessitates knowledge of how to balance one's life to keep symptoms under control as much as possible (Lubin, 1995).
- "Disease" refers to the state of unhealth related to biologic dysfunction. "Illness" is a person's personal perspective with regard to the impact or experiences related to the disease (Lubin, 1995).
- Health care professionals can assist the person to reduce the illness experiences.
- Assisting the person to realistically evaluate the effects of stress can promote stress reduction activities (Edelman & Mandle, 1990).

Management of Therapeutic Regimen, Ineffective

Management of Therapeutic Regimen, Ineffective: Family

Management of Therapeutic Regimen, Ineffective: Community

Management of Therapeutic Regimen, Ineffective

DEFINITION
Ineffective Management of Therapeutic Regimen: A pattern in which the individual experiences or is at risk to experience difficulty integrating into daily living a program for treatment of illness and the sequelae of illness that meets specific health goals.

DEFINING CHARACTERISTICS
Major (Must Be Present)
Verbalized desire to manage the treatment of illness and prevention of sequelae
Verbalized difficulty with regulation/integration of one or more prescribed regimens for treatment of illness and its effects or prevention of complications

Minor (May Be Present)
Acceleration (expected or unexpected) of illness symptoms
Verbalized that did not take action to include treatment regimens in daily routines
Verbalized that did not take action to reduce risk factors for progression of illness and sequelae

RELATED FACTORS
Treatment-Related
Related to:
Complexity of therapeutic regimen   Complexity of health care system
Financial cost of regimen   Side effects of therapy

Situational (Personal, Environmental)
Related to:
Decisional conflicts   Questions seriousness of problem
Insufficient knowledge   Questions susceptibility
Family conflicts   Questions benefits of regimen
Mistrust of regimen   Insufficient social support
Mistrust of health care personnel   Insufficient confidence
Health belief conflicts   Previous unsuccessful experiences
Related to barriers to comprehension secondary to:
Cognitive deficits   Fatigue
Hearing impairments   Motivation
Anxiety   Memory problems

Maturational

Child, adolescent
Related to fear of being different

Author's Note

Ineffective Management of Therapeutic Regimen represents a very useful diagnosis for nurses in most settings. Individuals and families experiencing a variety of health problems, acute or chronic, are usually faced with treatment programs that require changes in previous functioning or life-style. These changes or adaptations can be instrumental in influencing positive outcomes.

This diagnosis describes individuals or families who are experiencing difficulty in achieving positive outcomes. The nurse is the primary professional who, with the client, determines what choices are available and how success can be achieved. The primary nursing interventions are exploration of options available and teaching the client how to implement the selected option.

When an individual is faced with a complex regimen to follow or has compromised functioning that impedes successful management, the diagnosis *Risk for Ineffective Therapeutic Regimen* would be appropriate. In addition to teaching how to manage the regimen, the nurse must also assist the client to identify the adjustments needed because of a functional deficit.

Errors in Diagnostic Statements

Ineffective Management of Therapeutic Regimen related to a decision not to follow low-salt diet

When client makes a decision not to adhere to a therapeutic regimen, the nurse needs to explore with the client the circumstances surrounding this decision. More data need to be collected to determine if the client wants to adhere to the diet, or if the client understands the rationale for the diet. Did the client desire to adhere to the diet, but encounter difficulty? Did the client adhere to the diet but experience no positive effects? The nursing intervention strategies would differ with each of these three contributing factors. The following nursing diagnosis is an example of a client who desires to comply, but is having difficulty: *Ineffective Management of Therapeutic Regimen related to unplanned meals associated with frequent air travel schedule.*

Key Concepts

1. Successful management of a therapeutic regimen requires that the person make one or more changes in life-style. These changes or activities treat problems, prevent problems, and/or monitor for problems. Table II-16 illustrates examples of activities in each of the three types.
2. Self-efficacy is a theory that describes an individual's evaluation of his or her capabilities to manage stressful situations or to change behaviors to manage the situation (Bandura, 1982).
3. Successful management depends on the person believing that the behavior change will improve the situation (outcome expectancy) and that he or she can make the behavior change (self-efficacy expectancy) (Bandura, 1982).
4. Health education is the teaching–learning process of influencing client and family behavior through changes in knowledge, attitudes, and beliefs, and through the acquisition of psychomotor skills. The goal of patient teaching is to help the client assume responsibility for self-care.
5. Each person should be assessed for the knowledge and skill needed to monitor health status (*e.g.*, home blood glucose monitoring in diabetes), control or cure disease, or prevent disease (*e.g.*, diet, medication therapy, life-style changes), and prevent recurrence or complications (*e.g.*, postoperative leg exercises).

Table II-16 **Examples of Activities to Manage Therapeutic Regimen**

Therapeutic
Wound care
Medications
Specialized diet
Exercises

Preventive
Exercise program
Periodic evaluations
Balanced diet

Monitoring
Vital signs
Urine testing
Skin assessments

6. Inaccurate perceptions of health status usually involve misunderstanding of the nature and seriousness of the illness, susceptibility to complications, and the need for procedures for cure or control of illness.
7. Factors affecting learning or the learner (Redman & Thomas, 1992)
   a. Physical factors that affect learning include
      Presence of acute illness
      Fluid and electrolyte imbalance
      Nutritional status
      Illness or treatments that interfere with mental alertness (pain, medications)
      Illness or treatments that interfere with motor abilities (fatigue, equipment)
      Activity tolerance (endurance)
   b. Personal factors that affect learning include

Age	Past experiences or knowledge
Intelligence	Locus of control
Reading ability	Perception of
Level of motivation	Seriousness of condition
Level of anxiety	Susceptibility to complications
Denial of disease process	Prognosis
Depression	Ability to control progression or to cure
Stage of adaptation to illness	condition

   c. Socioeconomic factors that affect learning include

Language	Cultural background
Life-style	Transportation
Support system	Health care facility
Financial status	Drugstore
Past experiences with health care	

8. Factors resulting in ineffective teaching (Redman & Thomas, 1992)
   a. Inadequate or no assessment before teaching
   b. Assessment data not communicated or not considered when teaching (the most influential assessment factors are psychological status, physical stability, educational level, cultural background, socioeconomic status)
   c. Teaching not individualized
   d. Information not presented at a level consistent with the client's ability
   e. Tendency to talk down to client
   f. Use of misunderstood terms
   g. Fragmented presentation of information
   h. Too much information given, with important information hidden or lost among irrelevant information

    i. No repetition of information
    j. No feedback given in relation to process (or client is punished for not learning)
    k. No evaluation of client learning made

🏛 *Key Concepts*—*Older Adult*

1. The ability to manage one's therapeutic regimen profoundly influences one's self-esteem and independence. "Increasing geriatric clients' self-care capacity through education can be an effective way of meeting their self-esteem needs" (Rakel, 1991, p. 396).
2. It is a myth that older adults are unable to learn new concepts and skills. Some changes that occur during aging may deter learning, such as decreased visual acuity, decreased hearing, slowing of information processing, decreased attention span, difficulty in unlearning habits, fear of uncertainty or failure, decreased problem solving, and the need for a longer time and repetition to retain learning (Rakel, 1991).

TRANSCULTURAL CONSIDERATIONS

1. Because the dominant American culture is future oriented, it values living a life-style that promotes health and prevents disease. This value is challenged when a client or family of another culture is oriented to the present (Boyle & Andrews, 1995).
2. Individuals with an external locus of control believe that external factors or forces determine their health. This belief challenges the entire concept of health promotion (Andrews & Boyle, 1995).
3. Folk remedies are treatments or practices that cultural groups use to stay healthy or to treat illnesses. Spector (1985) questioned students of various cultures to determine health and illness behaviors. Table II-17 illustrates some of her findings.
4. Folk remedies are used to treat many illnesses, such as headaches, colds, rashes, coughs, sore throats, constipation, fever, warts, and menstrual cramps. Examples of folk remedies for headaches include (Spector, 1985): lie down and rest in complete darkness (Canadian); boil a beef bone, break up toast in the broth, and drink (German); cold or hot face cloth on forehead, rest (Irish); kerchief with ice around head (Italian); aspirin and hot liquids (Polish).
5. Some folk remedies may be misdiagnosed as abuse. Three folk practices of Southeast Asians leave marks on the body that can be taken for signs of violence or abuse. *Cao gio* is rubbing of the skin with a coin to produce dark blood or ecchymotic strips; it is done to treat colds and flulike symptoms. *Bat gio* is skin pinching on the temples to treat headaches or on the neck for sore throat; if petechiae or ecchymoses appear, the treatment is a success. *Poua* is burning of the skin with the tip of a dried, weedlike grass; it is believed the burning will cause the noxious element that causes the pain to exude (Andrews & Boyle, 1995).

Focus Assessment Criteria

Subjective Data

A. Assess for defining characteristics
    1. Determine present knowledge of
        Illness
            Severity   Susceptibility to complications
            Prognosis   Ability to cure it or control its progression
        Treatment/diagnostic studies
        Preventive measures
    2. What is the pattern of adhering to prescribed health behaviors?
        Complete
        Modified
        Not adhering

Table II-17   **Folk Remedies to Maintain Health**

Wine: It
Eat wholesome, balanced foods: It, P, S, A, BA, EB, FC, G, I, IC
Dress right for weather: BA, NA, EB, FC, FCC, G, IC
Cleanliness: BA, CC, EC, G, I, IC, N
Daily walks: EB, EC, S
Pray daily: BA, CC
Read: EB
Take baths: EC
Open bedroom windows at night: EC
Enough sleep: FCC, IC
Cod liver oil daily: FC, N, P, S
Exercise: FCC, IC, It
Take aspirin: G
Wear holy medals: IC
Brush teeth: I
Early to bed: It
Hard bread: It
Routine medical examination: S
Medical care when sick: EE, P
Rest: EC, FC, IC, N, P

(Spector, R. E. [1985]. *Cultural diversity in health and illness* [2nd ed.]. Norwalk, CT: Appleton-Century-Crofts.)

Code: A, Asian; BA, black African; CC, Canadian Catholic; EE, Eastern Europe, Jewish; EB, English Baptist; EC, English Catholic; FC, French Catholic; FCC, French Canadian Catholics; G, German Catholics; I, Iran Islam; IC, Irish Catholic; It, Italian; N, Norwegian; P, Polish; S, Swedish; NA, Native American.

---

3. Does anything interfere with adherence to the prescribed health behavior?
4. Learning needs (perceived by client, family)

B. Assess for related factors
   1. History of disease
      Onset   Effects on life-style (relationships, work, leisure activities,
      Symptoms   finances)
   2. Stage of adaptation to disease
      Disbelief   Anger
      Denial   Awareness
      Depression   Acceptance
   3. Learning ability (client, family)
      Level of education   Language spoken
      Ability to read   Language understood
   4. Cultural factors
      Traditions   Health care beliefs and practices
      Life-style   Values

Objective Data
A. Assess for related factors
   1. Ability to perform prescribed procedures
      Competency
      Accuracy
      Dexterity
   2. Level of cognitive and psychomotor development
      Age   Ability to read and write

3. Presence of sensory deficits
   Vision   Sense of taste (altered or lost)
   Hearing   Sense of touch
   Sense of smell (altered or lost)

Outcome Criteria

The person/family will
- Relate an intent to practice health behaviors needed or desired for recovery from illness and prevention of recurrence or complications
- Relate less anxiety, related to fear of the unknown, fear of loss of control, or misconceptions
- Describe disease process, causes and factors contributing to symptoms, and the regimen for disease or symptom control

---

Interventions

A. Identify causative or contributing factors that impede effective management
   1. Lack of trust
   2. Insufficient confidence (self-efficacy)
   3. Insufficient knowledge
   4. Insufficient resources

B. Build trust and strength (Zerwich, 1992)
   1. Gain entrance to family system.
      a. Behave as a guest.
      b. Do not take over.
      c. Gently ease in.
   2. Avoid impression of pressuring.
      a. Give space.
      b. Cease discussion when client shows indicators of closure or uneasiness.
   3. Listen to discover concerns, not to impose expectations.
   4. Attempt to discover a match between expressed needs and services the nurse can provide.
      a. Start where they are.
      b. Need a good "excuse" to continue relationship.
   5. Discover and affirm strengths.
   6. Accept people where they are.
      a. Avoid judging.
      b. Avoid setting expectations for others.
   7. Demonstrate persistence.
      a. Proceed slowly.
      b. Plan short, frequent visits.
   8. Demonstrate honesty, consistency, stability.
      a. Follow through on promises.
      b. Maintain preestablished contacts in person or by phone.
   9. Identify and emphasize strengths, such as:
      a. Survival skills
      b. Parent–child relationship
      c. Family caregiving abilities
   10. Consider cultural preferences or practices (Spector, 1985).
      a. What does your family do to maintain health?

   b. What does your family do to prevent illness?
   c. What home remedies do you or your family use?

C. Promote confidence and positive self-efficacy (Bandura, 1982)

   1. Explore with person(s) past successful management of problems.
   2. Emphasize their past successful coping.
   3. Tell stories of other "success."
   4. If appropriate, encourage opportunities to witness others successfully coping in a similar situation.
   5. Encourage participation in self-help groups.
   6. If high autonomic response (*e.g.*, rapid pulse, diaphoresis) is reducing feeling of confidence, teach short-term anxiety interrupters (Grainger, 1990).
      a. Look up.
      b. Control breathing.
      c. Lower shoulders.
      d. Slow thoughts.
      e. Alter voice.
      f. Give self directions (out loud, if possible).
      g. Exercise.
      h. "Scruff your face"—change facial expression.
      i. Change perspective: Imagine watching the situation from a distance.

D. Reduce or eliminate barriers to learning

   1. Assist meeting basic physiologic needs, if necessary.
   2. Support person in progressing through stages of psychosocial adaptation to illness.
      a. Stage of disbelief (denial)
         Orient person to hospital setting, routines affecting him.
         Teach with a focus on the present.
         Provide simple explanations of procedures as they are carried out.
         Help person feel safe, secure.
         Concentrate on one-to-one teaching, rather than group teaching.
         Teach family about the denial that person is having.
      b. State of developing awareness (guilt, anger)
         Listen carefully to person.
         Continue teaching with a present-tense focus.
         Allow hostility to be safely vented.
         Avoid arguing with person.
   3. Delay teaching until person is ready.
   4. Adapt teaching to person's physical and psychological status (Rakel, 1992).
      a. Comfort levels
      b. Fatigue levels
      c. Not concurrently with peaks of medications that alter perception or cognition
   5. Allow person to work through and express intense emotions before beginning to teach.
   6. Examine person's health beliefs and past experiences related to his illness and assess their impact on his desire to learn.

E. Reduce anxiety

   1. Encourage verbalization.
   2. Listen attentively.
   3. Meet person's expressed needs before giving other information.
   4. Develop trust with frequent, consistent interactions.
   5. Give correct, relevant information.
   6. Give nonthreatening information before more anxiety-producing information.
   7. Explain reason for and intended effect of treatment; emphasize the positive.
   8. Explore with person the effects of a new diagnosis, treatment, or surgery on his significant others.

9. Do not overwhelm person with too much information if anxiety is high or physical condition is unstable.
10. Allow person to maintain some control over himself and his routines by involving person in care.
11. Prepare person and family for what to expect concerning his environment, routines, the personnel giving care, sensations experienced, and so forth.

F. Promote personal/family learning
1. Individualize the teaching approach after a thorough assessment.
2. Plan and share necessity of learning outcomes with person/family.
3. Follow the principles of teaching/learning (refer to Key Concepts).
4. Explain and discuss (Rakel, 1992):
   a. Disease process, treatment regimen
   b. Treatment regimen (medications, diet, procedures, exercises, equipment use)
   c. Rational of regimen
   d. Expectations (client, family) of regimen
   e. Side effects of regimen
   f. Life-style changes needed
   g. Methods to monitor condition
   h. Follow-up care needed
   i. Signs/symptoms of complications
   j. Resources, support available
   k. Home environment alterations needed
5. Evaluate personal/family behaviors as evidence that learning outcomes have been achieved.

G. Proceed with referrals, as indicated
1. Community nursing services

Rationale

- A major determinant of self-efficacy is past successful coping in a similar situation (Bandura, 1982). In contrast, past unsuccessful management of a similar situation is a deterrent.
- In addition to past successful coping experiences, Bandura (1982) had identified three other factors that promote positive self-efficacy as:
  - Witnessing others successfully coping
  - Belief by others that they can successfully cope or manage
  - Not experiencing high autonomic arousal in response to the situation
- Zerwich (1992) has identified family caregiving competencies, which provide the essential groundwork to promote family self-help as building trust and strength.
- Vulnerable families have poor self-esteem and are "starved for validation" that they have capabilities (Zerwich, 1992).
- Research has shown that when family members are involved in care, an increase in client cooperation and positive adjustment to the experience result (Leske, 1993).
- Teaching should be routinely incorporated as an integral part of nursing care whenever a new diagnosis or change in regimen is made, or when the client faces an unfamiliar situation.
- An assessment before beginning teaching facilitates the meaningfulness, efficacy, and overall success of the teaching–learning process by defining *what* content should be present, *how* the content should be given, *when* the client is ready to learn, and *who* should be included in the process.
- Learning depends on physical and emotional readiness. The client needs to be relatively free of pain and extreme anxiety to learn. High anxiety decreases learning, whereas slight anxiety may increase learning.
- Client motivation is one of the most important variables affecting the amount of learning that takes place.

Management of Therapeutic Regimen, Ineffective: Family

DEFINITION

Ineffective Management of Therapeutic Regimen, Family: A pattern in which the family experiences or is at risk to experience difficulty integrating into daily living a program for treatment of illness and the sequelae of illness that meets specific health goals.

DEFINING CHARACTERISTICS

Major

Inappropriate family activities for meeting the goals of a treatment or prevention program

Minor

Acceleration (expected or unexpected) of illness symptoms of a family member

Lack of attention to illness and its sequelae

Verbalized desire to manage the treatment of illness and prevention of sequelae

Verbalized difficulty with regulation/integration of one or more prescribed regimens for treatment of illness and its effects or prevention of complications

Verbalized that family did not take action to reduce risk factors for progression of illness and sequelae

RELATED FACTORS

Refer to *Ineffective Management of Therapeutic Regimen*.

Author's Note

Refer to *Ineffective Management of Therapeutic Regimen*.

Errors in Diagnostic Statements

Refer to *Ineffective Management of Therapeutic Regimen*.

Key Concepts

Refer to *Ineffective Management of Therapeutic Regimen*.

Focus Assessment Criteria

Refer to *Ineffective Management of Therapeutic Regimen*.

Interventions

Refer to *Ineffective Management of Therapeutic Regimen*.

Management of Therapeutic Regimen, Ineffective: Community

DEFINITION

Ineffective Management of Therapeutic Regimen: Community: A pattern in which the community experiences or is at risk to experience difficulty integrating a program for treatment of illness and the sequelae of illness that meets specific health goals.

DEFINING CHARACTERISTICS
Major

Verbalized difficulty in meeting health needs in communities
Acceleration (expected or unexpected) of illness(es)
Morbidity, mortality rates above norm

RELATED FACTORS
Situational (Environmental)

Related to availability of community programs for (specify):

Prevention of diseases	Screening for diseases
Immunizations	Dental care
Accident prevention	Fire safety
Smoking cessation	Substance abuse
Alcohol abuse	Child abuse

Related to problem accessing program secondary to:
Inadequate communication
Limited hours
Lack of transportation
Insufficient funds
Related to complexity of population's needs
Related to lack of awareness of availability
Related to presence of environmental or occupational health hazards
Related to multiple needs of vulnerable groups (specify):
Homeless
Pregnant teenagers
Below poverty level
Home-bound individuals
Related to unavailable or insufficient health care agencies

Author's Note

This diagnosis describes a community that has evidence that a population is underserved because of lack of availability of, access to, or knowledge of health care resources. The community nurse using the results of a community assessment can identify at-risk groups and overall community needs. In addition, the nurse assesses health systems, transportation, social services, and access.

Key Concepts

Refer to Key Concepts under *Potential for Enhanced Community Coping* and *Ineffective Community Coping*.

Focus Assessment Criteria (Community Health Assessment [Helvie, 1991; Kriegler & Harton, 1992])

Subjective, Objective

A. Population

    1. Percentage of population in each age group (years)

0–5	45–54
5–14	55–64
15–24	65–75
25–34	75+
35–44	

    2. Gender and race distribution

    3. Vital statistics

       a. Births (mother's age, illegitimate)

       b. Death rate (neonates, infants, maternal, suicides, general)

B. Health perception–health maintenance pattern

    1. Vital statistics

       a. Communicable disease incidence

       b. Immunization percentages by age

       c. Ten leading causes of death

       d. Rate of chronic diseases

    2. Health care services (adequate, inadequate)

       a. Hospital services (general, maternity, psychiatric, pediatric, rehabilitation)

       b. Nursing home services

       c. Ambulatory services

       d. Occupational services

       e. School health services

       f. Health department services

       g. Community services

           Clinics (types, frequency)

       h. Home services (types, number of agencies)

    3. Protective services

       a. Police

       b. Fire

       c. Disaster response plan

       d. Ambulance service

       e. Environment protection services (air, water, industrial, wastes, food services, housing)

C. Nutritional–metabolic pattern

    1. Food sources (stores, markets, restaurants)

    2. Nutritional assistance programs (WIC, Meals on Wheels)

    3. Nutrition educational programs

D. Elimination pattern

    1. Sanitation (water supply, sewage disposal, trash and garbage disposal, rodent and vermin control)

    2. Ecologic concerns (recycling, hazardous wastes)

E. Activity–exercise pattern

    1. Transportation options

    2. Recreation and fitness facilities (types for various age groups)

F. Sleep–rest pattern

    1. Noise (traffic, airline, trains, industry)

G. Cognitive–perceptual pattern
  1. Process of community decisions (government, schools)
  2. Educational facilities (public, private, adult education, higher education, health education programs)
  3. Communication (publications, radio and TV stations, informal network)

H. Self-perception–self-concept pattern
  1. Population characteristics (ethnic origins, race)
  2. Social economic (primary occupations, average income level, percentage below poverty level, unemployment rate, percentage of homeowners vs. renters)

I. Role–relationship pattern (intergenerational, interracial, interethnic)
  1. Community-sponsored events

J. Sexuality–reproductive pattern
  1. Average size of family
  2. Reproduction (birth rate, teen pregnancies, prenatal care, abortion facilities)
  3. Birth control resources
  4. Educational programs (sex education, childbirth education classes, parenting classes)

K. Coping–stress tolerance pattern
  1. Assistance programs (federal, state)
  2. Community-based programs (self-help, telephone help-lines, crisis centers)

L. Value–belief pattern
  1. Religious distribution
  2. Religious outreach
  3. Social programs
    a. Fund raising
    b. Service organizations
    c. Senior citizen programs
    d. Handicap services
    e. Shelters
  4. Cultural–ethnic programs (services, social)

Outcome Criteria

The community will
- Identify community resources that are needed
- Promote the use of community resources for health problems

Interventions

A. Create a survey to determine:
  1. Health problem identification
  2. Awareness of health services
  3. Utilization of health services
  4. Interest in health promotion programs
  5. Recommendation for funding sources

B. Survey samples of the target population
  1. Mail survey
  2. One-to-one survey at community center, sports field, supermarket

3. Group survey (*e.g.*, church groups, clubs)
4. Key community leaders

C. Design survey for easy reading and answering (*e.g.*, circle the number that best describes your answer: 1—no concern; 2—medium; 3—high)
   1. How concerned are you about:
      a. Hypertension
      b. Stress
      c. Alcohol misuse

D. Organize the response data
   1. Rank-order entire sample
   2. Group responses of selected groups (*e.g.*, age, gender, income level, disabled)

E. Analyze the findings
   1. What are the overall health problems reported?
   2. What are the health concerns of
      a. Elderly population
      b. Households with children up to age 20 years
      c. Single-parent households
      d. Respondents younger than 45 years of age
      e. Individuals below the poverty level

F. Evaluate community resources
   1. What resources are available for the health problems identified?
   2. Are there utilization or access problems with the services?
   3. How does the population learn about services?
   4. Identify problems that do not have community services available.

G. If services are available but are underutilized, evaluate
   1. Hours of operation (convenient?)
   2. Location of services (access, esthetics)
   3. Efficiency and atmosphere
   4. Advertising strategies

H. If services are unavailable, pursue program development
   1. Examine and evaluate similar programs in other communities
      a. Basic information
      b. Purpose, goals
      c. Services available
      d. Funding
      e. Cost to participants
      f. Availability of services
      g. Accessibility of services
      h. Satisfaction (citizen, employees)
   2. Meet with appropriate persons to discuss findings (survey, on-site visits)
   3. Address the following:
      a. Presence of community support
      b. Available expertise and technology in community
      c. Financial support
   4. Identify appropriate community sources of assistance
      a. Hospital departments
      b. Health departments
      c. Industry
      d. Chamber of Commerce
      e. Health care professionals

      f. Schools of nursing
      g. Private foundations
      h. Public assistance agencies
      i. Professional societies
    5. Plan the program (refer to *Effective Community Coping* for Interventions for community planning)

I. Evaluate vulnerable population's access to health care and knowledge of risk factors
    1. Rural families, elderly
    2. Migrant workers
    3. New immigrants
    4. Homeless
    5. Below-poverty-level individuals, groups

J. Make a priority of ensuring that basic needs for food, shelter, clothing, and safety are met before attempting to address higher health needs

K. Provide information regarding illness prevention, health promotion, and health services to vulnerable populations
    1. Be sure reading material is appropriate for targeted group (*e.g.*, reading level, language, pictures)
    2. Use posters, flyers
    3. Select locations that are used regularly by the targeted population:
      a. Grocery, convenience stores
      b. Laundromat
      c. School activities
      d. Sporting events
      e. Community fairs
      f. Religious services, meetings
      g. Day care centers

Rationale

- In community base planning, it is necessary to conduct a needs assessment, set priorities, and establish objectives (Clemen-Stone, Eigasti, McGuire, 1991).
- Community involvement is necessary to validate which problems warrant attention and to ensure successful outcomes (Clemen-Stone et al., 1991).
- Incentives to mobilize the community to change are integrated into the planning.
- Evaluation of resources available is needed to match activities planned (Edelman & Mandle, 1990).
- Liaisons with community leaders and other sources of support are integral to successful program outcomes (Edelman & Mandle, 1990).

References/Bibliography

Andrews, M., & Boyle, J. (1995). *Transcultural concepts in nursing* (2nd ed.). Philadelphia: J. B. Lippincott.

Bandura, A. (1982). Self-efficacy mechanism in human agency. *American Psychology, 37*(3), 122–147.

Edelman, C. L., & Mandle, C. L. (1990). *Health promotion throughout the lifespan*. St. Louis: Mosby-Year Book.

Grainger, R. (1990). Anxiety interruptors. *American Journal of Nursing, 90,* 14–15.

Leske, J. (1993). Anxiety of elective surgical patients, family members. *AORN Journal, 57,* 1091–1103.

Lubin, J. M. (1995). *Chronic illness: Impact and interventions*. Boston: Jones & Bartlett.

Rakel, B. (1991). Knowledge deficit. In M. Maas, K. Buckwalter, & M. Hardy (Eds.). *Nursing diagnoses and interventions for the elderly.* Redwood City, CA: Addison-Wesley Nursing.

Rakel, B. A. (1992). Interventions related to teaching. In G. Bulechek & J. McCloskey (Eds.). *Nursing interventions* (2nd ed.). Philadelphia: W. B. Saunders.

Redman, B., & Thomas, S. (1992). Patient teaching. In G. Bulechek & J. McCloskey (Eds.). *Nursing interventions* (2nd ed.). Philadelphia: W. B. Saunders.

Spector, R. E. (1985). *Cultural diversity in health and illness* (2nd ed.). Norwalk, CT: Appleton-Century-Crofts.

Zerwich, J. (1992). Laying the groundwork for family self-help: Locating families, building trust and building strength. *Public Health Nursing, 9*(1), 15–21.

Community

Clemen-Stone, S., Eigasti, D., & McGuire, S. L. (1991). *Comprehensive family and community health nursing* (3rd ed.). St. Louis: Mosby-Yearbook.

Edelman, C. L., & Mandle, C. L. (1990). *Health promotion throughout the lifespan*. St. Louis: Mosby-Yearbook.

Helvie, C. O. (1991). *Community health nursing: Theory and practice*. New York: Springer.

Kriegler, N., & Harton, M. (1991). Community health assessment tool: A patterned approach to data collection and diagnosis. *Journal of Community Health Nursing, 9*, 229–234.

Mobility, Impaired Physical

DEFINITION

Impaired Physical Mobility: A state in which the individual experiences or is at risk of experiencing limitation of physical movement but is not immobile.

DEFINING CHARACTERISTICS (LEVIN, KRAINOVITCH, BAHRENBURG, & MITCHELL, 1989)

Major (80%–100%)

Compromised ability to move purposefully within the environment (*e.g.*, bed mobility, transfers, ambulation)

Range-of-motion (ROM) limitations

Minor (50%–80%)

Imposed restriction of movement

Reluctance to move

RELATED FACTORS

Pathophysiologic

Related to decreased strength and endurance secondary to:

(Neuromuscular impairment)

Autoimmune alterations (*e.g.*, multiple sclerosis, arthritis)

Nervous system diseases (*e.g.*, Parkinson's disease, myasthenia gravis)

Muscular dystrophy

Partial paralysis (spinal cord injury, stroke)

Central nervous system (CNS) tumor

Increased intracranial pressure

Sensory deficits

(Musculoskeletal impairment)

Fractures

Connective tissue disease (systemic lupus erythematosus)

Related to edema

Treatment-Related

Related to external devices (casts or splints, braces, IV tubing)
Related to insufficient strength and endurance for ambulation with (specify)

Prosthesis   Crutches   Walker

Situational (Personal, Environmental)

Related to:

Fatigue   Motivation   Pain

Maturational

Children
Related to abnormal gait secondary to:

Congenital skeletal deficiencies   Congenital hip dysplasia
Osteomyelitis   Legg-Calvé-Perthes disease

Older Adult

Related to decreased motor agility
Related to muscle weakness

Author's Note

Impaired Physical Mobility describes an individual with limited use of arm(s) or leg(s) or limited muscle strength. This diagnosis should not be used to describe complete immobility; in this case, *Disuse Syndrome* would be more applicable. Limitation of physical movement also can be the etiology of other nursing diagnoses, such as *Self-Care Deficit* and *Risk for Injury*.

Nursing interventions for *Impaired Physical Mobility* focus on strengthening and restoring function and preventing deterioration.

Errors in Diagnostic Statements

Impaired Physical Mobility related to traumatic amputation of left arm

Listing traumatic amputation of the left arm as a related factor does not describe the problem. Rather, the diagnostic statement should reflect how the loss of a left arm has affected functioning. A more appropriate diagnosis might be *Self-Care Deficit: Feeding related to insufficient knowledge of adaptations needed secondary to loss of left arm.*

Impaired Physical Mobility related to limited muscle strength secondary to cerebrovascular accident (CVA)

Limited muscle strength is a sign of *Impaired Physical Mobility*, not a related factor. The related factors should represent direction for nursing intervention, as reflected in the diagnosis *Impaired Physical Mobility related to insufficient knowledge of techniques needed to increase motor function secondary to upper motor neuron damage.*

Key Concepts

1. According to Miller (1995), "mobility is one of the most important aspects of physiological functioning because it is essential for the maintenance of independence."
2. Activity, mobility, and flexibility are integral to a person's life-style. Compromised mobility has a serious impact on self-concept and life-style (Christian, 1982).
3. There are three ROM categories—passive, active, and functional.
   a. *Passive ROM* keeps muscles and joints limber. One person passively moves another person's muscles (*e.g.*, the helper lifts and moves the person's legs).
   b. *Active ROM* exercise limbers and strengthens muscles and joints. The person actively uses his muscles (*e.g.*, while lying down, the person moves his legs).
   c. *Functional ROM* strengthens muscles and joints while performing necessary activity (*e.g.*, walking). Performed by individual himself.
4. Isometric exercise is when muscles contract or tense without joint movement. Isometric exercises are contraindicated for people with cardiac conditions because they cause

increased left ventricular function. When done, the muscle should be tensed for 5 to 15 seconds (Simpson, 1986).

5. Resistive exercises strengthen muscles by pushing against something or lifting against weights. Resistance can be applied by pushing against the client's leg as the person attempts to lift it (Maas, 1991).

🌀 *Key Concepts—Child*

See *Disuse Syndrome*.

🏛 *Key Concepts—Older Adult*

1. About one tenth of noninstitutionalized older adults report some limitation in mobility, and of the institutionalized elderly, over 90% are dependent in at least one activity of daily living (Miller, 1995). Problems with mobility are often the reason for nursing home admission or extensive in-home care. Assessment of mobility determines the extent of functional impairment as a result of disease or disability.

2. The effects of immobility in the older adult are particularly dangerous. Muscle weakness, atrophy, and decreased endurance are quick to occur, and the biochemical and physiologic effects such as nitrogen loss and hypercalciuria are important to consider (Hogue, 1985). Permanent functional loss is more likely with prolonged immobility, and older adults also are vulnerable to new morbidity such as pneumonia, pressure sores, falls and fracture, osteoporosis, incontinence, confusion, and depression. Every effort toward prevention and mobilization should be made.

3. The age-related changes in joint and connective tissue cause impaired flexion and extension movements, decrease flexibility, and reduce cushioning protection for joints (Whitbourne, 1985).

Focus Assessment Criteria

Subjective Data

A. Assess for defining characteristics

    1. History of symptoms (complaints of)

        Pain

        Muscle weakness

        Fatigue

            Attributed to?   Amount of time out of bed

            Induced by?   Amount of time sleeping or resting

B. Assess for related factors

    1. History of systemic disorders

        Neurologic

            CVA, head trauma, increased intracranial pressure

            Multiple sclerosis, polio, Guillain-Barré syndrome, myasthenia gravis

            Spinal cord injury, tumor, birth defect

        Cardiovascular

            Myocardial infarction   Congenital heart anomaly

            Congestive heart failure

        Musculoskeletal

            Osteoporosis   Arthritis   Fractures

        Respiratory

            Chronic obstructive pulmonary disease (COPD)   Orthopnea

            Dyspnea on exertion   Pneumonia

        Debilitating diseases

            Cancer   Renal disease   Endocrine disease

    2. History of symptoms that interfere with mobility

        Onset   Frequency

        Duration   Precipitated by what?

        Location   Relieved by what?

        Description   Aggravated by what?

3. History of recent trauma or surgery
    Fractures
    Head injury
    Abdominal surgery or injury
4. Current drug therapy
    Sedatives, hypnotics, CNS depressants
    Laxatives
    Other

Objective Data

A. Assess for defining characteristics
1. Dominant hand
    Right
    Left
    Ambidextrous
2. Motor function

Right arm	Strong	Weak	Absent	Spastic
Left arm	Strong	Weak	Absent	Spastic
Right leg	Strong	Weak	Absent	Spastic
Left leg	Strong	Weak	Absent	Spastic

3. Mobility

Ability to turn self	Yes	No	Assistance needed (specify)
Ability to sit	Yes	No	Assistance needed (specify)
Ability to stand	Yes	No	Assistance needed (specify)
Ability to get up	Yes	No	Assistance needed (specify)
Ability to transfer	Yes	No	Assistance needed (specify)
Ability to ambulate	Yes	No	Assistance needed (specify)

    Weight-bearing (assess both right and left sides)
        Full   As tolerated
        Partial   Non–weight-bearing
    Gait
        Stable
        Unstable
    Assistive devices
        Crutches   Wheelchair
        Cane   Prosthesis
        Braces   Other
        Walker
    Restrictive devices
        Cast or splint   Foley
        Traction   IV
        Braces   Monitor
        Ventilator   Dialysis
        Drain
    Range of motion (shoulders, elbows, arms, hips, legs)
        Full
        Limited (specify)
        None
4. Endurance (see *Activity Intolerance* for additional information)
    Assess
        Resting pulse, blood pressure, respirations
        Blood pressure, respirations, and pulse immediately after activity
        Pulse every 2 minutes until pulse returns to within 10 beats of resting pulse
        After activity, assess for presence of indicators of hypoxia (showing intensity, frequency, or duration of activity must be decreased or discontinued) as follows

Blood pressure
> Failure of systolic rate to increase
> Increase in diastolic of 155 mm Hg

Respirations
> Excessive rate increases Decrease in rate
> Dyspnea Irregular rhythm

Cerebral and other changes
> Confusion Pallor
> Weakness Change in equilibrium
> Uncoordination Cyanosis

B. Assess for related factors

1. Peripheral circulation
> Capillary refill time (normal, less than 3 seconds)
> Skin color, temperature, and turgor
> Peripheral pulses (rate, quality)
>> Brachial Posterior tibial
>> Radial Popliteal
>> Femoral Pedal

2. Motivation (as perceived by nurse and stated by person)
> Excellent
> Satisfactory
> Poor

Outcome Criteria

The person will
- Demonstrate the use of adaptive devices to increase mobility
- Use safety measures to minimize potential for injury
- Describe rationale for interventions
- Demonstrate measures to increase mobility
- Report an increase in strength and endurance of limbs

Interventions

A. Assess causative factors

1. Trauma (*e.g.*, cartilage tears, fractures, amputations)
2. Surgical procedure (*e.g.*, joint replacement, reduction of fractures, vascular surgery)
3. Debilitating disease (*e.g.*, diabetes, cancer, rheumatoid arthritis, multiple sclerosis, stroke)

B. Promote optimal mobility and movement

1. Increase limb mobility.
   a. Perform ROM exercises (frequency to be determined by condition of the individual):
   > Teach the client to perform active ROM exercises on unaffected limbs at least four times a day, if possible.
   > Perform passive ROM on affected limbs. Do the exercises slowly to allow the muscles time to relax, and support the extremity above and below the joint to prevent strain on joints and tissues.
   > During ROM, the client's legs and arms should be moved gently to within his pain tolerance; perform ROM slowly to allow the muscles time to relax.
   > For passive ROM, the supine position is the most effective. The individual who performs ROM himself can use a supine or sitting position.

Do ROM daily with bed bath, three to four times daily if there are specific problem areas. Try to incorporate into activities of daily living.
   b. Support extremity with pillows to prevent or reduce swelling.
   c. Medicate for pain as needed, especially before activity* (see *Altered Comfort*).
   d. Apply heat or cold to reduce pain, inflammation, and hematoma.*
   e. Apply cold to reduce swelling postinjury (usually first 48 hours).*
   f. Encourage the person to perform exercise regimens for specific joints as prescribed by physician or physical therapist (*e.g.*, isometric, resistive).
2. Position in alignment to prevent complications.
   a. Use a foot board.
   b. Avoid prolonged periods of sitting or lying in the same position.
   c. Change position of the shoulder joints every 2–4 hours.
   d. Use a small pillow or no pillow when in Fowler's position.
   e. Support the hand and wrist in natural alignment.
   f. If the client is supine or prone, place a rolled towel or small pillow under the lumbar curvature or under the end of the rib cage.
   g. Place a trochanter roll or sandbags alongside the hips and upper thighs.
   h. If the client is in the lateral position, place pillow(s) to support the leg from groin to foot, and a pillow to flex the shoulder and elbow slightly; if needed, support the lower foot in dorsal flexion with a sandbag.
   i. For upper extremities
      Arms abducted from the body with pillows
      Elbows in slight flexion
      Wrist in a neutral position, with fingers slightly flexed, and thumb abducted and slightly flexed
      Position of shoulder joints changed during the day (*e.g.*, adduction, abduction, range of circular motion)
3. Maintain good body alignment when mechanical devices are used.
   a. Traction devices
      Assess for correct position of traction and alignment of bones.
      Observe for correct amount and position of weights.
      Allow weights to hang freely, with no blankets or sheets on ropes.
      Assess for changes in circulation; check pulse quality, skin temperature, color of extremities, and capillary refill (should be less than 2 seconds).
      Assess for changes in circulation (numbness, tingling, pain).
      Assess for changes in mobility (ability to flex/extend unaffected joints).
      Assess for signs of skin irritation (redness, ulceration, blanching).
      Assess skeletal traction pin sites for loosening, inflammation, ulceration, and drainage; clean pin insertion sites (procedure may vary with type of pin and physician's order).
      Encourage isometrics* and prescribed exercise program.
   b. Casts
      Assess for proper fit of casts (they should not be too loose or too tight).
      Assess circulation to the encased area every 2 hours (color and temperature of skin, pulse quality, capillary refill less than 2 seconds).
      Assess for changes in sensation of extremities every 2 hours (numbness, tingling, pain).
      Assess motion of uninvolved joints (ability to flex and extend).
      Assess for skin irritation (redness, ulceration, or complaints of pain under the cast).
      Keep cast clean and dry; do not allow sharp objects to be inserted under cast; petal rough edges with adhesive tape; place soft cotton under edges that seem to be causing pressure points.
      Allow cast to air dry while resting on pillows to prevent dents.
      Observe cast for areas of softening or indentation.

* May require a primary care professional's order.

Exercise joints above and below cast if allowed (*e.g.*, wiggle fingers and toes every 2 hours).

Assist with prescribed exercise regimens and isometrics of muscles enclosed in casts.*

Keep extremities elevated after cast application to reduce swelling.

  c. Braces

Assess for correct positioning of braces.

Observe for signs of skin irritation (redness, ulceration, blanching, itching, pain).

Assist with exercises as prescribed for specific joints.

Have the client demonstrate correct application of the brace.

  d. Prosthetic devices

Observe for signs of skin irritation of the stump before applying prosthetic device (stump should be clean and dry; Ace bandage should be rewrapped and securely in place).

Have the client demonstrate the correct application of the prosthesis.

Assess for gait alterations or improper walking technique.

Proceed with health teaching, if indicated.

  e. Ace bandages

Assess for correct position of Ace bandage.

Apply Ace bandage with even pressure, wrapping from distal to proximal portions, and making sure that the bandage is not too tight or too loose.

Observe for "bunching" of the bandage.

Observe for signs of irritation of skin (redness, ulceration, excessive tightness).

Rewrap Ace bandage twice daily or as needed, unless contraindicated (*e.g.*, if the bandage is a postoperative compression dressing, it should be left in place).

When wrapping lower extremity, leave the heel exposed, using figure-8 technique.

  f. Slings

Assess for correct application; sling should be loose around neck and should support elbow and wrist above level of the heart.

Remove slings for ROM.*

Note: Some mechanical devices may be removed for exercises, depending on nature of injury or type and purpose of device. Consult with the physician to ascertain when the person may remove the device.

  4. Provide progressive mobilization.

  a. Assist slowly to sitting position.

  b. Allow client to dangle legs over the side of the bed for a few minutes before he stands up.

  c. Limit time to 15 minutes, three times a day, the first few times out of bed.

  d. Increase time out of bed, as tolerated by 15-minute increments.

  e. Progress to ambulation with or without assistive devices.

  f. If unable to walk, assist out of bed to a wheelchair or chair.

  g. Encourage ambulating for short, frequent walks (at least three times daily), with assistance if unsteady.

  h. Increase lengths of walks progressively each day.

  5. Encourage use of affected arm when possible.

  a. Encourage the person to use affected arm for self-care activities (*e.g.*, feeding himself, dressing, brushing hair).

  b. For post-CVA neglect of upper limb, see *Unilateral Neglect*.

  c. Instruct the person to use unaffected arm to exercise the affected arm.

  d. Use appropriate adaptive equipment to enhance the use of arms.

Universal cuff for feeding in individuals who have poor control in both arms, hands

---

* May require a primary care professional's order.

Large-handled or padded silverware to assist individuals with poor fine motor skills

Dishware with high edges to prevent food from slipping

Suction-cup aids to hold dishes in place to prevent sliding of plate

  e. Use a warm bath to alleviate early morning stiffness and improve mobility.
  f. Encourage the individual to practice handwriting skills, if able.
  g. Allow time for the individual to practice using affected limb.

C. Provide health teaching, as indicated

  1. Teach methods of transfer from bed to chair or commode and to standing position.
    a. Before transferring anyone, assess the number of personnel needed for assistance.
    b. The individual should be positioned on the side of the bed. His feet should be touching the floor, and he should be wearing stable shoes or slippers with nonskid soles.
    c. For getting in and out of bed, weight-bearing on the uninvolved or stronger side should be encouraged.
    d. Wheelchair should be locked before transfer. If using a regular chair, be sure it will not move.
    e. The person should be instructed to use the arm of the chair closer to him for support while standing.
    f. Place arm around the person's rib cage and keep back straight, with knees slightly bent.
    g. The person should be told to place his arms around the nurse's waist or rib cage, *not her neck.*
    h. Support the person's legs by bracing his with hers. (While facing the person, she should lock his knees with her knees.)
    i. Hemiplegic individuals should be instructed to pivot on the uninvolved foot.
    j. For individuals with lower limb weakness or paralysis, a sliding board transfer may be used.
        The person should wear pajamas so he will not stick to the board.
        The person needs good upper extremity strength to be able to slide his buttocks from the bed to the chair or wheelchair. (Wheelchairs should have removable arms.)
    k. When the person's arms are strong enough, he should progress to a sitting transfer without the board, if he can lift buttocks enough to clear bed and chair seat.
    l. If the person's legs give out, the nurse should guide him gently to the floor and *seek additional assistance.*
  2. Teach how to ambulate with adaptive equipment (*e.g.,* crutches, walkers, canes).
    a. Instruct the individual in weight-bearing status.
    b. Observe and teach the use of
        Crutches
            No pressure should be exerted on axilla; hand strength should be used.
            Type of gait varies with individual's diagnosis.
            Measure crutches 2–3 inches below axilla and tips 6 inches away from feet.
        Walkers
            Use arm strength to support weakness in lower limbs.
            Gait varies with individual's problems.
        Wheelchairs
            Practice transfers.
            Practice maneuvering around barriers.
        Prostheses (teach about the following)
            Stump wrapping before application of the prosthesis
            Application of the prosthesis
            Principles of stump care
            Importance of cleaning the stump, keeping it dry, and applying the prosthesis only when the stump is dry

c. Teach the individual safety precautions.

Protect areas of decreased sensation from extremes of heat and cold.

Practice falling and how to recover from falls while transferring or ambulating.

For decreased perception of lower extremity (post-CVA "neglect"), instruct the individual to check where limb is placed when changing positions or going through doorways; and check to make sure both shoes are tied, that affected leg is dressed with trousers, and that pants are not dragging.

Instruct individuals who are confined to wheelchair to shift position and lift up buttocks every 15 minutes to relieve pressure; maneuver curbs, ramps, inclines, and around obstacles; and lock wheelchairs before transferring.

d. Practice proper positioning, ROM (active or passive), and prescribed exercises.

e. Practice stair-climbing if individual's condition permits.

Rationale

- A regular exercise program including ROM, isometrics, and selected aerobic activities can help maintain integrity of joint function (Henderson, 1989).
- A warm-up period of local heat or gentle stretching before strengthening and endurance exercises allows muscles to become ready gradually for more intense work (Henderson, 1989).
- Exercises are needed to improve circulation and strengthen muscle groups needed for ambulation.
- Ambulatory aids must be used correctly and safely to ensure effectiveness and prevent injury.
- Promoting the client's feelings of control and self-determination may improve compliance with the exercise program.
- Exercise enhances independence. Incorporating ROM exercises into a person's daily routine encourages regular performance.
- Active ROM increases muscle mass, tone, and strength and improves cardiac and respiratory functioning. Passive ROM improves joint mobility and circulation.
- Prolonged immobility and impaired neurosensory function can cause permanent contractures.
- Prolonged bed rest or decreased blood volume can cause a sudden drop in blood pressure (orthostatic hypotension) as blood returns to peripheral circulation. Gradual progression to increased activity reduces fatigue and increases endurance (Kasper, 1993).
- Effective management of pain and depression is sometimes necessary. Inadequate pain relief may be a primary factor leading to depression in some individuals, but depression should not be discounted as a secondary feature of pain. Depression may require aggressive management, including drugs and other therapies (Kwentus, Harkins, & Lignon, 1985).

References/Bibliography

Christian, B. J. (1982). Immobilization: Psychosocial aspects. In C. Norris (Ed.). *Concept clarification in nursing*. Rockville, MD: Aspen Publications.

Henderson, L. (1989). Arthritis in motion: An exercise program for chronic arthritis patients. *Orthopedic Nursing, 8*(3), 41–45.

Hogue, C. (1985). Mobility. In E. Schneider (Ed.). *The teaching nursing home: A new approach to geriatric research, education, and clinical care*. New York: Raven Press.

Kasper, C. E. (1993). Alterations in skeletal muscle related to impaired physical mobility: An empirical model. *Research and Nursing Health, 16*, 265–273.

Kwentus, J., Harkins, S., & Lignon, N. (1985). Current concepts of geriatric pain and its treatment. *Geriatrics, 40*(4), 48–57.

Levin, R. F., Krainovitch, B. C., Bahrenburg, E., & Mitchell, C. A. (1989). Diagnostic content validity of nursing diagnoses. *Image, 21*(1), 40–44.

Maas, M. (1991). Impaired physical mobility. In M. Maas, K. Buckwalter, & M. Hardy (Eds.). *Nursing diagnoses and interventions for the elderly*. Redwood City, CA: Addison-Wesley Nursing.

Miller, C. A. (1995). *Nursing care of older adults* (2nd ed.). Glenview, IL: Scott, Foresman.

Simpson, W. (1986). Exercise: Prescriptions for the elderly. *Geriatrics, 41*(1), 95–100.

Whitbourne, S. K. (1985). Appearance and movement. In S. K. Whitbourne (Ed.). *The aging body*. New York: Springer-Verlag.

Noncompliance

DEFINITION

Noncompliance: The state in which an individual or group desires to comply but factors are present that deter adherence to health-related advice given by health professionals.

DEFINING CHARACTERISTICS
Major (Must Be Present)

Verbalization of noncompliance or nonparticipation or confusion about therapy and/or
Direct observation of behavior indicating noncompliance

Minor (May Be Present)

Missed appointments
Partially used or unused medications
Persistence of symptoms*
Progression of disease process*
Occurrence of undesired outcomes* (postoperative morbidity, pregnancy, obesity, addiction, regression during rehabilitation)

RELATED FACTORS
Pathophysiologic

Related to impaired ability to perform tasks because of disability secondary to:
Poor memory
Motor and sensory deficits
Related to increasing amount of disease-related symptoms despite adherence to advised regimen.

Treatment-Related

Related to:
Side effects of therapy
Previous unsuccessful experiences with advised regimen
Impersonal aspects of referral process
Nontherapeutic environment
Complex, unsupervised, or prolonged therapy
Financial cost of therapy

Situational (Personal, Environmental)

Related to barriers to access secondary to:
Mobility problems   Transportation problems
Financial issues   Inclement weather
Lack of child care
Related to concurrent illness of family member
Nonsupportive family, peers, community
Related to homelessness
Related to change in employment status
Related to change in health insurance coverage

* When these characteristics are considered to be the result of noncompliance, one is assuming that the therapy prescribed has been proved to be effective and is appropriate.

Related to barriers to comprehension secondary to:

Cognitive deficits	Anxiety
Visual deficits	Fatigue
Hearing deficits	Decreased attention span
Poor memory	Motivation

Author's Note

Compliance depends on various factors, including the person's motivation, perception of vulnerability, and beliefs about controlling or preventing illness; environmental variables; quality of health instruction; and ability to access resources (cost, accessibility).

The diagnosis *Noncompliance* describes a person desiring to comply but prevented from doing so by certain factors (*e.g.*, lack of understanding, inadequate finances, too-complex instructions). The nurse must attempt to reduce or eliminate these factors to ensure that interventions are successful.

A person's right to self-determination is protected through the process of informed consent. Informed consent has three conditions: the person must be capable of giving consent, must understand the advantages and disadvantages of consenting, and must not be coerced (Cassells & Redman, 1989). When a person refuses to comply with advice or instructions, it is important that the nurse assess for and validate that all required elements for an informed consent are present. The nurse is cautioned against using *Noncompliance* to describe a person who has made an informed autonomous decision not to comply. As Cassells and Redman (1989) state, "human dignity is respected by granting individuals the freedom to make choices in accordance with their own values." When an individual needs to change habits or life-style or perform certain activities to manage a health problem, the diagnosis *Risk for Ineffective Management of Therapeutic Regimen* is very useful.

Errors in Diagnostic Statements

Noncompliance related to reports of not following low-salt diet and resulting increased edema

The factors above would not have caused or contributed to noncompliance, but instead represent evidence of noncompliance. If the reason for the noncompliance is unknown, the diagnosis *Noncompliance related to unknown etiology, as evidenced by reports of (specify)* would be appropriate.

When the reasons are identified, the nurse must determine whether these factors can be reduced or eliminated. If the person has made an informed decision not to follow the prescribed diet, *Noncompliance* may not be the correct nursing diagnosis. Perhaps the nurse and client could examine the prescribed diet. Is it realistic? What is the probability that compliant behavior will improve quality of life?

Key Concepts

1. Compliance is a "positive behavior that clients exhibit when moving toward mutually defined therapeutic goals" (Conway-Rutkowski, 1982).
2. Compliance should be viewed on a continuum rather than as separate states, *e.g.*, compliance or noncompliance (Blevins & Lubkin, 1995).
3. Partnerships between the health care provider and the client involve choices and compromises. Some individuals desire a passive role, whereas others want complete autonomy.
4. Compliance involves a behavioral change, which is positively influenced by (Blevins & Lubkin, 1995; Dracup & Meleis, 1982; Hussey & Gilliland, 1989; Strauss et al., 1984):
   a. Initial and continuing trust in the health care professional
   b. Reinforcement by significant others
   c. Perception of own susceptibility to the disease

    d. Perception that the disease is serious

    e. Evidence that compliance works to control symptoms or the disease

    f. Side effects are tolerable

    g. Less interference with daily activities of individual or significant others

    h. More benefit provided by therapy than harm

    i. Positive sense of self

5. Compliance is negatively influenced by (Blevins & Lubkin, 1995; Hussey & Gilliland, 1989):

    a. Inadequate explanation

    b. Disagreement between client and provider

    c. Long duration of therapy

    d. High complexity or expense of regimen

    e. Large number and severity of side effects

6. Motivation, "the pre- and post-decisional processes which guide the initiation and maintenance of health behaviors," is an important factor for nurses to act on (Fleury, 1992). Aspects of motivation to consider include:

    a. What does the prescribed health behavior change mean to the client?

    b. What environmental factors may interfere with the new behavior?

    c. What future events may challenge the client's motivation?

    d. How will personal values affect the client's ability to remain motivated?

7. Self-efficacy, the client's beliefs about his or her ability to adopt, perform, and maintain a healthy behavior change, has also been shown to contribute to long-term compliance (Kavanagh & Gooley, 1993; Redland & Stuifbergen, 1993). A client's self-efficacy can be evaluated with questions, such as:

    a. How many days per week do you think you can take a walk?

    b. At what interval do you feel comfortable enough to breast feed your baby?

    c. How often do you think you can check your sugar?

8. Noncompliance that follows a period of compliant behavior is termed "relapse." "Relapse is believed to occur when nonsupportive environmental influences become so difficult for the person to contend with that the effort to perform the newly adopted behavior can no longer be sustained" (Redland & Stuifbergen, 1993). Causes of relapse can be any of the related factors already listed.

9. When evaluating noncompliance related to medication, the nurse must consider the following factors that may affect drug absorption, metabolism, effectiveness, side effects, and excretion: body weight, age, time of administration, route of administration, genetic factors, basal metabolic rate, interactions with other drugs and foods, presence of organ disease (*e.g.*, liver and kidneys), altered body chemistry (*e.g.*, hypokalemia), and infection. For example, serum theophylline levels are diminished in a person who smokes cigarettes.

🌐 *Key Concepts—Child*

1. The transfer of responsibility for self-care for a child with chronic illness is difficult when noncompliance results in increased risks to the child, anxiety to the parents, and costs to family (Wysocki & Wayne, 1992).

2. The child should progress gradually to self-care to increase self-confidence and reduce over-dependence (Wysocki & Wayne, 1992).

3. Compliance is lower during adolescence, when following a regimen competes with feelings of self-consciousness and concerns over peer reactions (Whatley, 1991).

4. Following a particular treatment regimen can be difficult and trying for an ill child and family. For example, certain drugs may affect behavior, alertness, or school performance (Scipien, Chard, Howe, & Barnard, 1990).

🏛 *Key Concepts—Older Adult*

1. Cargill (1992) identified factors influencing noncompliance in older adults as functional deficits, complicated regimens, cost, inconvenience, and side effects that decrease the person's functional status (*e.g.*, strength, alertness).

Focus Assessment Criteria

Subjective Data

A. Assess for defining characteristics
1. Unacceptable side effects of therapy

Unpleasant taste	Pain
Difficult swallowing	Too expensive
Time consuming or inconvenient	

2. Does family member report any of the above problems?
3. What does the client want from the nurse or physician?

B. Assess for related factors
1. What is the person's general health motivation?

Does client seek help when needed?	Does client intend to make the
Does client accept the diagnosis as valid?	advised life-style alterations?

2. What is the person's perception of his present state of health?
   Does client consider himself to be generally well?
   Is there fear of a specific illness?
   Does client believe his illness is severe?
3. How does the person view the advised treatment regimen?
4. Inability to repeat or demonstrate the prescribed behavior?

Exercise program	Drug names and schedule
Next appointment date	Treatment procedure

5. Situations that interfere with prescribed behavior?

Family demands	Travel (hotels, restaurants)
Stress	Lack of transportation
Occupations	

Objective Data

A. Assess for defining characteristics
1. Missed appointments
2. Evidence of noncompliance

Persistence of symptoms	With medications (pill count, serum drug levels)
Progression of disease	

B. Assess for related factors
1. Obstacles to self-care

Inability to read	Musculoskeletal deficits
Immaturity	Cognitive deficits
Memory lags	Pain

2. Evidence of obstacles in caregiving environment

Long waiting period	Hurried atmosphere

Outcome Criteria

The person will
- Describe reasons for suggested regimen
- Identify barriers to adhering to regimen
- Identify the behaviors desired to change or initiate change

Interventions

A. Determine person's understanding of
  1. Present or risk for health problem (prognosis, disability)
     a. His vulnerability to the problem
     b. The prevention or treatment measures available
     c. The effectiveness of preventive measures
     d. The effectiveness of treatment measures

B. Explore the person's feelings regarding
  1. Past attempts at compliance
  2. Present concerns regarding prevention or treatment modalities
  3. Which recommendations are feasible
  4. Level of guidance desired from professional
  5. Support from significant others

C. Encourage positive thinking about new health-related behaviors (Redland & Stuifbergen, 1993)
  1. Collaborate with clients to *set goals*.
     a. Short-term goals are most useful.
     b. Be flexible.
     c. Be realistic, considering the uniqueness of each individual.
     d. Avoid imposing your goals for him or her.
  2. Consider using a *contract*, a written statement of what behaviors are expected.
     a. Initially, use short-term contracts with family member, coworker, friend, or nurse.
     b. For the longer term, self-contracts work well; the client finds his own rewards and reinforces his own positive behavior changes.
  3. *Self-monitoring* is useful to determine positive and negative influences on compliance.
     a. Daily records
     b. Charts
     c. Diary of progress or symptoms, clinical values (*e.g.*, blood sugars, BPs), or dietary intake

D. Review present medication therapy (prescribed and over-the-counter)
  1. Discuss present therapy (names, dosages, time taken, side effects).
  2. Determine person's understanding of the need for medication.
     a. Emphasize life-long therapy when indicated (*e.g.*, hypertension, diabetes mellitus, lipid-lowering agents).
     b. Explain the complications of unmanaged diseases.
  3. Identify possible adverse interactions among drugs (consult pharmacist).
  4. Commit to work with person to reduce or eliminate side effects (*e.g.*, changing agents or dose).
  5. Ask person to call primary provider with problems rather than stopping the medication.
  6. Emphasize that unavoidable side effects are still better than the consequences of no therapy (*e.g.*, stroke, blindness, renal failure).

E. Assist to reduce side effects
  1. For gastric irritation, suggest that drug be taken with milk or food; may be advisable to eat yogurt (unless contraindicated).
  2. For drowsiness, take medication at bedtime or late in afternoon; consult primary provider for dose reduction.
  3. For leg cramps (hypokalemia), increase intake of foods high in potassium (oranges, raisins, tomatoes, bananas).
  4. For other side effects, consult pertinent references.
  5. Use long-acting intramuscular preparations whenever possible; this includes some antibiotics and antipsychotic medications.

6. Suggest the use combination pills if available (e.g., Maxzide [hydrochlorothiazide and triamterene] and Triavil [perphenazine and amitriptyline]).
7. When appropriate, be sure client is taking the fewest number of pills possible (check dosages to provide the largest dose available in the fewest number of pills).*
8. To decrease frequency of oral medications, suggest longer-acting drug preparations, including the transdermal patch (*e.g.*, nitroglycerin).
9. Encourage prescription of generic drugs for people with financial concerns. Determine if client needs assistance with health insurance reimbursement for drugs.
10. When treatments require more than one set of hands, evaluate home help situation.
11. When expensive equipment is involved for treatments at home, make appropriate referrals to social workers and local agencies.

F. If indicated, focus on emotional responses that interfere with compliance (*e.g.*, situational anxiety, depression, denial, relationship problems)

G. Initiate health teaching and referrals, as indicated
1. Teach importance of adhering to prescribed regimen.
2. Provide written drug information that is tailored to client's needs. Include drug names, dosages, number of tablets to be taken and when, purpose of drugs, potential side effects and adverse reactions, and directions for relief of side effects.
3. Offer praise for honesty about compliance and for sharing reasons. For example:
    "I'm glad you told me that you stopped Motrin because it made your stomach hurt. Now I understand why your hands still ache. Let's talk about ways we can get you some comfort." Or, "It's a good thing that you told me about your stopping the blood pressure pills. That explains your headaches and higher pressure today. Let's discuss how those pills made you feel."
4. At discharge from hospital or outpatient setting, provide written name and phone number of professional to call with questions or concerns about prescribed drug regimen.

Rationale

- Lack of understanding of the health problem, complications, and the client's own vulnerability contribute to noncompliance (Blevins & Lubkin, 1995).
- Involving the client in decision making places some sense of responsibility on the client for making sure the plan works, promoting compliance with treatment.
- Increasing the person's beliefs that the health behavior change is possible contributes to long-term compliance (Redland & Stuifbergen, 1993).
- Lack of understanding regarding reasons for drug therapy and options available contributes to noncompliance (Blevins & Lubkin, 1995).
- Open discussions about side effects can encourage the person to report problems before discontinuing treatment (Blevins & Lubkin, 1995).
- Coping problems take priority and prevent the person from incorporating health behavior changes (Blevins & Lubkin, 1995).
- Establishing a consensual regimen and goals validates that the client is the decision maker and the health care professional is the advisor (Blevins & Lubkin, 1995).
- Contracting engages a commitment to make changes and to be accountable for choices (Blevins & Lubkin, 1995).

🍃 Interventions—*Child Focus*

1. Discuss how child can participate in self-care according to developmental level (Wysocki & Wayne, 1992).
    a. Put stars on chart when exercises are complete.
    b. Draw up insulin.
    c. Select food choices.

---

* May require a primary care professional's order.

2. Establish accountability for child or family members.
3. Discuss conflicts (see *Altered Parenting*).
4. Elicit problems in compliance and possible solution or compromises (Wong, 1995).
5. Use age-related behavioral strategies (Wong, 1995).
   a. Earning tokens or stickers
   b. Contracting with positive reinforcers
   c. Disciplinary techniques (*e.g.*, time-out for younger children or withholding privileges for older children)
6. Establish method to monitor compliance (*e.g.*, frequent appointments, phone calls, postcards).

Rationale

- Compliance is increased when issues of expectations, responsibilities, and consequences are discussed (Wong, 1995).
- Attempts to engage the child in some aspect of self-care can increase independence, initiative, and self-confidence (Wysocki & Wayne, 1992).
- Contracting is an effective method with older children when they are involved in defining the rules of the agreement (Wong, 1995).

References/Bibliography

Blevins, D., & Lubkin, J. (1995). Compliance. In J. Lubkin (Ed.). *Chronic illness: Impact and interventions* (3rd ed.). Boston: Jones & Bartlett.

Campbell, M. K., DeVillis, B., Stretcher, V., Ammerman, A., Devillis, R., & Sandler, R. (1994). Improving dietary behavior: The effectiveness of tailored messages in primary care settings. *American Journal of Public Health, 84*, 783–787.

Cargill, J. M. (1992). Medication compliance in elderly people: Influencing variables and interventions. *Journal of Advanced Nursing, 17*(4), 422–426.

Cassells, J. M., & Redman, B. K. (1989). Preparing students to be moral agents in clinical nursing practice. *Nursing Clinics of North America, 24*, 463–473.

Charonko, C. (1992). Cultural influences in "noncompliant" behavior and decision making. *Holistic Nursing Practice, 6*(3), 73–78.

Conway-Rutkowski, B. (1982). The nurse, also an educator, patient advocate, and counselor. *Nursing Clinics of North America, 17,* 134–139.

DiMatteo, M. R., Sherbourne, C. D., Hays, R. D., Ordway, L., Kravitz, R. L., McGlynn, E. A., Kaplam, J., & Rogers, W. H. (1993). Physicians' characteristics influence patients' adherence to medical treatment: Results from the Medical Outcomes Study. *Health Psychology, 12*(2), 93–102.

Dracup, K. A., & Meleis, A. I. (1982). Compliance: An interactionist approach. *Nursing Research, 31*, 32–35.

Dunbar-Jacob, J. (1993). Contributions to patient adherence: Is is time to share the blame? *Health Psychology, 12*(2), 91–92.

Elpern, E. H., & Girzardas, A. M. (1993). Tuberculosis update: New challenges of an old disease. *Medical-Surgical Nursing, 2*, 176–183.

Fleury, J. (1992). The application of motivational theory to cardiovascular risk reduction. *Image, 24*, 229–239.

Hussey, L., & Gilliland, K. (1989). Compliance, low literacy and locus of control. *Nursing Clinics of North America, 24*, 605–611.

Kavanagh, D. J., & Gooley, S. (1993). Prediction of adherence and control in diabetes. *Journal of Behavioral Medicine, 16*, 509–522.

Redland, A. R., & Stuifbergen, A. K. (1993). Strategies for maintenance of health-promoting behaviors. *Nursing Clinics of North America, 28*, 427–442.

Scipien, G. M., Chard, M. A., Howe, J., & Barnard, M. U. (1990). *Pediatric nursing care.* St. Louis: C. V. Mosby.

Strauss, A. L., Corbin, J., Fagerhaugh, S., Glaser, B., Maines, D., Suczek, B., & Wiener, C. (1984). *Chronic illness and the quality of life* (2nd ed.). St. Louis: C. V. Mosby.

Whatley, J. H. (1991). Effects of health locus of control and social network on adolescent risk taking. *Pediatric Nursing, 17*(2), 239–240.

Wong, D. (1995). *Nursing care of infants and children* (5th ed.). St. Louis: Mosby-Yearbook.

Wysocki, T., & Wayne, W. (1992). Childhood diabetes and the family. *Practical Diabetology, 11*(2), 29–32

Nutrition, Altered: Less Than Body Requirements

Impaired Swallowing

Infant Feeding Pattern, Ineffective

Nutrition, Altered: Less Than Body Requirements

DEFINITIONS

Altered Nutrition: Less Than Body Requirements: The state in which an individual who is not NPO experiences or is at risk of experiencing reduced weight related to inadequate intake or metabolism of nutrients for metabolic needs.

DEFINING CHARACTERISTICS
Major (Must Be Present)

One who is not NPO reports or has: inadequate food intake less than recommended daily allowance (RDA) with or without weight loss and/or
Actual or potential metabolic needs in excess of intake with weight loss

Minor (May Be Present)

Weight 10% to 20%+ below ideal for height and frame
Triceps skin fold, mid-arm circumference, and mid-arm muscle circumference less than 60% standard measurement
Muscle weakness and tenderness
Mental irritability or confusion
Decreased serum albumin
Decreased serum transferrin or iron-binding capacity

RELATED FACTORS
Pathophysiologic

Related to increased caloric requirements and difficulty in ingesting sufficient calories secondary to:

Burns (postacute phase)	Cancer
Infection	Trauma
Chemical dependence	

Related to dysphagia secondary to:

Cerebrovascular accident (CVA)	Muscular dystrophy
Amyotrophic lateral sclerosis	Parkinson's disease
Cerebral palsy	Neuromuscular disorders

Related to decreased absorption of nutrients secondary to:

Crohn's disease	Lactose intolerance
Cystic fibrosis	

Related to decreased desire to eat secondary to altered level of consciousness
Related to self-induced vomiting, physical exercise in excess of caloric intake, or refusal to eat secondary to anorexia nervosa

Related to reluctance to eat for fear of poisoning secondary to paranoid behavior

Related to anorexia, excessive physical agitation secondary to bipolar disorder

Related to anorexia and diarrhea secondary to protozoal infection

Related to vomiting, anorexia, and impaired digestion secondary to pancreatitis

Related to anorexia, impaired protein and fat metabolism, and impaired storage of vitamins secondary to cirrhosis

Treatment-Related

Related to protein and vitamin requirements for wound healing and decreased intake secondary to:

Surgery	Wired jaw
Medications (chemotherapy)	Radiation therapy
Surgical reconstruction of mouth	

Related to inadequate absorption as a medication side effect of (specify)

Colchicine	Neomycin
Pyrimethamine	*para* Aminosalicylic acid
Antacid	

Related to decreased oral intake, mouth discomfort, nausea, and vomiting secondary to:

Radiation therapy	Tonsillectomy
Chemotherapy	

Situational (Personal, Environmental)

Related to decreased desire to eat secondary to:

Anorexia	Social isolation
Depression	Nausea and vomiting
Stress	Allergies

Related to inability to procure food (physical limitations, financial or transportation problems)

Related to inability to chew (damaged or missing teeth, ill-fitting dentures)

Related to diarrhea secondary to (specify)

Maturational

Infant/child

Related to inadequate intake secondary to:

Lack of emotional/sensory stimulation

Lack of knowledge of caregiver

Related to malabsorption, dietary restrictions, and anorexia secondary to:

Celiac disease

Lactose intolerance

Cystic fibrosis

Related to sucking difficulties (infant) and dysphagia secondary to:

Cerebral palsy

Cleft lip and palate

Related to inadequate sucking, fatigue, and dyspnea secondary to:

Congenital heart disease	Viral syndrome
Prematurity	

Author's Note

Nurses usually are the primary diagnosticians and prescribers for improving clients' nutritional status. Although *Altered Nutrition* is not a difficult diagnosis to validate, it can challenge the nurse in the area of interventions.

Food habits and nutritional status are influenced by many factors: personal, family, cultural, financial, functional ability, nutritional knowledge, disease and injury, and treatment regimens. *Altered Nutrition: Less Than Body Requirements* describes people who can ingest food, but eat an inadequate or imbalanced quality or quantity. For instance, the diet may have insufficient protein or excessive fat content. Quantity of intake may be insufficient because of increased metabolic requirements (*e.g.*, resulting from cancer or pregnancy) or interference with nutrient utilization (*e.g.*, impaired storage of vitamins in cirrhosis).

The nursing focus for *Altered Nutrition* is on assisting the person or family in improving nutritional intake. This diagnosis should not be used to describe individuals who are NPO or cannot ingest food. Those situations should be described by the collaborative problem of:

> *Potential Complication: Electrolyte imbalances*
> Negative nitrogen balance

Errors in Diagnostic Statements

Altered Nutrition: Less Than Body Requirements related to insulin deficiency, altered consciousness, and hypermetabolic state

This diagnosis represents a diabetic client experiencing diabetic ketoacidosis. In such a situation, nursing responsibility focuses on two major problems, managing the ketoacidosis with the physician and teaching the person and family how to prevent future episodes. Neither of these problems involves altered nutrition. The first is described by the collaborative problem *Potential Complication: Ketoacidosis*, for which the nurse would be responsible for monitoring for physiologic instability, initiating timely interventions, and evaluating the client's response. The second problem, described by the nursing diagnosis *Possible Ineffective Management of Therapeutic Regimen related to adherence to diabetic diet and insufficient knowledge of adaptation needed when sick*, would be investigated after the client was stable.

Altered Nutrition: Less Than Body Requirements related to parenteral therapy and NPO status

This diagnosis represents a situation with which nurses are intricately involved (parenteral therapy). However, from a nutritional perspective, what interventions do nurses prescribe to improve the nutritional status of an NPO client? Parenteral nutrition in a client who is NPO influences several actual or potential responses that nurses treat, representing both nursing diagnoses, such as *Risk for Infection* and *Altered Comfort*, and the collaborative problems *Potential Complication: Hypo/hyperglycemia* and *Potential Complication: Negative Nitrogen Balance*.

Impaired Swallowing related to tracheotomy tube

A tracheotomy represents a risk factor for the diagnosis *Risk for Aspiration*; a more specific diagnosis for the focus of nursing care would be *Risk for Aspiration related to increased secretions and loss of epiglottis protection secondary to tracheotomy*.

Key Concepts

1. For proper metabolic functioning, the body requires adequate carbohydrates, protein, fat, vitamins, minerals, electrolytes, and trace elements. Figure II-4 depicts the Food Pyramid developed by the United States Department of Agriculture. It recommends daily servings of five food groups. The sixth group—fats, oils, and sweets—is recommended to be eaten sparingly. This group should not exceed 30% of total calorie intake.
2. Overall, 25% of adult Americans are overweight (15% over ideal weight for height). Fifteen percent of adolescents are overweight. The range for children is 5%–25% (National Research Council, 1989).
3. Obesity is a risk factor for hypertension, non–insulin-dependent diabetes mellitus, coronary artery disease, and cancer of the breast, endometrium, cervix, ovary, colon, rectum, prostate, gallbladder, and biliary tract (Folson, 1993).
4. Studies report that American women consume less than the recommended daily allowance (RDA) of iron, calcium, and vitamins A and C (Lo, 1995).
5. Americans eat half of the RDA of fiber and 20% more fat than the RDA (Human Nutrition Information Service, 1992).

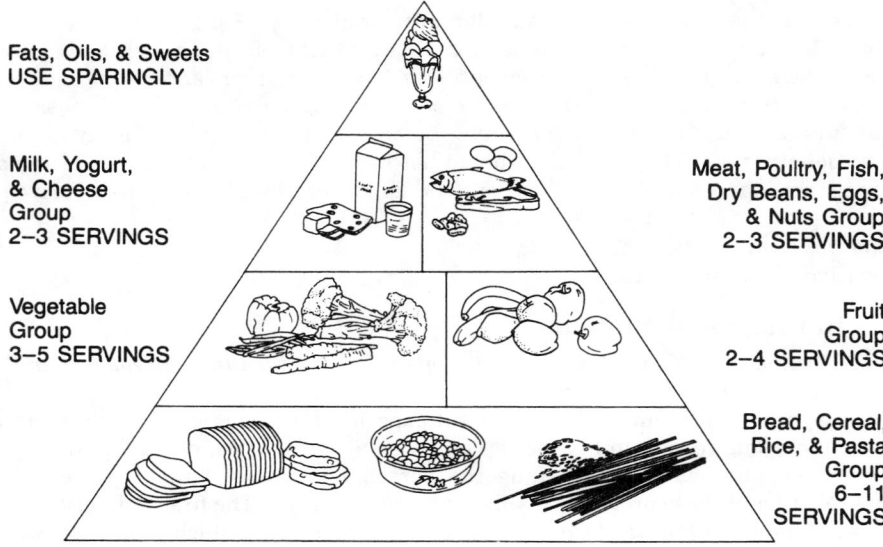

Fig. II-4 The food pyramid. (U.S. Department of Agriculture.)

6. The National Research Council (1989) compiled the dietary recommendations outlined in Table II-18.
7. Factors influencing nutrient requirements include age, activity, gender, health status (presence of disease, injuries), and nutrient metabolism (storage, absorption, use, excretion).
8. Factors influencing nutrient intake include personal (appetite, chewing and swallowing ability, functional ability, psychological status, culture) and structural (socialization, finances, ability to obtain and prepare food, kitchen facilities, transportation) (Miller, 1995).
9. The body requires a minimum level of nutrients for health and growth. During the life span, the nutritional needs of individuals vary, as indicated in Table II-19.
10. Tables II-20 and II-21 can be used to compare the individual's weight for height and anthropometric measurements.
11. The person with cancer experiences disease- and treatment-related nutritional problems, as indicated in the following list.

Disease-Related	Treatment-Related
Malabsorption	Stomatitis
Diarrhea	Diarrhea
Constipation	Nausea and vomiting
Anemia	Anorexia
Protein deficits	Fatigue
Fatigue	

🌎 *Key Concepts—Child*

1. Each growth period is characterized by changes in nutritional needs (see Table II-18).
2. Nonadolescent children should not be put on diets. The goal for growing children is to maintain weight, not lose weight. Healthy food choices of fruit, vegetables, low-fat snacks (*e.g.*, pretzels) can replace foods high in salt, fats, and sugar (Wilson, 1994).
3. Children at special risk for inadequate nutritional intake include those with
   a. Congenital anomalies (*e.g.*, tracheoesophageal fistula, cardiac or neurologic anomalies)
   b. Prematurity, intrauterine growth retardation
   c. Inborn errors of metabolism (*e.g.*, phenylketonuria)
   d. Malabsorption disorders
   e. Developmental disorders (*e.g.*, cerebral palsy)

Table II-18   **Dietary Recommendations of the National Research Council Report**

Reduce total fat intake to 30% or less of kcalories; saturated fatty acid intake to less than 10% of kcalories, and cholesterol to less than 300 mg daily*

Drink 8–10 glasses of water of noncaffeinated beverages.

Increase intake of starches and other complex carbohydrates.

Maintain protein intake at moderate levels.[†] Increase dry beans, fish.

Increase fiber intake 25–35 g daily.

Eat 2–4 servings of fruit daily.

Eat 3–5 servings of vegetables daily.

Limit total daily intake of salt (sodium chloride) to 6 g or less.[‡]

Maintain adequate calcium and iron intake.

Avoid taking dietary supplements in excess of the RDA in any one day.

Balance food intake and physical activity to maintain appropriate body weight.

For those who drink alcoholic beverages, limit consumption to the equivalent of less than 1 oz of pure alcohol in a single day.[§]

*The intake of fat and cholesterol can be reduced by substituting fish, poultry without skin, lean meats, and low-fat or nonfat dairy products for fatty meats and whole-milk dairy products; by choosing more vegetables, fruits, cereals, and legumes; and by limiting oils, fats, egg yolks, and fried and other fatty foods.
[†]Meet at least the RDA for protein, do not exceed twice the RDA.
[‡]Limit the use of salt in cooking, and avoid adding it to food at the table. Salty, highly processed salty, salt-preserved, and salt-pickled foods should be consumed sparingly.
[§]The Committee does not recommend alcohol consumption. One ounce of pure alcohol is the equivalent of two cans of beer, two small glasses of wine, or two average cocktails.
(National Research Council, Committee on Diet and Health of Food and Nutrition Board. [1989]. Diet and health: Implications for reducing chronic disease risk. *Nutrition Reviews, 47*, 142–149; *Healthy People 2000.* [1989]; Human Nutrition Information Service [1992]. *Food guide pyramid: A guide to daily food choices.* Leaflet No. 572. Washington, DC: U.S. Department of Agriculture.)

     f. Chronic illness (*e.g.*, cystic fibrosis, chronic infections, diabetes)

     g. Accelerated growth rates (*e.g.*, prematurity, infancy, adolescence)

     h. Parents who have inadequate attachment

4. Parents must follow sound feeding practices to prevent nutritional deficits in infancy (Anderson, 1989; Wong, 1995). Such practices include

     a. Feeding the infant breast milk or iron-fortified formula for the first year of life

     b. Adding solid foods by age 5–6 months

     c. Assessing the infant's cues for burping or satiation

     d. Holding the infant during the feeding versus propping the bottle

     e. Selecting foods appropriate to the infant's physiologic and motor development

     f. Preparing formula correctly

Key Concepts—Maternal

1. Nutritional needs change during pregnancy (refer to Table II-18).

2. Recommendations for total weight gain during pregnancy vary; the most common recommendation is 25–30 lb.

3. Naeye (1985) reported that the weight gain during pregnancy should be related to prepregnancy weight (*i.e.*, a mother of average weight can gain 20 lb, whereas a thin mother should gain 30 lb).

4. Dieting during pregnancy may result in insufficient maternal intake to provide the fetus with the necessary energy for growth. The fetus depends on the mother's dietary intake for growth and development, taking only iron and folate from maternal stores (May & Mahlmeister, 1994).

Key Concepts—Older Adult

1. In general, the elderly need the same kind of balanced diet as any other group, but with fewer calories. However, diets of elderly clients tend to be insufficient in iron, calcium, and vitamins (Drugay, 1986). The combination of long-established eating patterns, income, transportation, housing, social interaction, and the effects of chronic or acute disease influence the person's nutritional intake and health.

Table II-19 **Age-Related Daily Nutritional Requirements**

Age	Daily Nutritional Requirements
Infants	
Newborn	12–18 oz milk
2–3 months	20–30 oz milk
4–5 months	25–35 oz milk; strained vegetables and fruits; egg yolks
6–7 months	28–40 oz milk; above solids, plus meat
8–11 months	24 oz milk; 3 regular meals
1–2 years	24 oz milk; 100 calories/kg
Children	
Preschool (3–5 years)	90 calories/kg; 40 g protein Basic food groups Refer to Figure II-4

School (6–12 years)	80 calories/kg; 1.2 g/kg protein
	Basic food groups (as preschool)
	    1.5–2 g calcium
	    400 units vitamin D
	    1.5–3 liters water

Adolescent (13–17 years)	2200–2400 calories for girls
	3000 calories for boys
	Basic food groups (as preschool)
	    50–60 g protein
	    3 g calcium
	    400 units vitamin D

Adults	1600–3000 calorie range (based on physical activity, emotional state, body size, age, and individual metabolism) Basic food groups Refer to Figure II-4 Men need increased protein, ascorbic acid, riboflavin, and vitamins E and B_6 Women need the above and also increased iron and vitamins A and B_{12}

Pregnant women
  (2d and 3d trimesters)
	Daily calorie requirement
	    11–15 years, 2500
	    16–22 years, 2400
	    23–50 years, 2300
	Increase protein 10 g or 1 serving meat
	1.2–3.5 g calcium
	Increase vitamins A, B, and C
	30–60 mg iron

Lactating women	2500–3000 calories (500 over regular diet)
	Basic food groups
	  4 servings protein
	  5 servings dairy
	  4+ servings grain
	  5+ servings vegetables
	    2+ servings vitamin C-rich
	    1+ green leafy
	    2+ others
	Fluids 2–3 quarts (1 qt milk)
	Increase in vitamin A, C, niacin

Over 65 years	Basic food groups (same as adult) Caloric requirements decrease with age (1600–1800 for women, 2000–2400 for men), but dependent on activity, climate, and metabolic needs Ensure intake of essential amino acids, fatty acids, vitamins, elements, fiber, and water 60 mg ascorbic acid 40–60 mg protein 1000 mg calcium (1600 mg for women) 10 mg iron

Table II-20 **Weight for Height and Body Frame***

Height (Feet)	(Inches)	Small Frame	Medium Frame	Large Frame	Height (Feet)	(Inches)	Small Frame	Medium Frame	Large Frame
		Men					Women		
5	2	128–134	131–141	138–150	4	10	102–111	109–121	118–131
5	3	130–136	133–143	140–153	4	11	103–113	111–123	120–134
5	4	132–138	135–145	142–156	5	0	104–115	113–126	122–137
5	5	134–140	137–148	144–160	5	1	106–118	115–129	125–140
5	6	136–142	139–151	146–164	5	2	108–121	118–132	128–143
5	7	138–145	142–154	149–168	5	3	111–124	121–135	131–147
5	8	140–148	145–147	152–172	5	4	114–127	124–138	134–151
5	9	142–151	148–160	155–176	5	5	117–130	127–141	137–155
5	10	144–154	151–163	158–180	5	6	120–133	130–144	140–159
5	11	146–157	154–166	161–184	5	7	123–136	133–147	143–163
6	0	149–160	157–170	164–188	5	8	126–139	136–150	146–167
6	1	152–164	160–174	168–192	5	9	129–142	139–153	149–170
6	2	155–168	164–178	172–197	5	10	132–145	142–156	152–173
6	3	158–172	167–182	176–202	5	11	135–148	145–159	155–176
6	4	162–176	171–187	181–207	6	0	138–151	148–162	158–179

To Make an Approximation of Your Frame Size . . .

Extend your arm and bend the forearm upward at a 90° angle. Keep fingers straight and turn the inside of your wrist toward your body. If you have a caliper, use it to measure the space between the two prominent bones on *either* side of your elbow. Without a caliper, place thumb and index finger of your other hand on these two bones. Measure the space between your fingers against a ruler or tape measure. Compare it with these tables that list elbow measurements for *medium-framed* men and women. Measurements lower than those listed indicate you have a small frame. High measurements indicate a large frame.

Height in 10" Heels	Elbow Breadth	Height in 10" Heels	Elbow Breadth
	Men		Women
5'2"–5'3"	2½"–2⅞"	4'10"–4'11"	2¼"–2½"
5'4"–5'7"	2⅝"–2⅞"	5'0"–5'3"	2¼"–2½"
5'8"–5'11"	2¾"–3"	5'4"–5'7"	2⅜"–2⅝"
6'0"–6'3"	2¾"–3⅛"	5'8"–5'11"	2⅜"–2⅝"
6'4"	2⅞"–3¼"	6'0"	2½"–2¾"

*Weights at ages 25–59 years based on lowest mortality. Weight in pounds according to frame (in indoor clothing weighing 5 lb for men and 3 lb for women; shoes with 1" heels).

(Revised Height–Weight Tables derived from life insurance statistics prepared by the Metropolitan Life Insurance Company for men and women. Copyright 1983, Metropolitan Life Insurance Company.)

Table II-21 **Anthropometric Measurements (adult)***

Test	Sex	Reference	>90% Reference	90%–60% Reference	<60% Reference
Mid-Arm Circumference (MAC) (in cm)	Male	29.3	>26.3	26.3–17.6	<17.6
	Female	28.5	>25.7	25.7–17.1	<17.1
Mid-Arm Muscle Circumference (MAMC) (in cm)	Male	25.3	>22.8	22.8–15.2	<15.2
	Female	23.2	>20.9	20.9–13.9	<13.9
Triceps Skin Fold (TSF) (in mm)	Male	12.5	>11.3	11.3–7.5	< 7.5
	Female	16.5	>14.9	14.9–9.9	< 9.9

*If measurements are below 90% reference, nutritional support program may be indicated. (Jelliffe, D. B. [1986]. *The assessment of the nutritional status of the community*. World Health Organization Monograph No. 53. Geneva: World Health Organization.

2. The decreased energy needs of many older adults require a change in nutrient intake, as shown in the following:

	Age 25–50 years	Age Over 50 years
Carbohydrates	60%	55%
Protein	10%	20%
Fat	30%	25%
Kcal/day		
Female	2200	1900
Male	2900	2300

3. People receiving diuretics must be closely observed for adequate hydration (intake and output) and electrolyte balance, especially sodium and potassium. Potassium-rich foods should be regularly included in the diet.
4. Anemia due to iron deficiency usually occurs over a period of time and may be affected by chronic diseases and insufficient dietary iron intake. Increasing the intake of foods rich in vitamin C, folic acid, and dietary iron can improve the conditions necessary for optimal absorption of iron. Iron supplementation is often necessary.

TRANSCULTURAL CONSIDERATIONS

1. "For centuries diet has been used by many cultures in the treatment of specific disease conditions, the promotion of health during pregnancy, the fostering of growth and development for infants and children, and even the instillation of the magical hope of prolonging earthly life" (Boyle & Andrews, 1995, p. 333).
2. In some cultures, health is viewed as a state of balance among the body humors (blood, phlegm, black bile, and yellow bile). Illness is caused by a humoral imbalance that causes excessive dryness, cold, hot, or wetness. For example, an upset stomach is believed to be caused by eating too many foods identified as cold. Foods, herbs, and medicines are classified as hot or cold or wet or dry. They are used to restore the body to its natural balance. For example, bananas are classified as a cold food, whereas corn meal is a hot food (Boyle & Andrews, 1995).
3. Adult lactose intolerance has been reported among most of the populations of the world, "affecting 94% of Orientals, 90% of African blacks, 79% of American Indians, 75% of American blacks, 50% of Mexican Americans, and 17% of American whites" (Overfield, 1985).
4. Nutritional practices can be categorized as beneficial, neutral, or harmful. Beneficial and neutral practices should be encouraged. Harmful practices should be approached with sensitivity and their detrimental effects explained (Boyle & Andrews, 1995).
5. Group dining, which is encouraged in some settings (*e.g.*, rehabilitation, long-term, mental health), may be in conflict with certain cultures (*e.g.*, women eating with men) (Boyle & Andrews, 1995).
6. Food is used by many Italians to improve physical and psychological well-being. Wine is frequently drunk with meals (Giger & Davidhizar, 1991).
7. Maintaining a kosher diet for a Jewish client is possible even if the agency does not have a kosher kitchen. Fish with fins or scales will meet dietary requirements. Dairy products are also possible. Paper plates with disposable utensils are used so that meat and milk dishes are not mixed (Giger & Davidhizar, 1991).

Focus Assessment Criteria

Subjective Data

A. Assess for defining characteristics
    1. Weight/height ratio
        Weight 3 months ago   Ideal weight
        Current weight   Height

2. Usual intake
   Diet recall for 24 hours
   Is this the usual intake pattern?
   Is there sufficient intake of basic five food groups?
   Is there sufficient fluid intake?

B. Assess for related factors
   1. Appetite (usual, changes)
   2. Dietary patterns
      Food/fluid dislikes, preferences, taboos
      Religious dietary practices
   3. Activity level
      Occupation, exercise (type, frequency)
   4. Food procurement/preparation (who)
      Functional ability   Kitchen facilities
      Transportation   Income adequate for food needs
   5. Knowledge of nutrition
      Basic four food groups
      Recommended intake of carbohydrates, fats, salt
      Relationship of activity and metabolism
   6. Physiologic risk factors
      Medical conditions
      Surgical history
   7. Medications (prescribed, over-the-counter)
      Reports of
         Allergies   Dysphagia
         Nausea   Indigestion
         Vomiting   Chewing problems
         Anorexia   Constipation
         Fatigue   Diarrhea
         Sore mouth   Pain

Objective Data

A. Assess for defining characteristics
   1. General
      Appearance (muscle mass, fat distribution)   Hair, skin, nails
      Height and weight   Mouth, teeth
   2. Anthropometric measurements
      Mid-arm circumference   Triceps skin fold
      Mid-arm muscle circumference
   3. Laboratory studies
      Decreased serum albumin
      Decreased serum transferrin

B. Assess for related factors
   1. Ability to chew, swallow, feed self

Outcome Criteria

The client will:
- Ingest daily nutritional requirements in accordance with his activity level and metabolic needs
- Relate the importance of good nutrition

Interventions

A. Explain the need for adequate consumption of carbohydrates, fats, protein, vitamins, minerals, and fluids

B. Consult with a nutritionist to establish appropriate daily caloric and food type requirements for the client

C. Discuss with the client possible causes of decreased appetite

D. Encourage the client to rest before meals

E. Offer frequent, small meals instead of a few large ones; offer foods served cold

F. Restrict liquids with meals and avoid fluids 1 hour before and after meals

G. Encourage and help the client to maintain good oral hygiene

H. Arrange to have high-calorie and high-protein foods served at the times that the client usually feels most like eating

I. Take steps to promote appetite
   1. Determine the client's food preferences and arrange to have these foods provided, as appropriate.
   2. Eliminate any offensive odors and sights from the eating area.
   3. Control any pain and nausea before meals.
   4. Encourage the client's support people to bring allowed foods from home, if possible.
   5. Provide a relaxed atmosphere and some socialization during meals.

J. Give the client printed materials outlining a nutritious diet that includes the following
   1. High intake of complex carbohydrates and fiber
   2. Decreased intake of sugar, salt, cholesterol, total fat, and saturated fats
   3. Alcohol use only in moderation
   4. Proper caloric intake to maintain ideal weight

Rationale

- Food nutrients provide energy sources, build tissue, and regulate metabolic processes (Williams, 1992).
- Consultation can help ensure a diet that provides optimal caloric and nutrient intake (Williams, 1992).
- Factors such as pain, fatigue, analgesic use, and immobility can contribute to anorexia. Identifying a possible cause enables interventions to eliminate or minimize it (Skipper, Szeluga, & Groenwald, 1993).
- Fatigue further reduces an anorectic client's desire and ability to eat (Skipper et al., 1993).
- Even distribution of total daily caloric intake throughout the day helps prevent gastric distention, possibly increasing appetite (Skipper et al., 1993).
- Restricting fluids with meals helps prevent gastric distention (Skipper et al., 1993).
- Poor oral hygiene leads to bad odor and taste, which can diminish appetite (Williams, 1992).
- Presenting high-calorie and high-protein food when client is most likely to eat increases the likelihood of the client's consuming adequate calories and protein (Skipper et al., 1993).
- Diet planning focuses on avoiding nutritional excesses. Reducing fats, salt, and sugar can reduce the risk of heart disease, diabetes, certain cancers, and hypertension (Williams, 1992).

⊕ Interventions—*Child Focus*

1. Teach parents the age-related nutritional needs of their children (consult an appropriate textbook on pediatrics or nutrition for specific recommendations).
2. Discuss the importance of limiting high-salt, -sugar, or -fat snacks (*e.g.*, soda, candy, chips) to limit risks for cardiac disorders, obesity, and diabetes mellitus.
3. Advise how to substitute healthy snacks (*e.g.*, fresh fruits, plain popcorn, frozen fruit juice bars, fresh vegetables).
4. Assist to evaluate family's nutritional patterns.
5. Discuss strategies to make mealtime a social event and how to avoid mealtime struggles (Mahan & Arlin, 1992; Wong, 1995).
   a. Allow child to select one type of food they don't have to eat.
   b. Provide small servings (*e.g.*, one tablespoon of each food for every year of age).
   c. Make snacks as nutritiously important as meals (*e.g.*, hard-boiled eggs, raw vegetable sticks, peanut butter/crackers, fruit juices, cheese, fresh fruit).
   d. Offer a variety of foods.
   e. Encourage all members to share their day.
6. Elicit child in monitoring healthy eating (*e.g.*, create a chart where a child marks off intake of healthy foods daily).
7. Replace passive TV watching with a group activity (*e.g.*, Frisbee, biking, walking).

Rationale

- Nutritional requirements vary greatly for each age group. Periods of accelerated physical growth (*e.g.*, infancy, puberty) may necessitate doubling of iron, calcium, zinc, and protein intake (Wong, 1995).
- During periods of slow growth (*e.g.*, pre-school, primary school-age children) appetite is diminished (Mahan & Arlin, 1992).
- Increasing healthy snacks reduces the pressure for the child to eat a certain amount at mealtime (Wong, 1995).
- Family nutritional patterns are the primary influence in the development of food habits (*e.g.*, unhealthy snacks, excessive TV watching) (Mahan & Arlin, 1992).

⊘ Interventions—*Maternal*

1. Explain the physiologic changes and nutritional needs during pregnancy (see Table II-18).
2. Discuss the effects of alcohol, caffeine, and artificial sweeteners on developing fetus.
3. Explain the different nutritional requirements for pregnant girls aged 11–18 years, pregnant young women 19–24 years of age, and woman older than 25 years.
4. Determine if more calories are needed because of daily activity.

Rationale

- Explanations about metabolic changes can increase awareness of nutritional requirements (May & Mahlmeister, 1994).
- Studies have shown that alcohol consumption (2–4 drinks/day) can cause low birth weight. Larger amounts cause fetal alcohol syndrome (May & Mahlmeister, 1994).
- Caffeine has been proven to have little effect on pregnancy outcome, but moderation is recommended (Mahan & Arlin, 1992).
- Consumption of artificial sweeteners during pregnancy has not been found to be contraindicated, but moderation is suggested (Mahan & Arlin, 1992).
- Adolescent girls are in need of increased nutritional intake because of their own accelerated growth, and pregnancy increases the requirements even more (Mahan & Arlin, 1992).
- The resting caloric needs for pregnant women differ according to age (May & Mahlmeister, 1994):
  - 28.5 kcal/kg for 11–14 years
  - 24.9 kcal/kg for 15–18 years
  - 23.3 kcal/kg for 19–24 years
  - 21.9 kcal/kg for 25–50 years

- More calories are needed depending on activity level (May & Mahlmeister, 1995): multiply resting caloric needs by
  - 1.5 for light activity
  - 1.6 for moderate activity
  - 1.9 for heavy activity

Interventions—*Older Adult Focus*

1. Determine person's understanding of nutritional needs with:
   a. Aging
   b. Medication use
   c. Illness
   d. Activity
2. Assess if there are factors that interfere with procuring or ingesting foods (Miller, 1995; Rajcevich & Wakefield, 1991).
   a. Anorexia due to medications, grief, depression, illness
   b. Impaired mental status leading to inattention to hunger or selecting insufficient kinds/amounts of food
   c. Impaired mobility or manual dexterity (paresis, tremors, weakness, joint pain, or deformity)
   d. Voluntary fluid restriction for fear of urinary incontinence
   e. Small frame or history of undernutrition
   f. Inadequate income to purchase food
   g. Lack of transportation to buy food or facility to cook
   h. New dentures or poor dentition
   i. Dislike of cooking and eating alone
3. Explain decline in sensitivity to sweet and salty tastes.
4. If indicated, consult with home health nurse to evaluate home environment (*e.g.*, cooking facilities, food supply, cleanliness).
5. Access community agencies as indicated (*e.g.*, nutritional programs, community centers, home-delivered grocery services).

Rationale

- Nutritional requirements do not diminish, but overall caloric needs do with age. High-quality nutritious foods are very important (Miller, 1995).
- Multiple factors can interfere with access or ingestion of food, and strategies for improving nutrition should address specific factors (Mahan & Arlin, 1992).
- Older adults can consume excessive amounts of salt and sugar to compensate for loss of sensitivity to these tastes (Miller, 1995).
- A home assessment may provide more valid data when a nutritional problem is suspected (Miller, 1995).
- Certain medications or illnesses may require an adjustment in diet (*e.g.*, potassium, sodium, fiber).

■ Altered Nutrition: Less Than Body Requirements
Related to Anorexia Secondary to (Specify)

Outcome Criteria

The person will
- Increase oral intake as evidenced by (specify)
- Describe causative factors when known
- Describe rationale and procedure for treatments

Interventions

A. Assess causative factors
1. Diminished sense of taste or smell
2. Social isolation
3. Radiation therapy or chemotherapy
4. Altered body image or self-concept
5. Early satiety
6. Noxious stimuli (pain or painful or unpleasant procedures, fatigue, odors, nausea and vomiting)

B. Reduce or eliminate contributing factors, if possible
1. Diminished sense of taste or smell
   a. Explain to person the importance of consuming adequate amounts of nutrients.
   b. Teach person to use spices to help improve the taste and aroma of food (lemon juice, mint, cloves, basil, thyme, cinnamon, rosemary, bacon bits).
   c. Teach protein sources he may find more acceptable than red meat.
      Eggs and dairy products
      Chicken and turkey
      Fish (if not strong-smelling)
      Marinated meat (in wine, vinegar)
      Soy products (tofu)
   d. Chopped or ground meats/protein sources may be more acceptable.
   e. Mixing protein and vegetables may be more acceptable.
   f. Refer to meals as "snacks" to make them sound smaller.
2. Social isolation
   a. Encourage to eat with others (meals served in dining room or group area, at local meeting place such as community center, by church groups).
   b. Provide daily contact through phone calls by support system.
   c. See *Social Isolation* for additional interventions.
3. Noxious stimuli (pain, fatigue, odors, nausea, and vomiting)
   a. Pain
      Plan care so that unpleasant or painful procedures do not take place before meals.
      Schedule pain relief medications so optimal relief without drowsiness is achieved at meal time.
      Provide pleasant, relaxed atmosphere for eating (no bedpans in sight; don't rush); try a "surprise" (*e.g.*, flowers with meal).
      Arrange plan of care to decrease or eliminate nauseating odors or procedures near mealtimes.

  b. Fatigue

    Teach or assist individual to rest before meals.

    Teach individual to spend minimal energy in food preparation (cook large quantities and freeze several meals at a time; request assistance from others).

  c. Odor of food

    Teach him to avoid cooking odors—frying foods, brewing coffee—if possible (take a walk; select foods that can be eaten cold).

    Suggest using foods that require little cooking during periods of anorexia.

  d. Nausea and vomiting (Rhodes, 1990)

    Encourage frequent, small amounts of ice chips or cool, clear liquids (dilute tea, Jell-O water, flat ginger ale or cola) unless vomiting continues (adults 30–60 mL every ½–1 hour; children 15–30 mL every ½–1 hour).

    Consider giving medications by suppository, rather than by mouth.

    Decrease the stimulation of the vomiting center.

    Reduce unpleasant sights and odors.

    Provide good mouth care after vomiting.

    Teach to practice deep breathing and voluntary swallowing to suppress the vomiting reflex.

    Instruct to sit down after eating but not to lie down.

    Encourage to eat smaller meals and eat slowly.

    Reduce amount of food on tray to a minimum.

    Restrict liquids with meals to avoid overdistending the stomach; also avoid fluids 1 hour before and after meals.

    If possible, avoid the smell of food preparation.

    Try eating cold foods, which have less odor.

    Loosen clothing.

    Sit in fresh air, use a fan.

    Avoid lying down flat for at least 2 hours after eating (an individual who must rest should sit or recline so head is at least 4 inches higher than feet).

  4. See *Impaired Swallowing* for additional interventions.

C. Promote foods that stimulate eating and increase protein consumption (Skipper et al., 1993)

  1. Maintain good oral hygiene (brush teeth, rinse mouth) before and after ingestion of food.

  2. Offer frequent small feedings (6/day plus snacks) to reduce the feeling of a distended stomach.

  3. Allow individual to choose food items as close to actual eating time as possible.

  4. Arrange to have highest protein/calorie nutrients served at the time individual feels most like eating (*e.g.*, if chemotherapy is in early morning, serve in late afternoon).

  5. Encourage significant others to bring in favorite home foods.

  6. Instruct to

    a. Eat dry foods (toast, crackers) on arising.

    b. Eat salty foods, if permissible.

    c. Avoid overly sweet, rich, greasy, or fried foods.

    d. Try clear, cool beverages.

    e. Sip slowly through straw.

    f. Take whatever he feels he can tolerate.

    g. Eat small portions low in fat and eat more frequently.

7. Try commercial supplements available in many forms (liquids, powder, pudding); keep switching brands until some are found that are acceptable to individual in taste and consistency.
8. Teach techniques to individual and family for home food preparation.
   a. Add powdered milk or egg to milkshakes, gravies, sauces, puddings, cereals, meatballs, or milk to increase protein calorie content.
   b. Add blenderized or baby foods to meat juices or soups.
   c. Use fortified milk (*i.e.*, 1 cup instant nonfat milk to 1 qt fresh milk).
   d. Use milk or half-and-half instead of water when making soups and sauces; soy formulas can also be used.
   e. Add cheese or diced meat whenever able.
   f. Add cream cheese or peanut butter to toast, crackers, celery sticks.
   g. Add extra butter or margarine to soups, sauces, vegetables.
   h. Spread toast while hot.
   i. Use mayonnaise (100 cal/T) instead of salad dressing.
   j. Add sour cream or yogurt to vegetables or as dip.
   k. Use whipped cream (60 cal/T).
   l. Add raisins, dates, nuts, and brown sugar to hot or cold cereals.
   m. Have extra food (snacks) easily available.
9. Review high-calorie versus low-calorie foods. Avoid empty-calorie foods (*e.g.*, soda).
10. If lactose intolerant, explore alternate dairy source to drinking milk (*i.e.*, cheese, yogurt, acidophilus milk).

D. Initiate health teaching and referrals, as indicated
   1. Dietitian for meal planning
   2. Psychiatric therapy when indicated
   3. Community meal centers
   4. Support groups for anorectics

Rationale

- For most people, meals are social events. Loneliness at mealtime can reduce the incentive to prepare nutritious meals.
- The client should be given as much control as possible over his or her diet—for example, have the client make a list of food and fluid preferences and dislikes and try to incorporate these into the prescribed diet (Varella & Utermohlen, 1993).
- Maintaining good oral hygiene before and after meals decreases microorganisms that can cause foul taste and odor, inhibiting appetite.
- Fluid restrictions at meals can help prevent gastric overdistention and can enhance appetite.
- Nausea can be reduced by controlling environmental conditions and promoting positions that minimize abdominal pressure.
- Certain measures can increase the nutritional content of foods even when intake is limited.

■ Altered Nutrition: Less Than Body Requirements
Related to Difficulty or Inability to Procure Food

Altered ability to procure food is the inability to acquire food because of physical, economic, or sociocultural barriers.

Outcome Criteria

The person will
- Describe causative factors when known
- Identify a method to acquire food on a regular schedule

Interventions

A. Assess causative factors
1. Inadequate economic resources to obtain adequate nutrition
2. Sociocultural barrier
3. Physical inability to procure food, related to health problem such as chronic obstructive pulmonary disease, CVA, or quadriplegia

B. Eliminate or reduce contributing factors, if possible
1. Inadequate economic resources
   a. Assess eligibility for food stamps or other government-funded programs for low-income groups; consult with social service.
   b. Suggest cooperatives or local farmers' markets for shopping.
   c. Buy foods and meats on sale and freeze; use cheaper cuts and tenderize.
   d. Suggest foods that are low in cost and nutritionally high; decrease use of prepackaged or prepared items.
      Beans and legumes as protein source
      Powdered milk (alone or mixed half-and-half with whole milk)
      Seasonal foods when plentiful
   e. Encourage growing a small garden or participating in a community plot.
   f. Freeze or can fruits and vegetables in season (refer to county agricultural agent for information on canning and freezing).
2. Sociocultural barrier
   a. Introduce individual to locally available foodstuffs and instruct in their preparation.
   b. Suggest substitutions of locally available foodstuffs for those to which individual is accustomed.
   c. Refer to adult education home economics classes for food preparation.
   d. Assist individual in recognizing and using additional outlets and sources of food (grocery stores, meat and fruit markets).
   e. Encourage peer group meetings among people of similar backgrounds to allow learning and exchange of ideas.
   f. Acquaint with ethnic food store locations, if available.
3. Physical deficits
   a. Promote alternate methods of food procurement and preparation.
      Assess support systems for someone willing to purchase or prepare food for individual or take him to store.
      Supermarkets that deliver

Meals on Wheels or similar service
Homemaker
Group housing
Door-to-store bus service
Teach the individual or others to cook enough for six meals at one time and freeze; make own complete "frozen dinners."
   b. Aid person in planning daily activities to account for energy need in shopping for food and preparing meals.
Rest periods before and after activity
Rest periods during activity, if needed

C. Teach techniques for meal planning and preparation for one

1. Buy small cans of food (it may be more expensive, but spoiled food is costly).
2. When buying fruit, select three stages of ripeness (ripe, medium ripe, green).
3. Ask the grocer to break open family-sized packages of meat or fresh vegetables.
4. When you must buy in large quantity, make soups and stews with the extra.
5. Use powdered milk instead of fresh milk in recipes.
6. Buy fresh milk in pints or quarts.
7. Store large-quantity items (rice, flour, corn meal, dry milk, cereal) in glass jars. Place tightly sealed jars in the freezer for one night to kill any organisms and their eggs.
8. Experiment with stir-frying vegetables (*e.g.*, Chinese cabbage, celery) in a little chicken broth.
9. If freezer space is available, prepare four to six times as much as you need and freeze in individual portions, dating the packages.
10. Store half a loaf of bread well wrapped in freezer. (It will become stale in the refrigerator.)
11. Buy large bags of frozen vegetables, use small amounts, and close with twist ties.
12. Finely chop and freeze fresh herbs (parsley, dill, basil) in small freezer bags. Flatten so that small portions can be broken off after freezing.
13. Buy large quantities of meat and freeze in foil wrap (not freezer paper).

D. Initiate health teaching and referrals, as indicated

1. Refer to social worker, occupational therapist, or visiting nurse, as needed.
2. Refer to local extension office for information on vegetable gardening, community gardens, and techniques of freezing and canning foods.
3. Refer to dietitian for meal planning.

Rationale

- People who are impaired either physically or cognitively should receive the necessary support and supervision in selecting foods and in self-feeding.
- Activities needed to procure food depend on skills of cognition, balance, mobility, manual dexterity, and all five senses (Miller, 1995).
- Nurses need to be familiar with local resources available so referrals can be initiated (Miller, 1995).
- Individuals who have difficulty preparing meals can be assisted to reduce daily preparation time with specific planning (Mahan & Arlin, 1996).

References/Bibliography

Anderson, J. J. (1989). Families with infants. In R. L. Foster, M. M. Hunsberger, & J. J. T. Anderson (Eds.). *Family-centered nursing care of children*. Philadelphia: W. B. Saunders.

Boyle, J., & Andrews, M. (1995). *Transcultural concepts in nursing care* (2nd ed.). Philadelphia: J. B. Lippincott.

Drugay, M. (1986). Nutritional evaluation: Who needs it. *Journal of Gerontological Nursing, 12*(4), 14–18.

Folsom, A. R., Kaye, S. A., & Sellers, T. A. (1993). Body fat distribution and 5-year risk of death in older women. *Journal of the American Medical Association, 269*, 483–487.

Giger, J. N., & Davidhizar, R. E. (1991). *Transcultural nursing: Assessment and intervention*. St. Louis: Mosby-Year Book.

Human Nutrition Information Service. (1992). *Food guide pyramid: A guide to daily food choices*. Leaflet No. 572. Washington, DC: U.S. Department of Agriculture.

Light, I., & Contento, I. R. (1989). Changing the course: A school nutrition and cancer education curriculum developed by the American Cancer Society and the National Cancer Institute. *Journal of School Health, 59*, 205–209.

Lo, C. (1995). Nutritional requirements of women. In P. L. Carr, K. M. Freud, & S. Somati (Eds.). *The medical care of women*. Philadelphia: J. B. Lippincott.

Mahan, L. K., & Arlin, M. T. (1996). *Food, nutrition and diet therapy* (9th ed.). Philadelphia: W. B. Saunders.

May, K., & Mahlmeister, L. (1994). *Maternal and neonatal nursing: Family-centered care* (3rd ed.). Philadelphia: J. B. Lippincott.

Miller, C. A. (1995). *Nursing care of older adults* (2nd ed.). Glenview, IL: Scott, Foresman.

Naeye, R. L. (1985). Weight gain and outcome of pregnancy. *American Journal of Obstetrics and Gynecology, 153*, 3–9.

National Research Council, Committee on Diet and Health of Food and Nutrition Board. (1989). Diet and health: Implications for reducing chronic disease risk. *Nutrition Reviews, 47*, 142–149.

Overfield, T. (1985). *Biologic variation in health and illness: Race, age, and sex differences*. Menlo Park, CA: Addison-Wesley.

Rajcevich, K., & Wakefield, B. (1991). Altered nutrition: Less than body requirements. In M. Maas, K. Buckwalter, & M. Hardy (Eds.). *Nursing diagnoses and interventions for the elderly*. Redwood City, CA: Addison-Wesley Nursing.

Rhodes, V. (1990). Nausea, vomiting and retching. *Nursing Clinics of North America, 25*, 885–890.

Skipper, A., Szeluga, D., & Groenwald, S. (1993). Nutritional disturbances. In S. Groenwald, M. Frogge, M. Goodman, & C. Yarbo (Eds.). *Cancer nursing: Principles and practices*. Boston: Jones and Bartlett.

U.S. Department of Health and Human Services. (1989). *Healthy People 2000*. Washington, DC: Government Printing Office.

Varella, L., & Utermohlen, U. (1993). Nutritional support for the patient with renal failure. *Critical Care Nursing Clinics of North America, 5*(1), 79–96.

Williams, S. R. (1992). *Basic nutrition and diet therapy*. St. Louis: Mosby-Year Book.

Wilson, M. H. (1994) Feeding the healthy child. In F. Oski (Ed.). *Principles and practice of pediatrics* (2nd ed.). Philadelphia: J. B. Lippincott.

Wong, D. L. (1995). *Nursing care of infants and children* (5th ed.). St. Louis: C. V. Mosby.

Impaired Swallowing

DEFINITION

Impaired Swallowing: The state in which an individual has decreased ability voluntarily to pass fluids and/or solid foods from the mouth to the stomach.

DEFINING CHARACTERISTICS
Major (Must Be Present)

Observed evidence of difficulty in swallowing and/or
Stasis of food in oral cavity

Minor (May Be Present)

Coughing
Choking
Apraxia (ideational, constructional, or visual)

RELATED FACTORS
Pathophysiologic

Related to decreased/absent gag reflex, mastication difficulties, or decreased sensations
secondary to:
(Neurologic/neuromuscular disorders)

Cerebral palsy	Botulism
Muscular dystrophy	Poliomyelitis
Myasthenia gravis	Parkinson's disease
Guillain-Barré	Amyotrophic lateral sclerosis

Neoplastic disease (disease affecting brain and/or brain stem)
Cerebrovascular accident (CVA)
Right or left hemispheric damage to brain
Damage to 5th, 7th, 9th, 10th, or 11th cranial nerve
Related to tracheoesophageal tumors, edema

Treatment-Related

Related to surgical reconstruction of the mouth, throat, jaw, and/or nose
Related to decreased consciousness secondary to anesthesia
Related to mechanical obstruction secondary to tracheostomy tube
Related to esophagitis secondary to radiotherapy

Situational (Personal, Environmental)

Related to altered level of consciousness
Related to fatigue
Related to limited awareness, distractibility
Related to irritated oropharyngeal cavity
Related to decreased saliva

Maturational

Infants/children
Related to decreased sensations or difficulty with mastication
Older Adult
Related to reduction in saliva, taste

Author's Note

See *Altered Nutrition: Less Than Body Requirements*

Errors in Diagnostic Statements

See *Altered Nutrition: Less Than Body Requirements*

Key Concepts

1. Swallowing has an intellectual component as well as a physical one.
2. The swallowing process occurs in three stages with select cranial nerve involvement (Ter Matt & Tandy, 1991):
   a. *Stage 1*—Oral: Food is placed in oral cavity, the lips close, and swallowing is initiated as a reflex. The tongue maneuvers the food, and the soft palate and uvula close off the nasopharynx.

　　b. *Stage 2*—Pharyngeal: The food passes the anterior fossa arches and triggers the swallow reflex. The tongue prevents the food from returning to the oral cavity by elevation and contraction of the soft palate. Pharyngeal peristalsis begins, causing the food to move downward.

　　c. *Stage 3*—Esophageal: Pharyngeal peristalsis pushes the food downward. The larynx elevates and the cricopharyngeal muscles relax, allowing the food to move from the pharynx into the esophagus. The larynx wave pushes the food down the esophagus to the stomach.

3. The 5th, 7th, 9th, 10th, and 11th cranial nerves are involved in swallowing.
4. Impairment of cranial nerve function can cause the following swallowing problems (Ter Matt & Tandy, 1991):
　　a. Trigeminal (V)—loss of sensation and ability to move mandible.
　　b. Facial (VII)—Increased salivation; inability to pucker lips, pouching of foods.
　　c. Glossopharyngeal (IX)—diminished taste sensation, salivation, and gag reflex.
　　d. Vagus (X)—decreased peristalsis, decreased gag reflex.
　　e. Hypoglossal (XII)—poor tongue control, poor movement of food to the throat.
5. A cough reflex is essential for rehabilitation, but a gag reflex is not.
6. Do not confuse the ability to chew with the ability to swallow. See also *Altered Nutrition: Less Than Body Requirements*.

Focus Assessment Criteria

Subjective Data (Ter Matt & Tandy, 1991)

A. Assess for defining characteristics
　　1. History of problem with swallowing
　　　　a. Onset
　　　　b. History of nasal regurgitation, hoarseness, choking, or coughing
　　2. Problem foods or liquids
　　3. Nonproblem foods or liquids

B. Assess for related factors
　　1. CVA
　　2. Parkinson's disease
　　3. Multiple sclerosis
　　4. Brain lesions
　　5. Head trauma
　　6. Tracheoesophageal tumors
　　7. Oral surgery

Objective Data (Ter Matt & Tandy, 1991)

A. Assess for defining characteristics
　　1. Decreased or absent swallowing, cough, or gag reflex
　　2. Poor coordination of tongue
　　3. Observed choking or coughing with food or fluid

B. Assess for related factors
　　1. Facial muscle weakness
　　　　a. Drooling
　　　　b. Asymmetric
　　　　c. Poor lip closure
　　2. Impaired use of tongue
　　　　a. Decreased strength
　　　　b. Poor coordination
　　　　c. Inability to use
　　3. Chewing difficulties

4. Decreased saliva production
5. Thick cognition
6. Impaired cognition
   a. Poor short-term memory
   b. Distractibility
   c. Poor judgment

Outcome Criteria

The person will
- Report improved ability to swallow

The person and/or family will
- Describe causative factors when known
- Describe rationale and procedures for treatment

Interventions

A. Assess for causative or contributing factors
   1. Mechanical impairment of oropharyngeal structures
      a. Congenital anomalies
      b. Cleft lip/palate
      c. Cranial nerve damage (5th, 7th, 9th, 10th, and/or 11th)
      d. Surgical reconstruction of mouth
      e. CVA
      f. Altered level of consciousness
      g. Fatigue
      h. Reddened, irritated oropharyngeal cavity
      i. Decreased/absent gag reflex
   2. Muscle paralysis or paresis
      a. Post-CVA
      b. Cranial nerve damage
      c. Decreased/absent gag reflex (*e.g.*, postradiation)
   3. Impaired cognition or awareness
      a. Cortical damage
      b. Apraxia
      c. Aphasia

B. Reduce or eliminate causative/contributing factors in individuals with
   1. Mechanical impairment of mouth—assist the individual with moving the bolus of food from the anterior to the posterior of mouth.
      a. Place food in the posterior mouth where swallowing can be ensured, using
         A syringe with a short piece of tubing attached
         A glossectomy spoon
         Soft food of a consistency that can be manipulated by the tongue against the pharynx, such as gelatin, custard, or mashed potatoes
      b. Prevent/decrease thick secretions.
         Artificial saliva
         Papain tablets dissolved in mouth 10 minutes before eating
         Meat tenderizer made from papaya enzyme applied to oral cavity 10 minutes before eating
         Frequent mouth care
         Increase fluid intake
         Check medications for potential side effects of dry mouth/decreased salivation

2. Muscle paralysis or paresis
   a. Establish a visual method to communicate at bedside to staff that client is dysphagic.
   b. Plan meals when client is well rested; ensure that reliable suction equipment is on hand during meals. Discontinue feeding if client is tired.
   c. If indicated use modified supraglottic swallow technique (Emick-Herring & Wood, 1990).
      Position the head of the bed in semi- or high Fowler's position, with the neck flexed forward slightly and chin tilted down.
      Use cutout cup (remove and round out one third of side of foam cup).
      Take bolus of food and hold in strongest side of mouth for 1–2 seconds. Then immediately flex the neck with chin tucked against chest.
      Without breathing, swallow as many times as needed.
      When mouth is emptied, raise chin and clear throat.
   d. Offer highly viscous foods first at meal (*e.g.* mashed bananas, potatoes, gelatin, gravy).
   e. Offer thick liquids (*e.g.*, milk shakes, slushes, nectars, cream soups).
   f. Establish a goal for fluid intake.
   g. If drooling is present, use a quick-stretch stimulation just before each meal and toward the end of the meal (Emick-Herring & Wood, 1990).
      Digitally apply short, rapid, downward strokes to edge of bottom lip, mostly on affected side.
      Use a cold washcloth over finger for added stimulation.
   h. If a bolus of food is pocketed in the affected side, teach client how to use tongue to transfer food or apply external digital pressure to cheek to help remove the trapped bolus (Emick-Herring & Wood, 1990).
3. Impaired cognition or awareness
   a. General
      Remove feeding tube during training if increased gag reflex is present.
      Concentrate on solids rather than liquids, because liquids usually are less well tolerated.
      Keep extraneous stimuli at minimum while eating (*e.g.*, no television or radio, no verbal stimuli unless directed at task).
      Have person concentrate on task of swallowing.
      Have person sit up in chair with neck slightly flexed.
      Instruct person to hold breath while swallowing.
      Observe for swallowing and check mouth for emptying.
      Avoid overloading mouth, because this decreases swallowing effectiveness.
      Give solids and liquids separately.
      Progress slowly. Limit conversation.
      Provide several small meals to accommodate a short attention span.
   b. Person with aphasia, or left hemispheric damage
      Demonstrate expected behavior.
      Reinforce behaviors with simple, one-word commands.
   c. Person with apraxia, or right hemispheric damage
      Divide task into smallest units possible.
      Assist through each task with verbal commands.
      Allow to complete one unit fully before giving next command.
      Continue verbal assistance at each eating session until no longer needed.
      Incorporate written checklist as a reminder to person.

Note: Person may have both left and right hemispheric damage and require a combination of the above techniques.

C. Reduce the possibility of aspiration

1. Before beginning feeding, assess that person is adequately alert and responsive, is able to control mouth, has cough/gag reflex, and can swallow own saliva.

2. Have suction equipment available and functioning properly.
3. Position person correctly.
   a. Sit upright (60°–90°) in chair or dangle feet at side of bed if possible (prop pillows if necessary).
   b. Assume position 10–15 minutes before eating and maintain position for 10–15 minutes after finishing eating.
   c. Flex head forward on the midline about 45° to keep esophagus patent.
4. Keep individual focused on task by giving directions until he has finished swallowing each mouthful.
   a. "Take a breath."
   b. "Move food to middle of tongue."
   c. "Raise tongue to roof of mouth."
   d. "Think about swallowing."
   e. "Swallow."
   f. "Cough to clear airway."
   g. Reinforce voluntary action.
5. Start with small amounts and progress slowly as person learns to handle each step.
   a. Ice chips
   b. Part of eyedropper filled with water
   c. Whole eyedropper
   d. Use juice in place of water
   e. ¼ teaspoon semisolid
   f. ½ teaspoon semisolid
   g. 1 teaspoon semisolid
   h. Pureed food or commercial baby foods
   i. One-half cracker
   j. Soft diet
   k. Regular diet
   l. For person who has had a CVA, place food at back of tongue and on side of face he can control.
   m. Feed slowly, making certain previous bite has been swallowed.
   n. Some individuals do better with foods that hold together, such as soft-boiled eggs or ground meat and gravy.
6. If the above strategies are unsuccessful, consultation with physician may be necessary for alternative feeding techniques such as tube feedings or parenteral nutrition.

D. Initiate health teaching and referrals, as indicated
   1. Teach exercises to strengthen (Grober, 1984):
      a. Lips and facial muscles
         Alternate a tight frown with a broad smile with lips closed.
         Puff out cheeks with air and hold.
         Blow out of pursed lips.
         Practice pronouncing *u, m, b, p, w*.
         Suck hard on a popsicle.
      b. Tongue
         Lick a popsicle or lollipop.
         Push tip of tongue against roof of mouth and floor.
         Count teeth with tongue.
         Pronounce *la la la, ta ta ta, d, n, z, s*.
   2. Consult with speech pathologist.
   3. Consult with dietitian for meal planning.
   4. Explain to individual and significant others rationale of treatment and how to proceed with it.
   5. See *Altered Oral Mucous Membrane*.
   6. See *Altered Nutrition: Less Than Body Requirements*.

Rationale

- Interventions vary depending on the causative or contributing factors.
- A speech pathologist has the expertise needed to preform the dysphagia evaluation.
- The risk of aspiration can be reduced if all staff are alerted.
- Impaired reflexes increase the risk of aspiration.
- Fatigue can increase the risk of aspiration.
- Upright position uses the force of gravity to aid downward motion of food and decreases risk of aspiration.
- Straws and thin fluids hasten transit time and increase the risk of aspiration (Emick-Herring & Wood, 1990).
- Thicker fluids have a slower transit time and allow more time to trigger the swallow reflex (Emick-Herring & Wood, 1990).
- Poor tongue control with impaired oral sensation allows food into affected side (Emick-Herring & Wood, 1990).
- A confused client needs repetitive, simple instructions.
- Exercise can strengthen muscles to improve chewing and tongue movement of bolus to back of mouth to stimulate swallowing reflex (Porth, 1994).
- Avoid foods that do not form a bolus (*e.g.*, sticky foods, pureed foods, applesauce, dry foods) or do not stimulate the swallowing reflex (*e.g.*, thin liquids).

References/Bibliography

DiIorio, C., & Price, M. (1990). Swallowing: An assessment guide. *American Journal of Nursing, 90*(7), 38–48.

Emick-Herring, B., & Wood, P. (1990). A team approach to neurologically based swallowing disorders. *Rehabilitation Nursing, 15*, 126–132.

Grober, M. (Ed.). (1984). *Dysphagia*. Oxford, UK: Butterworth-Heinemann.

Porth, C. M. (1994). *Pathophysiology: Concepts of altered health states* (4th ed.). Philadelphia: J. B. Lippincott.

Ter Matt, M., & Tandy, L. (1991). Impaired swallowing. In M. Maas, K. Buckwalter & M. Hardy (Eds.). *Nursing diagnoses and interventions for the elderly*. Redwood City, Ca: Addison-Wesley Nursing.

Ineffective Infant Feeding Pattern

DEFINITION

Ineffective Infant Feeding Pattern: A state in which an infant (birth to 9 months) demonstrates an impaired ability to suck or coordinate the suck/swallow response, resulting in inadequate oral nutrition for metabolic needs.

DEFINING CHARACTERISTICS
Major (Must Be Present)

Inability to initiate or sustain an effective suck; inability to coordinate sucking, swallowing, and breathing

Actual metabolic needs in excess of oral intake with weight loss or need for enteral feeding supplement

Minor (May Be Present)

Inconsistent oral intake (volume, time interval, duration)
Oral motor developmental delay
Tachypnea with increased respiratory effort
Regurgitation or vomiting after feeding

RELATED FACTORS
Pathophysiologic

Related to increased caloric need secondary to:
Body temperature instability
Growth needs
Tachypnea with increased respiratory effort
Wound healing
Infection
Major organ system disease or failure
Related to muscle weakness/hypotonia secondary to:

Malnutrition   Congenital defects
Prematurity   Major organ system disease or failure
Acute/chronic illness   Neurologic impairment/delay
Lethargy

Treatment-Related

Related to hypermetabolic state and increased caloric needs secondary to:
Surgery
Painful procedures
Related to muscle weakness and lethargy secondary to:
Medications
Muscle relaxants (antiseizure medications, paralyzing agents in past, sedatives, narcotics)
Sleep deprivation
Related to oral hypersensitivity
Related to previous prolonged NPO state

Situational (Personal, Environmental)

Related to inconsistent caretakers (feeders)
Related to lack of knowledge or commitment of caretaker (feeder) to special feeding needs or regimen
Related to presence of noxious facial or absence of oral stimuli

Author's Note

Ineffective Infant Feeding Pattern describes an infant with sucking or swallowing difficulties. This infant experiences inadequate oral nutrition for growth and development, which is exacerbated when there is an increased caloric need, as in infection, illness, or stress. Nursing interventions assist infants and their caregivers with techniques to achieve nutritional intake needed for weight gain. In addition, the goal is that the intake eventually be exclusively oral.

Infants who have sucking or swallowing problems and who have not lost weight need nursing interventions to prevent weight loss. *Ineffective Infant Feeding Pattern* is clinically useful for this situation.

Errors in Diagnostic Statements

Risk for Ineffective Infant Feeding Pattern related to inconsistent oral intake with or without weight loss

Inconsistent oral intake is a defining characteristic for *Ineffective Infant Feeding Pattern*, not *Risk for Ineffective Infant Feeding Pattern*. *Ineffective Infant Feeding Pattern* may not be useful as a risk nursing diagnosis because this actual diagnosis exists whenever an infant has sucking or suck/swallow response difficulties, whether mild or severe. The diagnosis would be appropriate as *Ineffective Infant Feeding Pattern related to (specify contributing factors, e.g., lethargy) as evidenced by inconsistent oral intake*.

Key Concepts

1. There are two goals for infants with ineffective feeding patterns:
   a. The infant will receive adequate and appropriate calories (carbohydrate, protein, fat) for age with weight gain at a rate consistent with an individualized plan based on age and needs.
   b. The infant will take all feedings orally.
2. For an infant with an ineffective feeding pattern (with or without a demonstrable oral motor impairment), conversion from a catabolic state to an anabolic state with consistent weight gain from appropriate calories is a prerequisite for goal attainment.
3. Identification of contributing physiologic factors assists in evaluating and adapting the feeding plan. For example, fever increases caloric needs; mechanical ventilation can decrease caloric needs; infants with impaired renal function or fluid retention can experience weight gain without meeting nutritional metabolic needs; dysfunction in major organ systems or infection affect feeding patterns adversely and increase caloric needs.
4. Some infants with oral motor impairment or weakness feed adequately by mouth when their metabolic need for calories is normal. But in the presence of increased caloric need (*e.g.*, congestive heart failure, infection, major organ system dysfunction, wound healing, malnutrition), they are not able to take in adequate calories by increasing their volume intake sufficiently because of their ineffective feeding skills. Intervention with these infants is based on providing adequate calories, promoting oral feeding skills, and decreasing (if possible) caloric needs.
5. Knowledge of normal infant feeding patterns is necessary to promote effective feeding patterns. For example, a quiet, awake state is the ideal state for feeding; nonnutritive sucking preceding nutritive sucking can enhance feeding behaviors; there is a relation between sucking–swallowing–gastric emptying–bowel emptying during feeding; and so forth. Over time, each infant develops an effective feeding pattern that is unique (McCain, 1992).
6. In the neonate, options to promote breast-feeding (either by using previously pumped breast milk or feeding directly from the breast) should be explored with the mother by a lactation specialist. Many infants who initially have oral motor delays or lack of coordination of suck and swallow can successfully breast-feed with appropriate early intervention.
7. High-caloric formulas (up to 32 cal/oz) or calorie-enhanced breast milk can be safely administered to most infants, provided the preparation is consistent with the child's age and needs. For example, concentrating formula to increase calories can increase the protein load disproportionately; therefore, additives (carbohydrate or fat) are often used to increase calories safely. The appropriate use of high-calorie formulas can reduce the target volume/day goal for an infant, making it easier to attain the goal of total oral feedings. Serum protein, albumin, and renal function need to be assessed periodically when high-calorie formulas are used.
8. Enteral feedings are often required initially to ensure adequate caloric intake, weight gain, and anabolic state. Identifying a total plan for feeding from the beginning, which includes both enteral and oral feeding (or oral stimulation if feeding is not possible), is instrumental in promoting the goal of total oral feeding. Infants who are exclusively enterally fed in the first months of life, with no effort to develop oral feeding skills, can become behaviorally disinterested in oral feeding and may remain enterally fed indefinitely (VandenBerg, 1991).

Focus Assessment Criteria

Subjective Data

A. Assess for defining characteristics
   1. General
        Current weight and height
        Weight gain daily/weekly goal
        Calorie/kg daily goal
   2. Feeding history
        Previous oral feeding pattern (volume, time interval, duration)
        Previous enteral feeding pattern (continuous or bolus, NG, NJ, GT, GJ, volume, time interval, duration)
        Gastrointestinal tolerance of feedings (oral, enteral, emesis, stool pattern)

B. Assess for related factors
   1. Presence/absence of noxious stimuli to face and mouth (including NG/NJ feedings, endotracheal intubation, oral or NP suction, nasal cannula oxygen)
   2. Physiologic factors
        Hyperthermia or hypothermia   Oral motor developmental delay
        Infection   Gastroesophageal reflux
        Congestive heart failure   Colic
        Prematurity
        Prolonged NPO state with or without enteral feedings
        Neurologic dysfunction

Objective Data

A. Assess for related factors
   1. Elevated body temperature
   2. Increased respiratory rate and effort
   3. Strength and coordination of nonnutritive sucking
   4. Strength and coordination of nutritive sucking
   5. Impaired sleep patterns
   6. Irritability
   7. Lethargy

Outcome Criteria

The infant will:
- Receive adequate nutrition for growth appropriate to age and need
- Demonstrate increasing skill in oral feedings appropriate for developmental ability

---

Interventions

A. Assess the infant's feeding pattern and nutritional needs
   1. Assess volume, duration, and effort during feeding; respiratory rate and effort; signs of fatigue.
   2. Assess past caloric intake, weight gain, trends in intake and output, renal function, fluid retention.
   3. Identify physiologic risk factors.
   4. Identify physiologic ability to feed (VandenBerg, 1991):
        a. Can the infant stop breathing when sucking and swallowing?
        b. What happens to oxygen level, heart rate, respiratory rate when sucking/swallowing?

      c. Does the infant need rest periods? How long? Are there problems in initiating sucking/swallowing again?
  5. Assess nipple-feeding skills (Shaker, 1991):
      a. Does the infant actively suck with a bottle?
      b. Does the infant initiate a swallow in coordination with suck?
      c. Does the infant coordinate sucking, swallowing, and breathing?
      d. Is the feeding completed in a reasonable time?
  6. Collaborate with clinical dietitian to set calorie, volume, and weight gain goals.
  7. Collaborate with occupational therapist to identify oral motor skills and planned intervention, if needed.
  8. Collaborate with parent(s) about effective techniques used with this infant or other children, temperament, and responses to environmental stimuli.

B. Promote adequate caloric intake and anabolic state with consistent weight gain per goals (Hazinski, 1992)
  1. High-risk neonate: 120–150 cal/kg
  2. Normal neonate: 100–120 cal/kg

C. Provide specific interventions to promote effective oral feeding (McCain, 1992; Morris & Klein, 1987; VandenBerg, 1991)
  1. Encourage nonnutritive sucking not in response to noxious stimuli.
  2. Ensure nutritive sucking for identified amount of time (to prevent overtiring and unnecessary caloric expenditure).
  3. Choose nipple according to individual needs and successes; assess effects of changes in formula/breast milk temperature and thickness.
  4. Consider timing of feedings and competition in the environment.
  5. Specific interventions for facilitating feeding (McCain, 1992; Shaker, 1991):
      a. Position the infant in a semiupright position, with the trunk at approximately a 45°–60° angle (do not use a "head-back" position because it makes swallowing and sucking coordination more difficult).
      b. Stroke the infant's lips, cheeks, and tongue before feeding.
      c. Use nonnutritive sucking before feeding to promote an awake and alert state.
      d. Use fingers to provide inward and forward support for the infant's cheeks during feeding.
      e. Provide support for the base of the tongue (by placing fingers halfway between the chin and the throat, the nurse can provide a slight upward lift under the base of the tongue); *do not* provide strong upward pressure; steady support is most helpful; avoid moving fingers because it may interfere with the infant's own tongue movements.
  6. Implement specific interventions for oral motor delays (position, equipment, jaw/mouth manipulation) (Morris & Klein, 1987).
  7. Control adverse environmental stimuli and noxious stimuli to face and mouth.
  8. The following actions hinder, not help, the infant to feed (Shaker, 1991):
      a. Twisting or turning the nipple
      b. Moving the nipple up, down, around in the mouth
      c. Putting the nipple in and out of the mouth
      d. Putting pressure on the jaw or moving the infant's jaw up and down
      e. Positioning the infant in a head-back position
  9. Promote sleep and reduce unnecessary energy expenditure.
 10. If needed, plan for enteral feeding includes guidelines for increasing oral feeding and decreasing enteral feeding as the infant eats more effectively by mouth.
 11. Promote consistency in approach to feeding.
 12. As the infant ages, revise and change feeding plan (including calorie and weight goals) to encourage normal feeding patterns for age when possible. For example, change type of formula, add solid foods, and the like, when age appropriate.

D. Establish partnership with parent(s) in all stages of plan
  1. Clearly identify and negotiate mutual goals for intervention.
  2. Create a supportive environment for the parents to have the primary role in providing feeding-related intervention, when they are present. Whenever possible, nurses use the parents' approach when a parent is not present. In addition, when parents are not present, the nurses can support the parents' role by imitating their approach to the infant, and communicate the infant's responses to the parents at a later time.

E. Negotiate and identify plans for discharge with parents and incorporate into the overall feeding plan; provide ongoing information to parents about special needs and assist them in establishing needed resources (equipment, nursing care, other caretakers) when needed

Rationale

- Establishing parents as essential participants in the feeding plan gives them a role, a place, and a reason to be present so that a closer relationship with the child can be further developed.
- If the infant receives adequate calories, he or she will be physically more able to eat orally; if the parents support and value the way the calories are delivered and recognize milestones toward goal, the child will be more likely to receive adequate calories after discharge. In addition, interactions will be more rewarding for both infant and parent during the intervention period.
- Calm, quiet, dim environments offer less distraction; attempt to decrease the negative impact of painful or very stimulating experiences shortly before or after the feeding by timing feedings.
- Fever, infection, wound healing, malnutrition, and congestive heart failure increase caloric need beyond the goals listed for normal or high-risk neonates.
- For an infant with a demonstrable oral motor impairment, early intervention with an identified consistent approach to promoting oral feeding (equipment, body position, jaw and mouth manipulation, volume, time interval, duration) is essential for goal attainment.
- Identification of ineffective feeding patterns should be based on systematic assessment of the infant, in collaboration with other professionals. Behaviors that are cues to feeding dysfunction include ineffective coordination of suck/swallow/breathing, low energy or stamina, poor ability or inability to initiate sucking, disorganized rhythm in suck/swallow pattern, inadequate neurobehavioral control, and difficulty shifting back and forth from nonnutritive sucking and nutritive sucking (Morris & Klein, 1987; VandenBerg, 1991).
- Close collaboration with a clinical dietitian to assess, plan, set, and evaluate calorie goals, weight gain goals, calorie distribution, and formula preparation is necessary for infants at risk.
- Close collaboration with a professional skilled in the assessment of infant oral motor skills (*e.g.*, occupational therapist, speech therapist) is necessary to assess, plan, intervene, and evaluate progress toward appropriate oral motor skills in the infant with an oral motor impairment.
- Close collaboration with parents from the beginning about identified needs, negotiation of priorities, and development of interventions is crucial to establishing effective feeding patterns in the infant and strengthening the infant–parent relationship.
- Environmental factors, including light, noise, inconsistent caretakers (feeders), and noxious stimuli, contribute significantly to ineffective feeding patterns (Morris & Klein, 1987).
- Efforts to promote sleep and reduce energy expenditure (primarily by controlling environmental stimuli) can substantially improve the infant's strength and stamina during feeding.
- Nonnutritive sucking (pacifier) should not be exclusively used to comfort the infant during or after painful procedures or exposure to noxious stimuli. In addition, care and attention to reducing noxious stimuli to the face and mouth (type, frequency, intensity) should be initiated long before attempts to feed orally begin (Morris & Klein, 1987).

References/Bibliography

Hazinski, M. F. (1992). *Nursing care of the critically ill child.* St. Louis: C. V. Mosby.

McCain, G. (1992). Facilitating inactive awake states in preterm infants: A study of three interventions. *Nursing Research, 41,* 157–160.

Morris, S. E., & Klein, M. D. (1987). *Prefeeding skills.* Tucson: Therapy Skill Builders.

Shaker, C. S. (1991). Nipple feeding premature infants: A different perspective. *Neonatal Network, 8*(5), 9–17.

VandenBerg, K. (1991). Nippling management of the sick neonate in the NICU: The disorganized feeder. *Neonatal Network, 9*(1), 9–16.

Nutrition, Altered: More Than Body Requirements

DEFINITION

Altered Nutrition: More Than Body Requirements: The state in which the individual experiences or is at risk of experiencing weight gain related to an intake in excess of metabolic requirements.

DEFINING CHARACTERISTICS
Major (Must Be Present)

Overweight (weight 10% over ideal for height and frame), or
Obese (weight 20% or more over ideal for height and frame)
Triceps skin fold greater than 15 mm in men and 25 mm in women

Minor (May Be Present)

Reported undesirable eating patterns
Intake in excess of metabolic requirements
Sedentary activity patterns

RELATED FACTORS
Pathophysiologic

Related to altered satiety patterns secondary to (specify)
Related to decreased sense of taste and smell

Treatment-Related

Related to altered satiety secondary to:
    Medications (corticosteroids, antihistamines)
    Radiation (decreased sense of taste and smell)

Situational (Personal, Environmental)

Related to risk to gain more than 25–30 lb when pregnant
Related to lack of basic nutritional knowledge

Maturational

Adult/Older Adult
    Related to decreased activity patterns, decreased metabolic needs

Author's Note

Using this diagnosis to describe people who are overweight or obese places the focus of interventions on nutrition. Obesity is a complex condition with sociocultural, psychological, and metabolic implications. When the focus is primarily on limiting food intake, as with many weight-loss programs, the chance of permanent weight loss is slim. To be successful, a weight-loss program must focus on behavior modification and life-style changes.

The nursing diagnosis *Altered Nutrition: More Than Body Requirements* does not describe this focus. Rather, *Altered Health Maintenance related to intake in excess of metabolic requirements* better reflects the need to increase metabolic requirements through exercise and decrease intake. For some people who desire weight loss, *Ineffective Individual Coping related to increase in eating in response to stressors* could be a useful diagnosis in addition to *Altered Health Maintenance*.

The nurse should be cautioned against applying nursing diagnosis for an overweight or obese person who does not want to participate in a weight-loss program. A person's motivation for weight loss must come from within. Nurses can gently and expertly teach the hazards of obesity, but must respect a person's right to choose, the right of self-determination.

Altered Nutrition: More Than Body Requirements does have clinical usefulness in people at risk for or who have experienced weight gain because of pregnancy, taste or smell changes, or medications (*e.g.*, corticosteroids).

Errors in Diagnostic Statements

Altered Nutrition: More Than Body Requirements related to excessive calorie intake and sedentary life-style

As discussed in the Author's Note, *Altered Nutrition* does not describe the complex nature of obesity or overweight conditions. Obesity is not a nutritional problem, but rather a problem with coping and life-style choices. *Altered Health Maintenance* and *Ineffective Individual Coping* are more useful diagnoses for the focus of nursing interventions.

Altered Nutrition: More Than Body Requirements related to reports of gaining 50 lb with first pregnancy

A report of gaining 50 lb during first pregnancy should prompt the nurse to initiate a focus assessment to explore other variables. For example, the nurse could ask "What do you think contributed to your weight gain during your first pregnancy?" "What was the pattern of weight gain during each trimester?" The nurse also should discuss the difference between dieting during pregnancy versus a diet not excessive in simple carbohydrates or fat. After additional data collection, the following diagnosis possibly could prove valid: *Risk for Altered Nutrition: More Than Body Requirements related to lack of knowledge of nutritional needs during pregnancy and exercise needed and history of 50-lb weight gain during previous pregnancy*.

Key Concepts

1. Certain medications (*e.g.*, steroids, antihistamines, androgens, antipsychotics, antidepressants) can cause weight gain (Malseed, 1994).
2. Medications can affect taste (*e.g.*, amphetamines, clofibrate, lithium, griseofulvin, methicillin, phenindione, phenytoin, probucol) (Mahan & Arlin, 1992).

Focus Assessment Criteria

See *Altered Nutrition: Less Than Body Requirements*

Outcome Criteria

The person will
- Describe reasons why he is at risk for weight gain
- Describe reasons for increased intake with taste or olfactory deficits
- Discuss the nutritional needs during pregnancy
- Discuss the effects of exercise on weight control

Interventions

A. Assess for causative or contributing factors, such as
    1. Decreased sense of smell or taste
    2. Effects of medications
    3. History of weight gain over 30 lb during pregnancy

B. Explain the effects of decreased sense of taste and smell on perception of satiety after eating. Encourage the person to
    1. Evaluate intake by calorie counting, not feelings of satiety.
    2. If not contraindicated, spice foods heavily to satisfy decreased sense of taste. Experiment with seasonings (*e.g.*, dill, basil).
    3. When taste is diminished, concentrate on food smells.

C. Explain the rationale for increased appetite owing to use of certain medications (*e.g.*, steroids, androgens)

D. Discuss nutritional intake and weight gain during pregnancy
    1. See Key Concepts under *Altered Nutrition: Less Than Body Requirements*.

E. Assist to decrease unnecessary calorie intake and to increase metabolic activity
    1. Increase the client's awareness of actions that contribute to excessive food intake.
        a. Request that he write down all the food he ate in the past 24 hours.
        b. Instruct client to keep a diet diary for 1 week that specifies the following:
            What, when, where, and why eaten
            Whether he was doing anything else (*e.g.* watching TV, cooking) while eating
            Emotions before eating
            Others present (*e.g.* snacking with spouse, children)
        c. Review the diet diary to point out patterns (*e.g.* time, place, emotions, foods, persons) that affect food intake.
        d. Review high- and low-calorie food items.
    2. Teach behavior modification techniques to decrease caloric intake, such as:
        a. Eat only at a specific spot at home (*e.g.*, the kitchen table).
        b. Do not eat while performing other activities.
        c. Drink an 8-oz glass of water immediately before a meal.
        d. Decrease second helpings, fatty foods, sweets, and alcohol.
        e. Prepare small portions, just enough for one meal, and discard leftovers.
        f. Use small plates to make portions look bigger.
        g. Never eat from another person's plate.
        h. Eat slowly and chew food thoroughly.
        i. Put down utensils and wait 15 seconds between bites.
        j. Eat low-calorie snacks that must be chewed to satisfy oral needs (*e.g.*, carrots, celery, apples).
    3. Instruct to increase activity level to burn calories; encourage the following:
        a. Use the stairs instead of elevators.

    b. Park at the farthest point in parking lots and walk to buildings.

    c. Plan a daily walking program with a progressive increase in distance and pace.

Note: Urge the person to consult with a primary provider before beginning any exercise program.

F. Initiate referral to a community weight loss program, if indicated (*e.g.*, Weight Watchers)

Rationale

- The ability to lose weight while on corticosteroid therapy likely depends on limiting sodium intake and maintaining a reasonable caloric intake.
- Increased activity promotes weight loss.
- People with altered smell or taste may consume more food in an attempt to satisfy their taste (Mahan & Arlin, 1992).

References/Bibliography

Mahan, L. K., & Arlin, M. (1992). *Food, nutrition and diet therapy* (8th ed.). Philadelphia: W. B. Saunders.

Malseed, R. T. (1995). *Pharmacology: Drug therapy and nursing considerations* (4th ed.). Philadelphia: J. B. Lippincott.

Nutrition, Altered: Potential for More Than Body Requirements

DEFINITION

Altered Nutrition: Potential for More Than Body Requirements: The state in which an individual is at risk of experiencing an intake of nutrients that exceeds metabolic needs.

DEFINING CHARACTERISTICS

Reported or observed obesity in one or both parents

Rapid transition across growth percentiles in infants or children

Reported use of solid food as major food source before 5 months of age

Observed use of food as reward or comfort measure

Reported or observed higher baseline weight at beginning of each pregnancy

Dysfunctional eating patterns

Author's Note

This nursing diagnosis is similar to *Risk for Altered Nutrition: More Than Body Requirements*. It describes an individual who has a family history of obesity, is demonstrating a pattern of higher weight, and/or has had a history of excessive weight gain (*e.g.*, previous pregnancy). Until clinical research differentiates this diagnosis from other currently accepted diagnoses, use *Altered Health Maintenance (Actual* or *Risk for)* or *Risk for Altered Nutrition: More Than Body Requirements* to direct teaching to assist families and individuals to identify unhealthy dietary patterns.

Parenting, Altered

Parent–Infant Attachment, Risk for Altered

Parental Role Conflict

Parenting, Altered

DEFINITION

Altered Parenting: The state in which one or more caregivers demonstrate a real or potential inability to provide a constructive environment that nurtures the growth and development of his/her/their child (children).

DEFINING CHARACTERISTICS
Major (Must Be Present)

Inappropriate and/or non-nurturing parenting behaviors
Lack of parental attachment behavior

Minor (May Be Present)

Frequent verbalization of dissatisfaction or disappointment with infant/child
Verbalization of frustration of role
Verbalization of perceived or actual inadequacy
Diminished or inappropriate visual, tactile, or auditory stimulation of infant
Evidence of abuse or neglect of child
Growth and development lag in infant/child

RELATED FACTORS

Individuals or families who may be at risk for developing or experiencing parenting difficulties
Parent(s)

Single	Addicted to drugs
Adolescent	Terminally ill
Abusive	Acutely disabled
Emotionally disturbed	Accident victim
Alcoholic	

Child

Of unwanted pregnancy	Mentally handicapped
Of undesired gender	Hyperactive characteristics
With undesired characteristics	Terminally ill
Physically handicapped	

Situational (Personal, Environmental)

Related to interruption of bonding process secondary to:

Illness (child, parent)	Relocation
Incarceration	

Related to separation from nuclear family
Related to lack of knowledge

Related to inconsistent caregivers or techniques
Related to relationship problems (specify):

  Marital discord Step-parents

  Divorce   Live-in partner

  Separation   Relocation

Related to little external support and/or socially isolated family
Related to lack of available role model
Related to ineffective adaptation to stressors associated with

  Illness   Economic problems

  New baby   Substance abuse

  Elder care

Maturational

Adolescent

  Related to the conflict of meeting own needs over child's

  Related to history of ineffective relationships with own parents

  Related to parental history of abusive relationship with parents

  Related to unrealistic expectations of child by parent

  Related to unrealistic expectations of self by parent

  Related to unrealistic expectations of parent by child

  Related to unmet psychosocial needs of child by parent

Author's Note

The family environment should provide the basic needs for a child's physical growth and development: stimulation of the child's emotional, social, and cognitive potential; consistent, stable reinforcement to learn impulse control; reality testing; freedom to share emotions; and moral stability (Pfeffer, 1981). This environment nurtures a child to develop, as Pfeffer (1981) states, "the ability to disengage from the family constellation as part of a process of lifelong individualization." It is the role of parents to provide such an environment. Most parenting difficulties stem from lack of knowledge or inability to manage stressors constructively. The ability to parent effectively is at high risk when the child or parent has a condition that increases stress on the family unit (*e.g.*, illness, financial problems).

 Altered Parenting describes a parent experiencing difficulty creating or continuing a nurturing environment for a child. *Parental Role Conflict* describes a parent or parents whose previously effective functioning ability is challenged by external factors. In certain situations, such as illness, divorce, or remarriage, role confusion and conflict are expected. If parents do not receive assistance in adapting their role to external factors, *Parental Role Conflict* can lead to *Altered Parenting*.

Errors in Diagnostic Statements

Altered Parenting related to child abuse

 Child abuse is a sign of family dysfunction. Usually, each child abuse situation involves an abusing adult and a knowing nonabusing adult; the treatment plan must include both. Thus, the diagnosis *Ineffective Family Coping* would be more descriptive of this problem. *Altered Parenting* is most appropriate when an external factor challenges the parents. External factors do not cause child abuse; rather, emotional disturbances and ineffective coping do.

Key Concepts

1. In the past, because of living in extended families, young children observed and frequently assisted in the birth and care of infants. Today in the United States, because of our mobile society and the more isolated nuclear family life-style, young men and women

often approach parenthood with only a vague recollection of their own childhood, little knowledge of the birthing process, and limited, if any, experience in infant and child care.

2. Parenting is a learned behavior, and in general, people parent as they were parented.

3. Families acquire children through birth, adoption, and remarriage. Sometimes grandparents assume the parenting role for grandchildren because of the loss of parents, substance abuse, or a history of ineffective parenting (Janosik & Green, 1991).

4. Even though many parents anticipate the birth of their child with pleasure, most are unprepared for the changes that will occur. After a child is born, parental self-concepts develop. For a woman, her role as parent often overshadows her role as wife and individual. For a man, parenthood strengthens his role as husband and worker. Parenting often becomes a dominant role for women and a secondary role for men (Janosik & Green, 1991).

5. Situations that contribute to abuse are often related to ineffective individual or family coping. (See *Ineffective Family Coping: Disabling, as evidenced by child abuse.*)

6. Parenting behaviors are affected by perception of their child's vulnerability. Early life-threatening events (*e.g.*, illness, accident, prematurity) may lead to disturbed parent–child relationships, which may result in problematic psychosocial development. This phenomenon, termed the "vulnerable child syndrome," has important implications for nurses working with parents during the recovery phase of an illness.

Focus Assessment Criteria

Subjective/Objective Data

A. Assess for defining characteristics
    1. Attachment behavior
        Pregnancy
            Planned?   Was an abortion considered?
            Desired?   If yes, why was decision changed?
        Prenatal
            Verbalizes anticipation   Seeks prenatal care
            Selects name   Follows the regimen
            Plans layette
            Decides about infant feeding (breast or bottle)
        Intrapartum
            Participates in the decision and the birthing process
            Verbalizes positive feelings
            Attempts to see infant as soon as delivered
            Responds positively (happy) or negatively (sad, apathetic, disappointed, angry, ambivalent)
            Holds and talks to infant
            Uses baby's name
            Talks to baby's father
        Postpartum
            Verbalizes positive feelings
            Seeks proximity by holding infant closely; touches and hugs
            Smiles and gazes at infant; seeks eye-to-eye contact
            Seeks family resemblance (*i.e.*, "has my eyes," "sleeps like his father")
        Refers to infant by name and sex
        Expresses interest in learning infant care
        Performs nurturing behavior (*i.e.*, feeding, changing)
    2. Parent–child relationship
        Subjective
            Parental level of satisfaction with child
            Amount of play activities between mother and child

Amount of play activities between father and child
Amount of caretaking activities between mother and child
Amount of caretaking activities between father and child
Provisions for child development (toys, verbal stimulation)
Reasons for disciplining
Methods of discipline or punishment
Assess for presence of at-risk factors in parent and child (see Related Factors)
Objective
Child's affect (animated, warm, apathetic, cold, withdrawn)
Presence of touching/holding behavior
Presence of injuries
Explanation by child and parent
Correlation of explanation to injury
History of injuries (type, causes)
3. Observe
Parent–child interactions
Parental participation in caretaking activities
Parental comforting of child
Parental gathering and assimilation of information related to their child and themselves
Family communication patterns
Visiting patterns and changes in visiting patterns

B. Assess for related factors
1. Family structure/roles
Characteristics of the family: age and sex of family members, cultural and religious backgrounds, occupations of parents.
Roles of parents within and outside of family structure; identify potential for role conflicts
Demands of daily living (employment, financial)
Social support systems of parent(s)
Location of most relatives
Frequency of visits with relatives
Length of time lived at present residence
Patterns of parental socialization with friends and relatives
Interrelationship between parents
2. Parenting knowledge/experience
Parents' recall of their relationship with their parents or caretakers and types of discipline and punishment used
Experiences with previous pregnancies
Knowledge of developmental needs and demands
Parental expectations of child
3. What effects has having a child had on
Personal freedom   Marital relations
Leisure time   Career

Outcome Criteria

The parent/primary caregiver will
• Acknowledge a problem with parenting skills
• Provide a safe environment for child
• Describe resources available for assistance with improvement of parenting skills

Interventions

A. Encourage parents to express their frustrations regarding role responsibilities and/or parenting

   1. Convey empathy.
   2. Reserve judgment.

B. Explore parent's expectations of self, partner, child

   1. Help to develop realistic expectations
   2. Encourage discussion of feelings regarding unmet expectations.
   3. Discuss strategies that might increase the likelihood of expectations being met (*e.g.*, discussing with partner, child, setting personal goals).

C. Educate parents on normal growth and development and expected behaviors that are age related (refer to *Altered Growth and Development*)

D. Explore with parents the child's problem behavior (Herman-Staab, 1994)

   1. Frequency, duration
   2. Situational context (when, where, triggers)
   3. Consequences of problem behavior (parental attention, discipline, inconsistencies in response)
   4. Behavior desired by parents

E. Discuss positive parenting techniques (Herman-Staab, 1994)

   1. Convey to child that he or she is loved.
   2. Catch child being good; use good eye contact.
   3. Set aside "special time" when the parent guarantees a time with child without interruptions.
   4. Ignore minor transgressions by having no physical contact or eye contact or discussion about the behavior.
   5. Practice active listening. Describe what child is saying, reflect back the child's feelings, and do not judge.
   6. Use "I" statements when disapproving of behavior. Focus on the act as undesirable, not the child.

F. Explain the discipline technique of "time-out," which is a method to stop misconduct, convey disapproval, and provide both parent and child with time to regroup (Christophersen, 1992; Herman-Staab, 1994)

   1. Outline the procedure:
      a. Place or bring the child to a chair in a quiet place with few distractions (not the child's room or an isolated place).
      b. Instruct the child to stay in the chair. Set timer for 1 minute of quiet time for each year of age.
      c. Start the timer when the child is quiet.
      d. If the child misbehaves, cries, or gets off the chair, reset the timer.
      e. When the timer goes off, tell the child it is okay to get up.
   2. Explain to the child:
      a. This is not a game.
      b. Practice it once when then child is behaving.
      c. Explain rules and then ask the child questions to ensure understanding (if 3 years or older).
   3. Remember
      a. Do not warn child before sending for time out. If time out is appropriate, use it; do not threaten.
      b. If child laughs during time out, ignore it.

    c. Be sure no TV is on or can be seen.

    d. Do not look at or talk to or about him or her during time out.

    e. Do not act angry; remain calm.

    f. Keep yourself busy; let the child see you and what he or she is missing.

    g. Do not give up or give in.

G. If additional sources of conflict arise, refer to the specific nursing diagnosis (*e.g., Caregiver Role Strain, Fatigue, Altered Patterns of Sexuality*)

H. Take opportunities to role-model effective parenting skills; if relevant, share some of the frustrations you have experienced with your child in an attempt to normalize the frustrations

I. Clarify the strengths of the parents or family

J. Role-play asking for help or disciplining a child

K. Provide with general parenting guidelines

1. Practice open, honest dialogues. Never threaten (*e.g.,* "If you are bad I will not take you to the movies").

2. Do not lecture. Tell the child he was wrong and let it go. Spend time talking about pleasant experiences.

3. Compliment children on their achievements. Make each child feel important and special. Especially tell a child when he has been good; try not to focus on negative behavior.

4. Do not be afraid to hold and hug (boys as well as girls).

5. Set limits and keep them. Expect cooperation. Encourage the child to participate in activities that conform to your values. Do not be trapped by "But everybody else can."

6. Let the child help you as much as possible.

7. Discipline the child by restricting his activity. For a younger child, sit him in a chair for 3–5 minutes. If the child gets up, reprimand or spank him once and put him back. Continue until the child sits for the prescribed time. For an older child, restrict bicycle riding or movie-going (pick an activity that is important to him).

8. Make sure the discipline corresponds to the unacceptable behavior. Children should be allowed opportunities to make mistakes and to express anger verbally.

9. Spank, if necessary, only once (the first spank is for the child, the rest are for you). Stay in control. Try not to discipline when you are irritated.

10. Remember to examine what you are doing when you are not disciplining your child (*e.g.,* enjoying each other, loving each other).

11. Never reprimand a child in front of another person (child or adult). Take the child aside and talk.

12. Never decide you cannot control a child's destructive behavior. Examine your present response. Are you threatening? Do you follow through with the punishment or do you give in? Has the child learned you do not mean what you say?

13. Be a good model (the child learns from you whether you intend it or not). Never lie to a child even when you think it is better; the child must learn that you will not lie to him, no matter what.

14. Give each child a responsibility suited to his age, such as picking up toys, making beds, or drying dishes. Expect the child to complete the task.

15. Share your feelings with children (happiness, sadness, anger). Respect and be considerate of the child's feelings and of his right to be human.

L. Initiate health teaching and referrals as indicated

1. Community resources—counseling, social service, parenting classes

2. Support groups—self-help, church

Rationale

- Parents need confidence, as well as skill, to be comfortable in their new role. The nurse is in the enviable position of being able to assist families by providing them with information on parenting.
- Observations of parent–child interactions should be guided by attention to the reciprocal aspect to the interaction. Parenting behaviors may be hampered by an interactive "mismatch," evidenced when the infant is demanding and the parent lacks resilience or when the child's behavior is normal and the parents' expectations of the child are unrealistic.
- Certain levels of stress interfere with the parent's ability to show patience and understanding (Wong, 1995).
- Parents who are encouraged to discuss their parenting expectations and who agree to support each other's decisions have less family tension (Wong, 1995).
- Behavioral modification techniques can be implemented effectively only when parents are consistent (Wong, 1995).
- Discipline should be implemented at the time of the undesired behavior to increase effectiveness (Wong, 1995).
- Reasoning is not appropriate with young children, who are unable to "see the other side" (Wong, 1995).
- Ignoring problem behavior can minimize or eliminate it (Wong, 1995).
- The "time out" approach avoids many of the problems of other disciplinary approaches (*e.g.*, arguing, physical punishment, loss of control) (Wong, 1995)
- Children learn to be responsible adults by having responsibilities as children.

Parent–Infant Attachment, Risk for Altered

DEFINITION

Risk for Altered Parent–Infant Attachment: The state in which there is a risk for a disruption of a nurturing, protective, interactive process between a parent/primary caregiver and infant.

RISK FACTORS

Refer to Related Factors.

RELATED FACTORS
Pathophysiologic

Related to interruption of attachment process secondary to:
  Parental illness   Infant illness

Treatment-Related

Related to barriers to attachment secondary to:
  Lack of privacy   Intensive care monitoring
  Structured "visitation"   Equipment
  Restricted visitors

Situational (Personal, Environmental)

Related to unrealistic expectations (*e.g.*, of child, of self)

Related to unplanned pregnancy

Related to disappointment with infant (*e.g.*, gender, appearance)

Related to life event stressors associated with new baby and other responsibilities secondary to:

Health issues   Substance abuse

Mental illness   Relationship difficulties

Economic difficulties

Related to lack of knowledge and/or available role model for parental role

Related to physical disabilities of parent (*e.g.*, blindness, paralysis, deafness)

Related to being emotionally unprepared due to premature delivery of infant

Maturational

Adolescent

Related to difficulty delaying her own gratification for the gratification of the infant

Author's Note

This new diagnosis describes a parent or caregiver who is at risk for attachment difficulties with his or her infant. Barriers to attachment can be the environment, knowledge, anxiety, and the health of the parent or infant. This diagnosis is appropriate as a risk or high-risk diagnosis. If the nurse diagnoses a problem in infant–parent attachment, the diagnosis *Risk for Altered Parenting related to difficulties in parent–child attachment* would be more useful so that the nurse could focus on improving attachment and preventing destructive parenting patterns.

Errors in Diagnostic Statements

Risk for Altered Parent–Infant Attachment related to husband not being the biologic father of the infant

These related factors are certainly risk factors associated with attachment problems; however, this information is confidential and caution should be used to protect its disclosure. If it is shared during an assessment or interaction, the nurse should record it exactly in quotes in the progress notes. The nursing diagnosis can be written *Risk for Altered Parent–Infant Attachment related to possible rejection of infant by father*.

Key Concepts

1. The maternal–child relationship begins before conception by planning the pregnancy and its conception, as described by the following steps (Josten, 1981): planning the pregnancy, confirming the pregnancy, accepting the pregnancy, feeling fetal movement, accepting the fetus as an individual, giving birth, hearing and seeing the baby, touching and holding the baby, and caring for the baby.

2. Participation of the father in caregiving activities in American society has increased. Fathers who choose the traditional role (allowing the mother to be totally responsible for caretaking activities) must be assessed in their sociocultural context.

3. Attachment during the postpartum period is influenced by three factors: the characteristics of the baby—its appearance and behavior (alert); the characteristics of each parent (satisfaction with baby, beliefs about ability to care for baby, ability to console and comfort baby, frequency of interactions with baby); and support—the availability of a positive resource person (relative, neighbor) and the availability of follow-up for high-risk families.

4. The attachment process is impeded when the parent(s) and child are separated because of the condition of the infant or a parent (Klaus & Kennell, 1976). Neonatal intensive care units (NICU) should be structured so that the process of the parent–infant relationship

can be supported (Brown, Pearl, & Carrasco, 1991). Thurman (1991) describes a family-centered NICU as a setting adhering to the following parameters:

   a. Services are provided based on family identified and perceived needs.
   b. There is an adaptive fit between the family system and the service delivery system.
   c. Family empowerment is fostered while a stable ongoing support system is provided.
   d. The dynamism and complexity of the family system is recognized.

5. Mercer and Ferketich (1990) studied parental attachment of 121 high-risk women, 61 partners of high-risk women, 182 low-risk women, and 117 partners of low-risk women and found that the major predictor of parental attachment for all four groups was parental competence.

6. Parents of a premature infant or an infant with malformations may feel a sense of failure, leading to low self-esteem and subsequent difficulties with attachment (Klaus & Kennell, 1976).

7. No single behavior during pregnancy or in the postpartum period can be a conclusive sign of attachment difficulty. The presence of several characteristic signs should direct the nurse to gather more data.

8. Disorders of attachment may lead to manifestation of nonorganic failure to thrive—failure of a child to grow without an organic cause.

9. In multiple births, attachment takes longer because a mother can attach optimally only to one infant at a time. Mothers may feel differently about each infant of a multiple birth based on characteristics of the infants, such as health status or birth weight (Theroux, 1989).

Focus Assessment Criteria

Refer to *Altered Parenting* for assessment of attachment behaviors.

Outcome Criteria

The parent will
- Demonstrate increased attachment behaviors, such as holding infant close, smiling and talking to infant, and seeking eye contact with infant
- Be supported in his or her need to be involved in infant's care
- Begin to verbalize positive feelings regarding the infant

Interventions

A. Assess causative or contributing factors
   1. Maternal
      a. Unwanted pregnancy
      b. Prolonged or difficult labor and delivery
      c. Postpartum pain or fatigue
      d. Lack of positive support system (mother, spouse, friends)
      e. Lack of positive role model (mother, relative, neighbor)
      f. Inability to prepare emotionally for an unexpected delivery
   2. Parental inadequate coping patterns (one or both parents)
      a. Alcoholic
      b. Drug addict
      c. Marital difficulties (separation, divorce, violence)
      d. Change in lifestyle related to new role
      e. Adolescent parent
      f. Career change (*e.g.*, working woman to mother)
      g. Illness in family

3. Infant
   a. Premature, defective, ill
   b. Multiple birth

B. Eliminate or reduce contributing factors, if possible
   1. Illness, pain, fatigue
      a. Establish with mother what infant-care activities are feasible.
      b. Provide mother with uninterrupted sleep periods of at least 2 hours during the day and 4 hours during the night.
      c. Provide relief for discomforts.

      Episiotomy
         Evaluate degree of pain.
         Assess for hematomas and abscesses.
         Provide with comfort measures (ice, warm compresses, analgesics*).

      Hemorrhoids
         Prevent and treat constipation.
         Provide comfort measures (compresses with witch hazel, suppositories,* analgesics*).

      Breast engorgement of nursing mother
         Nurse as frequently as possible.
         Apply warm compresses (shower) before nursing.
         Apply cold compresses after nursing.
         Try hand massage, hand expressing, or breast pump between nursing.
         Offer mild analgesics.
         See *Ineffective Breast-feeding*.

      Breast engorgement of nonnursing mother
         Offer analgesics as ordered.
         Apply ice packs.
         Encourage use of a good supporting brassiere that covers the entire breast.

   2. Lack of experience or lack of positive mothering role model
      a. Explore with mother her feelings and attitudes concerning her own mother.
      b. Assist her to identify someone who is a positive mother and encourage her to seek that person's aid.
      c. Outline the teaching program available to her during hospitalization.
      d. Determine who will assist her at home initially.
      e. Identify community programs and reference material that can increase her learning about child care after discharge (see References/Bibliography).

   3. Lack of positive support system
      a. Identify parent's support system and assess its strengths (Zahr, 1991) and weaknesses.
      b. Assess the need for counseling.
         Encourage the parents to express feelings about the experience and about the future.
         Be an active listener to the parents.
         Observe the parents interacting with the infant.
         Assess for resources (financial, emotional) already available to the family.
         Be aware of resources available both within the hospital and in the community.
         Counsel the parents on assessed needs.
         Refer to hospital or community services.

   4. Barriers to practicing cultural beliefs that may affect the family unit during hospitalization
      a. Support mother–infant–family beliefs.

* May require a primary care professional's order.

b. Integrate culture and traditions into routine care.

c. Identify community resources.

5. Elimination of institutional barriers that inhibit individualizing of care

a. Sensitization of staff to practicing family-centered care

b. Use of families to review practice and policies

c. Cultural sensitization of staff

C. Provide opportunities for the process of mutual interaction

1. Promote bonding in the immediate postdelivery phase.

a. Encourage mother to hold infant following birth (may need a short recovery period).

b. Provide skin-to-skin contact if desired; keep room warm (72°–76°F) or use a heat panel over the infant.

c. Provide mother with an opportunity to breast-feed immediately after delivery, if desired.

d. Delay the administration of silver nitrate to allow for eye contact.

e. Give family as much time as they need together with minimum interruption from the staff (the "sensitive period" lasts from 30–90 minutes).

f. Encourage father to hold infant.

2. Facilitate the attachment process during the postpartum phase.

a. Check mother regularly for signs of fatigue, especially if she had anesthesia.

b. Offer flexible rooming-in to the mother; establish with her the amount of care she will assume initially and support her requests for assistance.

c. Discuss the future involvement of the father in the infant's care (if desired, plan opportunities for father to participate in his child's care during visits).

3. Provide support to the parents.

a. Listen to the mother's replay of her labor and delivery experience.

b. Allow for verbalization of feelings.

c. Indicate acceptance of feelings.

d. Point out the infant's strengths and individual characteristics to the parents.

e. Demonstrate the infant's responses to the parents.

f. Have a system of follow-up after discharge, especially for families considered at risk (*e.g.*, phone call or a home visit by the community health nurse).

g. Be aware of resources and support groups available within the hospital and the community and refer the family as needed.

4. Assess the need to support the parents' emerging confidence in child care.

a. Observe the parents interacting with the infant.

b. Support each parent's strengths.

c. Assist each parent in those areas in which they are uncomfortable (role modeling).

d. Offer classes in infant care (Mercer & Ferketich, 1990).

e. Have handouts and audiovisual aids available for parents to view at odd hours.

f. Assess for level of knowledge in the area of growth and development and provide information as needed (McCain, 1990).

g. Help parents understand infant's cues and temperament.

h. See References/Bibliography for recommended printed material on parenting and child care.

5. When immediate separation of the child from the parents is necessary because of prematurity or illness, provide for bonding/attachment experiences, as possible.

a. Invite parents to see and touch infant as soon as possible.

b. Encourage parents to spend prolonged time with infant.

c. Support activities such as skin-to-skin holding, containment of infant with parental hands in the isolette, basic caregiving activities.

d. If infant is transported to another facility and separated from mother:

Have staff make frequent calls to mother.

Encourage family to spend time in NICU and bring back verbal reports and pictures of infant.

Explore family and community resources to provide means of rejoining mother and infant as soon as possible.

D. For adoptive parents
1. Counsel adoptive mothers about the normality of a variety of emotions on first interaction with their adoptive infants.
2. Counsel adoptive mothers about the possibility of postadoption depression.
3. Encourage adoptive mothers to seek parenting classes before receiving their infant.

E. Initiate referrals, as needed
1. Consult with community agencies for follow-up visits if indicated.
2. Refer parents to pertinent organizations (see References/Bibliography).

Rationale

- Research indicates that there is a "sensitive period" during the newborn's first minutes and hours of life during which the child is beautifully equipped to meet and interact with the parents. Close contact at this time and in the days to follow is most beneficial to the bonding process (Klaus & Kennell, 1976).
- The period from birth to 3 days is an important period for the father–child relationship.
- Attachment is promoted by seeing, touching, and caring for the infant (Klaus & Kennell, 1976).
- When caring for families of high-risk neonates, foster attachment and reduce anxiety by letting parents know through frequent communication that they are welcome partners in their child's care (Kenner, 1992).
- In a longitudinal study of the interaction between 49 premature infants and their mothers, Zahr (1991) found that maternal rating of the infant's temperament and availability of support system were the most significant variables that correlated with a positive mother–infant interaction at 4 and 8 months postpartum.
- Parents are reluctant to form attachments to a sick infant because of their fear of loss. This reluctance creates tremendous guilt.
- Parents must be given the opportunity for grief work in the case of an ill or impaired infant before attachment can begin.
- The use of birthing rooms enhances the bonding process because of the decrease in interruptions.
- In a research study of 24 first-time adoptive mothers, Koepke, Anglin, Austin, and Delesalle (1991) found that adoptive mothers began developing affectional ties to their babies at much the same time and in as individual a way as birth mothers. Adoptive mothers may be as susceptible as birth mothers to periods of sadness and maternal depression.

Parental Role Conflict

DEFINITION

Parental Role Conflict: The state in which a parent or primary caregiver experiences or perceives a change in role in response to external factors (*e.g.*, illness, hospitalization, divorce, separation).

DEFINING CHARACTERISTICS
Major (Must Be Present)

Parent(s) express(es) concerns about changes in parental role
Demonstrated disruption in care and/or caretaking routines

Minor (May Be Present)

Parent(s) express(es) concerns/feelings of inadequacy to provide for child's physical and
emotional needs during hospitalization or in the home
Parent(s) express(es) concerns about effect of child's illness on other children
Parent(s) express(es) concerns about care of siblings at home
Parent(s) express(es) guilt about contributing to the child's illness through lack of knowledge, judgment, and so forth
Parent(s) express(es) concern about perceived loss of control over decisions relating to the
child
Parent(s) is (are) reluctant, unable, or unwilling to participate in normal caretaking activities, even with encouragement and support
Parent(s) verbalize(s), demonstrate(s) feelings of guilt, anger, fear, anxiety, and/or frustration

RELATED FACTORS
Situational (Personal, Environmental)

Related to separation from child secondary to:
> Birth of a child with a congenital defect and/or chronic illness
> Hospitalization of a child with an acute or chronic illness
> Change in acuity, prognosis, or environment of care (*e.g.*, transfer to or from an ICU)

Related to fear of involvement secondary to invasive or restrictive treatment modalities
(*e.g.*, isolation, intubation)
Related to interruption of family life secondary to:
> Home care of a child with special needs (*e.g.*, apnea monitoring, postural drainage,
> hyperalimentation)
> Frequent visits to hospital
> Addition of new family member (aging relative, newborn)

Related to change in ability to parent secondary to:

Illness of parent	Remarriage
Travel requirements	Dating
Work responsibilities	Death
Divorce	

Author's Note
See *Altered Parenting*

Key Concepts

1. The parental role is one of the most complex in our society because of the great number
   of role expectations and skills required for effective parenting.
2. Parenting behaviors are learned through role modeling, role rehearsal, and reference
   group interaction. External factors, both developmental (birth of a child) and situational
   (illness and/or hospitalization of a child), require the acquisition of new behaviors or the
   modification of existing parenting behaviors (Hymovich & Barnard, 1979). Difficulty in
   mastering the behaviors required for the role transition leads to role strain, uncertainty
   about what behaviors are required in the new role leads to lack of role clarity, and experiencing incompatibility between the new role expectations and already existing expectations leads to role conflict (Burr, 1972).

3. Parents experiencing their child's illness in an acute or a chronic situation are faced with the challenge of role transition to continue effective parenting on either a temporary or permanent basis. The parent must give up the role of parenting a well child and acquire the role of parenting a sick child (Jay, 1977).

4. Role conflicts can develop easily when a child receives home care from a parent or from a combination of parents and health care professionals. Role diffusion caused by the intrusion of treatments and/or providers into the home is a source of stress for the entire family and requires careful role negotiation on the part of parents and professionals (Hochstadt & Yost, 1989).

5. Clements, Copeland, and Loftus (1990) report in a study of 30 families with chronically ill children that parenting is more difficult at certain critical times: initial diagnosis; increase in physical symptoms; relocation of the child, such as rehospitalization; developmental changes for the child, such as the entrance into school; and the physical or emotional absence of one parent (*e.g.*, illness, pregnancy).

6. In a study of 45 mothers of acutely ill hospitalized children, Schepp (1991) found that predictability of events and anxiety influenced the mothers' coping effort. Mothers who knew what to expect were less anxious.

7. Using the Family Adaptation Model described by Patterson and McCubben (1983), Gallo (1991) postulates the following strategies for preventive intervention useful to nurses working with families adapting to childhood chronic illness:
   a. Focus on the family crisis.
   b. Assist family to gain a conscious grasp of the crisis to enhance problem-solving capability.
   c. Offer medical information and education about the problem.
   d. Help parents master physical care.
   e. Help parents overcome doubts of adequacy.
   f. Assist family members with interpersonal communication.
   g. Assist family in the development of social support and bridge access to community referral.

8. In reviewing 10 research studies of parental stress during hospitalization of their child in an intensive care unit, Jay and Youngblut (1991) found:
   a. Changes in parenting roles were very stressful to parents.
   b. There are differences between what mothers and fathers find stressful.
   c. Parents perceive that they sometimes experience unnecessary stress.

9. Caty, Ritchie, and Ellerton (1989) studied the coping strategies used by 32 mothers of hospitalized preschool children. The mothers described their most effective strategies in helping their child cope with a difficult situation as providing information and comfort.

Focus Assessment Criteria

Subjective Data

A. Assess family system
   1. Family structures/roles
      a. Characteristics of the family unit (as defined by the family) members, relationships, ages, sex, cultural and religious backgrounds
      b. Living accommodations, distance from hospital, transportation
      c. Roles of parents
      d. Employment, means of support
      e. Change (relocation, addition, deletion, economic)
   2. Family social support systems
      a. Presence of extended family
      b. Support from neighbors, church group, parent support group

B. Assess for related factors
   1. Recent changes, events

  a. Change in household members
  b. Occupation
  c. Marital status
 2. Child illness or hospitalization
  a. History of illness

   Acute or chronic   Resulting from an accident
   Congenital or acquired When diagnosis first made
   Knowledge of parents about diagnosis, prognosis, treatment
   Knowledge of child about diagnosis, prognosis, treatment

  b. Parent's knowledge/experiences

   Experience with own hospitalizations
   Experiences with previous hospitalizations of this child or other children
   Involvement with medical/nursing care in the home
   Knowledge of hospital systems
   Assertiveness
   Communication style and level
   Knowledge of child development and understanding of effect of hospitalization of child
   Understanding of need for this hospitalization
   Desired outcomes from current hospitalization
   Involvement in case management for child, if any

C. Assess for defining characteristics

 1. Plans for dealing with this hospitalization
  a. Visiting plans and travel arrangements
  b. Desired involvement in care
  c. Plans for acquiring information about child
  d. Plans for self-care
  e. Plans for payment of medical and hospital bills
  f. Plans for meeting other roles while child is hospitalized (*i.e.*, working, care of home and other children)
  g. Other emergent family situations that will have an impact on time and energy needed for parenting the ill child
 2. Concerns and fears

Objective Data

A. Assess for defining characteristics

 1. Parent–child interaction (observe each parent/caretaker)
  Involvement in caretaking
  Comforting of child
  Discipline of child
  Interpreting hospitalization/illness related events to child
  Support of child's development

Outcome Criteria

The parent and child will
• Express their feelings regarding the situation
The parent will
• Demonstrate control over decision making
• Identify sources of support

Interventions

A. Assess the present situation (Melnyk, 1991)
  1. Parents' and children's perceptions of and responses to situation
  2. Parental understanding of the impact of situation on children and their typical responses
  3. Changes in parenting practices and daily routines (employment or change in child care arrangements)
  4. Other related stressors (financial, job related)
  5. Level of conflict between parents
  6. Social support for both parents

B. Assist parents with gaining understanding of how their responses may affect children

C. Assist family to increase their self-determination, decision-making abilities, and self-efficacy (Dunst, Trivette, & Deal, 1988a)
  1. Emphasize parental responsibility for meeting needs and solving problems.
  2. Emphasize building on parental strengths.
  3. Provide active and reflective listening.
  4. Offer normative help that is congruent with parental appraisal of need.
  5. Promote acquisition of competencies.
  6. Use parent–professional collaboration as the mechanism for meeting needs.
  7. Allow locus of control to reside with the parent.
  8. Accept and support parental decisions.

D. Emphasize need to maintain an organized, predictable environment to promote feelings of security for children

E. Encourage children to express feelings openly

F. Consult school nurse

G. Encourage formation of and use of support groups for both parents and children

H. If parents are separating or divorcing
  1. Encourage parents to provide open and honest explanations about the reasons for divorce to allay guilt feeling of children.
  2. Emphasize that maintaining positive relationships between children and noncustodial parent is important for child's sense of self-esteem.
  3. Advise to seek counseling as individuals, couple, and family.

Rationale

- Nursing strategies based on an empowerment model are the most effective in helping parents resolve role conflict and move through role transition.
- These strategies can help parents acquire parenting behaviors that will be effective in the caring for their ill child in the hospital or the home on a temporary or long-term basis.
- Respecting parents as the experts in their child care promotes more confidence and collaboration with caregivers (Baker, 1994).

■ Parental Role Conflict
Related to Effects of Illness and/or Hospitalization of a Child

---

Outcome Criteria

Parent(s) will
- Demonstrate control over decision making concerning the child, collaborate with health professionals in making decisions about the health/illness care of the child
- Relate information about the child's health status and treatment plan
- Participate in caring for the child in the home/hospital setting to the degree he/she/they desire
- Verbalize feelings about the child's illness and the hospitalization
- Identify and use available support systems that allow parent time and energy to cope with ill child's needs

---

Interventions

A. Help parents adapt parenting behaviors to allow for continuation of parenting role during hospitalization and/or illness (Meleis, 1975; Miles, 1989)

1. Use role-supplementation strategies and role cues (Roy, 1967) to help parents adapt parenting role to meet the needs of the child.
2. Use role-model parenting behaviors appropriate to child's developmental stage and medical condition.
a. Instruct parents to continue limit-setting strategies and demonstrations of caring behaviors (*e.g.*, touching, hugging despite hospitalization and equipment).
3. Provide information to empower parents to adapt parenting role to the situation of hospitalization and/or the event of chronic illness of the child (Dunst, Trivette, Davis, & Wheeldreyer, 1988b).
4. Provide information about hospital routines and policies, such as visiting hours, mealtimes, division routines, medical and nursing routines, rooming-in, and the like (Flint & Walsh, 1988; Miles & Carter, 1983).
5. Introduce self and other health care workers involved in the child's care and explain the role of each member of the team.
6. Explain procedures and tests to parents; help them interpret these activities to the child; discuss child's age-appropriate range of responses.
7. Assess usual parenting role or interpretation of real or perceived parental role.
8. Assess parental knowledge about child's normal growth and development, safety issues, and the like, and offer supplemental information as appropriate (see *Altered Growth and Development*).
9. Teach parents special skills needed to provide for the physical and health care needs of the child.

B. Facilitate parents receiving information about the child's health status and treatment plan (Gallo, 1991; Jay & Youngblut, 1991; Schepp, 1991)

1. Foster open communication between self and parents, allowing time for questions, frequent repetition of information; provide direct and honest answers.

2. Facilitate open communication between parents and other members of the health care team.
3. Approach parents with new information; do not make them assume the responsibility for seeking out the information (Rushton, 1990).
4. When parents cannot be with their child, facilitate information-sharing through telephone calls; allow parents to call primary nurse or nurse caring for child.
5. Facilitate interdisciplinary communication so that all members of the health care team have congruent and consistent information to share with the family.
6. Minimize waiting time for parents whenever possible (Savedra, Tesher, & Ritchie 1987).
7. Assess parental understanding of the child's illness.
8. Explain and interpret medical terminology to parents to aid in their understanding of the child's condition. The list includes:
   a. What is the reason for the child's hospitalization?
   b. What is going to be done to the child during hospitalization?
   c. Will the child be awake for the procedures?
   d. Will the child feel pain or discomfort?
      Where will it hurt?
      What will be done for the discomfort?
   e. Will the child be changed in any way after the procedure? Is the change temporary or permanent?
   f. Who may visit the child? When?
   g. What may be brought to the hospital from home?
   h. How long will the child be in the hospital?
   i. Will there be any restrictions for the child at home?
9. Interpret hospital environment and events to parents.
10. Use role model interpretations of events to child; help parents interpret to child and other family members.
11. Respect confidentiality of information, share information about child with parents only, instruct other family members to obtain information from parents.
12. On an outpatient basis, parents continue to need information about medical and treatment plan as well as information about usual developmental issues of childhood (Meeropol, 1991).

C. Support continued decision making of parents concerning the child's care

1. Provide parents opportunity to help formulate plan of care for their child.
2. Use parents as source of information about the child, his or her usual behaviors, reactions, and preferences (Ogden-Burke, Castello, & Handley-Derry, 1989).
3. Recognize parents as "experts" about their child (Cardoso, 1991; Rushton, 1990).
4. Allow parents the choice to be present during treatments and procedures.
5. Involve parents in decisions about the child's care, giving them choices whenever possible.
6. Encourage both parents to share responsibility in decision making as appropriate to their usual pattern (Zaner & Bliton, 1991).

D. Allow parents to participate in caring for their child to the degree they desire (Biehler, 1992; Rushton, 1990)

1. Provide for 24-hour rooming-in for at least one parent and extended visiting for other family members.

2. Collaborate and negotiate with parents about parental tasks they wish to continue to do, tasks they wish others to assume, tasks they wish to share, and tasks they want to learn to do; continually assess changes in their desired involvement in care.

3. Assess parental ability to comfort the child; use comfort strategies that parents have indicated for the child (Jay & Youngblut, 1991; Miles & Carter, 1983).

4. Allow parents to have uninterrupted time with the child.

5. Provide consistent caregivers for the family through primary nursing; explain the primary nurse's role, responsibilities, and commitment to the parent and child (Miles & Carter, 1983; Rushton, 1990).

6. Explore with parents their personal responsibilities (*i.e.*, work schedule, sibling care, household responsibilities, responsibilities to extended family); assist them in establishing a schedule that allows sufficient caretaking time for the child and/or visiting time with the hospitalized child without frustration in meeting other role responsibilities (*e.g.*, if visiting is not possible until evening hours, delay child's bath time and allow parent to bathe child then).

E. Support parental ability to normalize the hospital/home environment for themselves and the child

1. Orient parents and child to hospital setting before admission, if possible, through prehospitalization or pretransfer tour (Miles & Carter, 1983).

2. Orient parents to the hospital environment: kitchen, playroom, tub room, treatment room, parent's lounge.

3. Orient parents on how to obtain needed supplies for self and child.

4. Orient parents to other hospital areas: cafeteria, chapel, gift shop, library, Ronald McDonald house.

5. Encourage parents to bring clothing and toys from home.

6. Allow parents to prepare home-cooked food or bring food from home if desired.

7. Encourage opportunities for families to eat meals together.

8. Provide for sibling visitation. Help parents prepare siblings for the visit (Flint & Walsh, 1988).

9. Construct daily routine around home routine as indicated by parent(s).

10. Provide privacy for parent–child interactions (*i.e.*, privacy for breast-feeding of infants, family time for teens and parents).

11. Provide parents with comfortable visiting and sleeping accommodations at the bedside, if possible, for easy access to the child.

12. Attempt to minimize stressors of the unit/division (*i.e.*, noise level, over-access by hospital personnel, unplanned patient care) that disrupt quiet/rest periods.

13. Provide age-appropriate developmental (school) and diversional activities for the child to provide for parenting opportunities.

14. Encourage opportunities for parents to take the child on leaves from the hospital, including visits home, as possible.

15. Use an interdisciplinary approach to care planning to minimize the length of hospitalization.

F. Help parents verbalize feelings about the child's illness and/or hospitalization and adaptation of the parenting role to the situation (Miles, 1979)

1. Encourage parents to express feelings and concerns about the child's illness and/or hospitalization and about the perceived need for parental role change (Myer, 1988; Rushton, 1990).

2. Provide opportunities for parents to be alone, not in the presence of the child, so they may feel free to express feelings, frustrations, fears.
3. Indicate acceptance of parental feelings.
4. Provide supportive climate in which parents feel comfortable sharing their concerns.
5. Identify members of the staff who have established a therapeutic relationship with the parents.
6. Provide opportunities for parents to talk about themselves, events related to hospitalization/illness, and real/perceived conflicts and changes in their role, whether temporary or permanent.
7. Facilitate process of adjustment to the diagnosis/prognosis and planning for future care.

G. Provide for physical and emotional needs of parents so that they have the energy and support to continue parenting during illness/hospitalization

1. Assess and facilitate parental ability to meet self-care needs (*i.e.*, rest, nutrition, activity, privacy) (Miles, 1989).
2. Allow parents an opportunity to determine the caregiving schedule to correspond with a schedule to meet their own needs.
3. Assess support systems: parent to parent, family, friends, minister, and so forth.
4. Assess, acknowledge, and facilitate family strengths.
5. Facilitate and reinforce effective coping strategies used by parents.
6. Continue to listen to parental concerns regarding the child and parental role.
7. Continue to assess additional stressors in the family setting.

H. Initiate referrals, if indicated

1. Chaplain, social service, community agencies (respite care), parent self-help groups.
2. Provide information to parents for self-referral (Austin, 1990; Myer, 1988).

Rationale

- Parents may be hampered in their acquisition of new effective parenting behaviors by feelings of anxiety, guilt, powerlessness, and diminished competence; and lack of information and/or unfamiliarity with hospital surroundings, personnel, and systems (Chan & Leff, 1982; Ogden-Burke et al., 1989).
- Nurses are in an exceptional position to use interventions to assist parents in acquiring effective parenting skills for their ill child by providing role cues (Roy, 1967) and role supplementation strategies such as role rehearsal and role modeling (Meleis, 1975).
- Nursing interventions that are instrumental in alleviating the environmental, situational, and personal stressors experienced by parents of a hospitalized child and that maximize the personal and environmental resources available to parents enhance role transition (Miles & Carter, 1983; Schepp, 1991).
- Support and enhancement of role transition for parents of an ill child can best be achieved in a setting that is guided by principles of family-centered care (Shelton, Geppson, & Johnson, 1987; Johnson, 1990) and by a nursing process that also is guided by this family-focused philosophy (Arango, 1990; Mott, 1990; Rushton, 1990).
- Based on the promotion of self-determination, decision-making capabilities, and self-efficacy, the family-centered empowerment model requires three beliefs: (1) parents are competent in or have the capacity to become competent in the care of their child; (2) parents must be given opportunities to display competencies in

the care of their children; and (3) parents need the necessary information to make informed decisions and to obtain resources to meet needs, and thus acquire control over their child's care (Dunst, Trivette, Davis, & Wheeldreyer, 1988).

- Nursing interventions based on this research should be oriented to preparing the mother for potential stressors in an effort to decrease anxiety, thus enabling mothers to spend more energy on normalizing the environment for their hospitalized children (Schepp, 1991).
- Parental stress may be mediated by (Jay & Youngblut, 1991)
  - Helping parents feel they are part of the team caring for their child and that they have all the information that is known about their child's condition
  - Allowing parents to comfort their child
  - Comforting the parent
  - Treating the child as an individual, such as using the child's name, approaching the child in an age-appropriate manner, and talking to the child even if the child is comatose
- Alexander, Powell, Williams, White, & Conlon (1988) found significantly higher anxiety levels in non–rooming-in parents of hospitalized children, especially as the duration of hospitalization increased.
- Knafl and Dixon (1984) reported that 24% of the fathers in their study reported role expansion as a result of the hospitalization of their child. Expansion included the responsibility for monitoring the child's care.
- Pass and Pass (1987) suggest providing parents with a list of questions they should be asking about their child's hospitalization.
- Alexander and coworkers (1988) found a significant level of high anxiety in non–rooming-in fathers with greater numbers of children at home, suggesting a shift in home responsibilities.

References/Bibliography

General

Cardoso, P. (1991). A parent's perspective family centered care. *Children's Health Care, 20,* 258–260.

Dunst, C. J., Trivette, C. M., & Deal, A. G. (1988a). *Enabling and empowering families: Principles and guidelines for practice.* Cambridge, MA: Brookline Books.

Hymovich, D. (1976). Parents of sick children, their needs and tasks. *Pediatric Nursing, 2*(6), 9–13.

Hymovich, D. (1981). Assessing the impact of chronic childhood illness on the family and parent coping. *Image, 13,* 71–74.

Johnson, B. (1990). The changing role of families in health care. *Children's Health Care, 19,* 234–241.

Johnson, S. H. (1986). *Nursing assessment and strategies for the family at risk: High-risk parenting* (2nd ed.). Philadelphia: J. B. Lippincott.

Koepke, J., Anglin, S. Austin, J., & Delesalle, J. (1991). Becoming parents: Feelings of adoptive mothers. *Pediatric Nursing, 17*(4), 337–340.

Pfeffer, C. R. (1981). Development issues among children of separation and divorce. In Stuart, I.R., & Abt, L.E. (Eds.). *Children of separation and divorce: Management and treatment.* New York: Van Nostrand Reinhold.

Shelton, T., Geppson, E., & Johnson, B. (1987). *Family-centered care for children with special health care needs.* Washington, DC: Association for Care of Children's Health.

Attachment

Affleck, G., & Tennen, H. (1991). The effect of newborn intensive care on parents' psychological well-being. *Children's Health Care, 20,* 6–13.

Brown, W., Pearl, L., & Carrasco, R. (1991). Evolving models of family-centered services in neonatal intensive care. *Children's Health Care, 20,* 50–52.

Josten, L. (1981). Prenatal assessment guide for illuminating possible problems with parenting. *Maternal–Child Nursing Journal, 6,* 113–117.

Mercer, R., & Ferketich S. (1990). Predictors of parental attachment during early parenthood. *Journal of Advanced Nursing, 15*(3), 268–280.

Thurman, K. (1991). Parameters for establishing family-centered neonatal intensive care services. *Children's Health Care, 20*(1), 34–40.

Zahr, L. (1991). Correlates of mother–infant interaction in premature infants from low socioeconomic background. *Pediatric Nursing, 17*(3), 259–263.

Zaner, R., & Bliton, M. (1991). Decisions in the NICU: The moral authority of parents. *Children's Health Care, 20*(1), 19–25.

Parenting, Altered

Adams, C., Eyler, F. D., & Behnke, M. (1990). Nursing interventions with mothers who are substance abusers. *Journal of Perinatal and Neonatal Nursing, 3*(4), 43–51.

Christopherson, E. R. (1992). Discipline. *Pediatric Clinics of North America, 39*, 395–411.

Herman-Staab, B. (1994). Screening, management and appropriate referral for pediatric behavior problems. *Nurse Practitioner, 19*(7), 40–49.

Janosik, E., & Green, E. (1991). *Family life: Process and practice.* Boston: Jones and Bartlett.

Kenner, C. A. (1992). Planning and implementing care. *Nurses' clinical guide: Neonatal care.* Springhouse, PA: Springhouse Corporation.

Klaus, M., & Kennell, J. (1976). *Maternal–infant bonding.* St. Louis: C. V. Mosby.

McCain, G. (1991). Parenting growing preterm infants. *Pediatric Nursing, 16*, 467–469.

Theroux, R. (1989). Multiple birth: A unique parenting experience. *Journal of Perinatal and Neonatal Nursing, 3*(1), 35–45.

Whitley, G. G. (1991). Altered parenting and the reconstituted family. *Journal of Child and Adolescent Psychiatric Mental Health Nursing, 4*(2), 72–77.

Younger, J. B. (1991). A model of parenting stress. *Research in Nursing and Health, 14*, 197–204.

Parental Role Conflict

Alexander, D., Powell, G. M., Williams, P., White, M., & Conlon, M. (1988). Anxiety levels of rooming-in and non-rooming-in parents of young hospitalized children. *Maternal–Child Nursing Journal, 17*(2), 79–98.

Arango, P. (1990). Family-centered care: Making it a reality. *Children's Health Care, 19*, 57–62.

Austin, J. (1990). Assessment of coping mechanisms used by parents and children with chronic illness. *American Journal of Maternal–Child Nursing, 15*(2), 98–102.

Baker, N. A. (1994). Avoid collisions with challenging families. *Maternal–Child Nursing Journal, 19*, 97–101.

Biehler, B. (1992). Impact of role sets on implementing self-care theory with children. *Pediatric Nursing, 18*(1), 30–34.

Burr, W. (1972). Role transitions: A reformation of theory. *Journal of Marriage and the Family, 17*, 407–415.

Caty, S., Ritchie J., & Ellerton, M. (1989). Helping hospitalized preschoolers manage stressful situations: The mother's role. *Children's Health Care, 18*, 202–209.

Chan, J. M., & Leff, P. T. (1982). Parenting the chronically ill child in the hospital: Issues and concerns. *Children's Health Care, 11*, 9–16.

Clements, D., Copeland, L., & Loftus, M. (1990). Critical times for families with a chronically ill child. *Pediatric Nursing, 16*(2), 157–161.

Dunst, C. J., Trivette, C. M., Davis, M., & Wheeldreyer, J. C. (1988b). Enabling and empowering families of children with health impairments. *Children's Health Care, 17*, 71–81.

Flint, N., & Walsh, M. (1988). Visiting policies in pediatrics: Parents' perceptions and preferences. *Journal of Pediatric Nursing, 3*, 237–245.

Gallo, A. (1991). Family adaptation in childhood chronic illness, *Journal of Pediatric Health Care, 5*, 78–85.

Hochstadt, N., & Yost, D. (1989). The health care–child welfare partnership: Transitioning medically complex children to the community. *Children's Health Care, 18*, 4–11.

Hymovich, D., & Barnard, M. (1979). *Family health care, volume two: Developmental and situational crises* (2nd ed.). New York: McGraw-Hill.

Jay, S. (1977). Pediatric intensive care: Involving parents in the care of their child. *Maternal–Child Nursing Journal, 6*, 195–204.

Jay S., & Youngblut, J. (1991). Parent stress associated with pediatric critical care nursing: Linking research and practice. *AACN Clinical Issues, 2*, 278–283.

Knafl, K., & Dixon, D. (1984). The participation of fathers in their children's hospitalization. *Issues in Comprehensive Pediatric Nursing, 7*, 269–281.

Meeropol, E. (1991). Parental needs assessment: A design for clinical nurse specialist practice. *Pediatric Nursing, 17*(5), 456–458.

Meleis, A. (1975). Role insufficiency and role supplementation: A conceptual framework. *Nursing Research, 24*, 264–271.

Melnyk, B. (1991). Changes in parent–child relationships following divorce. *Pediatric Nursing, 17*, 337–340.

Miles, M. (1989). Epilogue: The challenge of enhancing the parental role when a child is critically ill. *Maternal–Child Nursing Journal, 18*, 241–243.

Miles, M. S., & Carter, M. (1983). Assessing parental stress in intensive care units. *American Journal of Maternal–Child Nursing, 8*, 354–359.

Mott, S. (1990). *Nursing care of children and families: A holistic approach* (2nd ed.). Redwood City, CA: Addison-Wesley.

Myer, P. (1988). Parental adaptation to cystic fibrosis. *Journal of Pediatric Nursing, 2*, 20–28.

Ogden-Burke, S., Castello, E. A., & Handley-Derry, M. H. (1989). Maternal stress and repeated hospitalizations of children who are physically disabled. *Children's Health Care, 18*, 82–90.

Pass, M., & Pass, C. (1987). Anticipatory guidance for parents of hospitalized children. *Journal of Pediatric Nursing, 2*, 250–258.

Patterson, J., & McCubben, H. (1983). *Chronic illness, family stress and coping with catastrophe* (Vol. 2). New York: Brunner/Mazel.

Roy, M. C. (1967). Role cues and mothers of hospitalized children. *Nursing Research, 16*, 178–182.

Rushton, C. H. (1990). Strategies for family-centered care in the critical setting. *Pediatric Nursing, 16*, 195–199.

Savedra, M., Tesher, M., & Ritchie, J. (1987). Parent's waiting: Is it an inevitable part of the hospital experience? *Journal of Pediatric Nursing, 2*, 328–332.

Schepp, K. (1991). Factors influencing the coping effort of mothers of hospitalized children. *Nursing Research, 40*, 42–45.

Resources for the Consumer

Literature

Child care manual. ROCOM Press, P.O. Box 1577, Newark, NJ 07101.

Christophersen, E. R. (1977). *Little people: Guidelines for common sense childrearing.* Lawrence, KS: H & H Enterprises.

Mash, E. J. (1976). *Behavior modification approaches to parenting.* New York: Brunner/Mazel.

Parent resource directory. Washington, DC: Association for the Care of Children's Health.

Salk, L., & Kramer, R. (1973). *How to raise a human being.* New York: Warner Books.

Your child from 1 to 6. U.S. Department of Health and Human Services, Children's Bureau, Publication No. 30, Washington, DC 20014.

Organizations

Federation for Children with Special Needs, 312 Stuart Street, Boston, MA 02116.

LaLeche League International, 9616 Minneapolis Avenue, Franklin Park, IL 60131; also local chapters.

Parent Effectiveness Training, 531 Stevens Avenue, Solana Beach, CA 92075.

Parents for Parents, Inc., 125 Northmore Drive, Yorktown Heights, NY 10598.

Parents Helping Parents (PHP), 535 Race Street, Suite 220, San Jose, CA 95126, (408) 288-5010.

Parent Training and Information Centers (PTI's), U.S. Department of Education, 400 Maryland Ave SW, Washington, DC 20202 (202) 732-1032.

Parents Without Partners, 7910 Woodmount Avenue, Washington, DC 20014; also local chapters.

Sick Kids (Need) Involved People (SKIP), 216 Newport Drive, Severna Park, MD 21146, (301) 261-2602.

Local Counseling Services

Catholic Charities, Jewish Family Services, Christian Family Services, community agencies, and mental health centers.

Peripheral Neurovascular Dysfunction, Risk for

DEFINITION

Risk for Peripheral Neurovascular Dysfunction: A state in which an individual is at risk of experiencing a disruption in circulation, sensation, or motion of an extremity.

RISK FACTORS

Presence of risk factor (see Related Factors)

RELATED FACTORS

Pathophysiologic

Related to increased volume of (specify extremity) secondary to:

Bleeding (*e.g.*, trauma, fractures) Venous obstruction/pooling
Coagulation disorder Arterial obstruction

Related to increased capillary filtration secondary to:

Trauma Allergic response (*e.g.*, insect bites)
Severe burns (thermal, electrical) Venomous bites (*e.g.*, snake)

Hypothermia   Nephrotic syndrome
Frostbite
Related to restrictive envelope secondary to:
Circumferential burns of extremities   Excessive pressure

Treatment-Related

Related to increased volume secondary to:
Infiltration of intravenous infusion   Dislocated prosthesis (knee, hip)
Excessive movement   Nonpatent wound drainage system
Related to increased capillary filtration secondary to:
Total knee replacement   Total hip replacement
Related to restrictive envelope secondary to:
Tourniquet   Antishock trousers
Blood pressure cuff   Excessive traction
Cast   Circumferential dressings, Ace wraps
Brace   Air splints
Restraints   Premature or tight closure of fascial defects

Author's Note

This diagnosis represents a situation that nurses can prevent by identifying who is at risk and implementing measures to reduce or eliminate the causative or contributing factors. *Risk for Peripheral Neurovascular Dysfunction* can change to compartmental syndrome. *Potential Complication: Compartmental Syndrome* is inadequate tissue perfusion in a muscle, usually an arm or leg, caused by edema, which obstructs venous circulation and causes arterial occlusion. The nursing focus for compartmental syndrome is diagnosing its presence and notifying the physician. The medical interventions required to abate the problem are surgical ones such as evacuation of hematoma, repair of damaged vessels, or a fasciotomy. Refer to *Potential Complication: Compartmental Syndrome*, if indicated.

Errors in Diagnostic Statements

Risk for Peripheral Neurovascular Dysfunction related to thrombus in left leg.

This situation does not represent a high-risk situation that a nurse can prevent but, rather, a situation that requires nursing- and physician-prescribed interventions. The collaborative problem, *Potential Complication: Thrombus left leg*, would accurately describe this situation.

Risk for Peripheral Neurovascular Dysfunction related to cast

Although the cast is an influencing factor, this diagnosis implies that the cast is the problem. The problem is edema formation. The cast aggravates the condition because as edema increases the cast provides external compression. The diagnosis should contain both risk factors as *High Risk for Peripheral Neurovascular Dysfunction related to the effects of edema formation secondary to fractured tibia and compression effect of cast.*

Key Concepts

1. The most frequent cause of medical litigation in North America is failure to diagnose neurovascular compromise, which advances to compartmental syndrome (Bourne & Rorabeck, 1989).
2. After trauma or surgery or with certain therapeutic measures, obstruction of blood flow can be the result of:
   Edema   Embolus (air, fat, blood)
   Clot formation   Blood vessel trauma
   Pressure on the vessels (cast, tourniquet, restraints, constrictive nature of burned tissue)

3. Neurovascular compromise occurs when there is increased tissue pressure in a space-limiting envelope or site (Slye, 1991).
4. Factors that can limit a space are anatomic, such as skin or muscle fascia; pathophysiologic, such as circumferential burns of extremities; or treatment related, such as casts (Slye, 1991).
5. Factors that can increase tissue pressure or envelope content are bleeding, edema formation, or anything that decreases arterial pressure or increases venous pressure (Slye, 1991).
6. Vascular insufficiency and nerve compression from edema can reduce blood supply to an extremity and result in peripheral nerve damage (Slye, 1991). Permanent damage can result within 4–12 hours.
7. Compartments are areas of muscle, nerve, and blood vessels that are encased in inelastic boundaries of skin, muscle fascia, and bone. The body has 46 compartments, with 38 found in the arms or legs (Ross, 1991).
8. The effects of venous compression and the resulting signs and symptoms are outlined in Figure II-5.
9. Lower leg pain that is worse after running may indicate chronic compartmental syndrome. The achy, pounding leg pain occurs after muscles warm up (usually 5–10 minutes) and can persist for several minutes to hours (Landry, 1994).

Focus Assessment Criteria

Subjective Data

A. Assess for related factors
    1. History of
        Compromised peripheral circulation
        Peripheral thrombosis
    2. Tobacco use

Objective Data

A. Assess for related factors
    1. Edema
    2. Pressure on vessels
        Cast
        Restraints

Outcome Criteria

The individual will continue to demonstrate
- Palpable peripheral pulses
- Warm extremities
- Capillary refill less than 3 seconds

Interventions

A. Assess and evaluate neurovascular status at least every hour for first 24 hours; compare to unaffected limb, if possible
    1. Skin
        Temperature (cool, warm)
        Color (pale, dependent, rubor, flushed, cyanotic)
    2. Bilateral pulses (radial, posterior tibial, dorsalis pedis)
        Rate, rhythm

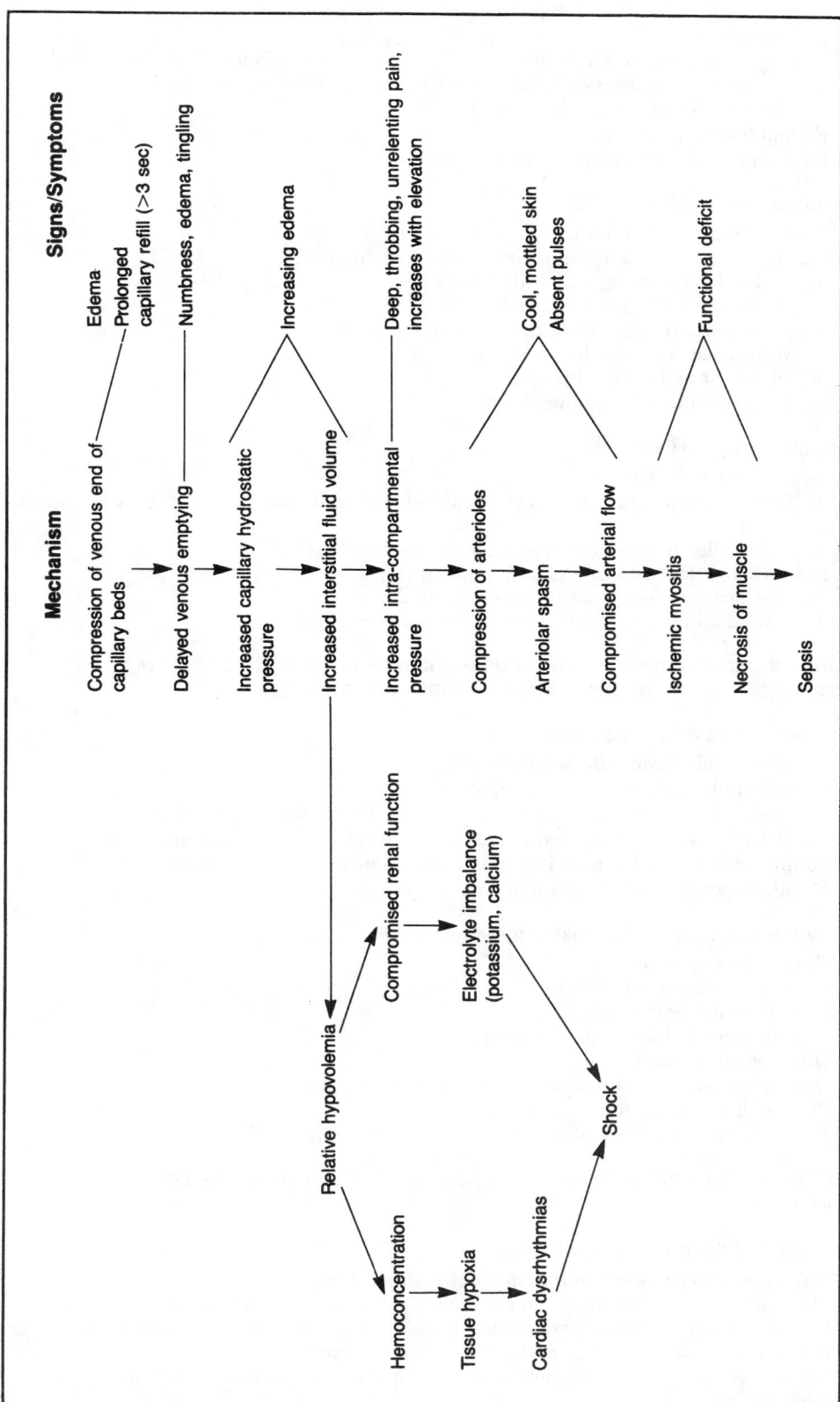

Fig. II-5 The effects of venous compression (Ross, 1991; Peck, 1991).

Volume
    0 = Absent, nonpalpable   +3 = Normal, easily palpable
    +1 = Thready, weak, fades in and out   +4 = Aneurysmal
    +2 = Present but diminished
  3. Edema (location, pitting)
  4. Capillary refill (normal less than 3 seconds)

B. For injured arms (Ross, 1991)
  1. Assess for movement ability.
    a. Hyperextension of thumbs, wrist, and four fingers
    b. Abduction (fanning out of) all fingers
    c. Touch thumb to small finger
  2. Assess sensation with pressure from a sharp point.
    a. Web space between thumb and index finger
    b. Distal fat pad of small finger
    c. Distal surface of the index finger

C. For injured legs (Ross, 1991)
  1. Assess for movement ability.
    a. Dorsiflex (upward movement) ankle and extend toes at metatarsal phalangeal joints.
    b. Plantarflex (downward movement) ankle and toes.
  2. Assess sensation with pressure from a sharp point.
    a. Web space between great toe and second toe
    b. Medial and lateral surfaces of the sole (upper third)

D. Instruct to report unusual, new, or different sensations, such as tingling, numbness, and/or decreased ability to move toes or fingers

E. Reduce edema or its effects on function
  1. Remove jewelry from affected limb.
  2. Elevate limbs unless contraindicated.
  3. Advise to move fingers or toes of affected limb two to four times per hour.
  4. Apply ice bags around injured site. Place a cloth between ice bag and skin.
  5. Monitor drainage (characteristics, amount) from wounds or incisional site.
  6. Maintain patency of the wound drainage system.

F. Notify the physician if the following occur
  1. Change in sensation
  2. Change in movement ability
  3. Pale, mottled, or cyanotic skin
  4. Capillary refill slower than 3 seconds
  5. Diminished or absent pulse
  6. Increasing pain or pain not controlled by medication
  7. Pain with passive stretching of muscle
  8. Pain increased with elevation

G. If foregoing signs or symptoms occur, discontinue elevation and ice application

H. Promote circulation in affected limb
  1. Ensure hydration is optimal to maximize circulation.
  2. Monitor traction apparatus and splints for pressure on vessels or nerves.
  3. If wrist or ankle restraints are used, monitor for pressure on vessels or nerves. Remove at least every hour and perform range-of-motion.
  4. Encourage active range-of-motion of unaffected body parts and ambulation, if permissible.

I. After hip or knee joint replacement
    1. Maintain correct positioning to prevent prosthetic dislocation
        a. Hip: keep in abduction at 45° or less
        b. Knee: slightly elevated from hip; do not flex or hyperextend
    2. Keep the affected joint in neutral position with rolls, pillows, or specified devices.

J. Initiate health teaching, as indicated
    1. Teach the client and family to watch for and report the following symptoms:
        a. Severe pain
        b. Numbness or tingling
        c. Swelling
        d. Skin discoloration
        e. Paralysis or reduced movement
        f. Cool, white toes or fingertips
        g. Foul odor, warm spots, soft areas, or cracks in the cast
    2. Emphasize the importance of follow-up evaluations.

Rationale

- Swelling that cannot be controlled causes increased tissue pressure and occlusion of the blood supply to nerve and muscle tissue, resulting in anoxia. This complication is compartmental syndrome.
- Dehydration or hypovolemia decreases circulating volume and tissue perfusion, thus increasing neurovascular compromise.
- Neurovascular compromise often begins as minor sensations; early detection can enable prompt intervention to prevent serious complications (Slye, 1991).
- A sudden change in temperature, drop in pressure, or absence of pulses indicates graft thrombosis. Changes in sensation or motor function can indicate compartmental syndrome (Dixon & Nunnelee, 1987).
- After a period of ischemia comes a period of increased capillary wall permeability. Restoration of arterial flow causes plasma and extracellular fluid to flow into the tissues, producing massive swelling in calf muscles. Pain and muscle tension result as the tissues are prevented from extending outward by the fascia and the inward pressure obliterates the circulation. The nerves become anoxic, causing paresthesias and motor deficits (Dixon & Nunnelee, 1987).
- Edema at the fracture site can compromise muscular vascular perfusion. Stretching of the damaged muscle causes pain. Sensory deficit is an early sign of nerve ischemia; the specific area of change indicates the affected compartment (Ross, 1991).
- Damaged tissue and muscles may not provide adequate support of the hip joint, resulting in displacement.
- Edema impairs circulation; however, if the extremity is elevated above heart level, this may decrease arterial blood flow. In a partial-thickness burn, edema may diminish blood flow and thus increase the depth of the burn wound (Schuman, 1991).
- Postoperative edema is expected in the newly vascularized limb. Careful assessment alerts the nurse to edema severe enough to cause compartmental syndrome. Treatment must be initiated within 8 hours to preserve function of the extremity (Dixon & Nunnelee, 1987).

References/Bibliography

Bourne, R. B., & Rorabeck, C. H. (1989). Compartmental syndrome of the lower leg. *Clinical Orthopaedics and Related Research, 240,* 97–104.

Dixon, M., & Nunnelee, J. (1987). Arterial reconstruction for atherosclerotic occlusive disease. *Journal of Cardiovascular Nursing, 1*(2), 36–49.

Landry, G. L. (1994). Sports medicine. In F. Oski (Ed.). *Principles and practice of pediatrics* (2nd ed.). Philadelphia: J. B. Lippincott.

Peck, S. (1991). Crush syndrome. *Orthopaedic Nursing, 9*(3), 33–40.

Ross, D. (1991). Acute compartment syndrome. *Orthopaedic Nursing, 10*(2), 33–38.

Schuman, L. (1991). Care of the patient with major burns. In R. B. Trofino (Ed.). *Nursing care of the burn injured patient.* Philadelphia: F. A. Davis.

Slye, D. A. (1991). Orthopedic complications. *Nursing Clinics of North America, 26,* 113–132.

Post-Trauma Response

Rape Trauma Syndrome

Post-Trauma Response

DEFINITION
Post-Trauma Response: A state in which the individual experiences a sustained painful response to one or more overwhelming traumatic events that have not been assimilated.

DEFINING CHARACTERISTICS
Major (Must Be Present)
Reexperience of the traumatic event, which may be identified in cognitive, affective, and/or sensory motor activities such as:
    Flashbacks, intrusive thoughts
    Repetitive dreams/nightmares
    Excessive verbalization of the traumatic event(s)
    Survival guilt or guilt about behavior required for survival
    Painful emotion, self-blame, shame, or sadness
    Vulnerability or helplessness, anxiety, or panic
    Fear of repetition, death, or loss of bodily control
    Angry outbursts/rage, startle reaction
    Hyperalertness or hypervigilance

Minor (May Be Present)
    Psychic/emotional numbness
        Impaired interpretation of reality, impaired memory
        Confusion, dissociation, or amnesia
        Vagueness about the traumatic event(s)
        Narrowed attention or inattention/daze
        Feeling of numbness, constricted affect
        Feeling detached/alienated
        Reduced interest in significant activities
        Rigid role-adherence or stereotyped behavior
    Altered life-style
        Submissiveness, passiveness, or dependency
        Self-destructiveness (*e.g.*, alcohol/drug abuse, suicide attempts, reckless driving, illegal activities)
        Thrill-seeking activities
        Difficulty with interpersonal relationships
        Development of phobia regarding trauma
        Avoidance of situations or activities that arouse recollection of the trauma
        Social isolation/withdrawal, negative self-concept
        Sleep disturbances, emotional disturbances
        Irritability, poor impulse control, or explosiveness
        Loss of faith in people or the world, feeling of meaninglessness in life
        Feeling of not achieving normally expected life goals
        Sense of foreshortened future or disturbance in orientation of the future
        Chronic anxiety or chronic depression
        Somatic preoccupation/multiple physiologic symptoms

RELATED FACTORS
Situational (Personal, Environmental)

Related to traumatic events of natural origin, including
> Floods
> Earthquakes
> Volcanic eruptions
> Storms
> Avalanches
> Epidemics (may be of human origin)
> Other natural disasters, which are overwhelming to most people

Related to traumatic events of human origin, such as

Wars	Concentration camp confinement
Airplane crashes	Torture
Serious car accidents	Assault
Large fires	Rape
Bombing	

Related to industrial disasters (nuclear, chemical, or other life-threatening accidents)

Author's Note

The diagnosis *Post-Trauma Response* represents a group of emotional responses to a traumatic event of either natural origin (*e.g.*, floods, volcanic eruptions, earthquakes) or human origin (*e.g.*, war, rape, torture). The emotional responses (*e.g.*, guilt, shame, fear, anger) interfere with interpersonal relationships and can precipitate self-destructive behavior (*e.g.*, alcohol/drug abuse, suicide attempts). The nurse may find it necessary to use additional diagnoses when specific interventions are indicated (*e.g.*, *Ineffective Family Coping, Risk for Self-Harm*).

The diagnosis *Rape Trauma Syndrome* was described in 1975 as encompassing an acute phase of disorganization and a long-term phase of reorganization. Based on the most recent definition of syndrome nursing diagnoses as a cluster of associated nursing diagnoses, this diagnosis does not represent a syndrome and would be more accurately labeled *Rape Trauma Response*. The inclusion of causative or contributing factors with this category is unnecessary, because the etiology is always rape. Thus, the second part of the diagnostic statement is omitted; however, the individual's report of the rape can be added to the statement. For example, *Rape Trauma Syndrome as evidenced by the report of a sexual assault and sodomy on June 22 and multiple facial bruises* (refer to ER record for description).

Errors in Diagnostic Statements

Post-Trauma Response related to expressions of survival guilt and recurring nightmares of auto accident

Survival guilt and nightmares of a traumatic event represent possible manifestations of post-trauma response, not related factors. The diagnosis should be restated as *Post-Trauma Response related to auto accident, as evidenced by recurring nightmares and expressions of survival guilt.*

Key Concepts

1. Trauma victims are identified as having specific health-related problems that need nursing care.
2. Trauma is defined in terms of the subjective experience of (an) overwhelming event(s) that cannot be dealt with or assimilated in the usual way.
3. Traumatic situations differ from ordinary experience in that they involve realistic danger of physiologic or psychological destruction that could mobilize fear of death.

4. A traumatic event may affect only a single person or many people at once, and it may be of human origin (*e.g.*, rape or wars) or natural origin (*e.g.*, avalanches or volcanic eruptions).
5. In general, traumatic events of natural origins are less severe or long-lasting compared with those of human origin (Green, 1990; Green & Lindy, 1994), because those of human origin are often perceived as resulting from indifference, negligence, or malice.
6. Despite different types of traumatic events, there are commonly shared human responses: reexperiencing the trauma, reduced psychic and emotional functioning, and altered adaptation pattern and life-style.
7. Horowitz (1986a, 1986b) conceptualized these phenomena and postulated a phasic tendency in human responses to traumatic events.
   a. The initial response to trauma is to survive and function in the immediate life-threatening situation by using all resources.
   b. The powerful coping method of "numbing" is used to reduce psychological and emotional impact.
   c. However, in an attempt to master the traumatic experience, intrusive recollection or reenactment of the trauma erupts into conscious awareness.
   d. There is a pattern of oscillation between "numbing" and intrusive reactions peculiar to each individual.
   e. Gradually, the individual works through the trauma by using a broader perception and rationale for the event and the aftermath.
   f. Finally, such an experience is assimilated into a meaningful whole that is congruent with basic beliefs and values.
8. Severity of trauma is associated with intensity, duration, and frequency of the traumatic experience. It involves a complex interaction of environmental conditions and the person's subjective experiences, such as degree of warning, threat to life, exposure to the grotesque, bereavement, displacement, and moral conflict about the role of the survivor.
9. Individual characteristics, such as early childhood experience, developmental phase, and character strength, may affect the outcome of responses to trauma.
   a. Unresolved childhood conflicts may be reactivated by the current trauma.
   b. Age can be a crucial factor, because trauma can interrupt a stage of human development.
   c. Individual coping resources are important when a person is confronted by a traumatic situation, and they influence the effectiveness of adaptation.
10. Cultural background also plays an important role in defining how a survivor deals with trauma (Kroll, 1989; Lebowitz & Roth, 1994).
11. Nurses need to explore their own feelings about traumas they encounter before attempting to intervene effectively with trauma victims.
12. The nurse may not see every symptom of trauma response, particularly when a victim is coping with "numbing."

🌀 *Key Concepts—Child*

1. A child's response to trauma depends on the nature and the extent of the trauma, the child's developmental age, and the response of significant others (Wong, 1995).

Focus Assessment Criteria

Subjective/Objective Data

A. Assess for defining characteristics
   1. History of the trauma*
      a. Ask if person was exposed to very stressful, disturbing situations like major earthquakes or floods, very serious accidents or fires, physical assault or rape, seeing

* May require a primary care professional's order.

other people killed or dead, being in war or heavy combat, or some other type of disaster during his or her life.
   b. List all traumas, including dates and duration.
2. The person's responses to the traumatic event(s)
   a. Ask about person's thoughts, feelings, or actions that he or she feels have been different since the traumatic experience, to assess signs and symptoms of reexperiencing or numbing responses.
   b. Ask if person's general life-style or pattern has changed since the traumatic event(s), to assess any readjustment difficulties.
3. Observe or consult with family members or other appropriate persons, as possible.
   a. Excessive verbalization of the traumatic events
   b. Preoccupation with trauma reminders, such as sorting through pictures or other trauma-related objects
   c. Use of denial, distortion, minimization, exaggeration, disavowal, fantasy, or avoidance
   d. Evidence of indifference or dissociation to stimuli (questions, noise, activities around him or her)
   e. Sudden or significant behavioral/personality changes since the traumatic event

---

Outcome Criteria

Short-Term Goals
The person will
- Report a lessening of reexperiencing the trauma or numbing symptoms
- Acknowledge the traumatic event and begin to work with the trauma by talking over the experience and expressing feelings such as fear, anger, and guilt
- Identify and make connection with support persons/resources

Long-Term Goals
The person will
- Assimilate the experience into a meaningful whole and go on to pursue his or her life, as evidenced by goal setting

---

Interventions

A. Determine if the person has experienced a traumatic event
   1. When interviewing the person, secure a quiet room where there will be no interruptions, but easy access to other staff in case of management problems.
   2. Be aware that talking about a traumatic experience may cause significant discomfort to the person.
   3. If the person becomes too anxious, the assessment should be discontinued and the person helped to regain control of the distress or provided with other appropriate intervention.

B. Evaluate the severity of the responses and the effects on current functioning level

C. Assist person to decrease extremes of reexperiencing or numbing symptoms
   1. Provide a safe, therapeutic environment where the person can regain control.
   2. Reassure the person that these feelings/symptoms are often experienced by the individuals who underwent such traumatic events.
   3. Stay with the person and offer support during an episode of high anxiety (see *Anxiety* for additional information).

4. Assist the person to control impulsive acting-out behavior by setting limits, promoting ventilation, and redirecting excess energy into physical exercise activity (*e.g.*, gym, walking, jogging). (See *Risk for Self-Harm* and *Risk for Violence* for additional information.)
5. Recognize that psychic/emotional numbness cushions the person's emotional impact.

D. Assist person to acknowledge the traumatic event and begin to work through the trauma by talking over the experience and expressing feelings such as fear, anger, and guilt

1. Provide a safe, structured setting for the person to describe the traumatic experience and to express feelings.
2. Explain that talking about the traumatic event may intensify the symptoms (*e.g.*, nightmares, flashbacks, painful emotions, feeling of numbness).
3. Assist the person to proceed at an individual pace.
4. Listen attentively with empathy and unhurried manner.
5. Assist to talk about trauma, to understand what has occurred, and to validate the reality of personal involvement.
6. Help to ventilate feelings associated with the traumatic event and to become aware of the link between the experience and anger, depression, or anxiety.
7. Assist to differentiate reality from fantasy and to look back and talk about the areas of his or her life that have been changed.
8. Recognize and support cultural and religious values in dealing with the traumatic event.

E. Assist person to identify and make connections with support people and resources

1. Help to identify his or her strength and resources.
2. Explore available support system.
3. Assist to make connections with support and resources according to his or her needs.
4. Assist to resume old activities and begin some new ones.

F. Assist family/significant others

1. Assist them to understand what is happening to the victim.
2. Encourage ventilation of their feelings.
3. Provide counseling sessions and/or link them with appropriate community resources, as necessary.

G. Provide nursing care appropriate to each individual's traumatic experience and needs (see *Rape Trauma Syndrome* for additional information, if relevant)

H. Provide or arrange follow-up treatment where person can continue to work through the trauma and to integrate the experience into a new self-concept

Rationale

- Short-term trauma crisis intervention should begin as soon as victims are identified.
- Careful recording of psychological responses assists in recording progress in therapy, planning treatment, or identifying those at greatest risk (DiVasto, 1985). Behavior can differ from individual to individual. Feelings can be fast and furious or slow, trance-like, mixed, or clear (Ruckman, 1992).
- Attempts to decrease extreme symptoms can help person regain some control (Charron, 1995).
- Interventions that focus on helping the person cope can reduce powerlessness (Charron, 1995).

- Assisting the person to recall the events and clarify the event puts that event in perspective and helps prevent repression (Bender, 1995).
- The process of working through the trauma may be interrupted when there is a lack of support or additional stresses.
- Victims need to work through trauma at their own pace.
- Unhurried, confident actions and eye contact help calm the victim and assure that he or she is alive and safe (Ruckman, 1992).
- Providing immediate and ongoing empathy and support prepares victims for referral to more in-depth psychological counseling (Tyra, 1993). Main issues in the acute stage are being in control, fear of being left alone, and having someone to listen (Ruckman, 1992).
- Follow-up counseling and long-term support therapy in the community should be arranged.

🌀 Interventions—*Child Focus*

1. Assist children to understand and to integrate the experience in accordance with their developmental stage
2. Assist to describe the experience and to express feelings (*e.g.*, fear, guilt, rage) in safe, supportive places, such as play therapy sessions.
3. Provide accurate information and explanations to the child in terms child can understand.
4. Evaluate risk for suicide, especially in male adolescents (see *Risk for Suicide* for assessment criteria).
5. Provide family counseling to promote family members' understanding of the child's needs.

Rationale

- Nursing assessment should include the child's symbolic or nonverbal language communication (Wong, 1995).
- Play therapy, such as writing, drawing, telling stories, or playing with dolls, should be offered so that the children can act out, express feelings, and/or communicate their experience safely (see Appendix IX).

References/Bibliography

American Psychiatric Association. (1994). *Diagnostic and statistical manual of mental disorders* (4th ed.). Washington, DC: Author.

Baum, A. (1990). Stress, intrusive imagery, and chronic distress. *Health Psychology, 9,* 653–675.

Bender, S. (1995). Crisis Intervention. In G. Stuart & S. Sundeen (Eds.). *Principles and practice of psychiatric nursing* (5th ed.). St. Louis: Mosby–Year Book.

Blanchard, E. B., Hickling, E. J., & Taylor, A. E. (1995). Psychiatric morbidity associated with motor vehicle accidents. *Journal of Nervous and Mental Disease, 183,* 495–504.

Boscarino, J. A. (1995). Post-traumatic stress and associated disorders among Vietnam veterans: The significance of combat exposure and social support. *Journal of Traumatic Stress, 8,* 317–335.

Charron, H. S. (1995). Anxiety disorders. In E. M. Vararolis (Ed.). *Foundations of psychiatric mental health nursing* (2nd ed.). Philadelphia: W. B. Saunders.

Davis, G. C., & Breslau, N. (1994). Post-traumatic stress disorder in victims of civilian trauma and criminal violence. *Psychiatric Clinics of North America, 17,* 289–299.

DiVasto, P. (1985). Measuring the aftermath of rape. *Journal of Psychosocial Nursing and Mental Health Services, 23*(2), 33–35.

Green, B. (1990). Buffalo Creek survivors in the second decade: Stability of stress symptoms. *American Journal of Orthopsychiatry, 60*(1), 43–54.

Green, B. L., & Lindy, J. D. (1994). Post-traumatic stress disorder in victims of disasters. *Psychiatric Clinics of North America, 17,* 301–309.

Hendin, H., & Haas, A. P. (1991). Suicide and guilt as manifestations of PTSD in Vietnam combat veterans. *American Journal of Psychiatry, 148,* 586–591.

Hogan, B. S. (1990). Caring for trauma victims: The emotional impact. *AACN Clinical Issues in Critical Care Nursing, 1,* 495–505.

Horowitz, M. J. (1986a). *Stress response syndromes* (2nd ed.). New York: Aronson.

Horowitz, M. J. (1986b). Stress response syndromes: A review of posttraumatic and adjustment disorders. *Hospital and Community Psychiatry, 37,* 241–248.

Koopman, C., Classen, C., & Cardena, E. (1995). When disaster strikes, acute stress disorder may follow. *Journal of Traumatic Stress, 8,* 29–46.

Kroll, J. (1989). Depression and posttraumatic stress disorder in Southeast Asian refugees. *American Journal of Psychiatry, 146,* 1592–1597.

Kubany, E. S. (1994). A cognitive model of guilt typology in combat-related PTSD. *Journal of Traumatic Stress, 7,* 3–19.

Lebowitz, L., & Roth, S. (1994). "I felt like a slut." The cultural context and women's response to being raped. *Journal of Traumatic Stress, 7,* 363–390.

Lifton, R. J. (1969). *Death in life: Survivors of Hiroshima.* New York: Vintage Books.

Mackey, T., Sereika, S. M., Weissfeld, L. A., Hacker, S. S., Zender, J. F., & Heard, S. L. (1992). Factors associated with long-term depressive symptoms of sexual assault victims. *Archives of Psychiatric Nursing, 6*(1), 10–25.

Mitchell, J. T., & Dyregrov, A. (1993). Traumatic stress in disaster workers and emergency personnel: Prevention and intervention. In J. P. Wilson & B. Raphael (Eds.). *International handbook of traumatic stress syndrome.* New York: Plenum Press.

Morrison, R. A. (1994). Early identification of chronic posttraumatic stress disorder by nurse clinicians. *Orthopaedic Nursing, 13*(4), 22–24.

Ruckman, L. (1992). Rape: How to begin healing. *AJN, 92,* 48–51.

San Blise, M. L. (1994). Crisis intervention: Aftershocks in the quake zone. *Journal of Psychosocial Nursing and Mental Health Service, 32*(55), 29–30.

Southwick, S. M., Bremner, D., & Krystal, J. H. (1994). Psychobiologic research in post-traumatic stress disorder. *Psychiatric Clinics of North America, 17,* 251–264.

Southwick, S. M., Morgan C. A. III, & Darnell, A. (1995). Trauma-related symptoms in veterans of Operation Desert Storm: A 2-year follow-up. *American Journal of Psychiatry, 152,* 1150–1155.

Symes, L. (1995). Post traumatic stress disorder: An evolving concept. *Archives of Psychiatric Nursing, 9*(4), 195–202.

Tanaka, K. (1991). Post-trauma response. In G. K. McFarland & M. D. Thomas (Eds.). *Psychiatric mental health nursing: Application of the nursing process.* Philadelphia: J. B. Lippincott.

Tyra, P. (1993). Older woman and rape. *Journal of Gerontological Nursing, 5,* 7–12.

Wong, D. (1995). *Nursing care of infants and children* (5th ed.). St. Louis: Mosby–Year Book.

Rape Trauma Syndrome

DEFINITION

Rape Trauma Syndrome: A state in which the individual experiences a forced, violent sexual assault (vaginal or anal penetration) against his or her will and without his or her consent. The trauma syndrome that develops from this attack or attempted attack includes an acute phase of disorganization of the victim and family's life-style and a long-term process of reorganization of life-style (Holmstrom & Burgess, 1975).

DEFINING CHARACTERISTICS
Major (Must Be Present)

Reports or evidence of sexual assault

Minor (May Be Present)

If the victim is a child, parents may experience similar responses

Acute Phase
    Somatic responses
        Gastrointestinal irritability (nausea, vomiting, anorexia)
        Genitourinary discomfort (pain, pruritus)
        Skeletal muscle tension (spasms, pain)
    Psychological responses
        Denial

Emotional shock
Anger
Fear—of being alone or that the rapist will return (a child victim fears punishment, repercussions, abandonment, rejection)
Guilt
Panic on seeing assailant or scene of the attack
Sexual responses
Mistrust of men (if victim is a woman)
Change in sexual behavior

Long-Term Phase

Any response of the acute phase may continue if resolution does not occur
Psychological responses
Phobias   Anxiety
Nightmares or sleep disturbances   Depression
Suicidal ideation

Author's Note
See *Post-Trauma Response*

Errors in Diagnostic Statements
See *Post-Trauma Response*

Key Concepts

1. In 1987, an estimated 91,111 cases of forcible rape occurred in the United States. National trends show a 21% increase in forcible rapes over the past 10 years (U.S. Department of Justice, 1989).
2. Rape is a crime using sexual expression to humiliate or degrade the victim (Foley & Darvies, 1987). The victim's right of privacy, sense of security, safety, and well-being are always violated (McCombie, 1980).
3. Rape is a crime that must be reported by health care providers (Brozan, 1985). It is estimated that only 4 of 10 rapes are reported (Smith-DiJulio, 1995).
4. Our past culture (and some cultures today) supported that (Heinrich, 1987)
   a. "A woman's rightful place in society is to fulfill man's destiny."
   b. "Women are property of men and are responsible for retaining value" (therefore, women who allow themselves to get raped are bad).
   c. "Women are important to men, as symbols of their power and status and as prizes of prowess."
5. Some myths about rape include (Heinrich, 1987)
   a. The rapist is a sexually unsatisfied man unable to control his urges.
   b. Committing rape is a one-time incident, representing a momentary lapse in judgment.
   c. Rapists are strangers.
   d. Rape is provoked by the victim.
   e. Only promiscuous women get raped.
   f. Rapes happen to women out alone at night. If a woman stays home, she will be safe.
   g. Women cannot be raped against their will—the rape can be avoided by resistance.
   h. Most rapes involve black men and white women.
   i. Women respect men for overpowering them; they may even enjoy the rape.
   j. Rapists are mentally ill or retarded and, therefore, are not responsible for their acts.
6. Victims, families, society, and caregivers who subscribe to these myths may not view themselves as victims or recognize the criminality of rape, may not seek help, or may be denied supportive interventions (Heinrich, 1987).
7. Burgess and Holmstrom (1974) categorize three main types of rape:
   a. *Rape:* Sex without consent in which the assailant uses confidence, coercion, or violence.
   b. *Accessory to sex:* Survivors collaborate in a secondary manner with the sexual activity, and consent or lack of consent is due to cognitive or personality development. (Mentally retarded people and children are susceptible.)

    c. *Sex-stress situation:* Sex is agreed on initially but then one party decides not to go through with it, usually because of exploitation, but this change of heart is not heeded.

8. Rape occurs in all age groups, all races, and all educational and economic groups (Smith-DiJulio, 1995).
9. Male rape victims (including homosexuals) are unlikely to report the rape, but are most likely to experience symptoms of rape trauma syndrome (Anderson, 1981–82; Kaufman, 1980; Smith-DiJulio, 1995).
10. The medical–legal examination serves to assess the condition of the victim and to gather documentary evidence. It consists of a general examination; oral, pelvic, and rectal examinations; a culture for sperm and venereal diseases; serum pregnancy test; blood typing; and a drug and alcohol screen. Obvious debris is placed in separate envelopes. Dried sperm is collected. The victim's pubic hair and head hair are combed, and samples are placed in separate envelopes. Fingernail scrapings are placed in separate envelopes for each hand (Heinrich, 1987).
11. Nurses need to explore their own feelings about rape before attempting to intervene effectively with rape trauma victims. The nurse's responses to rape victims can be anxiety and overcompensation, denial of the event, condescension, anger, coercing, blaming, helplessness, and/or overinvolvement.
12. The nurse may not see every symptom of rape trauma syndrome with each rape victim.
13. During the acute phase, hospital emergency rooms and crisis intervention centers are two places where the nurse may encounter the rape victim.
14. Nurses should consider conditions preexisting the rape trauma (*i.e.*, physical or psychiatric illnesses, substance abuse) that may lead to compound reactions.
15. Acute symptoms overlap with long-term symptoms of rape trauma syndrome.

🌀 *Key Concepts—Child*

1. An estimated 75% of sexual abuse victims are girls (Kauffman, Neill, & Thomas, 1986). The female adolescent is particularly at risk for sexual assault; it is estimated that more than 50% of rape victims are between 10 and 19 years of age (Wong, 1995).
2. The assailant of a child is most likely someone the child knows, and the assaults usually have occurred for a period of time within the child's own home or neighborhood (Pownall, 1985).
3. Adolescents, particularly boys, are more prone to commit suicide in the aftermath of rape (Collins, 1982).
4. Acquaintance rape is very prevalent among college-age women and is believed to be underrecognized and underreported (Ellis, 1994).
5. Greater emotional distress and long-term effects have been reported when the abuser of the child was known and trusted (Feinauer, 1989).
6. Adolescent girls frequently underreport acquaintance rape because they believe they may have contributed to the act in some way (*e.g.*, alcohol use) (Wong, 1995).

🌀 *Key Concepts—Maternal*

Refer to *Ineffective Family Coping—Domestic Violence*

🏛 *Key Concepts—Older Adult*

1. Incidences of rape frequently go unreported among the elderly (U.S. Department of Justice, 1987).
2. The elderly experience reactions to rape similar to those of other adult victims, but may have increased degrees of dependency, powerlessness, and depression (Davis & Brody, 1981; Fielo, 1987).

Focus Assessment Criteria

Subjective Data (Must Be Recorded)

A. Assess for defining characteristics

    1. History of the undesired sexual activity (child, adolescent, adult)*
        Time and place of event
        Identity or description of assailant

---

* The purpose of securing a history is to substantiate evidence of trauma and not to explore details of trauma. This should be done in an appropriate therapy session.

Sexual contact (type, amount, coercion, weapon)
Witnesses, if any
Activities that may alter evidence (changing clothes, bathing, urinating, douching)
Sexual history
    Date of last menses   Contraceptive use
    Menstrual history   Date of last sexual contact
    History of venereal disease
2. Response to the assault during acute phase
    Assess person and family for
        Somatic symptoms
        Psychological symptoms
        Sexual reactions
    Assess child for
        Understanding of the event
        Knowledge of the identity of the molester
        Possibility of previous assaults
    Assess parents, spouse, others for
        Understanding of the event
        Ability to help the victim cope
        Ability to cope
3. Response to the assault during long-term phase
    Assess person and family for reactions

Objective Data

A. Assess for injury (ecchymoses, lacerations, abrasions)
    Gastrointestinal system (mouth, anus, abdomen)
    Skeletal muscle system
    Genitourinary system

B. Assess the emotional responses
    Crying   Detachment
    Hysteria   Composure
    Withdrawal

Outcome Criteria

Short-Term Goals
The person will
• Share feelings
• Describe rationale and treatment procedures
• Identify members of support system and use them appropriately

Long-Term Goals
The person will
• Report sleeping well
• Report return to former eating pattern
• Report no or occasional somatic reactions
• Demonstrate calmness and relaxation
• Return to precrisis level of functioning

The child will
• Discuss the assault
• Express feelings concerning the assault and the treatment

The parents, spouse, or significant other will
• Discuss their response to the assault
• Return to precrisis level of functioning

Interventions

Psychological Responses

A. Assess for psychological responses (Jalowiec & Powers, 1981)
   1. General
      a. Phobias, nightmares
      b. Enuresis
      c. Denial, emotional shock
      d. Anger, fear, anxiety
      e. Depression, guilt
   2. Subjective
      a. Expressions of numbness, shame, self-blame
      b. Suicidal ideation
   3. Objective
      a. Crying
      b. Silence
      c. Trembling hands
      d. Excessive bathing (seen particularly with child or adolescent)
      e. Avoiding interaction with others (staff, family)
      f. Wearing excessive clothing (two or three pairs of pants or panties)

B. Assist to identify major concerns (psychological, medical, legal) and her or his perception of the help she or he needs
   1. Explain the care and examination she or he will experience.
      a. Conduct the examinations in an unhurried manner.
      b. Explain every detail before action.
      c. If this is the person's first pelvic examination, explain the position and the instruments.
      d. Discuss the possibility of pregnancy and a sexually transmitted disease, and treatments available.
   2. Explain the legal issues and police investigation (Heinrich, 1987).
      a. Explain the need to collect specimens for future possible court use.
      b. Explain that the choice to report the rape is the victim's.
      c. If the police interview is permitted
         Negotiate with victim and police for an advantageous time.
         Explain to victim what kind of questions will be asked.
         Remain with the victim during the interview; do not ask questions or offer answers.
         If the officer is insensitive, intimidating, offensive in manner or asks improper questions, discuss this with the officer in private. If the behavior continues, use proper channels and make a complaint.

C. Eliminate or reduce psychological responses, when possible
   1. Promote a trusting relationship.
      a. Stay with person during acute stage or arrange for other support.
      b. Brief person on police and hospital procedures during acute stage.
      c. Assist during medical examination and explain all procedures in advance.
      d. Help person to meet personal needs (bathing *after* examination and evidence has been acquired).
      e. Listen attentively to person's requests.
      f. Maintain unhurried attitude toward person and family.
      g. Avoid rescue feelings toward person.
      h. Maintain nonjudgmental attitude.
      i. Support person's beliefs and value system and avoid labeling.

   j. Initiate play therapy with a child to explain treatments and allow child to express feelings.
2. Whenever possible, provide crisis counseling within 1 hour of rape trauma event.
   a. Ask permission to contact the rape crisis counselor.
   b. Be flexible and individualize approach according to person's needs.
   c. Observe person's behavior carefully and record objective data.
   d. Encourage victim to verbalize thoughts, feelings, or perceptions of the event.
   e. Discuss her or his treatment as victim; express empathy.
   f. Assess person's verbal style (expressive, controlled).
   g. Discuss with person previous coping mechanism.
   h. Explore available support system; involve significant others if appropriate.
   i. Assess stress tolerance.
   j. Reassure person about manner in which she or he reacted.
   k. Explore with person her or his strengths and resources.
   l. Convey to person confidence in her or his ability to return to prior level of functioning.
   m. Assist person in decision making and problem solving; involve person in own treatment plan.
   n. Help restore person's dignity by calmly exploring together basis for feelings.
   o. Reassure person that these feelings/symptoms—fear of rapist, fear of death, guilt, loss of control, shame, short attention span, anger, anxiety, phobias, depression, flashbacks, embarrassment, and eating/sleeping pattern disturbances—are often experienced by rape trauma victims.
   p. Respect victim's right; honor wishes to restrict unwanted visitors and offer privacy when appropriate.
   q. Explain to person that this experience will disrupt her or his life, and that feelings that occurred during acute phase may recur; encourage person to proceed at her or his own pace.
   r. Offer explanation of any papers that need to be signed.
   s. Briefly counsel family and friends at their level.
      Share with them the immediate needs of the victim for love and support.
      Encourage them to express their feelings and ask questions.
3. Support person's efforts to overcome feelings.
   a. Change residence and/or telephone number.
   b. Use objects that symbolize safety (nightlight).
   c. Take a trip.
   d. Turn to support system.
   e. Plan a day at a time.
   f. Avoid highly stressful situations.
   g. Engage in diversional activities.
   h. Identify previous coping mechanisms that proved effective.

D. Fulfill medical–legal responsibilities by documentation (Heinrich, 1987)
   1. History of rape (date, time, place)
   2. Nature of injuries, use of force, weapons used, threats of violence or retribution, restraints used
   3. Nature of assault (fondling, oral, anal, vaginal penetration, ejaculation, use of condom)
   4. Postassault activities (douching, bathing/showering, gargling, urinating, defecating, changing clothes, eating, or drinking)
   5. Present state (use of drugs, alcohol)
   6. Medical history, tetanus immunization status, gynecologic history (last menstrual period), last voluntary intercourse
   7. Emotional state, mental status

8. Examination findings, smears/cultures taken, blood tests, evidence collected, and photographs (if appropriate)
9. Document to whom, when, and what evidence is delivered

E. Proceed with follow-up until victim is in control of reactions and feelings (Andrews, 1992)

1. Before person leaves hospital, provide card with information about follow-up appointments and names and telephone numbers of local crisis and counseling centers.
2. Plan home visit or telephone call.
3. Arrange for legal or pastoral counseling, if appropriate.
4. Recommend and make referrals to psychotherapist, mental health clinic, citizen action and community group advocacy-related services.

Sexual Responses

A. Assess responses (Furniss, 1983)

1. General
   a. Fear of intercourse
   b. Family's fear that assault will affect person's future sexual health
2. Subjective
   a. Mistrust of men
3. Objective
   a. Change in sexual behavior
   b. Lack of sexual desire (especially if victim never had intercourse before)

B. Promote helping relationship

1. Encourage person to express feelings openly.
2. Provide accepting atmosphere.
3. Reassure person that her or his symptoms are frequently experienced by rape trauma victims.
4. Offer feedback to person on feelings verbalized.
5. Encourage person to recognize positive responses or support from sexual partner or members of opposite sex.
6. Discuss with person possible fear of rejection by significant others.
7. Discuss potential anxiety about resuming sexual relations with partner.
8. Explore sexual concerns with person.

C. Proceed with referrals

1. Recommend couple therapy.
2. Recommend sexual counseling.

Somatic Responses

A. Assess for somatic responses

1. Gastrointestinal irritability
2. Genitourinary discomfort
3. Rectal discomfort
4. Skeletal muscle tension
5. Vaginal discharge
6. Bruising and edema
7. Reports of:
   a. Headaches
   b. Fatigue
   c. Itching
   d. Anorexia
   e. Nausea

f. Pain

g. Burning on urination

B. Eliminate or reduce somatic symptomatology

1. Gastrointestinal irritability

a. Anorexia

Offer small, frequent feedings.

Provide appealing foods.

Record intake.

Refer to *Altered Nutrition* if anorexia is prolonged.

b. Nausea

Avoid gas-forming foods.

Restrict carbonated beverages.

Observe for abdominal distention.

Offer antiemetic as per physician's order.

2. Genitourinary discomfort

a. Pain

Assess pain for quality and duration.

Monitor intake and output.

Inspect urine and external genitalia for bleeding.

Listen attentively to person's description of pain.

Give pain medication as per physician's order (see *Altered Comfort*).

b. Discharge

Assess amount, color, and odor of discharge.

Allow person time to wash and change garments after initial examination has been completed.

c. Itching

Encourage bathing in cool water.

Avoid use of detergent soaps.

Avoid touching area causing discomfort.

3. Skeletal muscle tension

a. Headaches

Avoid any sudden change of person's position.

Approach person in calm manner.

Slightly elevate bed (unless contraindicated).

Discuss with person pain-reducing measures that have been effective in the past.

b. Fatigue

Assess present sleeping patterns if altered (see *Sleep Pattern Disturbance*).

Discuss with person precipitating factors for sleep disturbance and try to eliminate these factors if possible.

Provide frequent rest periods throughout the day.

Avoid interruptions during sleep.

Avoid stress-producing situations.

c. Emotional responses

Provide person with emotionally secure environment.

Discuss person's daily routines and adhere to them as much as possible.

Avoid any sudden movements and approach in calm manner.

Provide frequent quiet periods throughout the day.

4. Generalized bruising and edema

a. Avoid constrictive garments.

b. Handle affected body parts gently.

c. Elevate affected body part if edema is present.

d. Apply cool, moist compress to edematous area the first 24 hours, then warm compress after 24 hours.

    e. Encourage person to verbalize discomfort.
    f. Record presence and location of bruises, lacerations, edema, or abrasions.

C. Proceed with health teaching with person and family

1. Gastrointestinal irritability: Explain to person side effects of diethylstilbestrol (DES): nausea and vomiting.
2. Genitourinary discomfort: Advise person against scratching area causing discomfort.
3. Skeletal muscle tension
    a. Explain to person potential causes of discomfort.
    b. Explain to person measures that may help release tension.
    c. Teach person relaxation methods (see Appendix X).
    d. Explain to person that these symptoms are often experienced by rape trauma victims.

Rationale

- The sooner intervention begins with a rape victim, the less psychological damage will be incurred (Aguilera & Messick, 1982). Many victims try to suppress the memory of the assault, so postponement of counseling even 1 day may weaken their pursuit of follow-up care. Immediate contact with a counselor may be a means of overcoming this reluctance (Dwyer, 1987).
- Because the victim's right to deny or consent to sexual activity has been violently violated, it is important to seek permission for subsequent care (Heinrich, 1987). It is important to tell the client as much as is practical or possible about what is happening, and why. Even in life-threatening situations, any sense of control that can be given to the victim is helpful (Beckman & Groetzinger, 1990).
- Careful recording of psychological responses assists in recording progress in therapy, planning treatment, or identifying those at greatest risk (DiVasto, 1985). Behavior can differ from individual to individual. Feelings can be fast and furious or slow, trance-like, mixed, or clear (Ruckman, 1992).
- The interventions for rape trauma syndrome are listed for usefulness under the three types of responses: psychological, sexual, and somatic. The nurse must assess and intervene with each response for each victim (DiVasto, 1985).
- Rape crisis centers provide rape victims and significant others with information concerning the medical examination, police interrogation, and court procedures; with escort service to hospital, police department, and courts; and with counseling.
- Rape crisis centers work in the community to educate the public on rape and rape prevention, improve the response of hospitals and the police to rape victims, and improve rape-related legislation.
- Short-term rape crisis intervention should begin during the acute phase.
- Follow-up intervention is usually counselor initiated.
- Nurses in community settings can teach primary prevention concepts by reviewing with clients measures to take to reduce the possibility of rape.
- Some destruction can be lessened if the victim's family and friends recognize symptoms as normal (Adams & Fay, 1989). Recovery can be greatly helped or hindered by the responses of others. Significant others are also faced with a crisis, a trauma, and the need for recovery (Adams & Fay, 1989).
- After rape, people have profound feelings of loss of control and victimization. Interventions focus on restoring a sense of control and safety (Smith-DiJulio, 1995).
- Emotional support and presence validates the person's worth and prevents escalation of anxiety (Smith-DiJulio, 1995).
- Crisis counseling can provide accurate information and ongoing assessment of emotional state (Smith-DiJulio, 1995).
- Detailed follow-up instructions are given because the person cannot assimilate the information at this time (Andrews, 1992).

- Follow-up counseling provides support over time and may lessen the intrapsychic impact of the rape experience (Smith-DiJulio, 1995).
- Providing accurate information about the medical–legal procedures and their relevance can reduce feelings of physical intrusion and loss of control (Parker & Campbell, 1995).
- Therapeutic alliances help the person ventilate feelings and fears (Francis, 1993).
- Helping the person identify methods to increase sense of safety can reduce panic levels of anxiety (Frances, 1993).
- When working with young rape trauma victims, nurses should be cognizant of individual developmental levels, because the impact of the event varies according to the child's developmental stage (Wong, 1995).
- The child's reaction depends on age, degree of physical trauma, relation to assailant, and parental (caretaker) reaction (Wong, 1995).
- Play therapy should be an integral part of the treatment regimen. (Guidelines for play therapy are presented in Appendix IX.) For rape victims, provide dolls that have genitalia for play therapy; rag dolls can have genitalia attached. The child can then act out the assault with dolls of appropriate sex (a boy victim can use two male dolls). Puppets are also beneficial for play therapy (Wong, 1995).

References/Bibliography

Adams, C., & Fay, J. (1989). *Free of the shadows*. Oakland: New Harbinger.

Aguilera, D. C., & Messick, J. M. (1982). *Crisis intervention: Theory and methodology* (4th ed.). St. Louis: C. V. Mosby.

Anderson, C. (1981–82). Males as sexual assault victims: Multiple levels of trauma. *Journal of Homosexuality, 7*, 145–159.

Andrews, J. (1992). Sexual assault: After care instructions. *Journal of Emergency Nursing, 18*, 152.

Beckman, C., & Groetzinger, L. (1990). Treating sexual victims. *Physician Assistant, 2*, 123–130.

Brozan, N. (1985, August 10). Rape trauma: Seeking court acceptance. *The New York Times*, p. 43.

Burgess, A. W., & Holmstrom, L. L. (1974). Rape trauma syndrome. *American Journal of Psychiatry, 131*, 981–986.

Collins, G. (1982, January 18). Counseling male rape victims. *The New York Times*, p. 27.

Davis, L., & Brody, E. (1981). *Rape and older women: A guide to prevention and protection*. Rockville, MD: U.S. Department of Health, Education and Welfare, Public Health Service, Alcohol, Drug Abuse, and Mental Health Administration, National Institute of Mental Health.

DiVasto, P. (1985). Measuring the aftermath of rape. *Journal of Psychosocial Nursing and Mental Health Services, 23*(2), 33–35.

Dwyer, J. (1987). Examination and treatment of the sexual assault victim. *Physician Assistant, 11*, 110–109.

Ellis, G. M. (1994). Acquaintance rape. *Perspectives in Psychiatric Care, 30*, 11–16.

Feinauer, L. (1989). Comparison of long-term effects of child abuse by type of abuse and by relationship of the offender to the victim. *American Journal of Family Therapy, 17*, 48–52.

Fielo, S. (1987). How does crime affect the elderly? *Geriatric Nursing, 8*(2), 80–83.

Foley, T., & Darvies, M. (1987). *Rape: Nursing care of victims*. St. Louis: C. V. Mosby.

Francis, S. (1993). Rape and sexual assault. In B. S. Johnson (Ed.). *Psychiatric–mental health nursing: Adaptation and growth*. Philadelphia: J. B. Lippincott.

Heinrich, L. (1987). Care of the female rape victim. *Nursing Practice, 12*(11), 9.

Holmstrom, L., & Burgess, A. W. (1975). Development of diagnostic categories: Sexual trauma. *American Journal of Nursing, 75*, 1288–1291.

Jalowiec, A., & Powers, M. J. (1981). Stress and coping in hypertensive and emergency room patients. *Nursing Research, 30*, 10–15.

Kaufman, A. (1980). Male rape victims: Non-institutionalized assault. *American Journal of Medicine, 137*, 221–223.

McCombie, S. (1980). *The rape crisis intervention handbook*. New York: Plenum Press.

Parker, B., & Campbell, J. C. (1995). Care of survivors of abuse and violence. In G. W. Stuart & S. J. Saudeen (Eds.). *Principles and practice of psychiatric nursing* (5th ed.). St. Louis: Mosby–Year Book.

Ruckman, L. (1992). Rape: How to begin the healing. *American Journal of Nursing, 9*, 48–51.

Smith-DiJulio, K. (1995). Evidence of maladaptive responses to crisis: Rape. In E. Varcarolis (Ed.). *Foundations of psychiatric–mental health nursing* (5th ed.). Philadelphia: W. B. Saunders.

U.S. Department of Justice, Federal Bureau of Investigation. (1989). *Uniform crime reports for the United States*. Washington, DC: U.S. Government Printing Office.

Children and Adolescents

Furniss, T. (1983). Mutual influences and interlocking professional–family process in the treatment of child sexual abuse and incest. *Child Abuse and Neglect, 7*, 207–223.

Kauffman, C. K., Neill, M. K., & Thomas, J. N. (1986). The abusive parent. In S. H. Johnson (Ed.). *High-risk parenting: Assessment and nursing strategies for families at risk.* Philadelphia: J. B. Lippincott.

Pownall, M. (1985). Health visiting: A family affair? . . . Sexual abuse of children. *Nursing Times, 81*(43), 58, 60–61.

Wong, D. L. (1995). *Nursing care of infants and children* (5th ed.). St. Louis: Mosby–Year Book.

Powerlessness

DEFINITION

Powerlessness: The state in which an individual or group perceives a lack of personal control over certain events or situations that affects outlook, goals, and life-style.

DEFINING CHARACTERISTICS
Major (Must Be Present)

Overt or covert (anger, apathy) expressions of dissatisfaction over inability to control a situation (*e.g.*, work, illness, prognosis, care, recovery rate) that is negatively affecting outlook, goals, and life-style

Minor (May Be Present)

Lack of information-seeking behaviors

Apathy	Unsatisfactory dependence on others
Anxiety	Acting-out behavior
Anger	Uneasiness
Violent behavior	Resignation
Depression	Passivity

RELATED FACTORS
Pathophysiologic

Any disease process, acute or chronic, can cause or contribute to powerlessness. Some common sources are

Related to inability to communicate secondary to cerebrovascular accident (CVA), Guillain-Barré syndrome, intubation

Related to inability to perform activities of daily living secondary to CVA, cervical trauma, myocardial infarction, pain

Related to inability to perform role responsibilities secondary to surgery, trauma, arthritis

Related to progressive debilitating disease secondary to multiple sclerosis, terminal cancer

Related to substance abuse

Situational (Personal, Environmental)

Related to change from curative status to palliative status

Related to feeling of loss of control and life-style restrictions secondary to: (specify)

Related to overeating patterns

Related to personal characteristics that highly value control (*e.g.*, internal locus of control)

Related to effects of hospital or institutional limitations

Related to life-style of helplessness
Related to fear of disapproval
Related to unmet dependency needs
Related to consistent negative feedback
Related to long-term abusive relationship

Maturational

Adolescent children
Related to child's rearing problems
Older Adult
Related to multiple losses secondary to aging (*e.g.*, retirement, sensory deficits, motor deficits, money, significant others)

Author's Note

Powerlessness is a feeling that all people experience to varying degrees in various situations. Stephenson (1979) has described two types of powerlessness. *Situational powerlessness* occurs in a specific event and is probably short-lived. *Trait powerlessness* is more pervasive, affecting general outlook, goals, life-style, and relationships. The nursing diagnosis *Powerlessness* may be more clinically useful when used to describe a person experiencing trait powerlessness rather than situational powerlessness.

Hopelessness differs from powerlessness in that a hopeless person sees no solution to his problem or no way to achieve what is desired, even if he feels in control of his life. A powerless person may see an alternative or answer to the problem, yet be unable to do anything about it because of perception of control and resources. Prolonged powerlessness may lead to hopelessness.

Errors in Diagnostic Statements

Powerlessness related to hospitalization

Hospitalization evokes varied responses in people and families, including anxiety, fear, and powerlessness. If the hospitalization is expected to be short, the diagnosis of *Anxiety related to unfamiliar environment, loss of usual routines, and invasion of privacy* may be useful to describe situational powerlessness. If the hospitalization is a readmission for a continuing problem, the use of *Powerlessness* may be more appropriate to describe trait powerlessness. The diagnosis should be restated as *Powerlessness related to readmission for pulmonary infection and effects of illness on career and marriage.*

Key Concepts

1. An individual's response to loss of control depends on the meaning of the loss, individual patterns of coping, personal characteristics (psychological, sociologic, cultural, spiritual), and the response of others.
2. Each individual, whether well or ill, has a desire for control. Feelings of powerlessness are sometimes appropriate.
   a. Powerlessness is precipitated by stressors in the here-and-now; however, the conflicts that emerge are often reminiscent of childhood issues (Drew, 1990).
3. When an individual does not expect to be able to control outcomes, attention to and retention of information is poor (Seeman, 1967).
4. Powerlessness is very closely related to, but not synonymous with, the concept of external versus internal locus of control.
   a. Locus of control is a rather stable personality trait, whereas powerlessness is situationally determined.

5. A person with internal locus of control believes he can affect his outcome by actively manipulating himself or the environment. Examples of internal behavior are participating in a regular exercise program, acquiring printed literature about a new diagnosis, or learning assertive skills.
6. A person with external locus of control believes that affecting his outcome is outside his control and attributes what happens to him to others or to fate. Examples of external behavior are losing weight because of fear of professional's response and blaming others for his present position (*e.g.*, depression, anger).
7. Internally controlled people motivate themselves, whereas externally controlled people usually need others to motivate them. Young children are usually externally controlled, but can be taught to be internally controlled. For example, a child can be taught to keep a daily chart record of the nutrients needed daily and his intake of them to assist him to understand the concept of good nutrition and to encourage him to take responsibility for his eating patterns.
8. Individuals possessing internal locus of control may experience the loss of decision-making ability more profoundly than individuals possessing external locus of control.
   a. Patients with an external locus of control seem to be more prone to development of powerlessness (Lubkin, 1995).
9. Powerlessness is part of a continuum with hopelessness and helplessness.
10. Simmons and West (1984–85) reported that older adults with high self-efficacy and occupational status had more difficulty with uncontrollable situations than their counterparts with lower self-efficacy. Younger adults were found to cope more effectively with uncontrollable situations if high efficacy, high income, and occupational status were present.
11. Miller (1985) postulates that if powerlessness is not contained, a cycle of lowered self-esteem and depression occurs, followed by hopelessness.
   a. Unrelieved states of powerlessness may lead to hopelessness and eventually may affect survival (Seligman, 1975).

🌹 *Key Concepts—Child*

1. Hospitalized children commonly experience powerlessness.
2. It may be difficult to differentiate the diagnosis *Powerlessness* from the diagnoses *Anxiety* and *Fear*, especially in children. Refer to Key Concepts—Child under the diagnoses *Anxiety* and *Fear*.

🏛 *Key Concepts—Older Adult*

1. The elderly are at high risk for powerlessness because multiple losses (previous roles, family, health, and functioning) may be encountered with the aging process. The added stressors of illness and institutionalization only compound feelings of powerlessness (O'Heath, 1991). Miller describes seven sources of power: physical strength and reserve, psychological stamina and support network, positive self-concept, energy, knowledge, motivation, and belief system (Miller, 1983; Spielman, 1986).
2. Internal locus of control and desired amount of control correlate with health status and high morale and life satisfaction (Chang, 1978; Fuller, 1978).
3. Personality traits, various effects of diseases, and environmental conditions affect powerlessness. For the elderly, disease states might place restrictions on mobility. Changes in environment (*e.g.*, relocating to an extended care facility) can remove opportunities for decision making and autonomy. Institutional policy may require physical or chemical restraints for certain agitated behaviors (Matteson & McConnell, 1988).
4. Late life changes in role, resources, and responsibility can contribute to feelings of loss of control (Richmond & Metcalf, 1986).
5. Extensive interactions with caregivers, rather than peers, can lead to a sense of powerlessness. This has implications for the older individual who, with an increased chance of multiple chronic illnesses, might be in the sick role for an extended period of time (Lambert & Lambert, 1981; Miller, 1995).

TRANSCULTURAL CONSIDERATIONS

1. The diagnosis of *Powerlessness* can be problematic with individuals from other cultures. In Latin cultures, the concept of fatalism (*e.g.*, what will be will be) may be a challenge to a nurse who is trying to initiate a life-style change for better health (Boyle & Andrews, 1995; Giger & Davidhizar, 1995).
2. The powerlessness associated with fatalism is accepted, and this usually does not constitute a problem for the person.
3. The nurse must distinguish his or her goal for the client from the client's goal. "Nurses should address those areas that are the greatest concern to clients and family members" (Andrews & Boyle, 1995, p. 235).

Focus Assessment Criteria

Because powerlessness is a subjective state, all inferences made concerning a person's feelings of powerlessness must be validated. The nurse assesses each individual to determine his usual level of control and decision making and the effects that losing elements of control have had on him.

Subjective Data
A. Assess for defining characteristics
  1. Decision-making patterns
      "How would you describe your usual method of making decisions (career, financial, health care)?"
      Make them alone
      Consult with others for advice (who?)
      Allow others to make them for me (spouse? children? others?)
  2. Individual and role responsibilities
      "What responsibilities did you have
        . . . as a school child and adolescent?"
        . . . at home?"
        . . . at work?"
        . . . in community and religious organizations?"

B. Assess for related factors
  1. Perception of control
      "How would you describe your ability—high, moderate, fair, or poor—to control or cure your present health problem?" (*e.g.*, diabetes mellitus, aphasia, activity intolerance, obesity)
      "To what do you attribute your (high, moderate, fair, poor) ability to control?"
        Preventive measures
          Good nutrition   Stress management
          Weight control   Exercise program
        Others
          Physician   Significant others
          Nurse   Peer group
        No control
          Fate
          Luck

Objective Data
A. Assess for defining characteristics
  1. Participation in grooming and hygiene care (when indicated)
      Actively seeks involvement
      Requires encouragement

Reluctant to participate
Refuses to participate
2. Information-seeking behaviors
Actively seeks information and literature from others concerning condition
Refuses to receive information
Requires encouragement to ask questions
Expresses lack of interest
3. Response to limits placed on decision-making and self-control behaviors

Acceptance	Increases attempts to exercise control
Apathy	Depression
Attempts to circumvent limits	Anger
Ignores limits	Withdrawal

Outcome Criteria

The person will
• Identify factors that can be controlled by him
• Make decisions regarding his care, treatment, and future when possible
• Verbalize ability to control/influence situations and outcomes

---

Interventions

A. Assess for causative and contributing factors

1. Lack of knowledge
2. Previous inadequate coping patterns (*e.g.*, depression; for discussion, see *Ineffective Individual Coping Related to Depression*)
3. Insufficient decision-making opportunities

B. Eliminate or reduce contributing factors, if possible

1. Lack of knowledge
   a. Increase effective communication between person and health care provider.
   b. Explain all procedures, rules, and options to person; avoid medical jargon.
      Help to anticipate realistic sensations that will occur during treatments (this provides reality-oriented cognitive images that bolster a sense of control and coping strategies).
   c. Allow time to answer questions; ask him to write questions down so that he does not forget them.
   d. Provide a specific time (10–15 minutes) each shift that person knows can be used to ask questions or discuss subjects as desired.
   e. Anticipate questions/interest and offer information.
      Help to anticipate events and outcomes
   f. While being realistic, point out positive changes in person's condition, such as serum enzymes decreasing after myocardial infarction or surgical incision healing well.
   g. Be an active listener by allowing person to verbalize concerns and feelings; assess for areas of concern.
   h. Provide consistent staffing.
   i. Single out one nurse to be responsible for 24-hour plan of care, and provide opportunities for person and family to identify with this nurse.
   j. Contact self-help support groups if available (*e.g.*, mastectomy, ostomy clubs, paraplegics).

   k. If contributing factors are pain or anxiety, provide information on how to use behavioral control techniques (*e.g.*, relaxation, imagery, deep breathing).

2. Provide opportunities for individual to control decisions.

   a. Allow person to manipulate surroundings, such as deciding what is to be kept where (shoes under bed, picture on window).

   b. If person desires, and as hospital policy permits, encourage person to bring personal effects from home (*e.g.*, pillows, pictures).

   c. Keep needed items within reach (call bell, urinal, tissues).

   d. Do not offer options if there are none (*e.g.*, a deep IM Z-track injection must be rotated).
      Offer options that are personally relevant.

   e. Discuss daily plan of activities and allow person to make as many decisions as possible about it.

   f. Increase decision-making opportunities as person progresses.

   g. Respect and follow individual's decision if you have given him options.

   h. Record person's specific choices on care plan to ensure that others on staff acknowledge preferences ("dislikes orange juice," "take showers," "plan dressing change at 7:30 before shower").

   i. Keep promises.

   j. Provide opportunity for person and family to express feelings.

   k. Provide opportunities for person and family to participate in care.

   l. Be alert for signs of paternalism/maternalism in health care providers (*e.g.*, making decisions for clients).

   m. Plan a care conference to allow staff to discuss methods of individualizing care; encourage each nurse to share at least one action that she discovered a particular individual liked.

   n. Shift emphasis from what one cannot do to what one can do.

   o. Set goals that are short-term, behavioral, practical, and realistic (walk 5 more feet every day; then in 1 week, client can walk to television room).

   p. Provide daily recognition of progress.

   q. Praise gains/achievements.

   r. Assist in identifying factors that are controllable and those that are not. Assist in realistically accepting what cannot be changed and altering what can.

   s. Emphasize positive aspects when the person becomes solely focused on fears of the worst (reduces fear by shifting perspective and allowing person to regain control).

   t. Allow person to experience outcomes that result from their own actions.

3. Assess the person's usual response to problems (see Focus Assessment Criteria).

   a. Internal control (seeks to change own behaviors or environment to control problems)

   b. External control (expects others or other factors—fate, luck—to control problems)

4. Provide person with internal locus of control the needed information to alter behavior or environment.

   a. Explain the problem as explicitly as the individual requests.

   b. Explain the relationship of prescribed behavior and outcome (*e.g.*, need for salt restriction, the physiologic effects of exercise, the effects of bed rest on impaired cardiac function).

5. Monitor a person with external locus of control to encourage participation.

   a. Have him keep a record for you (*e.g.*, his food intake for 1 week; weight loss chart; exercise program—type and frequency; medications taken).

   b. Use telephone contact to monitor if feasible.

   c. Provide explicit written directions to follow (*e.g.*, meal plans; exercise regimen—type, frequency, duration; speech practice lessons—for aphasia).

   d. Teach significant others methods to manipulate behaviors, if appropriate.

   e. Provide reward for each goal/step reached.

6. Assist client in deriving power from other sources.

    a. Give permission to use other power sources to both client and significant others (*e.g.*, prayer, stress reduction techniques).
    b. Self-help groups
    c. Support groups
    d. Offer referral to religious leader.
    e. Provide privacy and support for other measures client may request (*e.g.*, meditation, imagery, special rituals).

C. Initiate health teaching and referrals as indicated (social worker, psychiatric nurse/physician, visiting nurse, religious leader, self-help groups)

D. Evaluate the situation with the client
    1. Once the outcome criteria have been accomplished or feelings of powerlessness are diminishing, discuss the process used to relieve powerlessness. Explain how factors contributed to the powerlessness, review why certain strategies were effective, and discuss how person will manage feelings of powerlessness in the future.
    2. Advocate within the system to eliminate policies and routines that contribute to powerlessness.

Rationale

- To plan effective interventions, the nurse must determine whether the client usually seeks to change his own behaviors to control problems, or whether he expects others or external factors to control problems.
- Self-image changes negatively because of a restricted life-style, social isolation, unmet expectations, and dependence on others (Kersten, 1990).
- Individuals with chronic illness need to be assisted not to see themselves as helpless victims. People with a sense of hope, self-control, direction, purpose, and identity are better able to meet the challenges of their disease (Ledy, 1990).
- Self-concept can be enhanced when clients actively engage in decisions regarding health and life-style (Lee, Graydon, & Ross, 1991).
- Setting realistic goals can increase motivation and hope (Kersten, 1990).
- Loss of or decrease in power in one area may be counterbalanced by the introduction of a new source of power or by an increase in power in an existing area.
- Averill (1973) describes three types of control: behavioral, cognitive, and decisional. Interventions that allow people to participate in their care are enhancing their behavioral control. Interventions that provide the person with knowledge, solicit their input into situations, and provide feedback are examples of increasing a person's cognitive control. Interventions that allow the person to make choices are providing decisional control.
- Individuals with chronic illness need to be assisted not to see themselves as helpless victims. People with a sense of hope, self-control, direction, purpose, and identity are better able to meet the challenges of their disease (Ledy, 1990).
- Research has shown that 75% of clients with chronic obstructive pulmonary disease do not engage in thinking about the cause of their illness. People who do not engage in causal thinking may be in denial. This denial may produce a feeling of control, enabling them to be more functional. Contemplating causes may produce feelings of powerlessness, depression, and decreased functional status (Weaver & Narsavage, 1992).

Interventions—*Child Focus*

1. Provide opportunities for child to make decisions (*e.g.*, setting time for bath, holding still for injection)
2. Engage child in play therapy (see Appendix IX) before and after a traumatic situation (refer to *Altered Growth and Development* for specific interventions for age-related development needs).

Rationale

- The goals of nursing interventions to treat powerlessness include modifying the hospital environment to resemble the child's home and providing opportunities for acceptable control (Wong, 1995).
- Children can gain mastery over stressful situations by participating in play activities while ill or hospitalized (Wong, 1995). (See Appendix IX.)

References/Bibliography

Averill, J. (1973). Personal control over aversive stimuli and its relationship to stress. *Psychological Bulletin, 80,* 286.

Boyle, J., & Andrews, M. (1989). *Transcultural concepts in nursing care* (2nd ed.). Philadelphia: J. B. Lippincott.

Chang, B. (1978). Generalized expectancy, situational perception and morale among the institutionalized aged. *Nursing Research, 27,* 316–324.

Drew, B. L. (1990). Differentiation of hopelessness, helplessness, and powerlessness using Erik Erikson's "Roots of Virtue." *Archives of Psychiatric Nursing, 4,* 322–327.

Giger, J. N., & Davidhizar, R. E. (1995). *Transcultural nursing: Assessment and interventions* (2nd ed.). St. Louis: Mosby–Year Book.

Fuller, S. (1978). Inhibiting helplessness in elderly people. *Journal of Gerontological Nursing, 4,* 18–21.

Kersten, L. (1990) Changes in self concept during pulmonary rehabilitation; Part 1 and 2. *Heart and Lung, 19,* 456–470.

Lambert, V. A., & Lambert, C. E. (1981). Role theory and the concept of powerlessness. *Journal of Psychosocial Nursing and Mental Health Services, 19*(9), 11–14.

Ledy, N. (1990). A structural model of stress, psychosocial resources and symptomatic experiences in chronic physical illness. *Nursing Research, 39,* 230–236.

Lee, R., Graydon, J., & Ross, E. (1991). Effects of psychological well being, physical status and social support on oxygen dependent COPD patient's level of functioning. *Research in Nursing and Health, 14,* 323–328.

Lubkin, H. M. (1995). *Chronic illness: Impact and interventions* (3rd ed.). Boston: Jones & Bartlett.

Matteson, A. M., & McConnell, E. S. (1988). *Gerontological Nursing: Concepts and practice.* Philadelphia: W. B. Saunders.

Miller, C. (1995). *Nursing care of older adults* (2nd ed.). Philadelphia: J. B. Lippincott.

Miller, J. (1983). *Powerlessness: Coping with chronic illness.* Philadelphia: F. A. Davis.

Miller, J. F. (1985). Concept development of powerlessness: A nursing diagnosis. In J. F. Miller (Ed.). *Coping with chronic illness, overcoming powerlessness.* Philadelphia: F. A. Davis.

Miller, J. F. (1984). Development and validation of a diagnostic label: Powerlessness. In M. J. Kim & A. McLane (Eds.). *Classification of nursing diagnoses: Proceedings of the fifth national conference.* St Louis: C. V. Mosby.

O'Heath, K. (1991). Powerlessness. In M. Maas, K. Buckwalter, & M. Hardy (Eds.). *Nursing diagnoses and interventions for the elderly.* Redwood City, CA: Addison-Wesley Nursing.

Richmond, T. S., & Metcalf, J. A. (1986). Psychosocial responses to spinal cord injury. *Journal of Neuroscience Nursing, 18,* 183–187.

Seeman, M. (1967). Powerlessness and knowledge: A comparative study of alienation and learning. *Sociometry, 30*(1), 105–123.

Seligman, M. (1975). *Helplessness: On depression, development, and death.* San Francisco: W. H. Freeman.

Simmons, R., & West, G. (1984–85). Life changes, coping resources and health among the elderly. *International Journal of Aging and Human Development, 20,* 173–189.

Spielman, B. J. (1986). Rethinking paradigms in geriatric ethics. *Journal of Religion and Health, 25*(2), 79–83.

Stephenson, C. A. (1979). Powerlessness and chronic illness: Implications for nursing. *Baylor Nursing Educator, 1*(1), 17–28.

Weaver, T., & Narsavage, G. (1992). Physiological and psychological variables related to functional status in chronic obstructive pulmonary disease. *Nursing Research, 41,* 286–291.

Wong, D. L. (1995). *Nursing care of infants and children* (5th ed.). St. Louis: Mosby–Year Book.

Protection, Altered

Tissue Integrity, Impaired*

Skin Integrity, Impaired

Oral Mucous Membrane, Altered

Protection, Altered

DEFINITION

Altered Protection: The state in which an individual experiences a decrease in the ability to guard against internal or external threats, such as illness or injury.

DEFINING CHARACTERISTICS

Major (Must Be Present)

Deficient immunity
Impaired healing
Altered clotting
Maladaptive stress response
Neurosensory alterations

Minor (May Be Present)

Chills	Insomnia
Perspiring	Fatigue
Dyspnea	Anorexia
Cough	Weakness
Itching	Immobility
Restlessness	Disorientation
Pressure sores	

Author's Note

This broad diagnosis describes a person with compromised ability to defend against microorganisms and/or bleeding because of immunosuppression, myelosuppression, and/or abnormal clotting factors. Use of this diagnosis can entail several potential problems.

The nurse should be cautioned against substituting *Altered Protection* as a name for an immune system compromise, acquired immunodeficiency syndrome (AIDS), disseminated intravascular coagulation, diabetes mellitus, or other disorders. Rather, the nurse

---

* This diagnosis was developed and submitted to NANDA by the Clinical Nurse Specialist Group, Harper Hospital, in the Detroit Medical Center.

should focus on diagnoses describing the person's functional abilities that are or may be compromised by altered protection, such as *Fatigue, Risk for Infection*, and *Risk for Social Isolation*. The nurse also should address the physiologic complications of altered protection that require nursing and medical interventions for management, identifying appropriate collaborative problems.

For example, the nurse could use *Altered Protection* in each of these three cases: Mr. A, who has leukemia, leukopenia, and no evidence of infection; Mr. B, who is experiencing sickle cell crisis; and Mr. C, who has AIDS. The problem is that this diagnosis does not describe the specific focus of nursing, but instead describes situations in which more specific responses can be diagnosed. For Mr. A, the nursing diagnosis of *Risk for Infection related to compromised immune system* would apply. For Mr. B., the collaborative problem *Potential Complication: Sickle cell crisis* best describes his situation, which the nurse monitors and manages using physician- and nurse-prescribed interventions. The nursing diagnosis *Risk for Infection* and the collaborative problem *Potential Complication: Opportunistic infections* would apply for Mr. C.

As these examples show, in most cases the nursing diagnosis *Risk for Infection* and selected collaborative problems prove more clinically useful than *Altered Protection*.

Tissue Integrity, Impaired

DEFINITION

Impaired Tissue Integrity: A state in which an individual experiences or is at risk for damage to the integumentary, corneal, or mucous membranous tissues of the body.

DEFINING CHARACTERISTICS
Major (Must Be Present)

Disruptions of corneal, integumentary, or mucous membranous tissue or invasion of body structure (incision, dermal ulcer, corneal ulcer, oral lesion)

Minor (May Be Present)

Lesions (primary, secondary)	Dry mucous membrane
Edema	Leukoplakia
Erythema	Coated tongue

RELATED FACTORS
Pathophysiologic

Related to inflammation of dermal–epidermal junctions secondary to:
> Autoimmune alterations
>> Lupus erythematosus   Scleroderma
> Metabolic and endocrine alterations
>> Diabetes mellitus   Jaundice
>> Hepatitis   Cancer
>> Cirrhosis   Thyroid dysfunction
>> Renal failure

Bacterial (impetigo, folliculitis, cellulitis)
Viral (herpes zoster [shingles], herpes simplex, gingivitis, AIDS)
Fungal (ringworm [dermatophytosis], athlete's foot, vaginitis)
Related to decreased blood and nutrients to tissues secondary to:
Diabetes mellitus
Peripheral vascular alterations
Venous stasis
Arteriosclerosis
Anemia
Cardiopulmonary disorders
Nutritional alterations
Obesity   Emaciation
Dehydration   Malnutrition
Edema

Treatment-Related

Related to decreased blood and nutrients to tissues secondary to:
NPO status
Therapeutic extremes in body temperature
Surgery
Related to imposed immobility secondary to sedation
Related to mechanical trauma
Therapeutic fixation devices
Wired jaw   Casts
Traction   Orthopedic devices/braces
Related to effects of radiation on epithelial and basal cells
Related to effects of mechanical irritants or pressure secondary to:
Inflatable or foam donuts
Tourniquets
Footboards
Restraints
Dressings, tape, solutions
External urinary catheters
Nasogastric tubes
Endotracheal tubes
Oral prostheses/braces
Contact lenses

Situational (Personal, Environmental)

Related to chemical trauma secondary to:
Excretions
Secretions
Noxious agents/substances
Related to environmental irritants secondary to:
Radiation–sunburn   Humidity
Bites (insect, animal) Poison plants
Temperature   Parasites
Inhalants
Related to the effects of pressure of immobility secondary to:
Pain, fatigue, motivation, cognitive, sensory, or motor deficits
Related to inadequate personal habits (hygiene/dental/dietary/sleep)
Related to impaired mobility secondary to (specify)
Related to thin body frame

Maturational

Related to dry, thin skin and decreased dermal vascularity secondary to aging

Author's Note

Impaired Tissue Integrity is the broad diagnosis under which the more specific diagnoses of *Impaired Skin Integrity* and *Impaired Oral Mucous Membranes* fall. Because tissue is composed of epithelium, connective tissue, muscle, and nervous tissue, *Impaired Tissue Integrity* correctly describes some pressure ulcers that are deeper than the dermis. *Impaired Skin Integrity* should be used to describe disruptions of epidermal and dermal tissue only.

When a pressure ulcer is stage IV, necrotic, or infected, it may be more appropriate to label the diagnosis a collaborative problem, such as *Potential Complication: Stage IV pressure ulcer*. This would represent a situation that a nurse manages with physician- and nurse-prescribed interventions. When a stage II or III pressure ulcer needs a dressing that requires a physician's order in an acute care setting, the nurse should continue to label the situation a nursing diagnosis, because it would be appropriate and legal for a nurse to treat the ulcer independently in other settings (*e.g.*, in the community).

If an individual is immobile and multiple systems are threatened (respiratory, circulatory, musculoskeletal as well as integumentary), the nurse can use *Disuse Syndrome* to describe the entire situation. If an individual is at risk for damage to corneal tissue, the nurse can use a diagnosis such as *Risk for Impaired Corneal Tissue Integrity related to corneal drying and lower lacrimal production secondary to unconscious state*.

Errors in Diagnostic Statements

Impaired Skin Integrity related to surgical removal of skin/tissues

Impaired Skin Integrity should not be used as a new label for surgical incisions, tracheostomies, or burns. Surgical incisions disrupt the skin's protective mechanism, increasing vulnerability to microorganism invasion; a more clinically useful diagnosis would be *Risk for Infection related to surgical incision*.

Impaired Skin Integrity related to fecal diversion

Fecal diversions such as colostomy or ileostomy should not be renamed with the nursing diagnosis *Impaired Skin Integrity*. Instead, the nurse should assess the person's actual or potential responses to the surgical procedure that the nurse can treat. For example, the skin around an ostomy is at risk for erosion from effluent, calling for the diagnosis *Risk for Impaired Skin Integrity related to chemical irritation of effluent on adjacent skin*. If the adjacent skin exhibited lesions from irritants (chemical or mechanical), the diagnosis *Impaired Skin Integrity related to exposure to ostomy effluent, as evidenced by 2-cm ulcer left midline of stoma* would be appropriate.

Key Concepts

1. Tissues are groupings of specialized cells that unite to perform specific functions. The human body is composed of four basic types of tissue: epithelial, connective (including skeletal tissue and blood), muscle, and nervous.
2. The external covering of the body is composed of epithelial tissue, called the integument. Wherever the body exposes large openings to the outside (*e.g.*, the mouth), its outer covering changes from integument to an inner lining called the mucous membrane. Each layer of the integument has its counterpart in a complete mucous membrane. The integument includes both the skin and the subcutaneous tissue.
3. The skin is a complex organ consisting of two layers: the outer epidermis and the deeper dermis. The epidermis is approximately 0.04 mm thick, and the dermis is about 0.5 cm thick (Porth, 1994).
4. The epidermis functions as a barrier to protect inner tissues (from injury, chemicals, organisms); as a receptor for a range of sensations (touch, pain, heat, cold); as a regulator of body temperature through radiation (giving off heat), conduction (transfer of heat), and convection (movement of warm air molecules away from the body); as a regulator of water balance by preventing water and electrolyte loss; and as a receptor for vitamin D from the sun (Maklebust & Sieggreen, 1996).

5. Epidermal regeneration is depressed by a water-soluble mitotic inhibitor called chalone. Chalone levels are high during daytime stress and activity and lower during sleep. Healing is therefore promoted during rest and sleep (Maklebust & Sieggreen, 1996).
6. Beneath the avascular epidermis lies the highly vascularized dermis. The dermis contains epithelial tissue, connective tissue, muscle, and nervous tissue. The dermis is rich in collagen, which imparts toughness to the skin. Hair follicles extend into the dermis and serve as islands of cells for rapid reepithelialization of minor wounds. Sweat glands in the dermis contribute to control of body water and temperature. Small muscles within the dermis serve to produce goose pimples. Specialized dermal nerve endings for pain, touch, heat, and cold are irreplaceable once destroyed (Maklebust & Sieggreen, 1996).
7. The subcutaneous tissue, which lies beneath the dermis, stores fat for temperature regulation and contains the remainder of the sweat glands and hair follicles (Porth, 1994).
8. The skin's responses to antigens are capillary dilation (erythema), arteriole dilation (flare), and increased capillary permeability (wheal), which all contribute to localized edema, spasms, and pruritus.
9. Skin lesions can be described as primary or secondary. Primary lesions are the initial responses of the skin to an irritant. Secondary lesions result from changes that take place in primary lesions (Table II-22).

Table II-22 **Primary and Secondary Lesions**

Primary	Secondary
Macules Circumscribed, flat discolorations of the skin Examples: freckles, flat nevi	**Scales** Dead epidermal cells that thicken and flake off Examples: dandruff; psoriasis
Papules Circumscribed, elevated, superficial, solid lesions that are <1 cm Examples: elevated nevi, warts	**Crusts** Dried exudate on the surface of the skin produced when skin is damaged Examples: impetigo, infected dermatitis
Nodules Solid elevation, usually >1 cm in diameter, extend deeper into dermis than papules Examples: epitheliomas	**Fissures** Linear breaks in the tissue, sharply defined with abrupt walls Example: congenital syphilis, athlete's foot
Tumors >1 cm, solid lesions with depth; they may be above, level with, or beneath the skin Example: tumor stage of mycosis fungoides	**Erosion** Loss of epidermis that does not extend into the dermis Example: abrasion
Plaques Circumscribed, elevated, superficial, solid lesions that are >1 cm Examples: localized mycosis fungoides, neurodermatitis	**Ulcers** Localized areas of tissue destruction that may extend into the mucous membrane or through the epidermis, dermis, and underlying tissue Examples: venous ulcers of the legs, tertiary syphilis
Wheals Types of plaques; result is transient edema in dermis	**Scars** Formations of connective tissue replacing tissue lost through injury or disease Example: keloids
Vesicles Up to 1 cm, circumscribed elevations of the skin of mucous membrane containing serous fluid Examples: early chickenpox, contact dermatitis	
Bullae >1 cm, circumscribed elevations containing serous fluid Examples: pemphigus, second-degree burns	

10. Causes of tissue destruction can be mechanical, immunologic, bacterial, chemical, or thermal. Mechanical destruction includes physical trauma or surgical incision. Immunologic destruction occurs as an allergic response to an antigen. Bacterial destruction results from an overgrowth of organisms. Chemical destruction results when a caustic substance maintains contact with unprotected tissue. Thermal destruction occurs when tissue is exposed to temperature extremes that are incompatible with cell life (Maklebust & Sieggreen, 1996).

Wound Healing

1. Wound healing is a complex sequence of events initiated by injury to the tissues. The components of wound healing are coagulation of bleeding, inflammation, epithelialization, fibroplasia and collagen metabolism, collagen maturation and scar remodeling, and wound contraction (Hudson-Goodman, Girard, & Jones, 1990).
2. A wound must be considered in relation to the entire person. Major factors that affect wound healing are nutrition, vitamins, minerals, anemia, blood volume and tissue oxygenation, steroids and antiinflammatory drugs, diabetes mellitus, chemotherapy, and radiation.
3. Wound healing requires the following intrinsic factors (Pinchcofsky-Devin & Kaminski, 1986):
   a. Increased protein–carbohydrate intake sufficient to prevent negative nitrogen balance, hypoalbuminemia, and weight loss
   b. Increased daily intake of vitamins and minerals
   > Vitamin A, 10,000–50,000 IU
   > Vitamin B_1, 0.5–1.0 mg/1000 diet calories
   > Vitamin B_2, 0.25 mg/1000 diet calories
   > Vitamin B_6, 2 mg
   > Niacin, 15–20 mg
   > Vitamin B_{12}, 400 mg
   > Vitamin C, 75–300 mg
   > Vitamin D, 400 mg
   > Vitamin E, 10–15 IU
   > Traces of zinc, magnesium, calcium, copper, manganese
   c. Adequate oxygen supply and the blood volume and ability to transport it

🌀 *Key Concepts—Child*

1. A newborn commonly exhibits normal skin variations, such as mongolian spots, milia, and stork bites, which can be upsetting to parents but are clinically insignificant.
2. Several common conditions of the skin affect children in specific age groups. These include atopic, seborrheic, and diaper dermatitis in infancy and acne in adolescence.
3. Infants and young children have a thin epidermis and require special protection from the sun.

🏛 *Key Concepts—Older Adult*

1. Elastin, which gives the skin flexibility, elasticity, and tensile strength, decreases with age. It is found in tissues associated with body movement, such as the walls of major blood vessels, heart, lungs, and skin (Matteson & McConnell, 1988).
2. Found in all connective tissue, such as blood, lymph, and bone, collagen binds together and supports other tissues. The extracellular matrix of connecting tissue is composed primarily of collagen and elastin, and approximately 80% of the dermis consists of collagen. With aging, skin strength decreases owing to age-related loss of collagen from the dermis and the degeneration of the elastic properties of the remaining collagen.
3. Some older adults exhibit shiny, loose, thin, transparent skin primarily on the backs of the hands and the forearms. Subcutaneous fat decreases with aging, reducing the cushioning of bony prominences, putting elderly people at increased risk for pressure ulcers.

4. Age-related decrease in sebum secretion and the number of sebaceous glands cause drier, coarser skin that is more prone to fissures and cracks (Matteson & McConnell, 1988).

5. In older adults, cells are larger and proliferate more slowly, fibroblasts decrease in number, and dermal vascularity decreases. All these factors contribute to a slowed rate of wound healing.

6. With aging, the thermal threshold for sweating is raised and the sweat output is decreased.

7. Aging nails become dull, brittle, and thickened owing to decreased blood supply to the nailbed. Splitting of the nails can occur, increasing the risk of infection. Thickening of the toenails causes the distal portion of the nail to lift from the nailbed; debris collection creates a risk of fungal infection (Matteson & McConnell, 1988).

8. More than 90% of all older adults have some kind of skin disorder resulting from various causes (*e.g.*, malignancies, stress, metabolic diseases, vascular disorders, and toxic reactions to drugs). Any epidermal invasion carries the chance of infection. Immune system suppression increases the risk of systemic infection (Matteson & McConnell, 1988).

9. Sun exposure is the primary cause of age-related skin changes. The current generation of older adults might be more at risk than younger people, who have benefitted from sunscreens that have been popularized over the last decade or so. (The induction period for sun-caused cancers is 15–40 years.) Repeated sun exposure causes immediate sunburn erythema, thickening of the stratum corneum, and increased melanin production by melanocytes. Incidence of certain pathologic skin conditions (*e.g.*, premalignant cancers, basal cell epitheliomas, and squamous cell carcinomas) increases with sun exposure. Older adults also are at risk for secondary lesions (*e.g.*, scales, crusts, fissures, and ulcers), which predispose to localized or systemic infection.

10. Hypothermia is more common in older adults, particularly in those who show impaired regulation of skin blood flow. This impairment of the thermoregulatory skin vascular reflexes is probably due to degenerative neurologic changes affecting the autonomic nervous system.

11. Many conditions leading to malnutrition are common among older adults; therefore, it is not unusual to find protein depletion and vitamin and trace element deficiencies. Many of these deficiencies involve various cutaneous lesions and mucous membrane disruption. Hypoalbuminemia can contribute to the development of pressure ulcers and to delayed wound healing. Vitamin C seems to be of particular significance in wound healing (Allman, 1989).

TRANSCULTURAL CONSIDERATIONS

1. The darker the person's skin, the more difficult it is to assess for changes in color. A baseline must be established in daylight or with at least a 60-watt bulb. Baseline skin color should be assessed in areas with the least amount of pigmentation (*e.g.*, palms of hands, soles of feet, underside of forearms, abdomen, and buttocks) (Fuller & Schaller-Ayers, 1990).

2. All skin colors have an underlying red tone. Pallor in black-skinned individuals is seen as an ashen or gray tone. Pallor in brown-skinned individuals appears as a yellowish-brown color. Pallor can be assessed in mucous membranes, lips, nailbeds, and conjunctiva of the lower eyelids (Andrews & Boyle, 1995).

3. Assessment of capillary refill time can be done on the second or third finger, lips, or earlobes (Andrews & Boyle, 1995).

4. To assess for rashes and skin inflammations in dark-skinned individuals, the nurse should rely on palpation for warmth and induration, not observation (Giger & Davidhizar, 1995).

5. Mongolian spots are dark blue or black pigmentation seen on the skin of black, Asian, Native American, or Mexican American newborns. They are often mistaken for bruises. By adulthood they are lighter but visible (Giger & Davidhizar, 1995).

6. Some folk remedies may be misdiagnosed as injuries. Three folk practices of Southeast Asians leave marks on the body that can be taken for signs of violence or abuse. *Cao gio* is rubbing of the skin with a coin to produce dark blood or ecchymotic strips; it is done to treat colds and flulike symptoms. *Bat gio* is skin pinching on the temples to treat headaches or on the neck for a sore throat; if petechiae or ecchymoses appear, the treatment is a success. *Poua* is the burning of the skin with the tip of a dried weedlike grass; it is believed the burning will cause the noxious element that causes the pain to exude (Andrews & Boyle, 1995).

Focus Assessment Criteria

Subjective Data

A. Assess for related factors
- 1. History of symptoms
    - a. Onset
    - b. Precipitated by what?
    - c. Relieved by what?
    - d. Frequency?
- 2. History of exposure (if allergy is suspected)
    - a. Carrier of contagious disease
    - b. Chemicals, paints, cleaning agents, plants, animals
    - c. Heat or cold
- 3. Medical, surgical, and dental history; use of tobacco, alcohol
- 4. Current drug therapy
    - a. What drugs? How often? When was last dose taken?
    - b. Effects on symptoms
- 5. Factors contributing to the development or extension of tissue destruction (assess for)
    - a. Skin deficits

Dryness	Thinness
Edema	Excessive perspiration
Obesity	

        Aging skin (dry, thin, loss of elasticity, subcutaneous tissue)
    - b. Mucous membrane deficits

Mouth pain	Oral lesions or ulcers
Bleeding gums	Oral plaque
Coated tongue	Dryness
    - c. Corneal deficits

Absence of blink reflex	Diminished tearing
Corneal ulcers	Contact lens wear
Ptosis	Sensory deficits
Excessive tearing	
    - d. Impaired oxygen transport

        Edema

        Anemia

        Peripheral vascular disorders
        - Arteriosclerosis
        - Venous stasis
        - Cardiopulmonary disorders
    - e. Chemical/mechanical irritants

Radiation	Contact lenses
Casts, splints, braces	Oral prostheses
Incontinence (feces, urine)	
    - f. Nutritional deficits

Protein deficiencies	Vitamin deficiencies
Mineral and trace element deficiencies	Dehydration

g. Systemic disorders
   Infection
   Diabetes mellitus
   Cancer
   Hepatic or renal disorders
h. Sensory deficits
   Brain or cord injury
   Decreased level of consciousness
   Confusion
   Neuropathy
   Visual or taste alterations
i. Immobility

Objective Data

A. Assess for defining characteristics
   1. Skin

Color	Texture	Turgor
Pigment	Coarse	Good
Pallor	Thick	Poor
Cyanosis	Thin	
Jaundice		
Flushed		

Vascularity	Moisture	Temperature
Bruising	Dry	Cool, less than 98.6°F
Bleeding	Moist	Warm, greater than 98.6°F
Angioma	Normal	Normal
Petechiae		
Purpura		
Telangiectasis		

   2. Lesions (primary, secondary; see Table II-22)

Type	Shape
Location	Size
Distribution	Drainage
Color	

   3. Circulation
      a. Is erythema present?
      b. Does the skin blanch when pressure is applied?
      c. Do capillaries refill within 10 seconds after blocking?
      d. Does erythema subside within 30 minutes after pressure is removed?
   4. Edema
      a. Note degree and location
      b. Palpate over bony prominences for sponginess (indicates edema)
   5. Oral mucous membrane
   Refer to Focus Assessment Criteria for *Altered Oral Mucous Membrane*

Outcome Criteria

The person will
• Identify source of mechanical tissue destruction
• Identify rationale for treatment
• Participate in plan to promote wound healing
• Demonstrate progressive healing of tissue

Interventions

A. Identify causative/contributing factors

1. Removal of adhesives
2. Pressure dressings
3. Nasogastric tubes
4. Endotracheal tubes
5. Skeletal prominences with little overlying soft tissue
6. Hard supporting sleep or sitting surfaces
7. Prolonged sitting or lying in same position
8. Dragging across bed linens
9. Sitting in Fowler's position
10. Bladder and bowel incontinence (see *Incontinence*)
11. Profuse diaphoresis
12. Cognitive, sensory, motor deficits
13. Fixation devices
    a. Skeletal traction
    b. Oral prostheses
14. Contact lens wear

B. Reduce contributing factors to mechanical irritants to skin

1. Encourage highest degree of mobility to avoid prolonged periods of pressure.
2. For neuromuscular impairment
   a. Teach client/significant other appropriate measures to prevent pressure, shear, friction, maceration.
   b. Teach client to recognize early signs of tissue damage.
   c. Change position at least every 2 hours around the clock.
   d. Use 30-degree lateral side-lying position (Agency for Health Care Policy and Research [AHCPR], 1992).
   e. Frequently supplement full-body turns with minor shifts in body weight.
3. Keep client clean and dry.
4. Reduce environmental sources of pressure (drains, tubes, dressings).
5. Avoid stripping of epidermis when removing adhesives.
6. Use pressure-dispersing devices as appropriate.
7. Limit semi-Fowler's position in high-risk clients (limit elevation of head of bed to less than 30 degrees [AHCPR, 1992]).
8. Avoid use of knee gatch on bed.
9. Use lift sheet to reposition client.
10. Install overhead trapeze to allow clients increased mobility.
11. Use cornstarch to reduce friction (AHCPR, 1992).

C. Reduce causative factors if possible

1. For casts
   a. Monitor common pressure sites in relationship to cast application.
   b. Apply padding over bony prominence.
   c. Keep cast edges smooth and away from skin surfaces.
   d. Inspect for loose plaster and shifting of padding.

D. Protect skin around feeding tubes or endotracheal tubes with a protective barrier

1. Change dressing when moist.
2. Instruct to report discomforts.

E. Teach how to reduce mechanical irritation with contact lens use (Alexander, 1995)

1. Have person review care of lens.

2. If irritation occurs
   a. Remove lens.
   b. Clean with proper solution.
   c. Check for tears or chips.
   d. Reinsert lens after rewetting.

Rationale

- Contributing factors to tissue destruction can be intrinsic (*e.g.*, vulnerable skin, systemic disorders) or extrinsic (*e.g.*, mechanical, chemical). The more factors present, the more vulnerable the client.
- Principles of pressure ulcer prevention include reducing or rotating pressure on soft tissue. If pressure on soft tissue exceeds intracapillary pressure (approximately 32 mm Hg), capillary occlusion and resulting hypoxia can cause tissue damage.
- Exercise and mobility increase blood flow to all areas.
- Keeping the bed as flat as possible (lower than 30 degrees) and support feet with a foot board helps prevent shear, the pressure created when two adjacent tissue layers move in opposition. If a bony prominence slides across the subcutaneous tissue, the subepidermal capillaries may become bent and pinched, resulting in decreased tissue perfusion.
- Prolonged pressure of the cast on neurovascular structures and other body parts can cause necrosis, pressure sores, and nerve palsies (Mourad, 1980).
- Padding over bony prominences is essential to prevent pressure ulcers (Mourad, 1980).
- Rough or improperly bent plaster edges may cause damage to surrounding skin by friction. When an extremity is not elevated properly, cast edges press into the skin and cause pain (Mourad, 1980).
- Loose plaster or wrinkled padding can irritate skin under casts.
- The catheter can irritate skin and mucosa. Gastric juices can cause severe skin breakdown.
- Because contact lenses are foreign bodies, teaching should focus on prevention of infection and irritation (Alexander, 1995).
- If irritation continues, remove lens and contact eye specialist.
- Emphasize not to use tap water or saliva to lubricate lens.
- Emphasize need to follow disinfection procedures strictly, to rinse case daily and air dry, and to replace case every 3–6 months.

Skin Integrity, Impaired

DEFINITION

Impaired Skin Integrity: A state in which the individual experiences or is at risk for damage to the epidermal and dermal tissue.

DEFINING CHARACTERISTICS
Major (Must Be Present)

Disruptions of epidermal and dermal tissue

Minor (May Be Present)

Denuded skin   Lesions (primary, secondary)
Erythema   Pruritus

RELATED FACTORS

See *Impaired Tissue Integrity*

Author's Note

See *Impaired Tissue Integrity*

Errors in Diagnostic Statements

See *Impaired Tissue Integrity*

Key Concepts

See *Impaired Tissue Integrity*

Focus Assessment Criteria

See *Impaired Tissue Integrity*

Outcome Criteria

If able, the person will
- Participate in risk assessment
- Express willingness to participate in prevention of pressure ulcers
- Describe etiology and prevention measures
- Explain rationale for interventions
- Demonstrate skin integrity free of pressure ulcers

Interventions

A. Use a formal risk assessment scale to identify individual risk factors in addition to activity and mobility deficits (Bergstrom, Braden, Laguzza, & Holman, 1987; Gosnell, 1987; Norton, 1989)

Assess for
1. Skin deficits
   a. Dryness
   b. Edema
   c. Obesity
   d. Thinness
   e. Excessive perspiration
2. Impaired oxygen transport
   a. Edema
   b. Anemia
   c. Peripheral vascular disorders
   d. Arteriosclerosis
   e. Cardiopulmonary disorders
3. Chemical/mechanical/thermal irritants
   a. Radiation
   b. Incontinence (feces, urine)
   c. Casts, splints, braces
   d. Spasms

4. Nutritional deficits
   a. Protein deficiencies
   b. Vitamin deficiencies
   c. Mineral and trace element deficiencies
   d. Dehydration
5. Systemic disorders
   a. Infection
   b. Diabetes mellitus
   c. Cancer
   d. Hepatic or renal disorders
6. Sensory deficits
   a. Neuropathy
   b. Confusion
   c. Head injury
   d. Cord injury
7. Immobility

B. Attempt to modify contributing factors to lessen the possibility of development of a pressure ulcer

1. Incontinence of urine or feces
   a. Determine etiology of incontinence.
   b. Maintain sufficient fluid intake for adequate hydration (approximately 2500 mL daily, unless contraindicated); check mucous membranes in mouth for moisture and check urine specific gravity.
   c. Establish a schedule for emptying bladder (begin with every 2 hours).
   d. If person is confused, determine what his incontinence pattern is and intervene before incontinence occurs.
   e. Explain problem to individual and secure cooperation for plan.
   f. When incontinent, wash perineum with a liquid soap that does not alter skin pH.
   g. Apply a protective barrier to the perineal region (incontinence film barrier spray or wipes).
   h. Check person frequently for incontinence when indicated.
   i. For additional interventions, refer to *Altered Patterns of Urinary Elimination.*
2. Immobility
   a. Encourage range-of-motion exercise and weight-bearing mobility, when possible, to increase blood flow to all areas.
   b. Promote optimal circulation when in bed.
      Use repositioning schedule that relieves vulnerable area most often (*e.g.*, if vulnerable area is the back, turning schedule would be left side to back, back to right side, right side to left side, and left side to back); post "turn clock" at bedside.
      Turn person or instruct him to turn or shift weight every 30 minutes to 2 hours, depending on other causative factors present and the ability of the skin to recover from pressure.
      Frequency of turning schedule should be increased if any reddened areas that appear do not disappear within 1 hour after turning.
      Position person in normal or neutral position with body weight evenly distributed (Fig. II-6). Use 30 degree laterally inclined position when possible.
      Keep bed as flat as possible to reduce shearing forces; limit semi-Fowler's position for only 30 minutes at a time (AHCPR, 1992).
      Use foam blocks or pillows to provide a bridging effect to support the body above and below the high-risk or ulcerated area so that affected area does not touch bed surface. Do not use foam donuts or inflatable rings because these increase the area of pressure (AHCPR, 1992).

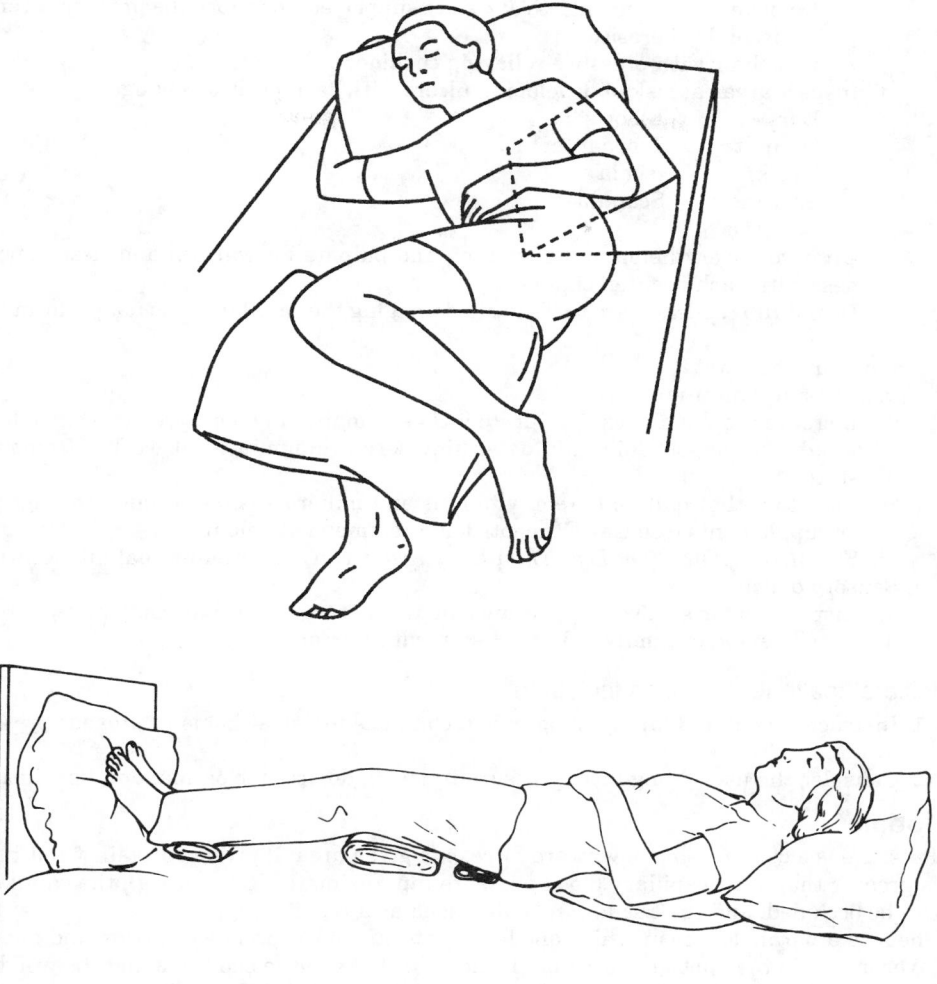

Fig. II-6 Positioning. (*Top*) Side-lying position. Pillows are used above and below the trochanter and lateral malleolus to relieve pressure. (Adapted from Maklebust, J. [December, 1991]). Pressure ulcer update. *RN,* 56–63. Original illustration by Jack Tandy. Used with permission.) (*Bottom*) Supine position. Pillows are used above and below the sacrum and above the heels to relieve pressure. A pillow above the knees prevents hyperextension of the knees and relieves pressure on the popliteal space.

Alternate or reduce the pressure on the skin surface with:
Foam mattresses (comfort only)
Triple-layered air mattresses (pressure relief)
Air-fluidized beds (pressure relief and moisture control)
Suspend heels off of bed surface (AHCPR, 1992).
c. Use enough personnel to lift person up in bed or chair rather than pull or slide skin surfaces. Have person wear long-sleeved top and socks to reduce friction on elbows and heels.
d. To reduce shearing forces, support feet with footboard to prevent sliding.
e. Promote optimum circulation when person is sitting.
Limit sitting time for person at high risk for ulcer development.
Instruct person to lift self using chair arms every 10 minutes, if possible, or assist person in rising up off the chair at least every hour, depending on risk factors present.

Do not elevate legs unless calves are supported, to reduce the pressure over the ischial tuberosities.

Pad chair with pressure-relieving cushion.

  f. Inspect areas at risk of developing ulcers with each position change.

Ears	Elbows
Occiput	Trochanter*
Heels*	Ischia
Sacrum	Scapula
Scrotum	

  g. Observe for erythema and blanching and palpate for warmth and tissue sponginess with each position change.

  h. Do not rub reddened areas. To avoid damaging the capillaries, do not perform massage.

3. Malnourished state

  a. Consult a dietitian.

  b. Increase protein and carbohydrate intake to maintain a positive nitrogen balance; weigh the person daily and determine serum albumin level weekly to monitor status.

  c. Ascertain that daily intake of vitamins and minerals is maintained through diet or supplements (see Key Concepts for recommended amounts).

  d. See *Altered Nutrition: Less Than Body Requirements* for additional interventions.

4. Sensory deficit

  a. Inspect person's skin daily, because he will not experience discomfort.

  b. Teach person or family to inspect skin with mirror.

C. Initiate health teaching, as indicated

1. Instruct person and family in specific techniques to use at home to prevent pressure ulcers.

2. Consider the use of long-term pressure-relieving devices for permanent disabilities.

Rationale

- Pressure is a compressing downward force on a given area. If pressure against soft tissue is greater than intracapillary blood pressure (approximately 32 mm Hg), the capillaries can be occluded, and the tissue can be damaged as a result of hypoxia.
- Shear is a parallel force in which one layer of tissue moves in one direction and another layer moves in the opposite direction. If the skin sticks to the bed linen and the weight of the sitting body makes the skeleton slide down inside the skin, the subepidermal capillaries may become angulated and pinched, resulting in decreased perfusion of the tissue.
- Friction is the physiologic wearing away of tissue. If the skin is rubbed against the bed linens, the epidermis can be denuded by abrasion.
- Maceration is a mechanism by which the tissue is softened by prolonged wetting or soaking. If the skin becomes waterlogged, the cells are weakened and the epidermis is easily eroded.
- Pressure relief is the one consistent intervention that must be included in all pressure ulcer treatment plans.
- A pressure-relieving surface must not be able to be fully compressed by the body. To be effective, a support surface must be capable of first being deformed and then redistributing the weight of the body across the surface. Comfort is not a valid criterion for determining adequate pressure relief. A hand check should be performed to determine if the product is effectively reducing pressure. The palm is placed under the pressure-reducing mattress; if the client can feel the hand or the caregiver can feel the client, the pressure is not adequate.
- Adequate nutrition (protein, vitamins, minerals) are vital for healing wounds, preventing infection, preserving immune function, and minimizing loss of strength (Maklebust & Sieggreen, 1996).

---

* Areas with little soft tissue over a body prominence are at greatest risk.

■ Impaired Skin Integrity
Related to the Effects of Pressure, Friction, Shear, Maceration

Outcome Criteria

The person will
• Identify causative factors for pressure ulcers
• Identify rationale for prevention and treatment
• Participate in the prescribed treatment plan to promote wound healing
• Demonstrate progressive healing of dermal ulcer

Interventions

A. Identify the stage of pressure ulcer development (National Pressure Advisory Panel, 1989; AHCPR, 1992)
   1. Stage I: Nonblanchable erythema of intact skin
   2. Stage II: Ulceration of epidermis and/or dermis
   3. Stage III: Ulceration involving subcutaneous fat
   4. Stage IV: Extensive ulceration penetrating muscle, bone, or supporting structure

B. Reduce or eliminate factors that contribute to the development or extension of pressure ulcers; refer to *Risk for Impaired Skin Integrity related to immobility*

C. Prevent deterioration of the ulcer
   1. Wash reddened area gently with a mild soap, rinse area thoroughly to remove soap, and pat dry.
   2. Avoid massage of bony prominence to stimulate circulation (AHCPR, 1992).
   3. Protect the healthy skin surface with one or a combination of the following.
      a. Apply a thin coat of liquid copolymer skin sealant.
      b. Cover area with moisture-permeable film dressing.
      c. Cover area with a hydrocolloid wafer barrier and secure with strips of 1-inch microscope tape; leave in place for 2–3 days.
   4. Increase dietary intake to promote wound healing.
      a. Initiate calorie count. Consult dietitian.
      b. Increase protein and carbohydrate intake to maintain a positive nitrogen balance: weigh the person daily and determine serum albumin level weekly to monitor status.
      c. Ascertain that daily intake of vitamins and minerals is maintained through diet or supplements (see Key Concepts for recommended amounts).
      d. See *Altered Nutrition: Less Than Body Requirements* for additional interventions.

D. Devise plan for pressure ulcer management using principles of moist wound healing (Maklebust & Sieggreen, 1996)
   1. Assess status of pressure ulcer. Measure size of wound bed for baseline data. Measure areas of tunneling or undermining. Assess color, odor, and amount of drainage from wound. Also assess color of skin surrounding wound bed.

2. Debride necrotic tissue (collaborate with physician).
3. Flush ulcer base with sterile saline solution. Avoid use of harsh antiseptic solutions.
4. Protect granulating wound bed from trauma and bacteria. Insulate wound surface.
5. Cover pressure ulcer with a sterile dressing that maintains a moist environment over the ulcer base (*e.g.*, film dressing, hydrocolloid wafer dressing, moist gauze dressing). Do not occlude ulcers on immunocompromised patients.
6. Avoid the use of drying agents (heat lamps, Maalox, Milk of Magnesia).
7. Monitor for clinical signs of wound infection.
8. Measure pressure ulcer weekly to determine progress of wound healing.

E. Consult with nurse specialist or physician for treatment of necrotic, infected, or deep pressure ulcers

F. Initiate health teaching and referrals, as indicated
1. Instruct person and family on care of ulcers (Maklebust & Magnan, 1992).
2. Teach the importance of good skin hygiene and optimum nutrition.
3. Refer to community nursing agency if additional assistance at home is needed.

Rationale

- See Rationale for *Impaired Skin Integrity*.
- Wound healing occurs most efficiently with the following extrinsic factors (Maklebust & Sieggreen, 1996).
  - Humidity affects the rate of epithelialization and the amount of scar formation. A moist environment provides the optimum conditions for rapid healing.
  - When wounds are left uncovered, epidermal cells must migrate under the scab and over the fibrous tissue below. When wounds are semioccluded and the surface of the wound remains moist, epidermal cells migrate more rapidly over the surface.
  - Moist wound healing may be promoted with the appropriate use of dressings. Wounds that are epidermal or dermal in depth may be mechanically protected and properly humidified by the use of semiocclusive film dressings or hydrocolloid barrier wafers. These dressings bathe the wound in serous exudate and do not adhere to the wound surface when they are removed. A physician's order may be required.
- Rationale of topical treatment (Doughty, 1990; Maklebust & Sieggreen, 1996):
  - Remove necrotic tissue. Necrotic tissue delays wound healing by prolonging the inflammatory phase.
  - Cleanse wound bed to decrease bacterial count. Bacterial counts >105 may produce infection by overwhelming the host.
  - Obliterate dead space in wound, which prevents premature closure and abscess formation.
  - Absorb excess exudate, which macerates surrounding skin and increases risk of infection in wound bed.
  - Maintain a moist wound surface, which promotes cellular migration. Dry wound surfaces delay epithelialization secondary to difficult cellular migration.
  - Insulate the wound surface, which enhances blood flow and increases epidermal migration.
  - Protect the healing wound from trauma and bacterial invasion. Open wounds are vulnerable to abrasion, contamination, drying, and shear mechanisms.

Oral Mucous Membrane, Altered

DEFINITION
Altered Oral Mucous Membrane: The state in which an individual experiences or is at risk of experiencing disruptions in the oral cavity.

DEFINING CHARACTERISTICS
Major (Must Be Present)
Disrupted oral mucous membranes

Minor (May Be Present)
Coated tongue	Leukoplakia
Xerostomia (dry mouth)	Edema
Stomatitis	Hemorrhagic gingivitis
Oral tumors	Purulent drainage
Oral lesions	

RELATED FACTORS
Pathophysiologic
Related to inflammation secondary to:
Diabetes mellitus	Periodontal disease
Oral cancer	Infection

Treatment-Related
Related to drying effects of:
- NPO more than 24 hours
- Radiation to head or neck
- Prolonged use of steroids or other immunosuppressives
- Use of antineoplastic drugs

Related to mechanical irritation secondary to:
- Endotracheal tube
- Nasogastric tube

Situational (Personal, Environmental)
Related to chemical irritants secondary to:
- Acidic foods
- Drugs
- Noxious agents
- Alcohol
- Tobacco

Related to mechanical trauma secondary to:
- Broken or jagged teeth
- Ill-fitting dentures
- Braces

Related to malnutrition
Related to dehydration
Related to mouth breathing
Related to inadequate oral hygiene
Related to lack of knowledge of oral hygiene
Related to decreased salivation

Author's Note

See *Impaired Tissue Integrity*

Errors in Diagnostic Statements

See *Impaired Tissue Integrity*

Key Concepts

1. Oral health directly influences many activities of daily living (eating, fluid intake, breathing) and interpersonal relations (appearance, self-concept, communication).
2. Many oral diseases begin quietly and are painless until significant involvement has taken place.
3. Common causes of decreased salivation are dehydration, anemia, radiation treatment to head and neck, vitamin deficiencies, removal of salivary glands, allergies, and side effects of drugs (*e.g.*, antihistamines, anticholinergics, phenothiazine, narcotics, chemotherapy).
4. Excessive use of hydrogen peroxide for mouth care may predispose to an oral yeast infection. Rinse afterward with normal saline (Pettigrew, 1989).
5. Lemon and glycerin swabs should be used only on clean, healthy mouths as a source of refreshment for an NPO client (Danielson, 1988).
6. Alcohol and tobacco are chronic irritants to oral mucosa and may lead to oral carcinoma.
7. Stomatitis is an inflammatory response of oral mucosal epithelial cells to the cytotoxic effects of chemotherapy and localized radiation therapy (Goodman, Ladd, & Purl, 1993).
8. Stomatitis occurs most frequently with antimetabolites and antitumor antibiotics (Goodman et al., 1993).
9. Chemotherapy or direct radiation can also cause xerostomia, which is a decrease in the quality and quantity of saliva (Goodman et al., 1993).

Key Concepts—Child

1. Oral candidiasis (thrush) is common in the newborn. It can be acquired by person-to-person transmission, from a maternal vaginal infection during delivery, or from use of contaminated nipples or other articles (Wong, 1995).
2. Teething may cause discomfort and make the gums appear red and swollen (Upton, 1989).

Key Concepts—Older Adult

1. Age-related changes in oral mucosa include loss of elasticity, atrophy of epithelial cells, and diminished blood supply to connective tissue (Miller, 1995).
2. Dry mouth and vitamin deficiencies in elderly people increase vulnerability to oral ulcerations and infection (Miller, 1995).
3. Elderly people commonly exhibit increased saliva viscosity and diminished saliva quantity (Lassila, 1987).

TRANSCULTURAL CONSIDERATIONS

1. In some ethnic groups, there is a bony protuberance in the mouth, either mandibular or palatine torus. This lump can be felt on either side of the mandible near the second premolar or on the midline of the palate. Palatine torus occurs in about 25% of people from various ethnic groups; mandibular torus occurs in up to 40% of Asians (Overfield, 1985).

Focus Assessment Criteria

Subjective Data

A. Assess for defining characteristics
   1. The person complains of
      a. Mouth pain, irritation, or burning

    b. Xerostomia (dry mouth)
    c. Bad taste or odor in mouth
    d. Chewing difficulties
    e. Change in tolerance to temperature of food (cold, hot)
    f. Change in tolerance to acidic or highly seasoned food
    g. Change in taste
    h. Inability to eat, drink, or swallow own saliva
    i. Poorly fitting dentures

B. Assess for related factors
  1. History
    a. Medical/surgical
    b. Medication use (prescribed, over-the-counter)
    c. Use of tobacco
        Type (cigarettes, pipe, cigars, snuff)
        Frequency (packs per day, how many years)
    d. Use of alcohol
        Type
        Amount (daily, weekly)
  2. Oral hygiene
    a. Frequency of dental checkups
    b. Personal hygiene
        "Describe your oral care procedure."
        Type of equipment (brush, floss)
        Frequency
    c. Possible barriers to performing oral care
        Unable to hold standard brush
        Unable to close hand
        Limited arm movement
        Semicomatose
        Lack of knowledge
  3. Nutritional status (refer to *Altered Nutrition* for specific assessment criteria)
    a. Daily intake of basic five food groups
    b. Daily fluid intake
    c. Difficulty in chewing or swallowing
    d. Are certain foods avoided? Why?

Objective Data
A. Assess for defining characteristics
  1. Lips
    a. Color
    b. Presence of
        Cracks   Blisters
        Fissures   Ulcers/lesions
  2. Tongue
    a. Color
    b. Presence of
        Masses   Cracks, dryness
        Lesions   Exudates
        Hairy extensions   Blisters
  3. Oral mucosa (gums, floor of mouth, inner cheeks, palate)
    a. Color, moisture
    b. Presence of
        Bleeding   Plaques
        Swelling   Lesions

4. Saliva

      Watery   Absent

      Thick

B. Assess for related factors

    1. Teeth

      a. Presence of

          Sharp edges   Looseness

          Chips   Missing teeth

          Cracks

    2. Dentures/prosthetics

      a. Condition

      b. Fit

      c. Presence of

          Sharp edges   Cracks

          Loose parts   Chips

Outcome Criteria

The person will
- Be free of oral mucosa irritation or exhibit signs of healing with decreased inflammation
- Demonstrate knowledge of optimal oral hygiene

Interventions

A. Assess for the presence of causative or contributing factors

    1. Poor oral hygiene, preexisting dental problems

    2. Malnourishment

    3. History of high alcohol intake and tobacco use

    4. Chemotherapeutic drugs with mucous membrane toxicity

    5. Radiation to head or neck

    6. Immunosuppression

    7. Dehydration

    8. Steroid therapy

    9. Antibiotics

B. Teach preventive oral hygiene to individuals at risk for development of stomatitis

    1. Refer to *Altered Oral Mucous Membrane Related to Inadequate Oral Hygiene* for specific instructions on brushing and flossing.

    2. Instruct person to

      a. Perform the regimen after meals and before sleep (if there is excessive exudate, perform regimen before breakfast also).

      b. Avoid mouthwashes with high alcohol content, lemon/glycerin swabs, or prolonged use of hydrogen peroxide.

      c. Rinse mouth with flavored saline solution.

      d. Apply lubricant to lips every 2 hours and PRN (*e.g.*, lanolin, A&D ointment, petroleum jelly).

      e. Inspect mouth daily for lesions and inflammation and report alterations.

    3. For person who is unable to tolerate brushing or swabbing, teach to irrigate mouth (every 2 hours and PRN).

      a. With normal saline, use an enema bag (labeled for oral use only) with a soft irrigation catheter tip.

    b. Place catheter tip in mouth and slowly increase flow while standing over a basin or having a basin held under chin.

    c. Remove dentures before irrigation and do not replace in person with severe stomatitis.

  4. Consult with physician for possible need of prophylactic antifungal or antibacterial agent.

  5. For individuals at risk for radiation-induced stomatitis (Goodman et al., 1993):

    a. Instruct to see dentist 2–3 weeks before initiation of therapy for diagnosis and treatment of infections and to ensure adequate time for healing.

    b. Consult with dentist for a regimen of daily fluoride treatments and oral hygiene.

    c. Continue to see dentist during treatment as needed and 2 months after treatment.

C. Promote healing and reduce progression of stomatitis

1. Inspect oral cavity three times daily with tongue blade and light; if stomatitis is severe, inspect mouth every 4 hours.
2. Ensure that oral hygiene regimen is done every 2 hours while awake and every 6 hours (every 4 hours if severe) during the night.
3. Use normal saline solution as a mouthwash.
4. Floss teeth only once in 24 hours.
5. Omit flossing if excessive bleeding occurs and use extreme caution with people with platelet counts of less than 50,000.

D. Reduce oral pain and maintain adequate food and fluid intake

1. Assess person's ability to chew and swallow.
2. Administer mild analgesic every 3 to 4 hours as ordered by physician.
3. Instruct individual to
    a. Avoid commercial mouthwashes, citrus fruit juices, spicy foods, extremes in food temperature (hot, cold), crusty or rough foods, alcohol, mouthwashes with alcohol.
    b. Eat bland, cool foods (sherbets).
    c. Drink cool liquids every 2 hours and PRN.
4. Consult with dietitian for specific interventions.
5. Refer to *Altered Nutrition: Less Than Body Requirements Related to Anorexia* for additional interventions.
6. Consult with physician for an oral pain relief solution.
    a. Xylocaine Viscous 2% oral, swish and expectorate every 2 hours and before meals (if throat is sore, the solution can be swallowed; if swallowed, Xylocaine produces local anesthesia and may affect the gag reflex).
    b. Mix equal parts of Xylocaine Viscous, 0.5 aqueous Benadryl solution, and Maalox, swish and swallow 1 oz of mixture every 2–4 hours PRN.
    c. Mix equal parts of 0.5 aqueous Benadryl solution and Kaopectate; swish and swallow every 2–4 hours PRN.

E. Initiate health teaching and referrals, as indicated

1. Teach person and family the factors that contribute to the development of stomatitis and its progression.
2. Teach diet modifications to reduce oral pain and to maintain optimal nutrition.
3. Have individual describe or demonstrate home care regimen.

Rationale

- The frequency of oral health maintenance varies according to an individual's health status and self-care ability. All people should have their teeth and mouths cleaned at least once after meals and at bedtime. High-risk people (*e.g.*, people with nasogastric tubes, cancer, and poorly nourished people) should have oral assessments daily. People in chronic care settings should have oral assessment *at least once* a week.
- Decreased salivary flow and increased viscosity of saliva reduce the removal of debris (food, bacteria) from the mouth (Pettigrew, 1989).

- Factors that contribute to stomatitis are poor oral hygiene, preexisting oral disease, irritants (spicy foods, citrus fruits, coarse foods [hard bread, pizza], ill-fitting dental prostheses, too-cold or too-hot foods, tobacco or alcohol), dehydration, malnutrition, and drug therapy (antibiotics, steroids) (Goodman et al., 1993).
- Proper hydration must be maintained to liquefy secretions and prevent drying of oral mucosa.
- Dry oral mucosa causes discomfort and increases the risk of breakdown and infection.

■ Risk for Altered Oral Mucous Membrane
Related to Inadequate Oral Hygiene or Inability to Perform Oral Hygiene

Outcome Criteria

The person will
- Demonstrate integrity of the oral cavity
- Be free of harmful plaque to prevent secondary infection
- Be free of oral discomfort during food and fluid intake

Interventions

A. Assess for the presence of causative or contributing factors
   1. Lack of knowledge
   2. Lack of motivation
   3. Impaired ability to use hands
   4. Fatigue
   5. Altered consciousness

B. Discuss the importance of daily oral hygiene and periodic dental examinations
   1. Explain the relationship of plaque to dental and gum disease.
   2. Evaluate the person's ability to perform oral hygiene.
   3. Allow person to perform as much of his oral care as possible.

C. Teach correct oral care
   1. Have person sit or stand upright over sink (if unable to get to sink, place an emesis pan under the chin).
   2. Remove and clean dentures and bridges daily.
      a. Fill wash bowl half full of water (place washcloth on bottom to keep denture from breaking if dropped).
      b. Brush dentures with a denture brush or stiff, hard toothbrush inside and outside; rinse in cool water before replacing.
      c. Stains and odors can be removed from dentures by soaking them overnight in 8 oz of water and 1 tsp of laundry bleach (avoid bleach on any appliance with metal).
      d. Hard deposits can be removed by soaking dentures in white (not brown) vinegar overnight.
      e. If commercial liquid denture cleaners are used, brushing is still required.

3. Floss teeth (every 24 hours).
   a. With a piece of dental floss approximately 25 inches long, floss each tooth by wrapping the floss around the second and third fingers of each hand.
   b. Beginning with the back teeth, insert the floss between each tooth gently to avoid injuring the gum.
   c. Wrap floss around tooth, making a C, and gently pull floss up and down over the back of each tooth.
   d. Repeat this in reverse to floss the front of the tooth.
   e. Remove the floss either by pulling straight up or by releasing one end and pulling the floss through (minor bleeding may occur).
   f. Allow the person to rinse.
   g. Floss holders can be used by the person or the nurse to make flossing easier (back teeth cannot be reached with a floss holder).
4. Brush teeth (after meals and before sleep).
   a. Use a soft toothbrush (avoid hard brushes) with a nonabrasive toothpaste or sodium bicarbonate (1 tsp in 8 oz of water; may be contraindicated in people with sodium restrictions).
   b. Brush back and forth or in a small circle, starting at the back of the mouth and brushing one or two teeth at a time.
   c. Gently brush tongue and inner sides of cheeks.
   d. Rinse with water.
5. Inspect mouth for lesions, sores, or excessive bleeding.

D. Perform oral hygiene on person who is unconscious or at risk for aspiration as often as needed
   1. Preparation
      a. Tell person what you are going to do.
      b. Turn person on his side, supporting back with pillow (protect bed with an absorbent pad).
      c. Place a tongue blade or bite block to keep mouth open.
      d. Wear gloves to protect self.
   2. Brushing procedure
      a. For people with their own teeth, brush following the procedure outlined in C, nos. 3 and 4.
      b. Use a solution instead of toothpaste:hydrogen peroxide and water (1:4), sodium bicarbonate (1 tsp:8 oz water), or normal saline solution (may be contraindicated in people with sodium restrictions).
      c. For people with dentures, remove dentures and clean according to procedure in C, no. 2.
      d. Leave dentures out for people who are semicomatose and store in water (in denture cup).
      e. If gums are inflamed, use moist cotton-tipped applicators or soft foam Toothettes.
      f. Use a bulb syringe to rinse mouth; aspirate rinse with suction or use an aspirating toothbrush.
      g. Move tongue blade or bite block for access to other areas; do not put fingers on tops or edges of teeth.
      h. Brush tongue and inner cheek tissue gently.
      i. Pat mouth dry and apply lip lubricant.
      j. Gums and teeth should be lightly wiped four to six times a day to prevent drying (*e.g.*, swab with mineral oil or saline but use sparingly to prevent aspiration).

E. Initiate health teaching and referrals, as indicated
1. Identify individuals who need toothbrush adaptations to perform own mouth care.
    a. Difficulty closing hand tightly (Danielson, 1988)
       Tape a wide elastic band to toothbrush tightly enough to hold brush snugly in hand.
    b. Limited hand mobility
       Enlarge toothbrush handle with a sponge hair roller, wrinkled aluminum foil, or a bicycle handlebar grip attached with a small amount of plaster of Paris.
    c. Limited arm movement
       Extend handle of standard toothbrush by attaching handle of an old toothbrush (after cutting off bristle end) to a new toothbrush with strong cord or plastic cement, or by attaching toothbrush to a plastic rod (the toothbrush can be curved by gently heating and then bending it).
2. Refer individuals with tooth and gum disorders to a dentist.

Rationale

- Refer also to *Altered Oral Mucous Membrane.*
- Factors that contribute to oral disease are alcohol and tobacco (excessive use), microorganisms, inadequate nutrition (quantity, quality), inadequate hygiene, and trauma (nasogastric tubes, ill-fitting dentures, sharp-edged teeth, sharp-edged prostheses, improper use of cleaning devices) (Harrell & Damon, 1989).
- Plaque is microbial flora found in the mouth and is the primary factor contributing to dental cavities and periodontal disease. Daily removal of plaque through brushing and flossing can help prevent dental decay and disease.

Interventions—*Child Focus*

1. Teach parents
    a. Provide their child with fluoride supplements if not present in concentrations over 0.7 parts per million (ppm) in drinking water.
    b. Avoid taking tetracycline drugs during pregnancy or giving to child under 8 years of age.
    c. Refrain from putting an infant to bed with a bottle of juice or milk.
    d. Provide child with safe objects for chewing during teething.
    e. Replace toothbrushes frequently (every 3 months).
    f. Schedule dental checkups every 6 months after the age of 2 years.
    g. Supervise and assist preschool child with brushing and flossing in front of mirror
       Talk to child when brushing
       "Ask child to 'tweet like a bird' to brush front teeth and 'roar as a lion' to brush back teeth" (Wong, 1995).
       Incorporate brushing and flossing teeth into bedtime rituals.
2. Teach child
    a. Why tooth care is important
    b. To avoid highly sugared liquids, foods, and chewing gum
    c. To drink water and extra fluid
    d. To brush teeth using fluoride toothpaste

Rationale

- The objective of oral hygiene is to remove plaque, which causes decay and periodontal disease (Wong, 1995).
- Flossing removes plaque from gum line.

- Fluoride makes enamel more resistant to caries by decreasing the effects of acid on surface (American Academy of Pediatrics, 1989).

Interventions—*Maternal Focus*

1. Stress the importance of good oral hygiene and continuation with dental examinations.
2. Remind to advise dentist of pregnancy.
3. Explain that gum hypertrophy and tenderness are normal during pregnancy.

Rationale

- Gum hypertrophy, tenderness, and bleeding may be present during a normal pregnancy (May & Mahlmeister, 1994).

Interventions—*Older Adult Focus*

1. Explain high-risk age-related factors (Miller, 1995).
   a. Degenerative bone disease
   b. Diminished oral blood supply
   c. Dry mouth
   d. Vitamin deficiencies
2. Explain that some medications cause dry mouth.
   Laxatives
   Antibiotics
   Antidepressants
   Anticholinergics
   Analgesics
   Iron sulfate
   Cardiovascular medications
3. Determine the presence of barriers to dental care.
   a. Financial
   b. Mobility
   c. Dexterity
   d. Lack of knowledge

Rationale

- Age-related changes and nutritional deficiencies increase vulnerability to oral ulcerations and infection (Miller, 1995).

References/Bibliography

Agency for Health Care Policy and Research [AHCPR] Panel for the Prediction and Prevention of Pressure Ulcers in Adults. (1992, May). *Pressure ulcers in adults: Prediction and prevention.* Clinical Practice Guidelines Number 3, AHCPR, Bulletin No. 92-0047. Rockville, MD: Agency for Health Care Policy & Research, Public Health Services, U.S. Department of Health and Human Services.

Alexander, K. (1995). *Primary eye care.* Philadelphia: J. B. Lippincott.

Allman, R. M. (1989). Pressure sores among the elderly. *New England Journal of Medicine, 320,* 850–853.

Andrews, M., & Boyle, J. (1995). *Transcultural concepts in nursing care* (2nd ed.). Philadelphia: J. B. Lippincott

Bergstrom, N., Braden, B. J., Laguzza, A., & Holman, V. (1987). The Braden Scale for predicting pressure sore risk. *Nursing Research, 36,* 205–210.

Bergstrom, N., Demuth, P. J., & Braden, B. (1987). A clinical trial of the Braden Scale for predicting pressure sore risk. *Nursing Clinics of North America, 22,* 417–428.

Doughty, D. (1990). Your patient: Which therapy? *Journal of Enterostomal Therapy, 17,* 154–159.

Fuller, J., & Schaller-Ayers, J. (1990). *Health assessment: A nursing approach.* Philadelphia: J. B. Lippincott.

Giger, J. N., & Davidhizar, R. E. (1991). *Transcultural nursing: Assessment and interventions.* St. Louis: Mosby–Year Book.

Gosnell, D. J. (1973). An assessment tool to identify pressure sores. *Nursing Research, 22,* 55.

Gosnell, D. J. (1987) Development of an instrument to assess client risk for pressure sores. In C. F. Waltz & O. Strickland (Eds.). *Measure-*

ment of clinical and education nursing outcomes: A compendium of tools for research, education, and practice. New York: Springer.

Hudson-Goodman, P., Girard, N., & Jones, M. B. (1990). Wound repair and the use of growth factors. Heart and Lung, 19, 379–384.

Maklebust, J. (1991). Impact of AHCPR pressure ulcers guidelines on nursing practice. Decubitus, 4(2), 46–50.

Maklebust, J., Brunckhorst, L., Cracchiolo-Caraway, A., Ducharme, M., Dundon, R., Panfilla, R., Parzuchowski, J., Sieggreen, M., & Walthall, S. (1988). Pressure ulcer incidence in high-risk patients managed on a special three layered air cushion. Decubitus, 1(4), 30–40.

Maklebust, J., & Magnan, M. (1992). Approaches to patient and family education for pressure ulcer management. Decubitus, 5(3), 43–47.

Maklebust, J. A., Mondoux, L. C., & Sieggreen, M. Y. (1986). Pressure relief characteristics of various support surfaces used in prevention and treatment of pressure ulcers. Journal of Enterostomal Therapy, 13(3), 85–89.

Maklebust, J., & Sieggreen, M. (1996). Pressure ulcers: Guidelines for prevention and nursing management (2nd ed.). Springhouse, PA: Springhouse.

Maklebust, J., Sieggreen, M. Y., & Mondoux, L. (1988). Pressure relieving capabilities: A comparison of the SoF-Care cushion and the Clinitron bed. Ostomy/Wound Management, 21, 32–41.

Matteson, M. A., & McConnell, E. S. (1988). Gerontological nursing: Concepts and practice. Philadelphia: W. B. Saunders.

May, K. A., & Mahlmeister, L. R. (1994). Maternal and neonatal nursing: Family-centered care (3rd ed.). Philadelphia: J. B. Lippincott.

Mourad, L. (1980). Nursing care of adults with orthopedic conditions. New York: John Wiley & Sons.

National Pressure Advisory Panel. (1989). Pressure ulcers: Incidence, economics, risk assessment, consensus development conference statement. West Dundee, IL: S-N Publications.

Norton, D. (1989). Calculating the risk: Reflections on the Norton scale. Decubitus, 2(3), 24–31.

Novotny, J. (1989). Adolescents, acne, and the side-effects of Accutane. Pediatric Nursing, 15, 247–248.

Overfield, T. (1985). Biologic variation in health and illness: Race, age, and sex differences. Menlo Park, CA: Addison-Wesley.

Pinchcofsky-Devin, G. D., & Kaminski, M. V. (1986). Correlation of pressure sores and nutritional status. Journal of the American Geriatric Society, 34, 435–440.

Porth, C. (1994). Pathophysiology: Concepts of altered health states (4th ed.). Philadelphia: J. B. Lippincott.

Upton, L. (1989). Growth and development of the infant. In R. L. Foster, M. M. Hunsberger, & J. J. T. Anderson (Eds.). Family-centered nursing care of children. Philadelphia: W, B. Saunders.

Wong, D. L. (1995). Nursing care of infants and children (5th ed.). St. Louis: Mosby–Year Book.

Oral Mucous Membrane

American Academy of Pediatrics, Committee on Nutrition. (1989). Fluoride supplementation. Pediatrics, 77, 758–761.

Danielson, K. H. (1988). Oral care and older adults. Journal of Gerontological Nursing, 14(11), 6–10.

Goodman, M, Ladd, L., & Purl, S. (1993). Integumentary and mucous membrane alterations. In S. Groenwald, M. Frogge, M. Goodman, & C. Yarbo (Eds.). Cancer nursing: Principles and practice. Boston: Jones and Bartlett.

Harrell, J. S., & Damon, J. F. (1989). Prediction of patient's need for mouth care. Western Journal of Nursing Research, 11, 748–756.

Lassila, V. P. (1987). Stimulated saliva and microbial growth in older adults. Special Care in Dentistry, 7, 157–160.

Miller, C. A. (1995). Nursing care of older adults (2nd ed.) Glenview, IL: Scott, Foresman.

Pettigrew, D. (1989). Investing in mouth care. Geriatric Nursing, 10(1), 22–24.

Western Consortium for Cancer Nursing Research. (1991). Development of a staging system for chemotherapy induced stomatitis. Cancer Nursing, 14(1), 6–12.

Relocation Stress [Syndrome]

DEFINITION

Relocation Stress [Syndrome]: A state in which an individual experiences physiologic and/or psychological disturbances as a result of transfer from one environment to another.

Other terms found in the literature that describe relocation stress include admission stress, postrelocation crisis, relocation crisis, relocation shock, relocation trauma, transfer stress, transfer trauma, translocation syndrome, and transplantation shock.

DEFINING CHARACTERISTICS*

Major (80%–100%)

Responds to transfer or relocation with

Loneliness	Depression
Apprehension	Anxiety

Increased confusion (older adult population)

Minor (50%–79%)

Change in former eating habits	Gastrointestinal disturbances
Change in former sleep patterns	Increased verbalization of needs
Demonstration of dependency	Need for excessive reassurance
Demonstration of insecurity	Restlessness
Demonstration of lack of trust	Sad affect

Unfavorable comparison of posttransfer to pretransfer staff
Verbalization of being concerned/upset about transfer
Verbalization of insecurity in new living situation

Vigilance	Withdrawal

Weight change

RELATED FACTORS

Pathophysiologic

Related to compromised ability to adapt to changes secondary to:
    (Decreased physical health status)
        Physical difficulties
    (Decreased psychosocial health status)
        Increased/perceived stress before relocation
        Depression
        Decreased self-esteem

Situational (Personal, Environmental)

Related to moderate to high degree of environmental change in new environment secondary to:
    Loss of privacy
    Decreased control of individual care
    Decrease and/or change in available caregivers
    Decrease/increase in patient monitoring equipment

* Harkulich, J., & Brugler, C. (1988). *Nursing diagnosis—translocation syndrome: Expert validation study*. Partial funding granted by the Peg Schlitz Fund, Delta Xi Chapter, Sigma Theta Tau International; Barnhouse, A. (1987). *Development of the nursing diagnosis of translocation syndrome with critical care patients*. Unpublished master's thesis, Kent State University, Kent, OH.

Physical differences between the two environments
Increased noise/activities in posttransfer environment
Inconsistencies in care
Decreased privacy due to changes in life-style
Related to negative history with previous transfers secondary to:
Involuntary move(s)
Frequent moves within short time spans
Transfers occurring at evening/nights
Related to concurrent, recent, and past interpersonal losses secondary to:
Negative experiences dealing with earlier separation(s) (for adults as well as children)
Loss of social and familial ties
Abandonment
Perceived/actual rejection by caregivers
Anticipation of lengthy and/or permanent stay in new environment
Threat to financial security
Change in relationship with family members
Related to little or no preparation for the impending move
Lack of predictability in new environment
Little or no time between when an individual is notified of an impending move and the actual move
Unrealistic expectations of individual/family members regarding facility and staff
Lack of decision making and control on behalf of the person who is moving

Maturational

School-age and adolescents
Related to losses associated with moving secondary to:
Fear of rejection
Loss of peer group
School-related problems
Decreased security in new adolescent peer group and school

Author's Note

This diagnosis has been accepted by NANDA as a syndrome diagnosis. *Relocation Stress* as a syndrome diagnosis does not fit the criterion for a syndrome diagnosis, which is a cluster of actual or risk nursing diagnoses as defining characteristics. The defining characteristics associated with *Relocation Stress* are observable or reportable cues consistent with *Relocation Stress*, not *Relocation Stress Syndrome*. The author recommends deleting "Syndrome" from the label.

Relocation represents a disruption for all individuals involved. It can occur with a transfer from one unit to another, or from one facility to another. It can involve a permanent move to a long-term care facility, or to a new home. All age groups involved are disturbed by the relocation. When physiologic and psychological disturbances compromise functioning, the nursing diagnosis *Relocation Stress [Syndrome]* is appropriate.

The most optimal nursing approach to relocation stress is to initiate preventive measures using *Risk for Relocation Stress* as the diagnosis.

Errors in Diagnostic Statements

Relocation Stress related to apprehension and sadness associated with impending family move

Sadness and apprehension are appropriate responses for children who are involved in a family move. Adolescents specifically are very disrupted because of peer relationships. Apprehension and sadness are not related factors but manifestations. The diagnosis should be written

Relocation Stress related to effects of family move on peer relationships, as evidenced by statements of sadness and apprehension.

Key Concepts

1. The process of relocation represents a transition for all relocated individuals (Puskar, 1986; Miller, 1995).
2. Relocation stress can occur with any type of move. Types of relocation include previous home to new home (house, apartment); home to institution (hospital, long-term care nursing facility); institution to home (especially after an extended illness); moves within an institution (from one bed to another bed in the same room, from one room to another room on the same unit/floor; from one room to another room on different units/floors) and between institutions (hospital to long-term care facility, long-term care nursing facility to a different long-term nursing facility).
3. Relocation stress typically occurs in the periods shortly before and/or after the move. Not all relocated individuals experience relocation stress, because the related factors are not present to the same degree in all individuals experiencing a relocation.
4. When a move is the result of a husband's change of employment, a relocated husband often finds satisfaction with his new job. The relocated wife seeks out new neighbors, friends, home, and community activities as a primary source of satisfaction. If previously employed, the wife often feels isolated over the unavailability of jobs in the new environment (Puskar, 1990b).
5. Relocated wives coped well when demonstrating active behaviors (problem solving, support seeking from family and friends, volunteer activities), rather than those wives who coped poorly with passive behaviors (eating, sleeping, crying, watching television, becoming angry at self and others) (Puskar, 1990b).

Critical Care Units

1. Relocation stress has been compared to separation anxiety due to separation from monitors and nurse and physician surveillance (Roberts, 1986).
2. Clients have feelings of interpersonal loss of the pretransfer staff and have missed the security and attention of the critical care unit (Hackett, Cassem, & Wishnie, 1968; Lethbridge, Somboom, & Shea, 1976).
3. Klein, Kliner, Zipes, Troyer, and Wallace (1968) reported the following in clients transferred from a coronary care unit: five of seven individuals exhibited emotional reactions and at least one cardiovascular complication to transfer, with concurrent increases in urine catecholamine excretion. After beginning a preparation program for transfer and continuity of care, no cardiovascular complications occurred.
4. Houser (1974) reported the following in a study of 12 clients transferred from a coronary care unit: 6 of 12 individuals required readmission for cardiovascular complications, and 5 of the 6 individuals had a high anxiety rating when transferred. Those individuals who did not discuss their feelings were most likely to experience complications after transfer. After instituting a program aimed at reducing transfer stress, clients had fewer complications, and the observed complications were less dangerous than those in the control group.
5. The incidence of psychophysiologic responses to relocation stress was higher for patients transferred during the afternoon and evening than for those transferred in the morning (Cassem, Hackett, Bascom, & Wishnie, 1970; Lethbridge et al., 1976).
6. In their study of 177 myocardial infarct clients in 6 hospitals, researchers reported some of the following previously unreported findings:
   a. The length of time for which the client had been notified of transfer was inversely related to the need for reassurance.
   b. Clients with abnormal blood pressures on admission to the coronary care unit were at higher risk for negative effects of transfer.
   c. Women had more physiologic indicators of stress with the relocation than men (Minckley et al., 1979).

Mentally Ill Clients

1. Clients who are more dependent are more likely to experience negative effects with relocation than less dependent individuals (Adshead, Nelson, Gooderally, & Gollogly, 1991).

2. Clients who are also physically frail are more accident prone in a new environment than more physically adept individuals (Adshead et al., 1991).

3. For many severely and chronically mentally ill clients, involuntary "transfers exacerbate their feelings of defeat and their sense that there was nothing helpful about the transfer" (Osborne et al., 1990, p. 226).

4. Decreasing a client's social acceptability (*e.g.*, transporting individual with restraints on) inhibits a person's integration in the new environment (Osborne et al., 1990).

🌀 *Key Concepts—Child*

1. When families need to relocate, their social attachment systems may be disrupted, thus affecting slight changes in their health status, daily functioning, and loneliness (Puskar, 1986).

2. Because of age and maturation, children of different ages experience relocation in different ways (Matter & Matter, 1988).

3. A relocated child's stress and frustration may lead to aggression, withdrawal, and/or deterioration in schoolwork, and may lead to future adjustment problems if the child is not well socialized in the new environment (Blair, Marchant, & Medway, 1984; Matter & Matter, 1988).

4. Relocated children and adults may experience pains of past separations that may arouse feelings of insecurity (Puskar & Dvorsak, 1991).

5. Toddlers and preschoolers often demonstrate changes in eating and sleeping patterns, along with minor disabilities when relocated (Puskar & Dvorsak, 1991).

6. Relocated adolescent boys may experience more difficulties with peers (diminished contact, rejection, teasing, meanness) in the new environment (Vernberg, 1990). However, relocated adolescent girls may verbalize more stress and loneliness (Raviv, Keinan, Abazoh, & Raviv, 1990).

🏛 *Key Concepts—Older Adult*

1. Contrary to many myths, the relocation of older adults to or within nursing homes is not correlated with increased mortality rates (Borup, Gallego, & Heffernam, 1979).

2. It is the process of relocation and not the event that affects physical and psychological well-being (Rosswurm, 1985).

3. Positive appraisal of relocation to a nursing home is associated with positive morale; a negative relocation appraisal is associated with negative morale (Gass, Gaustad, Oberst, & Hughes, 1992).

4. Highly educated nursing home residents have been found to view relocation more negatively than residents with less education (Gass et al., 1992).

5. Nursing home residents' view of relocation and later adaptation are reported to be related to psychological and physical health, prior and new support systems, morale, and functional independence (Beirne, Patterson, Galie, & Goodman, 1995; Gass et al., 1992).

6. Older adults may use a variety of coping strategies, ranging from aggressive anger to passive resignation, when relocated to a nursing home (Oleson & McGlynn Shadick, 1992).

7. Uncontrollable events in nursing home relocation generally stimulate emotion and cognitive-focused responses. Events that are at least somewhat controllable usually stimulate problem-solving and positive coping strategies (Oleson & McGlynn Shadick, 1992).

8. Any nursing interventions related to relocation stress should reflect the resident's effective coping strategies (Oleson & McGlynn Shadick, 1992).

9. Nursing interventions to minimize relocation stress may be refused (Oleson & McGlynn Shadick, 1992).

10. Living in a nursing home has been shown to be a cause of suicide in older adults. The person who is at risk for suicide when relocating to a nursing home is depressed and hopeless, with decreased life satisfaction and psychological well-being, as well as angry at the loss of control over his or her own life (Haight, 1995).

11. Lack of a confidante while in a nursing home has been correlated with suicidal ideation (Haight, 1995).

12. The presence of high self-esteem, arthritis, and a mean age of 85 years have also been found to be significant indicators of suicide risk in older adults in nursing homes (Haight, 1995).
13. The greatest incidence of relocation stress typically occurs in the periods shortly before and up to 3 months after the move (Beirne et al., 1995; Reinardy, 1995).

TRANSCULTURAL CONSIDERATIONS

1. Relocation stress is a transcultural phenomenon that occurs in all age groups. Of 33 nurses practicing in China, 100% reported that relocation stress exists; 23 nurses from 12 different countries also reported that relocation stress exists (Harkulich & Brugler, 1991). Israeli adolescents were also found to experience relocation stress after "moving house" (Raviv et al., 1990).

Focus Assessment Criteria

Subjective Data

A. Assess for defining characteristics
   1. The relocated person complains of:
      a. Lack of social contacts
      b. Dissatisfaction with new environment
      c. Decreased ability to make decisions
      d. Increased family conflicts
      e. Problems adjusting
      f. Alienation
      g. Loneliness
      h. Lack of preparation for the move(s)
      i. Increased fatigue
      j. Problems adjusting to new school/friends, and so forth
      k. Mistrust of support people/family/staff
      l. Loss of control
      m. Feelings of insecurity
      n. Anger toward people responsible for placement
      o. Anger at loss of control over own life
   2. Changes in
      a. Sleep patterns
      b. Nutritional intake
      c. Socialization
      d. Cognition
      e. Orientation

B. Assess for related factors
   1. History of:
      a. One or more changes in environment in last 3 months
      b. Multiple moves in last 5 years
      c. Traumatic experiences after previous moves
      d. Being in the same environment for over 40 years
   2. Sensory/perceptual problems (hearing/sight losses)
   3. Usual coping skills
   4. Previous responses to other life transitions/crises
   5. Perceived meaning of relocation
   6. Educational level
   7. Risk factors
      a. Moderate to severe confusion/disorientation

    b. Perceived poor health
    c. Lack of support/family/friends/staff
    d. Low self-esteem
    e. Functional deterioration
    f. Involuntary move
    g. Communication difficulties
    h. Lack of continuity of care
    i. Expression of dissatisfaction with life
    j. Lack of preparation for move(s)
    k. Lack of choices or input on the part of the relocating person
    l. Presence of multiple chronic illnesses
    m. Rapidly changing manifestation of emotion

Objective Data

A. Assess for defining characteristics
    1. Change in weight
    2. Sleep problems
    3. Change in eating patterns
    4. Change in cognition

Outcome Criteria*

Short-Term Goals
Family members will
*   Share in decision-making activities regarding the new environment
*   Express concerns regarding the move to a new environment
*   Verbalize one positive aspect of the relocation

Long-Term Goals
The family will
*   Report adjustment to the new environment without physiologic and/or psychological disturbances
*   Establish new bonds in the new environment
*   Become involved in activities in the new environment

Interventions

A. Encourage each family member to share feelings about the move
    1. Provide privacy for each individual.
    2. Encourage each family member to share feelings with each other.
    3. Discuss the possible and different effects of the move on each family member.
    4. Inform parents regarding potential changes in children's conduct with relocation, such as regression, withdrawal, acting-out behaviors, and changes with eating (breast/bottle-feeding).
    5. Instruct parents to obtain all pertinent documents regarding children's medical/dental history (*e.g.*, records of immunizations, communicable diseases, and dental work).
    6. Allow for some ritual(s) when leaving the old environment. Encourage reminiscing, which will bring closure for many family members.

---

* This diagnosis addresses relocation stress for individuals and families including children.

B. Teach parents techniques to assist their child/children with the move

    1. Remain positive about the move before, during, and after, with the acceptance that the child may not be optimistic.

    2. Instruct parents to explore various options with their children on how to communicate with friends/families in previous environment. Children's relationships with friends in the previous community are very important, especially for "peer reassurance" after relocation.

    3. Keep regular routines in the new environment and establish them as soon as possible.

    4. Acknowledge the difficulty of peer losses with the adolescent.

    5. Assess the following areas when counseling a relocated adolescent: perceptions about the move; concurrent stressors; usual and present coping skills; and family, peers, and community support groups.

    6. Access the organizations that the child previously belonged to (*e.g.*, Girl Scouts, sports).

    7. Assist children to focus on similarities between old and new environments (*e.g.*, clubs, Scouts, church groups).

    8. Plan a trip to school during a class and lunch period to reduce fear of unknown.

    9. Allow children some choices regarding room arrangements, decorating, and the like.

    10. Ask teacher or counselor at new school to introduce adolescent to a student who recently relocated to that school.

    11. Allow children to mourn their losses as a result of the move.

C. Initiate health teaching and referrals, as indicated

    1. Alert to possible need for counseling before, during, or after move.

    2. Furnish a written directory of relevant community organizations such as area churches, children's groups, Parents without Partners, senior citizens' groups, and Welcome Wagon or other local new neighbor groups.

    3. Instruct the family about appropriate community services.

Rationale

- Many researchers report that relocation stress is preventable (Brown, Cornwell, & Weist 1981; Mirotznik & Ruskin, 1985; Puskar, 1989; Wells & MacDonald, 1981). Therefore, eliminating and/or minimizing the causative, contributing, and risk factors can decrease the occurrence of relocation stress.
- It is important to assess individuals before relocation to identify those who are most at risk for relocation stress.
- Early relocation planning is paramount in ensuring a smooth transfer for all involved individuals (Brugler, Titus, & Nypaver, 1993).
- Children need early notification, predictability, and decision-making opportunities when an upcoming relocation is planned (Marsico & Puskar, 1986).
- Peer networks are important during adolescence because the relocated adolescent needs additional parental and peer reassurance (Vernberg, 1990).

■ **Relocation Stress**
Related to Changes Associated With Health Care
Facility Transfers or Admission to Long-Term Care
Facility

Outcome Criteria

Short-Term Goals
The person will
• Participate in decision-making activities regarding the new environment
• Voice concerns regarding the move to a new environment
• Describe realistic expectations of the new environment

Long-Term Goals
The person will
• Verbalize positive statements both in regard to acceptance of the new environment and reasons for leaving the previous environment
• Adjust to the new environment without physiologic and/or psychological disturbance
• Establish new bonds in the new environment
• Become involved in activities in the new environment

Interventions

A. Assess for factors that may contribute to relocation stress (see Related Factors and Focus Assessment Criteria)

B. Reduce or eliminate causative and contributing factors where possible to reduce relocation stress

   1. Environmental differences between old and new settings/minimal continuity of care in new environment
     a. Design a program to prepare the relocated residents and staff for the move, orienting to the physical layout many times until individuals feel familiar with the new environment.
     b. Provide visual presentations (through bulletin boards, posters, letters, and the like) and first-hand accounts of new environment for those individuals unable to view area before relocation.
     c. Seek input from former staff regarding patient and plan of care.
     d. Initially maintain person on same activity level and diet through pretransfer and posttransfer units.
     e. Transfer person to similar, proximal area when possible.
     f. Wean any monitoring equipment gradually before transfer.
     g. Transfer all personal items with the person, such as mobility aids, eyeglasses, hearing aids, dentures, prostheses, and belongings.
     h. Transfer person during daytime hours.
     i. Maintain similar heights of furnishings/beds.
     j. Clearly mark steps and other potential environmental hazards.
     k. Maintain people in familiar groups at mealtimes and in living arrangements.
     l. Promote a welcoming, warm, and clean receiving environment.

m. Allow time for discussions regarding living spaces that are being left and welcoming the new environment (Johnson & Hlava, 1994).

2. Involuntary relocation/lack of control in decision making
   a. Offer decision-making opportunities throughout relocation experience.
   b. Promote person's input regarding new environment when possible, such as use of decorations and arrangement of furniture.
   c. Present transfer from a critical care unit as indicator of improvement.
   d. Inform hospitalized person of signs of daily progress.
   e. Transfer in an unhurried manner.
   f. Establish mutual goals before relocation to nursing home.
   g. Provide opportunities for questions/answers with relocation preparation.
   h. Hold regular staff/resident meetings after relocation.

3. Recent or concurrent interpersonal loss
   a. Discuss adaptation to the relocation with family members.
   b. Assess responses of all family members to the relocation.
   c. Identify those family members who may need additional help with adjustment.
   d. Encourage family members to share their perceptions of relocation with each other.
   e. Offer the person help in maintaining contact with significant others by means such as telephone calls, writing letters, visits with previous roommates when applicable.
   f. Introduce person to nurse from posttransfer unit before transfer.
   g. Accompany to posttransfer unit.
   h. Provide follow-up visit of nurse from pretransfer unit to person on posttransfer unit.
   i. Encourage family members to visit person during and after relocation.
   j. Minimize number of transfers in the health care facility.
   k. Visit resident daily.
   l. Promote formation of friendships in new environment.
   m. Encourage family involvement in resident's care.
   n. Visit person in own home before nursing home placement.
   o. Support individual's effort to adjust to new environment.
   p. Assist in remembering past relocations that were positive (Johnson & Hlava, 1994).

4. Decreased physical and/or psychosocial state
   a. Promote discussion of feelings regarding relocation.
   c. Encourage use of problem-solving skills.
   d. Offer potential solutions to problems when person cannot do so.
   e. Promote sleep with use of previous bedtime routines, back rubs, white noise, music, warm milk, and minimization of noise in surrounding areas.
   f. Encourage positive eating habits with use of favorite foods, a pleasant eating environment, and any appropriate supplements.
   g. Orient fully to new environment.
   h. When possible, retain highly anxious person in pretransfer unit until anxiety decreases.
   i. Provide for spiritual needs (*e.g.*, visit from clergy, hanging religious symbols in new location, transporting to a religious ceremony).
   j. Use cues such as signs and arrows for the relocated.
   k. Assist person in learning to view the relocation more positively.
   l. Teach/mobilize coping strategies.
   m. Reassess relocation perceptions periodically.

C. Reduce the physiologic effects of relocation (refer to Key Concepts)

   1. Assess before relocation:
      a. Blood pressure, temperature
      b. Respiratory function
      c. Orientation
      d. Signs of infection
      e. Level of discomfort
   2. Identify individual at high risk for selected physiologic responses:
      a. Individual with musculoskeletal/neurologic deficits, advanced age, cardiovascular disorders,
      b. Changes in orientation
      c. Cardiovascular complications (*e.g.*, ischemia, dysrhythmias)
   3. Prevent or reduce the occurrence of
      a. Confusion
      b. Activity intolerance

D. Promote integration after transfer into a long-term care nursing facility

   1. Allow as many choices as possible regarding physical surroundings and daily routines.
   2. Encourage person or family to bring familiar objects from person's home.
   3. Orient to physical layout of environment.
   4. Introduce relocated individuals to new staff and fellow residents.
   5. Encourage to interact with other individuals in new facility.
   6. Assist in maintaining previous interpersonal relationships.
   7. Clearly state smoking rules and orient to areas where smoking is permitted.
   8. Promote the development or maintenance of a relationship with a confidante (Haight, 1995).

E. Initiate health teaching and referrals, as indicated

   1. Prepare person for relocation.
      a. Notify as early as possible to increase predictability regarding eventual relocation.
      b. Provide ongoing and structured in-client teaching regarding:
         Characteristics of postrelocation environment
         Staff capabilities
         Mechanisms for continuity of care
         Rationale for relocation and less constant professional attention when applicable
         Expectations of person in new environment
         Any increasing stages of activity/independence
      c. Include family in teaching.
   2. Offer information about positive health habits and resources during illness.
   3. Make appropriate professional referrals as needed, as well as suggesting a phone monitoring system such as "lifeline."
   4. Refer relocated families to community agencies related to newcomers and to mental health agencies when at risk for relocation stress syndrome (Puskar & Martsolf, 1994).

Rationale

- Open communication with the elderly both prerelocation and postrelocation, assessing their experiences with change and adjustment, coping history and style, and decisional control (Reinardy, 1995).

- With the influx of chronically mentally ill individuals into the community, it is important that their needs and problems be accurately assessed so that interventions and services can be planned and implemented to ensure a successful relocation and adjustment into the community (Murphy, Gass-Sternas, & Knight, 1995).
- Before nursing home placement of a loved one, family members should be assessed regarding their perceptions of nursing home placement. Areas of conflict and vulnerability can serve as the foci for family-centered nursing interventions (Johnson, Morton, & Knox, 1992).

References/Bibliography

Adshead, H., Nelson, H., Gooderally, V., & Gollogly, P. (1991). Guidelines for successful relocation. *Nursing Standard, 5*(28), 32–35.

Beirne, N. F., Patterson, M. N., Galie, M., & Goodman, P. (1995). Effects of a fast-track closing on a nursing facility population. *Health and Social Work, 20,* 117–123.

Blair, J. P., Marchant, K. H., & Medway, F. J. (1984). Aiding the relocated family and mobile child. *Elementary School Guidance and Counseling, 18,* 251–259.

Borup, J. H., Gallego, D. T., & Heffernam, P. G. (1979). Relocation and its effect on mortality. *The Gerontologist, 19,* 135–140.

Brown, M. M., Cornwell, J., & Weist, J. K. (1981). Reducing the risks to the institutionalized elderly: Part I. Depersonalization, negative effects, and medical care deficiencies. *Journal of Gerontological Nursing, 7,* 401–403.

Brugler, C., Titus, M., & Nypaver, J. (1993). Relocation stress syndrome: A patient and staff approach. *Journal of Nursing Administration, 23*(1), 45–50.

Cassem, N. H., Hackett, T. P., Bascom, C., & Wishnie, H. A. (1970). Reactions of coronary patients to the CCU nurse. *American Journal of Nursing, 70,* 319–325.

Gass, K. A., Gaustad, G., Oberst, M. T., & Hughes, S. (1992). Relocation appraisal, functional independence, morale, and health of nursing home residents. *Issues in Mental Health Nursing, 13,* 239–253.

Hackett, T. P., Cassem, N. H., & Wishnie, H. A. (1968). The coronary care unit: An appraisal of its psychological hazards. *New England Journal of Medicine, 279,* 1365–1370.

Haight, B. K. (1995). Suicide risk in frail elderly people relocated to nursing homes. *Geriatric Nursing, 16,* 104–107.

Harkulich, J., & Brugler, C. (1991). Relocation and the resident. *Activities, Adaptation and Aging, 15*(4), 51–60.

Harkulich, J. T., & Brugler, C. J. (1992). Relocation stress. In K. Gettrust & P. Brabec (Eds.). *Nursing diagnosis in clinical practice: Guides for care planning.* Louisville, KY: Delmar.

Houser, D. (1974). Safer care for the M.I. patient. *Nursing '74, 4*(7), 42–47.

Johnson, M. A., Morton, M. K., & Knox, S. M. (1992). The transition to a nursing home: Meeting the family's needs. *Geriatric Nursing, 13,* 299–302.

Johnson, R. A., & Hlava, C. (1994). Translocation of elders: Maintaining the spirit. *Geriatric Nursing, 15,* 209–212.

Klein, R. F., Kliner, V. A., Zipes, D. P., Troyer, W. G., & Wallace, A. G. (1968). Transfer from a coronary care unit: Some adverse responses. *Archives of Internal Medicine, 122,* 104–108.

Lethbridge, B., Somboom, O. P., & Shea, H. L. (1976). The transfer process. *Canadian Nurse, 72,* 39–40.

Manion, P. S., & Rantz, M. J. (1995). Relocation stress syndrome: A comprehensive plan for long-term care admissions. *Geriatric Nursing, 16,* 108–112.

Marsico, T., & Puskar, K. R. (1986). Family relocation: Helping children adjust. *Pediatric Nursing, 12*(2), 108–110.

Matter, D. E., & Matter, R. M. (1988). Helping young children cope with the stress of relocation: Action steps for the counselor. *Elementary School Guidance and Counseling, 23*(10), 23–29.

Miller, S. (1995). *After the boxes are unpacked.* Denver, CO: Focus on the Family.

Minckley, B. B., Burrows, D., Ehrat, K., Harper, L., Jenkin, S. A., Minckley, W. F., Page, B., Schramm, D. E., & Wood, C. (1979). Myocardial infarct stress-of-transfer inventory: Development of a research tool. *Nursing Research, 28,* 4–9.

Mirotznik, J., & Ruskin, A. P. (1985). Interinstitutional relocation and its effects on psychosocial status. *The Gerontologist, 25,* 265–269.

Murphy, L. N., Gass-Sternas, K., & Knight, K. (1995). Health of the chronically mentally ill wo rejoin the community: A community assessment. *Issues in Mental Health Nursing, 16,* 239–256.

Oleson, M., & McGlynn Shadick, K. (1993). Application of Moos and Schaefer's (1986) model to nursing care of elderly persons relocating to a nursing home. *Journal of Advanced Nursing, 18,* 479–485.

Osborne, O. H., Murphy, H. Leichman, S. S., Griffin, M., Hagerott, R. J., Ekland, E. S., & Thomas, M. D. (1990). Forced relocation of hospitalized psychiatric patients. *Archives of Psychiatric Nursing, 4,* 221–227.

Puskar, K. R. (1986). The usefulness of Mahler's phases of the separation–individuation process in providing a theoretical framework for understanding relocation. *Maternal–Child Nursing Journal, 15*(1), 15–22.

Puskar, K. R. (1989). Families on the move: Promoting health through family relocation adaptation. *Family Community Health, 11*(4), 52–62.

Puskar, K. R. (1990a). International relocation: Women's coping methods. *Health Care for Women International, 11*, 263–276.

Puskar, K. R. (1990b). Relocation support groups for corporate wives. *American Association of Occupational Health Nurses Journal, 38*(1), 25–31.

Puskar, K. R., & Dvorsak, K. G. (1991). Relocation stress in adolescents: Helping teenagers cope with a moving dilemma. *Pediatric Nursing, 17*, 295–298.

Puskar, K. R., & Martsolf, D. S. (1994). Adolescent geographic relocation: Theoretical perspective. *Issues in Mental Health Nursing, 15*, 471–481.

Raviv, A., Keinan, G., Abazoh, Y., & Raviv, A. (1990). Moving as a stressful life event for adolescents. *Journal of Community Psychology, 18*, 130–140.

Reinardy, J. R. (1995). Relocation to a new environment: Decisional control and the move to a nursing home. *Health and Social Work, 20*(1), 31–38.

Roberts, S. L. (1986). Transfer anxiety. In S. L. Roberts (Ed.). *Behavioral concepts and the critically ill patient* (2nd ed.). Norwalk, CT: Appleton-Century-Crofts.

Rosswurm, M. A. (1983). Relocation and the elderly. *Journal of Gerontological Nursing, 6*, 632–637.

Shedd, P. P., Kobokovich, L. J., & Slattery, M. (1995). Confused patients in the acute care setting: Prevalence, interventions and outcomes. *Journal of Gerontological Nursing, 21*(4), 5–12.

Vernberg, E. M. (1990). Experiences with peers following relocation during early adolescence. *American Journal of Orthopsychiatry, 60*, 466–472.

Wells, L., & MacDonald, G. (1981). Interpersonal networks and post-relocation adjustment of the institutionalized elderly. *The Gerontologist, 21*, 177–183.

Yow, P. A., Malachowski, J., & Fankhauser, K. (1994). Moving day doesn't begin (or end) on moving day. *Nursing Management, 25*(8), 54–57.

Respiratory Function, Risk for Altered*

Dysfunctional Ventilatory Weaning Response

Ineffective Airway Clearance

Ineffective Breathing Patterns

Impaired Gas Exchange

Inability to Sustain Spontaneous Ventilation

Respiratory Function, Risk for Altered

DEFINITION

Risk for Altered Respiratory Function (ARF): The state in which the individual is at risk of experiencing a threat to the passage of air through the respiratory tract and to the exchange of gases (O_2–CO_2) between the lungs and the vascular system.

RISK FACTORS

Presence of risk factors that can change respiratory function (see Related Factors).

RELATED FACTORS
Pathophysiologic

Related to excessive or thick secretions secondary to:
    Infection, inflammation, allergy, smoking, cardiac or pulmonary disease
Related to immobility, stasis of secretions, and ineffective cough secondary to:
    Diseases of the nervous system (*e.g.*, Guillain-Barré syndrome, multiple sclerosis, myasthenia gravis)
    Central nervous system (CNS) depression/head trauma
    Cerebrovascular accident (stroke)
    Quadriplegia

Treatment-Related

Related to immobility secondary to:
    Sedating effects of medications (specify)
    Anesthesia, general or spinal
Related to suppressed cough reflex secondary to (specify)
Related to effects of tracheostomy (altered secretions)

* This diagnosis is not currently on the NANDA list, but has been included for clarity or usefulness.

Situational (Personal, Environmental)

Related to immobility secondary to:

Surgery or trauma	Fatigue
Pain, fear, anxiety	Perception/cognitive impairment

Related to extreme high or low humidity
For infants, related to placement on stomachs for sleep

Author's Note

Nursing's many responsibilities associated with problems of respiratory function include preventing problems, reducing risk factors, reducing or eliminating contributing factors, monitoring respiratory status, and managing acute respiratory dysfunction.

Risk for Altered Respiratory Function has been added by the author to describe a state in which the entire respiratory system may be affected, not just isolated areas such as airway clearance or gas exchange. Allergy and immobility are examples of factors that affect the entire system and thus make it incorrect to say *Impaired Gas Exchange Related to Immobility*, because immobility also affects airway clearance and breathing patterns. The diagnoses *Ineffective Airway Clearance* and *Ineffective Breathing Patterns* can be used when the nurse can definitely alleviate the contributing factors that are influencing respiratory function, such as ineffective cough, immobility, or stress.

The nurse is cautioned not to use this diagnosis to describe acute respiratory disorders, which are the primary responsibility of medicine and nursing together (*i.e.*, collaborative problems). Such problems can be labeled *Potential Complication: Acute hypoxia* or *Potential Complication: Pulmonary edema*. When an individual's immobility is prolonged and threatens multiple systems—for example, integumentary, musculoskeletal, vascular, as well as respiratory—the nurse should use *Disuse Syndrome* to describe the entire situation.

Errors in Diagnostic Statements

Ineffective Breathing Patterns related to respiratory compensation for metabolic acidosis

This diagnosis represents the respiratory pattern associated with diabetic ketoacidosis. Nursing responsibilities for this situation include monitoring, early detection of changes, and rapid initiation of nursing and medical interventions. This case does not represent a situation for which nurses diagnose and are accountable to prescribe treatment. Rather, the collaborative problem *Potential Complication: Ketoacidosis* would represent the nursing accountability for the situation, not *Ineffective Breathing Patterns*.

Ineffective Airway Clearance related to mucosal edema and loss of ciliary action secondary to thermal injury

After sustaining burns of the upper airway, a person is at risk for pulmonary edema and respiratory distress. This potentially life-threatening situation requires both nurse- and physician-prescribed interventions. The collaborative problem *Potential Complication: Respiratory related to thermal injury* would alert nurses that close monitoring for respiratory complications, and management if they occur, are indicated.

Ineffective Airway Clearance related to decreased cough and gag reflexes secondary to anesthesia

The nursing focus for this client is on preventing aspiration through proper positioning and good oral hygiene, not on teaching effective coughing. Thus, the diagnosis should be restated as *Risk for Aspiration related to decreased cough and gag reflexes secondary to anesthesia*.

Key Concepts

1. Ventilation requires synchronous movement of the walls of the chest and abdomen. With *inspiration*, the diaphragm moves downward, the intercostal muscles contract, the chest wall lifts up and out, the pressure inside the thorax lowers, and air is drawn in. *Expiration* occurs as air is forced out of the lungs by the elastic recoil of the lungs and the relax-

ation of the chest and diaphragm. Expiration is diminished in the elderly and those with chronic pulmonary disease, increasing the likelihood of CO_2 retention.

2. Pulmonary function depends on
   a. Adequate perfusion (the passage of blood through pulmonary vessels)
   b. Satisfactory diffusion (the movement of oxygen and carbon dioxide across alveolar capillary membrane)
   c. Successful ventilation (the exchange of air between alveolar spaces and the atmosphere)

3. Oxygenation depends on the ability of the lungs to deliver oxygen to the blood and on the ability of the heart to pump enough blood to deliver the oxygen to the microcirculation of the cells.

4. In the presence of pulmonary dysfunction, pulmonary functions tests (PFTs) are essential to determine the nature and extent of dysfunction caused by obstruction, restriction, or both. *Obstructive* defects are caused by airway resistance. *Restrictive* defects are caused by a limitation in chest wall expansion. *Mixed* defects are a combination of obstructive and restrictive problems. Table II-23 describes obstructive and restrictive conditions that affect ventilation.

5. Although arterial blood gases and oxygen saturation studies are very helpful in diagnosing problems with oxygenation, *vital signs* and *mental function* are key guides to determining the seriousness of the problem (some patients can tolerate oxygen problems better than others). The effects of insufficient oxygenation (hypoxia or hypoxemia) on vital signs are:

Vital Signs	Early Hypoxia/Hypoxemia	Late Hypoxia/Hypoxemia
Blood pressures	Rising systolic/falling diastolics	Falling
Pulse	Rising, bounding, arrhythmic	Falling, shallow, arrhythmic
Pulse pressure	Widening	Widened/narrowed
Respirations	Rapid	Slowed/rapid

The effects of insufficient oxygenation on mental function are:

Early Hypoxia/Hypoxemia	Late Hypoxia/Hypoxemia
Irritability	Seizures
Headache	Coma or brain tissue swelling
Confusion	
Agitation	

6. A cough ("the guardian of the lungs") is accomplished by closure of the glottis and the explosive expulsion of air from the lungs by the work of the abdominal and chest muscles.

7. Breath-holding can result in a "Valsalva" maneuver: a marked increase in intrathoracic and intra-abdominal pressure, with profound circulatory changes (decreased heart rate, cardiac output, and blood pressure).

8. The terms tachypnea, hyperpnea, hyperventilation, bradypnea, and hypoventilation are frequently confused. These terms are defined as follows:
   Tachypnea: rapid, shallow respiratory rate
   Hyperpnea: rapid respiratory rate with increased depth
   Hyperventilation: increased rate or depth or respirations causing an alveolar ventilation that is above the body's normal metabolic requirements
   Bradypnea: slow respiratory rate
   Hypoventilation: decreased rate or depth of respiration, causing a minute alveolar ventilation that is less than the body's requirements

9. Hypoxia and hypoxemia contribute to coma and shock. Oxygen demand is greater during febrile illness, exercise, pain, and physical and emotional stress.

10. Oxygen should be administered carefully (less than 3 mL/minute) to people with a history of chronic CO_2 retention, because their drive to breathe is hypoxia.

11. Based on their investigations, researchers have recommended several different techniques to reduce suction-induced hypoxemia (Change, 1995). These techniques include use of:
    a. Oxygen saturation and cardiac rhythm monitors during and immediately after suctioning

Table II-23   **Conditions That Affect Ventilation**

Diagnosis	Basic Disturbance in Ventilation	Underlying Pathology
Obstructive Defects		
Asthma	Increased airway resistance	Bronchial edema, bronchospasm, and obstructive mucus
Bronchitis	Increased airway resistance	Same as above
Emphysema	Increased airway resistance	Loss in radial traction or respiratory airways due to destruction of alveolar septa
Restrictive Defects		
Kyphoscoliosis	Limitation on chest cavity expansion	Increase in elastic resistance of chest wall due to abnormal curvature of spine
Obesity	Same as above	Increase in elastic resistance of chest wall due to increase in adipose tissue, especially of abdomen
Muscular dystrophy	Same as above	Weakness of inspiratory muscles
Pneumoconiosis	Same as above	Increase in elastic resistance of lung due to fibroses of pulmonary tissue
Mixed Defect		
Pulmonary congestion	Increases in both airway resistance and limitation in expansion of chest cavity	Obstructive due to bronchial edema and compression of respiratory airway due to increased interstitial and intravenous fluid pressure. Restrictive due to increase in elastic resistance of lung due to increased interstitial and intravenous fluid pressure

(Fischbach, F. [1992]. *A manual of laboratory and diagnostic tests* [4th ed.] [p. 805]. Philadelphia: Lippincott–Raven Publishers.)

 b. Intermittent suction for less than 15 seconds (prolonged, continuous suction causes microatelectasis)

 c. Hyperinflation (increasing tidal volume to 11/2 time preset ventilation volume using a resuscitation bag or the sigh function of the ventilator)

 d. Preoxygenation (administering oxygen before suctioning)

 e. Hyperoxygenation (administering oxygen at greater oxygen concentrations than the preset ventilator level)

 f. Hyperventilation (increasing the respiratory rate without changing tidal volume)

12. Review of the literature indicates that the common practice of supine positioning to optimize ventilation may be erroneous. Because the right lung is larger, heavier, and more vascular, it is more likely to contribute more to arterial oxygen saturation than the left, making the right lateral position most desirable, so long as there is no unilateral lung disease present (in unilateral lung disease, the adage of "good lung down" defines the norm) (Lasater-Erhard, 1995).

☯ *Key Concepts—Child*

1. The characteristics of normal respiration in the newborn differ from those of older infants and children.

 a. Respirations are irregular and abdominal; to be accurate, count respirations for 1 full minute (Wong, 1995).

 b. The rate is between 30 and 50 breaths per minute (Wong, 1995).

 c. Periods of apnea, lasting less than 15 seconds, may occur (Wong, 1995).

 d. Obligate nasal breathing occurs through the first 3 weeks of life (Hunsberger, 1989).

2. Characteristics of the respiratory system of the infant and young child include:
   a. Abdominal breathing continues until the child is about 5 years of age (Hunsberger, 1989).
   b. Retractions are more often observed with respiratory illness because of increased chest wall compliance. Respiratory insufficiency may develop quickly in children (Hunsberger, 1989).
   c. Smaller airway diameter increases the risk of obstruction (Hunsberger, 1989).
   d. Infants and small children swallow sputum when it is produced (Wong, 1995).
3. Janson-Bjerklie, Ruma, Stulbarg, and Carrieri (1987) found that younger asthmatics appear to experience more intense dyspnea than older people at a given level of airway obstruction.
4. Huckabay and Daderian (1989) noted that pediatric clients who were given a choice in the selection of color of water in blow bottles performed significantly more breathing exercises than those who were not given a choice.
5. Ongoing research continues to suggest that air pollution contributes to respiratory problems in children (Braun-Fahrlander, Ackerman-Liebrich, Swartz, Gnehm, Rutishauser, & Wanner, 1992).
6. Recent studies have shown that the past common practice of placing infants on their stomach for sleep increases the incidence of sudden infant death syndrome (SIDS), making placement on back or side a safer option.

⚱ *Key Concepts—Maternal*

1. Increased levels of estrogen and progesterone increase tidal volume by decreasing pulmonary resistance (May & Mahlmeister, 1994).
2. Oxygen consumption is increased by 14%, half for fetus development and the rest for other increased needs (*e.g.*, uterus, breasts) (May & Mahlmeister, 1994).

⛩ *Key Concepts—Older Adult*

1. The age-related changes in the respiratory system have little effect on function in healthy adults unless they interact with risk factors such as smoking, immobility, or compromised immune system (Miller, 1995).
2. The following age-related changes in the respiratory system typically occur (Miller, 1995; Staab & Lyles, 1990):
   a. No change in total volume
   b. 50% increase in residual volume
   c. Compromised gas exchange in lower lung regions
   d. Reduced compliance of bony thorax
   e. Decreased strength of respiratory muscles and diaphragm
3. Age-related kyphosis and diminished immune response compromise respiratory function and increase the risk of pneumonia and other respiratory infections.
4. Adults age 65 years and older have a yearly death rate from pneumonia or influenza of 9/100,000. When smoking, exposure to air pollutants, or occupational exposure to toxic substances is present, the rate increases to 217/100,000. If two or more risk factors are present, the rate rises to 979/100,000 (Miller, 1995).

Focus Assessment Criteria

Subjective Data

A. Assess history of symptoms (*e.g.*, pain, dyspnea, cough)

       Onset? Precipitated by what?

       Description? Relieved by what?

       Effects on other body functions

          Gastrointestinal (nausea, vomiting, anorexia, constipation)?

          Genitourinary (impotence, kidney function)?

          Cardiovascular (angina, tachycardia/bradycardia, fluid retention)?

          Neurosensory (thought processes, headache)?

          Musculoskeletal (muscle fatigue, atrophy, use of accessory muscles?)

Effects on life-style
  Occupation   Social/sexual functions
  Role functions   Financial status
Effects on activity/exercise
Interventions used
  Controlled exercise program (what, how often)
  Relaxation techniques?
  Controlled breathing (specify how)

1. Current drug therapy
  Antibiotics? Bronchodilators? Steroids? Inhalers?
    What? How often? When was last dose taken?
    Effect on symptoms?
    For those using inhalers, have them demonstrate technique
    Flu vaccine taken? Type(s) _____ When _____

2. Medical/surgical history
  Cardiovascular disease
  Pulmonary disease
  Previous response to surgery/anesthesia

B. Assess for related factors

1. Presence of contributing or causative factors
  Smoking ("pack years": number of packs per day times number of smoking years)
  Allergy (medication, food, environmental factors—dust, pollen, other)
  Trauma, blunt or overt (chest, abdomen, upper airway, head)
  Surgery/pain
    Healing incision of chest/neck/head/abdomen
    Recent intubation
  Asthma/chronic obstructive pulmonary disease (COPD)/sinus problems
  Environmental factors
    Toxic fumes (cleaning agents, smoke)
    Extreme heat or cold
    Daily inspired air, work and home (humid, dry, level of pollution, level of pollens)
  Infection/inflammation

2. For infants only, history of:
  Prematurity? Low birth weight? Placement on stomach to sleep?
  Cesarean birth? Complicated delivery?
  Family history of SIDS?

Objective Data

A. Assess for defining characteristics

1. Mental status (more than one may apply)
  Alert   Drowsy
  Comatose   Confused
  Agitated

2. Respiratory status
  a. Airway
    Type
      Spontaneous nasal   Nasal endotracheal tube
      Spontaneous mouth breather   Oral endotracheal tube
      Oral airway   Tracheostomy
      Nasal airway
    Condition
      Clear
      Nasal flaring
      Loose secretions present

Bleeding (specify where, how much)
Thick secretions/encrustation present
Swelling (specify where)
Mechanical obstruction (packing/NG tube) present

b. Description

Spontaneous, labored or nonlabored
Controlled mechanical ventilation (CMV)
Spontaneous intermittent mechanical ventilations (SIMV)
Rate (per minute)
Baseline, bradypnea, tachypnea, hyperpnea
Rhythm

Regular	Uneven
Irregular	Periods of apnea
Smooth	

Depth

Decreased	Variable
Increased	Even
Asymmetric	Shallow/hypoventilation
Symmetric	

Type

Splinted/guarded	Kussmaul
Use of accessory muscles?	Cheyne-Stokes

c. Cough

Effective (brings forth sputum and clears lungs)
Ineffective (does not bring forth mucus or clear lungs)
Needs assistance with coughing
Description of cough

Raspy	Dry
Barking	None
Painful	Absent cough reflex
Productive	

d. Sputum

Color	Character	Amount	Odor
Clear	Frothy	Small	None
Yellow	Watery	Moderate	Foul
White	Tenacious	Copious	Yeastlike
Greenish	Hemoptysic (bloody)		
Reddish (bloody)			
Brown specks			

e. Breath sounds (detected by auscultation: compare right upper and lower lobes to left upper and lower lobes; listen to all four quadrants of the chest)

Within normal limits	Rales (crackles)
Diminished	Rhonchi (wheezes)
Absent	Rubs (squeaks)

3. Circulatory status

a. Pulse

Rate	Quality
Rhythm	Baseline

b. Blood pressure

Usual	Pulse pressure
Present	Baseline

c. Skin color

Within normal limits	Ashen
Pale	Ruddy
Cyanotic (central/peripheral)	

4. Diagnostic studies
  Chest x-ray   Oxygen saturation
  Blood gases

B. Assess for defining characteristics
   1. Nutritional status
     Within normal limits   Cachectic
     Obese

Outcome Criteria

The person will
- Perform hourly deep-breathing exercises (sigh) and cough sessions as needed
- Demonstrate satisfactory pulmonary function (adequate tidal volume, vital capacity, forced end-expiratory volume [FEV])
- Relate importance of daily pulmonary exercises

Interventions

A. Assess causative factors
   1. Pain, lethargy
   2. Medical order of bed rest
   3. Neuromuscular impairment
   4. Lack of motivation (to ambulate; to cough and deep breathe)
   5. Decreased level of consciousness
   6. Lack of knowledge
   7. Medications (narcotics, muscle relaxants, other CNS depressants)

B. Eliminate or reduce causative factors, if possible
   1. Assess for optimal pain relief with minimal period of fatigue or respiratory depression.
   2. Coordinate medication regimen with planned activities (*e.g.*, give PRN pain medication with least-sedating side effects 1 hour before physical therapy).
   3. Encourage ambulation as soon as consistent with medical plan of care.
      a. If unable to walk, establish a regimen for being out of bed in a chair several times a day (*i.e.*, 1 hour after meals and 1 hour before bedtime).
      b. Increase activity gradually, explaining that respiratory function will improve and dyspnea will decrease with practice.
   4. For neuromuscular impairment
      a. Vary the position of the bed, thereby gradually changing the horizontal and vertical position of the thorax, unless contraindicated.
      b. Assist to reposition, turning frequently from side to side (hourly if possible).
      c. Encourage deep-breathing and controlled-coughing exercises five times every hour.
      d. Teach individual to use blow bottle or incentive spirometer every hour while awake (with severe neuromuscular impairment, the person may have to be awakened during the night as well).
      e. For those with quadriplegia, teach person and caregivers the "quad cough" (caregiver places hand on client's diaphragm and thrusts upward and inward)
      f. For child, use colored water in blow bottle; have him blow up balloons.
      g. Ensure optimal hydration status.
   5. For the person with a decreased level of consciousness
      a. Position from *side to side* with set schedule (*e.g.*, left side even hours, right side odd hours); do not leave person lying flat on back.

    b. Position on right side after feedings (nasogastric tube feeding, gastrostomy) to prevent regurgitation and aspiration.

    c. Keep head of bed elevated 30 degrees unless contraindicated.

    d. See also *Risk for Aspiration*.

C. Prevent the complications of immobility

    See *Disuse Syndrome*

Rationale

- Lying flat causes the abdominal organs to shift toward the chest, thereby crowding the lungs and making it more difficult to breathe.
- Pulmonary function can be enhanced by interventions such as exercise conditioning to improve lung compliance, relaxation and breathing training, chest percussion, postural drainage, and psychosocial rehabilitation.
- Proper nutrition helps
  - Maintain immunologic competence necessary to fight off respiratory infections.
  - Provide calories for the energy needed for the work of breathing (energy requirements are increased in COPD).
  - Maintain muscles used in breathing
- Stasis of secretions can predispose to infection and atelectasis. People who are unable to mobilize secretions because of fatigue or viscosity need suctioning. Routine suctioning is not necessary for every client. Unnecessary suctioning can cause hypoxemia and airway collapse, and increase the risk of infection (Huddleston, 1990)
- Exercises and movement promote lung expansion and mobilization of secretions. Incentive spirometry promotes deep breathing by providing a visual indicator of the effectiveness of the breathing effort (Litwack, Saleh, & Schaltz, 1991).
- Adequate hydration liquefies secretions, enabling easier expectoration, and prevents stasis of secretions, which provide a medium for microorganism growth. It also helps decrease blood viscosity, which reduces the risk of clot formation (Huddleston, 1990).

■ Risk for Altered Respiratory Function
Related to Environmental Allergens

Outcome Criteria

The person will
- State causative allergens (if known) and describe methods of avoiding allergens
- Relate the emotional aspects of the allergic response
- Identify techniques to control emotional responses contributing to allergic response (*e.g.*, relaxation techniques, controlled breathing)
- Demonstrate and report decreased episodes of respiratory symptoms
- State the need to seek immediate medical attention for severe allergic response and demonstrate the use of hypodermic injection (for administration of epinephrine), if applicable

Interventions

A. Assess causative factors

    1. Chronic allergy (known allergens such as molds, dust, pollen, food, others)

2. Stinging insect
3. Nonspecific (unknown) allergen

B. Provide the following health teaching
1. For chronic allergy to molds
   a. Avoid barns, cut grass, leaves, weeds, decaying or rotting vegetation, firewood, house plants, damp basements, attics, and crawl spaces.
   b. Avoid eating marinated or aged foods (bread, flour, cheese, fruits, vegetables).
   c. Maintain household walls clean and dry.
      Be sure that there is adequate house drainage to keep walls dry.
      Check walls for black or grayish blue mold spots.
      Wash walls with chlorine bleach solution to remove mold.
   d. Reduce environmental allergens, especially in the bedroom.*
      Empty room to the bare walls, including closets (store contents elsewhere if possible).
      Scrub woodwork and floors.
      Thereafter, dust and vacuum well daily and clean thoroughly once a week.
      Keep bedroom furniture to a minimum (preferably wood, rather than stuffed furniture) and avoid wall-to-wall carpets.
      Choose waxed, hardwood floors (no carpets) if possible.
      Use pull shades rather than venetian blinds at windows; do not use curtains or draperies.
      Use closet to a minimum; keep it as dust free as the bedroom, and keep the door closed.
      Use bedroom for sleeping only; if it is a child's bedroom, encourage play elsewhere.
      Do not use stuffed toys.
      Keep animals with fur or feathers out of the area.
      Do not use fuzzy blankets or feather comforters; cotton bedspreads are preferred.
      Launder bed linens frequently.
      Have air and heat ducts and carpets professionally cleaned yearly.
   e. Keep dust down throughout the entire house.
      Use steam or hot-water heat if available.
      Maintain a clean filter in furnace; use air-conditioning, if possible.
      Cover hot-air furnace outlets with cheesecloth or have a filter installed; change filter frequently.
      Avoid any room while it is being cleaned, and do not handle any objects that may be dust collectors (such as books).
      Wear a mask while cleaning.
2. For chronic allergy to pollen
   a. Reduce exposure as much as possible to trees (April–May), grass (May–July), weeds (mid-May to first frost).
   b. Use air-conditioning with electrostatic filters.
   c. Stay inside on windy days, avoiding drafts and cross-ventilation.
   d. Use air conditioning in cars and avoid extended rides.
   e. Wear a dampened mask while cutting lawn.
   f. Avoid strong odors (scents and perfumes).
   g. Do not consume ice-cold beverages or food (can cause spasms).
   h. Avoid granaries, barns, decaying materials, cut grass, weeds, dry leaves, firewood.
   i. Try to arrange vacations during high-pollen season in a low-pollen area, such as the eastern seashore.

* It is difficult to keep one's home and work environment dust free, but special efforts can readily be made to keep the area where one sleeps free of dust.

　　　j. Be sure over-the-counter drugs such as antihistamines are approved by physician because some may have the opposite of the intended effect.

　3. To avoid stinging insects (bees, wasps, yellow jackets, hornets)

　　　a. Do not wear brightly colored clothing (choose lighter colors such as white, light green, khaki).

　　　b. Keep hair short or tied back; avoid hair sprays, perfumes, and floppy clothing.

　　　c. Wear shoes and socks.

　　　d. Avoid riding horses or bicycles in areas where bees or wasps are plentiful (*e.g.*, fields of clover, flowers).

　　　e. Avoid mowing lawns, trimming hedges, or pruning trees during the insect season.

　　　f. Carry an insect spray in the glove compartment of the car and keep one handy at home (attempts to swat or kill insects must be well planned, for a missed blow may infuriate the insect and make it more dangerous).

　　　g. If approached by a bee or wasp in the open, stay still or move back very slowly.

　　　h. Each spring, have home and garden searched for new hornets' or bees' nests and obtain professional assistance from an exterminator or fire department in eliminating them.

　4. For a severe allergic reaction in which hives, facial swelling, abnormal sensations of palate, tongue, or throat, or any respiratory symptoms appear, or *if there has been a previous severe reaction to any kind of sting*, carry out the following procedure:

　　　a. Remove stinger immediately.

　　　b. Keep as quiet as possible (avoid panic).

　　　c. Use emergency epinephrine injection if available.

　　　d. Call emergency medical services.

　　　e. Immediately apply ammonia or lemon to sting; follow with ice.

　5. Discuss the role of medication in reducing allergies.

　　　a. Point out that antihistamines prevent, but do not reverse, allergic responses; therefore, it is best to take them when expecting to encounter allergens or as soon as possible thereafter.

　　　b. Explain that there are new over-the-counter allergy medications that do not cause drowsiness (encourage checking with pharmacist).

　　　c. For those with more severe allergies, stress the need to see a physician (new, more effective medications, with fewer side effects are now available by prescription).

　6. Discuss the hazards of smoking and second-hand smoke exposure.

　7. Discuss healthy living habits

　　　a. Good nutrition

　　　b. Regular exercise

C. For people with asthma

　1. Explain asthma, airway response, and therapy goals.

　2. Explain the rationale for the medication and evaluate inhaler technique.

　3. Teach how to use a peak flow meter to manage symptoms.

　　　a. Teach proper technique and maintenance.

　　　b. Maintain daily chart of peak flows.

　　　c. Establish an evaluation system of peak flow readings and interventions needed (*e.g.*, medication, emergency room).

　4. Clarify the need to avoid cigarette smoke and other triggers (*e.g.*, animals, dander, strong perfumes). Explain use of protective masks.

　5. Clarify when primary provider should be contacted.

　　　a. When medications have to be increased to control symptoms

　　　b. Persistent cough, difficulty breathing with or without wheezing

　　　c. Peak flows less than 80% of normal

Rationale

- The effective management of asthma includes progressive pharmacologic management, environmental control, education, and regular follow-up (Bailey, Cheng, Lemanski, & Reed, 1994).
- Critical to effective management is a strong partnership between client and professionals.
- Peak flow monitoring and action plans can reduce severe asthma episodes (National Asthma Education Program, 1991).
- Medication overuse, substance abuse, and cigarette smoking are associated with increased risks for death (Centers for Disease Control and Prevention, 1995).

Interventions—*Child Focus*

1. Explain the need to control environmental antigens (see previous Interventions).
2. Provide the child with age-appropriate explanations of antigens to avoid.
3. Teach parents to avoid over-the-counter drugs and to consult with primary care professional.
4. Contract with parents to some level of smoking cessation.
   a. Complete smoking cessation
   b. No smoking in house
   c. No smoking in car
   d. No smoking when child is present
   e. No smoking in child's bedroom
5. Consult with school nurse for coordination of treatment plan and school activities.
6. Include all family members in educational sessions if possible.

Rationale

- Reduction and/or avoidance of environmental antigens can reduce exacerbations (Wong, 1995).
- Participation in school-related activities should be encouraged, but evaluation is needed for duration and intensity (Wong, 1995).
- Certain drugs (*e.g.*, aspirin, cough syrup, nonsteroidal antiinflammatory agents, antihistamines) can exacerbate symptoms (Wong, 1995).
- Cigarette smoke is a known trigger of asthma attacks (National Asthma Education Program, 1991).

Dysfunctional Ventilatory Weaning Response

DEFINITION

Dysfunctional Ventilatory Weaning Response (DVWR): A state in which an individual cannot adjust to lowered levels of mechanical ventilator support, which interrupts and prolongs the weaning process.

DEFINING CHARACTERISTICS

DVWR is a progressive state, and experienced nurses have identified three levels (Logan & Jenny, 1990). These defining characteristics occur in response to weaning.

Mild
Major

Restlessness
Slight increase in respiratory rate from baseline

Minor

Expressed feelings of increased oxygen need, breathing discomfort, fatigue, warmth
Queries about possible machine dysfunction
Increased concentration on breathing

Moderate
Major

Slight increase in blood pressure = 20 mm Hg or less from baseline
Slight increase in heart rate = 20 beats/minute or less from baseline
Increase in respiratory rate = 5 breaths/minute or less from baseline

Minor

Hypervigilance to activities
Inability to respond to coaching
Inability to cooperate
Apprehension
Diaphoresis
Eye-widening (wide-eyed look)
Decreased air entry heard on auscultation
Skin color changes: pale, slight cyanosis
Slight respiratory accessory muscle use

Severe
Major

Agitation
Significant deterioration in arterial blood gases from baseline
Increase in blood pressure greater than 20 mm Hg from baseline
Increase in heart rate greater than 20 beats per minute from baseline
Rapid, shallow breathing greater than 25 breaths/minute

Minor

Full respiratory accessory muscle use
Shallow, gasping breaths
Paradoxical abdominal breathing
Adventitious breath sounds
Cyanosis
Profuse diaphoresis
Uncoordinated breathing with the ventilator
Decreased level of consciousness

RELATED FACTORS
Pathophysiologic

Related to muscle weakness and fatigue secondary to:
Unstable hemodynamic status
Decreased level of consciousness
Anemia
Infection
Metabolic or acid–base abnormalities
Fluid and/or electrolyte imbalance
Related to ineffective airway clearance
Severe disease process
Chronic respiratory disease
Chronic neuromuscular disability
Multisystem disease
Chronic nutritional deficit
Debilitated condition

Treatment-Related

Related to obstructed airway
Related to muscle weakness and fatigue secondary to:
Excess sedation, analgesia
Uncontrolled pain
Related to inadequate nutrition (deficit in calories, excess carbohydrates, inadequate fats
and protein intake)

Related to prolonged ventilator dependence more than 1 week
Related to previous unsuccessful ventilator weaning attempt(s)
Related to too-rapid pacing of the weaning process

Situational (Personal, Environmental)

Related to insufficient knowledge of the weaning process
Related to excessive energy demands (self-care activities, diagnostic and treatment procedures, visitors)
Related to inadequate social support
Related to insecure environment (noisy, upsetting events, busy room)
Related to fatigue secondary to interrupted sleep patterns
Related to inadequate self-efficacy
Related to moderate to high anxiety related to breathing efforts
Related to fear of separation from ventilator
Related to feelings of powerlessness
Related to feelings of hopelessness

Author's Note

DVWR is a specific diagnosis within the category of *Risk for Altered Respiratory Function*. *Ineffective Airway Clearance, Ineffective Breathing Patterns*, and *Impaired Gas Exchange* can also be encountered in the weaning situation, either as indicators of lack of weaning readiness or as factors related to the onset of DVWR. DVWR is a separate client state. Its distinctive etiologies and treatments arise from the process of separating the client from the mechanical ventilator.

The process of weaning is an art and a science. Because weaning is a collaborative process, the nurse's ability to gain the client's trust and willingness to work is an important determinant of the weaning outcomes, especially with long-term clients. This trust is fostered by the knowledge and self-confidence nurses display, and by their ability to deal with clients' specific concerns (Jenny & Logan, 1991).

Errors in Diagnostic Statements

Dysfunctional Weaning Response related to increase in blood pressure, heart rate, respiratory rate, and agitation during weaning

This diagnosis does not indicate the reasons for weaning problems. The related factors are evidence of *Dysfunctional Weaning Response*, not causative and contributing factors. The diagnosis should be written with the related factors if they are known, or "unknown etiology" if not known.

Many of the following assessments and interventions apply to the prevention of moderate and severe responses as well as the treatment phases of managing the diagnosis.

Key Concepts

1. Weaning is the process of assisting patients to breathe spontaneously without mechanical ventilation, and weaning success has been defined as spontaneous breathing for 24 hours without ventilatory support, with or without an artificial airway (Knebel, Shekleton, Burns, Clochesy, Goodnough Hanneman, & Ingersoll, 1994, pp. 416, 419).

2. Ventilator weaning is a multidisciplinary effort in which the presence of knowledgeable nurses affects the outcomes positively (Thorens, Kaelin, Jolliet, & Chevrolet, 1995). Experienced nurses agree that weaning is a collaborative process shared with the client that has both a physical and a psychological aspect. For ventilator-dependent clients, it can be a very stressful experience (Logan & Jenny, 1991). Recent work on clients' perceptions of ventilator weaning describe their concerns, which include physical discomfort, nurse caring behaviors, feelings of altered self, and the clients' physical emotional, and cognitive work involved in weaning (Jenny & Logan, in press).

3. There are ventilator-associated complications that may occur with prolonged ventilation (Tobin, 1994). A long period of intubation and mechanical ventilation places clients at risk for postoperative pulmonary complications (Brooks-Brunn, 1995). Systematic daily assessment of the oropharyngeal cavity is necessary for ventilated clients, especially those who are orally intubated, to detect or prevent lesions and infection (Treloar & Stechmiller, 1995). Raymond (1995) recommends that normal saline instillation before suctioning should not be a routine practice, but should be done only after assessing the need based on quality of secretions, quality of breath sounds, quality and effectiveness of cough, and oxygenation and ventilatory status.

4. Various criteria have been proposed for determining weaning readiness (Burns, Burns, & Truwit, 1994; Morganroth, Morganroth, Nett, & Petty, 1984; Yang & Tobin, 1991). These criteria are measures of oxygenation, respiratory muscle strength, and the ability to ventilate sufficiently to maintain an adequate arterial carbon dioxide level ($Paco_2$) (Witta, 1990). However, gaps exist in our current knowledge of client responses to ventilator weaning and in the prediction of outcomes. Goodnough Hanneman (1994) suggests that one reason that weaning predictors do not have adequate predictive power may be that the interrelationship of cardiopulmonary pathophysiologic determinants of outcomes is not reflected by independent predictive criteria (*e.g.*, pulmonary mechanics). The ongoing use of a systematic assessment tool may help tailor the process to the client's current status and prevent a premature weaning trial or a dysfunctional weaning response (Burns, Burns, & Truwit, 1994).

5. Because of the controversies over predictive tests and weaning methods (Burns, Clochesy, Goodnough Hanneman, Ingersoll, Knebel, & Shekleton, 1995; Pierson, 1995; Yang & Tobin, 1991), nurses rely on the approaches used in their own setting.

6. Outcomes after short-term mechanical ventilation differ from those after long-term ventilation. Psychological outlook, ventilatory drive, respiratory muscle strength and endurance, minute volume requirements, and nutritional status appear to have little bearing on short-term ventilator weaning (Goodnough Hanneman et al., 1994).

7. The physiologic inspiratory work of breathing includes three components:
   a. Compliance work to expand the elastic forces of the lung
   b. Tissue resistance work to overcome the viscosity of the lung and thoracic cage
   c. Airway resistance work to overcome the resistance to the flow of air into and out of the lungs (Clochesy, Breu, Cardin, Rudy, & Whittaker, 1993)
   Mechanical ventilation increase the work of breathing by decreasing airway diameter and increasing its length, thus increasing resistance. During the weaning process, the clinician manipulates pressure/volume changes to promote reconditioning of the respiratory muscles without causing excessive fatigue (Witta, 1990).

8. Dysfunctional ventilatory weaning response can involve respiratory inspiratory muscle fatigue, which can take up to 24–48 hours for recovery. The fatigue increase dyspnea, which in turn creates anxiety, triggering more fatigue and increased breathlessness.

Focus Assessment Criteria

Subjective Data

A. Assess for defining characteristics
   1. Concerns about starting or continuing weaning process
      Readiness   Previous experience
      Expectations   Possibility of failure
   2. Feelings about comfort, rest, energy status
   3. Knowledge of weaning process
      Collaborative role
      Assistance available

B. Assess for related factors
   1. Medication history
   2. Tobacco, alcohol use

Objective Data

A. Assess for defining characteristics

    1. Respiratory status: Complete respiratory assessment (see Focus Assessment Criteria in *Respiratory Function, Risk for Altered*)

        Level of consciousness

        Baseline skin color

        Type and amount of secretions

        Airway clearance

        Presence or absence of adventitious breath sounds

        Use of accessory muscles of respiration

        Arterial blood gases

        Vital signs

B. Assess for related factors

    1. Presence of respiratory disease, acute and chronic diseases

    2. Mechanical ventilator information

        Ventilator settings and size of endotracheal or tracheostomy tube

        Ventilation history, including reason for ventilation

        Length of time on the ventilator

        Whether weaning has been attempted before, and if so, with what results

    3. Current hemodynamic, nutritional, infection, and pain status

---

Outcome Criteria

The person will
- Achieve progressive weaning goals
- Spontaneous breathing for 24 hours without ventilatory support *or*
- Demonstrate a positive attitude toward the next weaning trial: collaborate willingly with the weaning plan, communicate comfort status during the weaning process, attempt to control the breathing pattern, and try to control emotional responses
- Be tired from the work of weaning, but not exhausted

Interventions

A. If applicable, assess causative factors for previous unsuccessful weaning attempts

    1. Inadequate energy substrates: oxygen, nutrition, and rest

    2. Inadequate comfort status

    3. Excessive activity demands

    4. Decreased self-esteem, confidence, feelings of control

    5. Lack of knowledge of the clients' role

    6. Lack of trust relationship with staff

    7. Negative emotional state

    8. Adverse weaning environment

B. Determine readiness for weaning (Geisman, 1989)

    1. Respiratory rate less than 25 breaths/minute

    2. Oxygen concentration of 40% or less on the ventilator

    3. Negative inspiratory pressure less than -20

    4. Positive expiratory pressure over $+30$

    5. Spontaneous tidal volume over 5 mL/kg

    6. Vital capacity over 10–15 mL/kg

7. Rested, controlled discomfort
8. Willingness to try weaning

C. If readiness for weaning is determined to be present, engage client in establishing the plan
1. Explain the weaning process.
2. Jointly negotiate progressive weaning goals.
3. Create a visual display of goals that allows for symbols to indicate progression (*e.g.*, bar or line graph to indicate increasing time off ventilator).
4. Explain that these goals will be reexamined daily with the individual.
5. Refer to unit protocols for specific weaning procedures.

D. Explain client's role in the weaning process
1. From the time of the initial intubation, promote the understanding that mechanical ventilation is a temporary mechanism.
2. Share the nurses' expectations of their collaborative work role when person is judged ready to wean.
3. Help the person to understand the importance of communicating comfort status and trying to reach the current weaning goals, and that rest will be allowed throughout the process.

E. Strengthen feelings of self-esteem, self-efficacy, and control
1. Reinforce self-esteem, confidence, and control through normalizing strategies such as grooming, dressing, mobilizing, and social conversation about things of interest to the person.
2. Permit as much control as possible through informing person of the situation and his progress, permitting shared decision making about details of care, observing client's preferences as far as possible, and improving comfort status.
3. Increase confidence by praising successful activities, encouraging a positive outlook, reviewing positive progress to date. Explain that people usually succeed in weaning and reassure client that you will be with him every step of the way.
4. Demonstrate confidence in client's ability to wean.
5. Maintain client's confidence by adopting a weaning pace* that ensures success and minimizes setbacks.

F. Promote trust in the staff and environment
1. Establish a trust relationship by communicating interest and concern for the person's well-being.
2. Help client to get to know you by sharing information about yourself.
3. Demonstrate competence and confidence in your own ability to manage the weaning process.
4. Maintain a calm manner and a relaxed atmosphere.
5. Explain what you are doing and why, to reduce the person's vigilance and feelings of uncertainty.
6. Note concerns that adversely affect comfort and confidence (family members, topics of conversation, room events, or previous weaning failures) and discuss them openly. Reduce their occurrence, if possible.

G. Reduce negative effects of anxiety and fatigue
1. Monitor status frequently to avoid undue fatigue and anxiety. Use of a systematic comprehensive tool is advantageous. A pulse oximeter is a noninvasive and unobtrusive way to monitor oxygen saturation levels.

---

* May require a primary care professional's order.

   2. Provide regular periods of rest before fatigue is advanced, by reducing activities and maintaining or increasing ventilator support and/or oxygen in consultation with a physician.

   3. Encourage emotional calmness and breath control by reassuring, presenting, and reinforcing that client can and will succeed.

   4. Consider use of alternative therapies such as music, hypnosis, and biofeedback.

   5. If the individual is becoming agitated, talk him down while remaining at the bedside, and coach him to regain breathing control. Monitor oxygen saturation and vital signs closely during this intervention.

   6. If weaning trial is discontinued, address person's perceptions of weaning failure. Reassure client that the trial was good exercise and a useful form of training. Remind client that the work is good for the respiratory muscles and will improve future performance.

H. Create a positive weaning environment that increases the person's feelings of security

   1. Provide a room with a quiet atmosphere, low activity, and no chatter within the person's hearing.

   2. Delegate the most skilled staff to wean individuals who have experienced moderate to severe responses or who are at high risk for doing so.

   3. Remain visible in the room to reinforce feelings of safety.

   4. Reassure the person that help is immediately available, if needed.

   5. Monitor visitors' effects on the individual and help the visitors to understand how they can best assist the person.

   6. Facilitate the presence of supportive visitors when possible during the weaning process. Rearrange visiting from active-weaning periods for visitors who upset the person.

   7. Ensure that clients are included in discussions that they are likely to overhear.

I. Promote optimal energy resources

   1. Assist person to cough and deep breathe regularly, and use prescribed bronchodilators, humidification, and suctioning to improve air entry.

   2. Ensure that nutritional support falls within current guidelines for ventilated and weaning clients.

   3. Provide sufficient rest periods to prevent undue fatigue.

   4. Use ventilator support at night if necessary to increase sleep time, and try to avoid unnecessary awakening.

   5. Monitor the disease processes to determine the body systems' stability.

J. Control activity demands

   1. Coordinate necessary activities to promote adequate time for rest or relaxation.

   2. Ensure that all staff follow the individualized care plan.

   3. Coach in breath control by regular demonstrations of slow, deep, rhythmic patterns of breathing. Help client to synchronize breathing with the ventilator.

   4. If person's concentration starts to create tension and increase anxiety, provide distraction in the form of supportive visitors, radio, television, or conversation.

K. Optimize comfort status to increase participation

   1. Identify strengths and resources, such as supportive family members or friends or a sense of humor, that can be mobilized to enhance coping and weaning efforts.

   2. Advocate for additional resources, such as analgesia, sedation, or room changes, that will increase client's comfort and willingness to work.

   3. Coordinate analgesia schedule with the weaning schedule.

   4. Wean in a sitting position or reverse Trendelenburg position, if not contraindicated.

   5. Start weaning trial when the person is rested, usually in the morning after a night's sleep.

   6. Use of a bedside fan may reduce feelings of dyspnea.

L. Negotiate elements of the weaning process with other clinicians to maximize the probability of weaning success
   1. The starting time
   2. The pace of the weaning
   3. Adherence to the care plan
   4. Diversional activities (*e.g.*, trips outside the unit)
   5. Scheduling of activities and rest periods

Rationale

- Successful weaning work depends on clients' adequate energy resources, careful utilization of their available energy, and skilled withdrawal of the ventilator support within the limits of the person's ability to tolerate additional breathing work. Fatigue is enhanced by altered or depleted energy reserve (Burns, 1991). Thus, energy conservation techniques are crucial to all weaning approaches (Jenny & Logan, in press; Logan & Jenny, 1990).
- To maintain adequate energy levels, nutritional support is necessary. It should avoid creating the complications of lipogenesis, overfeeding, and excessive carbohydrate loading to prevent excessive levels of carbon dioxide and respiratory acidemia (McMahon, Benotti, & Bistrian, 1990).
- As ventilator support is withdrawn, clients have to work harder. Their work of weaning involves control of their breathing, communication of their comfort status, cooperation with the therapeutic regimen, and trying to control their emotional responses to feelings of fatigue and anxiety (Jenny & Logan, 1991).
- Weaning setbacks are common, and require client support. During prolonged weaning, the client must be psychologically motivated to wean. Music therapy appears to have a beneficial effect in promoting relaxation in mechanically ventilated clients (Chlan, 1995). Feelings of powerlessness, hopelessness, and depression are combated with active decision making with the person, explanation of the sensations experienced, positive feedback, and the conveyance of hopefulness, encouragement, and support (Logan & Jenny, 1991; Witta, 1990). Additional optional interventions for weaning include use of active listening, humor, physical restraint, spiritual support, and pressure ulcer prevention (McCloskey & Bulechek, 1996, p. 682).
- Successful weaning is both an art and a science. The art of weaning depends on using subjective clinical judgment about the individual situation. Weaning as a science involves the theories of oxygen exchange, carbon dioxide exchange, and mechanical efficiency (Henneman, 1991). Nurses are a critical factor in imparting a positive outlook, creating a secure environment, enhancing clients' feelings of self-esteem and self-confidence, and helping clients deal with setbacks through their ability to combine the art and science of weaning (Jenny & Logan, 1994).

Risk for Dysfunctional Ventilatory Weaning Response

DEFINITION

Risk for Dysfunctional Ventilatory Weaning Response: The state in which an individual is at risk for experiencing an inability to adjust to lowered levels of mechanical ventilator support during the weaning process, related to physical and/or psychological unreadiness to wean.

RISK FACTORS
Pathophysiologic

Related to airway obstruction
Related to muscle weakness and fatigue secondary to:

Impaired respiratory functioning

Unstable hemodynamic status

Anemia

Dysrhythmia

Decreased level of consciousness

Mental confusion

Infection

Fever

Metabolic abnormalities

Acid–base abnormalities

Fluid and/or electrolyte imbalance

Severe disease process

Multisystem disease

Treatment-Related

Related to ineffective airway clearance
Related to excess sedation, analgesia
Related to uncontrolled pain
Related to fatigue
Related to inadequate nutrition (deficit in calories, excess carbohydrates, inadequate fats and protein intake)
Related to prolonged ventilator dependence (more than 1 week)
Related to previous unsuccessful ventilator weaning attempt(s)
Related to too-rapid pacing of the weaning process

Situational (Personal, Environmental)

Related to muscle weakness and fatigue secondary to:

Chronic nutritional deficit

Obesity

Ineffective sleep patterns

Related to knowledge deficit related to the weaning process
Related to inadequate self-efficacy related to weaning
Related to moderate to high anxiety related to breathing efforts
Related to fear of separation from ventilator
Related to feelings of powerlessness
Related to depressed mood
Related to feelings of hopelessness
Related to uncontrolled energy demands (self-care activities, diagnostic and treatment procedures, visitors)
Related to inadequate social support
Related to insecure environmental (noisy, upsetting events, busy room)

Author's Note

See *Dysfunctional Ventilatory Weaning Response*

Errors in Diagnostic Considerations

See *Dysfunctional Ventilatory Weaning Response*

Key Concepts

1. Clients at high risk for ventilator weaning are those who for one reason or another do not meet the traditional criteria for readiness to wean, such as:
   a. Respiratory rate less than 25 breaths/minute
   b. Oxygen concentration of 40% or less on the ventilator
   c. Negative inspiratory pressure less than −20
   d. Positive expiratory pressure over +30
   e. Spontaneous tidal volume over 5 mL/kg

   f. Vital capacity over 10–15 mL/kg
   g. Adequate arterial blood gases for client
   h. Rested, controlled discomfort
2. Although weaning as early as possible is important to avoid muscle deconditioning and complications related to prolonged endotracheal intubation and tracheostomy, premature attempts may be counterproductive because of the adverse physiologic and psychological effects.
3. Because weaning is a collaborative process, the nurse's ability to gain the client's trust and willingness to work is an important determinant of the weaning outcomes, especially with long-term clients. This trust is fostered by the knowledge and self-confidence nurses display, and their ability to deal with the persons's specific concerns (Jenny & Logan, 1991).
4. Weaning collaboration involves specific roles for both the nurses and the clients. The nurse must know the clients, manage their energy, and assist them with the work of weaning. Clients' collaborative work requires a trust relationship, and the belief that they will be protected during the weaning process.
5. Respiratory muscles must be stressed to a certain point of fatigue and then allowed to rest. The critical point of fatigue and duration of rest have not been documented in the literature, and this judgment depends on clinical expertise (Slutsky, 1993).
6. Dysfunctional ventilatory weaning is usually multifactorial. Marini (1991) notes that at the bedside, the subjective assessment of the weaning trial by an experienced clinician remains the most reliable predictor of weaning success or failure. Close monitoring of the client's weaning work is needed to prevent serious respiratory fatigue, which can require up to 24–48 hours' recovery before the person can proceed.
7. A dysfunctional weaning response to a weaning trial can have an impact also on the client's motivation and self-efficacy, creating doubt about the ability to wean and weakening the resolve to work (Jenny & Logan, 1991).

Focus Assessment Criteria

See *Dysfunctional Ventilatory Weaning Response*

Outcome Criteria

The person will demonstrate
- A willingness to start weaning
- A positive attitude about ability to succeed

The person will
- Maintain emotional control
- Collaborate with planning of the weaning

Interventions

A. Assess for causative and contributory factors of inadequate self-efficacy about weaning readiness
   1. Desire for continued need for ventilator support
   2. Excuses for delaying the start of weaning
   3. Concern about ability to adjust to lowered level of ventilator support or about the probability of success of weaning
   4. Agitated when weaning is mentioned
   5. Elevation of blood pressure, pulse, and respirations when weaning is discussed

B. Reduce risk factors
1. Negotiate with the medical staff for a delayed start and a weaning plan with a slow pace that ensures success at each stage
2. See *Dysfunctional Ventilatory Weaning Response*, Interventions, section E.

Rationale

- Experienced critical care nurses agree that weaning readiness involves both physical and psychological preparedness (Logan & Jenny, 1991). Despite ongoing research to evaluate objective criteria for weaning the "challenge to wean" client, a growing consensus is that a more holistic evaluation of ventilator dependence is required (Witta, 1990).
- A critical strategy in weaning at-risk individuals is the development of a weaning plan that maximizes the chances of success in meeting progressive weaning goals and decreases the chances for failure. This plan is designed to eliminate or reduce the intensity of the risk factors and/or compensate for those factors that cannot be altered.
- An initial step in the weaning plan is the careful preparation of clients. This includes teaching them about their collaborative weaning role, maximizing their energy resources and physical rest, enhancing their psychological willingness to proceed, and reinforcing their belief that they can perform the work of weaning (Carrieri-Kohlman, 1991; Jenny & Logan, 1994). Clients may have difficulty expressing their thoughts, so nurses must use multiple communication methods and persist until an effective method is found (Knebel, 1991).
- See also Rationale for *Dysfunctional Ventilatory Weaning Response*.

References/Bibliography

Brooks-Brunn, J. A. (1995). Postoperative atelectasis and pneumonia: Risk factors. *American Journal of Critical Care, 4*, 340–349.

Burns, S. M. (1991). Preventing diaphragm fatigue in the ventilated patient. *Dimensions of Critical Care Nursing, 10*, 13–20.

Burns, S. M., Burns, J. E., & Truwit, J. D. (1994). Comparison of five clinical weaning indices. *American Journal of Critical Care, 3*, 342–353.

Burns, S. M., Clochesy, J. M., Goodnough Hanneman, S. K., Ingersoll, G. E., Knebel, A. R., & Shekleton, M. (1995). Weaning from long-term mechanical ventilation. *American Journal of Critical Care, 4*, 4–22.

Carrieri-Kohlman, V. (1991). Dyspnea in the weaning patient: Assessment and intervention. *AACN Clinical Issues in Critical Care Nursing, 2*, 464–473.

Chlan, L. L. (1995). Psychophysiologic responses of mechanically ventilated patients to music: A pilot study. *American Journal of Critical Care, 4*, 233–238.

Clochesy, J. M., Breu, C., Cardin, S., Rudy, E. B., & Whittaker, A. A. (1993). *Critical care nursing*. Philadelphia: W. B. Saunders.

Geisman, L. K. (1989). Advances in weaning from mechanical ventilation. *Critical Care Nursing Clinics of North America, 1*, 697–705.

Goodnough Hanneman, S. K. (1994). Multidimensional predictors of success or failure with early weaning from mechanical ventilation after cardiac surgery. *Nursing Research, 43*, 4–10.

Goodnough Hanneman, S. K., Ingersoll, G.E., Knebel, A. R., Shekleton, M. E., Burns, S. M., & Clochesy, J. M. (1994). Weaning from short-term mechanical ventilation: A review. *American Journal of Critical Care, 3*, 421–432.

Henneman, E. A. (1991). The art and science of weaning from mechanical ventilation. *AACN Focus on Critical Care, 18*, 490–501.

Jenny, J., & Logan, J. (In press). Caring and comfort metaphors used by critical care patients. *Image*.

Jenny, J., & Logan, J. (1991). Analyzing expert nursing practice to develop a new nursing diagnosis: Dysfunctional ventilatory weaning response. In R. M. Carroll-Johnson (Ed.). *Classification of nursing diagnoses: Proceedings of the ninth conference*. Philadelphia: J. B. Lippincott.

Jenny, J., & Logan, J. (1994). Promoting ventilator independence. *Dimensions of Critical Care Nursing, 13*, 29–37.

Knebel, A. R. (1991). Weaning from mechanical ventilation: Current controversies. *Heart and Lung, 20*, 321–331.

Knebel, A. R., Shekleton, M. E., Burns, S. M., Clochesy, J. M., Goodnough Hanneman, S. K., & Ingersoll, G. L. (1994). Weaning from mechanical ventilation: Concept development. *American Journal of Critical Care, 3*, 416–420.

Logan, J., & Jenny, J. (1990). Deriving a new nursing diagnosis through qualitative research: Dysfunctional ventilatory weaning response. *Nursing Diagnosis, 1*(1), 37–43.

Logan, J., & Jenny, J. (1991). Interventions for the nursing diagnosis Dysfunctional Ventilatory Weaning Response: A qualitative study. In

R. M. Carroll-Johnson (Ed.). *Classification of nursing diagnosis: Proceedings of the ninth conference.* Philadelphia: J. B. Lippincott.

Marini, J. J. (1991). Editorials. *New England Journal of Medicine, 324,* 1496–1498.

McCloskey, J. C., & Bulechek, G. (Eds.). (1996). *Nursing interventions classification (NIC).* St Louis: Mosby–Year Book

McMahon, M. M., Benotti, P. N., & Bistrian, B. R. (1990). A clinical application of exercise physiology and nutritional support for the mechanically ventilated patient. *Journal of Parenteral Enteral Nutrition, 14,* 538–542.

Morganroth, M. L., Morganroth, J. L., Nett, L., & Petty, T. L. (1984). Criteria for weaning from prolonged mechanical ventilation. *Archives of Internal Medicine, 144,* 1012–1016.

Pierson, D. J. (1995). Weaning from mechanical ventilation: Why all the confusion? *Respiratory Care, 40,* 228–232.

Raymond, S. J. (1995). Normal saline instillation before suctioning: Helpful or harmful? A review of the literature. *American Journal of Critical Care, 4,* 267–271.

Slutsky, A. S. (1993). ACCP consensus conference: Mechanical ventilation. *Chest, 104,* 1833–1859.

Thorens, J. B., Kaelin, R. M., Jolliet, P., & Chevrolet, J. C. (1995). Influence of the quality of nursing on the duration of weaning from mechanical ventilation in patients with chronic obstructive pulmonary disease. *Critical Care Medicine, 23,* 1807–1815.

Tobin, M. J. (1994). Mechanical ventilation. *New England Journal of Medicine, 330,* 1056–1061.

Treloar, D. M., & Stechmiller, J. K. (1995). Use of a clinical assessment tool for orally intubated patients. *American Journal of Critical Care, 4,* 355–360.

Witta, K. (1990). New techniques for weaning difficult patients from mechanical ventilation. *AACN Clinical Issues, 1,* 260–266.

Yang, K. L., & Tobin, M. J. (1991). A prospective study of indexes predicting the outcome of trials of weaning from mechanical ventilation. *New England Journal of Medicine, 324,* 1445–1451.

Ineffective Airway Clearance

DEFINITION

Ineffective Airway Clearance: The state in which the individual experiences a threat to respiratory status related to inability to cough effectively.

DEFINING CHARACTERISTICS
Major (Must Be Present)

Ineffective or absent cough
Inability to remove airway secretions

Minor (May Be Present)

Abnormal breath sounds
Abnormal respiratory rate, rhythm, depth

RELATED FACTORS

See *Risk for Altered Respiratory Function*

Key Concepts

See *Risk for Altered Respiratory Function*

Focus Assessment Criteria

See *Risk for Altered Respiratory Function*

> **Outcome Criteria**
>
> The person will
> - Not experience aspiration
> - Demonstrate effective coughing and increased air exchange

Interventions

The nursing interventions for the diagnosis *Ineffective Airway Clearance* represent interventions for any individual with this nursing diagnosis, regardless of the related factors.

A. Assess for causative or contributing factors

    1. Inability to maintain proper position

    2. Ineffective cough

    3. Pain or fear of pain

    4. Viscous secretions (dehydration)

    5. Fatigue, weakness, drowsiness

    6. Chronic, nonrelieved cough

B. Reduce or eliminate factors, if possible

    1. Inability to maintain proper position

       a. Refer to *Risk for Aspiration*

    2. Ineffective cough

       a. Instruct person on the proper method of controlled coughing

           Breathe deeply and slowly while sitting up as high as possible

           Use diaphragmatic breathing

           Hold the breath for 3–5 seconds and then slowly exhale as much of this breath as possible through the mouth (lower rib cage and abdomen should sink down)

           Take a second breath, hold, slowly exhale, and cough forcefully from the chest (not from the back of the mouth or throat), using two short forceful coughs

    3. Pain or fear of pain

       a. Assess present analgesic regimen.

           Administer pain medications as needed.

           Coordinate analgesic doses with coughing sessions (*e.g.*, give doses ½–1 hour before coughing sessions)

           Assess its effectiveness: Is the individual too lethargic? Is the individual still in pain?

           Note time when person appears to have best pain relief with optimal level of alertness and physical performance: *This is the time for active breathing and coughing exercises*.

       b. Provide emotional support.

           Stay with person for the entire coughing session.

           Explain the importance of coughing after pain relief.

           Reassure person that suture lines are secure and that splinting by hand or pillow will minimize pain of movement.

       c. Use appropriate comfort measures for site of pain.

           Splint abdominal or chest incisions with hand, pillow, or both.

       d. For sore throat

           Assess for adequate humidity in the inspired air.

           Consider warm saline gargle every 2–4 hours.

Consider use of anesthetic lozenge or gargle, especially before coughing sessions.*

Examine throat for exudate, redness, and swelling and note if it is associated with fever.

Explain that a sore throat is common after anesthesia and should be a short-term problem.

e. Maintain good body alignment to prevent muscular pain and strain.

Acquire and use extra pillows on both sides of person, especially the affected side, for support.

Position person to prevent slouching and cramping positions of the thorax and abdomen; reassess positioning frequently.

f. Assess person's understanding of the use of analgesia to enhance breathing and coughing effort.

Teach person during periods of optimal level of consciousness.

Continually reinforce rationale for plan of nursing care. ("I will be back to help you cough when the pain medicine is working and you can be most effective.")

4. Viscous (thick) secretions

a. Maintain adequate hydration (increase fluid intake to 2–3 quarts a day if not contraindicated by decreased cardiac output or renal disease).

b. Maintain adequate humidity of inspired air.

5. Fatigue, weakness, drowsiness

a. Plan and bargain for rest periods ("Work to cough well now; then I can let you rest.").

b. Vigorously coach and encourage coughing, using positive reinforcement ("You worked hard; I know it's not easy, but it is important.").

c. Be sure coughing session occurs at peak comfort period after analgesics, but not peak level of sleepiness.

d. Allow for rest after coughing and before meals.

e. For lethargy or decreased level of consciousness, stimulate person to breathe deeply on an hourly basis. ("Take a deep breath.")

6. For chronic, nonrelieved coughing

a. Minimize irritants in the inspired air (*e.g.*, dust, allergens).

b. Provide periods of uninterrupted rest.

c. Administer prescribed medications—cough suppressant, expectorant—as ordered by physician (withhold food and drink immediately after administration of medications for best results).

d. Relieve mucous membrane irritation through humidity (inhaling steam from shower, or sitting over pot of steaming water with a towel over the head, loosens thick secretions and soothes the membranes).

Rationale

- Uncontrolled coughing is tiring and ineffective, leading to frustration.
- Deep breathing dilates the airways, stimulates surfactant production, and expands the lung tissue surface, thus improving respiratory gas exchange. Coughing loosens secretions and forces them into the bronchus to be expectorated or suctioned. In some clients, "huffing" breathing may be effective and is less painful.
- Sitting high shifts the abdominal organs away from the lungs, enabling greater expansion.
- Diaphragmatic breathing reduces the respiratory rate and increase alveolar ventilation.
- Increasing the volume of air in lungs promotes expulsion of secretions.
- Thick secretions are difficult to expectorate and can cause mucus plugs, which can lead to atelectasis.

* May require a primary care professional's order.

- Good oral hygiene promotes a sense of well-being and prevents mouth odor.
- The secretions must be sufficiently liquid to enable expulsion.
- Pain or fear of pain can inhibit participation in coughing and breathing exercises. Adequate pain relief is essential.
- Coughing exercises are fatiguing and painful. Emotional support provides encouragement; warm water can aid relaxation (Mumford, Schlesinger, & Glass, 1982).

🐚 Interventions—*Child Focus*

1. Instruct parents on the need for child to cough, even if painful.
2. Allow adult and older child to listen to lungs; describe if clear or if rales are present.
3. Consult with respiratory therapist for assistance, if needed.

Rationale

- Explaining and demonstrating the benefits of coughing can increase parent and child cooperation (Wong, 1995).

Ineffective Breathing Patterns

DEFINITION

Ineffective Breathing Patterns: The state in which the individual experiences an actual or potential loss of adequate ventilation related to an altered breathing pattern.

DEFINING CHARACTERISTICS
Major (Must Be Present)

Changes in respiratory rate or pattern (from baseline)
Changes in pulse (rate, rhythm, quality)

Minor (May Be Present)

Orthopnea   Dysrhythmic respirations
Tachypnea, hyperpnea, hyperventilation   Splinted/guarded respirations

RELATED FACTORS

See *Risk for Altered Respiratory Function*

Author's Note
See *Risk for Altered Respiratory Function*

Errors in Diagnostic Statements
See *Risk for Altered Respiratory Function*

Key Concepts

1. Hyperventilation is overbreathing with a reduction in P_{CO_2} and respiratory alkaloses (Porth, 1994).

2. Causes of hyperventilation syndrome are organic (drug effects, central nervous system lesions), physiologic (response to high altitude, heat, exercise), emotional (anxiety, hysteria, anger, depression), and habitual faulty breathing habits (rapid, shallow breathing) (Porth, 1994).
3. Symptoms of hyperventilation syndrome are headache, dyspnea, numbness and tingling sensations, light-headedness, chest pain, palpitations, and occasionally syncope (Porth, 1994).
4. Panic can manifest with hyperventilation, and people with panic disorders can hyperventilate (Porth, 1994).

Outcome Criteria

The person will
- Demonstrate an effective respiratory rate
- Relate relief of symptoms
- Relate the causative factors, if known, and relate adaptive ways of coping with them

---

Interventions

A. Assess history of symptoms and causative factors
    1. Previous episodes—when, where, circumstances
    2. Causes
        a. Organic
        b. Physiologic
        c. Emotional
        d. Faulty breathing habits

B. Remove or eliminate causative factors
    1. Explain the cause
    2. Stay with person
    3. If fear or panic has precipitated the episode:
        a. Remove cause of fear, if possible.
        b. Reassure that measures are being taken to ensure safety.
        c. Distract person from thinking about his anxious state by having him maintain eye contact with you (or perhaps with someone else he trusts); say, "Now look at me and breathe slowly with me like this."
        d. Consider use of paper bag as means of rebreathing expired air (expired CO_2 will be reinspired, thereby slowing respiratory rate).
        e. See *Fear*.
    4. Reassure person they can control their breathing.
    5. Consult with respiratory therapist for training to overcome faulty breathing patterns.

Rationale

- Interventions are focused on slowing breathing pattern and educating the person to control response (Porth, 1994).

Impaired Gas Exchange

DEFINITION

Impaired Gas Exchange: The state in which the individual experiences an actual or potential decreased passage of gases (oxygen and carbon dioxide) between the alveoli of the lungs and the vascular system.

DEFINING CHARACTERISTICS
Major (Must Be Present)

Dyspnea on exertion

Minor (May Be Present)

Tendency to assume three-point position (sitting, one hand on each knee, bending forward)

Pursed-lip breathing with prolonged expiratory phase

Confusion/agitation

Lethargy and fatigue

Increased pulmonary vascular resistance (increased pulmonary artery/right ventricular pressure)

Decreased gastric motility, prolonged gastric emptying

Decreased oxygen content, decreased oxygen saturation, increased PCO_2, as measured by blood gas analysis

Cyanosis

RELATED FACTORS

See *Risk for Altered Respiratory Function*

Author's Note

Respiratory problems that nurses treat as nursing diagnoses are *Ineffective Airway Clearance*, *Ineffective Breathing Pattern*, *Risk for Altered Respiratory Function*, *Dysfunctional Ventilatory Weaning Response*, and *Activity Intolerance*. If these nursing diagnoses are treated, then it follows that gas exchange should improve. If gas exchange does not improve, then the problem is a collaborative problem and should be labeled as such (*e.g., Potential Complication: Hypoxemia* or *Potential Complication: Respiratory Insufficiency*). In this case, the nursing role is monitoring to detect changes in status. If respiratory status worsens, the nurse manages the situation using nursing- and medical-prescribed interventions.

Some nurses are tempted to use *Impaired Gas Exchange* to describe the problem of COPD. Labeling COPD as *Impaired Gas Exchange* does not help in determining nursing interventions. What does the nurse do for *Impaired Gas Exchange?* . . . the nurse helps the person by treating the *Ineffective Airway Clearance*, *Ineffective Breathing Patterns*, and *Activity Intolerance*, and preventing *Altered Respiratory Function*. The nurse would also assess for functional health patterns that have been or may be affected by decreased oxygenation as sleep, emotional status, and nutrition.

Inability to Sustain Spontaneous Ventilation

DEFINITION

Inability to Sustain Spontaneous Ventilation: A state in which an individual is unable to maintain adequate breathing to support life. This is measured by deterioration of arterial blood gases, increased work of breathing, and decreasing energy.

DEFINING CHARACTERISTICS
Major

Dyspnea
Increased metabolic rate

Minor

Increased restlessness
Apprehension
Increased use of accessory muscles
Decreased tidal volume
Increased heart rate

Decreased PO_2
Increased PCO_2
Decreased cooperation
Decreased SaO_2

Author's Note

This diagnosis represents respiratory insufficiency with corresponding metabolic changes that are incompatible with life. This situation requires rapid nursing and medical management, specifically resuscitation and mechanical ventilation. Inability to sustain spontaneous ventilation is not appropriate as a nursing diagnosis—it is hypoxemia, a collaborative problem. Hypoxemia is insufficient plasma oxygen saturation due to alveolar hypoventilation, pulmonary shunting, or ventilation–perfusion inequality. As a collaborative problem, the definitive treatments are prescribed by physicians; however, both nursing- and medical-prescribed interventions are required for management. The nursing accountability is to monitor status continuously and to manage changes in status with the appropriate interventions, using protocols.

References/Bibliography

Bailey, W. C., Cheng, F., Lemanski, R., & Reed, C. E. (1994). Asthma update: Better diagnosis, close control. *Patient Care, 11,* 64–67.

Braun-Fahrlander, C., Ackerman-Liebrich, U., Swartz, J., Gnehm, H., Rutishauser, M., & Wanner, H. (1992). Air pollution in preschool children. *American Review of Respiratory Disease, 145,* 42–47.

Brooks-Brunn, J. (1995). Postoperative atelectasis and pneumonia: Risk factors. *American Journal of Critical Care, 4,* 340–351.

Centers for Disease Control and Prevention. (1995). Asthma: United States 1982–1992. *Morbidity and Mortality Weekly Report, 43*(51), 952–955.

Change, V. (1995). Protocol for prevention of complications of endotracheal intubation. *Critical Care Nurse, 13*(4), 19–26.

Clark, J., Votteri, B., & Ariagno, R. (1992). Non-invasive assessment of blood gases. *American Review of Respiratory Disease, 145,* 220–232.

Earwood, G. L. (1996). Managing Adult asthma in primary care setting. *Journal of American Academy of Nurse Practitioners, 8*(1), 33–39.

Fishbach, F. (1996). *A manual of laboratory and diagnostic tests* (5th ed.). Philadelphia: Lippincott–Raven Publishers.

Haldfeldt, K., Siebeck, M., Thetter, O., & Schweiberer, L. (1995). The effect of thoracic surgery on pulmonary function. *American Journal of Critical Care, 4,* 352–354.

Huckabay, L., & Daderian, A. (1989). Effect of choices on breathing exercises post open heart surgery. *Dimensions of Critical Care Nursing, 9,* 190–201.

Huddleston, V. B. (1990). Pulmonary problems. *Critical Care Nursing Clinics of North America, 2*, 527–536.

Hunsberger, M. (1989). Nursing strategies: Altered respiratory function. In R. L. Foster, M. M. Hunsberger, & J. J. T. Anderson (Eds.). *Family-centered nursing care of children.* Philadelphia: W. B. Saunders.

Janson-Bjerklie, S., Ferketich, S., Benner, P., & Becker, G. (1992). Clinical markers of asthma severity risk: Importance of subjective as well as objective factors. *Heart and Lung, 21,* 265–272.

Janson-Bjerklie, S., Ruma, S., Stulbarg, M., & Carrieri, V. (1987). Predictors of dyspnea intensity in asthma. *Nursing Research, 36,* 179–183.

Lasater-Erhard, M. (1995). The effect of patient position on arterial oxygen saturation. *Critical Care Nurse, 13*(4), 31–35.

Litwack, K., Saleh, D., & Schaltz, P. (1991). Postoperative pulmonary complications. *Critical Care Nursing Clinics of North America, 3,* 77–82.

May, K. A., & Mahlmeister, L. R. (1994). *Maternal and neonatal nursing: Family-centered care* (3rd ed.). Philadelphia: J. B. Lippincott.

Miller, C. A. (1995). *Nursing care of older adults* (2nd ed.). Glenview, IL: Scott, Foresman.

Mumford, E., Schlesinger, H., & Glass, G. (1982). The effects of psychological interventions in recovery from surgery and heart attacks: An analysis of the literature. *American Journal of Public Health, 72,* 141–151.

National Asthma Education Program, Expert Panel. (1991). *Guidelines for the diagnosis and management of asthma.* DHHS Publication No. 91-3042A. Bethesda, MD: National Heart, Lung and Blood Institute.

Porth, C. (1994). *Pathophysiology: Concepts of altered health states* (4th ed.). Philadelphia: J. B. Lippincott.

Staab, A., & Lyles, M. (1990). *Manual of geriatric nursing.* Glenview, IL: Scott, Foresman.

Wake, M., Fehring, R., & Fadden, T. (1991). Multinational validation of anxiety, hopelessness, and ineffective airway clearance. *Nursing Diagnosis, 2*(2), 57–64.

Webster, J., & Kadah, H. (1991). Unique aspects of respiratory disease in the aged. *Geriatrics, 46*(7), 31–43.

Wong, D. L. (1995). *Nursing care of infants and children* (5th ed.). St. Louis: Mosby–Year Book.

Role Performance, Altered

DEFINITION

Altered Role Performance: The state in which an individual experiences or is at risk of experiencing a disruption in the way he or she perceives his or her role performance.

DEFINING CHARACTERISTICS
Major (Must Be Present)

Conflict related to role perception or performance

Minor (May Be Present)

Change in self-perception of role

Denial of role

Change in others' perception of role

Change in physical capacity to resume role

Lack of knowledge of role

Change in usual patterns of responsibility

Author's Note

The nursing diagnosis *Altered Role Performance* has a defining characteristic of "conflict related to role perception or performance." All individuals have multiple roles. Some of these roles are prescribed, such as gender and age; some acquired, such as parent and occupation; and some transitional, such as elected office or team member.

Various factors affect a person's roles, including developmental stage, societal norms, cultural beliefs, values, life events, illness, and disabilities. When a person has difficulty with role performance, it may be more useful to describe the effect of the difficulty on functioning, rather than to describe the problem as *Altered Role Performance*. For example, a person who has experienced a cerebrovascular accident (CVA) may undergo a change from being the primary breadwinner to becoming unemployed. In this situation, the nursing diagnosis *Grieving related to loss of role as financial provider secondary to effects of CVA* would be appropriate. In another example, if a woman became unable to continue her household responsibilities because of illness and these responsibilities were assumed by the other family members, the situations that may arise would better be described as *Risk for Self-Concept Disturbance related to recent loss of role responsibility secondary to illness* and *Risk for Impaired Home Maintenance Management related to lack of knowledge of family members*.

A conflict in a family regarding others meeting role obligations or expectations can represent related factors for the diagnosis *Altered Family Processes related to conflict regarding expectations of members meeting role obligations*.

Until clinical research defines this diagnosis and the associated nursing interventions, use "altered role performance" as a related factor for another nursing diagnosis (*e.g., Anxiety, Grieving,* or *Self-Concept Disturbance*).

Self-Care Deficit Syndrome*

Feeding Self-Care Deficit

Bathing/Hygiene Self-Care Deficit

Dressing/Grooming Self-Care Deficit

Toileting Self-Care Deficit

Instrumental Self-Care Deficit*

Self-Care Deficit Syndrome

DEFINITION
Self-Care Deficit Syndrome: The state in which the individual experiences an impaired motor function or cognitive function, causing a decreased ability in performing each of the five self-care activities.

DEFINING CHARACTERISTICS
Major (One Deficit Must Be Present in Each Activity)

1. Self-feeding deficits
   - Unable to cut food or open packages
   - Unable to bring food to mouth
2. Self-bathing deficits (includes washing entire body, combing hair, brushing teeth, attending to skin and nail care, and applying makeup)
   - Unable or unwilling to wash body or body parts
   - Unable to obtain a water source
   - Unable to regulate temperature or water flow
   - Inability to perceive need for hygienic measures
3. Self-dressing deficits (including donning regular or special clothing, not nightclothes)
   - Impaired ability to put on or take off clothing
   - Unable to fasten clothing
   - Unable to groom self satisfactorily
   - Unable to obtain or replace articles of clothing
4. Self-toileting deficits
   - Unable or unwilling to get to toilet or commode
   - Unable or unwilling to carry out proper hygiene
   - Unable to transfer to and from toilet or commode
   - Unable to handle clothing to accommodate toileting
   - Unable to flush toilet or empty commode

*These diagnoses are not currently on the NANDA list but have been included for clarity or usefulness.

5. Instrumental self-care deficits
    Difficulty using telephone
    Difficulty accessing transportation
    Difficulty laundering, ironing   Difficulty managing money
    Difficulty preparing meals   Difficulty with medication administration
    Difficulty shopping

RELATED FACTORS
Pathophysiologic

Related to lack of coordination secondary to (specify)
Related to spasticity or flaccidity secondary to (specify)
Related to muscular weakness secondary to (specify)
Related to partial or total paralysis secondary to (specify)
Related to atrophy secondary to (specify)
Related to muscle contractures secondary to (specify)
Related to comatose state
Related to visual disorders secondary to (specify)
Related to nonfunctioning or missing limb(s)
Related to regression to an earlier level of development
Related to excessive ritualistic behaviors
Related to somatoform deficits (specify)

Treatment-Related

Related to external devices (specify) (casts, splints, braces, IV equipment)
Related to postoperative fatigue and pain

Situational (Personal, Environmental)

Related to cognitive deficits   Related to fatigue
Related to pain   Related to confusion
Related to decreased motivation   Related to disabling anxiety

Maturational

Older Adult
    Related to decreased visual and motor ability, muscle weakness

Author's Note

Self-care encompasses the activities needed to meet daily needs, commonly known as activities of daily living (ADLs), which are learned over time and become lifelong habits. Self-care activities involve not only what is to be done (hygiene, bathing, dressing, toileting, feeding), but how much, when, where, with whom, and how it is done (Miller, 1995).

In every person, the threat or reality of a self-care deficit evokes panic. Many people report that they fear loss of independence more than death. A self-care deficit affects the core of one's self-concept and self-determination. For this reason, the nursing focus for self-care deficit should not be on providing the care measure, but rather on identifying adaptive techniques to allow the person the maximum degree of participation and independence possible.

The diagnosis *Total Self-Care Deficit* once was used to describe a person's inability to complete feeding, bathing, toileting, dressing, and grooming (Carpenito, 1983; Gordon, 1982). The intent of specifying "Total" was to describe a person with deficits in several ADLs. Unfortunately, sometimes its use invites, according to Magnan (1989, personal communication), "preconceived judgments about the state of an individual and the nursing interventions required." The person may be viewed as in a vegetative state, requiring only minimal custodial care. *Total Self-Care Deficit* has been eliminated because its language does not denote potential for growth or rehabilitation.

Currently not on the NANDA list, the diagnosis *Self-Care Deficit Syndrome* has been added here to describe a person with compromised ability in all five self-care activities. For this person, the nurse assesses functioning in each of the five areas and identifies the level of participation of which the person is capable. The goal is to maintain the current level of functioning and/or to increase participation and independence. The syndrome distinction clusters all five self-care deficits together to enable grouping of interventions when indicated, while also permitting specialized interventions for a specific deficit.

The danger of applying a *Self-Care Deficit* diagnosis lies in the possibility of prematurely labeling a person as unable to participate at any level, eliminating a rehabilitation focus. It is important that the nurse classify the person's functional level to promote independence. (Refer to the functional level classification scale in Focus Assessment Criteria.) Continuous reevaluation also is necessary to identify changes in the person's ability to participate in self-care.

Errors in Diagnostic Considerations

Toileting Self-Care Deficit related to insufficient knowledge of ostomy care

The diagnosis *Toileting Self-Care Deficit* describes a person who cannot get to, sit on, or rise up from the toilet, or perform clothing and hygiene activities related to toileting. Insufficient knowledge of ostomy care does not apply to this diagnosis. Depending on presence of risk factors or signs and symptoms, the diagnosis of *Ineffective Management of Therapeutic Regimen related to insufficient knowledge of ostomy care* would apply to this situation.

Dressing Self-Care Deficit related to inability to fasten clothing

Inability to fasten clothing represents a sign or symptom of *Dressing Self-Care Deficit*, not a related factor. Using a focus assessment, the nurse needs to determine the contributing factors (*e.g.*, insufficient knowledge of adaptive techniques needed).

Self-Care Deficit Syndrome related to cognitive deficits

As a syndrome diagnosis, no related factors are indicated and, in fact, are not very useful for treatment. Instead, the nurse should write the diagnosis as *Self-Care Deficit Syndrome: Feeding (1), Bathing (4), Dressing/Grooming (4), Toileting (5), Instrumental (2).* The number code indicates the present level of functioning needed. The outcome criteria should represent improved or increased functioning.

Key Concepts

1. The concept of self-care emphasizes each person's right to maintain individual control over his own pattern of living. (This applies to both the ill individual and the well individual.) (Tracey, 1992).
2. It is acceptable for a limited time to be dependent on others to provide basic physiologic and psychological needs.
3. Regression in ability to perform self-care activities may be a defense mechanism to threatening situations.
4. Neglect of an extremity refers to the memory loss of the presence of an extremity (*e.g.*, a person who has had a stroke or brain injury resulting in partial paralysis may ignore the arm or leg on the affected side of the body).
5. The following key elements promote relearning of self-care tasks:
   a. Providing a structured, consistent environment and routine
   b. Repeating instructions and tasks
   c. Teaching and practicing tasks during periods of least fatigue
   d. Maintaining a familiar environment and teacher
   e. Using patience, determination, and a positive attitude (by both learner and teacher)
   f. Practice, practice, practice
6. Lubkin (1995) describes four principles to motivate as:
   a. Uncover hidden resources
   b. Increase underutilized abilities
   c. Initiate positive life patterns
   d. Flourish within existing limitations

Endurance

1. The endurance or ability of the individual to maintain a given level of performance is influenced by the ability to use oxygen to produce energy (related to the optimal functioning of the heart and respiratory and circulatory systems) and the functioning of the neurologic and musculoskeletal systems. Thus, individuals with alterations in these systems have increased energy demands or a decreased ability to produce energy.
2. Stress is energy consuming; the more stressors an individual has, the more fatigue he experiences. Stressors can be personal, environmental, disease-related, and treatment-related. Examples of possible stressors follow.

Personal	Environmental	Disease-Related	Treatment-Related
Age	Isolation	Pain	Walker
Support system	Noise	Anemia	Medications
Life-style	Unfamiliar setting	Diagnostic studies	

3. The signs and symptoms of decreased oxygen in response to an activity (*e.g.*, self-care, mobility) are
    Sustained increased heart rate 3–5 minutes after ceasing the activity, or a change in the pulse rhythm
    Failure of systolic blood pressure reading to increase with activity, or a decrease in value
    Decrease or excessive increase in respiratory rate and dyspnea
    Weakness, pallor, cerebral hypoxia (confusion, incoordination)
4. Refer to Key Concepts under *Activity Intolerance* for additional information.

🌀 *Key Concepts—Child*

1. The infant and young child depend on a caregiver for assistance with ADLs.
2. Parents/caregivers can facilitate a child's mastery of self-care skills. The desired outcome is that the child participates in his care to the maximum of his abilities (Wong, 1995).
3. The nurse should assess each child's unique ability to engage in self-care activities to promote control over self and environment.

🏛 *Key Concepts—Older Adult*

1. Age-related changes do not in themselves cause self-care deficits. Older adults do, however, have an increased incidence of chronic diseases that can compromise functional ability (*e.g.*, arthritis, cardiac disorders, visual impairment).
2. Comparing statistics from 1961 to 1981 reveals a substantial improvement in overall functioning among older adults (Palmer & Tonis, 1980).
3. About 70% of people age 65 years and older rate their health as excellent. Only 20% of adults age 65–74 and 24% older than age 75 years report limitations in activity due to chronic illness (U.S. Department of Health and Human Services, 1987).
4. Older adults with dementia have varying degrees of difficulty with self-care activities depending on memory deficits, ability to follow directions, and judgment (Miller, 1995).
5. Sixty-three percent of older nursing home residents cannot perform basic ADLs because of cognitive impairment (Miller, 1995)
6. Caregivers frequently promote excess disability and a quicker deterioration in the elderly because they believe independent behavior is atypical (Miller, 1995).

TRANSCULTURAL CONSIDERATIONS

1. In some cultures, family members may show their concern for the sick family member by doing as much as possible for him or her (*e.g.*, feeding him or her, bathing). This practice may prevent the client from actively participating in a rehabilitation program (Andrews & Boyle, 1995).
2. "All culture groups have rules, often unspoken, about who touches whom, when and where" (Andrews & Boyle, 1995, p. 19).

Focus Assessment Criteria

Subjective/Objective

A. Evaluate each ADL using the following scale:

        0 = Completely independent
        1 = Requires use of assistive device
        2 = Needs minimal help
        3 = Needs assistance and/or some supervision
        4 = Needs total supervision
        5 = Needs total assistance or unable to assist

B. Assess for defining characteristics

    1. Self-feeding abilities

Swallowing	Selecting foods
Chewing	Seeing
Using utensils and cutting food	Opening cartons
Drinking from cup	

    2. Self-bathing abilities
        Undressing to bathe
        Reaching water source
        Differentiating water temperatures
        Obtaining equipment (water, soap, towels)
        Washing body parts
        Performing oral care

    3. Self-dressing/grooming abilities

Putting on or taking off clothing	Cleaning/trimming nails
Selecting appropriate clothing	Brushing teeth
Washing and styling hair	Plugging in cord
Shaving	Retrieving appropriate clothing
Using deodorant	Fastening clothing

    4. Self-toileting abilities

Getting to toilet and undressing	Redressing
Sitting on toilet	Performing hygiene (washing hands)
Rising from toilet	Can use tampon/sanitary napkin
Cleaning self/flushing toilet	

    5. Instrumental ADLs
        Telephone
            Ability to dial   Ability to talk, hear
            Ability to answer
        Transportation
            Ability to drive
            Access to transportation
        Laundry
            Availability of washer
            Ability to wash, iron
            Ability to put away
        Food procurement and preparation
            Ability to cook
            Ability to select foods
            Ability to shop
        Medications
            Ability to remember
            Ability to administer

    6. Finances
        Ability to write checks, pay bills
        Ability to handle cash transactions (simple, complex)

C. Assess for related factors
  1. Mental status
     Ability to remember
     Judgment
     Ability to follow directions
     Ability to identify/express needs
     Ability to anticipate needs (food, laundry)
     Social supports
        Support people
        Availability of help with transportation, shopping, money management, laundry, housekeeping, food preparation
        Community resources
  2. Motivation
  3. Endurance

Outcome Criteria

The person will
- Identify preferences in self-care activities (*e.g.* time, products, location)
- Demonstrate optimal hygiene after assistance with care
- Participate physically and/or verbally in feeding, dressing, toileting, bathing activities

---

Interventions

A. Assess for causative or contributing factors
  1. Visual deficits
  2. Impaired cognition
  3. Decreased motivation
  4. Impaired mobility
  5. Lack of knowledge
  6. Inadequate social support
  7. Excessive ritualistic behavior
  8. Disabling anxiety
  9. Irrational fears
  10. Regression to an earlier level of development

B. Promote optimal participation
  1. Assess present level of participation.
  2. Determine areas for potential increase in participation in each self-care activity.
  3. Explore the person's goals.
  4. Allow ample time to complete activities without help. Promote independence, but assist when person is unable to perform an activity.
  5. Demonstrate how to perform an activity that is problematic.

C. Promote self-esteem and self-determination
  1. Determine preferences for
     a. Schedule
     b. Products
     c. Methods
     d. Clothing selection
     e. Hair styling

2. During self-care activities, provide choices and request preferences.
3. Do not focus on disability.
4. Offer praise for independent accomplishments
5. Do not allow to use disability as a manipulative tool. Withdraw attention if person continues to focus on limitations (Townsend, 1994).

D. Evaluate ability to participate in each self-care activity (feeding, dressing, bathing, toileting)
1. Assign a number value to each activity (refer to the coding scale in Focus Assessment Criteria).
2. Reassess ability frequently and revise code as appropriate.

E. Refer to interventions under each diagnosis—Feeding, Bathing, Dressing, Toileting, and Instrumental Self-Care Deficit—as indicated

Rationale
- Enhancing a client's self-care abilities can increase his sense of control and independence, promoting overall well-being (Tracey, 1992).
- Regardless of handicap, people should be given privacy and treated with dignity while performing self-care activities.
- Self-care does not imply allowing the person to do things for himself as planned by the nurse but, rather, encouraging and teaching the person to make his own plans for optimal daily living.
- Mobility is necessary to meet self-care needs and to maintain good health and self-esteem.
- Cleanliness is important for comfort, for positive self-esteem, and for social interactions with others.
- Inability to care for oneself produces feelings of dependency and poor self-concept. With increased ability for self-care, self-esteem increases.
- Disability often causes denial, anger, and frustration. These are valid emotions that must be recognized and addressed.
- Optimal education promotes self-care. To teach effectively, the nurse must determine what the learner perceives as his own needs and goals, determine what the nurse feels are the learner's needs and goals, and then work to establish mutually acceptable goals.
- Offering the individual choices and including him in planning his own care reduces feelings of powerlessness; promotes feelings of freedom, control, and self-worth; and increases the person's willingness to comply with therapeutic regimens.

Feeding Self-Care Deficit

DEFINITION
Feeding Self-Care Deficit: A state in which the individual experiences an impaired ability to perform or complete feeding activities for himself or herself.

DEFINING CHARACTERISTICS
Unable to cut food or open food packages
Unable to bring food to mouth

RELATED FACTORS

See *Self-Care Deficit Syndrome*

Errors in Diagnostic Statements

See *Self-Care Deficit Syndrome*

Key Concepts

See *Self-Care Deficit Syndrome*

Focus Assessment Criteria

See *Self-Care Deficit Syndrome*

Outcome Criteria

The person will
- Demonstrate increased ability to feed self *or*
- Report that he is unable to feed self
- Demonstrate ability to make use of adaptive devices, if indicated
- Demonstrate increased interest and desire to eat
- Describe rationale and procedure for treatment
- Describe causative factors for feeding deficit

Interventions

A. Assess causative factors
   1. Visual deficits (blindness, field cuts, poor depth perception)
   2. Affected or missing limbs (casts, amputations, paresis, paralysis)
   3. Cognitive deficits (dementia, trauma, cerebrovascular accident [CVA])

B. Provide opportunities to relearn or adapt to activity
   1. Common nursing interventions for feeding
      a. Ascertain from person or family members what foods the person likes or dislikes.
      b. Have meals taken in the same setting: pleasant surroundings that are not too distracting.
      c. Maintain correct food temperatures (hot foods hot, cold foods cold).
      d. Provide pain relief, because pain can affect appetite and ability to feed self.
      e. Provide good oral hygiene before and after meals.
      f. Encourage person to wear dentures and eyeglasses.
      g. Assist to the most normal eating position suited to his physical disability (best is sitting in a chair at a table).
      h. Provide social contact during eating.
      i. See *Altered Nutrition: Less Than Body Requirements*.
   2. Specific interventions for people with sensory/perceptual deficits
      a. Encourage to wear prescribed corrective lenses.
      b. Describe location of utensils and food on tray or table.
      c. Describe food items to stimulate appetite.

    d. For perceptual deficits, choose different-colored dishes to help distinguish items (*e.g.*, red tray, white plates).

    e. Ascertain usual eating patterns and provide food items according to preference (or arrange food items in clocklike pattern); record on care plan the arrangement used (*e.g.*, meat, 6 o'clock; potatoes, 9 o'clock; vegetables, 12 o'clock).

    f. Encourage eating of "finger foods" (*e.g.*, bread, bacon, fruit, hot dogs) to promote independence.

    g. Avoid placing food to blind side of person with field cut, until visually accommodated to surroundings; then encourage him to scan entire visual field.

3. Specific interventions for people with missing limbs

    a. Provide for eating environment that is not embarrassing to individual, and allow sufficient time for the task of eating.

    b. Provide only the amount of supervision and assistance necessary for relearning or adaptation.

    c. To enhance maximum amount of independence, provide necessary adaptive devices:

        Plate guard to avoid pushing food off plate

        Suction device under plate or bowl for stabilization

        Padded handles on utensils for a more secure grip

        Wrist or hand splints with clamp to hold eating utensils

        Special drinking cup

        Rocker knife for cutting

    d. Assist with set-up if needed, opening containers, napkins, condiment packages; cutting meat; buttering bread.

    e. Arrange food so person has adequate amount of space to perform the task of eating.

4. Specific interventions for people with cognitive deficits

    a. Provide isolated, quiet atmosphere until person is able to attend to eating and is not easily distracted from the task.

    b. Supervise feeding program until there is no danger of choking or aspiration.

    c. Orient person to location and purpose of feeding equipment.

    d. Avoid external distractions and unnecessary conversation.

    e. Place person in the most normal eating position he is physically able to assume.

    f. Encourage person to attend to the task, but be alert for fatigue, frustration, or agitation.

    g. Provide one food at a time in usual sequence of eating until person is able to eat the entire meal in normal sequence.

    h. Encourage person to be tidy, to eat in small amounts, and to put food in unaffected side of mouth if paresis or paralysis is present.

    i. Check for food in cheeks.

    j. Refer to *Impaired Swallowing* for additional interventions.

5. For a person who is not eating because of fears of being poisoned:

    a. Allow person to open cans of foods.

    b. Serve food family style, so he can witness others eating.

C. Initiate health teaching and referrals, as indicated

1. Assess to ensure that both person and family understand the reason and purpose of all interventions.

2. Proceed with teaching as needed.

    a. Maintain safe-eating methods.

    b. Prevent aspiration.

    c. Use appropriate eating utensils (avoid sharp instruments).

    d. Test temperature of hot liquids and wear protective clothing (*e.g.*, paper bib).

    e. Teach use of adaptive devices.

Rationale

- Eating has physiologic, psychological, social, and cultural implications. Providing control over meals promotes overall well-being.

Bathing/Hygiene Self-Care Deficit

DEFINITION

Bathing/Hygiene Self-Care Deficit: A state in which the individual experiences an impaired ability to perform or complete bathing/hygiene activities for himself or herself.

DEFINING CHARACTERISTICS

Self-bathing deficits (including washing entire body, combing hair, brushing teeth, attending to skin and nail care, and applying makeup)

Unable or unwilling to wash body or body parts

Unable to obtain a water source

Unable to regulate temperature or water flow

Inability to perceive need for hygienic measures

RELATED FACTORS

See *Self-Care Deficit Syndrome*

Author's Note
See *Self-Care Deficit Syndrome*

Errors in Diagnostic Statements
See *Self-Care Deficit Syndrome*

Key Concepts
See *Self-Care Deficit Syndrome*

Focus Assessment Criteria

See *Self-Care Deficit Syndrome*

Outcome Criteria

The person will
- Perform bathing activity at expected optimal level *or*
- Report satisfaction with accomplishments despite limitations
- Relate feeling of comfort and satisfaction with body cleanliness
- Demonstrate ability to use adaptive devices
- Describe causative factors of bathing deficit

Interventions

A. Assess causative factors
  1. Visual deficits (blindness, field cuts, poor depth perception)
  2. Affected or missing limbs (casts, amputations, paresis, paralysis, arthritis)
  3. Cognitive deficits (aging, trauma, CVA)

B. Provide opportunities to relearn or adapt to activity
  1. General nursing interventions for inability to bathe
    a. Bathing time and routine should be consistent to encourage greatest amount of independence.
    b. Encourage person to wear prescribed corrective lenses or hearing aid.
    c. Keep bathroom temperature warm; ascertain individual's preferred water temperature.
    d. Provide for privacy during bathing routine.
    e. Keep environment simple and uncluttered.
    f. Observe skin condition during bathing.
    g. Provide all bathing equipment within easy reach.
    h. Provide for safety in the bathroom (nonslip mats, grab bars).
    i. When person is physically able, encourage use of either tub or shower stall, depending on which facility is at home (the person should practice in the hospital in preparation for going home).
    j. Provide for adaptive equipment as needed.
        Chair or stool in bathtub or shower
        Long-handled sponge to reach back or lower extremities
        Grab bars on bathroom walls where needed to assist in mobility
        Bath board for transferring to tub chair or stool
        Safety treads or nonslip mat on floor of bathroom, tub, and shower
        Washing mitts with pocket for soap
        Adapted toothbrushes
        Shaver holders
        Hand-held shower spray
    k. Provide for relief of pain that may affect ability to bathe self.*
  2. Specific interventions for bathing for people with visual deficits
    a. Place bathing equipment in location most suitable to individual.
    b. Avoid placing bathing equipment to blind side if person has a field cut and is not visually accommodated to surroundings.
    c. Keep call bell within reach if person is to bathe alone.
    d. Give the visually impaired individual the same degree of privacy and dignity as any other person.
    e. Verbally announce yourself before entering or leaving the bathing area.
    f. Observe the person's ability to locate all bathing utensils.
    g. Observe the person's ability to perform mouth care, hair combing, and shaving tasks.
    h. Provide place for clean clothing within easy reach.
  3. Specific interventions for bathing for people with affected or missing limbs
    a. Bathe early in morning or before bed at night to avoid unnecessary dressing and undressing.
    b. Encourage to use a mirror during bathing to inspect the skin of paralyzed areas.
    c. Encourage the person with amputation to inspect remaining foot or stump for good skin integrity.
    d. For limb amputations, bathe stump twice a day and be sure it is dry before wrapping it or applying prosthesis.
    e. Provide only the amount of supervision or assistance necessary for relearning the use of extremity or adaptation to the handicap.
    f. For lack of sensation, encourage use of the affected area in the bathing process (an individual tends to forget the existence of body parts in which there is no sensation).

* May require a primary care professional's order.

4. Specific interventions for bathing for people with cognitive deficits
    a. Provide a consistent time for the bathing routine as part of a structured program to help decrease confusion.
    b. Keep instructions simple and avoid distractions; orient to purpose of bathing equipment, put toothpaste on toothbrush.
    c. If person is unable to bathe the entire body, have him bathe one part until he does it correctly; give positive reinforcement for success.
    d. Supervise activity until person can safely perform the task unassisted.
    e. Encourage attention to the task, but be alert for fatigue that may increase confusion.
    f. Apply firm pressure to the skin when bathing; it is less likely to be misinterpreted than a gentle touch.
    g. Use a warm shower or bath to help a confused or agitated person to relax.

C. Initiate health teaching and referrals, as indicated
    1. Communicate to staff and family the person's ability and willingness to learn.
    2. Teach use of adaptive devices.
    3. Ascertain bathing facilities at home and assist in determining if there is any need to make adaptations; refer to occupational therapy or social service for help in obtaining needed home equipment.
    4. Teach to use tub or shower stall, depending on type of facility at home.
    5. If person is paralyzed, instruct him or his family to demonstrate complete skin check on key areas for redness (buttocks, bony prominences).
    6. Teach to maintain a safe bathing environment.

Rationale

- Inability to perform self-care produces feelings of dependency and poor self-concept. With increased ability for self-care, self-esteem increases (Tracey, 1992).

Dressing/Grooming Self-Care Deficit

DEFINITION

Dressing/Grooming Self-Care Deficit: A state in which the individual experiences an impaired ability to perform or complete dressing and grooming activities for himself or herself.

DEFINING CHARACTERISTICS

Self-dressing deficits (including donning regular or special clothing, not nightclothes)
    Impaired ability to put on or take off clothing
    Unable to fasten clothing
    Unable to groom self satisfactorily
    Unable to obtain or replace articles of clothing

RELATED FACTORS

See *Self-Care Deficit Syndrome*

Errors in Diagnostic Statements

See *Self-Care Deficit Syndrome*

Key Concepts

See *Self-Care Deficit Syndrome*

Focus Assessment Criteria

See *Self-Care Deficit Syndrome*

Outcome Criteria

The person will
- Demonstrate increased ability to dress self *or*
- Report the need for having someone else assist him in performing the task
- Demonstrate ability to learn how to use adaptive devices to facilitate optimal independence in the task of dressing
- Demonstrate increased interest in wearing street clothes
- Describe causative factors for dressing deficits
- Relate rationale and procedures for treatments

Interventions

A. Assess causative factors
   1. Visual deficits (blindness, field cuts, poor depth perception)
   2. Affected or missing limbs (casts, amputations, arthritis, paresis, paralysis)
   3. Cognitive deficits (aging, trauma, CVA)

B. Provide opportunities to relearn or adapt to activity
   1. General nursing interventions for self-dressing
      a. Encourage person to wear prescribed corrective lenses or hearing aid.
      b. Promote independence in dressing through continual and unaided practice.
      c. Choose clothing that is loose fitting, with wide sleeves and pant legs and front fasteners.
      d. Allow sufficient time for dressing and undressing because the task may be tiring, painful, or difficult.
      e. Plan for person to learn and demonstrate one part of an activity before progressing further.
      f. Lay clothes out in the order in which they will be needed to dress.
      g. Provide dressing aids as necessary (some commonly used aids include dressing stick, Swedish reacher, zipper pull, buttonhook, long-handled shoehorn, and shoe fasteners adapted with elastic laces, Velcro closures, or flip-back tongues; all garments with fasteners may be adapted with Velcro closures).
      h. Encourage person to wear ordinary or special clothing rather than nightclothes.

     i. Increase participation in dressing by medicating for pain 30 minutes before it is time to dress or undress, if indicated.*

     j. Provide for privacy during dressing routine.

     k. Provide for safety by ensuring easy access to all clothing and by ascertaining individual's performance level.

2. Specific interventions for dressing for people with visual deficits

     a. Allow person to ascertain the most convenient location for clothing and adapt the environment to accomplish the task best (*e.g.*, remove unnecessary barriers).

     b. Verbally announce yourself before entering or leaving the dressing area.

     c. If person has a field cut, avoid placing clothing to the blind side until he is visually accommodated to surroundings; then encourage him to turn head to scan entire visual field.

     d. Apply adaptive devices (*e.g.*, hand splints) before dressing activity.

     e. Consult or refer to physical or occupational therapy for teaching application of prosthetics to missing limbs.

3. Specific interventions for dressing for people with cognitive deficits (Beck, Heacock, Mercer, Walton, & Shook, 1991)

     a. Keep verbal communication simple.

         Ask yes/no questions.

         Use one-step requests (*e.g.*, "put your sock on").

         Praise after each step.

         Be specific and concise.

         Call by name.

         Use same word for same thing (*e.g.*, "shirt").

         Dress bottom half, then top half.

     b. Prepare an uncluttered environment.

         Ensure good lighting.

         Make bed, minimize visual clutter.

         Lay clothes face down.

         Place in order that they will be used.

         Allow resident a choice from only two pieces.

         Place matching clothes together on hangers.

         Remove dirty clothes from dressing area.

     c. Provide nonverbal cues.

         Hand one clothing item at a time in correct order.

         Place shoes beside correct foot.

         Use gestures to explain.

         Point or touch body part to be used.

         If person cannot complete all the steps, always allow him to finish the dressing step, if possible—zipper pants, buckle belt.

         Decrease assistance gradually.

C. Initiate health teaching and referrals, as indicated

1. Assess understanding and knowledge of individual and family for above instructions and rationale.

2. Proceed with teaching as needed.

     a. Communicate the individual's ability and willingness to learn to staff and family members.

     b. Teach use of adaptive devices and techniques that are specific to each disability.

     c. Teach to maintain a safe dressing environment.

     d. Attempt to be noncritical in correcting errors.

---

* May require a primary care professional's order.

Rationale

- Optimal personal grooming promotes psychological well-being (Tracey, 1992).

Toileting Self-Care Deficit

DEFINITION

Toileting Self-Care Deficit: A state in which the individual experiences an impaired ability to perform or complete toileting activities for himself or herself.

DEFINING CHARACTERISTICS

Unable or unwilling to get to toilet or commode
Unable or unwilling to carry out proper hygiene
Unable to transfer to and from toilet or commode
Unable to handle clothing to accommodate toileting
Unable to flush toilet or empty commode

RELATED FACTORS

See *Self-Care Deficit Syndrome*

Author's Note

See *Self-Care Deficit Syndrome*

Errors in Diagnostic Statements

See *Self-Care Deficit Syndrome*

Key Concepts

See *Self-Care Deficit Syndrome*

Focus Assessment Criteria

See *Self-Care Deficit Syndrome*

Outcome Criteria

The person will
- Demonstrate increased ability to toilet self *or*
- Report that he is unable to toilet self
- Demonstrate ability to make use of adaptive devices to facilitate toileting
- Describe causative factors for toileting deficit
- Relate rationale and procedures for treatment

Interventions

A. Assess causative factors

    1. Visual deficits (blindness, field cuts, poor depth perception)

    2. Affected or missing limbs (casts, amputations, paresis, paralysis)

    3. Cognitive deficits (aging, trauma, CVA)

B. Provide opportunities to relearn or adapt to activity

    1. Common nursing interventions for toileting difficulties

        a. Encourage to wear prescribed corrective lenses or hearing aid.

        b. Obtain bladder and bowel history from individual or significant other (see *Altered Bowel Elimination* or *Altered Patterns of Urinary Elimination*).

        c. Ascertain communication system person uses to express the need to toilet.

        d. Maintain bladder and bowel record to determine toileting patterns.

        e. Provide for adequate fluid intake and balanced diet to promote adequate urinary output and normal bowel evacuation.

        f. Promote normal elimination by encouraging activity and exercise within the person's capabilities.

        g. Avoid development of "bowel fixation" by less frequent discussion and inquiries about bowel movements.

        h. Be alert to possibility of falls when toileting person (be prepared to ease him to floor without causing injury to either of you).

        i. Achieve independence in toileting by continual and unaided practice.

        j. Allow sufficient time for the task of toileting to avoid fatigue (lack of sufficient time to toilet may cause incontinence or constipation).

        k. Avoid use of indwelling catheters and condom catheters to expedite bladder continence (if possible).

    2. Specific interventions for toileting for people with visual deficits

        a. Keep call bell easily accessible so person can quickly obtain help to toilet; answer call bell promptly to decrease anxiety.

        b. If bedpan or urinal is necessary for toileting, be sure it is within person's reach.

        c. Avoid placing toileting equipment to the blind side of an individual with field cut (when he is visually accommodated to surroundings, you may suggest he search entire visual field for equipment).

        d. Verbally announce yourself before entering or leaving toileting area.

        e. Observe person's ability to obtain equipment or get to the toilet unassisted.

        f. Provide for a safe and clear pathway to toilet area.

    3. Specific interventions for toileting for people with affected or missing limbs

        a. Provide only the amount of supervision and assistance necessary for relearning or adapting to the prosthesis.

        b. Encourage person to look at affected area or limb and use it during toileting tasks.

        c. Encourage useful transfer techniques taught by occupational or physical therapy (the nurse should familiarize herself with planned mode of transfer).

        d. Provide the necessary adaptive devices to enhance the maximum amount of independence and safety (commode chairs, spill-proof urinals, fracture bedpans, raised toilet seats, support side rails for toilets).

        e. Provide for a safe and clear pathway to toilet area.

    4. Specific interventions for toileting for people with cognitive deficits

        a. Offer toileting reminders every 2 hours, after meals, and before bedtime.

        b. When person is able to indicate the need to toilet, begin toileting at 2-hour intervals, after meals, and before bedtime.

        c. Answer call bell immediately to avoid frustration and failure to be continent.

        d. Encourage wearing ordinary clothes (many confused individuals are continent while wearing regular clothing).

    e. Avoid the use of bedpans and urinals; if physically possible, provide a normal atmosphere of elimination in bathroom (the toilet used should remain constant to promote familiarity).

    f. Give verbal cues as to what is expected of the individual, and give positive reinforcement for success.

    g. Work to achieve daytime continence before expecting nighttime continence (nighttime incontinence may continue after daytime continence has returned).

    h. See *Altered Patterns of Urinary Elimination* for additional information on incontinence.

C. Initiate health teaching and referrals, as indicated

    1. Assess the understanding and knowledge of the individual and significant others of foregoing interventions and rationale.

      a. Communicate person's ability and willingness to learn to staff and family.

      b. Maintain a safe toileting environment.

      c. Reinforce knowledge of transferring techniques.

      d. Teach use of adaptive devices.

      e. Ascertain home toileting needs and refer to occupational therapy or social services for help in obtaining necessary equipment.

Rationale

- Inability to perform self-care produces feelings of dependency and poor self-concept. With increased self-care ability, self-esteem increases (Tracey, 1992).
- The client's maximum involvement in toileting activities can reduce the embarrassment associated with assistance with toileting (Tracey, 1992).

Instrumental Self-Care Deficit

DEFINITION

Instrumental Self-Care Deficit: A state in which the individual experiences an impaired ability to perform certain activities or access certain services essential for managing a household.

DEFINING CHARACTERISTICS

Observed or reported difficulty in one or more of the following:

Using a telephone
Accessing transportation
Laundering, ironing
Preparing meals
Shopping (food, clothes)
Managing money
Medication administration

RELATED FACTORS

See *Self-Care Deficit Syndrome*

Author's Note

Instrumental Self-Care Deficit is not currently on the NANDA list, but has been added here for clarity and usefulness. This diagnosis describes problems in performing certain activities or accessing certain services needed to live in the community (*e.g.*, phone use, shopping, money management). This diagnosis is important to consider in discharge planning and during home visits by community nurses.

Errors in Diagnostic Statements

Instrumental Self-Care Deficit related to possible inability to plan meals and manage laundry

When a nurse suspects that a client or family may have compromised ability to engage in certain activities needed to live in and run a household, the nurse should label the diagnosis *Possible Instrumental Self-Care Deficit* and add related factors representing why the nurse suspects the diagnosis (*e.g., related to difficulty remembering routine tasks* or *related to poor planning skills*). The nurse detecting evidence of memory or judgment difficulties could interpret this as a risk factor for *Risk for Instrumental Self-Care Deficit*.

Key Concepts

1. Brody (1985) identified that to live in the community an individual not only had to perform or have assistance with six ADLs, but also had to perform or have assistance with additional activities.
2. Instrumental ADLs include housekeeping, food preparation and procurement, shopping, laundry, ability to self-medicate safely, ability to manage money, and access to transportation (Miller, 1995).
3. Instrumental ADLs are more complex tasks than ADLs.
4. Maintaining people in the community, rather than in nursing homes, has significant financial benefit. In 1981, 25% of all health care expenditures for older adults in the United States went to nursing homes, but only 5% of the elderly population were receiving care in these facilities. Medicaid covers about 90% of public spending for nursing home care (Miller, 1995).
5. Maintaining people in the community, rather than in a nursing home, also maintains autonomy, strengthens family life, and affirms the value of older adults in our society.

Focus Assessment Criteria

See *Self-Care Deficit Syndrome*

Outcome Criteria

The person/family will
- Demonstrate use of adaptive devices (*e.g.*, phone, cooking aids)
- Describe a method to ensure adherence to medication schedule
- Report ability to call on and answer telephone
- Report regular laundering by self or others
- Report daily intake of two nutritious meals
- Identify transportation options to stores, physician, house of worship, social activities
- Demonstrate management of simple money transactions
- Identify individuals who will assist with money matters

Interventions

A. Assess for causative and contributing factors

1. Visual, hearing deficits
2. Impaired cognition
3. Impaired mobility
4. Lack of knowledge
5. Inadequate social support

B. Assist to identify self-help devices

1. Grooming–dressing aids (see *Impaired Physical Mobility*)
2. Kitchen/eating aids
    a. One-side built-up dishes
    b. Built-up handles on cutlery (use plastic foam curlers)
    c. Bulldog clip to secure a straw in glass
    d. Built-up corner of cutlery board to hold and anchor food or pot (*e.g.*, to butter toast, mash potatoes)
    e. Mounted jar opener
    f. Nonslip material applied under dishes (same strips used to prevent slipping in bath tub)
    g. Two-sided suction holder to hold dishes in place
3. Communication/security
    a. Motion-activated lights near walkway/entrance
    b. Night-light for path to bathroom
    c. Light next to bed
    d. Specially adapted phones (amplified, big buttons)

C. Promote self-care and safety for person with cognitive deficit

1. Evaluate activities that are achievable.
2. Teach safety techniques.
    a. Turn lights on before dark.
    b. Use night-lights.
    c. Keep environment simple, uncluttered.
    d. Use clocks, calenders as cues.
    e. Mark on calender (using picture symbols) reminders for shopping, laundry, cleaning, doctor's appointments, and the like.
3. For laundry, teach to:
    a. Separate dark and light clothes.
    b. Use pictures to illustrate steps for washing clothes.
    c. Mark cup with line to indicate amount of soap needed.
    d. Minimize ironing.
    e. Use an iron with automatic shutoff mechanism.
4. Evaluate ability to procure, select, and prepare nutritious food daily.
    a. Prepare a permanent shopping list with cues for essential foods, products.
    b. Teach to review list before shopping and check items needed, and in the store, check off items selected. (Use a pencil that can be erased to reuse list.)
    c. Teach how to shop for single-person meals (refer to *Altered Nutrition* for specific techniques).
    d. If possible, teach to use a microwave to reduce the risk of heat-related injuries or accidents.
5. Teach hints to improve adherence to medication schedule.
    a. Have someone place medications in a commercial pill holder divided into 7 days.
    b. Take out exact amount of pills for the day. Divide them in small cups, each labeled with time of day.
    c. If needed, draw a picture of the pills and the quantity on each cup.
    d. Teach to take pills from cup to a small plastic bag when planning to be away from home.
6. Teach who to call for instructions if a dose is missed.

D. Determine available sources of transportation
   1. Neighbors, relatives
   2. Community center
   3. Church group
   4. Social service agency

E. Determine available sources of social support
   1. Discuss the possibility of bartering for services (*e.g.*, wash neighbor's clothes in exchange for shopping help).
   2. Identify a person who can provide immediate help (*e.g.*, neighbor, friend, hot line).
   3. Identify sources for help with laundry, shopping, money matters.

F. Initiate health teaching and referrals, as indicated
   1. Discuss the importance of identifying the need for assistance.
   2. Refer to community agencies for assistance (*e.g.*, Department of Social Services, area agency on aging, senior neighbors, public health nursing).

Rationale

- Interventions are focused to assist the person and family in maintaining as much functional independence as possible (Miller, 1995).
- Community resources can assist the person when caregivers are unavailable (Miller 1995).

References/Bibliography

Andrews, M., & Boyle, J. (1995). *Transcultural concepts in nursing care* (2nd ed.). Philadelphia: J. B. Lippincott.

Beck, C., Heacock, P., Mercer, S., Walton, C., & Shook, J. (1991). Dressing for success. *Journal of Psychosocial Nursing, 29*(7), 30–35.

Brody, E. (1985). Parent care as a normative family stress. *The Gerontologist, 25*(1), 19–29.

Carpenito, L. J. (1983). *Nursing diagnosis: Application to clinical practice*. Philadelphia: J. B. Lippincott.

Gordon, M. (1982). *Manual of nursing diagnosis*. New York: McGraw-Hill.

Lubkin, I. M. (1995). *Chronic illness: Impact and interventions* (3rd ed.). Boston: Jones & Bartlett.

Miller, C. A. (1995). *Nursing care of older adults* (2nd ed.). Glenview, IL: Scott, Foresman.

Palmer, M., & Tonis, J. (1980). *Manual for functional training*. Philadelphia: F. A. Davis.

Townsend, M. (1994). *Nursing diagnoses in psychiatric nursing* (3rd ed.). Philadelphia: F. A. Davis.

Tracey, C. (1992). Hygiene assistance. In G. Bulechek & J. McCloskey (Eds.). *Nursing interventions: Essential nursing treatments*. Philadelphia: W. B. Saunders.

U. S. Department of Health and Human Services. (1987, October). *Current estimates from the National Health Interview Survey, United States, 1986*. Hyattsville, MD: Author.

Wong, D. L. (1995). *Nursing care of infants and children* (5th ed.). St. Louis: Mosby–Year Book.

Self-Concept Disturbance*

Body Image Disturbance

Personal Identity Disturbance

Self-Esteem Disturbance

Chronic Low Self-Esteem

Situational Low Self-Esteem

Self-Concept Disturbance

DEFINITION

Self-Concept Disturbance: The state in which the individual experiences or is at risk of experiencing a negative state of change about the way he feels, thinks, or views himself. It may include a change in body image, self-ideal, self-esteem, role performance, or personal identity.

DEFINING CHARACTERISTICS

Because a self-concept disturbance may include a change in any one or combination of its five component parts (body image, self-ideal, self-esteem, role performance, personal identity), and because the nature of the change causing the alteration can be so varied, there is no "typical" response to this diagnosis. Reactions may include:

Refusal to touch or look at a body part
Refusal to look into a mirror
Unwillingness to discuss a limitation, deformity, or disfigurement
Refusal to accept rehabilitation efforts
Inappropriate attempts to direct own treatment
Denial of the existence of a deformity or disfigurement
Increasing dependence on others
Signs of grieving: weeping, despair, anger
Refusal to participate in own care or take responsibility for self-care (self-neglect)
Self-destructive behavior (alcohol, drug abuse)
Displaying hostility toward the healthy
Withdrawal from social contacts
Changing usual patterns of responsibility
Showing change in ability to estimate relation of body to environment

*This diagnosis is not currently on the NANDA list but has been included for clarity or usefulness.

RELATED FACTORS

A self-concept disturbance can occur as a response to a variety of health problems, situations, and conflicts. Some common sources follow.

Pathophysiologic

Related to change in appearance, life-style, role, response of others secondary to:

Chronic disease   Severe trauma

Loss of body parts   Pain

Loss of body functions

Situational (Personal, Environmental)

Related to feelings of abandonment or failure secondary to:

Divorce, separation from, or death of a significant other

Loss of job or ability to work

Related to immobility or loss of function

Related to unsatisfactory relationships (parental, spousal)

Maturational

Middle age

Loss of role and responsibilities

Older adult

Loss of role and responsibilities

Author's Note

Self-concept reflects self-view, encompassing body image, esteem, role performance, and personal identity. In constant evolution and change, self-concept is influenced by interactions with the environment and other people, and by the person's perceptions of how others view him or her.

Self-Concept Disturbance represents a broad diagnostic category under which fall more specific nursing diagnoses. Initially, the nurse may not have sufficient clinical data to validate a more specific diagnosis, such as *Chronic Low Self-Esteem* or *Body Image Disturbance*; thus, *Self-Concept Disturbance* can be used until data can support a more specific diagnosis.

Self-esteem is one of the four components of Self-concept. *Self-Esteem Disturbance* is the general diagnostic category. *Chronic Low Self-Esteem* and *Situational Low Self-Esteem* represent specific types of *Self-Esteem Disturbances*, and thus involve more specific interventions. Initially, the nurse may not have sufficient clinical data to validate a more specific diagnosis, such as *Chronic Low Self-Esteem* or *Situational Low Self-Esteem*. Refer to the major defining characteristics under these categories for validation.

Situational Low Self-Esteem is an episodic event; repeated occurrence and/or the continuation of negative self-appraisals over time can lead to *Chronic Low Self-Esteem* (Willard, personal communication, 1990).

Errors in Diagnostic Statements

Self-Concept Disturbance related to substance abuse

Although a relation exists between negative self-concept and alcohol and/or drug abuse, listing substance abuse as a related factor does not describe the nursing focus. If the person acknowledged a substance abuse problem and expressed a desire for assistance, the diagnosis *Ineffective Individual Coping related to inability to constructively manage stressors without alcohol or drugs* could be appropriate. If the person denied a problem, the diagnosis *Ineffective Denial related to lack of acknowledgment of substance abuse/dependency* would apply—if the nurse will be addressing the denial. A nurse with data that suggest or confirm *Self-Concept Disturbance* should explore contributing factors (*e.g.,* guilt influenced by social stigma). The nurse can use "unknown etiology" until focus assessment identifies contributing factors.

Body Image Disturbance related to mastectomy

Mastectomy can produce various responses, including grief, anger, and negative feelings about self. A woman undergoing breast surgery for cancer is at high risk for both *Body Image Disturbance* and *Self-Esteem Disturbance*. Thus, the diagnosis *Risk for Self-Concept Disturbance related to perceived negative effects of changed appearance and diagnosis of cancer* would be most appropriate. A nurse with data to support *Self-Concept Disturbance* should record it as an actual diagnosis with these same related factors and including "as evidenced by" to specify signs and symptoms of or manifestations (*e.g., Self-Concept Disturbance related to perceived negative effects of changed appearance and diagnosis of cancer, as evidenced by reports of negative feelings about "new self" and determination not to let husband see her*).

Key Concepts

1. Both the client and the nurse have their own personal self-concept. To deal effectively with others, the nurse must be aware of her own behavior, feelings, attitudes, and responses.
2. Self-concept involves a person's feelings, attitudes, and values and affects his reactions to all experiences.
3. A person's self-concept evolves from infancy through old age. With aging, new skills and challenges emerge. Successful completion of developmental tasks contributes to a positive self-concept (Fuller & Schaller-Ayers, 1990).
4. A person's self-concept is influenced by interactions with others, the sociocultural milieu, and developmental task completion (Fuller & Schaller-Ayers, 1990).
5. The concept of self includes components of body image, self-ideal, self-esteem, role performance, and personal identity (Stuart & Sundeen, 1995).
   Body image: The sum of the conscious and unconscious attitudes the individual has toward his body. It includes present and past perceptions (see no. 6 for expansion).
   Self-ideal: The individual's perception of how he should behave based on certain personal standards, aspirations, goals, or values.
   Self-esteem: The individual's personal judgment of his own worth obtained by analyzing how well his behavior conforms to his self-ideal. High self-esteem is a feeling rooted in unconditional acceptance of self, despite mistakes, defeats, and failures, as an innately worthy and important being.
   Role performance: Sets of socially expected behavior patterns associated with an individual's function in various social groups. Ascribed roles are assigned roles over which the person has no choice. Assumed roles are those selected or chosen by the individual.
   Personal identity: The organizing principle of the personality that accounts for the unity, continuity, consistency, and uniqueness of the individual. It connotes autonomy and includes self-perceptions of sexuality. Identity formation begins in infancy and proceeds throughout life, but is the major task of the adolescent period.
6. Body image consists of three components: body reality, body ideal, and body presentation (Price, 1990).
   Body reality: The body as it really exists, constrained by the effects of human genetics and the wear and tear of life in the external environment (as it might be described in a formal physician's examination). It changes both as a result of the aging process and because we use and abuse it. Abrupt changes in body reality are associated with trauma, malignancy, infection, and malnutrition. Body reality is at once a part of the environment and the frequent point of contact between body image threat and body image change.
   Body ideal: This is the picture in our heads of how we should like the body to look and to perform. Body ideal includes norms of body contour, body space, and boundaries. It is profoundly influenced by societal and cultural norms, by advertising,

and by the changing attitudes toward fitness and health. Body ideal is threatened by changes in body reality, but disorders of body ideal (*e.g.*, anorexia nervosa) may also directly affect the equilibrium.

Body presentation: Body reality only rarely meets our body ideal standards, and in the effort to make these two balance, body presentation is used. This is how the body is literally presented to the outside environment, the way we dress, groom, walk, talk, pose our limbs, and use props such as walking sticks or hearing aids. Fashion (working through body ideal) may drastically affect the way in which body presentation changes. Equally, paralysis or loss of limb (body reality) also affects facility in body presentation. Much of the presentation is for public consumption, laden with symbolic value.

7. Disturbances in the components of self-concept are described as follows:

Body image: Viewing oneself differently as a result of actual or perceived changes in body structure or function

Self-ideal: A change in self-expectations/striving

Self-esteem: Lack of confidence in ability to accomplish that which is desired

Role performance: Inability to perform those functions and activities expected of a particular role in a given society

Personal identity: Disturbance in perception of self ("Who am I?")

8. Intrusive procedures can threaten an individual's sense of wholeness. The nurse should provide a great deal of emotional support during procedures that increase a person's sense of vulnerability.

9. Body image changes constantly. There is often a time lag between the actual body change and the change in body image. The nurse must be aware that during this lag the individual may reject both the diagnosis and the education and treatment prescribed.

10. Body image is influenced during pregnancy in relation to biologic, psychological, and role changes.

Loss of Body Part/Function

1. Individuals have a concept of self that includes feelings about self, worth, attractiveness, lovableness, and capabilities (Peretz, 1970). One's mental image of one's own body and person is assaulted after a physical injury. This injury or loss involves the grieving process.

2. The grieving process in response to a recent disability has been described as (Friedman-Campbell & Hart, 1984):

    a. Shock–denial

    Denies injury or severity of the injury

    Minimally allows self to think of loss to protect self

    Intellectually accepts the loss but denies it emotionally

    b. Developing awareness

    Realizes the impact of the loss on self

    Experiences acute somatic feelings of loss

    Displaces anger

    Is preoccupied with guilt and blaming

    Mourns the loss and withdraws

    Shuns change and clings to routines

    c. Managing loss of body function

    Begins to deal with the impact of the loss on self

    Frees self slowly from the bondage of the loss

    Readjusts to changed environment

    Invests in new relationships

3. Physically disabled people are faced with many challenges that require adjustments and change. Everyday stressors challenge the physically disabled more profoundly (*e.g.*, food preparation, time management) (Swanson, Cronin-Stubbs, & Sheldon, 1989).

Self-Esteem

1. Self-esteem evolves from a comparison between the self-concept and self-ideal. The greater the congruency, the higher the self-esteem (Stuart & Sundeen, 1995).
2. Self-esteem derives from the person's own perceptions of competency and efficacy and from appraisals of others. In general, people hold positive self-enhancing beliefs about themselves, the world, and the future. These biased perceptions are considerably more positive than objective evidence indicates (Taylor, 1989).
3. High self-esteem is rooted in unconditional self-acceptance as an innately worthy person (Stuart & Sundeen, 1995). Such people tend to attribute failures or threatening events to external causes beyond their control—unlike people with low self-esteem, who tend to attribute failure or threatening events to internal causes (Tenner & Herzberger, 1987).
4. Low self-esteem may be an indicator of susceptibility to depression. Low self-esteem can be a trait in some individuals that is stable over time. For others it can be initiated by a broad range of stressful situations (Tenner & Herzberger, 1987).
5. As self-esteem declines, so does a person's belief that he can exert control over his environment. Likewise, as personal control is perceived to decrease, so does self-esteem (Taft, 1985). Attributing failure to a lack of ability (internal cause) leads to decreased expectations and motivation (Antaki & Bruoin, 1982).
6. In response to a threat to a person's self-concept, self-esteem is protected through three cognitive processes:
   a. Searching for meaning in the experience
   b. Regaining mastery over the event; exerting personal control
   c. Self-enhancement ("How am I managing as compared with others?") (Taylor, 1989).
7. The following behaviors are associated with low self-esteem: rigidity; procrastination; repetitive, unnecessary apologies; minimizing one's abilities; emphasizing deficits; expecting failure; self-destructive behaviors; approval-seeking behavior; inability to accept compliments; disregard for one's own opinions; difficulty in forming close relationships; and inability to say "no" when appropriate (Miller, 1995).

🌀 *Key Concepts—Child*

1. Self-concept is learned. A child's concept of self, for example, emerges as a result of changes occurring during earlier developmental stages (Whiting, 1986).
2. To develop and maintain self-esteem, a child needs to feel worthwhile, different in some way, and superior to and more lovable than any other child (Wong, 1995).
3. Self-esteem increases as a child develops meaningful relationships and masters developmental tasks. Early adolescence is a time of risk to self-esteem as the adolescent strives to define an identity and sense of self within a peer group (Stuart & Sundeen, 1995).
4. A child's development of body image is based on his own body, which is influenced by present and past perceptions of his body, physiologic functioning, developmental maturation, and the response of others to him (Stuart & Sundeen, 1995).
5. Adolescence is probably the critical period of development for body image formation, as pubertal changes force alteration of the adolescent's body image (Stuart & Sundeen, 1995).
6. The development of a positive body image by age is charted below (Drapo, 1986):

Age	Developmental Task
Birth–1 year	Learns to tolerate small frustrations
	Learns to trust
1–3 years	Learns to like body
	Learns mastery of
	Motor skills
	Language skills
	Bowel training
3–6 years	Learns initiative
	Learns sex typing
	Identifies with parent models
	Increases skills (motor, language)

6–12 years	Develops a sense of industry
	Has a clear sex role identification
	Learns peer interaction
	Develops academic skills
Adolescence	Establishes self-identity and sexual role
	Uses abstract thought
	Develops personal value system

7. A child learns to see himself in the way he is seen by his parents and or significant others (Stuart & Sundeen, 1995).
8. To develop a healthy personality, a child needs a positive and accurate body image, realistic self-ideal, positive self-concept, and high self-esteem (Stuart & Sundeen, 1995).
9. Experiences with and restrictions imposed by chronic illness or disability may interfere with development of healthy self-esteem (Scipien, Chard, Howe, & Barnard, 1990).
10. Obese children and adolescents are at particular risk for developing body image or self-esteem disturbance (Wong, 1995).
11. Negative self-concepts have been associated with self-destructive health behaviors in children and adolescents, such as overeating, alcoholism, smoking, and drug abuse (Winkelstein, 1989).
12. Mastery describes positive coping with stress. Successful coping enhances self-esteem (Johnson, 1993).

Key Concepts—Older Adult

1. According to Miller (1995), self-esteem is "one of the characteristics most highly associated with both depression and happiness" in older adults.
2. Self-esteem depends on interactions with others and on others' opinions. In Western societies, a generally negative view of aging can contribute to an older adult's decreased self-esteem.
3. Many variables interact to produce a decline in self-esteem in older adults, including negative societal attitudes, decreased social interactions, and decreased power and control over the environment (Taft, 1985).
4. Meisenhelder (1985) reported that the following people exert the most significant influence on self-esteem in older adults: spouse, peers (most important for men), authority figures (most important for women), people they live with, and people in the immediate social, work, and church environments.
5. Environmental factors in long-term care facilities that can influence self-esteem of elderly residents include decor, social roles, choices available, architectural design, space, and privacy (Miller, 1995).
6. Older adults with poor health, high degree of disability, and daily pain report the lowest self-esteem (Hunter, Linn, & Harris, 1981–82).

TRANSCULTURAL CONSIDERATIONS

1. In the Latin culture, the man is the head of the household and has authority over his family. The man must provide for and protect his family. Self-image and family image are intertwined. Anything that challenges the ability of a man to provide for his family challenges his very core or self-concept (Andrews & Boyle, 1995).

Focus Assessment Criteria

Self-Concept Disturbance is manifested in a variety of ways. An individual may respond with an alteration in another life process (see *Spiritual Distress, Fear, Ineffective Individual Coping*). The nurse should be aware of this and use the assessment data to ascertain the dimensions affected.

It may be difficult for the nurse to identify the cues and make the inferences necessary to diagnose a self-concept disturbance. Each individual reacts differently to loss, pain, disability, and disfigurement. Therefore, the nurse should determine an individual's usual reactions to problems and feelings about himself before attempting to diagnose a change.

Subjective Data

A. Assess for defining characteristics
   1. Self views
      "Describe yourself."
      "What do you like most/least about yourself?"
      "What do others like?"
      "What do you/others want to change about you?"
      "What do you enjoy?"
      "Has being ill affected how you see yourself?"
   2. Identity
      "What personal achievements have given you satisfaction?"
      "What are your future plans?"
   3. Role responsibilities
      "What do you do for a living? Job responsibilities? Home responsibilities?"
      "Are these satisfying?"
      If the person has had a role change, how has it affected life-style and relationships?
   4. Somatic problems
      "Do you feel fearful, anxious, or nervous?"
      "Ever feel like you are falling apart? Dizziness? Aches and pains? Shortness of breath? Palpitations? Urinary frequency? Nausea/vomiting? Sleep problems? Fatigue? Loss of sexual interest?"
   5. Affect and mood
      "How do you feel now?"
      "How would you describe your usual mood?"
      "What things make you happy/upset?"
      "Have you ever thought of harming yourself?"
   6. Body image
      "What do you like most/least about your body?"
      "What parts are most important to you?"
      "Before you were sick, how did you feel about people who were sick or disabled?"
      "What do you understand to be your health problem?"
      "What limitations do you think will result?"
      "How do you feel about this illness/disability?"
      "Has it changed the way you feel about yourself or the way others respond to you?"
      Children may be able to draw self-portraits.

B. Assess for related factors
   1. Stress management
      "How do you manage stress?"
      "To whom do you go for help with a problem?"
      Substance abuse?
      Exercise
      Religious convictions
      Problem-solving approach
   2. Support system
      "Any problems in current relationships?"
      "How does your family feel about your illness?" "Do they understand?"
      "Does your family regularly discuss problems?"
      "What other supports do you have? Church? Friends?"

Objective Data

A. Assess for defining characteristics

1. General appearance
    Facial expression
    Affect
    Hygiene (cleanliness)
    Grooming (clothes, hair, makeup; do these reflect modern trends?)
    Dress (condition, appropriateness)
    Body posture/language (eye contact, head and shoulder flexion, gait/stride)

2. Thought processes/content

Orientation	Suspicious
Feelings of depersonalization	Homicidal/suicidal ideation
Rambling	Sexual preoccupation

    Delusions (grandeur, persecution, reference, influence, or bodily sensations)
    Difficulty concentrating
    Slowed thought processes
    Poor memory or may even be missing large portions of personal history
    Impaired judgment
    Anxiety

3. Behavior

Irritability	Hyperactivity
Aggressiveness	Delinquency

    School problems (truancy, low/drop in grades)
    Problems on job (lateness, decreased productivity, accident prone, burnout symptoms)
    Social withdrawal
    Ability for self-care
    Sexual behavior (increase, decrease, promiscuity)

4. Communication patterns
    With significant others

Relates well	Dependent
Hostile	Demanding

    Physical impairment to communication (*e.g.*, deafness, aphasia, trach)
    Cultural variations in communication (*e.g.*, use of gestures, touch)

5. Decision-making ability
    Indecisive
    Procrastination

6. Nutritional status
    Appetite
    Eating patterns
    Weight (gain/loss)

7. Rest–sleep pattern
    Recent change
    Early wakefulness
    Insomnia

Outcome Criteria

The person will
- Appraise self-situations in a realistic manner without distortions
- Verbalize and demonstrate increased positive feelings
- Demonstrate healthy adaptation, coping skills

Interventions

Nursing interventions for the variety of problems that might be associated with a diagnosis of *Self-Concept Disturbance* are very similar.

A. Contact the client frequently and treat him with warm, positive regard

B. Encourage the client to express feelings and thoughts about the following
   1. Condition
   2. Progress
   3. Prognosis
   4. Effects on life-style
   5. Support system
   6. Treatment

C. Provide reliable information and clarify any misconceptions

D. Help the client to identify positive attributes and possible new opportunities

E. Assist with hygiene and grooming, as needed

F. Encourage visitors

G. Help the client identify strategies to increase independence and maintain role responsibilities
   1. Prioritizing activities
   2. Using mobility aids and assistive devices, as needed

H. Discuss with client's support system the importance of communicating the client's value and importance to them

I. Assess for signs and symptoms. Use the Focus Assessment Criteria to isolate signs and symptoms. Refer to the Defining Characteristics of *Self-Esteem Disturbance, Body Image Disturbance*, and *Altered Role Performance*. After confirmation, use Interventions under the diagnosis

J. Initiate health teaching, as indicated
   1. Teach person what community resources are available, if needed (*e.g.*, mental health centers, such self-help groups as Reach for Recovery, Make Today Count).
   2. Refer to specific health teaching issues under *Body Image Disturbance, Self-Esteem Disturbance* (*Chronic* and *Situational*).

Rationale

- Frequent contact by the caregiver indicates acceptance and may facilitate trust. The client may be hesitant to approach the staff because of negative self-concept (Dudas, 1993).
- Encouraging the client to share feelings can provide a safe outlet for fears and frustrations and can increase self-awareness (Dudas, 1993).
- Misconceptions can needlessly increase anxiety and damage self-concept.
- The client may tend to focus only on the change in self-image and not on the positive characteristics that contribute to the whole concept of self. The nurse must reinforce these positive aspects and encourage the client to reincorporate them into his new self-concept (Dudas, 1993).
- Participation in self-care and planning can aid positive coping.
- Frequent visits by support people can help the client feel that he is still a worthwhile, acceptable person, which should promote a positive self-concept.

- A strong component of self-concept is the ability to perform functions expected of one's role, thus decreasing dependency and reducing the need for others' involvement.
- Communication of client's values enhances self-esteem and promotes adjustment (Dudas, 1993).
- Optimism enhances social relationships and enables a person to make more effective use of social supports to maintain self-esteem. Supportive friends and family can bolster self-esteem by reinforcing a sense of personal control through suggestions and resources and a sense of confidence (Taylor, 1989).

🌸 Interventions—*Child Focus*

1. Allow the child to bring his or her own experiences into the situation (Johnson, 1995) (*e.g.*, "Some children say that an injection feels like a insect sting; some say they don't feel anything. After we do this, you can tell me how it feels.").
2. Avoid using "good" or "bad" to describe behavior. Be specific and descriptive (*e.g.*, "You really helped me by holding still, thank you for helping.") (Johnson, 1995).
3. Connect a previous experiences with the present one (*e.g.*, "The x-ray camera will look different from the last time. You will have to hold real still again. The table will move, too.") (Johnson, 1995).
4. Convey optimism with positive self-talk (*e.g.*, "I am so busy today. I wonder if I will get all my work done? I bet I can"; or, "When you come back from surgery you will need to stay in bed. What would you like to do when you come back?").
5. Help the child plan playtime with choices. Encourage crafts that produce an end product.
6. Encourage interactions with peers and supportive adults.
7. Encourage to decorate room with crafts and personal items.

Rationale

- It is more helpful to be specific and descriptive when praising a child, rather than describing behavior as "good" or "bad" (Johnson, 1995).
- Allowing the child to describe their experience supports that the child is unique (Johnson, 1995).
- The nurse can provide information that helps the child make sense of the situation by linking the present or future experience to past experience (Johnson, 1995).
- Positive self-talk denotes optimism to the child (Johnson, 1995).
- Allowing the child choices and productive play can enhance self-concept.

Body Image Disturbance

DEFINITION

Body Image Disturbance: The state in which an individual experiences or is at risk to experience a disruption in the way he perceives his body image.

DEFINING CHARACTERISTICS
Major (Must Be Present)

Verbal or nonverbal negative response to actual or perceived change in structure and/or function (*i.e.*, shame, embarrassment, guilt, revulsion)

Minor (May Be Present)

Not looking at body part
Not touching body part
Hiding or overexposing body part
Change in social involvement
Negative feelings about body; feelings of helplessness, hopelessness, powerlessness, vulnerability
Preoccupation with change or loss
Refusal to verify actual change
Depersonalization of part or loss
Self-destructive behaviors (*i.e.*, mutilation, suicide attempts, overeating/undereating)

RELATED FACTORS
Pathophysiologic

Related to changes in appearance secondary to
Chronic disease
Loss of body part
Loss of body function
Severe trauma
Related to unrealistic perceptions of appearance secondary to
Psychoses
Anorexia nervosa
Bulimia

Treatment-Related

Related to changes in appearance secondary to
Hospitalization
Surgery
Chemotherapy
Radiation

Situational (Personal, Environmental)

Related to physical trauma secondary to
Sexual abuse
Rape (perpetrator known or unknown)
Assault
Related to effects of (specify) on appearance
Obesity   Immobility
Pregnancy

Author's Note

See *Self-Concept Disturbance*

Errors in Diagnostic Statements

See *Self-Concept Disturbance*

Key Concepts

See *Self-Concept Disturbance*

Focus Assessment Criteria

See *Self-Concept Disturbance*

Outcome Criteria

The person will
- Implement new coping patterns
- Verbalize and demonstrate acceptance of appearance (grooming, dress, posture, eating patterns, presentation of self)
- Demonstrate a willingness and ability to resume self-care/role responsibilities
- Initiate new or reestablish contacts with existing support systems

Interventions

A. Establish a trusting nurse–client relationship
1. Encourage person to express his feelings, especially about the way he feels, thinks, or views himself.
2. Acknowledge person's feelings of hostility, grief, fear, and dependency and teach strategies for coping with emotions.
3. Explore belief system (*e.g.*, does pain, suffering, loss mean punishment?)
4. Encourage person to ask questions about his health problem, his treatment, his progress, his prognosis.
5. Provide reliable information and reinforce information already given.
6. Clarify any misconceptions the person has about himself, his care, or his caregivers.
7. Avoid negative criticism.
8. Provide privacy and a safe environment.
9. Use therapeutic touch with person's consent.

B. Promote social interaction
1. Assist person to accept help from others.
2. Avoid overprotection, but limit the demands made on the individual.
3. Encourage movement.
4. Prepare significant others for physical and emotional changes.
5. Support family as they adapt.
6. Encourage visits from peers and significant others.
7. Encourage contact (letters, telephone) with peers and family.
8. Encourage involvement in unit activities.
9. Provide opportunity to share with people going through similar experiences.
10. Discuss the importance of communicating the client's value and importance to them with his or her support system (Dudas, 1993)

C. Provide specific interventions in selected situations
1. Loss of body part or function
   a. Assess the meaning of the loss for the individual and significant others, as related to visibility of loss, function of loss, and emotional investment.
   b. Explore and clarify misconceptions, myths regarding loss or ability to function with loss.
   c. Expect the individual to respond to the loss with denial, shock, anger, and depression.
   d. Be aware of the effect of the responses of others to the loss; encourage sharing of feelings between significant others.
   e. Validate feelings by allowing the individual to ventilate his feelings and to grieve.
   f. Use role-playing to assist with sharing; if person says, "I know my husband will not want to touch me with this colostomy," take the husband's role and discuss her colostomy, then switch roles so she can act out her feelings about her husband's response.

    g. Explore realistic alternatives and provide encouragement.

    h. Explore strengths and resources with person.

    i. Assist with the resolution of a surgically created alteration of body image.

        Replace the lost body part with prosthesis as soon as possible.

        Encourage viewing of site.

        Encourage touching of site.

        Encourage activities that encompass new body image (*e.g.*, shopping for new clothes).

    j. Teach about the health problem and how to manage.

    k. Begin to incorporate person in care of operative site.

    l. Gradually allow person to assume full self-care responsibility, if feasible.

    m. Teach person to monitor own progress (Miller, 1995).

    n. Refer to *Sexual Dysfunction* for additional information, if indicated.

2. Changes associated with chemotherapy (Cooley, Yeomans, & Cobb, 1986; Dudas, 1993)

    a. Discuss the possibility of hair loss, absence of menses, temporary or permanent sterility, decreased estrogen levels, vaginal dryness, mucositis.

    b. Encourage to share concerns, fears, and their perception of the impact of these changes on their life.

    c. Explain where hair loss may occur (head, eyelashes, eyebrows, axillary hair, pubic and leg hair).

    d. Explain that hair will grow back after treatment, but may change in color and texture.

    e. Select a wig before hair loss, wear it before hair loss. Consult a beautician for tips on how to vary the look (*e.g.*, combs, clips).

    f. Encourage the wearing of scarves, turbans when wig is not on.

    g. Teach to minimize the amount of hair loss by

        Avoiding excessive shampooing, using a conditioner twice weekly

        Patting hair dry gently

        Avoiding electric curlers, dryers, and curling irons

        Avoiding pulling hair with bands, clips, or bobby pins

        Avoiding hair spray and hair dye

        Using wide-tooth comb, avoiding vigorous brushing

    h. Refer to American Cancer Society for information about new or used wigs. Inform the client that the wig is a tax-deductible item.

    i. Discuss the difficulty that others (spouse, friends, coworkers) may have with visible changes.

    j. Encourage the person to initiate calls and contacts with others who may be having difficulty.

    k. Encourage the person to ask for assistance of friends, relatives. Ask person if the situation were reversed, what he or she would want to do to help a friend.

    l. Allow significant others opportunities to share their feelings and fears.

    m. Assist significant others to identify positive aspects of the client and ways this can be shared.

    n. Provide information about support groups for couples.

3. Anorexia nervosa, bulimia nervosa

    a. Differentiate between body image distortion and body image dissatisfaction.

    b. Refer to *Altered Nutrition: Less Than Body Requirements related to anorexia* for additional interventions.

4. Psychoses—refer to *Altered Thought Process* for specific information, interventions.

5. Sexual abuse—refer to *Ineffective Family Coping* for specific information, interventions.

6. Sexual assault—refer to *Rape Trauma Syndrome* for specific information, interventions.

7. Assault—refer to *Post-Trauma Response* for specific information, interventions.

D. Initiate health teaching, as indicated
   1. Teach what community resources are available, if needed (*e.g.*, mental health centers, self-help groups such as Reach for Recovery, Make Today Count).
   2. Teach wellness strategies (see *Health-Seeking Behaviors*).

Rationale

- Frequent contact by the caregiver indicates acceptance and may facilitate trust. The client may be hesitant to approach the staff because of negative self-concept; the nurse must reach out (Dudas, 1993).
- Social interactions can reaffirm that the individual is acceptable and that previous support system is still intact (Stuart & Sundeen, 1995).
- Expressing feelings and perceptions increases the client's self-awareness and helps the nurse plan effective interventions to address his needs. Validating the client's perceptions provides reassurance and can decrease anxiety (Dudas, 1993).
- Identifying personal attributes and strengths can help the client focus on the positive characteristics that contribute to the whole concept of self rather than only on the change in body image. The nurse should reinforce these positive aspects and encourage the client to reincorporate them into his or her new self-concept (Dudas, 1993).
- Open, honest discussions—expressing that changes will occur but that they are manageable—promote feelings of control.
- Participation in self-care and planning promotes positive coping with the change.
- Professional counseling is indicated for a client with poor ego strengths and inadequate coping resources.
- Increased social interaction through involvement in groups enables a person to receive social and intellectual stimulation, which enhances self-esteem (Taft, 1985).

🌹 Interventions—*Child Focus*

1. For hospitalized child
   a. Prepare child for hospitalization, if possible, with an explanation and a visit to the hospital to meet personnel and examine the environment.
   b. Provide familiarities/routines of home as much as possible (*e.g.*, favorite toy or blanket, story at bedtime).
   c. Provide nurturance (*i.e.*, hug).
   d. Provide child with opportunities to share fears, concerns, anger (see Appendix IX for play therapy guidelines).
      Acknowledge the normality of these fears, concerns, anger.
      Correct child's misconceptions (*e.g.*, that he is being punished; that his parents are angry).
      Encourage family to stay with or visit child, despite the child's crying when they leave; teach them to provide accurate information about when they will return to reduce fears of abandonment.
      Allow parents to help with care.
      Ask child to draw a picture of himself or herself and then ask for a verbal description.
   e. Assist child to understand his experiences.
      Provide child with an explanation ahead of time, if possible.
      Explain sensations and discomforts of condition, treatments, and medications.
      Encourage crying.
   f. Maintain sense of intactness during periods of immobility.
      Encourage movement, no matter how slight.
      During bath, ask child to identify body parts: "Where is your leg?"
      Allow child access to mirror to provide visualization of body.
2. Discuss with parents how body image develops and what interactions contribute to their child's self-perception.
   a. Teach the names and functions of body parts.

    b. Acknowledge changes (*e.g.*, height).
    c. Allow some choices for what to wear.
3. Ask child to draw a picture of his or her body just after a bath (naked). Ask to describe picture.
4. For adolescents
    a. Discuss with parents the adolescent's need to "fit in."
        Do not dismiss adolescent's concerns too quickly.
        Be flexible and compromise when possible (*e.g.*, clothes are temporary, tattoos are not).
        Negotiate a time period to think about options and alternatives (*e.g.*, 4–5 weeks).
        Provide with reasons for denying a request. Elicit adolescent's reasons. Compromise if possible (*e.g.*, parents want curfew at 11:00; adolescent wants 12:00; compromise 11:30).
    b. Provide opportunities to discuss concerns when parents are not present.
    c. Ask to describe best features and those they dislike.
    d. Prepare for impending developmental changes.

Rationale

- Attempts to retain the "normality" of the child's world can help to increase feeling of security (Wong, 1995).
- Play therapy puts the child in control by providing opportunities to make choices (Wong, 1995).
- Interventions that provide expressive outlets for tension and fear can help maintain the child's integrity (Wong, 1995).
- Opportunities for choices and success enhance self-esteem and coping (Johnson, 1993).

Interventions—*Maternal Focus*

1. Encourage the woman to share her concerns.
2. Attend to each concern if possible, or refer her to others for assistance.
3. Discuss the challenges and changes that pregnancy and motherhood bring.
4. Encourage her to share expectations: her own and those of her significant others.
5. Assist her to identify sources for love and affection.
6. Provide anticipatory guidance to both parents-to-be concerning
    a. Fatigue and irritability
    b. Appetite swings
    c. Gastric disturbances (nausea, constipation)
    d. Back and leg aches
    e. Changes in sexual desire and activity (*i.e.*, sexual positions as pregnancy advances)
    f. Mood swings
    g. Fear (for self, for unborn baby, of loss of attractiveness, of inadequacy as a mother)
7. Encourage the mutual sharing of concerns between spouses.

Rationale

- Open, honest discussions—expressing that changes will occur but that they are manageable—promote feelings of control.
- Support can be given more freely and more realistically if others are prepared (Dudas, 1993).
- Pregnancy disrupts the adolescent from becoming comfortable with her body image (Johnson, 1993).

Personal Identity Disturbance

DEFINITION

Personal Identity Disturbance: The state in which an individual experiences or is at risk of experiencing an inability to distinguish between self and nonself.

DEFINING CHARACTERISTICS

See Defining Characteristics for *Self-Concept Disturbance* or *Altered Growth and Development*

> **Author's Note**
>
> This nursing diagnosis is a subcategory under *Self-Concept Disturbance*. Until clinical research defines and differentiates this subcategory from others, refer to *Self-Concept Disturbance* or *Altered Growth and Development* for assessment criteria and interventions.

Self-Esteem Disturbance

DEFINITION

Self-Esteem Disturbance: The state in which an individual experiences or is at risk of experiencing negative self-evaluation about self or capabilities.

DEFINING CHARACTERISTICS

Overt or covert
    Self-negating verbalization*
    Expressions of shame or guilt*
    Evaluates self as unable to deal with events*
    Rationalizes away/rejects positive feedback and exaggerates negative feedback about
        self*
    Inability to set goals
    Indecisiveness
    Lack of/poor problem-solving ability
    Exhibits signs of depression (sleeping, eating)

* Source: Norris, J., & Kunes-Connell M. (1987). Self-esteem disturbance: A clinical validation study. In A. McLane (Ed.). *Classification of nursing diagnoses: Proceedings of the seventh conference.* St. Louis: C. V. Mosby.

Seeks approval/reassurance excessively

Poor body presentation (posture, eye contact, movements)

Self-abusive behavior (mutilation, suicide attempts, nail biting, substance abuse, becoming a victim)

Hesitant to try new things/situations*

Denial of problems obvious to others*

Projection of blame/responsibility for problems*

Rationalizes personal failures*

Hypersensitivity to slight criticism*

Grandiosity*

RELATED FACTORS

Self-Esteem Disturbance can be either an episodic event or a chronic problem. Failure to resolve a problem or multiple sequential stresses can result in chronic low self-esteem (CLSE). Those factors that occur over time and are associated with CLSE are indicated by "CLSE" in parentheses.

Pathophysiologic

Related to change in appearance secondary to
    Loss of body parts
    Loss of body functions
    Disfigurement (trauma, surgery, birth defects)

Situational (Personal, Environmental)

Related to unmet dependency needs

Related to feelings of abandonment secondary to
    Death of significant other
    Child abduction/murder
    Separation from significant other

Related to feelings of failure secondary to
    Loss of job or ability to work
    Increase/decrease in weight
    Unemployment
    Financial problems
    Premenstrual syndrome
    Relationship problems
        Marital discord
        Separation
        Step-parents
        In-laws

Related to assault (personal, or relating to the event of another's assault—*e.g.*, same age, same community)

Related to failure in school

Related to history of ineffective relationship with own parents (CLSE)

Related to history of abusive relationships (CLSE)

Related to unrealistic expectations of child by parent (CLSE)

Related to unrealistic expectations of self (CLSE)

Related to unrealistic expectations of parent by child (CLSE)

Related to parental rejection (CLSE)

Related to inconsistent punishment (CLSE)

* Source: Norris, J., & Kunes-Connell M. (1987). Self-esteem disturbance: A clinical validation study. In A. McLane (Ed.). *Classification of nursing diagnoses: Proceedings of the seventh conference.* St. Louis: C. V. Mosby.

Related to feelings of helplessness and/or failure secondary to institutionalization
    Mental health facility   Orphanage
    Jail   Halfway house
Related to history of numerous failures (CLSE)

Maturational

Infant/toddler/preschool
    Related to lack of stimulation or closeness (CLSE)
    Related to separation from parents/significant others (CLSE)
    Related to continual negative evaluation by parents
    Related to inadequate parental support (CLSE)
    Related to inability to trust significant other (CLSE)
School aged
    Related to failure to achieve grade level objectives
    Related to loss of peer group
    Related to repeated negative feedback
Adolescent
    Related to loss of independence and autonomy secondary to (specify)
    Related to disruption of peer relationships
    Related to scholastic problems
    Related to loss of significant others
Middle aged
    Related to changes associated with aging
Older adult
    Related to losses (people, function, financial, retirement)

Author's Note
See *Self-Concept Disturbance*

Errors in Diagnostic Statements
See *Self-Concept Disturbance*

Key Concepts
See *Self-Concept Disturbance*

Focus Assessment Criteria
See *Self-Concept Disturbance*

Chronic Low Self-Esteem

DEFINITION
Chronic Low Self-Esteem: The state in which an individual experiences a long-standing negative self-evaluation about self or capabilities.

DEFINING CHARACTERISTICS*
Major (80%–100%)

Long-standing or chronic
   Self-negating verbalization
   Expressions of shame/guilt
   Evaluates self as unable to deal with events
   Rationalizes away/rejects positive feedback and exaggerates negative feedback about self
   Hesitant to try new things/situations

Minor (50%–79%)

   Frequent lack of success in work or other life events
   Overly conforming, dependent on others' opinions
   Poor body presentation (eye contact, posture, movements)
   Nonassertive/passive
   Indecisive
   Excessively seeks reassurance

RELATED FACTORS

See *Self-Esteem Disturbance*

Author's Note
See *Self-Concept Disturbance*

Errors in Diagnostic Statements
See *Self-Concept Disturbance*

Key Concepts
See *Self-Concept Disturbance*

Focus Assessment Criteria

See *Self-Concept Disturbance*

Outcome Criteria

The individual will
- Modify excessive and unrealistic self-expectations
- Verbalize acceptance of limitations
- Verbalize nonjudgmental perceptions of self
- Identify positive aspects of self
- Cease self-abusive behavior
- Report freedom from symptoms of depression
- Begin to take verbal and behavioral risks

---

* Source: Norris, J., & Kunes-Connell M. (1987). Self-esteem disturbance: A clinical validation study. In A. McLane (Ed.). *Classification of nursing diagnoses: Proceedings of the seventh conference.* St. Louis: C. V. Mosby.

Interventions

A. Assist the person to reduce his present anxiety level
  1. Be supportive, nonjudgmental.
  2. Accept silence, but let him know you are there.
  3. Orient as necessary.
  4. Clarify distortions; do not use confrontation.
  5. Be aware of your own anxiety and avoid communicating it to the individual.
  6. Refer to *Anxiety* for further interventions.

B. Enhance the person's sense of self
  1. Be attentive.
  2. Respect his personal space.
  3. Validate your interpretation of what he is saying or experiencing ("Is this what you mean?").
  4. Help him to verbalize what he is expressing nonverbally.
  5. Assist to reframe and redefine negative expressions (*e.g.*, not "failure," but "setback").
  6. Use communication that helps to maintain his own individuality ("I" instead of "we").
  7. Pay attention to person, especially new behavior.
  8. Encourage good physical habits (healthy food and eating patterns, exercise, proper sleep).
  9. Provide encouragement as a task or skill is attempted.
  10. Provide realistic positive feedback on accomplishments.
  11. Teach person to validate consensually with others.
  12. Teach and encourage esteem-building exercises (self-affirmations, imagery, mirror work, use of humor, meditation/prayer, relaxation).
  13. Respect need for privacy.
  14. Assist in establishing appropriate personal boundaries.
  15. Provide consistency among staff (Miller, 1995).

C. Promote use of coping resources (Stuart & Sundeen, 1995)
  1. Identify areas of personal strength of the person.
     a. Sports, hobbies, crafts
     b. Health, self-care
     c. Work, training, education
     d. Imagination, creativity
     e. Writing skills, math
     f. Interpersonal relationships
  2. Share your observations with the person
  3. Provide opportunities for person to engage in the activities.

D. Assist person in expressing thoughts and feelings
  1. Use open-ended statements and questions.
  2. Encourage expression of both positive and negative statements.
  3. Use movement, art, and music as means of expression.
  4. If person has impaired reality-testing ability, refer to *Altered Thought Processes* for further interventions.

E. Provide opportunities for positive socialization
  1. Encourage visits/contact with peers and significant others (letters, telephone).
  2. Be a role model in one-to-one interactions.
  3. Involve in activities, especially when strengths can be used.
  4. Do not allow person to isolate self (refer to *Social Isolation* for further interventions).
  5. Involve in supportive group therapy.
  6. Teach social skills as required (refer to *Impaired Social Interaction* for further interventions).
  7. Encourage participation with others sharing similar experiences.

F. Set limits on problematic behavior such as aggression, poor hygiene, ruminations, and suicidal preoccupation. Refer to *Risk for Suicide* and/or *Risk for Violence* if these are assessed as problems.

G. Provide for development of social and vocational skills
    1. Reinforce confidence as person demonstrates new skills.
    2. Refer for vocational counseling.
    3. Involve in volunteer organizations.
    4. Encourage participation in activities with age-related others.
    5. Arrange for continuation of education (*e.g.*, literacy class, GEDs, vocational training, art/music classes).

H. Assist in self-exploration as anxiety and trust permit
    1. Identify positive self-evaluation.
    2. Assess self-appraisal.
    3. Address unrealistic self-expectations (*e.g.*, "I should").
    4. Encourage work on family of origin issues (healing) with one or combination of (Whitfield, 1990):
        Professional counselor   Self-help workbooks
        Self-help groups
    5. Assist person with forgiveness issues (self, others, God).
    6. Refer to *Situational Low Self-Esteem* for specific interventions.

Rationale

- Individuals with low self-esteem are usually anxious, fearful people. Anxiety levels must be mild or moderate before other interventions can be effective (Johnson, 1993).
- Strategies are focused on helping the person reexamine negative feelings about himself or herself and to identify positive attributes (Wilson & Kneisel, 1996).
- Providing opportunities for the person to be successful increase self-esteem (Stuart & Sundeen, 1995).
- Client collaboration is necessary for him to assume ultimate responsibility for his own behavior (Stuart & Sundeen, 1995).
- Conveying acceptance of the person's feelings promotes self-acceptance.

Situational Low Self-Esteem

DEFINITION

Situational Low Self-Esteem: The state in which an individual who previously had positive self-esteem experiences negative feelings about self in response to an event (loss, change).

DEFINING CHARACTERISTICS*
Major (80%–100%)

Episodic occurrence of negative self-appraisal in response to life events in a person with a previous positive self-evaluation

Verbalization of negative feelings about self (helplessness, uselessness)

* Source: Norris, J., & Kunes-Connell M. (1987). Self-esteem disturbance: A clinical validation study. In A. McLane (Ed.). *Classification of nursing diagnoses: Proceedings of the seventh conference.* St. Louis: C. V. Mosby.

Minor (50%–79%)

Self-negating verbalizations
Expressions of shame/guilt
Evaluates self as unable to handle situations/events
Difficulty making decisions
Self-neglect
Social isolation

RELATED FACTORS

See *Self-Esteem Disturbance*

Author's Note

See *Self-Concept Disturbance*

Errors in Diagnostic Statements

See *Self-Concept Disturbance*

Key Concepts

1. Qualities of a healthy personality are (Stuart & Sundeen, 1995, p. 382)
   a. Positive and accurate body image
   b. Realistic self-ideal
   c. Positive self-concept
   d. High self-esteem
   e. Satisfying role performance
   f. Clear sense of identity
2. Individuals with healthy personalities can experience a change in their positive self-perception in response to a profound event or a series of negative experiences (Stuart & Sundeen, 1995).
3. Responses to a situation that challenges a person's previously positive view of self are feelings of being weak, helpless, or hopeless; fear, vulnerability; of being fragile, incomplete, worthless, and inadequate (Stuart & Sundeen, 1995).

Outcome Criteria

The person will
- Identify source of threat to self-esteem and work through that issue
- Identify positive aspects of self
- Express a positive outlook for the future
- Analyze his own behavior and its consequences
- Identify ways of exerting control and influencing outcomes
- Resume previous level of functioning

Interventions

A. Assist the individual in identifying and expressing feelings
1. Be empathetic, nonjudgmental.
2. Listen. Do not discourage expressions of anger, crying, and so forth.
3. What was happening when he began feeling this way?
4. Clarify relationships between life events.

5. Encourage putting the traumatic event (assault) in context of life experiences as a whole while supporting common-sense safety precautions.

B. Assist in identifying positive self-evaluations

1. How has he handled other crises?
2. How does he manage anxiety—through exercise, withdrawal, drinking/drugs, talking?
3. Reinforce adaptive coping mechanisms.
4. Examine and reinforce positive abilities and traits (*e.g.*, hobbies, skills, school, relationships, appearance, loyalty, industriousness).
5. Help individual accept both positive and negative feelings.
6. Do not confront defenses.
7. Communicate confidence in person's ability.
8. Involve person in mutual goal setting.
9. Have clients write positive true statements about themselves (for their eyes only); have them read the list daily as a part of their normal routine (Grainger, 1990).
10. Reinforce use of esteem-building exercises (self-affirmations, imagery, meditation/prayer, relaxation, use of humor).

C. Explore relation between behavior and self-appraisals

1. Encourage examination of current behavior and its consequences (*e.g.*, dependency, procrastination, isolation).
2. Assist in mutually identifying faulty perceptions.
3. Explore person's concept of success/failure and loss/punishment, and assist in putting things into proper perspective.
4. Assist in identifying unrealistic expectations.
5. Help to identify negative automatic thoughts. ("I will never be able to do this.")
6. Examine if person is overgeneralizing. ("If I can't do this, then I'm a failure at everything.")
7. Assist person in identifying own responsibility and control in a situation (*e.g.*, when continually blaming others for problems).

D. Assess and mobilize current support system

1. Does he live alone? Employed?
2. Does he have available friends and relatives?
3. Is religion a support?
4. Has he previously used community resources?
5. Refer to vocational rehabilitation for retraining.
6. Support returning to school for further training.
7. Assist in involving in local volunteer organizations (senior citizens employment, Foster Grandparents, local support groups).
8. Arrange continuation of school studies for students.

E. Assist individual in learning new coping skills

1. Teach about how people respond to a life change.
2. Let him know he is not alone.
3. Assist in identifying options (*e.g.*, saying no, time off).
4. Refer to Appendix VII, Guidelines for Problem-Solving and Crisis Intervention.
5. Refer to Appendix X, Stress Management Techniques.
6. Encourage a trial of new behavior.
7. Reinforce the belief that the individual does have control over the situation.
8. Obtain a commitment to action.

F. Assist person in managing specific problems

1. Rape—refer to *Rape-Trauma Syndrome*.
2. Loss—refer to *Grieving*.
3. Hospitalization—refer to *Powerlessness* and *Parental Role Conflict*.

4. Ill family member—refer to *Altered Family Processes*.
5. Change or loss of body part—refer to *Body Image Disturbance*.
6. Depression—refer to *Ineffective Individual Coping* and *Hopelessness*.
7. Domestic violence—refer to *Ineffective Family Coping*.

Rationale

See *Chronic Low Self-Esteem*

😉 Interventions—*Child Focus*

1. Provide opportunities for child to be successful and needed.
2. Personalize the child's environment with pictures, possessions, and crafts he made.
3. Provide structured and unstructured playtime.
4. Ensure continuation of academic experiences in the hospital and home.
   a. Provide uninterrupted time for school work.

Rationale

See *Self-Concept Disturbance*

🏛 Interventions—*Older Adult Focus*

1. Acknowledge person by name.
2. Use a tone of voice that you use for your peer group.
3. Avoid words associated with infants (*e.g.*, "diapers").
4. Ask about family pictures, personal items, and past experiences.
5. Avoid attributing disabilities to "old age."
6. Knock on door of bedrooms and bathrooms.
7. Allow enough time to accomplish tasks at own pace.

Rationale

- Because self-esteem depends partially on the responses of others, caregivers must reflect respect for the aged as competent adults (Miller, 1995

References/Bibliography

Antaki, C., & Bruoin, C. (Eds.). (1982). *Attributions and psychological change*. London: Academic Press.

Andrews, M., & Boyle, J. (1995). *Transcultural concepts in nursing care* (2nd ed.). Philadelphia: J. B. Lippincott.

Cooley, M. E., Yeomans, A., & Cobb, S. (1986). Sexual and reproductive issues for women with Hodgkin's disease. *Cancer Nursing, 9,* 248–255.

Drapo, P. J. (1986). Mental retardation. In B. S. Johnson (Ed.). *Adaptation and growth*. Philadelphia: J. B. Lippincott.

Dudas, S. (1993). Altered body image and sexuality. In S. Groenwald, M. Frogge, M. Goodman, M., & C. Yarbo (Eds.). *Cancer nursing: Principles and practices*. Boston: Jones and Bartlett.

Friedman-Campbell, M., & Hart, C. A. (1984). Theoretical strategies and nursing interventions to promote psychological adaptation to spinal cord injuries and disability. *Journal of Neurosurgical Nursing, 16,* 335–342.

Fuller, J., & Schaller-Ayers, J. (1990). *Health assessment: A nursing approach*. Philadelphia: J. B. Lippincott.

Grainger, R. (1990). How to feel good about being you. *American Journal of Nursing, 90*(4), 14.

Harper, J., & Marshall, E. (1992). Adolescents' problems and their relationship to self-esteem. *Adolescence, 26,* 799–807.

Hunter, K., Linn, M., & Harris, R. (1981–82). Characteristics of high and low self-esteem in the elderly. *International Journal of Aging and Human Development, 14,* 117–126.

Johnson, B. S. (1993). *Psychiatric–mental health nursing* (3rd ed.). Philadelphia: J. B. Lippincott.

Johnson, B. S. (1995). *Child, adolescent and family psychiatric nursing*. Philadelphia: J. B. Lippincott.

Meisenhelder, J. B. (1985). Self-esteem: A closer look at clinical interventions. *International Journal of Nursing Studies, 22,* 127–135.

Miller, C. A. (1995). *Nursing care of older adults* (2nd ed.). Glenview, IL: Scott, Foresman.

Miller, S. (1987). Promoting self-esteem in the hospitalized adolescent: Clinical interventions. *Issues of Comprehensive Pediatric Nursing, 10,* 187–194.

Norris, J., & Kunes-Connell, M. (1985). Self-esteem disturbance. *Nursing Clinics of North America, 20,* 745–761.

Peretz, D. (1970). Reaction to loss. In A. C. Carr & D. Peretz (Eds.). *Loss and grief: Psychological management in medicine.* New York: Columbia University Press.

Polatajko, H. J. (1991). The effect of a sensory integration program on academic achievement, motor performance, and self-esteem in children identified as learning disabled: Results of a clinical trial. *Occupational Therapy Journal of Research, 11,* 155–176.

Price, B. (1990). A model for body-image care. *Journal of Advanced Nursing, 5,* 585–593.

Scipien, G. M., Chard, M. A., Howe, J., & Barnard, M. U. (1990). *Pediatric nursing care.* St. Louis: C. V. Mosby.

Stuart, G., & Sundeen, S. (1995). *Principles and practice of psychiatric nursing* (5th ed.). St. Louis: Mosby–Year Book.

Swanson, B., Cronin-Stubbs, R., & Sheldon, J. (1989). The impact of psychosocial factors on adapting to physical disability: A review of the research literature. *Rehabilitation Nursing, 14*(2), 64–68.

Taft, L. B. (1985). Self-esteem in later life: A nursing perspective. *Advances in Nursing Science, 8,* 77–84.

Taylor, S. (1989). *Positive illusions.* New York: Basic Books.

Tenner, H., & Herzberger, S. (1987). Depression, self-esteem and the absence of self-protective attributional biases. *Journal of Personality and Social Psychology, 52*(2), 72–80.

Whitehead, J. R. (1991). Effects of fitness test type, teacher, and gender on exercise intrinsic motivation and physical self-worth. *Journal of School Health, 61*(1), 11–16.

Whitfield, C. (1990). *A gift of myself.* Deerfield Beach, FL: Public Health Communications.

Whiting, S. M. A. (1986). Development of the person. In B. S. Johnson (Ed.). *Adaptation and growth.* Philadelphia: J. B. Lippincott.

Wilson, H. S., & Kneisel, C. R. (1996). *Psychiatric nursing* (5th ed.). Redwood City, CA: Addison-Wesley Nursing.

Winkelstein, M. L. (1989). Fostering positive self-concept in the school-age child. *Pediatric Nursing, 15,* 229–233.

Wong, D. L. (1995). *Nursing care of infants and children* (5th ed.). St. Louis: Mosby–Year Book.

Risk for Self-Harm*

Risk for Self-Abuse

Risk for Self-Mutilation

Risk for Suicide*

Risk for Self-Harm

DEFINITION
Risk for Self-Harm: A state in which an individual is at risk for inflicting direct harm on himself or herself. This may include one or more of the following: self-abuse, self-mutilation, suicide.

DEFINING CHARACTERISTICS
Major
Expresses desire or intent to harm self
Expresses desire to die or commit suicide
Past history of attempts to harm self

Minor
Reported or observed

Depression
Poor self-concept
Hallucinations/delusions
Substance abuse
Poor impulse control
Agitation

Hopelessness
Helplessness
Lack of support system
Emotional pain
Hostility

RELATED FACTORS
Risk for Self-Harm can occur as a response to a variety of health problems, situations, and conflicts. Some sources are listed.

Pathophysiologic
Related to feelings of helplessness, loneliness, or hopelessness secondary to:
Disabilities
Terminal illness
Chronic illness
Chronic pain
Chemical dependency

* These diagnoses are not currently on the NANDA list but have been included for clarity or usefulness.

Substance abuse
Mental impairment (organic or traumatic)
Psychiatric disorder
Schizophrenia   Personality disorder
Bipolar disorder   Adolescent adjustment disorder
Post-trauma syndrome   Somatoform disorders

Treatment-Related

Related to unsatisfactory outcome of treatment (medical, surgical, psychological)
Related to prolonged dependence on
Dialysis   Chemotherapy/radiation
Insulin injections   Ventilator

Situational (Personal, Environmental)

Related to:
Depression
Ineffective individual coping skills
Parental/marital conflict
Substance abuse in family
Child abuse
Real or perceived loss secondary to:
Finances/job   Separation/divorce
Status/prestige   Death of significant others
Threat of abandonment   Someone leaving home
Related to wish for revenge on real or perceived injury (body or self-esteem)

Maturational

Adolescent
Related to feelings of abandonment
Related to peer pressure
Related to unrealistic expectations of child by parents
Related to depression
Related to relocation
Related to significant loss
Older Adult
Related to multiple losses secondary to:
Retirement
Social isolation
Significant loss
Illness

Author's Note

Risk for Self-Harm represents a broad diagnosis that can encompass self-abuse, self-mutilation, and/or risk for suicide. Although initially they may appear the same, the distinction lies in the intent. Self-mutilation and self-abuse are pathologic attempts to relieve stress (temporary reprieve), whereas suicide is an attempt to die (to relieve stress permanently) (Carscadden, 1992, personal communication). *Risk for Self-Harm* can also be a useful early diagnosis when insufficient data are present to differentiate one from the other.

Risk for Suicide currently is not on the NANDA list, but has been added here for clarity. *Risk for Violence to Self* is included under *Risk for Violence*. The term *violence* is defined as a swift and intense force or a rough or injurious physical force. As the reader knows, suicide can be either violent or nonviolent (*e.g.*, overdose of barbiturates). Using the term "violence" in this diagnostic context unfortunately can lead to nondetection of a person at risk for suicide because of the perception that the person is not capable of violence.

Risk for Suicide clearly denotes a person as high risk for suicide and in need of protection. Treatment of this diagnosis involves validating the risk, contracting with the person, and providing protection. Treatment of the person's underlying depression and hopelessness should be addressed with other applicable nursing diagnoses (*e.g., Ineffective Individual Coping, Hopelessness*).

Errors in Diagnostic Statements

Risk for Suicide related to recent diagnosis of cancer

In this situation, the recent diagnosis of cancer in itself is not a risk factor for suicide. The person must be depressed and severely stressed and exhibit suicidal intentions. The nurse must not automatically label a person as suicidal based on a single crisis or severe physical disability. All *Risk for Self-Harm* diagnostic statements should contain both verbal and nonverbal cues to suicidal intent (*e.g., Risk for Suicide related to remarks about life being unbearable and reports of giving belongings away*).

Key Concepts

1. Violence, whether directed toward oneself or others, can elicit strong reactions from people. Nurses, whose profession encompasses caregiving, health promotion, and nurturance, must examine their own attitudes, responses, and behavior toward the violent.
2. Because much of the practice of self-harm is a "shame-based" problem, the condition is more likely to be underreported rather than overreported. Identification is difficult because so many become extremely adept at hiding the causes of their injuries.
3. Found in all economic and educational backgrounds, self-mutilation is found in some men but mainly in women, and usually appears in the early teenage years. It is frequently associated with long-term effects of physical, psychological, and sexual abuse during childhood.
4. Often repetitive and chronic in nature, the self-harm often distorts or disrupts the client–therapist relationship and increases the need for and length of hospitalizations. These hospitalizations often further exacerbate the problem. Hospitalization usually increases the clients' dependency and decreases their accountability.
5. Basics of dysfunctional family dynamics
   a. Characteristics
      Little nurturance given
      Avoids showing feelings
      Maintains rigid rules
      Usually abusive (physical/psychological/sexual)
   b. Family members exhibit
      Denial   Need/expectation of perfection
      Minimization   Need for control of self/others
      Blame
   c. Child grows up with
      Fear of rejection   Fear of losing control
      Fear of abandonment   Feelings of hopelessness and helplessness
   d. As a child and later as an adult, that individual will have difficulty in
      Trusting
      Asking for wants and needs
      Identifying and expressing feelings
      Disregarding internalized messages that create poor self-concept
6. There are various levels or stages in impending self-harm. The transition from one level to another may be rapid or slowly progressive. The individual may or may not be aware of the stages and the transition. Awareness of the stages and characteristics of each facilitates intervention. The earlier the stage, the clearer the thinking, the less intense are the feelings, and the more control the individual has. An individual can easily identify stages once the defining characteristics are learned (Carscadden, 1993a).

a. Beginning stage ("thinking" stage)

Person often unaware of this stage

May have been ruminating

May have encountered a "trigger," which set off a memory tap or ignited a flash-back

Advancement into this stage might produce

Change in concentration/attention	Mild heart palpitations
Small tremor	Slight tightening of muscles
Change in facial color	

b. Climbing stage ("feeling" stage)

Stage many individuals become aware of first

Feelings begin to intensify

Tremor increases, may become a shake	Muscles tense to fight or flight
Unable to concentrate	May experience shortness of breath
Heart begins to race	Perspiration may occur

c. Crisis stage ("behavior" stage)

Concentration will be extremely limited and focused on intent to relieve pent-up feelings

May "numb out" or disassociate

Agitation may increase or become extremely calm

Sudden moves, flurried activity

Physical touch may be perceived as real threat

Individual often sees no alternative but self-harm at this point

d. Postcrisis stage

May experience mixed emotions: whatever relief the self-harm provides, but also guilt, shame, or frustration at having failed expectations

May cry or withdraw

Often the worst stage for the person because of the negative response from others, including many caregivers

7. The person who has delusions or hallucinations (schizophrenia or drug induced) presents a different rationale for self-harm. Delusions and hallucinations must be brought under control. Safety for the person in the meantime is essential and a top priority.

Suicide

1. Self-harm ranges from injurious acts to reduce stress to direct acts of suicide. Self-abuse or mutilation behavior has the potential to be harmful and result in death. Self-injurers are very aware that their actions have a potential of resulting in death if they miscalculate (*e.g.*, how many pills, how much cutting or burning; availability of help; their own degree of control to stop once started) (Carscadden, 1993a). With direct self-destructive behavior, usually referred to as suicidal, the intent is death, and the individual is aware.

2. Suicidal behavior is an attempt to escape from intolerable life stressors that have accumulated over time. It is accompanied by intense feelings of hopelessness (Shneidman, 1989).

3. The lack of healthy coping skills and the use of avoidant behaviors such as alcohol and drugs are frequently correlated with suicidal behavior (Stillion & McDowell, 1991).

4. A suicidal crisis happens both to the individual and to the person's support system.

5. Suicide may be seen as a viable alternative both by the individual and by significant others.

6. Depression, low self-esteem, helplessness, and hopelessness are positively related to suicide. The greater the degree of hopelessness, the greater the risk for suicide (Stillion & McDowell, 1991). Loss clearly increases the risk of suicide. Cumulative losses increase the risk dramatically (Stillion & McDowell, 1991).

7. People exhibiting poor reality testing, delusions, and poor impulse control are at high risk. Alcohol and drugs tend to lower impulse control.
8. Changes in behavior (*e.g.*, giving away possessions) may signal an increase in risk. Individuals may appear to be better just before an attempt. This may be due to feelings of relief after making a decision.
9. Demographic factors can serve the caregiver, identifying people who are at high risk for suicidal behavior (Jacobs, 1989).
   a. Older white men have the highest suicidal rate in the United States. The risk increases linearly as the person ages (Mellick, Buckwalter, & Stolley, 1992).
   b. Adolescents also represent a high-risk group.
   c. More women attempt suicide, but men complete suicide more often.
   d. Unemployment and frequent job changes are associated with an increased risk.
   e. Alcohol is associated with a high risk.
   f. The greater the satisfaction with social relationships, the lower the risk will be; thus, divorce, separation, and widowhood increase the risk.
      Previous attempts place people in a high-risk group because they are likely to repeat the attempt.
10. The suicide rate among psychiatric inpatients markedly exceeds the general suicide rate (Modestin & Kopp, 1988).
11. The more resources are available, the more likely the crisis can be effectively managed. This includes personal support systems, employment, physical and mental abilities, finances, and housing.
12. Some individuals use suicide attempts as a way to cope with stress. The more frequent the attempts and the more lethal, the higher is the current risk. Suicidal ideation moves from the general to the specific, with more detailed plans representing a higher risk. A precipitating event may occur before an attempt. The difference between a negative life event and one that may lead to a suicide attempt is that with the latter, the person has already engaged in significant suicidal ideation (Stillion & McDowell, 1991).
13. Long-term suicide risk exists for some people. This can be assessed best by evaluating
   a. Their coping strategies when confronted with stress
   b. Their life-style—is it stable or unstable?
   c. The specificity and lethality of the plan
14. Use verbal and nonverbal clues to assess risk, because seriously suicidal people may deny suicidal thoughts.
15. Prediction of suicide risk is not an exact science. Some of the errors that can be made result from:
   a. Overreliance on mood as an indicator; not all people who commit suicide are clinically depressed
   b. Reliance on intuition; many people can totally conceal their intention
   c. Failure to assess support system
   d. Countertransference, particularly the failure of the therapist to acknowledge negative feelings that are aroused (Maltsberger, 1986)
16. Levels of risk can be assessed as low or high. Not all of the following parameters are necessarily present in any one individual (Hatton & Valente, 1977).
   a. High

Adolescent or older than 45 years	Male
Divorced, separated, widowed	Isolated socially
Professional worker	Unemployed or lack of stable job
Chronic or terminal illness	history
Delusions/hallucinations	Severe depression
Hopelessness/helplessness	Severe anxiety
Intoxicated or addicted	Multiple attempts
Frequent or constant suicidal thoughts	With a specific plan, method is
Means—readily available	highly lethal

b. Low

25–45 years of age or younger than 12 years

Married

Blue-collar worker

No serious medical problems

No specific plan, or has a plan with low lethality

Female

Socially active

Employed

Infrequent substance abuse

Thoughts are fleeting (if person has a vague plan)

✿ *Key Concepts—Child*

1. Preteen and early adolescence is often the age at which self-harm begins to manifest itself.
2. Adults must be in tune with changes in behavior and changes in apparel and be highly suspicious of multiple "accidents."
3. Suicide is the second leading cause of death during adolescence. A significant trend is the rise among people in the younger age groups (U.S. Bureau of the Census, 1984).
4. Suicide in children (ages 5–14 years) tends to be more impulsive than in any other age groups. Hyperactivity also seems to contribute to the impulsive nature of the act (Stillion & McDowell, 1991).
5. A number of environmental risk factors contribute to child and adolescent suicide; however, the leading risk factor is parental conflict, abuse, and neglect (Stillion & McDowell, 1991).
6. Recognition of depression in adolescents is often difficult because they mask their feelings with bored and angry behavior. Some of the symptoms include being sad or blue, withdrawal from social activities, trouble concentrating, somatic complaints, changes in sleep or eating patterns, and feelings of guilt or inadequacy (Pallikkathayil & Flood, 1991).
7. Suicidal adolescents rarely have close friends and exhibit poor peer relationships (Stillion & McDowell, 1991).
8. Gay youths are estimated to be two to three times more likely to attempt suicide than their heterosexual peers. As many as 30% of suicides annually are believed to be gay teens (Fekar & Koslap-Petraco, 1991).
9. Suicide is the leading cause of death among adolescents. A frequent factor is lack of or loss of a meaningful relationship (Johnson, 1993).

⛩ *Key Concepts—Older Adult*

1. White men older than 60 years of age have a suicide rate twice the rate in all other age groups. They constitute 18.5% of the population but commit 23% of all suicides (U.S. Bureau of the Census, 1984).
2. The self-esteem of older men is negatively affected by retirement, loss of vigor, and loss of a meaningful role (Boxwell, 1988).
3. The elderly tend to complete suicide when attempted. The rate of attempts to completion is 4:1, whereas for younger people the ratio is approximately 200:1 (McIntosh, 1985).
4. Alcohol contributes to depression. Depression increases alcohol use. Both are significant risk factors for suicide in older adults (Blazer, 1982).
5. Depressed older adults usually talk less about suicide than younger adults, but use more violent means and are more successful (Miller, 1995).
6. Suicidal potential often is overlooked because of the prevalent view that older adults are in general passive and nonviolent. In addition, complaints about depression and hopelessness may be subtle and thus easily ignored in older adults (Miller, 1995).
7. Older adults communicate their intentions less frequently and they use more lethal means (Mellick, Buckwalter, & Stolley, 1992). Families, senior citizen centers, clergy, and physicians are the network that can most readily identify the potential problem.

TRANSCULTURAL CONSIDERATIONS

1. Acceptance of sudden, violent death is difficult for family members in most societies (Andrews & Boyle, 1995).
2. Suicide is strictly forbidden under Islamic law. Church funerals are not permitted for suicide victims in some religions (*e.g.*, Catholicism).
3. Suicide or any violent death is believed by the Northern Cheyenne Indians to prevent the spirit from entering the spirit world (Andrews & Boyle, 1995).
4. Suicide of elderly Eskimos, who could no longer contribute to the sustenance of the tribe, was expected (Giger & Davidhizar, 1995).

Focus Assessment Criteria

The nurse must be able to differentiate between the diagnoses of *Risk for Suicide* and *Risk for Self-Mutilation* or *Self-Abuse*. Although initially they may appear (in action) or sound (in statements) the same, the distinction lies in the intent. Self-mutilation and self-abuse are pathologic attempts to relieve stress (temporary reprieve), whereas suicide is an attempt to die (to relieve stress permanently). The perspicacious nurse will be able in the assessment to gather data that enable her to distinguish which diagnosis is appropriate for the client. It is prudent to remember that some clients may become so self-harmful that they eventually die, even though they are not intentionally suicidal.

Subjective Data

A. Assess for risk factors

    1. Psychological status

      a. Present concerns

          What are you thinking about?

          How are you feeling?

          Do you want to hurt yourself?

          Can you tell me the reason?

          How would you hurt yourself?

          Are you wanting to die or just have the pain (thoughts/feelings) go away?

          Assess for a suicide plan

               Method: Is there a specific plan (*e.g.*, pills, wrist-slashing, shooting), plans for rescue?

               Availability: Is the method accessible? Is access easy or difficult?

               Specificity: How specific is plan?

               Lethality: How lethal is the method?

      b. Assess for feelings of

Hopelessness	Anger/hostility
Helplessness	Guilt/shame
Isolation/abandonment	Impulsivity

      c. Chemical dependency/substance abuse. Assess if person is suffering from withdrawal or is under the influences.

          What drug/alcohol have you used?

          When did you last use it?

          How often do you use?

          How are you feeling?

          Are you hearing/seeing anything that concerns you?

      d. History of psychiatric problems

          Diagnosis

               Schizophrenic/affective—are delusions and/or hallucinations present?

                    Are you hearing voices?

                    What are they telling you?

                    Are you seeing anything that is frightening or upsetting you?

Bipolar disorder—what phase of cycle is person in?
Post-trauma syndrome
How recent was the trauma?
What effects has it had on the person?
Personality disorder—currently in therapy with a counselor?
Treatment and compliance with it
Previous history of self-harm
Methods   Recency
Lethality   Number of times
Outpatient follow-up support system
2. Medical status
a. Acute or chronic illness—how is it affecting life?
b. Has the person consulted a physician in past 6 months?
c. How many physicians have and currently are treating the person, and for what condition?
d. Prescribed drugs
What is person using?
Is it taken according to directions?
e. Nonprescribed drugs
What is person using?   How often?
How much?   Reason?
3. Sources of stress in past environment
a. Job change/loss
b. Failure in work/school
c. Threat of financial loss
d. Divorce/separation
e. Death of significant other
f. Illness/accident
g. Alcohol/drug use in family
h. Parental rejection
i. Dysfunctional family dynamics
j. Physical, psychological, sexual abuse
k. Unrealistic expectations
Of child by parent
Of parent by child
Of self
l. Severe trauma
4. Sources of stress in current environment
a. Any of the above (past environment)
b. Threat of criminal prosecution
c. Alcohol/drug use by person
d. Role change/responsibilities
e. Any threat to self-concept (real or perceived)
5. Assess person's awareness
a. Acknowledgment or denial—does the person admit self-harm or claim to have "accidents"?
b. What are the payoffs or reasons for self-harm?
Nonverbal communication—gains someone's attention and coerces others for their needs
Makes others believe—physical evidence of pain
Demonstrates the feeling of hopelessness
Demonstrates outside what feels like inside (ugly, scarred, garbage)
Deserves it—bad, ugly, evil, crazy
Release of pain and anger—use of self-harm is a safety valve to prevent suicide
(Re)establish control over one's body
Verifies there is still life—physical evidence of life in flow of blood

   c. Can the person identify specifics in the process?
         Personal triggers
               Sensory input
               Situations
               Particular types of people or places
         Experiences flashbacks or nightmares?
         Does the person disassociate or "numb out?"
         Can person identify levels or stages before the act of self-harm?
   d. Motivation to cease self-harm
         Wants to stop and is willing to work toward that end
         Wants the emotional pain to stop, sees self-harm as part of that pain and is
               considering change
         Unwilling to give up self-harm behavior
 6. Coping strategies (past and present)
   a. Assess ability of individual and family to cope with repeated stressors
   b. Available resources
   c. Level of impulse control
   d. Taking unnecessary risks
 7. Support system
   a. Who is relied on during periods of stress?
         Are they available
         What is their reaction to current situation?
               Denial   Helplessness/frustration
               Not receptive to helping   Concern and willingness to help
               Anger/guilt
   b. Personal and financial resources
         Employment   Housing
         Finances

Objective Data

A. Assess for risk factors

 1. General appearance
         Facial expression   Apparel
         Posture
 2. Behavior during interview
         Agitated   Hostile
         Restless   Cooperative
         Withdrawn   Disassociated
 3. Communication pattern
         Allusive   Hopeless/helpless (subjective)
         Denial   Suicidal expressions
         Delusional   Indecisive
         Hallucinates   Pressured speech
         Misinterprets   Difficulty concentrating
         Supersensitive (subjective)
 4. Nutritional status
         Appetite   Bulimic behavior
         Weight (anorectic, obese)
 5. Sleep–rest pattern
         Afraid of dark   Easily awakened
         Difficulty falling asleep   Sleeps too much
         Difficulty staying asleep   Nightmares
 6. Physical manifestations
         Tremors   Heart palpitations
         Agitation   Tightness of chest
         Hyperalertness   Buzzing in head

Shortness of breath   Fists clench
Perspiration   Complains of various aches and pains; stomach, head,
Change in facial color   muscles

7. Evidence of self-harm
   a. Be highly suspicious if
         There have been repeated accidents
         Person wears long sleeves in hot weather
         Person is reluctant to uncover parts of body
   b. Look for
         Scars   Lumps/bumps
         Open cuts   Reddened, irritated areas
         Sores   Areas that do not heal as expected
         Burn marks   Clumps or patches of missing hair
   c. Body parts often affected
         Wrists, arms, legs, feet
         Head, face, eyes, neck
         Chest, abdomen
         Genitals
   d. Behaviors of self-mutilation
         Cutting   Picking
         Slashing   Gouging
         Stabbing   Head smashing
         Scratching   Hitting (*e.g.*, fists against walls)
         Burning (cigarettes, lighters, matches, stove, clothes iron, curling iron)
         Use of corrosives (*e.g.*, drain cleaner)
   e. Behaviors of self-abuse
         Head banging
         Slapping
         Picking
         Scratching
         Nonlethal use of drugs/poison
         Anorectic/bulimic behaviors
         Swallowing foreign objects (glass, needles, safety pins, straight pins, various
             hardware, *e.g.*, nails, screws)
         Hair pulling
         Excessive rubbing
         Noncompliance with treatment for serious physical conditions (*e.g.*, diabetes).

Outcome Criteria

The person will
- Acknowledge self-harm thoughts
- Admit to use of self-harm behavior if it occurs
- Make a commitment to control behaviors
- Be able to identify personal triggers
- Learn properly to identify and tolerate uncomfortable feelings
- Choose alternatives that are not harmful

The person with impaired/altered thought processes will
- Acknowledge self-harm thoughts
- Admit to use of self-harm behavior if it occurs
- Attempt to identify stressors
- Cooperate with interventions used to decrease thoughts and control behavior

Interventions

A. Establish a trusting nurse–client relationship
   1. Demonstrate an acceptance of the individual as a worthwhile person through the use of nonjudgmental statements and behavior.
   2. Direct questions in a caring, concerned manner.
   3. Encourage expression of thoughts and feelings.
   4. Actively listen or provide support by just being there if the person is silent.
   5. Be aware of the individual's supersensitivity.
   6. Label the behavior, not the person.
   7. Be honest in your interactions.
   8. Assist in recognizing the presence of hope and the element of alternatives.
   9. Provide reasons for procedures or interventions necessary.
   10. Maintain individual's dignity throughout your therapeutic relationship.

B. Validate reality
   1. Schizophrenia or drug-induced psychosis
      a. Tell the person "you are safe."
      b. Use quiet, calming voice.
      c. Use "talk downs" when a hallucinogenic drug has been taken. If agitation increases, stop immediately.
      d. Orient individual as required. Point out sensory/environmental misperception without belittling his fears or indicating disapproval of verbal expressions.
      e. Reassure that this will pass.
      f. Watch for signs of increase in delusional thinking and/or frightening hallucinations (increased anxiety, agitation, irritability, pacing, hypervigilance).
   2. Post-trauma or dysfunctional
      a. Tell the person "you are not bad, crazy, hopeless."
      b. Say you believe them when they tell you their personal history; many grew up in denial or minimization.
      c. Let the person know she is not the only one.

C. Help reframe old thinking/feeling patterns (Carscadden, 1993a)
   1. Encourage the belief that change is possible.
   2. Assist in identifying thought–feeling–behavior concept.
   3. Help assess payoffs and drawbacks to self-harm.
   4. Rename words that have a negative connotation (*e.g.*, "setback," not "failure").
   5. Encourage identification of personal triggers.
   6. Assist in exploring viable alternatives.
   7. Help in looking at feelings of ambivalence about recovery.
   8. Encourage becoming comfortable with and using feelings.

D. Facilitate the development of new behavior
   1. Validate good coping skills already in existence.
   2. Provide role modeling in your own behavior and interactions.
   3. Encourage the use of positive affirmations, meditation and relaxation techniques, and other esteem-building exercises.
   4. Promote the concept of being helpful instead of helpless.
   5. Encourage journaling, keeping a diary of triggers, thoughts, feelings, and alternatives that work or do not work.
   6. Assist in developing body awareness as a method of ascertaining triggers and determining levels of impending self-harm.
   7. Introduce "contracting" to individual.
   8. Assist in role-playing to problem-solve situations/relationships.
   9. Promote development of healthy self-boundaries for the individual.

E. Provide an environment that demotes self-harm
   1. Structure time and activities.
      a. Provide a scheduled day that meets the individual's need for activity and rest.
      b. Encourage assistance to and activities with others without competitiveness.
      c. Relieve pent-up tension and purposeless hyperactivity with physical activity (*e.g.*, brisk walk, dance therapy, aerobics).
   2. Reduce excessive stimuli.
      a. Provide a quiet, serene atmosphere.
      b. Establish firm, consistent limits while giving individual as much control/choice as possible within those boundaries.
      c. Intervene at earliest stages to assist in person regaining control, preventing escalation, and allowing treatment in the least restrictive manner.
      d. Keep communication simple. Agitated people are unable to process complicated communication.
      e. Provide an area where individual can retreat to decrease stimuli (*e.g.*, time-out room, quiet room; person on hallucinogens needs a darkened, quiet room with a nonintrusive observer).
      f. Remove potentially dangerous objects from environment (if in crisis stage).
   3. Reduce triggers as much as possible.
      a. Assess problem areas and assist in problem solving with individual.
         Is person afraid of dark? Allow a small light on at night.
         Is person afraid of being alone? Put in a double room with roommate.
   4. Promote the use of alternatives.
      a. Stress that there are always alternatives.
      b. Stress that self-harm is a choice, not something uncontrollable.
      c. Allow opportunities for verbal expression of thoughts and feelings.
      d. Provide acceptable physical outlets (*e.g.*, yelling, pounding pillow, tearing up newspapers, using clay or Play-Doh, taking a brisk walk).
      e. Provide for less physical alternatives (*e.g.*, relaxation tapes, soft music, warm bath, diversional activities).

F. Determine present level of impending self-harm
   1. Beginning stage (thought stage)
      a. Provide soothing touch if permissible by person (predetermined).
      b. Remind individual that this is an "old tape" and to replace with new thinking and belief patterns.
      c. Provide unintrusive, calming alternatives.
   2. Climbing stage (feeling stage)
      a. Remind individual to consider other alternatives.
      b. Give as much control to the person as possible to support his accountability.
         Are you in control?   In what way can I help?
         Would you like me to assist?
      c. Provide more intense interventions at this stage.
      d. Encourage person to turn over any potential items of self-harm.
   3. Crisis stage (behavior stage)
      a. Give positives if individual chooses an alternative and does not self-harm.
      b. Ask person to put down any object of harm if he possesses one.
      c. Continue to emphasize there are always alternatives.
      d. Restrain only if individual becomes out of control.
      e. Release from restraints as soon as possible to give responsibility back to person. "Are you in control now?" "Are you feeling safe?"
      f. Remain calm and caring throughout the crisis period.
      g. Attend to practical issues in a nonpunitive, nonjudgmental manner.
   4. Postcrisis stage
      a. Give positive reinforcements if individual did not self-harm.
      b. Assist to problem-solve on how to divert self before crisis stage.

    c. Assess degree of injury/harm if individual did not choose alternative.
    d. Provide assistance or medical care, as necessary.
    e. Pay as little attention as possible to the act of self-harm and focus on prior stages (*i.e.*, "Can you remember what triggered you?" "What kinds of things were going through your mind?" "What do you think you might have done instead?").
    f. Return individual to normal activities/routine as soon as possible.

G. Initiate support systems to community, when/where indicated
  1. Teach family
    a. Constructive expression of feelings
    b. How to recognize levels of impending self-harm
    c. How to assist with appropriate interventions
    d. How to deal with self-harm behavior/results
  2. Supply phone number of 24-hour emergency hot lines
  3. Referral to counseling
    a. Individual therapist
    b. Family counseling
    c. Peer support group
  4. Referral to
    a. Leisure/vocational counseling
    b. Halfway houses
    c. Other community resources

Rationale
- Frequent contact by the caregiver indicates acceptance and may facilitate trust. The client may be hesitant to approach the staff because of negative self-concept; the nurse must reach out.
- Expressing feelings and perceptions increases the client's self-awareness and helps the nurse plan effective interventions to address his needs. Validating the client's perceptions provides reassurance and can decrease anxiety.
- The nurse must be aware that the person may express or exhibit ambivalence about stopping the self-harm behavior. This coping mechanism probably served a useful purpose. Often, unless the payoffs cease or until the payoffs for not harming are greater or more important, the behavior will continue.
- It is important that the act of self-harm is not rewarded with reinforcements (negative or positive). Treatment of the injury should be done in a matter-of-fact manner, much like removing a splinter, but also providing the person with dignity. Returning to activities/schedules as quickly as possible restores responsibility to the individual.
- Control of environment is a basic, but not to be discounted, intervention. A structured schedule provides boundaries and security, enhancing the sense of safety. A quiet environment reduces reactivity, enhances calm feelings, and decreases the likelihood of confusion and fear. Gross motor activity in a protected environment can lessen aggressive drives, whereas rest periods promote opportunities for relaxation, calm the emergency response, and reconnect body/mind/heart.
- The therapeutic alliance promotes client responsibility for behavioral restraint while supplementing internal controls. Ventilation of feelings may assist in resolving feelings regardless of the discomfort involved, and decreases the need for physical action.
- Making a contract with the individual
  - Gets the subject out in the open
  - Conveys the attitude of acceptance of the person as a worthwhile individual
  - Presents element of choice, the possibility and importance of thinking through situations before acting
  - Provides individual with a degree of control as he shares responsibility for own safety
- Maladaptive behaviors can be replaced with healthy ones to manage stress and anxiety (Stuart & Sundeen, 1993).

- Social isolation perpetuates feelings of low self-esteem and self-destructive behavior (Stuart & Sundeen, 1993).
- Behavior must be supervised until self-control has been demonstrated (Stuart & Sundeen, 1993).

Risk for Self-Abuse

DEFINITION

Risk for Self-Abuse: A state in which an individual is at risk to perform a deliberate act on the self, without the intent to kill, that may or may not cause harm to the body.

DEFINING CHARACTERISTICS
Major

Expresses a desire or intent to harm self
Evidence of self-abuse, including:
    Head banging
    Slapping
    Picking
    Scratching
    Nonlethal use of drugs/poison
    Anorectic/bulimic behaviors
    Swallowing foreign objects, (glass, needles, safety pins, straight pins, various hardware, *e.g.*, nails, screws)

RELATED FACTORS

See *Risk for Self-Harm*

Author's Note
See *Risk for Self-Harm*

Errors in Diagnostic Statements
See *Risk for Self-Harm*

Key Concepts
See *Risk for Self-Harm*

Risk for Self-Mutilation

DEFINITION

Risk for Self-Mutilation: A state in which an individual is at risk to perform a deliberate act on the self with the intent to injure, not kill, that produces immediate tissue damage to the body.

DEFINING CHARACTERISTICS
Major

Expresses desire or intent to harm self
Past history of attempts to harm self, including:

Cutting	Scratching
Slashing	Picking
Stabbing	Gouging

RELATED FACTORS

See *Risk for Self-Harm*

Author's Note
See *Risk for Self-Harm*

Errors in Diagnostic Statements
See *Risk for Self-Harm*

Key Concepts
See *Risk for Self-Harm*

Risk for Suicide

DEFINITION

Risk for Suicide: A state in which an individual is at risk for killing himself or herself.

DEFINING CHARACTERISTICS
Major (Must be Present)

Suicidal ideation
Previous suicidal attempts

Minor
See *Risk for Self-Harm*

RELATED FACTORS
See *Risk for Self-Harm*

Key Concepts
See *Risk for Self-Harm*

Focus Assessment Criteria

Information must be gathered from the individual and at least one significant other.

The nurse must not be reluctant to ask questions about suicide. People with no suicidal thoughts cannot be led to suicidal thoughts through questioning. Questions to assess a person's risk for suicide should focus on encouraging sharing of feelings and perceptions of the future. Questions such as "Have you ever thought of committing suicide?" are not useful because they usually evoke a "yes" or "no" answer with no description of the person's feelings.

Subjective Data
A. Assess for risk factors
    1. Psychological status
       a. Present concerns
           What are you thinking about?   What brought you here?
           What is on your mind?
       b. Assess for feelings of
           Hopelessness   Helplessness/hopelessness
           Isolation/abandonment   Guilt, shame
           Low self-esteem   Suicide as a viable alternative
           Anger, hostility
       c. Suicidal ideation
           Do you ever think
             Life is not worth living?
             About escaping from your problems?
             About harming yourself?
             How you would harm yourself?
             Under what circumstances you would act on your plan?
           Assess for a suicide plan
             Method: Is there a specific plan (*e.g.*, pills, wrist-slashing, shooting); plans
                for rescue?
             Availability: Is the method accessible? Is access easy or difficult?
             Specificity: How specific is plan?
             Lethality: How lethal is the method?
       d. Recent changes in behavior
           Verbal threats   Truancy/poor school performance
           Self-injurious behavior   Sleep disturbance
           Giving away possessions
       e. History of psychiatric problems
           Delusions/hallucinations
           Outpatient treatment
           Previous attempts
             Number   Lethality
             Recency
           Hospitalization
    2. Medical status
       a. Acute or chronic illness—how is it affecting life?
       b. Has person consulted physician in past 6 months?

   c. History of alcoholism/drug abuse?
   d. History of depression
3. Sources of stress in current environment
   a. Job change/loss
   b. Failure in work/school
   c. Threat of financial loss
   d. Divorce/separation
   e. Death of significant other
   f. Illness/accident
   g. Threat of criminal prosecution
   h. Alcohol/drug use in family
   i. Presence of firearms or other means of self-destruction
   j. Parental conflict/abuse
4. Coping strategies (past and present)
   a. Assess ability of individual and family to cope with repeated stresses
   b. Available resources
   c. Level of impulse control
   d. Taking unnecessary risks (drugs, alcohol)
5. Support system
   a. Who is relied on during periods of stress?
           Are they available?
           Their reaction to current situation
               Denial of problem   Helplessness, frustration
               Not receptive to helping now   Concern and willingness to help
               Anger, guilt
   b. Personal and financial resources
           Employment   Financial problems
           Housing
   c. Peer relationships

Objective Data

A. Assess for risk factors
   1. General appearance
           Facial expression   Dress
           Posture
   2. Behavior during interview
               Withdrawn   Quiet
               Hostile   Cooperative
               Hopeless
   3. Communication pattern (subjective/objective)
           Content
               Appropriate
               Suspicions
               Denial of problem
               Delusions (grandeur, persecution)
               Suicidal thoughts ("I may as well be dead"; "I wish I were dead")
               Tangential/allusive
               Hopelessness ("It's hopeless; it's the end of the road")
               Negative cognitive set
               Rigidity of thought
               Overgeneralization
           Pattern of speech
               Appropriate   Ideas loosely connected
               Jumps from one topic to another Unable to see alternatives (tunnel
               Blocking of ideas   vision)
               Unable to come to a decision

Rate of speech
  Appropriate   Excessive
  Reduced   Pressured
Reaction of significant others
  Ignoring suicidal expressions
  Leaving or turning away following expression
  Anger at expressions
4. Activities of daily living
  Capable of caring for self
  Impaired ability to care for self
5. Nutritional status
  Weight (increased, decreased)   Appetite
6. Sleep–rest pattern
  Recent change   Early wakefulness
  Insomnia   Sleeps too much
7. Personal hygiene
  Cleanliness   Clothes (condition, appropriateness)
  Grooming
8. Motor activity
  Within normal limits
  Decreased   Increased
  Repetitive   Agitated
9. Evidence of self-harm
  Wrist slashes   Eye enucleation
  Burns on body   Gunshot wound
  Broken bones   Overdose

Outcome Criteria

The person will
• Not commit suicide
• State the desire to live
• Verbalize feelings of anger, loneliness, hopelessness
• Identify persons to contact if suicide thoughts occur
• Identify alternative coping mechanisms

Interventions

A. Assist the person in reducing his present risk for self-destruction
  1. Assess level of present risk (Table II-24).
    a. High
    b. Moderate
    c. Low
  2. Assess level of long-term risk.
    a. Life-style
    b. Lethality of plan
    c. Usual coping mechanisms
  3. Provide a safe environment based on level of risk.
    Immediate management for high-risk person
    a. Acutely suicidal people should be admitted to a closely supervised environment.
    b. Although it is impossible to create a completely safe environment, removal of dangerous objects and close observation convey a nonverbal message of concern to the individual. Restrict glass, nail files, scissors, nail polish remover, mirrors, needles,

Table II-24 **Assessing the Degree of Suicidal Risk**

		Intensity of Risk	
Behavior or Symptom	Low	Moderate	High
Anxiety	Mild	Moderate	High, or panic state
Depression	Mild	Moderate	Severe
Isolation/withdrawal	Some feelings of isolation, no withdrawal	Some feelings of hopelessness, and withdrawal	Hopeless, withdrawn, and self-deprecating, isolation
Daily functioning	Effective Good grades in school* Close friends No prior suicide attempt Stable job	Moody Variable grades* Some friends Prior suicidal thoughts	Depressed Poor grades* Few or not close friends Prior suicide attempts Erratic or poor work history
Life-style	Stable	Moderately stable	Unstable
Alcohol/drug use	Infrequently to excess	Frequently to excess	Continual abuse
Previous suicide attempts	None or of low lethality (few pills)	One or more (pills, superficial wrist slash)	One or more (entire bottle of pills, gun, hanging)
Associated events	None, or an argument	Disciplinary action* Failing grades* Work problems Family illness	Relationship breakup Death of a loved one Loss of job Pregnancy*
Purpose of act	None, or not clear	Relief of shame or guilt To punish others To get attention	Wants to die Escape to join deceased Debilitating disease
Family's reaction and structure	Supportive Intact family Good coping and mental health No history of suicide	Mixed reaction Divorced/separated Usually copes and understands	Angry and unsupportive Disorganized Rigid/abusive Prior history of suicide in family
Suicide plan (method, location, time)	No plan	Frequent thoughts, occasional ideas about a plan	Specific plan

* Applies only to children and adolescents
(Adapted from Hatton, C. L., & McBride, S. (1984). *Suicide: Assessment and intervention.* Norwalk, CT: Appleton-Century-Crofts; and Jackson, D. B., & Saunders, R. B. (1993). *Child health nursing.* Philadelphia: Lippincott-Raven Publishers.)

    razors, soda cans, plastic bags, lighters, electric equipment, belts, hangers, knives, tweezers, alcohol, guns.

  c. Meals should be provided in a closely supervised area, usually on the unit or in individual's own room.

      Ensure adequate food and fluid intake.

      Use paper/plastic plates and utensils.

      Check to be sure all items are returned on the tray.

  d. When administering oral medications, check to ensure that all medications are swallowed.

  e. Designate a staff member to provide checks on the person as designated by institution's policy. Provide relief for the staff member.

  f. Restrict the individual to the unit unless specifically ordered by physician. When off unit, provide a staff member to accompany the person.

  g. Instruct visitors on restricted items. Ensure that they do not give the person food in a plastic bag, for example.

  h. Restricted items may be used by individual in presence of staff, depending on level of risk. Acutely suicidal people should not be allowed access to such items.

  i. The acutely suicidal person may be required to wear a hospital gown to prevent elopement. As risk decreases, client may be allowed own clothing.

  j. Room searches should be done periodically according to institution policy.

  k. Use seclusion and restraint if necessary (refer to *Risk for Violence* for discussion).

  l. Notify police if the person elopes and is at risk for suicide.

  m. When the individual is being constantly observed, he is not to be allowed out of sight, even though privacy is lost.

4. Notify all staff that this person is at risk for self-harm.

  a. Use both written and oral communication.

5. Make a no-suicide contract with the individual (include family if person is at home).

  a. Use a written contract.

  b. Mutual agreement

    "I will not kill myself" or "I will not accidentally or intentionally take medicine except according to instructions." "I will talk to a staff member about my thoughts when suicidal ideas increase."

B. Help build self-esteem

1. Be nonjudgmental and empathetic.
2. Be aware of own reactions to the situation.
3. Provide genuine praise.
4. Encourage interactions with others.
5. Divert attention to external world (*e.g.*, odd jobs).
6. Convey sense that he is not alone (use group or peer therapy).
7. Seek out person for interactions.
8. Set limits by informing of rules.
9. Use firm, consistent approach.
10. Provide planned daily schedules to people with low impulse control.

C. Assist in identifying and contacting support system

1. Inform family and significant others.
2. Enlist support.
3. Do not provide false reassurance that behavior will not recur.
4. Point out vague or unclear messages from individual or support system.
5. Encourage an increase in social activity.

D. Assist individual in developing positive coping mechanisms

1. Refer to *Anxiety, Ineffective Individual Coping*, and *Hopelessness* for further interventions.
2. Encourage appropriate expression of anger and hostility.

    3. Set limits on ruminations about suicide or previous attempts.

    4. Assist in recognizing predisposing factors: "What was happening before you started having these thoughts?"

    5. Facilitate examination of life stresses and past coping mechanisms.

    6. Explore alternative behaviors.

    7. Anticipate future stresses and assist in planning alternatives.

    8. Use appropriate behavior modification techniques for noncompliant, resistive people.

    9. Help identify negative thinking patterns and direct person to practice altering these patterns.

    10. Involve person in planning the treatment goals and evaluating progress.

E. **Initiate health teaching and referrals, when indicated**

    1. Provide teaching that prepares person to deal with life stresses (relaxation, problem-solving skills, how to express feelings constructively).

    2. Refer for peer or group therapy.

    3. Refer for family therapy, especially when child or adolescent is involved.

    4. Teach family limit-setting techniques.

    5. Teach family constructive expression of feelings.

    6. Instruct significant others in how to recognize an increase in risk: change in behavior, verbal or nonverbal communication, withdrawal, signs of depression.

    7. Supply phone number of 24-hour emergency hotlines.

    8. Refer to vocational training if appropriate.

    9. Refer to halfway houses or other agencies, as appropriate.

    10. Refer to ongoing psychiatric follow-up.

    11. Refer to senior citizen centers or other agencies to increase leisure time activities.

    12. Initiate referral for family intervention after a completed suicide.

Rationale

- Suicidal behavior can be assessed by evaluating biologic, psychological, cognitive, and environmental risk factors, suicidal ideation, and precipitating events (Stillion & McDowell, 1991).
- Suicidal individuals are usually ambivalent about the decision. Staff can work with the positive goals to effect a change in attitude (Shneidman, 1989).
- To assess more accurately the risk for suicide, the caregiver must question the person directly. Ask simple, straightforward questions. The more specific, more lethal, and more available the means, the higher is the present risk. The most lethal methods in our culture are shooting and hanging. The least lethal is wrist-slashing.
- Interventions are based on the type of risk the person presents. Long-term treatment is often more difficult to institute than emergency care.
- Caregivers can become immobilized or drained by the acutely suicidal person. Feelings of hopelessness are often communicated to the caregiver (Gibbs, 1990).
- Making a contract with the individual
  - Gets the subject out in the open
  - Conveys the attitude of acceptance of the person as a worthwhile individual
  - Presents element of choice, the possibility and importance of thinking through situations before acting
  - Provides individual with a degree of control as he shares responsibility for own safety

❊ Interventions—*Child Focus*

1. Take all suicide threats seriously.

2. Assume that the child understands the finality of death (*e.g.*, "What does it mean to die?"; "Have you ever seen a dead animal on the road? Can it get up and run?").

3. Engage parents, friends, school personnel, and the individual in behavior contracts to "keep safe."

4. Explore feelings and reason for suicidal feelings.

5. Consult with a psychiatric expert regarding the most appropriate environment for treatment.
6. Participate in programs in school to teach about the symptoms of depression and signs of suicidal behavior.
7. With adolescents, explore (Johnson, 1993; Wilson & Kneish, 1996):
   a. Family problems
   b. Mental status
   c. Strength of support systems
   d. Disruption of friendship or romantic alliance
   e. The seriousness of the attempt
   f. Presence of performance failure (*e.g.*, examination, course).
   g. Recent or upcoming change (change of school, relocation).
8. Convey empathy regarding problems and/or losses.
9. Be alert for symptoms of a masked depression (*e.g.*, boredom, restlessness, irritability, difficulty concentrating, somatic preoccupation, excessive dependence on or isolation from others, especially adults) (Johnson, 1993).

Rationale

- "All threats or gestures to hurt oneself must be taken seriously regardless of the child's developmental age" (Johnson, 1995, p. 259).
- Treatment strategies depend on child's living situation, psychiatric history, and support system available (Johnson, 1995).
- Parents, friends, and school personnel should be enlisted to help.
- Suicidal threats and ideation signal a crisis that requires specific care (Johnson, 1995).
- Suicide attempts or threats may not represent a true desire to die, but it definitely represent a cry for help (Johnson, 1995).
- Children who attempt suicide may have a marked depression (Wilson & Kneish, 1996).
- Certain stressors are especially significant for adolescents who are developmentally preoccupied with status, peers, and appearances (Wilson & Kneish, 1996).

References/Bibliography

Andrews, M., & Boyle, J. (1995). *Transcultural concepts in nursing care* (2nd ed.). Philadelphia: J. B. Lippincott.

Blazer, D. G. (1982). *Depression in late life*. St. Louis: C. V. Mosby.

Boxwell, A. (1988). Geriatric suicide, the preventable death. *Nurse Practitioner, 13*(6), 10–14.

Carscadden, J. S. (1993a). *On the cutting edge: A guide for working with people who self injure*. London, Ontario: London Psychiatric Hospital.

Carscadden, J. S. (1993b). *Above the cutting edge: A workbook for people who want to stop self injury*. London, Ontario: London Psychiatric Hospital.

Fekar, C. R., & Koslap-Petraco, M. (1991). What about gay teenagers? (letter). *American Journal of Diseases of Children, 145*, 252.

Gibbs, A. (1990). Aspects of communication with people who have attempted suicide. *Journal of Advanced Nursing, 15,* 1245–1249.

Giger, J. N., & Davidhizar, R. E. (1995). *Transcultural nursing: Assessment and interventions* (2nd ed.). St. Louis: Mosby–Year Book.

Hatton, C., & Valente, S. (1977). Assessment of suicidal risk. In C. Hatton (Ed.). *Suicide: Assessment and intervention*. New York: Appleton-Century-Crofts.

Jacobs, D. (1989). Evaluation and care of suicidal behavior in emergency settings. In D. Jacobs &

H. Brown (Eds.). *Suicide: Understanding and responding*. Madison, CT: International University Press.

Johnson, B. S. (1993). *Psychiatric–mental health nursing* (3rd ed.). Philadelphia: J. B. Lippincott.

Johnson, B. S. (1995). *Child, adolescent and family psychiatric nursing*. Philadelphia: J. B. Lippincott.

Maltsberger, J. (1986). *Suicide risk*. New York: University Press.

Mellick, E., Buckwalter, & Stolley (1992). Suicide among elderly white men: Development of a profile. *Journal of Psychosocial Nursing, 30*(2), 29–34.

McIntosh, J. L. (1985). Suicide among the elderly: Levels and trends. *American Journal of Orthopsychiatry, 55*(4), 288–293.

Miller, C. A. (1995). *Nursing care of older adults* (2nd ed.). Glenview, IL: Scott, Foresman.

Modestin, J., & Kopp, N. (1988). A study of clinical suicide. *Journal of Nervous and Mental Disease, 176,* 668–673.

Pallikkathayil, L., & Flood, M. (1991). Adolescent suicide. *Nursing Clinics of North America, 26,* 623–630.

Shneidman, E. (1989). Overview: A multidimensional approach to suicide. In D. Jacobs & H. Brown (Eds.). *Suicide: Understanding and responding.* Madison, CT: International University Press.

Stillion, J., & McDowell, E. (1991). Examining suicide from a life span perspective. *Death Studies, 15*, 327–354.

Stuart, G. W., & Sundeen, S. J. (1995). *Principles and practice of psychiatric nursing* (5th ed.). St. Louis: Mosby–Year Book.

U.S. Bureau of the Census. (1984). *Statistical abstracts of the United States: 1985* (105th ed.). Washington, DC: Government Printing Office.

Wilson, H. S., & Kneish, C. R. (1996). *Psychiatric nursing* (5th ed.). Redwood, CA: Addison-Wesley Nursing.

Sensory–Perceptual Alterations

DEFINITION

Sensory–Perceptual Alterations: A state in which the individual/group experiences or is at risk of experiencing a change in the amount, pattern, or interpretation of incoming stimuli.

DEFINING CHARACTERISTICS
Major (Must Be Present)

Inaccurate interpretation of environmental stimuli and/or negative change in amount or pattern of incoming stimuli

Minor (May Be Present)

Disoriented in time or place
Disoriented about people
Altered ability to problem-solve
Altered behavior or communication pattern
Restlessness
Reports auditory or visual hallucinations
Fear
Anxiety
Apathy
Irritability

RELATED FACTORS

Many factors in an individual's life can contribute to sensory–perceptual alterations. Some common factors are listed below.

Pathophysiologic (Sensory Organ Alterations)

Related to misinterpretations secondary to:
  (Sensory organ alterations)
    Visual, gustatory, auditory, olfactory, and tactile deficits
  (Neurological alterations)

Cerebrovascular accident (CVA)	Neuropathies
Encephalitis meningitis	Tumors

  (Metabolic alterations)

Fluid and electrolyte imbalance	Acidosis
Renal failure	Alkalosis

(Impaired oxygen transport)
  Cerebral
  Cardiac
  Respiratory
  Anemia
Related to mobility restrictions secondary to:
Paraplegia
Quadriplegia

Treatment-Related

Related to chemical changes secondary to:
  Medications (*e.g.*, sedatives, tranquilizers, steroids, anticonvulsants, antihistamines, cardiac glycosides, anticholinergics)
  Surgery (*e.g.*, glaucoma, cataract, detached retina)
Related to physical isolation (*e.g.*, reverse isolation, communicable disease, prison)
Related to immobility
Related to mobility restrictions (*e.g.*, bed rest, traction, casts, Stryker frame, CircOlectric bed)

Situational (Personal, Environmental)

Related to
  Pain
  Stress
  Sleep interpretations
Related to environmental barriers
  Noise
  Lights
  Lack of privacy
  Constant changes
  Excess activity
  Frequent demands
  Unfamiliar
Related to monotonous environment
Related to loss of socialization
Related to loss of control

Author's Note

Sensory–Perceptual Alterations describes a person with altered perception and cognition influenced by physiologic factors (*e.g.*, pain, sleep deprivation, immobility, or excessive or decreased meaningful environmental stimuli). Keep in mind that the diagnosis *Altered Thought Processes* also can manifest with altered perception and cognition. To differentiate between the two diagnoses, remember that *Sensory–Perceptual Alterations* applies when barriers or factors interfere with a person's ability to interpret stimuli accurately; in contrast, when personality or mental disorders interfere with this ability, *Altered Thought Processes* would be a more accurate diagnosis.

The diagnosis *Sensory–Perceptual Alterations* encompasses six subcategories: *Visual, Auditory, Kinesthetic, Gustatory, Tactile*, and *Olfactory*. Use of these subcategories can pose some problems in clinical situations; for example, for a person with a visual deficit, how does the nurse intervene with a diagnosis such as *Sensory–Perceptual Alterations: Visual related to effects of glaucoma*? What would the outcome criteria be? The nurse should assess for the individual's response to the visual loss and specifically label the response, not the deficit.

Sensory–Perceptual Alterations is more clinically useful without the addition of the sensory deficit. Examples of responses to sensory deficits may be:

Visual:	*Risk for Injury*
	Self-Care Deficit
Auditory:	*Impaired Communication*
	Social Isolation
Kinesthetic:	*Risk for Injury*
Olfactory:	*Altered Nutrition*
Tactile:	*Risk for Injury*
Gustatory:	*Altered Nutrition*

Errors in Diagnostic Statements

Sensory–Perceptual Alterations related to impairment of sensory tracts secondary to spinal cord injury

   A person suffering spinal cord injury experiences several responses related to loss of sensation, which can be described and addressed by diagnoses such as *Risk for Injury, Diversional Activity Deficit*, and *Sensory–Perceptual Alterations*. If the nursing focus is to increase meaningful sensory input because of loss of sensation, immobility, and position restrictions, the diagnosis should be recorded as *Sensory–Perceptual Alterations related to decreased visual field when prone and inadequate tactile stimulation.*

Sensory–Perceptual Alterations: Visual related to altered sensory reception

   Visual deficits can contribute to a variety of responses, including fear, high risk for injury, self-care deficits, and sensory deprivation. Using *Sensory–Perceptual Alterations* to rename a visual or hearing deficit fails to clarify a problem that the nurse can treat.

Key Concepts

1. "Perception is the process of integrating, classifying, discriminating, and assigning meaning to stimuli. The individual is oriented to surroundings through the ability to receive and organize information. Stimuli are gathered through sensory receptors" (Drury & Akins, 1991, p. 369).
2. Any situation or condition that compromises a person's senses—sight, hearing, olfactory, tactile, taste, or kinesthesia—or one's ability to interpret can cause sensory–perceptual alterations (Drury & Akins, 1991).
3. "Behavioral characteristics of sensory–perceptual alterations develop suddenly, over 1–2 days of hospitalization, and usually last only hours to several weeks" (Wilson, 1993, p. 751). The number and severity of the behavioral manifestations may vary from mild disorientation to frank psychoses (Wilson, 1993).
4. Manifestations of sensory–perceptual alterations may be continuous or have a diurnal pattern. For example, certain behaviors may occur only at night (Wilson, 1993).
5. Changes in a person's sensory perception affect his ability to interface with his environment (Drury & Akins, 1991).
6. All individuals attempt to control the degree and variety of stimuli to a level that is comfortable for them (Drury & Akins, 1991).
7. Individuals need to experience change, complexity, and stimulus to (Drury & Akins, 1991)
   a. Maintain the functions of attention, concentration, arousal, and consciousness
   b. Maintain internalized order and reality
   c. Promote cognitive activity and socialization
8. Immobility reduces the quality and quantity of sensory information available to the person. In addition, the person has reduced ability to interact with the environment (Porth, 1994).
9. Immobility in an acute care setting also exposes the person to sensory overload with repetitive and meaningless sounds (*e.g.*, intercoms, monitors, hospital personnel) (Porth, 1994).
10. Sensory overload produces the problem of sensory bombardment and also blocks out meaningful stimuli, thus concurrently producing sensory deprivation.

11. A disruption in the quality or quantity of incoming stimuli can affect an individual's physiologic, emotional, cognitive, and affective domains.
12. An illness state may decrease the efficiency of the sensory organs and thus alter a person's capacity for adequate reception and perception of information.
13. Refer to Key Concepts for *Altered Thought Processes* for additional information.

🌀 *Key Concepts*—*Child*

1. The newborn has well-developed sensory abilities that have an important effect on growth and development (Wong, 1995):
    a. Newborns demonstrate discrimination between patterns, sizes, and shapes, but lack accommodation to distance.
    b. Newborns respond to sound stimuli by alerting, crying, and the startle reaction.
    c. Newborns differentiate between bitter and sweet taste.
    d. Newborns perceive tactile stimulation, particularly on the face (Anderson, 1989; Wong, 1995).
2. Piaget calls the first 2 years of life the sensorimotor period. This period is characterized by integration and organization of information derived through sensorimotor experiences (Scipien, Chard, Howe, & Barnard, 1990).
3. Children with sensory–perceptual alterations have the same basic needs as other children. However, their experiences must be adapted to promote optimal development (Hunsberger, 1989).

🏛 *Key Concepts*—*Older Adult*

1. Older adults need more time to process visual information when in unfamiliar situations; they also need more light to identify and process the input, and take longer to respond to changes in illumination (Miller, 1995).
2. Insufficient time to process auditory and visual input can lead to sensory overload.
3. Older adults are more prone to development of sensory deprivation because of loneliness, physical isolation, and the increased incidence of chronic disabilities experienced during this life stage.
4. There is a fourfold increase in the incidence of sensory–perceptual alteration after the age of 40 years, with the highest occurrence among people older than 70 years of age (Lipowski, 1990).
5. Wilson (1993) reported that the overall incidence of sensory perceptual alterations in hospitalized elderly varied from 24% to 80%.

Focus Assessment Criteria

Subjective Data

A. Assess for defining characteristics
    1. History of symptoms
        a. The person reports

Difficulty concentrating	Fatigue or irritability
Anxiety	Unusual sensations

        b. Onset and description

Precipitated by?	Frequency?
Relieved by?	

B. Assess for related factors
    1. Recent surgery
    2. Recent hospitalization
    3. Neurologic impairment
    4. Sensory organ deficit
    5. Change in biorhythm pattern
    6. Mobility restrictions
    7. Social isolation

8. Substance abuse (drugs, alcohol)
9. Medications

Objective Data

A. Assess for related factors

1. Sensory acuity
   a. Visual
      Snellen chart
      Newspaper clippings and large lettered index cards
      Aids (contact lenses, glasses)
   b. Auditory
      Observation of client during normal conversation
      Use of hearing aids
   c. Tactile
      Thermal sensation   Sensitivity
   d. Olfactory/gustatory
2. Miscellaneous
   Sensory deprivation (isolation, lack of visitors)
   Sensory overload (noise, personnel)
   Physiologic alterations
   Medication (side effects, toxic levels)
   Sleep deprivation
   Fluid, electrolyte, nutritional imbalances
   Crisis, fears, losses

Subjective/Objective Data

A. Assess risk level

1. Refer to Table II-25.
2. Because all individuals in certain environments are at risk for sensory–perceptual alterations, the tool shown in Table II-25 identifies which individuals are at high risk. The higher the score, the higher the risk (Wilson, 1993).

Outcome Criteria

The person will
- Demonstrate decreased symptoms of sensory overload, as evidenced by (specify)
- Identify and eliminate the potential risk factors, if possible
- Describe the rationale for the treatment modality

Interventions

A. Identify high-risk individuals

See Focus Assessment Criteria

B. Reduce or eliminate causative and contributing factors, when possible

1. Excessive noise or light
   a. Cover nonessential blinking lights at bedside with tape.
   b. Dim lights at night.
   c. Encourage use of blindfolds.
   d. Decrease noise output.
      Shut off nonessential alarms.
      Encourage use of earplugs.
      If possible, limit the use of flasher and the like during sleep hours.

Table II-25 **Sensory–Perceptual Alteration Risk Assessment Tool**

Prehospital Status	*Current Status*

Prehospital Status

A. Age greater than 80   Score A. ☐
☐ No = 0 ☐ Yes = 1

B. Gender   Score B. ☐
☐ 0 = female ☐ 1 = male

C. Documented history of cognitive impairment
☐ 0 = no impairment   Score C. ☐
☐ 1 = impaired

D. Auditory function   Score D. ☐
☐ 0 = no impairment
☐ 1 = using corrective aid or assist device
☐ 3 = not using corrective aid or assist device
Acute change—auditory ☐ No = 0 Yes = 1

E. Vision   Score E. ☐
☐ 0 = no impairment
☐ 1 = using corrective aid or assist device
☐ 3 = not using corrective aid or assist device
Acute change—vision ☐ No = 0 ☐ Yes = 1

F. Verbal ability   Score F. ☐
☐ 0 = no impairment
☐ 1 = using corrective aid or assist device
☐ 3 = not using corrective aid or assist device
Acute change—verbal ☐ No = 0 ☐ Yes = 1

G. Self-care ability   Score G. ☐
☐ 0 = independent
☐ 1 = requires the assistance of another
     person
Acute change—self-care
☐ No = 0 ☐ Yes = 1

H. Mobility   Score H. ☐
☐ 0 = independent
☐ 1 = requires assist device
☐ 2 = requires human assistance
Acute change—mobility
☐ No = 0 ☐ Yes = 1

I. Fracture on admission   Score I. ☐
☐ No = 0 ☐ Yes = 1

J. Elimination pattern   Score J. ☐
☐ 0 = normal or independent
☐ 1 = uncontrolled, incontinent, dependent
Acute change—elimination pattern
☐ No = 0 ☐ Yes = 1

Current Status

A. Admission priority   Score A. ☐
☐ 1 = elective ☐ 2 = emergent or urgent

B. Predisposition   Score B. ☐
☐ 0 = home ☐ 1 = institutional setting

C. Cognitive status rating   Score C. ☐
☐ 0 = SPMSQ* score 0–2
     or intact cognitive function per assessment
☐ 1 = SPMSQ score 3–10
     or impaired cognitive function per
     assessment
SPMSQ Score ☐

D. Chemical agent variations   Score D. ☐
1. # chemicals before hospitalization (BH) ☐
2. # of chemicals BH that are current   ☐
3. Difference 1 and 2   ☐
4. # new chemicals since admission   ☐
5. Receiving narcotics
   ☐ No = 0 ☐ Yes = 1   ☐
6. Receiving neuroleptics
   ☐ No = 0 ☐ Yes = 1   ☐

E. Blood chemistry   Score E. ☐
☐ 0 = within normal limits
☐ 1 = lab values out of normal range

F. Symptomatic infection   Score F. ☐
☐ No = 0 ☐ Yes = 1

G. Pain   Score G. ☐
☐ 0 = no pain
☐ 1 = controlled pain
     (rated 1–3 on scale of 0–10)
☐ 2 = uncontrolled pain
     (rated 4 or greater on scale of 0–10)

H. Visitation by significant others   Score H. ☐
☐ 0 = continuous presence
☐ 1 = significant others visit 2–3 times a day
☐ 2 = Less than two visits per day

I. Room type   Score I. ☐
☐ 0 = Window with view to outdoors
     and exposure to light changes
☐ 1 = Window with view into unit
     or outdoors walls or buildings
☐ 2 = No windows

Add the Prehospitalization and Current Status risk factor scores. Grand total risk score ☐

* SPMSQ = Short Portable Mental Status Questionnaire.
  Lisa D. Brodersen, Copyright 1993 Revised 2/1/95. Used with author's permission. Cardio MAC Iowa Health Institute, Des Moines IA.

Turn off unnecessary equipment.

Position person away from direct source of noise, if possible.

Curtail nonessential personnel conversation.

Avoid loud noises.

Discourage television after 10 P.M.

e. Share with person the source of the noise.

f. Discuss the use of a radio with earplugs to provide soft, relaxing music.

g. Share with personnel the need to reduce noise and provide individuals with uninterrupted sleep of at least 2 to 4 hours' duration.

h. Discuss the advantages of turning hearing aid off during high noise times.

2. Unfamiliar environment

a. Attempt to reduce fears and concerns by explaining equipment, its purpose, and noises.

b. Encourage person to share his perceptions of noises.

c. Enlist the aid of an interpreter to explain the environment to person who does not speak English.

C. Promote reorientation

1. Orient to all three spheres (person, place, time).

a. Address person by name.

b. Introduce yourself frequently.

c. Identify the place.

d. Identify the time.

"Good morning, Mr. Jones. I am Mary Smith. I will be your nurse today."

"Where are you, Mr. Jones? You are in the hospital."

"Today is May sixth and it is eight-thirty in the morning."

2. Explain all activities.

a. Offer simple explanations of each task.

b. Provide subjective and objective descriptions of sensations that will be experienced.

c. Allow person to handle equipment related to the task.

d. Allow him to participate in task, such as washing his face.

e. Acknowledge when you leave and when you will return.

D. Promote movement

1. Encourage to remain out of bed as much as possible (eat meals in chair).

2. Teach to perform isometric and isotonic exercises when in bed.

3. Encourage to change his position frequently, even if it is just lifting one side off a surface by rolling slightly.

4. To encourage walking, choose a destination to reach or give the walk a purpose (walking to the lounge for breakfast).

E. Use measures to prevent injury

1. Keep side rails in place and bed in lowest position.

2. Place call bell in convenient location.

3. Refer to *Risk for Injury* for additional interventions.

F. Assist person to differentiate reality from fantasy

1. Refer to *Altered Thought Processes related to inability to evaluate reality* for additional interventions.

Rationale

- Promoting regular and varied sensory stimulation can help prevent alterations from prolonged sensory deprivation.
- "Care givers should be aware that their actions and activity patterns may add to the environmental chaos or become a positive contribution to the therapeutic milieu" (Drury & Akins, 1991, p. 379).

- The quality and quantity of sensory input are reduced by immobility or confinement.
- Explaining what sensory stimuli the person will experience before the experience reduces distress, tension, and confusion (Christman & Kirckhoff, 1992).
- Wearing hearing aids in an excessively noisy environment (*e.g.*, clinic, intensive care unit) also can cause sensory overload.

References/Bibliography

Anderson, J. J. (1989). Development and adaptations of the family with an infant. In R. L. Foster, M. M. Hunsberger, & J. J. T. Anderson (Eds.). *Family-centered nursing care of children*. Philadelphia: W. B. Saunders.

Christman, N., & Kirckhoff, K. (1992). Preparatory sensory information. In G. Bulechek & J. McCloskey (Eds.). *Nursing interventions: Essential nursing treatments*. Philadelphia: W. B. Saunders.

Drury, J., & Akins, J. (1991). Sensory–perceptual alterations. In M. Maas, K. Buckwalter, & M. Hardy (Eds.). *Nursing diagnoses and interventions for the elderly*. Menlo Park, CA: Addison-Wesley Nursing.

Hunsberger, M. (1989). Nursing strategies: Sensory and communication alterations. In R. L. Foster, M. M. Hunsberger, & J. J. T. Anderson (Eds.). *Family-centered nursing care of children*, Philadelphia: W. B. Saunders.

Liposwski, Z. (1990). *Delirium: Acute confusional states*. New York, Oxford University Press. As reported in Wilson, L. D. (1993). Sensory perceptual alteration: Diagnosis, prediction and intervention in the hospitalized adult. *Nursing Clinics of North America, 28*, 747–765.

Miller, C. A. (1995). *Nursing care of the older adult* (2nd ed.). Philadelphia: J. B. Lippincott.

Porth, C. (1994) *Pathophysiology: Concepts of altered health status* (4th ed.). Philadelphia: J. B. Lippincott.

Scipien, G. M., Chard, M. A., Howe, J., & Barnard, M. U. (1990). *Pediatric nursing care*. St. Louis: C. V. Mosby.

Wilson, L. D. (1993). Sensory perceptual alteration: Diagnosis, prediction and intervention in the hospitalized adult. *Nursing Clinics of North America, 28*, 747–765.

Wong, D. L. (1995). *Nursing care of infants and children* (5th ed.). St. Louis: Mosby–Year Book.

Sexuality Patterns, Altered

Sexual Dysfunction

Sexuality Patterns, Altered

DEFINITION
Altered Sexuality Patterns: The state in which an individual experiences or is at risk of experiencing a change in sexual behaviors or sexual health.

DEFINING CHARACTERISTICS
Major (Must Be Present)
Actual or anticipated negative changes in sexual behaviors, sexual health, sexual functioning, or sexual identity

Minor (May Be Present)
Expression of concern about sexual behaviors, health, functioning, or sexual identity
Inappropriate sexual verbal or nonverbal behavior
Changes in primary and/or secondary sexual characteristics

RELATED FACTORS
Altered sexual patterns can occur as a response to various health problems, situations, and conflicts. Some common sources are listed.

Pathophysiologic
Related to biochemical effects on energy, libido secondary to:
  (Endocrine)
    Diabetes mellitus   Hyperthyroidism
    Decreased hormone production Addison's disease
    Myxedema   Acromegaly
  (Genitourinary)
    Chronic renal failure
  (Neuromuscular and skeletal)
    Arthritis   Amyotrophic lateral sclerosis
    Multiple sclerosis
    Disturbances of the nerve supply to the brain, spinal cord, sensory nerves, or autonomic nerves
  (Cardiorespiratory)
    Peripheral vascular disorders   Chronic respiratory disorders
    Myocardial infarction   Congestive heart failure
  (Cancer)
Related to fears associated with (specify) (sexually transmitted diseases [STDs])
  HIV/AIDS   Human papilloma virus
  Herpes   Chlamydia
  Syphilis   Gonorrhea
Related to effects of alcohol on performance

Related to decreased vaginal lubrication secondary to (specify)
Related to fear of premature ejaculation
Related to (specify) phobia (*e.g.*, pregnancy, cancer, STD)

Treatment-Related

Related to effects of:
Medications (Table II-26)
Radiation therapy
Related to altered self-concept from change in appearance (trauma, radical surgery)

Table II-26   **Drugs That Alter Sexuality**

Drug	Effect on Sexuality
Alcohol	In small amounts, may increase libido and decrease sexual inhibitions In large amounts, impairs neural reflexes involved in erection and ejaculation Chronic use causes impotence and sterility in men; decreased desire and orgasmic dysfunction in women
Amyl nitrate	Peripheral vasodilator reputed to cause intensified orgasms when inhaled at time of orgasm May cause loss of erection, hypotension, and syncope
Antidepressants	Peripheral blockage of nervous innervation to sex organs Significant percentage of impotence and ejaculatory dysfunction
Antihistamines	Block parasympathetic nervous innervation of sex organs Sedative effect may decrease desire Decrease in vaginal lubrication
Antihypertensives	Libido may be decreased in both sexes Some antihypertensives cause impotence and ejaculatory problems in up to 50% of men
Antispasmodics	Inhibit parasympathetic innervation of sex organs May cause impotence
Chemotherapeutics	Combination therapy may cause azoospermia or oligospermia in men and temporary or permanent menopause in women; fertility may be temporarily or permanently altered; libido may be decreased and body image altered
Cocaine	Short-term use is reported to enhance sexual experience Chronic use causes loss of desire and sexual dysfunction in both sexes
Hormones	Estrogen suppresses sexual function in men Testosterone may increase libido in both sexes, but causes virilization in women Chronic use of anabolic steroids causes testicular atrophy, decreased testosterone, and decreased sperm production; may cause permanent sterility
Marijuana	May decrease sexual inhibitions Chronic use may cause decreased libido and impotence
Narcotics	Chronic use causes decreased libido in both sexes Testosterone levels and amount of semen decreased Erectile and ejaculatory dysfunction common
Oral contraceptives	Remove fear of pregnancy May cause decreased libido
Sedatives/tranquilizers	Initially and in low doses may enhance sexual pleasure due to relaxation and decrease of inhibitions Long-term use decreases libido and may cause orgasmic dysfunction and impotence

Situational (Personal, Environmental)

Related to partner problem (specify)

Unwilling	Not available
Uninformed	Abusive
Separated, divorced	

Related to no privacy

Related to stressors secondary to:

Job problems	Value conflicts
Financial worries	Relationship conflicts

Related to misinformation or lack of knowledge

Related to fatigue

Related to fear of rejection secondary to obesity

Related to pain

Related to fear of sexual failure

Related to fear of pregnancy

Related to depression

Related to anxiety

Related to guilt

Related to fear of STDs

Related to history of unsatisfactory sexual experiences

Maturational

Adolescent

Related to ineffective role models

Related to negative sexual teaching

Related to absence of sexual teaching

Adult

Related to adjustment to parenthood

Related to menopause

Related to values conflict

Related to effects of pregnancy on energy levels and body image

Related to effects of aging on energy levels and body image

Author's Note

The diagnoses *Altered Sexuality Patterns* and *Sexuality Dysfunction* are difficult to differentiate. *Altered Sexuality Patterns* represents a broad diagnosis, of which sexual dysfunction can be one part. *Sexual Dysfunction* may be used most appropriately by a nurse with advanced preparation in sex therapy. Until *Sexual Dysfunction* is well differentiated from *Altered Sexuality Patterns*, it should not be used by most nurses.

Errors in Diagnostic Statements

Altered Sexuality Patterns related to reports of absent libido

Report of absent libido represents a symptom of *Altered Sexuality Patterns*, not a "related to" statement. If further assessment revealed the person's dissatisfaction with present sexual patterns, the nurse could record the diagnosis *Altered Sexuality Patterns related to unknown etiology, as evidenced by reports of absent libido*. The use of "unknown etiology" in this diagnostic statement prompts focus assessments to determine contributing factors (*e.g.*, stress, medication side effects).

Sexual Dysfunction related to impotence secondary to spinal cord injury

How would the nurse treat this diagnosis? A nurse planning to explore feelings and provide information and referrals would not be treating sexual dysfunction. Instead, the nursing focus would be best described in the diagnosis *Anxiety related to effects of spinal cord injury on sexual function and insufficient knowledge of causes and community resources available.*

Key Concepts

1. Sexual health is the integration of somatic, emotional, intellectual, and social aspects of sexual being in ways that are enriching and that enhance personality, communication, and love (World Health Organization [WHO], 1975).
2. Sexual behaviors are the behaviors an individual uses to communicate feelings and attitudes about sexuality to others. They include behaviors used in release of sexual tension, either alone or with another person to attain sexual satisfaction, or for procreation (Wilmoth, 1993).
3. All people are sexual beings. Sexuality is an integral part of identity (WHO, 1975).
4. Sexuality encompasses how a person feels about himself or herself and how a person interacts with others.
5. Sexual function refers to psychological and physiologic ability to perform in a sexually satisfying manner, with or without a partner.
6. Sexuality and sexual function are influenced by age, marital and/or relationship status, sexual orientation, personal value system, sexual knowledge, resources (social, economic, geographic), culture, physical health, and emotional health (Katzun, 1992; Smith, 1993).
7. Research shows that many individuals with a serious illness experience decreased sexual desire, decreased frequency of sexual activity, and/or decreased satisfaction with sexual function (Fitzsimmons, Verderber, & Shively, 1993; Thranov & Klee, 1994).
8. The characteristics of a sexually healthy person are (Lion, 1982):
   a. A positive body image despite the body's packaging
   b. Acceptance of sexual and body functions as normal and natural
   c. Accurate knowledge about human sexuality and sexual functioning
   d. Recognition and acceptance of own sexual feelings
   e. Effective interpersonal relationships
   f. Acceptance of mistakes/imperfections in self and others
9. Sexuality is not restricted solely to the young and healthy.
10. Sexual expression is not limited to sexual intercourse; it includes closeness and touch, as well as other forms of verbal and nonverbal communication (Steinke & Bergen 1986).
11. Individuals must have the opportunity to make their own educated decisions regarding sexuality and sexual expression. Individuals decide what is comfortable in expression of their sexuality (Sanford, 1989).

The Nurse's Role in Discussing Sexuality

1. Sexuality is as important as other aspects of human health and should be incorporated into nursing assessments and other aspects of nursing care (Smith, 1993; Wilmoth, 1994b; Woods, 1984).
2. The nurse must become educated regarding sexuality and sexual health through the life span. It is important for the nurse to examine her own beliefs and feelings concerning sexuality, sexual function, and what is considered sexually normal and abnormal.
3. Many nurses have difficulty providing care in the area of sexuality and do not address sexual concerns unless the client asks specific questions. Research indicates, however, that many clients wish nurses and other health care professionals would *initiate* discussion of sexuality (Krueger, Hassell, Goggins, Ishimatsu, Pablico, & Tuttle, 1979; Matocha & Waterhouse, 1993; Waterhouse, 1993).
4. The PLISSIT model (Annon, 1976) is helpful for the nurse generalist providing care in the area of sexuality:
   a. **Permission:** Convey to the person and significant others a willingness to discuss sexual thoughts and feelings (*e.g.*, "Some people with your diagnosis have concerns about how their illness will affect their sexual functioning. Is this a concern for you or your partner?").
   b. **Limited Information:** Provide the person and significant other with information on the effects certain situations (*e.g.*, pregnancy), conditions (*e.g.*, cancer), and treatments (*e.g.*, medications) can have on sexuality and sexual function.
   c. **Specific Suggestions:** Provide specific instructions that can facilitate positive sexual functioning (*e.g.*, changes in coital positions).

d. **Intensive Therapy:** Refer people who need more help to an appropriate health care professional (*e.g.*, sex therapist, surgeon).

5. Giving a person "permission" to discuss sexual concerns is by far the most important aspect of nursing care in the area of sexuality. The nurse should give permission by:
   a. Including sexuality in the initial health history and addressing questions on sexuality in a manner similar to questions on bowel and bladder function. This helps the person see that nurses view sexuality as a routine part of human health.
   b. Offering to discuss sexual concerns at appropriate times during the client's hospitalization/visit (Wilmoth, 1994a).

6. The nurse should assure the person of the confidentiality of all data on sexuality and obtain permission from the person before making a referral for a sexual problem.

7. If a diagnosis of *Altered Sexuality Patterns* or *Sexual Dysfunction* is made, the diagnosis, goals, and general interventions should be marked on the care plan and the name of the nurse providing care for this diagnosis indicated. Details of the assessment and interactions should not be included on the chart to ensure confidentiality.

Contraception and Sexually Transmitted Diseases

1. Research has shown that use of mechanical barrier methods (condom, diaphragm, vaginal sponge, cervical cap) and/or chemical barriers containing nonoxynol-9 (foam, jelly, cream) are effective in reducing the transmission of HIV and other STDs (Hatcher et al., 1994).

2. Use of the intrauterine device, oral contraceptives, Norplant, Depo-provera, or sterilization provide *no* protection from STDs. Clients using these methods must be counseled to use a chemical or mechanical barrier method to protect themselves from disease.

💬 *Key Concepts—Child*

1. Sex role identification begins in infancy and is determined by adolescence.
   a. Infants are able to identify body parts by the end of the first year.
   b. Toddlers learn gender differentiation.
   c. Preschoolers frequently engage in masturbation and sex play with peers (*e.g.*, comparing genitals).
   d. School-agers continue to gain awareness about their sex role identity. Although masturbation and sex play are common in young school-agers, the older school-aged child becomes involved in purposeful sexual behavior (*e.g.*, hugging, kissing members of opposite sex) (Rew, 1989; Wong, 1995).
   e. Adolescents experience altered body image in response to the physical changes of puberty. The key developmental task of adolescence is identity formation, which is influenced by sexual maturation and assuming a sex role (Wong, 1995).

2. Parents are the primary force in sexuality education in a child's life. This includes what is not said as well as what is said (Gordon & Gordon, 1983).

3. Formal sex education, presented from a lifespan approach, is best offered during middle childhood. Topics should include information about sexual maturation and the process of reproduction (Wong, 1995).

4. Sexually transmitted diseases are a major cause of morbidity during adolescents and young adults. Ten million people younger than 25 years of age are afflicted (U.S. Department of Health and Human Services, 1993).

5. Risky behavior by adolescents and young adults increases their vulnerability to STDs, pelvic inflammatory disease, infertility, AIDS, and chronic incurable conditions such as hepatitis B virus (HBV) infection, human papilloma virus (HPV) infection, and genital herpes.

📖 *Key Concepts—Maternal*

1. Pregnant women have varying degrees of sexual desire during pregnancy.
   a. Some women are very sexually excitable.
   b. Some women are not very desirous of sex.
   c. Libido changes by large degrees during different stages of pregnancy.

    d. A woman's body image affects her sexuality. (If thinness is an attribute, then many pregnant women are confused about changing size.)

    e. A woman's attitude toward her body can influence her partner's sexual attraction toward her.

2. The postpartum period is a time of self-doubt. For the first 6 weeks, a new mother feels lost, overwhelmed, tired, depressed, ignorant, and isolated. Her self-esteem as well as her sexuality may suffer.

3. A new father may experience his own adjustments postnatally, which can be manifested by a lack of interest in sex. He may feel inadequate to care for the child and may experience jealousy of the closeness of mother and infant. He may be disturbed by the woman's postpartum body, and/or may view her as changed since she moved into the "mother" role (May, 1987).

🏛 *Key Concepts—Older Adult*

1. The elderly person is psychologically and physically capable of engaging in sexual activity regardless of changes in sexual anatomy and physiology due to aging.

2. Sexual activity is often beneficial for the elderly, reducing anxiety while providing intimacy and improving quality of life (Nay, 1992; Wallace, 1992).

3. Women experience decreased breast tone, thinning and loss of elasticity of the vaginal wall, decreased vaginal lubrication, and shortening of vaginal length due to the loss of circulating estrogen (Miller, 1995).

4. Men experience decreased production of spermatozoa, decreased ejaculatory force, and smaller, less firm testicles. Direct stimulation may be required to achieve an erection; however, the erection may be maintained for a longer time (Miller, 1995).

5. The need for intimacy and touch is especially important for the elderly, who may be experiencing diminishing meaningful relationships.

6. Past sexual function (enjoyment, interest, frequency) are predictors of sexual activity in the elderly. To be capable of sexual activity in old age, the individual must participate in sexual activity throughout life.

7. Adult children and caregivers commonly view sexual activities of older adults as "immoral, inappropriate and negative" (Convey, 1989).

8. The sexual functioning of older adults is most influenced by myths and misunderstanding. According to Miller (1995), "Because sex is so closely identified with youthfulness, the stereotype of sexless seniors is widely believed."

Medications and Sexuality

1. Drugs can influence sexual functioning positively and negatively (see Table II–26).

2. The person has the right to be educated about all medication side effects, including those affecting sexuality.

TRANSCULTURAL CONSIDERATIONS

1. People of some cultures are very hesitant to discuss sexuality (*e.g.*, Hispanic, American Indian).

2. Horn (1993) reports that black women view child-bearing as a validation of their femaleness. White teenage girls approve of prevention of pregnancy; Indian teenage girls value pregnancy (Horn, 1993).

3. Some cultures view the postpartum period as a state of impurity. Certain foods and practices are taboo (*e.g.*, intercourse). The woman may be secluded during the period of postpartum bleeding. Some cultures end the seclusion with a ritual bath (*e.g.*, Navajo, Hispanic, Orthodox Jewish) (Andrews & Boyle, 1995).

4. American Indian women "believe in the importance of monthly menstruation for maintaining harmony and physical well-being" (Andrews & Boyle, 1995, p. 113).

Focus Assessment Criteria

Guidelines for Taking a Sexual History (Woods, 1984)

1. Discuss sexuality in a private, relaxed setting to ensure confidentiality.
2. Do not judge the individual by your own beliefs/practices.
3. Permit the individual to refuse to answer.
4. Clarify vocabulary; use slang terms if needed to convey meaning.
5. Assess only those areas pertinent for this client at this time.
6. Strive to be open, warm, objective, unembarrassed, and reassuring.
7. Keep in mind that it is more appropriate to assume that the client has had some sexual experience than to assume none.
8. Several sessions may be necessary to complete the interview.

Subjective Data

A. Assess background

Age, sex, marital/relationship status	Religious and cultural background
Sexual orientation/preference	Job and financial status
Quality of relationship with significant other	Medical and surgical history
Communication patterns with significant others	Drug and alcohol use (present and
Number of children and siblings	past)

B. Assess for defining characteristics

1. How has your (health problem) affected your ability to function as a (wife/mother/partner/father/husband) (Wilmoth, 1994a)?
2. How has your (health problem) affected the way you feel about yourself as a (man/woman) (Wilmoth, 1994a)?
3. What aspects of your sexuality have been affected by your (health problem) (Wilmoth, 1994a)?
4. How has your (health problem) affected your ability to function sexually (Wilmoth, 1994a)?
5. Sexual function
   Usual pattern
   Present pattern
   Satisfaction (individual, partner)
   Erection problems for man (attaining, sustaining)
   Ejaculation problems for man (premature, retarded, retrograde)
   Altered lubrication in woman
   Altered orgasm in woman
6. Sexual problem
   Description
   Onset (when, gradual/sudden)
   Pattern over time (increased, decreased, unchanged)
   Person's concept of cause
   Knowledge of problem by others (partner, physician, others)
   Past diagnostic studies and treatments
   Expectations
7. School-aged child
   a. Knowledge
      "What is the difference between boys and girls?"
      "What do you know about having babies?"
      "Who taught you? At what age?"
   b. Body changes
      "Is your body changing in any way? How? Why?"
      "How do you feel about these changes?"

   c. Masturbation

   "Almost everyone touches their body; how do you feel about this?"

8. Adolescent

   a. Knowledge and attitudes

   "What are your parents' attitudes toward sex, nudity, and touching?"

   "How are subjects discussed in your home?"

   "How does pregnancy occur?"

   "What are some methods of birth control?"

   "What do you know about sexually transmitted diseases?"

   b. Body changes

   "Is your body changing in any ways? How? Why?"

   "How do you feel about these changes?"

   c. Sexual activity

   "Some young people are sexually active and others choose not to be sexually active; what are your beliefs about this?"

   "Are you sexually active? Is so, describe the type of birth control and safe sex practices you use."

   "Some teens are attracted to people of their gender; have you experienced these feelings?" (Lion, 1982; Smith, 1993).

C. Assess for related factors

   1. Sexual knowledge and attitudes

   Source of sexual information

   Knowledge of anatomy and physiology

   Childhood sexual experiences (parental influence, religious influence, masturbation)

   Attitudes concerning sexual variations

   Myths and taboos

   Menstruation, menopause

   Birth control methods

   STD transmission

Objective Data

A. Assess for related factors

   1. Menstrual/reproductive history
   2. Fertility status
   3. Genitourinary/gynecologic assessment
   4. Surgical/congenital alterations
   5. Primary/secondary sexual characteristics
   6. Dress, grooming
   7. General health status

Outcome Criteria

The person will

- Identify impact of stressors, loss, or change on sexual functioning
- Modify behavior to reduce stressors
- Resume previous sexual activity or engage in alternate satisfying sexual activity
- Identify factual limitations on sexual activity caused by health problem
- Identify appropriate modifications in sexual practices in response to these limitations
- Report satisfying sexual activity

Interventions

A. Assess for causative or contributing factors, which may include

See Related Factors

B. Explore the client's patterns of sexual functioning, encouraging him or her to share concerns; assume that all clients have had some sexual experience, and convey a willingness to discuss feelings and concerns

C. Discuss the relationship between sexual functioning and stressors

1. Clarify relation between stressors and problem in sexual functioning.
2. Explore options available for reducing the impact of the stressor on sexual functioning (*e.g.*, increase sleep, increase exercise, modify diet, explore stress reduction methods).

D. Reaffirm the need for frank discussion between sexual partners

1. Explain how the client and partner can use role playing to discuss concerns about sex.
2. Reaffirm the need for closeness and expressions of caring through touching, massage, and other means.
3. Suggest that sexual activity need not always culminate in vaginal intercourse, but that the partner can reach orgasm through noncoital manual or oral stimulation.

E. With acute or chronic illness:

1. Eliminate or reduce causative or contributing factors, if possible. Teach the importance of adhering to medical regimen designed to reduce or control disease symptoms.
2. Provide limited information and specific suggestions.
   a. Provide appropriate information to patient and partner concerning actual limitations on sexual functioning caused by the illness (limited information).
   b. Teach possible modifications in sexual practices to assist in dealing with limitations caused by illness (specific suggestions).
   c. See Table II–27 for more details.
3. Provide opportunities for the person to discuss the impact of limited activity tolerance on sexuality.
   a. Promote an atmosphere of openness, understanding, and acceptance.
   b. Some people with chronic obstructive pulmonary disease may fear that sexual activity will increase dyspnea and, therefore, avoid it altogether. Others may simply give up before or during sexual activity because of shortness of breath and associated frustration.
   c. Providing some common-sense information may be all that is needed for people to resume satisfying sexual relations.
   d. Explain that attempting lovemaking while fatigued, during a chest infection, after a large meal, or after indulgence in large amounts of alcohol increases the likelihood of failure.
   e. Suggest that planned lovemaking during midday or early evening when energy levels are highest may be more satisfying than late-night relations when the person is already fatigued.

F. Facilitate adaptation to change in or loss of body part by

1. Assessing the stage of adaptation of the person and partner to the loss (denial, depression, anger, resolution; see *Grieving*)
2. Encouraging adherence to the medical regimen to promote maximum recovery
3. Encouraging the couple to discuss the strengths of their relationship and to assess the influence of the loss on these strengths
4. Clarifying the relationship between loss or change and the problem in sexual functioning

Table II-27 **Disorders That Alter Sexuality**

Health Problem	Sexual Complication	Nursing Intervention
Diabetes mellitus	Men: Erectile difficulties due to diabetic neuropathies or microangiopathy	LI: Encourage proper metabolic control. SS: Eventually may require penile implant; refer to urologist.
	Women: Decreased desire; decreased vaginal lubrication	LI: Encourage proper metabolic control; teach signs and symptoms of vaginitis. SS: Suggest use of water-soluble lubricating jelly.
Chronic obstructive pulmonary disease	Activity intolerance due to exertional dyspnea; coughing and expectoration	LI: Teach controlled breathing; plan intercourse for time of peak effect from medications; avoid sex after large meal or physical exertion, or immediately after awakening; plan for nonhurried, relaxed, low-stress encounters.
	Anxiety	SS: Suggest positions that minimize chest pressure (sitting or side-lying); explain that waterbeds also help decrease exertion during sex.
Arthritis		LI: Explain that arthritis has no effect on physiologic aspects of sexual functioning.
	Pain, joint stiffness, fatigue	SS: Suggest that the couple plan intercourse for time of peak medication effects; promote joint relaxation by taking warm bath/shower alone/with partner; perform mild range-of-motion exercises.
	Decreased libido from steroid medications	LI: Teach that decreased desire is a common side effect of medication.
Transurethral resection of the prostate (TURP) to treat benign prostatic hypertrophy	Retrograde ejaculation due to damage to internal bladder sphincter	LI: Explain that erection and orgasm will still occur, but ejaculate will be decreased or absent; urine will be cloudy.
Cardiovascular disease	Anxiety, fear of performance, fear of chest pain, death, decreased desire, decreased arousal, decision of partner to stop sexual activity	LI: Explain that infarction has no direct effect on physiologic sexual functioning; activity usually is safe 5–8 weeks postinfarction, based on Index of Sexual Readiness (ability to take brisk walk, climb two flights of stairs without chest pain). Teach to avoid sexual activity after large meal, drinking alcohol, or in room with extremes in temperature. Point out that some medications may cause sexual dysfunction (see Table II-26). SS: Encourage nonsexual touching; suggest positions that conserve energy (side-to-side lying, supine lying position, or sitting in chair with partner on top); explore option of masturbation; assure that oral–genital sex does not place additional strain on heart. Warn to avoid anal sex, because anal penetration stimulates vagus nerve and decreases cardiac function.
Chronic renal failure (CRF)	Chronic/recurrent uremia can produce state of depression, decreased sexual desire and arousal	LI: Acknowledge that stress of disease and dialysis may cause decreased desire; encourage nonsexual touching without pressure to perform.
	Untreated CRF causes cessation of ovulation and menses in women and causes atrophy of	Reassure that these problems are usually reversible with dialysis. Warn that birth control should be continued because fertility

(continued)

Table II-27   **Disorders That Alter Sexuality**   *(continued)*

Health Problem	Sexual Complication	Nursing Intervention
	testicles, decreased spermato-genesis, decreased plasma testosterone, and erectile dysfunction in men. Dialysis may restore ovulation and menses in women and return testosterone levels to normal in men; sexual desire may return to predisease levels with treatment.	may return. Explain that sexual dysfunction may be a product of emotional stress and the physiologic components of the disease. SS: Explain that measurement of nocturnal penile tumescence can distinguish between organic and psychological causes of sexual dysfunction in men.
Total abdominal hysterectomy with bilateral salpingo-oophorectomy	Loss of circulating estrogen	LI: Teach signs and symptoms of menopause, use of water-soluble vaginal lubricants. Encourage discussion with physician about estrogen replacement creams. Explain that in most cases intercourse may be resumed after 6-week postoperative visit.
	Postoperative psychological adjustment or change in sexual identity, grieving, loss of reproductive capacity	Explore the meaning of uterine and ovarian loss to the woman. Assure her that the surgery will not change her ability to respond and function sexually.
Enterostomal surgery Anterior–posterior resection	Women: Loss of uterus and ovaries; shortening of vagina	LI: See above. SS: Suggest coital positions that decrease depth of penetration (*e.g.,* side-to-side lying, man on top with legs outside the woman's, woman on top).
	Men: Erectile dysfunction, decrease in amount/force of ejaculate or retrograde ejaculation due to interruption of sympathetic and parasympathetic nerve supply **Note:** Amount of rectal tissue removed appears to determine degree of dysfunction	LI: Explain that erectile dysfunction may be temporary or permanent. Encourage use of touch and other noncoital means of sexual communication.
Colostomy/ ileostomy	Alteration in sexual self-concept, body image	LI: Allow person to express feelings about change in body appearance; encourage communication with partner.
	Decrease in desire, arousal, and orgasm	LI: Teach that fatigue and decreased desire are common after surgery. Discuss ways to increase sexual attractiveness; suggest wearing sexy lingerie or other clothing to hide appliance.
	Anxiety over spillage, odor	Teach to empty bag before sexual activity; encourage to maintain a sense of humor, because accidents will sometimes occur.
	Erectile dysfunction in men (varies with age and type of surgery)	Encourage alternate ways to express sexuality if intercourse is not possible.
Spinal cord injury	Sexual disability depends on level and type of cord injury: after injury, separation of genital sexual functioning and cerebral eroticism	LI: Discuss sexual options available; depend on extent of injury (*e.g.,* a waterbed to amplify pelvic movements). Encourage continued use of contraceptives, as appropriate.

(continued)

Table II-27 **Disorders That Alter Sexuality** *(continued)*

Health Problem	Sexual Complication	Nursing Intervention
	Men with complete upper motor neuron injury may not be able to ejaculate	SS: Discuss alternate positions (*e.g.,* partner on top). Encourage experimentation with vibrators, massage, and other means of sexual expression. May be a candidate for a penile implant. May have urinary tract infection. Refer to a urologist.

Note: Much information is available on the sexual implications of spinal cord injury. The reader is referred to available literature on this subject.

Health Problem	Sexual Complication	Nursing Intervention
Cancer	Sexual implications depend on site of disease and treatment	LI: Encourage expression of anxiety and fear; encourage grieving.
	May feel guilty about desiring touch, need for sexual activity	Assure that sexual expression, even when one has cancer, is natural, and that need for intimacy often increases during this time.
	Changes in role function and sexually defined gender roles	Encourage discussion between partners about this; encourage negotiation about role changes, which may be temporary.
	Fear of being contagious	Assure person and partner that the disease cannot be transmitted through sexual activity.
	Change in body image	Discuss purchase of wig, false eyelashes before hair loss; suggest sexy lingerie, other ways to pamper oneself to increase feelings of sexual desirability and attractiveness.
	Fatigue	Explain that severe fatigue may hinder sexual desire and that fatigue does not indicate rejection of partner. Encourage verbal and nonverbal communication between person and partner.
Chemotherapy	Alkylating agents, antimetabolites, and antitumor antibiotics: Amenorrhea, oligospermia, azoospermia, decreased desire, ovarian dysfunction, erectile dysfunction	LI: Encourage discussion about changes in body appearance/function. Explore option of sperm banking. Urge to continue use of contraceptives. False-positive Pap smear possible.
	Vinca alkaloids: Retrograde ejaculation, erectile dysfunction, decreased desire, ovarian dysfunction, temporary decrease in sexual desire/arousal	Encourage nonsexual touching; rest; avoidance of alcoholic beverages, narcotics and sedatives before sexual activity; use of water-soluble lubricants to decrease vaginal irritation; avoidance of oral and anal sex during periods of neutropenia.
	Genetic teratogenicity and mutagenicity	Encourage the couple to seek genetic counseling before conception.
Radiation therapy	Most side effects are site dependent; however, side effects such as fatigue, neutropenia, anorexia generally are present in all people	LI: Teach to plan sexual activity after rest periods and to use positions that require less exertion for the patient. Encourage nonsexual touching and communication. Teach that patient is not radioactive during external treatment. Teach site-specific side effects and impact on sexual functioning.

LI = limited information; SS = specific suggestion.

G. Teach possible modifications in sexual practices to assist in dealing with limitations caused by illness (specific suggestions), for example
   1. Modifications in positions
   2. Use of pillows for comfort and/or balance
   3. Techniques to control drainage or odor
   4. Use of attractive lingerie to cover affected part

H. Provide referrals as indicated, which may include
   1. Enterostomal therapist
   2. Physician
   3. Nurse specialist
   4. Sex therapist

Rationale
- Many clients are reluctant to discuss sexuality issues. The proper approach can encourage the client to share feelings and concerns.
- Explaining that impaired sexual functioning has a physiologic basis can reduce feelings of inadequacy and decreased self-esteem, which actually may help improve sexual function.
- Role-playing helps a person gain insight by placing himself or herself in another's position, and allows more spontaneous sharing of fears and concerns.
- Both partners probably have concerns about sexual activity. Repressing these feelings negatively influences the relationship.
- Sexual pleasure and gratification is not limited to intercourse. Other expressions of caring may prove more meaningful.
- Sexual gratification is an individual matter. It is not limited to intercourse, but includes closeness, touching, and giving pleasure to others.
- Providing accurate information on the effect of cord injury on sexual functioning can prevent false hope or give real hope, as appropriate.
- Certain sexual problems necessitate continuing therapy and the advanced knowledge of specialists.

■ Altered Sexuality Patterns
Related to Prenatal and Postpartum Changes

Outcome Criteria
The person will
- Share concerns
- Express increased satisfaction with sexual patterns

Interventions
A. Assess the sexual patterns during and after pregnancy (Reeder, Mastroianni, & Martin, 1992; May & Mahlmeister, 1994)

Prenatal
   1. Has the pregnancy made many changes in your life and sexual relationship?

2. Are there any concerns or worries about your sexual relationship during pregnancy or afterward?
3. What has your physician said about sex during pregnancy?
4. How does the pregnancy make you feel? (asked of both partners)
5. How do you feel about changes in appearance?
6. How do you feel about changes in emotions?
7. How do you feel about one another's experience of the pregnancy?
8. What are your feelings about sex during pregnancy? Cultural influences?
9. What have you heard about what you should or should not do sexually during pregnancy?
10. Have you experienced any physical difficulties with intercourse during pregnancy?
11. How do you think having a baby will change your life? How do you plan to manage these changes?
12. How do you feel physically?
13. What medications do you take?
14. Have you had any recent changes in your health?

Postpartum
1. Are you still bleeding?
2. Have you resumed sexual activity?
3. Are you concerned about conceiving again?
4. Has breast-feeding altered your sexual relationship?
5. How has the baby affected your sexuality?
6. Is your episiotomy healed and comfortable during intercourse?
7. Have you experienced a lack of lubrication since delivery?
8. Do you ever have time alone with your partner?

B. Assess contributing factors
　　1. Body changes
　　2. Change in sex drive
　　3. Fatigue
　　4. Emotional lability
　　　　a. Anxieties about taking on parental responsibilities
　　　　b. Grief about separating from childhood
　　　　c. Anxiety about outcome of pregnancy
　　　　d. Ambivalence about having a baby
　　　　e. Guilt about desiring sex when pregnancy has been achieved (religious, social pressure)
　　　　f. Fear of dependency
　　　　g. Fear of loss of current status (career, freedom)
　　　　h. Self-doubt
　　5. Fear of damaging fetus
　　6. Dyspareunia in pregnancy
　　7. Dyspareunia in postpartum
　　8. Guilt because of baby
　　　　a. Afraid to let go and enjoy sex lest something happen to baby
　　　　b. Woman may feel envious of all the care the infant receives. She may feel more infantile herself and less like a sexual woman.
　　9. Influence of others
　　　　a. Relatives (mother, in-laws)
　　　　　　Attitudes related to pregnancy and child care
　　　　　　Cultural attitudes toward sex during pregnancy and toward mothers as sexual beings

b. Partner
   Intrusion on time together
c. Baby: intrusion on time (nursing, care)
10. Fear of pregnancy (post delivery)
11. Breast-feeding
   a. Breast-feeding and orgasm are influenced by same hormones. Nursing women often feel confused and ashamed at sensuous feelings aroused during nursing.
   b. See *Ineffective Breast-Feeding.*

C. Reduce or eliminate contributing factors
   1. Body changes
      a. Provide literature or suggested reading list for person to read to establish knowledge of normality of pregnancy and changes.
      b. Refer to community resources.
      c. Refer to early pregnancy classes.
      d. Refer to childbirth preparation classes.
      e. View video about sex during pregnancy.
      f. Suggest alternative sexual positions for later pregnancy to prevent abdominal pressure.

Side-lying	Woman on hands and knees
Woman kneeling	Woman on top
Woman standing	Woman astride man

      g. Discuss postpartum changes.
         Provide literature.
         Give reassurance about these changes.
            Episiotomy
            Lochia—how long it will last, how it will change
            Lubrication
            Uterine resolution
            Flabby abdominal musculature
            Breast engorgement
            Breast leakage during lovemaking
         Reassure that this is a temporary state and will resolve in 2–3 months.
         Refer to postpartum exercise class.
   2. Change in sex drive
      a. Reassure that sexual attitudes change throughout pregnancy from feeling very desirous of sex to wanting only to be cuddled.
      b. Support acceptance of whatever pleasuring may be desired. Encourage flexibility and alternative sexual patterns (*e.g.*, oral sex, mutual masturbation, fondling, stroking, massage, vibrators).
      c. Encourage honest communication with partner concerning desires or changes in interest.
   3. Fatigue
      a. Acknowledge this as factor, especially during first trimester and again during last month.
      b. Fatigue can be a major contributor to postpartum sexual problem.
      c. Encourage person to make time for her relationship, in sexual as well as other contexts.
      d. Encourage to ask for help, hire a sitter, and so forth.
   4. Emotional lability
      a. Encourage woman and/or partner to discuss emotions.
         i. Postpartum emotional changes can be intense. They can be hormonally influenced but are aggravated by fatigue and loss of identity.

    ii. Conflicting feelings are common. Woman and partner need opportunity to vent these feelings.

        Resentment of partner is common; this will certainly affect sexual rapport.

        Resentment of infant can create intense guilt. May cause woman to cling more to child and reject others, or she may become depressed and less responsive to infant and partner.

        Expression and acceptance of their feelings is imperative.

  b. Listen—allow time for person to elaborate on feelings.

  c. Reassure that these feelings are normal.

  d. Refer to reading material.

  e. Refer to other pregnant couples for verification.

  f. Relate your own experiences, if appropriate.

  g. Refer to therapy, if indicated.

5. Fear of damaging fetus

  a. Reassure that unless problems exist (preterm labor, previous early loss, bleeding or rupture of membrane), intercourse is allowed until labor begins.

  b. Refer to physician for reassurance.

  c. Explore misinformation. Use anatomic charts to show protection of baby in uterus.

  d. Inform that orgasm causes contractions that are not harmful and will subside.

6. Dyspareunia in pregnancy

  a. Explore what pain is experienced and when.

  b. Suggest alternative positions:

    Woman on top   Posterior–vaginal entry

    Side-lying

  c. Suggest use of water-soluble lubricant.

  d. Refer to physician if pain continues.

7. Dyspareunia in postpartum

  a. Explore what pain is experienced and under what circumstances.

  b. Assess healing of episiotomy.

    The incision heals on the surface after 1 week.

    Dissolvable stitches can take up to a month to resolve; there may be tenderness and swelling until then.

    Nerves can remain sensitive and tender for as long as 6 months.

  c. Suggest varied positions.

  d. Suggest use of water-soluble lubricant (nursing women report reduced vaginal lubrication during entire nursing experience).

  e. Teach person to identify her pelvic floor muscles and strengthen them with exercise.

    "For posterior pelvic floor muscles, imagine you are trying to stop the passage of stool and tighten your anus muscles without tightening your legs or your abdominal muscles."

    "For anterior pelvic floor muscles, imagine you are trying to stop the passage of urine, tighten the muscles (back and front) for 4 seconds, and then release them; repeat ten times, four times a day" (can be increased to four times an hour if indicated).

  f. Instruct person to stop and start the urinary stream several times during voiding.

  g. Refer to physician if pain continues.

8. Guilt due to baby
   a. Encourage discussion; reassure that these feelings are normal; allow time to elaborate.
   b. Expression of these feelings often creates a release and relaxation.
   c. Include partner in discussion (both may have similar feelings they have not felt free to express to one another).
   d. Refer to postpartum support groups.
   e. Refer to psychological or social assistance if pathology is observed.
   f. Encourage couple to allow themselves to get help in caring for infant. They need time alone. Arrange a "date" where they can be alone, with no threat of intrusion of a crying baby. They may then be able to rediscover their sexuality.

9. Influence of others
   a. Encourage discussion of mother/woman relationship.
      Does woman see her mother as a sexual being?
      Does she now feel confused about her roles as mother versus sex partner?
   b. Reassure that identity confusion is common.
   c. Refer to postpartum discussion groups.
   d. Allow to express feelings concerning changes in life.
   e. Include partner in discussion (perhaps at a later time)—let both parties talk about adjustment and pressures that interfere with relating sexually and otherwise.
   f. Interview partners separately. (This may allow an opening-up that may be difficult with the other person present.)

10. Fear of pregnancy
    a. Encourage discussion.
    b. Explore contraceptive choices.
    c. Refer to nurse practitioner or gynecologist for contraception.
    d. Inform patient that breast-feeding does not provide effective contraception and that prepregnancy contraceptive devices may no longer fit.
       Warn that although some oral contraceptives can be used while nursing, they usually significantly reduce milk supply.

D. Initiate health teaching and referrals

1. Teach couples to abstain from intercourse and seek the advice of their health care provider if any of the following situations are present (Zlatnik & Burmeistey, 1982):
   a. Vaginal bleeding
   b. Premature dilation
   c. Multiple pregnancy
   d. Engaged fetal head or lightening
   e. Placenta previa
   f. Rupture of membranes
   g. History of premature delivery
   h. History of miscarriage
   i. If any of the above are present, the couple should not engage in *any* sex play. Orgasm even without intercourse is contraindicated in most circumstances. Couples should be instructed to ask *very specific* questions about what is allowed and what is not allowed.
2. Refer to suggested references for printed material.
3. Refer to counselor if resolution is not achieved.

Rationale

- Barring complications, a pregnant woman is free to engage in sexual activity with her partner to the extent that it is comfortable and desired.
- Exploring sexual patterns, concerns, and fears can provide opportunities to correct misinformation and to open dialogue between partners (May & Mahlmeister, 1994).
- Pregnancy is a time of stress for both man and woman; to deny physical closeness at a time when both partners are struggling can add to tension and alienation.
- The client may worry about his or her partner's acceptance; the partner may be afraid of hurting the client and needs to know that the fetus is not harmed by sexual activity.
- Fathers will have their own adjustment postnatally. They may feel lost, displaced, or left out of the constant direct attention an infant requires. They may have confusing feelings of resentment, especially as infant suckles the breast.
- Intercourse and orgasm are safe for most women except those with high-risk pregnancies (May & Mahlmeister, 1994).
- Alternate sexual positions can prevent abdominal pressure or deep penetration (May & Mahlmeister, 1994).
- Preparation of the woman and her partner for the changes associated with pregnancy, labor, and delivery and postpartum can clarify misinformation and reduce anxiety (Reeder, Martin, & Koniak, 1992).
- Helping the couple understand what factors affect libido (*e.g.*, fatigue) can reduce feelings of rejection (Reeder et al., 1992).
- Communication problems are the most common type of martial problems. Couples are encouraged to share their sexual needs and preferences (Reeder et al., 1992).

■ Risk for Altered Sexuality Patterns
Related to Fear of Pregnancy and/or Sexually Transmitted Diseases (STDs)

Outcome Criteria

The person will
- Report proper use of contraceptive methods
- Report use of methods to reduce risk of acquiring HIV, HBV, or other STDs
- Report satisfaction with contraceptive method and sexuality patterns
- Not experience an unplanned pregnancy or acquire an STD

Interventions

A. Assess for causative or contributing factors, such as
   1. Lack of exposure to or understanding of information on contraception and STDs
   2. Newly sexually active

3. Change in sexual partner
4. Multiple/sequential sexual partners
5. Intravenous drug use by self or partner

B. Eliminate or reduce causative or contributing factors, if possible
1. Stress genuine risk of pregnancy or STD with unprotected sexual activity.
   a. Clarify the confidentiality of you discussion.
   b. Directly ask, "Do you use condoms? Every time?"
   c. Emphasize that one sexual experience without a condom can transmit an STD.
   d. Clearly outline that some STDs are not curable (*e.g.*, HPV, HBV).
   e. Explain that many STDs have no symptoms initially.
2. Encourage abstinence from sexual activity, or thoughtful consideration in choice and number of sexual partners.
   a. Discuss the hazards of casual sex.
   b. Role play with individual on how to say no, how to discuss previous sexual partners, how to request condom use.
   c. Clarify that each sexual partner exposes one to all previous sexual partners of this person.
   d. Explain that herpes and HPV can be contracted even with condom use (*e.g.*, pubic to pubic contact).

C. Provide limited information and specific suggestions
1. Discuss advantages and disadvantages of various contraceptive methods.
   a. Effectiveness of pregnancy prevention
   b. Effectiveness of disease prevention
2. Provide specific information on chosen contraceptive method, including written/graphic material and return demonstration if appropriate.
3. Teach to abstain from sexual activity if partner has symptoms of an STD.
4. Teach danger of infertility, morbidity, or death from contracting an STD (see *Risk for Infection*).

D. Provide referrals, as indicated
1. Physician
2. Nurse practitioners
3. Family planning clinic

Sexual Dysfunction

DEFINITION

Sexual Dysfunction: The state in which an individual experiences or is at risk of experiencing a change in sexual function that is viewed as unrewarding or inadequate.

DEFINING CHARACTERISTICS
Major (Must Be Present)
Verbalization of problem with sexual function
Meets *DSM IV* criteria for Sexual Dysfunction

Minor (May Be Present)
Fears future limitations on sexual performance
Misinformed about sexuality
Lacks knowledge about sexuality and sexual function
Value conflicts involving sexual expression (cultural, religious)
Altered relationship with significant other
Dissatisfaction with sex role (perceived or actual)

Author's Note
See *Altered Sexuality Patterns*

References/Bibliography

Andrews, M., & Boyle, J. (1995). *Transcultural concepts in nursing care* (2nd ed.). Philadelphia: J. B. Lippincott.

Annon, J. S. (1976). The PLISS + model: A proposed conceptual scheme for the behavioral treatment of sexual problems. *Journal of Sex Education and Therapy, 2*, 211–215.

Bing, E., & Colman, L. (1977). *Making love during pregnancy*. New York: Bantam Books.

Brenner P., & Greenberg, M. (1977). The impact of pregnancy on marriage. *Medical Aspects of Human Sexuality, 2*, 15–22.

Convey, H. L. (1989). Perceptions and attitudes toward sexuality of the elderly during middle ages. *The Gerontologist, 29*(1), 93–100.

DiIorio, C., Parsons, M., Lehr, S., Adame, D., & Carlone, J. (1993). Factors associated with use of safer sex practices among college freshmen. *Research in Nursing and Health, 16*, 343–350.

Falicov, C. J. (1973). Sexual adjustment during first pregnancy and postpartum. *American Journal of Obstetrics and Gynecology, 117*, 991–1000.

Fischman, S. H., Rankin, E. A., Soeken, K. L., & Lenz, E. R. (1986). Changes in sexual relationships in postpartum couples. *Journal of Obstetrics, Gynecology and Neonatal Nursing, 15*, 58–63.

Fitzsimmons, L., Verderber, A., & Shively, M. (1993). Research connections: Post-cardiac surgery patterns of social and sexual activity. *Journal of Cardiovascular Nursing, 7*, 88–90.

Friday, N. (1980). *My mother myself*. New York: Dell.

Genevie, L., & Margolies, C. (1987). *The motherhood report*. New York: Macmillan.

Gordon, S., & Gordon, J. (1983). *Raising a child conservatively in a sexually permissive world*. New York: Simon & Schuster.

Hatcher, R. A., Guest, F., Stewart, F., Stewart, G. K., Trussell, J., Bowen, S. C., & Cates, W. (1994). *Contraceptive technology* (16th ed.). New York: Irvington Publishers.

Horn, B. (1993). Cultural beliefs and teenage pregnancy. *Nurse Practitioner, 8*(8), 35, 39, 74.

Johnston, J. M., & Amico, J. (1986). A prospective longitudinal study of the release of oxytocin and prolactin in response to infant suckling in long term lactation. *Journal of Clinical Endocrinology and Metabolism, 62*, 653–657.

Katzun, L. (1990). Chronic illness and sexuality. *American Journal of Nursing, 90*, 57–59.

Keverne, E. B., Levy, F., Poindron P., & Lindsay, D. R. (1983). Vaginal stimulation: An important determinant of maternal bonding in sheep. *Science, 219*, 81–83.

Kimball, C. D. (1987). Do opioid hormones mediate appetites and lovebonds? *American Journal of Obstetrics and Gynecology, 156*, 1463–1466.

Krueger, J. C., Hassell, J., Goggins, D. B., Ishimatsu, T., Pablico, M. R., & Tuttle, E. J. (1979). Relationship between nurse counseling and sexual adjustment after hysterectomy. *Nursing Research, 28*, 145–150.

Lion, E. (1982). *Human sexuality in nursing process*. New York: John Wiley & Sons.

Masters, W. H., & Johnson, V. E. (1966). *Human sexual response*. Boston: Little, Brown.

Matocha, L. K., & Waterhouse, J. K. (1993). Current nursing practice related to sexuality. *Research in Nursing and Health, 16*, 371–378.

May, K. (1987). Men's sexuality during the childbearing years. *Holistic Nursing Practice, 1*(4), 60–66.

May, K. A., & Mahlmeister, L. R. (1994). *Maternal and neonatal nursing: Family-centered care* (3rd ed.). Philadelphia: J. B. Lippincott.

McNally, A. S., Robinson, I. C. A., Houston, M. J., & Howie, P. W. (1983). Release of oxytocin and prolactin in response to suckling. *British Medical Journal, 286*, 257–259.

Metcalfe, M. C., & Fischman, S. H. (1985). Factors affecting the sexuality of patients with head and neck cancer. *Oncology Nursing Forum, 12*, 21–25.

Miller, C. A. (1995). *Nursing care of the older adult* (2nd ed.). Glenview, IL: Scott, Foresman.

Nay, R. (1992). Sexuality and aged women in nursing homes. *Geriatric Nursing, 15*(6), 312–314.

Reeder, S., Martin, L., & Koniak, D. (1992). *Maternity nursing: Family, newborn, and women's health care* (17th ed.). Philadelphia: J.B. Lippincott.

Reeder, S., Mastroianni, L., & Martin, L. (1983). *Maternity nursing*. Philadelphia: J. B. Lippincott.

Rew, L. (1989). Promoting healthy sexuality. In R. L. Foster, M. M. Hunsberger, & J. J. T. Anderson (Eds.). *Family-centered nursing care of children*. Philadelphia: W. B. Saunders.

Sanford, N. D. (1989). Providing sensitive health care to gay and lesbian youth. *Nurse Practitioner, 14*, 33–47.

Smith, M. (1993). Pediatric sexuality: Promoting normal sexual development in children. *Nurse Practitioner, 18*, 37–44.

Steinke, E., & Bergen, B. (1986). Sexuality and aging. *Journal of Gerontological Nursing, 12*, 6–10.

Thranov, I., & Klee, M. (1994). Sexuality among gynecologic cancer patients: A cross-sectional study. *Gynecologic Oncology, 52*, 14–19.

U. S. Department of Health and Human Services. (1993). 1993 Sexually transmitted diseases treatment guidelines. *Morbidity and Mortality Weekly Report, 42*(RR-14), 1–102.

Wallace, M. (1992). Management of sexual relationships among elderly residents of long-term care facilities. *Geriatric Nursing, 15*(6), 308–311.

Waterhouse, J. (1993). Discussing sexual concerns with health care professionals. *Journal of Holistic Nursing, 11*, 125–134.

Waterhouse, J., & Metcalfe, M. (1991). Attitudes toward nurses discussing sexual concerns with patients. *Journal of Advanced Nursing, 16*, 1048–1054.

Wilmoth, M. C. (1993). Development and testing of the sexual behaviors questionnaire. *Dissertation Abstracts International, 54*, 6137B–6138B.

Wilmoth, M. C. (1994a). Strategies for becoming comfortable with sexual assessment. *Oncology Nursing News, 12*(2), 6–7.

Wilmoth, M. C. (1994b). Nurses' and patients' perspectives on sexuality: Bridging the gap. *Innovations in Oncology Nursing, 10*, 34–36.

Woods, N. F. (1984). *Human sexuality in health and illness* (3rd ed.). St. Louis: C. V. Mosby.

World Health Organization. (1975). *Education and treatment in human sexuality: The training of health professionals*. Report of a WHO Meeting, Technical Report Series No. 572. Geneva: WHO.

Zlatnick, F. J., & Burmeistey, L. F. (1982). Reported sexual behavior in late pregnancy. *Selected Medicine, 27*(3), 627–632.

Sleep Pattern Disturbance

DEFINITION

Sleep Pattern Disturbance: The state in which the individual experiences or is at risk of experiencing a change in the quantity or quality of his rest pattern that causes discomfort or interferes with desired life-style.

Defining Characteristics

Adults

Major (Must Be Present)

Difficulty falling or remaining asleep

Minor (May Be Present)

Fatigue on awakening or during the day
Dozing during the day
Agitation
Mood alterations

Children

Sleep disturbances in children are frequently related to fear, enuresis, or inconsistent responses of parents to child's requests for changes in sleep rules, such as requests to stay up late.

Reluctance to retire	Desire to sleep with parents
Frequent awakening during the night	

RELATED FACTORS

Many factors in an individual's life can contribute to sleep pattern disturbances. Some common factors are listed.

Pathophysiologic

Related to frequent awakenings secondary to:
(Impaired oxygen transport)

Angina	Respiratory disorders
Peripheral arteriosclerosis	Circulatory disorders

(Impaired elimination; bowel or bladder)

Diarrhea	Retention
Constipation	Dysuria
Incontinence	Frequency

(Impaired metabolism)

Hyperthyroidism	Hepatic disorders
Gastric ulcers	

Treatment-Related

Related to difficulty assuming usual position secondary to (specify):
Related to excessive daytime sleeping secondary to medications

Tranquilizers	Soporifics
Sedatives	Monoamine oxidase inhibitors
Hypnotics	Barbiturates
Antidepressants	Corticosteroids
Antihypertensives	Amphetamines

Situational (Personal, Environmental)

Related to excessive hyperactivity secondary to:

Bipolar disorder	Attention-deficit disorder
Panic anxiety	

Related to excessive daytime sleeping
Related to depression
Related to inadequate daytime activities
Related to pain
Related to anxiety response
Related to discomforts secondary to pregnancy
Related to life-style disruptions
   Occupational
   Emotional
   Social
   Sexual
   Financial
Related to environmental changes (specify)
   Hospitalization (noise, disturbing roommate, fear)
   Travel
Related to fears
Related to circadian rhythm changes

Maturational

Child
    Related to fear of dark
Adult women
    Related to hormonal changes (*e.g.*, perimenopausal)

Author's Note

The inability to rest and sleep has been described as "one of the causes, as well as one of the accompaniments of disease" (Henderson, 1969). Sleep disturbances can result from physiologic, psychological, social, environmental, and maturational changes or problems.

The nursing diagnosis *Sleep Pattern Disturbance* must be differentiated from sleep disorders, which are chronic conditions (*e.g.*, sleep apnea, narcolepsy) usually not treatable by a nurse generalist. *Sleep Pattern Disturbance* should be used to describe temporary changes in usual sleep patterns and/or those which a nurse can prevent or reduce (*e.g.*, disruptions for treatments, anxiety response).

Errors in Diagnostic Statements

Sleep Pattern Disturbance related to apnea

This diagnosis requires monitoring and comanagement by nurses and physicians; thus, it should be written as the collaborative problem *Potential Complication: Sleep apnea*.

Sleep Pattern Disturbance related to hospitalization

This diagnosis does not reflect the treatment needed. The effects of hospitalization on sleep should be specified, such as in *Sleep Pattern Disturbance related to changes in usual sleep environment, unfamiliar noises, and interruptions for assessments*.

Key Concepts

1. Sleep involves two distinct stages: REM (rapid eye movement) and NREM (non-rapid eye movement). NREM sleep constitutes about 75% of total sleep time; REM sleep accounts for the remaining 25% (Rechtschaffen & Kales, 1968).
2. The entire sleep cycle is completed in an interval of 70–100 minutes; this cycle repeats itself four or five times during the course of the sleep pattern (Cohen & Merritt, 1992).
3. Sleep is a restorative and recuperative process that facilitates cellular growth and the repair of damaged and aging body tissues. During NREM sleep, metabolic, cardiac, and respiratory rates decrease to basal levels and blood pressure decreases. There is profound muscle relaxation, bone marrow mitotic activity, and accelerated tissue repair and protein synthesis. During REM sleep, the sympathetic nervous system accelerates, with erratic increases in cardiac output and heart and respiratory rate. Perfusion to gray matter doubles, and cognitive and emotional information is stored, filtered, and organized (Williams & Jackson, 1982).
4. The active phase of the sleep cycle, REM sleep is characterized by increased irregular vital signs, penile erections, flaccid musculature, and the release of adrenal hormones. REM sleep occurs approximately four to five times a night and is essential to a person's sense of well-being. REM sleep is instrumental in facilitating emotional adaptation; a person needs substantially more REM sleep after periods of increased stress or learning (Sebilia, 1981).
5. Perception of the quality of one's sleep is influenced by the percentage of time in bed at night actually spent asleep, or *sleep efficiency*. Studies report that younger people typically report a sleep efficiency of 80%–95%, whereas older people report 67%–70% (Dement, Richardson, Prinz, Carskadon, Kripke, & Czeisler, 1985; Hayashi & Endo, 1982).
6. Monroe (1967) reported a high correlation between what people report about their sleep patterns and what polysomnographic evaluation (EEG, EMG, EOG) reveals. The subjects

in this study were young and healthy; it is not known if the same results could be replicated with ill adults.

7. Sleep deprivation results in impaired cognitive functioning (memory, concentration, judgment) and perception, reduced emotional control, and increased suspicion, irritability, and disorientation. It also lowers the pain threshold and decreases production of catecholamines, corticosteroids, and hormones (Berger & Oswald, 1962; Fuller & Schaller-Ayers, 1990).

8. The average amount of sleep needed according to age follows (William, 1971):

Age	Hours of Sleep
Newborn	14 to 18
6 months	12 to 16
Over 6 months to 4 years	12 to 13
5 to 13 years	7 to 8.5
13 to 21 years	7 to 8.75
Adults younger than 60	6 to 9
Adults older than 60	7 to 8

9. Hammer (1991) identified three subcategories of *Sleep Pattern Disturbance:* latency or difficulty falling asleep, interrupted, and early A.M. awakening.

10. Individuals with depression report early-morning awakenings and inability to return to sleep. Anxious people complain of insomnia and multiple awakenings throughout the night (Hammer, 1991).

11. Hypnotics contribute to sleep disturbances by:
   a. Requiring increasing dosage due to tolerance
   b. Depressing central nervous system (CNS) function
   c. Producing paradoxic effects (nightmares, agitation)
   d. Interfering with REM and deep sleep stages
   e. Causing daytime somnolence owing to a very long half-life

Key Concepts—Child

1. Children exhibit a wide variation in the amount and distribution of sleep (Wong, 1995).
2. Sleep affects a child's growth and development as well as the family unit as a whole (Hunsberger, 1989).
3. As children mature, the number of hours spent in sleep decreases. Moreover, there is a change in the quality of sleep with maturity. Sleep is characterized as being deep and restful 50% of the time in an infant, versus 80% of the time in the older child (Wong, 1995).

Key Concepts—Maternal

1. Discomforts related to enlarging uterus can interfere with usual sleep positions (Reeder, Martin, & Koniak, 1992).

Key Concepts—Older Adult

1. Research has found that sleep efficiency declines with advancing age, so more time is needed in bed to achieve restorative sleep. Sleep time decreases with age (*e.g.*, 6 hours by age 70 years). There is a decrease in stages 3 and 4 and REM sleep with aging (Hammer, 1991).
2. Sleep pattern disturbances are the most frequent complaint among older adults (Hammer, 1991).
3. Older adults have more difficulty falling asleep, are more easily awakened, and spend more time in the drowsiness stage and less time in the dream stages (Miller, 1995).
4. Miller (1995, p. 347) reports that "approximately one-third of adults complain of some type of sleep disturbance, usually involving primary symptoms of daytime sleepiness, difficulty falling asleep, and frequent arousals during the night."

Focus Assessment Criteria

Subjective Data

A. Assess for defining characteristics

    1. Sleep patterns (present, past)

        Rate sleep on a scale of 1–10 (10 = rested, refreshed)

        Usual bedtime and arising time

        Difficulty in getting to sleep, staying asleep, awakening

    2. Sleep requirements

        To establish the amount of sleep an individual needs, have him go to bed and sleep until he wakes in the morning (without an alarm clock). This should be done for a few days and the average of the total sleeping hours calculated—with the subtraction of 20–30 minutes, which is the time most people need to fall asleep.

    3. History of symptoms

        Complaints of

            Sleeplessness

            Anxiety

            Irritability

            Depression

            Fear (nightmares, dark, maturational situations)

        Onset and duration

        Location

        Description

            Precipitated by what?

            Relieved by what?

            Aggravated by what?

B. Assess for related factors

    1. Interruptions

        Noise

        Travel schedule

        Need to void

    2. Lack of usual sleep aids or rituals

        Warm bath   Position

        Drink or food (milk, wine)   Toy, book

        Pillows

    3. Naps (frequency, length)

    4. Side effects of medication

    5. Alcohol, caffeine use

    6. Intrinsic causes

        Sleep apnea   Alzheimer's dementia

        Psychophysiologic insomnia   Depression

        Unrelieved pain   Thyroid, hepatic, or renal disease

        Nocturnal dyspnea   Chronic brain syndrome

        Parkinsonism

Objective Data

A. Assess for defining characteristics

    1. Physical characteristics

        Drawn appearance (pale, dark circles under eyes, puffy eyes)

        Yawning

        Dozing during the day

        Decreased attention span

        Irritability

Outcome Criteria

The person will
- Describe factors that prevent or inhibit sleep
- Identify techniques to induce sleep
- Report an optimal balance of rest and activity

Interventions

Because a variety of factors can disrupt sleep patterns, the nurse should consult the index for specific interventions to reduce certain factors (*e.g.*, pain, anxiety, fear). The following suggests general interventions for promoting sleep and specific interventions for selected clinical situations.

A. Identify causative contributing factors
  1. Pain (see *Altered Comfort*)
  2. Fear (see *Fear*)
  3. Stress or anxiety (see *Anxiety*)
  4. Immobility or decreased activity
  5. Pregnancy
  6. Urinary frequency or incontinence (see *Altered Patterns of Urinary Elimination*)
  7. Unfamiliar or noisy environment
  8. Temperature (too hot/cold)
  9. Insufficient daily stimulation or activity

B. Reduce or eliminate environmental distractions and sleep interruptions
  1. Noise
     a. Close door to room.
     b. Pull curtains.
     c. Unplug telephone.
     d. Use "white noise" (*e.g.*, fan, quiet, music, tape of rain, waves).
     e. Eliminate 24-hour lighting.
     f. Provide night-lights.
     g. Decrease the amount and kind of incoming stimuli (*e.g.*, staff conversations).
     h. Cover blinking lights with tape.
     i. Reduce the volume of alarms and televisions.
     j. Place with compatible roommate if possible.
  2. Interruptions
     a. Organize procedures to provide the fewest number of disturbances during sleep period (*e.g.*, when individual awakens for medication, also administer treatments and obtain vital signs).
     b. Avoid unnecessary procedures during sleep period.
     c. Limit visitors during optimal rest periods (*e.g.*, after meals).
     d. If voiding during the night is disruptive, have person limit his nighttime fluids and void before retiring.

C. Increase daytime activities, as indicated
  1. Establish with person a schedule for a daytime program of activity (walking, physical therapy).
  2. Discourage naps longer than 90 minutes.
  3. Encourage naps in the morning.
  4. Limit amount and length of daytime sleeping if excessive (*i.e.*, more than 1 hour).
  5. Provide others to communicate with person and stimulate wakefulness.

D. Promote sleep in agency
1. Assess with person, family, or parents the usual bedtime routine—time, hygiene practices, rituals (reading, toy)—and adhere to it as closely as possible.
2. Encourage or provide evening care.
a. Bathroom or bedpan
b. Personal hygiene (mouth care, bath, shower, partial bath)
c. Clean linen and bedclothes (freshly made bed, sufficient blankets)
3. Use sleep aids.
a. Warm bath
b. Desired bedtime snack (avoid highly seasoned and high-roughage foods)
c. Reading material
d. Back rub or massage
e. Milk
f. Soft music or tape-recorded story
g. Relaxation/breathing exercises
4. Use pillows for support (painful limb, pregnant or obese abdomen, back).
5. Discourage naps longer than 90 minutes.
6. Ensure that the person has at least four to five periods of at least 90 minutes each of uninterrupted sleep every 24 hours.
7. Document the amount of the person's uninterrupted sleep each shift.

E. Reduce the potential for injury during sleep
1. Use side rails if needed.
2. Place bed in low position.
3. Provide adequate supervision.
4. Provide night-lights.
5. Place call bell within reach.
6. Ensure that an adequate length of tubing is available for turning (IV tubing, Levin tube).

F. Provide health teaching and referrals, as indicated
1. Teach an at-home sleep routine (Miller, 1995):
a. Maintain a consistent daily schedule for waking, sleeping, and resting (weekdays, weekends).
b. Arise at the usual time even after not sleeping well; avoid staying in bed when awake.
c. Use bed only for activities associated with sleeping.
d. If awakened and cannot return to sleep, get out of bed and read in another room for 30 minutes.
e. Avoid caffeine-containing foods and beverages (*e.g.*, chocolate, tea, coffee) during afternoon and evening.
f. Avoid alcohol.
g. Try a bedtime snack of foods high in L-tryptophan (*e.g.*, milk, peanuts).
2. Teach the importance of regular exercise (walking, running, aerobic dance and exercise) for at least one-half hour three times a week (if not contraindicated) to reduce stress and promote sleep.
3. Explain that hypnotic medications are not for long-term use owing to the risk for development of tolerance and interference with daytime functioning.
4. Explain to person and significant others the causes of sleep/rest disturbance and possible ways to avoid or minimize these causes.
5. Refer a person with a chronic sleep problem to a sleep disorders center.

Rationale

- Sleep cycle includes REM, NREM, and wakefulness. A person typically goes through four or five complete sleep cycles each night. Awakening during a cycle may cause him to feel not well rested in the morning (Cohen & Merritt, 1992).

- Although many believe that a person needs 8 hours of sleep each night, no scientific evidence supports this belief. Individual sleep requirements vary greatly. In general, a person who can relax and rest easily requires less sleep to feel refreshed. With age, total sleep time usually decreases—especially stage IV sleep—and stage I sleep increases (Cohen & Merritt, 1992).
- Sleep is difficult without relaxation. The unfamiliar hospital environment can hinder relaxation (Cohen & Merritt, 1992).
- To feel rested, a person usually must complete an entire sleep cycle (70–100 minutes) four or five times a night (Cohen & Merritt, 1992).
- Sedative and hypnotic drugs begin to lose their effectiveness after a week of use, requiring increasing dosages and leading to the risk of dependence.
- A familiar bedtime ritual may promote relaxation and sleep (Cohen & Merritt, 1992).
- Warm milk contains L-tryptophan, which is a sleep inducer (Hammer, 1991).
- Caffeine and nicotine are CNS stimulants that lengthen sleep latency and increase nighttime wakening (Miller, 1995).
- Alcohol induces drowsiness but suppresses REM sleep and increases the number of awakenings (Miller, 1995).
- Early-morning naps produce more REM sleep than do afternoon naps. Naps over 90 minutes long decrease the stimulus for longer sleep cycles in which REM sleep is obtained (Thelan, Davie, & Urden, 1990).
- Researchers have reported that the chief deterrents to sleep in critical care clients were activity, noise, pain, physical condition, nursing procedures, lights, vapor tents, and hypothermia (Dlin, Rosen, & Dickstein, 1971).
- Environmental noise that cannot be eliminated or reduced can be masked with "white noise" (*e.g.*, fan, soft music, tape-recorded sounds [rain, ocean waves]) (Miller, 1995).
- Irregular sleeping patterns can disrupt normal circadian rhythms, possibly leading to sleep difficulties.

Interventions—*Child Focus*

1. Explain night to the child (stars and moon).
2. Discuss how some people (nurses, factory workers) work at night.
3. Explain that when night comes for them, day is coming for other people somewhere else in the world.
4. If a nightmare occurs, encourage the child to talk about it, if possible. Reassure child that it is a dream, even though it seems very real. Share with child that you have dreams too.
5. Provide child with a night-light or a flashlight to use to give child control over the dark.
6. Reassure child that you will be nearby all night.
7. Explain the possible problems of sleeping with child.

Rationale

- Sleep problems commonly are related to feeding, resistance to separation, and normal fears (Hunsberger, 1989).
- Children need to understand nighttime and be assisted to prepare for it. Preparation for bedtime involves switching the child from activity to bedtime gradually. It is a time for calmness, reassurance, and closeness.
- Children should be helped to learn that their beds are safe places to be in.

Interventions—*Maternal Focus*

1. Explain some reasons for sleeping difficulties during pregnancy (*e.g.*, leg cramps, backache).
2. Teach how to position pillows in side-lying position (one between legs, one under abdomen, one under top arm, one under head).
3. Teach to avoid caffeine and large meal within 2 to 3 hours of bedtime.
4. Teach to exercise daily and take a warm bath at bedtime.

Rationale

- Interventions that reduce discomfort of enlarging uterus can promote sleep (Reeder et al., 1992).
- See Rationale for generic Interventions

🏛 Interventions—*Older Adult Focus*

1. Explain the effects of alcohol on sleep (*e.g.*, nightmares, frequent awakenings).
2. Explain that sleeping pills (prescribed or over-the-counter) are not effective after 1 month and that they interfere with the quality of sleep and daytime functioning.
3. Instruct to avoid over-the-counter sleeping pills because of their antihistamine effects.
4. If sleeping pills are needed for a few days, advise to consult primary care provider for a type with a short half-life.

Rationale

- Older adults have increased sensitivity to hypnotics and sleeping medications and experience more adverse effects (*e.g.*, constipation, confusion, and interference with quality of sleep).
- Alcohol and caffeine may cause insomnia, as do certain drugs such as steroids, theophylline, β-blockers, and chronic use of sedatives or hypnotics (Haponik, 1994).

References/Bibliography

Berger R. J., & Oswald, I. (1962). Effects of sleep deprivation on behavior, subsequent sleep and dreaming. *Journal of Mental Science, 108,* 457.

Cohen, F., & Merritt, S. (1992). Sleep promotion. In G. Bulechek & J. McCloskey (Eds.). *Nursing interventions: Essential nursing treatments* (2nd ed.). Philadelphia: W. B. Saunders.

Dement, W., Richardson, G., Prinz, P., Carskadon, M., Kripke, D., & Czeisler, C. (1985). Changes of sleep and wakefulness with age. In C. E. Finch & E. L. Schneider (Eds.). *Handbook of the biology of aging* (2nd ed.). New York: Van Nostrand Reinhold.

Dlin, B., Rosen, H., & Dickstein, K. (1971). The problems of sleep and rest in the intensive care unit. *Psychosomatics, 12,* 155.

Fuller, J., & Schaller-Ayers, J. (1990). *Health assessment: A nursing approach.* Philadelphia: J. B. Lippincott.

Hammer, B. (1991). Sleep pattern disturbance. In M. Maas, K. Buckwalter, & M. Hardy (Eds.). *Nursing diagnoses and interventions for the elderly.* Redwood City, CA: Addison-Wesley Nursing.

Haponik, E. (1994). Sleep problems. In W. Hazzard, E. Bieman, J. Bless, W. Ettinger, & J. Halter (Eds.). *Principles of geriatric medicine and gerontology.* New York: McGraw-Hill.

Hayashi, Y., & Endo, S. (1982). All-night sleep polygraphic recordings of healthy aged persons: REM and slow-wave sleep. *Sleep, 5,* 277–283.

Henderson, V. (1969). *Basic principles of nursing care.* New York: Macmillan.

Hunsberger, M. (1989). Promoting healthy sleep patterns. In R. L. Foster, M. M. Hunsberger, & J. J. T. Anderson (Eds.). *Family-centered nursing care of children.* Philadelphia: W. B. Saunders.

Miller, C. A. (1995). *Nursing care of older adults* (2nd ed.). Glenview, IL: Scott, Foresman.

Monroe, L. J. (1967). Psychological and physiological differences between good and poor sleepers. *Journal of Abnormal Psychology, 72,* 225–264.

Rechtschaffen, A., & Kales, A. (1968). *A manual of standardized terminology, techniques and scoring system for sleep stages of human subjects.* NIHM Publication 204. Washington, DC: U.S. Government Printing Office.

Reeder, S., Martin, L., Koniak, D. (1992). *Maternity nursing: Family, newborn and women's health care* (7th ed.). Philadelphia: J. B. Lippincott.

Sebilia, A. (1981). Sleep deprivation and biological rhythms in the critical care unit. *Critical Care Nurse, 3,* 19.

Thelan, L., Davie, J., & Urden, L. (1990). *Textbook of critical care nursing.* St. Louis: C. V. Mosby.

White, M. A. (1990). Sleep onset latency and distress in hospitalized children. *Nursing Research, 39,* 134–139.

William, D. (1971). Sleep and disease. *American Journal of Nursing, 71,* 2321–2324.

Williams, R. L., & Jackson, D. (1982). Problems with sleep. *Heart and Lung, 11,* 262.

Wong, D. L. (1995). *Nursing care of infants and children* (5th ed.). St. Louis: Mosby–Year Book.

Resources for the Consumer

Sleep and aging (GPO 885-270), National Institute of Aging, U.S. Government Printing Office, Washington, DC 20402.

The sleep book. AARP Books, Dept. L078, 1865 Miner St., Des Plaines, IL 60018.

Association of Sleep Disorders Centers, 604 Second St. SW, Rochester, MN 55902; (507) 287-6006 (provides list of accredited sleep disorder centers).

Social Interactions, Impaired

DEFINITION

Impaired Social Interaction: The state in which individual experiences or is at risk of experiencing negative, insufficient, or unsatisfactory responses from interactions.

DEFINING CHARACTERISTICS
Major (Must Be Present)

Reports inability to establish and/or maintain stable, supportive relationships
Dissatisfied with social network

Minor (May Be Present)

Avoidance of others
Interpersonal difficulties at work
Others report problematic patterns of interaction
Feelings of being misunderstood
Feelings of rejection
Blames others for interpersonal problems
Social isolation
Superficial relationships

RELATED FACTORS

Impaired social interactions can result from a variety of situations and health problems that are related to the inability to establish and maintain rewarding relationships. Some common sources are listed.

Pathophysiologic

Related to embarrassment, limited physical mobility or energy secondary to:

Loss of body function   Loss of body part
Terminal illness

Related to communication barriers secondary to:

Hearing deficits   Speech impediments
Mental retardation   Chronic mental illness
Visual deficits

Treatment-Related

Related to surgical disfigurement
Related to therapeutic isolation

Situational (Personal, Environmental)

Related to alienation from others secondary to:

Constant complaining	High anxiety
Rumination	Impulsive behavior
Overt hostility	Delusions
Manipulative behaviors	Hallucinations
Mistrust or suspicions	Disorganized thinking
Illogical ideas	Dependent behavior
Egocentric behavior	Strong unpopular beliefs
Emotional immaturity	Depressive behavior
Aggressive responses	

Related to language/cultural barriers
Related to lack of social skills
Related to change in usual social patterns secondary to:
   Divorce
   Relocation
   Death

Maturational

Child/adolescent
   Related to inadequate sensory stimulation
   Related to altered appearance
   Related to speech impediments
Adult
   Related to loss of ability to practice vocation
Older Adult
   Related to change in usual social patterns secondary to:
      Death of spouse   Functional deficits
      Retirement

Author's Note

Social competence refers to a person's ability to interact effectively with others. Interpersonal relationships assist a person through life experiences, both positive and negative. Positive relationships with others require positive self-concept, social skills, social sensitivity, and acceptance of the need for independence. To interact satisfactorily with others, a person must acknowledge and accept his or her limitations and strengths (Maroni, 1989).

A person without positive mental health usually does not have social sensitivity, and thus is uncomfortable with the interdependence necessary for effective social interactions. A person with poor self-concept may constantly sacrifice his or her needs for those of others or may always put personal needs before the needs of others.

The diagnosis *Impaired Social Interactions* describes a person who exhibits ineffective interactions with others. If extreme and/or prolonged, this problem can lead to a diagnosis of *Social Isolation*. The nursing focus for *Impaired Social Interactions* is on increasing the person's sensitivity to the needs of others and teaching reciprocity.

Errors in Diagnostic Statements

Impaired Social Interactions related to verbalized discomfort in social situations

In this diagnosis, the person's report of discomfort represents a diagnostic cue, not a related factor. The nurse performs a focus assessment to determine reasons for the person's discomfort; until these reasons are known, the diagnosis *Impaired Social Interactions related to unknown etiology* can be recorded.

Key Concepts

1. Blumer (1995) described three premises of human conduct and interactions:
   a. Life experiences have different meanings for each person. Individuals respond toward situations and people on the basis of these meanings or significance.
   b. Individuals learn meanings from social interactions with others.
   c. During encounters, individuals interpret the situation and apply their previous meanings or modify them.
2. Social competence is the ability of the individual to interact effectively with his or her environment.
3. Effective reality testing, ability to problem solve, and a variety of coping mechanisms are necessary for the individual to be socially competent.

4. Both the individual and the environment contribute to impaired functioning. A person may be able to function in one environment or situation, but not in others.
5. Adequate social functioning is most often associated with conjugal living and a stable occupation.

Chronic Mental Illness

1. Chronic mental illness is characterized by recurring episodes over a long period. The extent to which the individual is impaired in role performance varies. The extent of impairment is related to social inadequacy.
2. Altered thought processes may interfere with the individual's ability to engage in appropriate social or occupational role behavior.
3. Dependency is one of the most consistent features presented. It may be seen through multiple readmissions requiring a large amount of clinician's time, resistance to discharge, resistance to any change including medication, and refusal to leave home.
4. The origins of impaired social interactions in the chronically mentally ill vary. For some, it is the result of poor reality testing. If a person is unable to perceive reality accurately, it is difficult to manage everyday problems. For others, it may be the result of social isolation or the loss of interpersonal skills because of long-term institutionalization.
5. The chronically mentally ill person usually has no friends, is socially isolated, and engages in little community activity (Varcarolis, 1994)
6. Deinstitutionalization has decreased the number of institutionalized individuals and decreased the median length of hospital stay, thus changing the character of today's chronically ill population. There is now an emerging group of individuals 18–35 years of age who are distinctly different from the older institutionalized adults, in that their lives reflect a transient existence and multiple hospital admissions, versus stable, long-term residence in a state hospital (Bachrach, 1982).
7. Chronically mentally ill people often lose their jobs, not because of an inability to do job tasks, but because of deficits in emotional and interpersonal functions (Anthony, 1980). Research in social skills training has shown that posthospital adjustment is improved by skill-building programs (Manderino & Bzdek, 1987).

🌸 *Key Concepts*—*Child*

1. A child is significantly affected when a parent is emotionally disturbed. Emotionally disturbed parents may not be able to meet the physical or safety needs of their children (Krone, 1986).
2. Young children depend on their parents to interpret the world for them. Parents with impaired social interaction and/or *Altered Thought Processes* may not accurately interpret experiences for the child (Krone, 1986).
3. Impaired social interaction may result in *Social Isolation*. Also, see the nursing diagnosis *Altered Parenting*.
4. Adolescents with substance abuse problems use the substance to achieve popularity and/or for stress reduction. Poor personal and social competence are also present (Johnson, 1995).
5. Young people with chronic mental illness exhibit problems with impulse control (*e.g.*, suicidal gestures, legal problems, alcohol/drug intoxication), disturbances in affect (*e.g.*, anger, argumentativeness, belligerence), and poor reality testing, especially when under stress. The population varies from system-dependent, poorly motivated people to system-resistant people with low frustration tolerance and refusal to acknowledge problems (Pepper, Ryglewicz, & Kirshner, 1982).
6. Despite the variations, children and adolescents with chronic mental illness have several factors in common (Pepper et al., 1982).
   a. Difficulty in maintaining stable, supportive relationships—most have transient, unstable relationships with marginally functional people.
   b. Repeated errors in judgment—seen in their inability to learn from their experiences and the inability to transfer knowledge from one situation to another.
   c. Vulnerability to stress—those experiencing stress are at greater risk for relapse.

d. Patterns of social interaction are demanding, hostile, and manipulative, which produce negative reactions among caregivers.

🏛 *Key Concepts—Older Adult*

1. Effective social interactions depend on positive self-esteem. No data suggest that older adults have diminished self-esteem compared with younger adults (Miller, 1995).
2. In older adults, common threats to self-esteem include devaluation, dependency, functional impairments, and decreased sense of control (Miller, 1995).
3. Depression-related affective disturbances of daily life occur in 27% of older adults. Major depression occurs in 2% of community-living older adults and in 12% of older people living in nursing homes (Parmelee, Katz, & Lawton, 1989).
4. Depressed older adults lose interest in social activities and do not display positive interactions when they do interact.

Focus Assessment Criteria

Subjective Data

A. Assess for defining characteristics
  1. Availability and responses of others
     a. Family and significant others

Fearful	Angry
Frustrated	Embarrassed
Guilty	Hopeless

  2. Relationships
     a. Does he have friends?
     b. Does he initiate friendships?
     c. Does he initiate contact or wait for friends to contact him?
     d. Is he satisfied with social interactions?
     e. What is the reason for dissatisfaction with his social network?
  3. Coping skills
     a. How does he respond to stress, conflict?

Substance abuse	Substance abuse (drugs, alcohol, food)
Aggression (verbal or physical)	Withdrawal
Suicidal ideation or gestures	

  4. Legal history
     a. Arrests and convictions

B. Assess for related factors
  1. Interaction patterns and skills
     a. Job-related
        Job-seeking and interviewing skills
           Able to identify own job-related assets
           Dresses appropriately
           Asks appropriate questions
           Identifies employment sources
           Ability to complete an application
           Realistic employment expectations
        Employment status
           Employed
           Unemployed
        Employment history
           Length of employment
           Reasons for leaving (problems with coworkers or supervisors)
           Frequency of job changes
        Interactions with coworkers
           Contacts outside work

 b. Living arrangements
    Ability to live cooperatively with others
       Ability to participate with others in group tasks, such as food preparation, cleaning
       Performs assigned tasks
       Adequacy of personal hygiene
       How does he handle conflict?
       Dependability
    Residential patterns
       Where?—family, group home, boarding house, institution
       How long?
       Frequency of relocation
       Reasons for relocation
    Obstacles to community functioning
       Poor personal hygiene   Legal problems
       Expects self-reliance   Unemployed
       Lacks leisure-time activities   Unstable, transient residences
       Inappropriate behavior in public   Social isolation
 c. Leisure/recreation
    "What do you do with your free time?"
    "Who do you share your time with?"
    Attendance at any structured activity?
    What interferes with participating in recreational activities?
    Preference for individual or group activity?
2. Recent life changes (Krauss & Slavinsky, 1982)
 a. Explore each of the following:
    Emergencies (*e.g.*, police, fire)
    Health (*e.g.*, others in household)
    Financial (*e.g.*, increase or decrease in income, increased debt)
    Job (*e.g.*, change in responsibility)
    Relationships (*e.g.*, new, broken)
    Treatment (*e.g.*, change in medications, therapist)
    Maturational (*e.g.* menopause)

Objective Data

A. Assess for related factors
 1. General appearance
  a. Facial expression (*e.g.*, sad, hostile, expressionless)
  b. Dress (*e.g.*, meticulous, disheveled, seductive, eccentric)
  c. Personal hygiene
     Cleanliness   Clothes (appropriateness, condition)
     Grooming
 2. Communication pattern
  a. During interview
       Quiet   Egocentric
       Hostile   Withdrawn
       Apathetic   Cooperative
       Elated   Hyperactive
  b. Content
       Appropriate   Religiosity
       Rambling   Worthlessness
       Suspicious   Delusions
       Denial of problem   Obsessions
       Exaggerated   Homicidal or suicidal plans
       Sexually preoccupied

c. Pattern of speech

Appropriate	Indecisive
Circumstantial (unable to get to the point)	Neologisms
Blocking (unable to finish an idea)	Word salad
Jumps from one topic to another	

d. Rate of speech

Appropriate	Reduced
Excessive	Pressured

3. Relationship skills
   a. Able to listen and respond appropriately
   b. Has conversational skills
   c. Does not seek interactions
   d. Withdrawn/preoccupied with self
   e. Lives cooperatively with others
   f. Shows dependency, passivity
   g. Demanding/pleading
   h. Hostile
   i. Barriers to satisfactory relationships

Social isolation	Thought disturbances
Severe depression	Chronic mental illness
Panic attacks	Preoccupation with illness

Outcome Criteria

The person will
- Identify problematic behavior that deters socialization
- Substitute constructive behavior for disruptive social behavior (specify)

The family will
- Describe strategies to promote effective socialization

Interventions

A. Provide support for the maintenance of basic social skills and reduce social isolation (refer to *Social Isolation* for further interventions)
   1. Provide an individual, supportive relationship.
      a. Assist person in managing life stresses.
      b. Focus on present and reality.
      c. Help to identify how stress precipitates problems.
      d. Support healthy defenses.
      e. Help to identify alternative courses of action.
      f. Assist in analyzing approaches that work best.
   2. Provide supportive group therapy.
      a. Focus on here and now.
      b. Establish group norms that discourage inappropriate behavior.
      c. Encourage testing of new social behavior.
      d. Use snacks or coffee to decrease anxiety during sessions.
      e. Role-model certain accepted social behaviors (*e.g.,* responding to a friendly greeting versus ignoring it).
      f. Foster development of relationships among members through self-disclosure and genuineness.
      g. Use questions and observations to encourage people with limited interaction skills.
      h. Encourage members to validate their perception with others.

   i. Identify strengths among members and ignore selected weaknesses.

   j. Activity groups, drop-in socialization centers can be used for some individuals.

  3. Monitor medication compliance.

   a. Use small groups or scheduled individual sessions.

   b. Question individual about side effects and symptom exacerbation (do not expect person to self-monitor).

  4. Be assertive with people who are unmotivated or passive.

   a. Contact the person when he fails to attend a scheduled appointment, job interview, and the like.

   b. Do not wait for person to initiate participation.

  5. Hold people accountable for their own actions.

   a. Treat as responsible citizens.

   b. Allow decision making, but may have to outline limits.

   c. Do not allow them to use their illness as an excuse for their behavior.

   d. Set consequences and enforce when necessary, including encounters with law.

   e. Help to see how their behaviors or attitudes contribute to their frequent interpersonal conflicts.

  6. Allow individual to be dependent as necessary.

  7. Use a wide variety of agencies and services (medical, psychiatric, vocational, social, residential).

   a. Services must be coordinated by one agency (individual will not be able to coordinate for self).

   b. Case managers have been successful in providing linkage.

   c. Programs must be flexible and culturally relevant.

B. Decrease problematic behavior

  1. Impaired reality testing (refer to *Altered Thought Processes*)

  2. Lack of leisure-time activities (refer to *Diversional Activity Deficit*)

   a. Companionship program

   b. Day treatment centers

  3. Social isolation (refer to *Social Isolation*)

  4. Hostility and violent outbursts (refer to *Anxiety* and *Risk for Violence*)

  5. Suicidal threats or attempts (refer to *Risk for Suicide*)

  6. Manipulation

   a. Use limit setting (refer to section on anger in *Anxiety*).

   b. Be aware of own reactions.

C. Provide for development of social skills

  1. Identify the environment in which social interactions are impaired.

   a. Living

   b. Learning

   c. Working

  2. Provide instruction in the environment where person is expected to function when possible (*e.g.*, accompany to job site, work with person in own residence).

  3. Develop an individualized social skill program. Examples of some social skills are grooming–personal hygiene, posture, gait, eye contact, beginning a conversation, listening, and ending a conversation. Include modeling, behavior rehearsal, and homework (Manderino & Bzdek, 1987).

  4. Combine verbal instructions with demonstration and practice.

  5. Be firm in setting parameters of appropriate social behaviors, such as punctuality, attendance, managing illnesses with employers, dress, and so forth.

  6. Use group as a method of discussing work-related problems.

  7. Use sheltered workshops and part-time employment depending on person's level where success can best be achieved.

8. Give positive feedback; make sure it is specific and detailed. Focus on no more than three behavioral connections at a time; too-lengthy feedback adds confusion and increases anxiety.
9. Convey a "can-do" attitude.
10. Role-play aspects of social interactions (McFarland, Wasli, & Gerety, 1992, p. 150):
    a. How to initiate a conversation
    b. How to continue a conversation
    c. How to terminate a conversation
    d. How to refuse a request
    e. How to ask for something
    f. How to interview for a job
    g. How to ask someone to participate in an activity (*e.g.*, going to the movies)

D. Assist family and community members in understanding and providing support
    1. Provide factual information concerning mental illness, treatment, and progress to family members. Gently help family accept the fact of the illness in the person.
    2. Validate family members' feelings of frustration in dealing with daily problems.
    3. Provide guidance on overstimulating or understimulating environments.
    4. Allow families to discuss their feelings of guilt and how their behavior affects the person. Refer to a family support group, if available.
    5. Develop an alliance with family.
    6. Arrange for periodic respite care.
    7. Provide support to landlords, shopkeepers, and anyone else with whom person has contact.
        a. Provide information on mental illness.
        b. Teach them relationship skills needed to manage person (*e.g.*, direct, firm, simple directions; use of modeling).
        c. Give person name and number he can call when problems arise.
        d. Provide this education as the need arises with specific individuals.

E. Explore strategies for handling difficult situations (*e.g.*, disrupted communications, altered thoughts, alcohol and drug use) (Stuart & Sundeen, 1995)
    1. Discuss feelings among members.
    2. Establish a cooperative plan.
    3. Plan regular activities to strengthen marital–parental coalition.
    4. Identify when stress reduction is needed.

F. Initiate health teaching and referrals, as indicated
    1. Teach the person (McFarland & Wasli, 1992)
        a. Responsibilities of his or her role as a client (making requests clearly known, participating in therapies)
        b. To outline activities of the day and to focus on accomplishing them
        c. How to approach others to communicate
        d. To identify which interactions encourage others to give him or her consideration and respect
        e. To identify how he or she can participate in formulating family roles and responsibility to comply
        f. To recognize signs of anxiety and methods to relieve them
        g. To identify his or her positive behavior and to experience satisfaction with himself in selecting constructive choices
    2. Teach basic coping skills necessary to live independently (home management, personal hygiene, financial management, transportation skills).
    3. Teach or refer for assertive skill training.
    4. Teach or refer to anger management.

   5. Teach basic conversational skills.
   6. Teach job-seeking skills.
   7. Teach parenting skills.
   8. Refer to a variety of social agencies; however, coordination and continuity should be maintained by one agency.
   9. Refer for supportive family therapy as indicated.
   10. Refer families to local self-help groups.
   11. Provide numbers for crisis intervention services.

Rationale

- The person needs continual encouragement to test new social skills and to explore new social situations (Rawlins, Williams, & Beck, 1993).
- The nurse role-models appropriate social skills and uses groups as other examples of social skills (Rawlins et al., 1993).
- Effective social skills can be learned with guidance, demonstration, practice, and feedback (Stuart & Sundeen, 1995).
- Role playing provides a opportunity to rehearse problematic issues and to receive feedback. Consequences of responses can be explored safely (Stuart & Sundeen, 1995).
- Interventions for the family are very important for successful rehabilitation of a chronically mentally ill family member (Johnson, 1995).
- Both the individuals and families are under stress. The individual's behaviors that strain the family include his or her excessively demanding behavior, social withdrawal, lack of conversation, and minimal leisure interests. The family also affects the individual's ability to survive in the community by either supportive or nonsupportive behaviors.
- Passivity or lack of motivation is a part of the illness and thus should not simply be accepted by the caregivers. Caregivers must use an assertive approach in which the treatment is "taken to the person" rather than waiting for him to participate (Varcarolis, 1994).
- Helping the family learn strategies to handle problem behavior provides a sense of control over their lives (Stuart & Sundeen, 1995).

🌹 Interventions—*Child Focus*

1. If impulse control is a problem (Johnson, 1995):
   a. Set firm, responsible limits
   b. Don't lecture.
   c. State them simply and back them up.
   d. Maintain routines.
   e. Limit play to one playmate to learn appropriate play skills (*e.g.*, relative, adult, quiet child).
   f. Gradually increase number of playmates.
   g. Provide immediate and constant feedback.
2. Discuss selective parenting skills.
   a. Reward small increments of desired behavior.
   b. Contract appropriate age-related consequences (*e.g.*, time-out, loss of activity [use of car, bicycle]).
3. Teach parents to
   a. Avoid harsh criticism
   b. Not to disagree in front of child
   c. To establish eye contact before giving instructions and ask child to repeat back what was said
4. Teach older child to self-monitor target behaviors and to develop self-reliance.
5. If antisocial behavior is present, help to (Johnson, 1995):
   a. Describe behaviors that interfere with socialization
   b. Role-play alternate responses
   c. Limit social circle to a manageable size
   d. Elicit peer feedback for positive and negative behavior

6. Assist the adolescent to decrease social deficits (Johnson, 1995):
   a. Assertiveness
   b. Anger management
   c. Problem solving
   d. Refusal skills
   e. Stress management
   f. Values clarification

Rationale

- Failure to control impulses disrupts socialization (*e.g.*, family, peers, school) (Johnson, 1995).
- Families can be helped to learn effective parenting skills to enhance the child's success (Wong, 1995).
- Skills that reduce social deficits can increase social acceptance and increase control and self-esteem (Johnson, 1995).

References/Bibliography

Anthony, W. A. (1980). *The principles of psychiatric rehabilitation.* Baltimore: University Park Press.

Bachrach, L. (1982). Young adult chronic patients: An analytical review of the literature. *Hospital and Community Psychiatry, 33,* 189–197.

Blumer, H. (1969). Symbolic interaction: Perspective and method. In H. S. Wilson & C. R. Kneisle (Eds.). *Psychiatric nursing* (5th ed). Redwood City, CA: Addison-Wesley Nursing.

Johnson, B. S. (1995). *Child, adolescent, and family psychiatric nursing.* Philadelphia: J. B. Lippincott.

Krauss, J., & Slavinsky, A. (1982). *The chronically ill psychiatric patient and the community.* Oxford: Blackwell Scientific.

Krone, C. H. (1986). The emotionally disturbed parent. In S. H. Johnson (Ed.). *High-risk parenting: Nursing assessment and strategies for the family at risk.* Philadelphia: J. B. Lippincott.

Manderino, M., & Bzdek, V. (1987). Social skill building. *Journal of Psychosocial Nursing, 25*(9), 18–22.

Maroni, J. (1989). Impaired social interactions. In G. McFarland & E. McFarlane (Eds.). *Nursing diagnosis and interventions.* St. Louis: C. V. Mosby.

McFarland, G., Wasli, E., & Gerety, E. (1992). *Nursing diagnoses and process in psychiatric mental health nursing* (2nd ed.). Philadelphia: J. B. Lippincott.

Miller, C. A. (1995). *Nursing care of older adults* (2nd ed.). Glenview, IL: Scott, Foresman.

Parmelee, P. A., Katz, I. R., & Lawton, M. P. (1989). Depression among institutionalized aged. *Journal of Gerontology: Medical Sciences, 44*(1), 22–29.

Pepper, B., Ryglewicz, H., & Kirshner M. (1982). The uninstitutionalized generation: A new breed of psychiatric patient. In B. Pepper & H. Ryglewicz (Eds.). *New directions for mental health services: The young adult chronic patient No. 14.* San Francisco: Jossey-Bass.

Rawlins, R. P., Williams, S. R., & Beck, C. K. (1993). *Mental health–psychiatric nursing: A holistic life-cycle approach* (3rd ed.). St. Louis: Mosby–Year Book.

Stuart, G. W., & Sundeen, S. L. (1995). *Principles and practice of psychiatric nursing* (5th ed.). St. Louis: Mosby–Year Book.

Varcarolis, E. M. (1994). *Foundations of psychiatric–mental health nursing* (2nd ed.). Philadelphia: W. B. Saunders.

Wong, D. (1995). *Nursing care of infants and children* (5th ed.). St. Louis: Mosby–Year Book.

Social Isolation

DEFINITION

Social Isolation: The state in which the individual or group experiences or perceives a need or desire for increased involvement with others but is unable to make that contact.

DEFINING CHARACTERISTICS

Because social isolation is a subjective state, all inferences made concerning a person's feelings of aloneness must be validated, because the causes vary and people show their aloneness in different ways.

Major (Must Be Present)

Expressed feelings of aloneness, rejection
Desire for more contact with people
Reports insecurity in social situations*
Describes a lack of meaningful relationships

Minor (May Be Present)

Time passing slowly ("Mondays are so long for me.")
Inability to concentrate and make decisions
Feelings of uselessness   Uncommunicative*
Feeling of rejection   Withdrawn*
Sad, dull affect*   Poor eye contact*
Preoccupied with own thoughts and memories*
Underactivity (physical or verbal)
Appearing depressed, anxious, or angry
Failure to interact with others nearby

RELATED FACTORS

A state of social isolation can result from a variety of situations and health problems that are related to a loss of established relationships or to a failure to generate these relationships. Some common sources follow.

Pathophysiologic

Related to fear of rejection secondary to:
　　Obesity
　　Cancer (disfiguring surgery of head or neck, superstitions of others)
　　Physical handicaps (paraplegia, amputation, arthritis, hemiplegia)
　　Emotional handicaps (extreme anxiety, depression, paranoia, phobias)
　　Incontinence (embarrassment, odor)
　　Communicable diseases (acquired immunodeficiency syndrome, hepatitis)
　　Psychiatric illness (schizophrenia, bipolar affective disorder, personality disorders)

Situational (Personal, Environmental)

Related to death of a significant other
Related to divorce
Related to disfiguring appearance

* Elsen, J., & Blegen, M. (1991). Social isolation. In M. Maas, K. Buckwalter, & M. Hardy, M. (Eds.). *Nursing diagnoses and interventions for the elderly*. Redwood City, CA: Addison-Wesley Nursing.

Related to fear of rejection secondary to:

Obesity	Hospitalization or terminal illness (dying process)
Extreme poverty	Unemployment

Related to moving to another culture (*e.g.*, unfamiliar language)
Related to loss of usual means of transportation
Related to history of unsatisfactory relationships secondary to:

Drug abuse	Unacceptable social behavior
Alcohol abuse	Delusional thinking
Immature behavior	

Maturational

Child
   Related to protective isolation or a communicable disease
Older Adult
   Related to loss of usual social contacts

Author's Note

In 1994 NANDA added a new diagnosis, *Risk for Loneliness*. Although this diagnosis is only in stage I of a four-stage developmental process, it more accurately adheres to the NANDA definition of "response to." Social isolation is not a response but instead a cause or contributing factor to loneliness. In addition, A person can experience loneliness even with many people around.

   This author recommends deleting *Social Isolation* from clinical use and using *Loneliness* or *Risk for Loneliness*.

Spiritual Distress

Spiritual Well-Being, Potential for Enhanced

Spiritual Distress

DEFINITION

Spiritual Distress: The state in which the individual or group experiences or is at risk of experiencing a disturbance in the belief or value system that provides strength, hope, and meaning to life.

DEFINING CHARACTERISTICS
Major (Must Be Present)

Experiences a disturbance in belief system

Minor (May Be Present)

Questions meaning of life, death, suffering
Questions credibility of belief system
Demonstrates discouragement or despair
Chooses not to practice usual religious rituals
Has ambivalent feelings (doubts) about beliefs
Expresses that he has no reason for living
Feels a sense of spiritual emptiness
Shows emotional detachment from self and others
Expresses concern—anger, resentment, fear—over meaning of life, suffering, death
Requests spiritual assistance for a disturbance in belief system

RELATED FACTORS
Pathophysiologic

Related to challenge to belief system or separation from spiritual ties secondary to:

Loss of body part or function	Pain
Terminal illness	Trauma
Debilitating disease	Miscarriage, stillbirth

Treatment-Related

Related to conflict between (specify prescribed regimen) and beliefs

Abortion	Isolation
Surgery	Amputation
Blood transfusion	Medications
Dietary restrictions	Medical procedures

Situational (Personal, Environmental)

Related to death or illness of significant other
Related to embarrassment at practicing spiritual rituals

Related to barriers to practicing spiritual rituals
    Restrictions of intensive care   Lack of privacy
    Confinement to bed or room   Lack of availability of special foods/diet
Related to beliefs opposed by family, peers, health care providers
Related to divorce, separation from loved on

Author's Note

Wellness represents a response to a person's potential for personal growth, involving utilization of all of a person's resources (social, psychological, cultural, environmental, spiritual, and physiologic) (Bruhn, Cordova, Williams, & Fuentes, 1977). Nurses profess to care for the whole client, but several studies report that nurses commonly avoid addressing the spiritual dimension of clients, families, and communities (DeYoung, 1984; Martin, Burrows, & Pomilio, 1978).

    To promote positive spirituality with clients and families, the nurse must possess positive spirituality. For the nurse, self-evaluation must precede assessment of spiritual concerns, and assessment of spiritual health should be confined to the context of nursing. The nurse can assist people with spiritual concerns or distress by providing resources for spiritual help, by listening nonjudgmentally, and by providing opportunities for meeting spiritual needs (Stoll, 1984). The nurse should be cautioned against establishing practice patterns that routinely result in referring all spiritual needs of clients and families to religious or spiritual leaders.

Errors in Diagnostic Statements

Spiritual Distress related to critical illness and doubts about religious beliefs
    Critical illness can challenge a person's spiritual beliefs and can evoke feelings of guilt, anger, disappointment, and helplessness. However, critical illness does not represent a specific contributing factor or cue to the presence of spiritual distress. Until related factors are known, the nurse can record the diagnosis as *Spiritual Distress related to unknown etiology, as evidenced by expressions of doubt about religious beliefs*. The nursing focus will be on actively listening to the person's feelings and fears.

Key Concepts

1. All people have a spiritual dimension, regardless of whether they participate in formal religious practices (Burkhardt, 1994; Carson, 1989). An individual is a spiritual person even when disoriented, confused, emotionally ill, irrational, or cognitively impaired.
2. The individual's spiritual nature must be considered as part of their total care, along with the physical and psychosocial dimensions (Carson, 1989; Wald & Bailey, 1990). Research indicates that most clients feel religion is very important in times of crisis (Sodestrom & Martinson, 1987).
3. The spiritual may include, but is not limited to, religion; spiritual needs include religion, values, relationships, transcendence, and affective feeling and communication (Emblen & Halstead, 1993); creativity and self-expression may also be important to spirituality (Wald & Bailey, 1990). Other descriptions of spirituality include inner strength, meaning and purpose, and knowing and becoming (Burkhardt, 1994).
4. Health care systems often give spiritual concerns low priority in care planning and delivery. This is less true in hospice organizations, where the spiritual component of care is more likely to be recognized and included (Millison, 1995; Wald & Bailey, 1990).
5. Religion influences attitudes and behavior related to right and wrong, family, child-rearing, work, money, politics, and many other functional areas (Taylor, Lillis, & LeMone, 1989).
6. To deal effectively with a person's spiritual needs, the nurse must recognize her or his own beliefs and values, acknowledge that these values may not be applicable to others, and respect the person's beliefs when helping him meet perceived spiritual needs (Taylor et al., 1989).

7. The value of prayers or spiritual rituals to the believer is not affected by whether they can be scientifically "proved" to be beneficial.

8. Research indicates that many nurses feel inadequately prepared to provide spiritual care, and that fewer than 15% include spirituality in nursing care (Piles, 1990). "Among the reasons that nurses fail to provide spiritual care are the following: (1) they view religion as a private matter; (2) they feel that spirituality is a private matter concerning only an individual and his Creator; (3) they are uncomfortable about their own religious beliefs or deny having spiritual needs; (4) they lack knowledge about spirituality and the religious beliefs of others; (5) they mistake spiritual needs for psychosocial needs; and (6) they view meeting the spiritual needs of clients as a family or pastoral responsibility, not as a nursing responsibility" (Andrews & Boyle, 1995, p. 360).

9. To assist people in spiritual distress, the nurse must know certain beliefs and practices of the various spiritual groups found in this country. Table II-28 provides information on the beliefs and practices that are most directly related to health and illness. It is intended as a reference only. Major religions, denominations, and spiritual groups are arranged alphabetically. Denominations with similar practices and restrictions are grouped together. No attempt is made to discuss the broad beliefs and philosophies of the selected groups; see References/Bibliography for texts supplying such in-depth information.

🌀 *Key Concepts—Child*

1. Children's spiritual needs include love and relatedness, forgiveness, meaning, and purpose (Van Heukelem, 1982).

2. Spiritual beliefs are influenced by moral and cognitive development (Wong, 1995).

3. Children learn faith and religion from the practices of parents/significant others (Wong, 1995).

🏛 *Key Concepts—Older Adult*

1. The White House Council on Aging in 1971 described spiritual concerns as "the human need to deal with sociocultural deprivations, anxieties and fears, death and dying, social alienation, and philosophy of life" (Moberg, 1984; Ryan, 1985).

2. The National Interfaith Coalition on Aging describes spiritual well-being as "the affirmation of life in a relationship with God, self, community, and environment that nurtures and celebrates wholeness" (Ryan & Patterson, 1987).

3. Factors that contribute to spiritual distress and put elderly people at risk include questions concerning life after death as the person ages, separation from formal religious community, and a value–belief system that is continuously challenged by losses and suffering (Matteson & McConnell, 1988; Patterson, 1984).

4. About 75% of all elderly people are members of religious organizations. This does not necessarily mean that they attend their formal services and meetings regularly (Matteson & McConnell, 1988).

5. Elderly people tend to participate in formal religious groups less than younger people. Nonorganizational participation increases dramatically with age, and the desire to participate in the church activities remains constant throughout their lives. Elderly people may find religious services difficult to attend and participate in owing to physical impairments. Factors such as lack of transportation, inaccessible toileting facilities, poor acoustics and sound systems for hearing-impaired, and small-print hymn books or prayer books can diminish active involvement in formal religious activities (Inlay & Smith, 1984; Mindel & Vaughan, 1978).

6. Older adults must complete Erikson's developmental stage of Ego Integrity versus Despair to achieve life satisfaction. The older person may reflect on his life, expressing that he has lived in accordance with his value system, and may express contentment with his life. These behaviors demonstrate fulfillment of the need for meaning and purpose in life (Matteson & McConnell, 1988).

(text continues on page 863)

Table II-28 **Overview of Religious Beliefs**

Agnostic

BELIEFS

It is impossible to know if God exists (specific moral values may guide behavior)

Amish

ILLNESS

Usually taken care of within family

TEXTS

Bible

Ausbund (16th century German hymnal)

BELIEFS

Rejection of all government aid
Rejection of modernization
Legally exempt from immunizations

Armenian

See Eastern Orthodox

Atheist

BELIEFS

God does not exist (specific moral values may guide behavior)

Baha'i

ILLNESS

Religion and science are both important
Usual hospital routines and treatments are usually acceptable

DEATH

Burial mandatory; internment near place of death

BELIEFS

Purpose of religion is to promote harmony and peace
Education very important

Baptist, Churches of God, Churches of Christ, and Pentecostal (Assemblies of God, Foursquare Church)

ILLNESS

Some practice laying on of hands, divine healing through prayer
May request Communion
Some prohibit medical therapy
May consider illness divine punishment or intrusion of Satan

DIET

No alcohol (mandatory for most)
No coffee, tea, tobacco, pork, or strangled animals (mandatory for some)
Some fasting

BIRTH

Opposes infant baptism

TEXT

Bible

BELIEFS

Some practice glossolalia (speaking in tongues)

Buddhism

ILLNESS

Considered trial that develops the soul
May wish counseling by priest
May refuse treatment on holy days (1/1, 1/16, 2/15, 3/21, 4/8, 5/21, 6/15, 8/1, 8/23, 12/8, 12/31)

(continued)

Table II-28 **Overview of Religious Beliefs** *(continued)*

DIET

Strict vegetarianism (mandatory for some)

Discourages use of alcohol, tobacco, and drugs

DEATH

Last-rite chanting by priest

Death leads to rebirth, may wish to remain alert and lucid

TEXTS

Buddha's sermon on the "eightfold path"

The Tripitaka, or "three baskets" of wisdom

BELIEFS

Cleanliness is of great importance

Suffering is universal

Christian Science

ILLNESS

Caused by errors in thought and mind

May oppose drugs; IV fluid; blood transfusions; psychotherapy; hypnotism; physical examinations; biopsies; eye, ear, and blood pressure screening; and other medical and nursing interventions

Accepts only legally required immunizations

May desire support from a Christian Science reader or treatment by a Christian Science nurse or practitioner (a list of these nonmedical practitioners and nurses may be found in the *Christian Science Journal*)

Healing is spiritual renewal

DEATH

Autopsy permitted only in cases of sudden death

TEXT

Bible

Science and Health With Key to the Scriptures by Mary Baker Eddy

Church of Christ

See Baptist

Church of God

See Baptist

Confucian

ILLNESS

The body was given by one's parents and should therefore be well cared for

May be strongly motivated to maintain or regain wellness

BELIEFS

Respect for family and older people very important

Cults (variety of groups, usually with living leader)

ILLNESS

Most practice faith healing

May reject modern medicine and condemn health personnel as enemies

Therapeutic compliance and follow-up are usually poor

Illness may represent wrong thinking or inhabitation by Satan

BELIEFS

Expansion of cult through conversions important

May depend on cult environment for definition of reality

Eastern Orthodox (Greek Orthodox, Russian Orthodox, Armenian)

ILLNESS

May desire Holy Communion, laying on of hands, anointing, or sacrament of Holy Unction

Most oppose euthanasia and favor every effort to preserve life

Russian Orthodox men should be shaved only if necessary for surgery

Table II-28 **Overview of Religious Beliefs** (continued)

DIET

May fast Wednesdays, Fridays, during Lent, before Christmas, or for 6 hours before Communion (seriously ill are exempted)

May avoid meat, dairy products, and olive oil during fast (seriously ill are exempted)

BIRTH

Baptism 8–40 days after birth, usually by immersion (mandatory for some)

May be followed immediately by confirmation

Greek Orthodox only: If death of infant is imminent, nurse should baptize infant by touching the forehead with a small amount of water three times

DEATH

Last rites and administration of Holy Communion (mandatory for some)

May oppose autopsy, embalming, and cremation

TEXTS

Bible

Prayer book

RELIGIOUS ARTICLES

Icons (pictures of Jesus, Mary, saints) are very important

Holy water and lighted candles

Russian Orthodox wears cross necklace that should be removed only if necessary

OTHER

Greek Orthodox opposes abortion

Confession at least yearly (mandatory for some)

Holy Communion four times yearly: Christmas, Easter, 6/30, and 8/15 (mandatory for some)

Dates of holy days may differ from Western Christian calendar

Episcopal

ILLNESS

May believe in spiritual healing

May desire confession and Communion

DIET

May abstain from meat on Fridays

May fast during Lent or before Communion

BIRTH

Infant baptism is mandatory (nurse may baptize infant when death is imminent by pouring water on forehead and saying, "I baptize you in the name of the Father, the Son, and the Holy Spirit")

DEATH

Last rites optional

TEXTS

Bible

Prayer book

Friends (Quaker)

No minister or priests; direct, individual, inner experience of God is vital

DIET

Most avoid alcohol and drugs and favor practice of moderation

DEATH

Many do not believe in afterlife

BELIEFS

Pacifism important; many are conscientious objectors to war

Greek Orthodox

See Eastern Orthodox

(continued)

Table II-28 **Overview of Religious Beliefs** *(continued)*

Hinduism

ILLNESS

May minimize illness and emphasize its temporary nature

Viewed as result of karma (actions/fate) of previous life

Caused by body and spirit not being in harmony or by tension in interpersonal relationships

Belief in healing responses triggered by treatment

Strong belief in alternative healing practices (*e.g.,* herbal treatments, faith healing)

DIET

Various doctrines, many vegetarian; many abstain from alcohol (mandatory for some); beef and pork are forbidden

Prefers fresh, cooked foods

DEATH

Believe in immortality of the soul

Seen as rebirth; may wish to be alert; chant prayer

Priest may tie sacred thread around neck or wrist, or body—do not remove

Water is poured into mouth, and family washes body

Cremation preferred—must be soon after death

BELIEFS

Physical, mental, and spiritual discipline, and purification of body and soul emphasized

Believe in the world as a manifestation of *Brahman,* one divine being pervading all things.

TEXTS

Vedas	Ramayana
Upanishad	Mahabharata
Bhagavad-Gita	Puranas

WORSHIP

Daily prayers, usually in home

Quiet meditation

Rituals may include use of water, fire, lights, sounds, natural objects, special postures, and gestures

Jehovah's Witness

ILLNESS

Opposes blood transfusions and organ transplantation (mandatory)

May oppose other medical treatment and all modern science

Opposes faith healing

Opposes abortion

DIET

Refuses foods to which blood has been added; may eat meats that have been drained

TEXT

Bible

Judaism

ILLNESS

Medical care emphasized

Rabbinical consultation necessary for donation and transplantation of organs

May oppose surgical procedures on the Sabbath (sundown Friday to sundown Saturday); seriously ill are exempted

May prefer burial of removed organs or body tissues

May oppose shaving

May wear skull cap and socks continuously, believing head and feet should be covered

DIET

Fasting for 24 hours on holy days of Yom Kippur (in September or October) and Tishah-b'Ab (in August)

Matzo replaces leavened bread during Passover week (in March or April)

Table II-28 **Overview of Religious Beliefs** *(continued)*

May observe strict Kosher dietary laws (mandatory for some) that prohibit pork, shellfish, and the eating of meat and dairy products at same meal or with same dishes (milk products, served first, can be followed by meat in a few minutes; reverse is not Kosher); seriously ill are exempted

BIRTH

Ritual circumcision 8 days after birth (mandatory for some)

Fetuses are buried

DEATH

Ritual burial; society members wash body

Burial as soon as possible

May oppose cremation

Many oppose autopsy and donation of body to science

Most do not believe in afterlife

Generally oppose prolongation of life after irreversible brain damage

TEXTS

Torah (first five books of Old Testament)

Talmud

Prayer book

RELIGIOUS ARTICLES

Menorah (seven-branched candlestick)

Yarmulke (skull cap, may be worn continuously)

Tallith (prayer shawl worn for morning prayers)

Tefillin, or phylacteries (leather boxes on straps containing scripture passages)

Star of David (may be worn around neck)

BELIEFS

Observation of the Sabbath (Friday evening to Saturday evening) may require not writing, traveling, using electrical appliances, or receiving treatment

Krishna

DIET

Vegetarian diet; no garlic or onions

No drugs, alcohol; herbal tea only

DEATH

Cremation mandatory

TEXTS

Vedas

Srimad-Bhagavatam

BELIEFS

Continual practice of mantra (chant)

Belief in reincarnation

Lutheran, Methodist, Presbyterian

ILLNESS

May request Communion, anointing and blessing, or visitation by minister or elder

Generally encourages use of medical science

BIRTH

Baptism by sprinkling or immersion of infants, children, or adults

DEATH

Optional last rites or scripture reading

TEXTS

Bible

Prayer book

(continued)

Table II-28   **Overview of Religious Beliefs**   *(continued)*

Mennonite

ILLNESS

Opposes laying on of hands

May oppose shock treatment and drugs

TEXTS

Bible

18 articles of the Dondecht Confession of Faith

BELIEFS

Shun modernization

No participation in government, pensions, or health plans

Methodist

See Lutheran

Mormon (Church of Jesus Christ of Latter-Day Saints)

ILLNESS

May come through partaking of harmful substances such as alcohol, tobacco, drugs, etc.

May be seen as a necessary part of the plan of salvation

May desire Sacrament of the Lord's Supper to be administered by a Church Priesthood holder

Divine healing through laying on of hands

Church may provide financial support during illness

DIET

Prohibits alcohol, tobacco, and hot drinks (tea and coffee)

Sparing use of meats

BIRTH

No infant baptism

Infants are born innocent

DEATH

Cremation is opposed

TEXTS

Bible

Book of Mormon

RELIGIOUS ARTICLES

Special undergarment may be worn by both men and women and should not be removed except during serious illness, childbirth, emergencies, etc.

BELIEFS

Abortion is opposed

Vicarious baptism for deceased who were not baptized in life

Muslim (Islamic, Moslem) and Black Muslim

ILLNESS

Opposes faith healing

May be noncompliant because of fatalistic view (illness is God's will)

Group prayer may be helpful—no priests

Favors every effort to prolong life

DIET

Pork prohibited

May oppose alcohol and traditional black American foods (corn bread, collard greens)

Fasts sunrise to sunset during Ramadan (9th month of Muslim year—falls different time each year on Western calendar); seriously ill are exempted

BIRTH

Circumcision practiced with accompanying ceremony

Aborted fetus after 30 days is treated as human being

Table II-28   **Overview of Religious Beliefs**   *(continued)*

DEATH

Confession of sins before death, with family present if possible; may wish to face toward Mecca

Family follows specific procedure for washing and preparing body, which is then turned to face Mecca

May oppose autopsy and organ transplants

Funeral usually within 24 hours after death

TEXTS

Koran (scriptures)

Hadith (traditions)

PRAYER

Five times daily—on rising, midday, afternoon, early evening, and before bed—facing Mecca and kneeling on prayer rug

Ritual washing after prayer

BELIEFS

All activities (including sleep) restricted to what is necessary for health

Personal cleanliness very important

All Muslims: gambling and idol worship prohibited

Pentecostal
See Baptist

Presbyterian
See Lutheran

Quakers
See Friends

Roman Catholic
ILLNESS

Allowed by God because of man's sins, but not considered personal punishment

May desire confession (penance) and Communion

Anointing of sick for all seriously ill patients (some patients may equate this with "Last Rites" and assume they are dying)

Donation and transplantation of organs permitted

Burial of amputated limbs (mandatory for some)

DIET

Fasting or abstaining from meat mandatory on Ash Wednesday and Good Friday (seriously ill are exempted); optional during Lent and on Fridays

Fasts from solid food for 1 hour and abstains from alcohol for 3 hours before receiving Communion (mandatory; seriously ill are exempted)

BIRTH

Baptism of infants and aborted fetuses mandatory (nurse may baptize in case of imminent death by sprinkling water on the forehead and saying, "I baptize you in the name of the Father, of the Son, and of the Holy Ghost")

DEATH

Anointing of sick (mandatory)

Extraordinary artificial means of sustaining life are unnecessary

TEXTS

Bible

Prayer book

RELIGIOUS ARTICLES

Rosary, crucifix, saints' medals, statues, holy water, lighted candles

OTHER

Attendance at mass required (seriously ill are exempted) on Sundays or late Saturday and on holy days (1/1, 8/15, 11/1, 12/8, 12/25, and 40 days after Easter)

Sacrament of Penance at least yearly (mandatory)

Opposes abortion

(continued)

Table II-28   **Overview of Religious Beliefs**   *(continued)*

Russian Orthodox
See Eastern Orthodox

Seventh-Day Adventist (Advent Christian Church)
ILLNESS

May desire baptism or Communion
Some believe in divine healing
May oppose hypnosis
May refuse treatment on the Sabbath (sundown Friday to sundown Saturday)
Healthful diet and life-style are stressed

DIET

No alcohol, coffee, tea, narcotics, or stimulants (mandatory)
Some abstain from pork, other meat, and shellfish

BIRTH

Opposes infant baptism

TEXT

Bible, especially Ten Commandments and Old Testament

Shinto
ILLNESS

May believe in prayer healing
Great concern for personal cleanliness
Physical health may be valued because of emphasis on joy and beauty of life
Family extremely important in giving care and providing emotional support

BELIEFS

Worships ancestors, ancient heroes, and nature
Traditions emphasized
Esthetically pleasing area for worship important

Sikhism
DIET

Frequently vegetarian; may exclude eggs and fish

RELIGIOUS ARTICLES

Men may wear uncut hair, a wooden comb, an iron wrist band, a short sword, and short trousers. These
symbols should not be disturbed.

DEATH

Cremation mandatory, usually within 24 hours after death

TEXT

Guru Grant Sahab

Taoist
ILLNESS

Illness is seen as part of the health/illness dualism
May be resigned to and accepting of illness
May consider medical treatment as interference

DEATH

Seen as natural part of life
Body is kept in house for 49 days
Mourning follows specific ritual patterns

TEXT

Tao-te-ching by Lao-tzu

BELIEFS

Esthetically pleasing area for meditation important

Table II-28 **Overview of Religious Beliefs**   *(continued)*

Unitarian Universalist

ILLNESS

Reason, knowledge, and individual responsibility are emphasized, so may prefer not to see clergy

BIRTH

Most do not practice infant baptism

DEATH

Prefers cremation

Zen

Meditation using lotus position (many hours and years are spent in meditation and contemplation): goal is to discover simplicity

ILLNESS

May wish consultation with Zen master

---

7. Those who have not sought religion early in life will not automatically become more religious in later life (Inlay & Smith, 1984; Nelsen, 1981).

8. A common coping method for elderly people, prayer increases feelings of self-worth and hope by reducing the sense of aloneness and abandonment. In addition to private prayer and meditation, television and radio often provide adjunct stimulus for spiritual life. Estimates indicate that 60% of viewers of religious television programs are older than age 50 years and are primarily women (Bearon & Koenig, 1990; Carson, 1989; Inlay & Smith, 1984).

9. The elderly may rely on spiritual life more than most young people because of other limitations in their lives. The spiritual realm allows for satisfying connectedness with others (Giuri, 1980; Hall, 1985). An older individual can counterbalance some of the negative, isolating aspects of aging by identifying with tradition and institutional values. Private religion can help to motivate and provide purpose to life.

10. Older adults commonly intertwine their religious beliefs with beliefs about health and illness. The nurse must assess these beliefs appropriately to facilitate the person's understanding of his illness in the context of his religion (Bearon & Koenig, 1990).

11. Three phases of suffering in the frail elderly can explain spiritual distress:
    a. Mute suffering, which revolves around a feeling of abandonment, belief that prayers are not answered, and self-isolation
    b. The cry of lament, which can be explained as an interpretation that bad things are happening because of earlier mistakes in life
    c. Liberation for change, which allows the person to transcend loneliness and to approach hope through suffering (Bearon & Koenig, 1990; Patterson, 1984; Shea, 1986)

12. Older adults commonly report a sense of increased power and control from religion and spiritual resources (Stevenson, 1982).

13. Spiritual well-being can be described as harmony and interconnection of relationships. These relationships are either time- or person-related, such as ultimate other (describes a love of God), other/nature (expresses mutual love and concern), self (values inner self), past (recognizes influence in past sociocultural and religious practices), present (finds meaning and purpose in life experiences), and future (hopes in ultimate integration). In reviewing the above, it seems likely that older adults who have achieved passage through developmental phases or tasks can use their spirituality to work through Erikson's stage of Ego Integrity versus Despair. A strong sense of satisfaction with self and life conveys an inner harmony (Hungelmann, Kenkel-Rossi, Klassen, & Stollenwerk, 1985).

14. DeYoung (1984) reported a study in which 76% of older adults in nursing homes expressed a sense of spiritual well-being. About 25% of the subjects reported that a nurse had helped them with their spiritual needs, but 79% were against nursing involvement in their spiritual lives. Reasons cited included differing beliefs and the nurse's need to focus on physical care.

TRANSCULTURAL CONSIDERATIONS

1. Religious beliefs, an integral component of culture, may influence a client's explanation of the causes of illness, perception of its severity, and choice of healer. In times of crisis, such as serious illness and impending death, religion may be a source of consolation for the client and family and may influence the course of action believed to be appropriate (Andrews & Boyle, 1995; p. 353).
2. Belonging to a specific cultural group does not imply that the person subscribes to the dominant religion of that culture. In addition, even when an individual identifies with a particular religion, the person may not accept all its beliefs or practices (Andrews & Boyle, 1995).
3. The nurse's role is not "to judge the religious virtues of individuals but rather to understand those aspects related to religion that are important to the client and family members (Andrews & Boyle, 1995; p. 355). Table II-28 was compiled with the intent to assist nurses with this understanding.

Focus Assessment Criteria

Subjective Data

A. Assess for defining characteristics
1. What is your source of spiritual strength or meaning? What is your source of peace, comfort, faith, well-being, hope, or worth?
2. How do you practice your spiritual beliefs?
3. Are there any practices that are important for your spiritual well-being?
4. Do you have a spiritual leader?
5. Has being ill or hurt affected your spiritual beliefs?

B. Assess for related factors
1. How can I help you maintain your spiritual strength (*e.g.*, contact spiritual leader, provide privacy at special times, request reading materials)?

Objective Data

A. Assess for defining characteristics
1. Current practices
    The presence of religious or spiritual articles (clothing, medals, texts)
    Visits from spiritual leader
    Visits to place of worship or meditation
    Requests for spiritual counseling or assistance
2. Response to interview on spiritual needs
    Grief   Doubt
    Anxiety   Anger
3. Participation in spiritual practices
    Rejection or neglect of previous practices
    Increased interest in spiritual matters

Outcome Criteria

The person will
*   Express his feelings related to change in beliefs
*   Describe spiritual belief system positively
*   Express desire to perform religious/spiritual practices
*   Describe satisfaction with meaning and purpose of illness/suffering/death

Interventions

A. Assess for causative and contributing factors

1. Failure of spiritual beliefs to provide explanation/comfort during crisis of illness/suffering/impending death
2. Doubting quality or strength of own faith to deal with current crisis
3. Anger toward God/spiritual beliefs for allowing/causing illness/suffering/death

B. Eliminate or reduce causative and contributing factors, if possible

1. Feeling threatened and vulnerable because of symptoms or possible death.
   a. Inform patients and families about the importance of finding meaning in illness.
   b. Suggest using prayer, imagery, and meditation to view selves as survivors rather than victims (Carson & Green, 1992).
2. Failure of spiritual beliefs to provide explanation/comfort during crisis of illness/suffering/impending death
   a. Communicate your concern seriously by being available to listen to feelings, questions, and so forth.
   b. Give "permission" to discuss spiritual matters with nurse by bringing up subject of spiritual welfare, if necessary.
   c. Use questions about past beliefs and spiritual experiences to assist person in putting this life event into wider perspective.
   d. Assist person to begin problem-solving process and move toward new spiritual understandings if necessary.
   e. Offer to contact usual or new spiritual leader.
   f. Offer to pray/meditate/read with client if you are comfortable with this, or arrange for another member of health care team if more appropriate.
   g. Provide uninterrupted quiet time for prayer/reading/meditation on spiritual concerns.
3. Doubting quality of own faith to deal with current illness/suffering/death
   a. Be available and willing to listen when client expresses self-doubt, guilt, or other negative feelings.
   b. Silence and/or touch may be useful in communicating the nurse's presence and support during times of doubt or despair.
   c. Suggest process of "life review" to identify past sources of strength or spiritual support.
   d. Suggest guided imagery or meditation to reinforce faith/beliefs.
   e. Offer to contact usual or new spiritual leader.
4. Anger toward God/spiritual beliefs for allowing or causing illness/suffering/death
   a. Express to person that anger toward God is a common reaction to illness/suffering/death.
   b. Help client recognize and discuss feelings of anger.
   c. Allow client to problem solve to find ways to express and relieve anger.
   d. Offer to contact usual spiritual leader.
   e. Offer to contact other spiritual support person (*e.g.*, pastoral care, hospital chaplain) if person cannot share feelings with usual spiritual leader.

Rationale

- The client may view anger at God and a religious leader as a "forbidden" topic, and may be reluctant to initiate discussions of spiritual conflicts.
- Spirituality influences attitudes and behavior related to right and wrong, family, child rearing, work, money, politics, and many other functional areas (Taylor et al., 1989).
- According to Stoll (1984, p. 347), "prayer, private or with a significant other, is overwhelmingly reported as the most meaningful spiritual coping strategy and religious practice."
- The nature of the spiritual care an individual receives may directly affect the speed and quality of the individual's recovery, or the quality of the individual and family's dying experience (Carson & Green, 1992; Stiles, 1990).

- The physical environment often influences spirituality, so nurses should provide appropriate settings whenever possible, considering such aspects as quiet, nature, music, art, and the like.
- Research shows that people with higher levels of spiritual well-being tend to experience lower levels of anxiety (Kaczorowski, 1989). For many people, spiritual activities provide a direct coping action (Sodestrom & Martinson, 1987) and may positively influence adaptation to illness (Carson & Green, 1992).
- The nurse should function as an advocate in recognizing and respecting the individual's spiritual needs, which may sometimes be overlooked or ignored by other health professionals.

Interventions—*Child Focus*

1. Encourage children to maintain bedtime or before-meal prayer rituals.
2. If compatible with the child's religious beliefs
   a. Share religious picture book and other religious articles.
   b. Consult with family for appropriate books or objects (*e.g.*, medals, statues).
3. Explore child's feelings regarding illness as punishment for wrongdoing (Wong, 1995).

Rationale

- Continuance of activities that are usually parts of their lives can help the child cope with threatening situations (Wong, 1995).
- Because this society has a Judeo-Christian orientation, the nurse must be sensitive to other religious backgrounds (*e.g.*, Buddhist, Hindu, Moslem).
- Often illness or injury is viewed as punishment for real or imagined wrongdoing (Wong, 1995).

■ Spiritual Distress
Related to Conflict Between Religious or Spiritual Beliefs and Prescribed Health Regimen

Outcome Criteria

The person will
- Express religious or spiritual satisfaction
- Express decreased feelings of guilt and fear
- Relate he is supported in his decision about his health regimen
- State that conflict has been eliminated or reduced

Interventions

A. Assess for causative and contributing factors (see Table II-28)

1. Lack of information about or understanding of spiritual restrictions
2. Lack of information about or understanding of health regimen
3. Informed, true conflict
4. Parental conflict concerning treatment of child
5. Lack of time for deliberation before emergency treatment or surgery

B. Eliminate or reduce causative and contributing factors, if possible
   1. Lack of information about spiritual restrictions
      a. Have spiritual leader discuss restrictions and exemptions as they apply to those who are seriously ill or hospitalized.
      b. Provide reading materials on religious and spiritual restrictions and exemptions.
      c. Encourage person to seek information from and discuss restrictions with others in spiritual group.
      d. Chart results of these discussions.
   2. Lack of information about health regimen
      a. Provide accurate information about health regimen, treatments, medications.
      b. Explain the nature and purpose of therapy.
      c. Discuss possible outcomes without therapy; be factual and honest, but do not attempt to frighten or force person to accept treatment.
   3. Informed, true conflict
      a. Encourage individual and physician to consider alternate methods of therapy* (*e.g.*, use of Christian Science nurses and practitioners; special surgeons and techniques for surgery without blood transfusions).
      b. Support individual making informed decision—even if decision conflicts with own values.
         Consult own spiritual leader.
         Change assignment so that person can be cared for by nurse with compatible beliefs.
         Arrange for discussions among health care team to share feelings.
   4. Parental conflict over treatment of child
      a. If parents refuse treatment of child, follow interventions under 3a and 3b, above.
      b. If treatment is still refused, physician or hospital administrator may obtain court order appointing temporary guardian to consent to treatment.*
      c. Call spiritual leader to support parents (and possibly child).
      d. Encourage expression of negative feelings.
   5. Emergency treatment
      a. Consult family if possible.
      b. Delay treatment, if possible, until spiritual needs have been met (*e.g.*, receiving last rites before surgery);* send spiritual leader to treatment room or operating room, if necessary.
      c. Anticipate reaction and provide support when individual chooses to accept or is forced to accept spiritually unacceptable therapy.
         Depression, withdrawal, anger, fear
         Loss of will to live
         Reduced speed and quality of recovery

Rationale

- The nurse's role is as an advocate for the family.
- Interventions focus on providing information about all alternatives and the consequences of each option (Quintero, 1993).
- The nurse should be the link between the family and other members of the health care team (Quintero, 1993).
- Court orders to save a child's life remove the parent's right to refuse (Wong, 1995).

* May require a primary care professional's order.

■ Spiritual Distress
Related to (Specify), as Evidenced by Inability to Practice Spiritual Rituals

---

Outcome Criteria

The person will
- Continue spiritual practices not detrimental to health
- Express decreasing feelings of guilt and anxiety
- Express satisfaction with spiritual condition

Interventions

A. Explore whether the client desires to engage in an allowable religious or spiritual practice or ritual; if so, provide opportunities for him to do so

B. Express your understanding and acceptance of the importance of the client's religious or spiritual beliefs and practices

C. Assess for causative and contributing factors
  1. Hospital or nursing home environment
  2. Limitations related to disease process or treatment regimen (*e.g.*, cannot kneel to pray owing to traction; prescribed diet differs from usual religious diet)
  3. Fear of imposing on or antagonizing medical and nursing staff with requests for spiritual rituals
  4. Embarrassment over spiritual beliefs or customs (especially common in adolescents)
  5. Separation from articles, texts, or environment of spiritual significance
  6. Lack of transportation to spiritual place or service
  7. Spiritual leader unavailable because of emergency or lack of time

D. Eliminate or reduce causative and contributing factors, if possible
  1. Limitations imposed by the hospital or nursing home environment
      a. Provide privacy and quiet as needed for daily prayer, for visit of spiritual leader, and for spiritual reading and contemplation.
          Pull curtains or close door.
          Turn off television and radio.
          Ask desk to hold calls if possible.
          Note spiritual interventions on Kardex and include in care plan.
      b. Contact spiritual leader to clarify practices and perform religious rites or services, if desired.
          Communicate with spiritual leader concerning person's condition.
          Address Roman Catholic, Orthodox, and Episcopal priests as "Father," other Christian ministers as "Pastor," and Jewish rabbis as "Rabbi."
          Prevent interruption during visit, if possible.
          Offer to provide table or stand covered with clean white cloth.
          Chart visit and patient's response.
      c. Inform about religious services and materials available within the institution.

2. Limitations related to disease process or treatment regimen
   a. Encourage spiritual rituals not detrimental to health (see Table II-28).

   Assist individuals with physical limitations in prayer and spiritual observances (*e.g.*, help to hold rosary; help to kneeling position, if appropriate).

   Assist in habits of personal cleanliness.

   Avoid shaving if beard is of spiritual significance.

   Allow to wear religious clothing or jewelry whenever possible.

   Make special arrangements for burial of resected limbs or body organs.

   Allow family or spiritual leader to perform ritual care of body.

   Make arrangements as needed for other important spiritual rituals (*e.g.*, circumcisions).

   b. Maintain diet with spiritual restrictions when not detrimental to health (see Table II-28).

   Consult with dietitian.

   Allow fasting for short periods if possible.*

   Change therapeutic diet as necessary.*

   Have family or friends bring in special food, if possible.

   Have members of spiritual group supply meals to the person at home.

   Be as flexible as possible in serving methods, times of meals, and so forth.

3. Fear of imposing or embarrassment
   a. Communicate acceptance of various spiritual beliefs and practices.
   b. Convey nonjudgmental, respectful attitude.
   c. Acknowledge importance of spiritual needs.
   d. Express willingness of health care team to help in meeting spiritual needs.
   e. Provide privacy and ensure confidentiality.

4. Separation from articles, texts, or environment of spiritual significance
   a. Question individual about missing religious or spiritual articles or reading material (see Table II-28).
   b. Obtain missing items from clergy in hospital, spiritual leader, family, or members of spiritual group.
   c. Treat these articles and books with respect.
   d. Allow person to keep spiritual articles and books within reach as much as possible, or where they can be easily seen.
   e. Protect from loss or damage (*e.g.*, medal pinned to gown can be lost in laundry).
   f. Recognize that articles without overt religious meaning may have spiritual significance for individual (*e.g.*, wedding band).
   g. Use spiritual texts in large print, in Braille, or on tape when appropriate.
   h. Provide opportunity for individual to pray with others or be read to by members of own religious group or member of the health care team who feels comfortable with these activities.

   Jews and Seventh-Day Adventists would find Psalms 23, 34, 42, 63, 71, 103, 121, and 127 appropriate.

   Christians would also appreciate I Corinthians 13, Matthew 5:3–11, Romans 12, and the Lord's Prayer.

* May require a primary care professional's order.

5. Lack of transportation
   a. Take person to chapel or quiet environment on hospital grounds.
   b. Arrange transportation to church or synagogue for individual in home.
   c. Provide access to spiritual programming on radio and television when appropriate.
6. Spiritual leader unavailable because of emergency or lack of time
   a. Baptize critically ill newborn of Greek Orthodox, Episcopal, or Roman Catholic parents (see Table II-28).
   b. Perform other mandatory spiritual rituals if possible.

Rationale

- For a client who places a high value on prayer or other spiritual practices, these practices can provide meaning and purpose and can be a source of comfort and strength (Carson, 1989).
- Conveying a nonjudgmental attitude may help reduce the client's uneasiness about expressing his beliefs and practices (Sodestrom & Martinson, 1987).
- Privacy and quiet provide an environment that enables reflection and contemplation.
- The nurse—even one who does not subscribe to the same religious beliefs or values of the client—can still help him meet his spiritual needs.
- These measures can help the client maintain spiritual ties and practice important rituals (Carson, 1989).
- Many religious prohibit certain behaviors; complying with restrictions may be an important part of the client's worship.

Spiritual Well-Being, Potential for Enhanced

DEFINITION

Potential for Enhanced Spiritual Well-Being: An individual who experiences affirmation of life in a relationship with a higher power (as defined by the person), self, community, and environment that nurtures and celebrates wholeness (The National Interfaith Coalition on Aging, 1980).

DEFINING CHARACTERISTICS (CARSON, 1989)

Inner strength that nurtures
Sense of awareness	Sacred source
Trust relationships	Inner peace
Unifying force	

Intangible motivation and commitment directed toward ultimate values of love, meaning, hope, beauty, and truth
Trust relations with or in the transcendent that provide bases for meaning and hope in life's experiences and love in one's relationships
Has meaning and purpose to existence

RISK FACTORS

Refer to Related Factors.

RELATED FACTORS

Because this is a diagnosis of positive functioning, the use of related factors is not warranted.

> **Author's Note**
> Refer to *Spiritual Distress*.

Key Concepts

1. "Growth in spirituality is a dynamic process in which an individual becomes increasingly aware of the meaning, purpose and values in life" (Carson, 1989, p. 26). Spiritual growth is a two-directional process: horizontal and vertical. "The horizontal process increases the person's awareness of the transcendent values inherent in all relationships and activities of life" (Carson, 1989, p. 26). The vertical process moves the person into a closer relationship with a higher being, as conceived by the person. Carson illustrates that it is possible to develop spirituality through the horizontal process and not the vertical. For example, a person can define his or her spirituality in terms of relationships, art, or music without a relationship with a higher being, just as an individual can focus his or her spirituality on a higher being and may not express spirituality through other avenues.
2. Faith is necessary for spiritual growth to occur, particularly for a relationship to a higher being. Hope is also critical for spiritual development and is integral to the horizontal and vertical processes (Carson, 1989).
3. Research suggests that human immunodeficiency virus–positive individuals who are spiritually well and who find meaning and purpose in life are also hardier (Carson & Green, 1992).
4. Regardless of a person's religion or lack of belief in any, the process of spiritual growth is similar. The religious foundations that guide the growth are very different. "When people are together on the level of spirituality, they meet on the level of the heart. On this level, all people are one. There is only one God, and it would seem logical that people's experiences of the transcendent would be similar. When the experiences are reframed into religious dogma, that is when disagreements begin" (Carson, 1989, p. 46).
5. Spirituality has been found to be especially important to caregivers of victims of chronic illness, and nurses can work to enhance spiritual well-being for these individuals (Kaye & Robinson, 1994).

Focus Assessment Criteria

Subjective

A. Person communicates
   1. A trust relationship with or in the transcendent that provides bases for meaning and hope in life's experiences
   2. Meaning and purpose to existence
   3. An inner strength that nurtures
   4. An inner peace

> **Outcome Criteria**
>
> The person will
> - Maintain previous relationship with his or her higher being
> - Continue spiritual practices not detrimental to health
> - Express continued spiritual harmony and wholeness

Interventions

A. Support the person's spiritual practices

1. Refer to Interventions to reduce barriers to spiritual practices under *Spiritual Distress related to (specify) as evidenced by inability to practice spiritual rituals.*

References/Bibliography

Andrews, M., & Boyle, J. (1995). *Transcultural concepts in nursing care* (2nd ed.). Philadelphia: J. B. Lippincott.

Bauer, T., & Barron, C. R. (1995). Nursing interventions for spiritual care: Preferences of the community-based elderly. *Journal of Holistic Nursing, 13*, 268–279.

Bearon, L., & Koenig, H. (1990). Religious cognitions and use of prayer in health and illness. *The Gerontologist, 30*, 249–253.

Bruhn, J. G., Cordova, F. D., Williams, J. A., & Fuentes, R. G. (1977). The wellness process. *Journal of Community Health, 2*, 234–240.

Burkhardt, M. A. (1994). Becoming and connecting: Elements of spirituality for women. *Holistic Nursing Practice, 8*, 12–21.

Carson, V. B. (1989). *Spiritual dimensions of nursing practice*. Philadelphia: W. B. Saunders.

Carson, V. B., & Green, H. (1992). Spiritual well-being: A predictor of hardiness in patients with acquired immunodeficiency syndrome. *Journal of Professional Nursing, 8*, 209–220.

DeYoung, S. (1984). Perceptions of the institutionalized elderly regarding the nurse's role in supporting spiritual well-being. In R. Fehring (Ed.). *Proceedings of the conference on spirituality*. Milwaukee, WI: Marquette University.

Emblen, J. D., & Halstead, L. (1993). Spiritual needs and interventions: Comparing the views of patients, nurses and chaplains. *Clinical Nurse Specialist, 7*, 175–182.

Giuri, A. (1980). Aging and the spiritual life. *Spiritual Life, 26*, 41–46.

Hall, C. M. (1985). Religion and aging. *Journal of Religion and Health, 24*, 70–78.

Hungelmann, J., Kenkel-Rossi, E., Klassen, L., & Stollenwerk, R. M. (1985). Spiritual well-being in older adults, harmonious interconnectedness. *Journal of Religion and Health, 24*, 147–153.

Inlay, S. C., & Smith, D. R. (1984). Aging and religious participation. *Journal of Gerontology, 39*, 357–363.

Kaczorowski, J. M. (1989). Spiritual well-being and anxiety in adults diagnosed with cancer. *The Hospice Journal, 5*(3/4), 105–115.

Kaye, J., & Robinson, K. M. (1994). Spirituality among caregivers. *Image: The Journal of Nursing Scholarship, 26*, 218–221.

Martin, C., Burrows, C., & Pomilio, J. (1978). Spiritual needs of patients survey. In S. Fish & J. A. Shelly (Eds.). *Spiritual care: The nurse's role*. Downers Grove, IL: Intervarsity Press.

Matteson, A. M., & McConnell, E. S. (1988). *Gerontological nursing: Concepts and practice*. Philadelphia: W. B. Saunders.

Millison, M. B. (1995). A review of the research on spiritual care and hospice. *The Hospice Journal, 10*, 3–17.

Mindel, C. H., & Vaughan, C. E. (1978). A multidimensional approach to religiosity and disengagement. *Journal of Gerontology, 33*, 103–108.

Moberg, D. O. (1984). Subjective measures of spiritual well-being. *Review of Religious Research, 25*, 351–364.

Nelsen, H. M. (1981). Life without afterlife: Toward a congruency of belief across generations. *Journal of Scientific Study in Religion, 20*, 109–118.

Patterson, R. A. (1984). The search for meaning: A pastoral response to suffering. *Hospital Progress, 65*, 46–49.

Peri, T. C. (1995). Promoting spirituality in persons with acquired immunodeficiency syndrome: A nursing intervention. *Holistic Nursing Practice, 10*, 68–76.

Piles, C. L. (1990). Providing spiritual care. *Nurse Educator, 15*(1), 36–41.

Quintero, C. (1993). Blood administration in pediatric Jehovah's Witness. *Pediatric Nursing, 19*(1), 46–48.

Ryan, E. (1985). Selecting an instrument to measure spiritual distress. *Oncology Nursing Forum, 12*(2), 93–94, 99.

Ryan, J. (1984). The neglected crisis. *American Journal of Nursing, 84*, 1257–1258.

Ryan, M. C., & Patterson, J. (1987). Loneliness in the elderly. *Journal of Gerontological Nursing, 13*(5), 6–12.

Shea, G. (1986). Meeting the pastoral care needs of an aging population. *Health Progress, 67*(5), 36–37, 68.

Sodestrom, K. E., & Martinson, I. M. (1987). Patients' spiritual coping strategies: A study of nurse and patient perspectives. *Oncology Nursing Forum, 14*(2), 41–46.

Stevenson, J. S. (1982). Construction of a scale to measure load, power and margin in life. *Nursing Research, 31*, 222–225.

Stiles, M. K. (1990). The shining stranger: Nurse–family spiritual relationship. *Cancer Nursing, 13*, 235–245.

Stoll, R. I. (1984). Spiritual assessment: A nursing perspective. In R. Fehring (Ed.). *Proceedings of the conference on spirituality*. Milwaukee, WI: Marquette University.

Taylor, C., Lillis, C., & LeMone, P. (1989). *Fundamentals of nursing: The art and science of nursing care*. Philadelphia: J. B. Lippincott.

Van Heukelem, J. (1982). Assessing the spiritual needs of children and their families. In J. A. Shelley (Ed.). *The spiritual needs of children*. Downers Grove, IL: Intervarsity Press.

Wald, F. S., & Bailey, C. (1990). Nurturing the spiritual component in care for the terminally ill. *CARING Magazine, 9*(11), 64–68.

Whaley, L. F., & Wong, D. L. (1993). *Essentials of pediatric nursing* (4th ed.). St. Louis: C. V. Mosby.

Wong, D. (1995). *Nursing care of infants and children* (5th ed.). St. Louis: Mosby–Year Book.

Thought Processes, Altered

DEFINITION
Altered Thought Processes: A state in which an individual experiences a disruption in such mental activities as conscious thought, reality orientation, problem solving, judgment, and comprehension related to coping, personality, and/or mental disorder.

DEFINING CHARACTERISTICS
Major (Must Be Present)
Inaccurate interpretation of stimuli, internal and/or external

Minor (May Be Present)
Cognitive defects, including problem solving, abstraction, memory deficits
Suspiciousness
Delusions
Hallucinations
Phobias
Obsessions
Distractibility
Lack of consensual validation
Confusion/disorientation
Ritualistic behavior
Impulsivity
Inappropriate social behavior

RELATED FACTORS
Pathophysiologic
Related to physiologic changes secondary to:
    Drug or alcohol withdrawal
Related to biochemical alterations
Related to acute primary brain pathology (*e.g.*, traumatic brain injury)
Related to degenerative brain pathology (*e.g.*, Alzheimer's dementia)

Situational (Personal, Environmental)
Related to emotional trauma
Related to abuse (physical, sexual, mental)
Related to torture
Related to childhood trauma
Related to repressed fears
Related to panic level of anxiety
Related to continued low levels of stimulation

Related to decreased attention span and ability to process information secondary to:
Depression
Fear
Anxiety
Grieving

Maturational

Older Adult
Related to isolation, late-life depression

Author's Note

Altered Thought Processes describes a person with altered perception and cognition that interferes with daily living. Causes are psychological disturbances (*e.g.*, depression, personality disorders, bipolar disorders). For this diagnosis, the focus of nursing is on reducing disturbed thinking and/or promoting reality orientation.

The nurse should be cautioned against using this diagnosis as a "waste basket" diagnosis for all clients with disturbed thinking or confusion. Frequently, confusion in an elderly person is erroneously attributed to aging. Confusion in the elderly can be caused by a single factor (*e.g.*, dementia, medication side effects, metabolic disorder) or by depression related to multiple factors associated with aging. Depression causes impaired thinking more frequently than dementia in older adults (Miller, 1995). Refer to *Confusion* for additional information.

Errors in Diagnostic Statements

Altered Thought Processes related to depression

When a person exhibits signs and symptoms of depression and impaired cognition, use of *Altered Thought Processes* would seem appropriate. However, the impaired cognition associated with depression should be viewed as a manifestation of depression, rather than as a response to be treated. Depression is a state that represents ineffective coping; thus, the following diagnosis would be more clinically useful: *Ineffective Individual Coping related to unknown etiology, as evidenced by slowed affect, reports of constant sadness, little motivation, and memory difficulties*. Because the central issue in depression is low self-esteem, the nurse uses a focus assessment to determine factors that are causing or contributing to low self-esteem (*e.g.*, disabilities, losses, feelings of rejection).

Altered Thought Processes related to loss of memory

Loss of memory can be present in many situations (*e.g.*, depression, dementia, anxiety, sensory deprivation, psychiatric disorders, endocrine disorders). The nursing focus would vary, depending on the contributing factors. For example, loss of memory with head injuries usually is very anxiety producing; thus, a diagnosis of *Anxiety* would be more useful. Loss of memory that poses a danger would be associated with *Risk for Injury*. If *Altered Thought Processes* were appropriate for this person, the diagnosis should be restated as *Altered Thought Process related to* (specify, *e.g.*, *effects of hypoxia secondary to cerebrovascular accident), as evidenced by loss of memory*.

Key Concepts

1. Thought is a functioning process of the brain that integrates every individual's daily living experiences. Cognitive processes are the mental processes related to reasoning, comprehension, judgment, and memory. Cognitive function is influenced by physiologic functions, stimuli from the environment, and the person's emotional state (Porth, 1994).
2. The cognitive processes of remembering and perception are influenced by the individual's current needs and interests as well as his store of knowledge.
3. Development of cognitive abilities follows a systematic pattern of maturational experiences and requires varied perceptual stimulation.

4. A disruption in the quality and quantity of incoming stimuli can affect an individual's thought processes.
5. What a person thinks about an event influences both feelings and behavior. Any changes in thoughts, feelings, or behavior result in changes in the other two (Potocki & Everly, 1989).
6. People attempt to gain control over a situation by assigning meaning; sometimes this is a rational explanation, and sometimes it is irrational (Sideleau, 1987).
7. Over time, irrational beliefs lead to chronic dissatisfaction; the person's thinking patterns become characterized by "shoulds" and "musts" (Sideleau, 1987).
8. Helping the person to restructure irrational belief is based on the use of objective, reality-based data. Three basic questions are raised (Everly, 1989):
   a. What is the evidence?
   b. What is another explanation?
   c. So what if it happens?
9. Actual events frequently become reorganized and reinterpreted individually so that they may be substantially changed and distorted during the process of remembering.
10. The ability to conceptualize develops relatively slowly and requires contact with others; the development of concrete concepts precedes the development of abstract concepts.
11. Suicide may be a possible risk for these individuals because of the potential for multiple losses and disruptions to their life, such as loss of social supports through course of illness, low self-esteem enhancing delusions and hallucinations as illness recedes, hopelessness associated with a severe illness, and so forth.

Reality

1. Reality testing is the objective evaluation and judgment of the world outside the self, differentiated from one's thoughts and feelings.
2. Reality testing is determined by early life experiences and by significant people in one's life.
3. Delusions—fixed false beliefs—and hallucinations originate during extreme emotional stress; they represent attempts to decrease panic (Varcarolis, 1994).
4. Delusions include those of:
   a. *Grandeur:* An exaggerated sense of importance of identity or of ability
   b. *Persecution:* A sense that one is being harassed
   c. *Reference:* Belief that the behavior of others refers to oneself
   d. *Influence:* Exaggerated sense of power over others
   e. *Control:* Sense that one is being manipulated by others
   f. *Bodily sensations:* Belief that one's organs are diseased, despite contrary evidence
   g. *Infidelity:* Belief, due to pathologic jealousy, that one's lover is unfaithful
5. Delusions arise when the person attempts to alter reality. First, he denies his own feelings, then projects those feelings onto the environment, and finally he must explain this to others (Dixon, 1969).
6. The fundamental feelings being projected by suspicious and grandiose clients are inadequacy and worthlessness.
7. Hallucinations are perceptions that arise from within the person's own thoughts; he actually hears, sees, feels, or tastes the phenomenon.
8. Hallucinations meet underlying needs (*e.g.*, loneliness, anxiety, self-worth), and until a person can substitute other activities, he may be unwilling to "give these up" (Schwartzman, 1976). Hallucinations occur most frequently in the auditory mode.
9. The person may spend much time in his fantasy world, which leads to a lack of consensual validation of language. Not only are the connections between words disturbed, but the words often have a different meaning to the person than is generally accepted.
10. Disorganized thinking often leads to regression in behavior, disturbed communication, and difficulty in interactions with others.
11. Illusions are mistaken or misinterpreted sensory perceptions. They occur most commonly in acute delirium and in organic brain syndromes.

Focus Assessment Criteria

Acquire data from client and significant others.

Subjective Data

A. Assess the history of the individual

   1. Life-style

      Interests

      Strengths and limitations

      Work history

      Coping patterns (past and present)

      Education

      Previous level of functioning and handling stress

      Use of alcohol/drugs

   2. Support system (availability)

   3. History of medical problems and treatments (medications)

   4. Activities of daily living (ability and desire to perform)

   5. Family

      Quality of relationships

      History of mental illness

      Beliefs about symptoms

   6. Involvement with cultural, religious, or ethnic groups

      Quality of support

      Beliefs about mental illness

B. Assess for defining characteristics

   1. Feelings of

      Extreme sadness and worthlessness   Mistrust or suspiciousness of others

      Guilt for past actions   Others making him do and say things

      Apprehension in various situations   Excessive self-importance

      Being rejected or isolated   Depersonalization

      Living in an unreal world

   2. Fears

      That others will harm him   Of thoughts racing

      Of falling apart   Of being held prisoner

      That mind is being controlled by external agents   Body is rotting or not there

      Of being unable to cope

   3. Hallucinations (visual, auditory, gustatory, olfactory, tactile—includes an objective component)

      Circumstances   Positive or negative

      Number/day, type, particulars, and details   Antecedents

      Frequency, time of day   Consequences

      Duration   Ability to control them

   4. Depression (Miller, 1995)

      Difficulties with memory   Consistent sadness

      Lack of motivation   Apathetic responses

      Inability to concentrate

   5. Delusions

      Fixed or fleeting

      Thought broadcasting (others can hear person's thoughts)

      Thought insertion (others putting thoughts into person's mind)

      Physical complaints of fatigue, anorexia, constipation, insomnia, dysphagia

      Delusions of foreboding gloom, diminished self-esteem, money, death, guilt

   6. Orientation

      Person

         "What is your name?"

         "What is your occupation?"

Time
"What season is it?"
"What month is it?"
Place
"Where are you?"
"Where do you live?"
7. Problem-solving ability
"What would you do if the phone rang?"
"What is the difference between the doctor and the president?"
8. Memory: immediate, recent, remote
9. Reality testing
Degrees of realness person feels regarding the experiences in relation to actual reality
Extent to which person will act on these experiences
10. Unusual sensations and thought productions

Precipitating factors	Routine time of occurrence
Frequency and duration	Description in individual's own words

Objective Data (Includes a Subjective Component)

A. Assess for defining characteristics
1. General appearance
Facial expression (alert, sad, hostile, expressionless)
Dress (meticulous, disheveled, seductive, eccentric)
2. Behavior during interview

Withdrawn	Quiet
Hostile	Negativism
Apathetic	Level of attention/concentration
Cooperative	Level of anxiety

3. Communication pattern
Content

Appropriate	Homicidal plans
Sexual preoccupations	Suicidal ideas
Rambling	Lacking content
Suspicious	Obsessions

Denying problem
Delusions (grandeur, persecution, reference, influence, control, or bodily sensations)
Religiousness
Worthlessness

Pattern of speech

Appropriate	Word salad
Loose connection of ideas	Unable to come to conclusion, be decisive
Blocking (unable to finish idea)	
Jumps from one topic to another	Clang association
Circumstantial (unable to get to point)	Echolalia
Neologisms	

Rate of speech

Appropriate	Reduced
Excessive	Pressured

Affect
Blunted
Bright
Flat
Sad
Gestures, mannerisms, facial grimaces
Posture

Affect congruent with content of speech
Affect appropriate to verbal content
Affect inappropriate to verbal content

4. Interaction skills
    With nurse

Inappropriate	Shows dependency
Relates well	Demanding/pleading
Withdrawn/preoccupied	Hostile

With significant others
Relates with all (some) family members
Does not seek interaction
Hostile toward one (all) members
Does not have visitors

5. Motor activity

Within normal limits	Waxy flexibility
Agitated	Echopraxia
Decreased/stuporous	Stereotyped behavior

6. Activities of daily living

Time management	Initiation and sequencing of activities
Task organization	Safety issues

Outcome Criteria

The person will
- Recognize changes in thinking/behavior
- Identify situations that occur before hallucinations/delusions
- Use coping strategies to deal effectively with hallucinations/delusions (specify)
- Maintain reality orientation
- Communicate clearly with others
- Participate in unit activities (specify)
- Express delusional material less frequently

Interventions

A. Promote communication that enhances the person's sense of integrity

1. Encourage open, honest dialogue.
    a. Approach in a calm, nurturing manner.
    b. Persevere, be consistent, be hopeful.
    c. Be open and share with the person. Use his or her name throughout conversations.
    d. Discuss expectations and demands.
    e. Recognize when person is testing the trustworthiness of others.
    f. Avoid making promises that cannot be fulfilled.
    g. Offer set periods of time during each shift when you can meet; initial staff contact should be minimal and brief with a suspicious person. Increase time as suspiciousness decreases.
    h. Explain if appointments cannot be kept.
    i. Verify your interpretation of what person is experiencing. ("I understand you are fearful of others.")
    j. Be an attentive listener; note both verbal and nonverbal messages.
    k. Help individual verbalize what person indicates nonverbally.
    l. Use terminology that is familiar and evokes little anxiety.
    m. Speak clearly and audibly.
    n. Recognize the importance of body posture, facial expression, and tone of voice.

o. Present information in a matter-of-fact way that is least likely to be misinterpreted; do not use humor or bantering with suspicious people.

p. Use communication that helps person maintain his own individuality (*e.g.*, "I" instead of "we").

q. Eliminate whispered comments or incomplete explanations that encourage fantasy interpretation.

r. Tell person about all the various meetings in which their case will be discussed with other health professionals.

s. Give brief explanations before doing any unfamiliar procedures with the person (*e.g.*, medications, invasive procedures, treatments).

2. Maintain client's personal space.

a. Do not touch person until you have developed an ongoing trusting relationship.

b. Talk to the person in open space; avoid small rooms or offices.

c. Face at a 45-degree angle.

3. Minimize distress by reassuring person that these symptoms are part of the illness but can recede as the illness improves.

4. Try to understand the client's private world and what it means.

5. Minimize number of staff assigned to care for client to help establish a rapport.

6. Try to maintain client in quiet, well-lit areas.

B. Assist person to differentiate between own thoughts and reality

1. Validate the presence of hallucinations.

a. Observe for verbal and nonverbal cues—inappropriate laughter, delayed verbal response, eye movements, moving lips without sound, increased motor movements, grinning.

"Are you hearing/seeing something now?"

"What's happening now?"

b. Assist person in observing thoughts and feelings as they relate to the underlying needs being met.

"Has this happened before?"   "You were lonely?"

"What were you doing/thinking?"

c. Assist person to analyze the hallucinations.

How often do they occur (frequency)

Intensity or clarity of the hallucinations (intensity)

How long do the episodes last (duration)

Where and when the incidents occur and what happens just before the incidents (antecedents)

What happens after the hallucinations (consequences)

Describe the hallucinations in detail.

Probe for presence of alternative hallucinations (*e.g.*, person may have different voices giving different messages).

2. Help person to self-regulate or control hallucinations (Hamera, Peterson, & Handley, 1991; Johnson, 1993; Williams, 1989)

a. Identify triggers that increase anxiety.

b. Discuss the use of a control strategy (refer to B5a–c, for behavioral, cognitive, or physiologic strategies).

c. Teach to dismiss the hallucinations ("Tell the voices to go away").

d. Explain the effects of using competing stimuli (*e.g.*, music, humming for voices).

3. Focus on here-and-now.

a. Accept the person's experiences and perceptions of reality (Baker, 1995).

b. Understand the language used to describe their experiences. There is often a variety of symbols and feelings involved (Baker, 1995).

c. Encourage person to validate his thoughts by sharing them with significant others.

d. Avoid derogation or belittling when person misinterprets stimuli or is delusional; do not laugh or make fun of him.

    e. Encourage person to identify and focus on his strengths, not his weaknesses.

    f. Encourage differentiation of stimuli arising from inner sources from those from outside (*e.g.*, in response to "I hear voices," say: "Those are the voices of people on TV" or "I hear no one speaking now; they are your own thoughts").

    g. Avoid the impression that you confirm or approve reality distortions; tactfully express doubt without arguing or debating.

    h. Focus on feelings behind the reality distortions rather than the content.

    i. Focus on reality-oriented aspects of the communication (*e.g.*, if person states, "The TV is controlling my mind," the nurse can say, "How does it make you feel when others try to control you?").

    j. Set limits for discussing repetitive delusional material. ("You've already told me about that; let's talk about something realistic.")

    k. Teach person to relearn to focus attention on real things and people.

    l. Identify the underlying needs being met by the delusions/hallucinations.

    m. Help person become aware that his needs are being expressed in fantasy and teach more appropriate ways to meet these needs (*e.g.*, aggression expressed through delusion of persecution can be put into constructive activity, such as hammering metal objects).

    n. Do not automatically dismiss physical complaints; however, do not express undue concern.

    o. Provide positive reinforcement when person talks about feelings and reality-based experiences.

    p. When person is experiencing illusions, remove object causing the illusion; dismantle it, if possible, explaining in reassuring tones what it is, and allow person to examine it if he or she desires.

    q. Minimize episodes of illusions by allowing person to have sense-related objects from home, providing a night-light, explaining strange equipment/objects and allowing person to handle them, and matching surroundings to the person's sensory level (*i.e.*, reducing sensory overload or increasing sensory stimuli).

4. Assist in restricting irrational thoughts (refer to *Anxiety*).

5. Explore various strategies that help people cope with their symptoms (*i.e.*, hallucinations, delusions) (Frederick & Cotanch, 1995; Westacott, 1995; Gardner & Thompson, 1994).

    a. Behavioral control strategies

        Increasing or decreasing activity level

        Postural change

        Avoidance mechanisms

            Avoiding potentially unpleasant situations

            Use of specific and restricted social withdrawal

        Engaging in leisure activities

            Reading   Shopping

            Drawing   Hobbies

            Yard work

        Monaural inclusion/single ear plug to reduce hallucinations

            Humming

            Gargling

    b. Cognitive control strategies

        Passive and active attention diversion

        Actively suppressing disturbing thoughts and voices

        Thought stopping

        Dismissing the voices/thoughts

        Problem solving

        Distraction

            Listening to radio   Singing

            Watching TV   Praying

        Improving self-image

    c. Physiologic control strategies

Drug or alcohol use	Sleep
Relaxation	Anxiety management
Exercise	Taking PRN medications

  6. Encourage and support client to take an active part in the treatment program by initiating coping strategies, challenging symptoms, and looking for alternative views on how they interpret events, situations, and so forth (Tarrier, Harwood, & Yusopoff, 1990).

C. Assist the person with disordered thinking in communicating more effectively

1. Ask for the meaning of what is said; do not assume that you understand.
2. Validate your interpretation of what is being said ("Is this what you mean?").
3. Clarify all global pronouns—we, they ("Who is *they?*").
4. Refocus when person changes the subject in the middle of an explanation or thought.
5. Tell the person when you are not following his train of thought.
6. Do not mimic or restate words or phrases that you do not understand.
7. Teach the person to validate consensually with others.
8. When it is necessary to confront the person about the behavior, use the components of DISC: *d*escribe the behavior of the person, *i*ndicate the desired behavior, *s*pecify nursing actions, and describe the positive and negative *c*onsequences. ("Your yelling is disrupting people. I suggest you spend some time alone in your room until you gain control of yourself. I'll check on you in 15 minutes; if you haven't gained control by then, I'll give you some medication to help you settle.")

D. Encourage a more mature level of functioning

1. Assist person to set limits on his own behavior.
   a. Discuss alternative methods of coping (*e.g.*, taking a walk instead of crying).
   b. Confront person with the attitude that regression is not acceptable behavior.
   c. Help delay gratification (*e.g.*, "I want you to wait 5 minutes before you repeat your request for help in making your bed").
   d. Encourage person to achieve realistic expectations.
   e. Pace expectations to avoid frustration.
2. Encourage and support person in the decision-making process.
   a. Help person review options and the advantages and disadvantages of each option.
   b. Assist in structuring daily living activities (*e.g.*, help schedule bath time before activity hour).
   c. Compliment the person who assumes more responsibility.
   d. Show patience and understanding when a mistake is made. Assist to develop a plan from which to learn from mistake.
   e. Provide opportunity for person to contribute to his own treatment plan.
   f. Help establish future goals that are realistic; examine problems in achieving a goal and suggest various alternatives.
3. Assist person to differentiate between needs and demands.
   a. Explain the difference between needs and demands (*e.g.*, food and clothing are needs; expectations that others dress and feed him, if he can do it, are demands).
   b. Assist to examine the effects of his behavior on others; encourage a change in behavior if it evokes negative responses.
   c. Teach negotiation to achieve needs and goals.
   d. Help person ask for what he wants and tell others how he feels.
   e. Help person realize that failure of others to meet his needs and demands is not always related to their regard for him.
4. Use cognitive behavioral therapy either individually or in groups.
   a. Help the person to recognize that the symptoms are causing the problems and that he or she can do something about them.
   b. Assist in developing strategies to deal with symptoms.
   c. Encourage the person to challenge symptoms.

E. Provide person with opportunities for positive socialization
   1. Help him share on a one-to-one basis.
      a. Be warm, honest, and sincere in interactions.
      b. Demonstrate that you accept him.
      c. Recognize that some people deny the need for close relationships.
      d. Be sensitive to behaviors that indicate resistance to interpersonal involvement.
      e. Help person know that you recognize his uneasiness in social situations. ("It must be difficult for you.")
      f. Use touch judiciously if person fears closeness.
      g. Encourage the person to discuss reality-based issues and topics.
   2. Help person recognize behaviors that stimulate rejection.
      a. Identify activities that reduce interpersonal anxiety (*e.g.*, exercise, controlled-breathing exercises; see Appendix X).
      b. Set limits firmly and kindly on destructive behavior.
      c. Allow expression of negative emotions, verbally or in constructive activity.
      d. Avoid argument or debate about delusional ideas or destructive behavior.
      e. Help person accept responsibility for responses he elicits from others.
      f. Encourage discussion of problems in relating after visits with family members.
      g. Help person test new skills in relating to others in role-playing situations.
   3. Refer to impaired socialization for further interventions.
   4. Help person to limit delusional and hallucinatory activity to private situations. When able to accomplish this, provide positive reinforcement of his ability for self-control.

F. Promote physical well-being and prevent injury
   1. Explain and monitor medication regimen.
      a. Assess person's ability to remember to take medications.
      b. Assist person to remember to take medications by color coding each bottle with a sticker and writing out the times of the day that medications are prescribed for, with the appropriate color of sticker next to the time.
      c. Teach about the purpose of medications and their side effects.
      d. Encourage person to report all physical symptoms.
      e. Encourage person to take prescribed medication, especially antipsychotic (*e.g.*, lithium).
      f. Check to ensure that medication was swallowed. If you have doubts about patient taking oral medications (*e.g.*, failure to improve), change to concentrate form.
      g. Extremely suspicious and hostile people should begin on concentrate, so that you will not have to check mouth and increase distrust.
      h. Do not mix medications with food.
      i. Discuss dangers of mixing medications with alcohol.
   2. Monitor nutritional intake.
      a. Observe eating habits (amount, selection, frequency, food preferences and dislikes, appetite).
      b. Note weight gain or loss.
      c. Discuss adequate nutrition in relation to activity level.
      d. Allow person to choose food he especially likes; contract with individual who eats predominantly snack foods (*e.g.*, "If you eat one egg you can order a doughnut").
      e. Note delusions regarding food or body that might interfere with nutritional intake.
      f. Encourage increased calorie intake for hyperactive person.
      g. Provide finger foods that can be eaten on-the-run (*e.g.*, sandwiches).
      h. Allow choices in foods (may prefer to eat food brought in by family, in unopened packages, fruit, and the like).
      i. Refer to *Altered Nutrition* for additional interventions.
   3. Assess ability for self-care activities.
      a. Identify areas of physical care for which person needs assistance (sleep and rest, nutrition, bathing, dressing, elimination, exercise).
      b. Note person's motivation and interest in appearance.

c. Teach skills required to assume responsibility for self-care.
d. Assist person in planning his daily routines to foster independence and responsibility.
e. Monitor for sleep disturbances.
f. Provide a single room for extremely suspicious person.
g. Suggest leaving the light on.
h. Give nonstimulating drinks with a snack at bedtime.
i. Assess the need for a sleeping medication.
j. If appropriate, arrange to give last dose of antipsychotic medication at bedtime (*e.g.*, b.i.d. medication—give A.M. and h.s.).
k. Refer to *Self-Care Deficit* for additional interventions.
4. Assess sleep–rest patterns (altered thought processes can disrupt sleep–rest patterns and disrupted sleep–rest patterns can worsen altered thought processes).
a. Structure times for sleep, rest, and diversional activities.
b. Explore techniques that may promote sleep (*e.g.*, warm milk, bath, reading).
c. Monitor sleep–rest patterns by graph until no longer a problem.
5. Monitor stimuli and their effects on the person.
a. Teach the person to gauge the effects stimuli have on his or her thoughts.
b. Explore strategies that mitigate the effects of the stimuli (distraction, physical activity, removing oneself from the stimuli).
c. Focus on one activity at a time.
6. Encourage physical activity.

G. Reduce the potential for violence to self and others

1. Provide a minimally stimulating environment.
a. Reduce incidence of bright colors and loud noises.
b. Be short, concise, and matter-of-fact.
c. Be consistent.
d. May need to assign staff responsible for developing trusting relationship.
e. Avoid large groups.
2. Provide activities in which he will be successful.
a. Avoid competitive sports.
b. Suspicious people are often good managers.
c. Involve in activities for a short period.
3. Allow ventilation of hostility (as long as it is not combative/destructive).
a. Be nonjudgmental.
b. Do not personalize.
4. Assess for signs indicative of aggression ("Those Russian spies are going to attack me tonight"). Refer to *Risk for Violence* for further interventions.
5. Identify cues to suicide.
a. Sudden changes in mood or behavior
b. Report of plan to harm himself
c. Report of voices directing person to harm himself or others
d. Observe closely for changes in behavior; increase vigilance.
e. Share with personnel the individual's potential for self-harm.
f. Refer to *Risk for Suicide* for further interventions.
6. Interview family and note approaches that have been beneficial in the past in controlling aggression.
7. Reduce anxiety and develop a sense of safety through a climate of care and concern.

H. Initiate health teaching and referrals, as indicated

1. Anticipate difficulties in adjusting to community living; discuss concerns about returning to community and elicit family reaction to individual's discharge.
2. Provide health teaching that prepares person to deal with life stresses (methods of relaxation, problem-solving skills, how to negotiate with others, how to express feelings constructively).

3. Review signs and symptoms of recurrent illness that indicate impending maladjustment.
4. Refer to other professions for assistance.
   a. To occupational therapist to learn leisure-time activities
   b. To industrial therapist to improve or learn new job skills
   c. To social worker to discuss living arrangements, financial problems, or family negotiations
5. Supply telephone number and address of local mental health clinic.
6. Inform individual of social agencies that offer help in adjusting to community living.
   a. General social agencies
      Mental health and mental retardation centers
      Mental Health Association
      HELP (alternative to mental health center)
      Family Service (family counseling)
      Drug rehabilitation centers
   b. Specific social agencies
      Alcoholics Anonymous
      Gray Panthers
      Suicide Crisis Intervention Center
      Synanon
      Contact
7. Educate family and significant others concerning person's illness and successful coping strategies. Support them emotionally.

Rationale

- Effective caregivers are self-confident, honest, flexible, hopeful, and tolerant of uncertainty, error, and madness (Johnson, 1993).
- Leaving a hallucinating person alone increases fear and deepens their preoccupation (Johnson, 1993).
- The nurse provides a healthy role model with appropriate verbal and nonverbal responses (Johnson, 1993).
- Physiologic control strategies alter the physiologic state to reduce autonomic arousal.
- Cognitive control strategies involve mental processes to distract from symptoms.
- Behavioral control strategies are responses that can distract from the symptoms.
- The person can be helped to regain contact with reality by gently introducing conversation or activities that are oriented to the here-and-now (Johnson, 1993).
- Interventions that require the person to engage in active mental work (*e.g.*, must give a verbal response) are effective (Williams, 1989).
- Helping the person identify what specific situations trigger hallucinations gives insight into possible prevention strategies (Hamera et al., 1991).
- Honesty provides insight and discourages the person from discounting his or her feelings.
- Encouraging self-care promotes independence and increase self-esteem.
- Hostility can arise from therapeutic relationships because of the intensity of the closeness and fear of rejection (Johnson, 1993).
- Families can be helped to improve their interpersonal functioning and to handle behavior and feelings effectively (Varcarolis, 1994).
- Environmental stress increases anxiety and distorts reality (Varcarolis, 1994).

Interventions—*Child Focus*

1. For children with thought disturbance, assess for signs of dissociative disorder (Johnson, 1995).
   a. Abusive history (physical, sexual)
   b. Amnestic periods
   c. Switching between alternate personalities
   d. Affect disturbances
   e. Abrupt behavioral changes
2. Refer for multidiscipline evaluation.

Rationale
- Recognition, evaluation, and treatment of dissociative disorders are critical. The child is afforded proper treatment early and abuse is terminated. Family dysfunction can be addressed with a plan for family recovery (Johnson, 1995).

Memory, Impaired

DEFINITION
Impaired Memory: The state in which an individual experiences a temporary or permanent inability to remember or recall bits of information or behavioral skills.

DEFINING CHARACTERISTICS
Major
    Observed or reported experiences of forgetting
    Inability to determine if a behavior was performed
    Inability to learn or retain new skills or information
    Inability to perform a previously learned skill
    Inability to recall factual information
    Inability to recall recent or past events

RELATED FACTORS
Pathophysiologic
    Related to central nervous system changes secondary to:
        Degenerative brain disease
        Lesion
        Head injury
        Cerebrovascular accident
    Related to reduced quantity and quality of information processed secondary to:
        Visual deficits   Hearing deficits
        Poor physical fitness   Fatigue
        Learning habits   Intellectual skills
        Educational level
    Related to nutritional deficiencies (*e.g.*, vitamins C and B_{12}, folate, niacin, thiamine)

Treatment-Related
    Related to effects of medication (specify) on memory storage

Situational (Personal, Environmental)
    Related to self-fulfilling expectations
    Related to excessive self-focusing and worrying secondary to:
        Grieving   Anxiety
        Depression
    Related to alcohol consumption
    Related to lack of motivation
    Related to lack of stimulation

Related to difficulty concentrating secondary to:

Stress

Distractions

Lack of intellectual stimulation

Pain

Sleep disturbances

Author's Note

This diagnosis is useful when the person can be helped to function better because of improved memory. If the person's memory cannot be improved because of cerebral degeneration, this diagnosis is not appropriate. Instead, the nurse should evaluate the effects of impaired memory on functioning, such as *Self-Care Deficits* or *Risk for Injury*. The focus of interventions would be on improving self care or protection, not improving memory.

Key Concepts

1. "Memory is viewed as a continuum of processing, ranging from shallow to deep levels, and the duration of a particular memory depends on the depths of the processing" (Miller, 1995, p. 91).
2. There are three stages of memory (Miller, 1995):
   a. Sensory memory—awareness of information obtained through vision, hearing, taste, smell, and touch, which lasts only a few seconds.
   b. Short-term memory—working memory, contains small amounts of information (*e.g.*, a telephone number)
   c. Long-term memory—memory bank; can be retrieved whenever it is needed
3. Memory function worries people more than any other cognitive function. When an older person forgets, it is interpreted it as a sign of disease; when a younger person forgets, it is attributed to too many things being on one's mind.
4. When concentration is difficult, relaxation and imagery have improved memory and learning (Miller, 1995).

Key Concepts—*Older Adult*

1. Short-term memory shows a slight decline with aging (Miller, 1995).
2. Benign senescent forgetfulness is minor degrees of memory loss that is not progressive and does not produce dysfunction in daily living (Kane, Ouslander, & Abrass, 1994).
3. If memory deficits progress and other areas of intellectual functioning are affected, dementia should be considered (Kane et al., 1994).

Focus Assessment Criteria

(Acquire from client and significant others)

Subjective

A. Assess for defining characteristics
   1. Remote events: "Where were you born?" "Where did you go to grade school?" "What was your first job?" "When were you married?"
   2. Recent past events: "Do you live with anyone?" "Do you have any grandchildren?" "What are the names of your grandchildren?" "When was the last time you went to the doctor?"
   3. Immediate memory, retention: State three unrelated facts and ask the person to repeat the information immediately and again after 5 minutes.
   4. Immediate memory, general grasp, and recall: Have the person read a short story and then summarize the information.
   5. Immediate memory, recognition: Ask a multiple-choice question and ask the person to choose the correct answer.

6. Ability to remember:

Self-care activities	To shop for necessities
To take medications	Appointments
To pay bills	

Outcome Criteria

The individual will
• Identify three techniques to improve memory

Interventions

A. Discuss the person's beliefs about memory deficits
   1. Correct misinformation.
   2. Explain that negative expectations can result in memory deficits.

B. Explain that if one wants to improve one's memory, both the intent to remember and the knowledge about techniques for remembering are needed (Miller, 1995)

C. If the person has difficulty concentrating, explain the favorable effects of relaxation and imagery (refer to Appendix X for specific guidelines)

D. Teach the person two or three of the following methods for improving memory skills (Miller, 1995)
   1. Write things down (*e.g.*, use lists, calendars, and notebooks).
   2. Use auditory cues (*e.g.*, timers, alarm clocks) in conjunction with written cues.
   3. Use environmental cues (*e.g.*, you might remove something from its usual place, then return it to its normal location after it has served its purpose as a reminder).
   4. Have specific places for specific items and keep the items in their proper place (*e.g.*, keep keys on a hook near the door).
   5. Put reminders in appropriate places (*e.g.*, place shoes to be repaired near the door).
   6. Use visual images ("A picture is worth a thousand words"). Create a picture in your mind when you want to remember something; the more bizarre the picture, the more likely it is that you will remember.
   7. Use active observation—pay attention to details of what's going on around you, and be alert to the environment.
   8. Make associations, or mental connections (*e.g.*, Spring ahead and fall back" for changing clocks to and from daylight savings time).
   9. Make associations between names and mental images (*e.g.*, Carol and Christmas carol).
   10. Rehearse items you want to remember by repeating them aloud or writing the information on paper.
   11. Use self-instruction—say things aloud (*e.g.*, "I'm putting my keys on the counter so I remember to turn off the stove before I leave").
   12. Divide information into small "chunks" that can be remembered easily (*e.g.*, to remember an address or a zip code, divide it into groups ["seven hundred sixty, fifty five"]).
   13. Organize information into logical categories (*e.g.*, shampoo and hair spray, toothpaste and mouthwash, soap and deodorant).
   14. Use rhyming cues (*e.g.*, "In 1492, Columbus sailed the ocean blue").
   15. Use first-letter cues and make associations (*e.g.*, to remember to buy carrots, apples, radishes, pickles, eggs, and tea bags, remember the word *carpet*).

16. Make word associations (*e.g.*, to remember the letters of your license plate, make a word, such as "camel" for CML).
17. Search the alphabet while focusing on what you're trying to remember (*e.g.*, to remember that someone's name is Martin, start with names that begin with "A" and continue naming names through the alphabet until your memory is jogged for the correct one).
18. Make up a story to connect things you want to remember (*e.g.*, if you have to go to the cleaners and post office, create a story about mailing a pair of pants).

E. Explain that when one is trying to learn or remember something
   1. Minimize distractions.
   2. Do not rush.
   3. Maintain some form of organization of routine tasks.
   4. Carry a note pad or calendar or use written cues.

F. When teaching (Miller, 1995; Stanley & Beare, 1995)
   1. Eliminate distractions.
   2. Present information as concretely as possible.
   3. Use practical examples.
   4. Allow learner to pace the learning.
   5. Use visual, auditory aids.
   6. Provide advance organizers; outlines, written cues.
   7. Encourage use of aids.
   8. Make sure glasses are clean and lights are soft white.
   9. Correct wrong answers immediately.
   10. Encourage verbal responses.

Rationale

- Memory is significantly influenced by many personal and environmental factors, such as level of education and expectations. For example, if society expects older people to be forgetful, it can become a self-fulfilling prophecy.
- Older adults can benefit from cognitive exercises to improve memory (Baltes, 1993).
- Memory impairment can be improved when information is meaningful and logical rather than abstract (Rakel, 1991).

Interventions—*Older Adult Focus*

1. Provide accurate information about age-related changes.
2. Explain the difference between age-related forgetfulness and dementia.

Rationale

- Individuals and family members may equate any memory problems with Alzheimer's disease.
- Providing accurate information can allay fears.

References/Bibliography

Baker, P. (1995). Accepting the inner voices. *Nursing Times, 91*(31), 59–61.

Baltes, P. B. (1993). The aging mind: Potential and limits. *Gerontologist, 33*, 580–594.

Burrow, S. (1994). Nurse-aid management of psychiatric emergencies: 1. *British Journal of Nursing, 3*(1), 34–37.

Dixon, B. (1969). Intervening when the patient is delusional. *Journal of Psychiatric Nursing, 7*(1), 25–34.

Everly, G. (1989). *A guide to the treatment of human stress response.* New York: Plenum Press.

Frederick, J., & Cotanch, P. (1995). Self-help techniques for auditory hallucinations in schizophrenia. *Issues in Mental Health Nursing, 16*, 213–324.

Gardner, B., & Thompson, S. (1994). Strategic thinking . . . enable people with schizophrenia to learn self-help methods. *Nursing Times, 90*(1), 32–34.

Glick, O. J. (1993). Normal thought processes: An overview. *Nursing Clinics of North America, 28*, 715–727.

Hamera, Peterson, & Handley. (1991). Patient self-regulation and functioning in schizophrenia. *Hospital and Community Psychiatry, 42,* 630–631.

Johnson, B. S. (1993). *Psychiatric–mental health nursing: Adaptation and growth* (3rd ed.). Philadelphia: J. B. Lippincott.

Johnson, B. S. (1995). *Child, adolescent and family psychiatric nursing.* Philadelphia: J. B. Lippincott.

Kane, R., Ouslander, J. G., & Abrass, I. B. (1994). *Essentials of clinical geriatrics* (3rd ed.). New York: McGraw-Hill.

Miller, C. (1995). *Nursing care of older adults* (2nd ed.). Glenview, IL: Scott, Foresman.

Porth, C. M. (1994). *Pathophysiology: Concepts of altered health states* (4th ed.). Philadelphia: J. B. Lippincott.

Potocki, E., & Everly, G. (1989). Control and the human stress response. In G. Everly (Ed.). *A guide to the treatment of human stress response.* New York: Plenum Press.

Rakel, B. (1991). Knowledge deficit. In M. Maas, K. Buckwalter, & M. Hardy (Eds.). *Nursing diagnoses and interventions for the elderly.* Redwood City, CA: Addison-Wesley Nursing.

Schwartzman, S. T. (1976). The hallucinating patient and nursing intervention. *Journal of Psychiatric Nursing, 13*(6), 23–28, 33–36.

Sideleau, B. (1987). Irrational beliefs and interventions. *Journal of Psychosocial Nursing, 25*(3), 18–24.

Stanley, M., & Beare, P. G. (1995). *Gerontological nursing.* Philadelphia: F. A. Davis.

Tarrier, N., Harwood, S., & Yusopoff, L. (1990). Coping strategy enhancement (CSE): A method of treating residual schizophrenic symptoms. *Behavioral Psychotherapy, 18,* 282–293.

Varcarolis, E. (1994). *Foundations of psychiatric–mental health nursing* (2nd ed.). Philadelphia: W. B. Saunders.

Westacott, M. (1995). Strategies for managing auditory hallucinations. *Nursing Times, 91*(3), 35–37.

Williams, C. A. (1989). Perspectives on the hallucinatory process. *Issues in Mental Health Nursing, 10,* 99–119.

Tissue Perfusion, Altered (Specify) (Renal, cerebral, cardiopulmonary, gastrointestinal)

Tissue Perfusion, Altered Peripheral

Tissue Perfusion, Altered (Specify) (Renal, cerebral, cardiopulmonary, gastrointestinal)

DEFINITION

Altered Tissue Perfusion: The state in which the individual experiences or is at risk of experiencing a decrease in nutrition and respiration at the cellular level because of a decrease in capillary blood supply.

Author's Note

Tissue perfusion depends on many physiologic factors within the body systems and in cellular structures and functions. A person's response to altered tissue perfusion can disrupt some or all functional health patterns and can cause physiologic complications. For example, a person with chronic renal failure will be at risk for fluid/electrolyte imbalances, acidosis, nutritional problems, edema, fatigue, pruritus, and self-concept disturbances. Does the diagnosis *Altered Renal Tissue Perfusion* describe these varied responses, or does it simply rename renal failure or renal calculi?

The use of any *Altered Tissue Perfusion* diagnosis other than *Peripheral* merely provides new labels for medical diagnoses, labels that do not describe the nursing focus or accountability. The following represent examples of *Altered Tissue Perfusion* diagnoses with associated goals from the literature:

- *Altered Tissue Perfusion related to hypovolemia secondary to GI bleeding*
  Goal: *Tissue perfusion improves, as evidenced by stabilized vital signs*
- *Altered Cerebral Tissue Perfusion related to increased intracranial pressure*
  Goal: ICP is no greater than 15 mm Hg and clinical signs of ICP are decreased
- *Altered Tissue Perfusion related to vaso-occlusive nature of sickling secondary to sickle cell crisis*
  Goal: Demonstrates improved tissue perfusion, as evidenced by adequate urine output, absence of pain, strong peripheral pulses

All the above outcomes represent criteria that nurses use to assess the client's status to determine the appropriate nursing and medical interventions indicated. Thus, these situations represent the following collaborative problems, respectively: *PC: GI bleeding, PC: Increased ICP* and *PC: Sickling crisis.*

The diagnosis *Altered Tissue Perfusion (Renal, cerebral, cardiopulmonary, gastrointestinal)* was approved by NANDA in 1980. Currently, it does not conform to the NANDA definition approved in 1990 (refer to Chap. 2). When using these diagnoses, nurses cannot be accountable for prescribing the interventions for outcome achievement. Instead of using *Altered Tissue Perfusion,* the nurse should focus on the nursing diagnoses and collaborative problems applicable due to altered renal, cardiac, cerebral, pulmonary, or GI tissue perfusion.

Altered Peripheral Tissue Perfusion can be a clinically useful nursing diagnosis if used to describe chronic vascular insufficiency or potential thrombophlebitis. (In contrast, acute embolism and thrombophlebitis represent collaborative problems.) A nurse focusing on preventing thrombophlebitis in a postoperative client would write the diagnosis *Risk for Altered Peripheral Tissue Perfusion related to postoperative immobility and dehydration*.

Errors in Diagnostic Statements

Altered GI Tissue Perfusion related to esophageal bleeding varices

Because this diagnosis actually represents a situation that nurses monitor and manage with nursing and medical interventions, the diagnosis should be rewritten as the collaborative problem *Potential Complication: Esophageal bleeding varices*.

Altered Cerebral Tissue Perfusion related to cerebral edema secondary to intracranial infections

This diagnosis represents merely a new label for encephalitis, meningitis, or abscess. Instead, the nurse should specify collaborative problems to clearly describe and designate the nursing accountability: *Potential Complication: Increased intracranial pressure* and *Potential Complication: Septicemia*. In addition, certain nursing diagnoses may be indicated (*e.g., Risk for Infection Transmission, Altered Comfort*).

Altered Peripheral Tissue Perfusion related to deep vein thrombosis

Deep vein thrombosis is a medical diagnosis that evokes responses for which nurses are accountable: monitoring for and managing, with physician- and nurse-prescribed interventions, physiologic complications (*e.g.*, embolism, stasis ulcers). This situation would be represented by collaborative problems such as *Potential Complication: Embolism*. In addition, the nurse would intervene independently to prevent complications of immobility and teach how to prevent recurrence, applying nursing diagnoses such as *Disuse Syndrome* and *Risk for Altered Health Maintenance related to insufficient knowledge of risk factors*.

Tissue Perfusion, Altered Peripheral

DEFINITION

Altered Peripheral Tissue Perfusion: The state in which an individual experiences or is at risk of experiencing a decrease in nutrition and respiration at the peripheral cellular level because of a decrease in capillary blood supply.

DEFINING CHARACTERISTICS
Major (Must Be Present)

Presence of one of the following types (see Key Concepts for definitions)
 Claudication (arterial) Aching pain (arterial or venous)
 Rest pain (arterial)
Diminished or absent arterial pulses (arterial)
Skin color changes
 Pallor (arterial) Reactive hyperemia (arterial)
 Cyanosis (venous)

Skin temperature changes
  Cooler (arterial)
  Warmer (venous)
Decreased blood pressure (arterial)
Capillary refill longer than 3 seconds (arterial)

Minor (May Be Present)

Edema (venous)
Change of sensory function (arterial)
Change of motor function (arterial)
Trophic tissue changes (arterial)
  Hard, thick nails
  Loss of hair
  Nonhealing wound

RELATED FACTORS
Pathophysiologic

Related to compromised blood flow secondary to:
  (Vascular disorders)

Arteriosclerosis	Leriche's syndrome
Hypertension	Raynaud's disease/syndrome
Aneurysm	Varicosities
Arterial thrombosis	Buerger's disease
Deep vein thrombosis	Sickle cell crisis
Collagen vascular disease	Cirrhosis
Rheumatoid arthritis	Alcoholism

  Diabetes mellitus
  Hypotension
  Blood dyscrasias (platelet disorders)
  Renal failure
  Cancer/tumor

Treatment-Related

Related to immobilization
Related to presence of invasive lines
Related to pressure sites/constriction (Ace bandages, stockings)
Related to blood vessel trauma or compression

Situational (Personal, Environmental)

Related to pressure of enlarging uterus on peripheral circulation
Related to pressure of enlarged abdomen on pelvic and peripheral circulation
Related to vasoconstricting effects of tobacco
Related to decreased circulating volume secondary to dehydration
Related to dependent venous pooling
Related to hypothermia
Related to pressure of muscle mass secondary to weight lifting

Author's Note
See *Altered Peripheral Tissue Perfusion*

Errors in Diagnostic Statements
See *Altered Peripheral Tissue Perfusion*

Key Concepts

1. Cellular nutrition and respiration depend on adequate blood flow through the microcirculation.
2. Adequate cellular oxygenation depends on the following processes (Porth, 1994):
   a. The ability of the lungs to exchange air adequately (O_2–CO_2)
   b. The ability of the pulmonary alveoli to diffuse oxygen and carbon dioxide across the cell membrane to the blood
   c. The ability of the red blood cells (hemoglobin) to carry oxygen
   d. The ability of the heart to pump with enough force to deliver the blood to the microcirculation
   e. The ability of intact blood vessels to deliver blood to the microcirculation
3. Hypoxemia (decreased oxygen content of the blood) results in cellular hypoxia, which causes cellular swelling and contributes to tissue injury.
4. *Arterial* blood flow is enhanced by a *dependent* position and inhibited by an *elevated* position (gravity pulls blood downward, away from the heart).
5. Tissue perfusion depends on many physiologic factors within the systems of the body and in the structures and functions of the cells. When an alteration in peripheral tissue perfusion exists, the nurse must take into account the nature of the alteration in perfusion. The two major components of the peripheral vascular system are the arterial and the venous systems. Signs, symptoms, etiology, and nursing interventions are different for problems occurring in each of these two systems and, therefore, are addressed separately.
6. Changes in arterial walls increase the incidence of stroke and coronary artery disease (Baxendale, 1992).
7. High levels of circulating lipids increase the risk of coronary heart disease, peripheral vascular disease, and stroke (Baxendale, 1992).

 ### *Key Concepts—Older Adult*

1. Age-related vascular changes include stiffened blood vessels, which cause increased peripheral resistance, impaired baroreceptor functioning, and diminished ability to increase organ blood flow (Adelman, 1988).
2. These age-related changes cause the veins to become thicker, more dilated, and less elastic. Valves of the large leg veins become less efficient. Age-related reduction in muscle mass and inactivity further reduces peripheral circulation (Miller, 1995).
3. Physical deconditioning or lack of exercise accentuates the functional consequences of age-related changes in cardiovascular functioning. Factors that can contribute to deconditioning include acute illness, mobility limitations, cardiac disease, depression, and lack of motivation (Miller, 1995).

Focus Assessment Criteria

See Tables II-29 and II-30

Subjective Data

A. Assess for defining characteristics
   1. Symptoms
      Pain (associated with, time of day)   Pallor, cyanosis, paresthesias
      Temperature change   Change in motor function

B. Assess for related factors
   1. Medical history
      See Related Factors
   2. Risk factors
      Smoking (never, quit, number of years)   Immobility
      History of phlebitis   Sedentary life-style
      Family history for heart disease, peripheral vascular disease, stroke, kidney disease, or diabetes mellitus
      Stress

Table II-29 **Arterial Insufficiency vs. Venous Insufficiency: A Comparison of Subjective Data**

Symptom	Arterial Insufficiency	Venous Insufficiency
Pain		
Location	Feet, muscles of legs, toes	Ankles, lower legs
Quality	Burning, shocking, prickling, throbbing, cramping	Aching, tightness
Quantity	Increase in severity with increased muscle activity	Varies with fluid intake, use of support hose, and decreased muscle activity
Chronology	Brought on predictably by exercise	Greater in evening than in morning
Setting	Use of affected muscle groups	Increases during course of day with prolonged standing or sitting
Aggravating factors	Exercise Extremity elevation	Immobility Extremity dependence
Alleviating factors	Cessation of exercise Extremity dependence	Extremity elevation Compression stockings or Ace wraps
Paresthesia	Numbness, tingling, burning, decreased sensation	No change unless arterial system or nerves are affected

    3. Medications
         Type   Presence of side effects
         Dosage

Objective Data
A. Assess for defining characteristics
    1. Skin
         Temperature (cool, warm)
         Color (pale, dependent rubor, flushed, cyanotic, brown discolorations)
         Ulcerations (size, location, description of surrounding tissue)

Table II-30 **Arterial Insufficiency vs. Venous Insufficiency: A Comparison of Objective Data**

Sign	Arterial Insufficiency	Venous Insufficiency
Temperature	Cool skin	Warm skin
Color	Pale on elevation, dependent rubor (reactive hyperemia)	Flushed, cyanotic Typical brown discoloration around ankles
Capillary filling	>3 sec	Nonapplicable
Pulses	Absent	Present unless there is concomitant arterial disease
Movement	Decreased motor ability with nerve and muscle ischemia	Motor ability unchanged unless edema is severe enough to restrict joint mobility
Ulceration	Occurs on foot at site of trauma or at tips of toes (most distal to be perfused) Ulcers are deep with well-defined margins Surrounding tissue is shiny and taut with thin skin	Occurs around ankle (area of greatest pressure from chronic venous stasis due to valvular incompetence) Ulcers shallow with irregular edges Surrounding tissue edematous with engorged veins

2. Bilateral pulses (radial, posterior tibial, dorsalis pedis)
   Rate, rhythm
   Volume
       0 = Absent, nonpalpable   +3 = Normal, easily palpable
      +1 = Thready, weak, fades in and out   +4 = Aneurysmal
      +2 = Present but diminished
3. Paresthesia (numbness, tingling, burning)
4. Edema (location, pitting)
5. Capillary refill (normal less than 3 seconds)
6. Motor ability (normal, compromised)

Outcome Criteria

The individual will
- Define peripheral vascular problem in own words
- Identify factors that improve peripheral circulation
- Identify necessary life-style changes
- Identify medical regimen, diet, medications, activities that promote vasodilation
- Identify factors that inhibit peripheral circulation
- Report decrease in pain
- State when to contact physician or health care professional

---

Interventions

A. Assess causative and contributing factors
1. Underlying disease
2. Inhibited arterial blood flow
3. Inhibited venous blood flow
4. Fluid volume excess or deficit
5. Hypothermia or vasoconstriction
6. Activities related to symptom/sign onset

B. Promote factors that improve arterial blood flow
1. Keep extremity in a dependent position.
2. Keep extremity warm (do not use heating pad or hot water bottle, because the individual with a peripheral vascular disease may have a disturbance in sensation and will not be able to determine if the temperature is hot enough to damage tissue; the use of external heat may also increase the metabolic demands of the tissue beyond its capacity).
3. Reduce risk for trauma.
   a. Change positions at least every hour.
   b. Avoid leg crossing.
   c. Reduce external pressure points (inspect shoes daily for rough lining).
   d. Avoid sheepskin heel protectors (they increase heel pressure and pressure across dorsum of foot).
   e. Encourage range-of-motion exercises.
   f. Discuss cessation of smoking (see *Altered Health Maintenance Related to Tobacco Use*).

C. Promote factors that improve venous blood flow
1. Elevate extremity above the level of the heart (may be contraindicated if severe cardiac or respiratory disease is present).
2. Avoid standing or sitting with legs dependent for long periods of time.
3. Consider the use of Ace bandages or below-knee elastic stockings to prevent venous stasis.

4. Reduce or removal external venous compression, which impedes venous flow.
   a. Avoid pillows behind the knees or Gatch bed, which is elevated at the knees.
   b. Avoid leg crossing.
   c. Change positions, move extremities, or wiggle fingers and toes every hour.
   d. Avoid garters and tight elastic stockings above the knees.
5. Measure baseline circumference of calves and thighs if individual is at risk for deep venous thrombosis, or if it is suspected.

D. Discuss the implications of condition and choices

1. Encourage to share feeling, concerns, and understanding of his or her risk factors, disease process, and effect on life.
2. Assist to select life-style behaviors that he or she chooses to change (Burch, Todd, Crosby, Ventura, Lohr, & Grace, 1991).
   a. Avoid multiple changes.
   b. Consider personal abilities, resources, and overall health.
   c. Be realistic and optimistic.

E. Plan a daily walking program (Burch et al., 1991)

1. Instruct individual in reasons for program.
2. Teach individual to avoid fatigue.
3. Instruct to avoid increase in exercise until assessed by physician for cardiac problems.
4. Reassure individual that walking does not harm the blood vessels or the muscles; "walking into the pain," resting and resuming walking, assists in developing collateral circulation.
5. Start slowly.
6. Emphasize that it is not the speed or distance but the action of walking that is important.
7. Assist to set goals and the steps to achieve them (*e.g.*, will walk 30 minutes daily).
   a. Will walk 10 minutes daily.
   b. Will walk 10 minutes daily and 20 minutes three times a week.
   c. Will walk 20 minutes daily.
   d. Will walk 20 minutes daily and 30 minutes three times a week.
8. Suggest a method to self-monitor progress (*e.g.*, graph, checklist).

F. Initiate health teaching, as indicated

1. Teach to (Helt, 1991):
   a. Avoid long car or plane rides (get up and walk around at least every hour).
   b. Keep dry skin lubricated (cracked skin eliminates the physical barrier to infection).
   c. Wear warm clothing during cold weather.
   d. Wear cotton or wool socks.
   e. Use gloves or mittens if hands are exposed to cold (including home freezers).
   f. Avoid dehydration in warm weather.
   g. Give special attention to feet and toes.
      Wash feet and dry well daily.
      Do not soak feet.
      Avoid harsh soaps or chemicals (including iodine) on feet.
      Keep nails trimmed and filed smooth.
   h. Inspect feet and legs daily for injuries and pressure points.
   i. Wear clean socks.
   j. Wear shoes that offer support and fit comfortably.
   k. Inspect the inside of shoes daily for rough lining.
2. Briefly explain the relation of certain risk factors to the development of atherosclerosis (Baxendale, 1992; Burch et al., 1991; Hart, 1993):
   a. Smoking

Vasoconstriction	Increased lipidemia
Decreased oxygenation of the blood	Increased platelet aggregation
Elevated blood pressure	

  b. Hypertension

Constant trauma of pressure causes vessel lining damage that promotes plaque formation and narrowing.

  c. Hyperlipidemia

Promotes atherosclerosis.

  d. Sedentary life-style

Decreases muscle tone and strength.

Decreases circulation.

  e. Excess weight (>10% of ideal)

Fatty tissue increases peripheral resistance.

Fatty tissue is less vascular.

  3. Teach methods to relieve pain.

  a. Assume dependent position for ischemic pain.

  b. Elevate extremities for relief of venous aching.

  c. Phantom pain after an amputation may be relieved by massaging or tapping stump or opposite limb.

  d. Use other nursing measures such as relaxation or distraction to assist in pain relief.

  e. If pain is not relieved by these methods, refer to a physician.

  f. Teach symptoms/signs of underlying disease and when to call the physician or health care professional.

Rationale

- *Venous* blood flow is enhanced by an *elevated* position and inhibited by a *dependent* position (gravity pulls blood downward, away from the heart).
- Immobility and venous stasis predispose to thrombus and embolus production.
- The effects of nicotine on the cardiovascular system contribute to coronary artery disease, stroke, hypertension, and peripheral vascular disease (Hart, 1993).
- Lack of exercise inhibits the pumping action of the muscles, which enhances circulation. In the presence of peripheral vascular disease, exercise promotes collateral circulation development (Skelton, 1992).
- Overweight status increases cardiac workload, thus causing hypertension (Cunningham, 1992).
- Older client may have life-style patterns of inactivity, smoking, and high-fat diet that put the client at risk; the client should be counseled to change (Burch et al., 1991).
- Attaining short-term goals can foster motivation for continuing the process of change (Burch et al., 1991).
- Daily foot care can reduce tissue damage and help prevent or detect early further injury and infection (Helt, 1991).
- Well-fitting shoes help prevent injury to skin and underlying tissue (Helt, 1991).
- Tight garments and certain leg positions constrict leg vessels, further reducing circulation (Helt, 1991).
- Community resources can assist the client with weight loss, smoking cessation, diet, and exercise programs.

References/Bibliography

Adelman, B. (1988). Peripheral vascular disease. In J. W. Rowe & R. W. Besdive (Eds.). *Geriatric medicine.* Boston: Little, Brown.

Baxendale, L. (1992). Pathophysiology of coronary artery disease. *Nursing Clinics of North America, 27,* 143–151.

Burch, K., Todd, K., Crosby, F., Ventura, M., Lohr, G., & Grace, M. L. (1991). PVD: Nurse patient interventions. *Journal of Vascular Nursing, 9*(4), 13–16.

Cunningham, S. (1992). The epidemiologic basis of coronary disease prevention. *Nursing Clinics of North America, 27,* 153–170.

Hart, B. P. (1993). Vascular consequences of smoking and benefits of smoking cessation. *Journal of Vascular Nursing, 11*(2), 48–51.

Helt, J. (1991). Foot care and footwear to prevent amputation. *Journal of Vascular Nursing, 9*(4), 2–8.

Maves, M. (1992). Mutual goal setting. In G. Bulecheck & J. McCloskey (Eds.). *Nursing interventions*. Philadelphia: W. B. Saunders.

Miller, C. A. (1995). *Nursing care of older adults* (2nd ed.). Glenview, IL: Scott, Foresman.

Patient Education Committee, Society for Vascular Nursing. (1992). *Venous disease*. Norwood, MA: Society for Vascular Nursing.

Porth, C. M. (1994). *Pathophysiology: Concepts of altered health states* (4th ed.). Philadelphia, J. B. Lippincott.

Sieggreen, M. (1987). Healing of physical wounds. *Nursing Clinics of North America, 22*, 439–448.

Sieggreen, M. (1989). Nursing management of adults with arterial disorders; Nursing management of adults with venous and lymphatic disorders. In P. Beare & J. Myers (Eds.). *Principles and practice of adult health nursing*. St. Louis: C. V. Mosby.

Skelton, N. K. (1992). Medical implications of obesity: Losing pounds and gaining years. *Postgraduate Medicine, 92*, 151–162.

Unilateral Neglect

DEFINITION

Unilateral Neglect: The state in which an individual is unable to attend to or "ignores" the hemiplegic side of the body and/or, on the affected side, objects, persons, or sounds in the environment.

DEFINING CHARACTERISTICS
Major (Must Be Present)

Neglect of involved body parts and/or extrapersonal space (hemispatial neglect), and/or
Denial of the existence of the affected limb or side of body (anosognosia)

Minor (May Be Present)

Left homonymous hemianopsia
Difficulty with spatial–perceptual tasks
Hemiplegia (usually of the left side)

RELATED FACTORS
Pathophysiologic

Related to the impaired perceptual abilities secondary to:

Cerebrovascular accident   Brain injury/trauma
Cerebral tumors   Cerebral aneurysms

Author's Note

Unilateral Neglect represents a disturbance in the reciprocal loop that occurs most often in the right hemisphere of the brain. This diagnosis also could be viewed as a syndrome diagnosis, *Unilateral Neglect Syndrome*. As mentioned in Chapter 3, syndrome diagnoses encompass a cluster of nursing diagnoses related to the situation. The nursing interventions for *Unilateral Neglect Syndrome* would focus on *Self-Care Deficit, Anxiety*, and *Risk for Injury*.

Errors in Diagnostic Statements

Unilateral Neglect related to lack of grooming and hygiene for right side of face, head, and right arm

Lack of grooming on one side of the body can be an indicator of *Unilateral Neglect* if neurologic disease or damage is present; it is not a related factor. When writing the diagnostic statement, the nurse should ask herself or himself, "How does the nurse treat unilateral neglect?" Because the nursing focus is on teaching adaptive techniques, phrasing the diagnosis *Unilateral Neglect related to lack of knowledge of adaptive techniques* would be appropriate. If *Unilateral Neglect* were viewed as a syndrome diagnosis, the appropriate diagnostic statement would be *Unilateral Neglect Syndrome*. No "related to" is needed with a syndrome diagnosis because the label includes the etiology. The interventions would have the same focus, reducing neglect by using adaptive techniques.

Key Concepts

1. Unilateral neglect is also called hemi-inattention, unilateral asomatognosia (unilateral spatial agnosia, Anton-Babinski syndrome), anosognosia, and atopognosia.
2. The most common cause of unilateral neglect is right hemispheric brain damage; specifically, lesions in the right parietal lobe cause this defect much more frequently than lesions in the left lobe (Heilman & Valenstein, 1972).
3. The neglect phenomena has been demonstrated with unilateral lesions in an area identified as the reciprocal loop (the cortical–limbic–reticular loop). Heilman and Van Den Abell (1980) postulated that any lesion that disrupts this system produces neglect, and that this neglect is a manifestation of a deficit in the orienting response, which is thought to be related to the reticular activating system.
4. The right parietal lobe attends to stimuli presented to both the right and left sides; in a lesion of the left parietal lobe, the right parietal lobe could continue attending to the ipsilateral (same side) or contralateral (right-sided) stimuli. However, because the left parietal lobe cannot attend to ipsilateral stimuli as well as the right parietal lobe can, lesions of the right parietal lobe are more likely to induce a profound contralateral sensory inattention than lesions of the left parietal lobe (Heilman & Van Den Abell, 1980).
5. Severe and persistent neglect of the left hemisphere usually occurs after combined injury to frontal, parietal, and deep structures (Hier, Mondlock, & Caplan, 1983).
6. Unilateral neglect is characterized by an unawareness or denial of the affected half of the body, often extending to the extrapersonal space.
7. The extent of sensory loss does not correlate with the severity of neglect (Mitchell, Hodges, Muwaswes, & Walleck, 1988).
8. Homonymous hemianopsia (loss of vision on the contralateral side) usually occurs with unilateral neglect. However, unilateral neglect and hemianopsia are two separate phenomena, and either can be present without the other. When they occur together, the person has more difficulty compensating for the loss.
9. Anosognosia (ignorance of paralysis) and dressing apraxia may occur in lesions of either hemisphere, but have been observed more frequently in lesions of the nondominant hemisphere.
10. The person with a parietal lobe injury demonstrates problems with body schema, spatial judgment, and sensory interpretation.
11. In addition, the person with this type of brain injury may exhibit some or all of the following characteristics that complicate the neglect syndrome:
    a. Impulsiveness
    b. Short attention span
    c. Lack of insight into the extent of the disability
    d. Diminished learning skills
    e. Inability to recognize faces
    f. Decrease in concrete thinking
    g. Confusion

12. Prognosis for recovery from many of the behavioral abnormalities associated with right hemisphere stroke is more favorable after hemorrhage as opposed to after infarction (Hier et al., 1983).
13. Early recognition of the existence and extent of these syndromes allows more accurate planning of goals.

🌀 Key Concepts—Child

1. Children at greatest risk for development of unilateral neglect are those with acquired hemiplegia (*e.g.*, from stroke). Strokes may occur in children with congenital heart disease, sickle cell anemia, meningitis, or head trauma (Painter & Bergman, 1990).

🏛 Key Concepts—Older Adult

1. Most people who experience unilateral neglect are older adults, simply because the incidence of stroke is greatest in the elderly population.

Focus Assessment Criteria

Subjective/Objective Data

A. Assess for defining characteristics
    1. Person's perception of the problem
    2. Effects on activities of daily living (ADLs)
       a. Bathing, grooming, and hygiene
           Does the person

Wash the affected side of his body?	Comb only part of his hair?
Shave both sides of his face?	Apply makeup to both sides
Brush all his teeth?	of face?
Put dentures in straight?	Put eyeglasses on straight?

       b. Feeding
           Does the person
           Pocket food on the affected side of his mouth?
           Eat only half of his food (*i.e.*, eat only food on the unaffected side of plate/tray)?
       c. Dressing
           Does the person
           Dress the affected limbs?
       d. Mobility/positioning
           When sitting in a wheelchair, does the person lean or tilt toward the unaffected side?
           Does the affected arm dangle off the lapboard?
           Are the head and eyes turned toward the unaffected side?
           When propelling the wheelchair or when ambulating, does the person bump or run into objects on affected side?
       e. Safety
           Does the person
           Attempt to walk or transfer out of the chair or bed when unable to ambulate?
           Have sensation in the affected limbs?
           Frequently injure the affected arm or hand (cuts, bumps, bruises)?
           Feel pain when injured?
           Realize when injury occurs?
           Scan the entire visual field?
           Turn head to the affected side to compensate?
           Respond to stimuli presented from the affected side?
       f. Does the affected arm dangle at the side and get caught in the wheelchair spokes, side rails, doorways, and so forth?

Outcome Criteria

The person will
- Demonstrate an ability to scan the visual field to compensate for loss of function/sensation in affected limbs
- Identify safety hazards in the environment
- Describe the deficit and the rationale for treatment

Interventions

A. Assist the person to recognize the perceptual deficit
1. Initially adapt the environment to the deficit:
   a. Position person, call light, bedside stand, television, telephone, and personal items on the unaffected side.
   b. Position bed with unaffected side toward the door.
   c. Approach and speak to person from his uninvolved side.
   d. If you must approach person from affected side, announce your presence as soon as you enter the room to avoid startling the person.
   e. When working with the person's affected extremity, position the unaffected side near a wall to minimize distractions.
2. Gradually change the person's environment as you teach him to compensate and learn to recognize the forgotten field; move furniture and personal items out of the visual field (Baggerly, 1992).
3. Provide a simplified, well lighted, uncluttered environment (Baggerly, 1992).
   a. Provide a moment between activities.
   b. Provide concrete cues: "You are on your side facing the wall."
4. Provide a full-length mirror to help with vertical orientation and to diminish the distortion of the vertical and horizontal plane, which manifests itself in the patient leaning toward the affected side.
5. Use verbal instructions, rather than mere demonstrations. Keep instructions simple.
6. For a person in a wheelchair, obtain a lapboard (preferably Plexiglas); position the affected arm on the lapboard with the fingertips at midline. Encourage person to look for the arm on the board.
7. For an ambulatory person, obtain an arm sling to prevent the arm from dangling and causing shoulder subluxation.
8. When the person is in bed, elevate affected arm on a pillow to prevent dependent edema.
9. Constantly cue the person to the environment.
10. Encourage to wear a watch, favorite ring, or bracelet on affected arm to draw attention to it.

B. Assist the person with adaptations needed for self-care and other ADLs
1. Encourage to wear prescribed corrective lenses or hearing aids.
2. For bathing, dressing, and toileting
   a. Instruct to attend to affected extremity/side first when performing ADLs.
   b. Instruct client always to look for affected extremity when performing ADL, to know where it is at all times.
   c. Teach to perform dressing and grooming tasks in front of a mirror.
   d. Suggest color-coded markers sewn or placed inside shoes or clothes to help distinguish right from left.
   e. Encourage client to integrate affected extremity during bathing and to feel extremity by rubbing and massaging it.

f. Use adaptive equipment as appropriate.

g. Refer to *Self-Care Deficit* for additional interventions.

3. For feeding

a. Set up meals with a minimum of dishes, food, and utensils.

b. Instruct client to eat in small amounts and place food on unaffected side of mouth.

c. Instruct client to use tongue to sweep out "pockets" of food from affected side after every bite.

d. After meals/medications, check oral cavity for pocketed food/medication.

e. Provide oral care t.i.d. and PRN.

f. Initially place food in the person's visual field; gradually move food out of field and teach person to scan entire visual field.

g. Use adaptive feeding equipment as appropriate.

h. Refer to *Self-Care Deficit: Feeding* for additional interventions.

i. Refer to *Altered Nutrition: Less Than Body Requirements related to swallowing difficulties* if person has difficulty in chewing and swallowing food.

C. Teach measures to prevent injury

1. Retrain person to scan his entire environment.

a. Instruct to turn head past midline to view scene on the affected side.

b. Perform activities that require turning the head.

c. Remind client to scan when ambulating or propelling a wheelchair.

2. Use tactile sensation to reintroduce affected arm/extremity to the person.

a. Have person stroke involved side with uninvolved hand and watch the arm or leg while stroking it.

b. Rub different-textured materials to stimulate sensations (hot, cold, rough, soft).

3. Instruct the person to keep the affected arm and/or leg in view.

a. Position arm on lapboard. (Plexiglas lapboards allow person to view affected leg, thereby helping to integrate the leg into the body schema.)

b. Provide an arm sling for an ambulatory person.

c. Instruct client to take extra care around sources of heat or cold and moving machinery or parts to protect affected side from injury.

D. Initiate health teaching and referrals

1. Assess to ensure that both person and family understand the cause of unilateral neglect and the purpose and rationale of all interventions.

2. Proceed with teaching as needed.

a. Explain unilateral neglect.

b. Instruct family on how to facilitate the person's relearning techniques (*e.g.*, cueing, scanning visual field).

c. Teach use of adaptive equipment, if appropriate.

d. Teach principles of maintaining a safe environment.

Rationale

• Adapting the environment minimizes sensory deprivation. Initially, however, attempts should be made to have the person attend to both sides (Baggerly, 1992).

• Reminders can help the client adapt to the environment.

• Rapid movements can precipitate anxiety (Baggerly, 1992).

• Cues can help with adjustment to position changes (Baggerly, 1992).

• Clients know that something is wrong but may attribute it to being "disturbed" (Baggerly, 1992).

• Tactile stimulation of the affected parts promotes their integration into the whole body (Baggerly, 1992).

• Scanning can help prevent injury and increase awareness of entire space.

• Decreased sensation or motor function increases the vulnerability to injury.

• The client may need specific reminders to prevent him from ignoring nonfunctioning body parts.

References/Bibliography

Baggerly, J. (1992). Sensory perceptual problems following stroke. *Nursing Clinics of North America, 26,* 997–1005.

Burt, M. M. (1970). Perceptual deficits in hemiplegia. *American Journal of Nursing, 70,* 1026–1029.

Heilman, K. M., & Valenstein, E. (1972). Frontal lobe neglect in man. *Neurology, 22,* 660–664.

Heilman, K. M., & Van Den Abell, T. (1980). Right hemisphere dominance for attention: The mechanism underlying hemispheric asymmetries of inattention (neglect). *Neurology, 30,* 327–330.

Hier, D., Mondlock B., & Caplan, L. (1983). Behavioral abnormalities after right hemisphere stroke. *Neurology, 33,* 337–344.

Mitchell, P. H., Hodges, L. C., Muwaswes, M., & Walleck, C. A. (1992). *AANN's neuroscience nursing* (2nd ed.). Norwalk, CT: Appleton & Lange.

Painter, M. J., & Bergman, I. (1990). Neurology. In R. E. Behrman & R. Kliegman (Eds.). *Nelson's essentials of pediatrics.* Philadelphia: W. B. Saunders.

Weinberg, J., Diller, L., Gordon, W., Gerstman, L., Lieberman, A., Lakin, P., Hodges G., & Erachi, O. (1979). Training sensory awareness and spatial organization in people with right brain damage. *Archives of Physical Rehabilitation, 60,* 491–496.

Urinary Elimination, Altered Patterns of

Maturational Enuresis*

Functional Incontinence

Reflex Incontinence

Stress Incontinence

Total Incontinence

Urge Incontinence

Urinary Retention

Urinary Elimination, Altered Patterns of

DEFINITION
Altered Patterns of Urinary Elimination: The state in which the individual experiences or is at risk of experiencing urinary elimination dysfunction.

DEFINING CHARACTERISTICS
Major (Must Be Present)

Reports or experiences a urinary elimination problem, such as

Urgency	Dribbling
Frequency	Bladder distention
Hesitancy	Large residual urine volumes
Nocturia	Incontinence
Enuresis	

RELATED FACTORS
Pathophysiologic

Related to incompetent bladder outlet secondary to congenital urinary tract anomalies

Related to decreased bladder capacity or irritation to bladder secondary to:

Infection	Glucosuria
Trauma	Carcinoma
Urethritis	

* This diagnosis is not currently on the NANDA list but has been included for clarity or usefulness.

Related to diminished bladder cues or impaired ability to recognize bladder cues secondary to:

Cord injury/tumor/infection   Diabetic neuropathy
Brain injury/tumor/infection   Alcoholic neuropathy
Cerebrovascular accident   Tabes dorsalis
Demyelinating diseases   Parkinsonism
Multiple sclerosis

Treatment-Related

Related to effects of surgery on bladder sphincter secondary to:
Postprostatectomy
Extensive pelvic dissection
Related to diagnostic instrumentation
Related to decreased muscle tone secondary to:
General or spinal anesthesia
Drug therapy (iatrogenic)

Antihistamines   Immunosuppressant therapy
Epinephrine   Diuretics
Anticholinergics   Tranquilizers
Sedatives   Muscle relaxants
Post-indwelling catheters

Situational (Personal, Environmental)

Related to weak pelvic floor muscles secondary to:
Obesity   Childbirth
Aging   Recent substantial weight loss
Related to inability to communicate needs
Related to bladder outlet obstruction secondary to fecal impaction/chronic constipation
Related to decreased bladder muscle tone secondary to dehydration
Related to decreased attention to bladder cues secondary to:
Depression   Delirium
Intentional suppression (self-induced deconditioning)   Confusion
Related to environmental barriers to bathroom secondary to:
Distant toilets
Poor lighting
Unfamiliar surroundings
Bed too high
Side rails
Related to inability to access bathroom on time secondary to:
Caffeine/alcohol use
Impaired mobility

Maturational

Child
Related to small bladder capacity
Related to lack of motivation

Author's Note

Altered Patterns of Urinary Elimination probably is too broad a diagnosis for effective clinical use. For this reason, the nurse should use a more specific diagnosis, such as *Stress Incontinence*, whenever possible. When the etiologic or contributing factors for incontinence have not been identified, the nurse could temporarily write a diagnosis of *Altered Patterns of Urinary Elimination related to unknown etiology, as evidenced by incontinence.*

The nurse performs a focus assessment to determine whether the incontinence is transient, in response to an acute condition (*e.g.*, infection, medication side effects), or established in response to various chronic neural or genitourinary conditions (Miller, 1995). In addition, the nurse should differentiate the type of incontinence: functional, reflex, stress, urge, or total. The diagnosis *Total Incontinence* should not be used unless all other types of incontinence have been ruled out.

Errors in Diagnostic Statements

Altered Patterns of Urinary Elimination related to surgical diversion

This diagnosis represents a new label for urostomy, and does not focus on the nursing accountability. A person with a urostomy should be assessed for its effect on functional patterns and on physiologic functioning. For this person, the collaborative problems *Potential Complication: Stomal obstruction* and *Potential Complication: Internal urine leakage*, as well as nursing diagnoses such as *Risk for Body Image Disturbance* and *Risk for Altered Health Maintenance*, could be applicable.

Altered Patterns of Urinary Elimination related to renal failure

This diagnosis renames renal failure and is inappropriate as a nursing diagnosis. For this reason, the diagnosis *Fluid Volume Excess related to acute renal failure* also would be incorrect. Renal failure causes or contributes to various actual or potential nursing diagnoses, such as *Risk for Infection* and *Risk for Altered Nutrition*, and collaborative problems, such as *Potential Complication: Fluid/electrolyte imbalances* and *Potential Complication: Metabolic acidosis*.

Total Incontinence related to effects of aging

The physiologic effects of aging on the urinary tract system can negatively influence functioning when other risk factors also are present (*e.g.*, mobility problems, dehydration, side effects of medications, decreased awareness of bladder cues). This nursing diagnosis projects a biased view of anticipated incontinence in an elderly person, with associated use of indwelling catheters, diapers, and/or bed pads. When this equipment is used, the nurse is not treating incontinence, but rather managing urine. The use of such equipment is a short-term solution. For these situations, *Risk for Infection* and *Risk for Impaired Skin Integrity* would apply. When an elderly person has an incontinent episode, the nurse should proceed cautiously before applying the nursing diagnosis label of "incontinence." If factors exist that increase the likelihood of recurrence and the client is motivated, the diagnosis *Risk for Functional/Urge Incontinence related to* (specify—*e.g.*, dehydration, mobility difficulties, decreased bladder capacity) could apply. This diagnosis would focus nursing interventions on preventing incontinence, rather than expecting it as inevitable. For an elderly person with the combination of functional and urge incontinence, the nurse would focus on assisting the person to increase bladder capacity and reduce barriers to bathrooms, using the diagnosis *Functional/Urge Incontinence related to age-related effects on bladder capacity, self-induced fluid limitations, and unstable gait.*

Key Concepts

1. The three components of the lower urinary tract that assist to maintain continence are (Porth, 1994)
   a. Detrusor muscle in the bladder wall, which allows bladder expansion to increase with volume of urine
   b. Internal sphincter or proximal urethra, which, when contracted, prevents urine leakage
   c. External sphincter, which by voluntary control provides added support during stressed situations (*e.g.*, overdistended bladder)
2. Innervation of the bladder arises from the spinal cord at the levels of S2–S4. The bladder is under parasympathetic control. Voluntary control over urination is influenced by the cortex, midbrain, and medulla.

3. The female urethra is 3–5 cm long. The male urethra is approximately 20 cm long. Continence is maintained primarily by the urethra, but the cerebral cortex is the principal area for suppression of the desire to micturate.

4. Capacity of the normal bladder (without experiencing discomfort) is 250–400 mL. The desire to void occurs when there is 150–250 mL of urine in the bladder.

5. The sitting position for the female and the standing position for the male allow optimal relaxation of the external urinary sphincter and perineal muscles.

6. Bladder tissue tone can be lost if the bladder is distended to 1000 mL (atonic bladder) or continuously drained (Foley catheter).

7. Mechanisms to stimulate the voiding reflex or Credé's method may be ineffective if the bladder capacity is less than 200 mL.

8. Alcohol, coffee, and tea have a natural diuretic effect and are bladder irritants.

9. Injury to the spinal cord above S2–S4 produces a spastic or reflex bladder tone. Injury to the spinal cord below S2–S4 produces a flaccid or atonic bladder.

10. Lesions affecting inhibitory centers in the brain or the pathways transmitting inhibitory impulses to the bladder result in an uninhibited bladder.

Infection

1. Stasis or pooling of urine contributes to bacterial growth. Bacteria can travel up the ureters to the kidney (ascending infection).

2. Recurrent bladder infections cause fibrotic changes in the bladder wall with resultant decrease in bladder capacity.

3. Urinary stasis, infections, alkaline urine, and decreased urine volume contribute to the formation of urinary tract calculi.

Incontinence

1. Incontinence is transient in as many as 50% of individuals presenting with the problem, and of the remaining group, about two thirds can be cured or markedly improved with treatment (Resnick & Yalla, 1985). There are many effective corrective measures for the management of urinary tract disease in the elderly, and a positive approach should be taken to minimize the incidence of urinary incontinence (Urinary Incontinence Guideline Panel, 1992).

2. The daily cost of caring for incontinence in nursing homes nationwide is $2.9 million. An estimated one half of the 1.4 million home residents receiving Medicaid benefits are incontinent (Cella, 1988).

3. Incontinence can be transient or reversible. Causes of transient incontinence are acute confusion, urinary tract infection, atrophic vaginitis, side effects of medication, metabolic imbalance, impaction, mobility problems (Wyman, 1988), urosepsis, depression, and pressure sores (Smith & Newman, 1991).

4. It is important to determine the natural history of the incontinent pattern. A new onset of incontinence is likely to be due to an external precipitating factor outside of the urinary tract (*e.g.*, medications, acute illness, inaccessible toilets, impaired mobility preventing getting to the toilet on time), which can often be easily corrected. Incontinence can be either transient (reversible) or established (controllable). Controllable incontinence cannot be cured, but urine removal can be planned (Urinary Incontinence Guideline Panel, 1992).

5. Certain medications are associated with incontinence. Narcotics and sedatives diminish awareness of bladder cues. Adrenergic agents cause retention by increasing bladder outlet resistance. Anticholinergics (antidepressants, some antiparkinsonian medications, antispasmodics, antihistamines, antiarrhythmics, opiates) cause chronic retention with overflow. Diuretics rapidly increase urine volume and can cause incontinence if voiding cannot be delayed (Miller, 1995; Wyman, 1988).

6. People with diabetes mellitus, which can contribute to increased residual urine, frequency, and urgency, may be less aware of bladder fullness.

7. Social isolation of incontinent people can be self-imposed because of fear and embarrassment, or imposed by others because of odor and esthetics.

8. Depression can prevent the person from recognizing or responding to bladder cues and thus contributes to incontinence.

Intermittent Catheterization

1. This method maintains the tonicity of the bladder muscle, prevents overdistention, and provides for complete emptying of the bladder.
2. The initial removal of more than 500 mL of urine from a chronically distended bladder can cause severe hemorrhage, which results when bladder veins, previously compressed by the distended bladder, rapidly dilate and rupture when bladder pressure is abruptly released. (After the initial release of 500 mL of urine, alternate the release of 100 mL of urine with 15-minute catheter clamps).
3. The accumulation of more than 500–700 mL of urine in a bladder should not be permitted.
4. In individuals with spinal injuries at the T4 level or above, it is necessary to empty the bladder completely regardless of high volumes (>500 mL) owing to the risk of autonomic dysreflexia. Interruption of the sympathetic nervous system causes the veins not to dilate rapidly.

Total Incontinence

1. A cognitively impaired person with total incontinence requires caregiver-directed treatment. In institutional settings, indwelling and external catheters or disposal or washable diapers or pads are beneficial to the caregivers, but detrimental to the incontinent person. Aids and equipment should be considered only after other means have been attempted. In the home setting, the caregiver's needs may take precedence over the cognitively impaired person's. Urinary incontinence is cited as the major reason for seeking institutional care for people living at home (Miller, 1995).

Key Concepts—Older Adult

1. Urinary incontinence affects 5%–15% of elderly people living in the community, and its prevalence increases to about 40% in hospitalized clients and 50% in the institutionalized clients (Resnick & Yalla, 1985). One of the major problems of incontinence in the elderly is that it may be overlooked and not adequately evaluated by professionals, and, as a result, appropriate treatment is denied. Elderly people themselves may not admit to the problem because of attitudes about the inevitability of complications such as incontinence.
2. Age-related physiologic changes result in decreased bladder capacity, incomplete emptying, contractions during filling, and increased residual urine (Miller, 1995).
3. Older adults can comfortably store 250–300 mL of urine, compared with a storage capacity of 350–400 mL in younger adults.
4. The sensation to void is delayed in older adults, which shortens the interval between the initial perception of the urge and the actual need to void, resulting in urgency (Miller, 1995). Any factor that interferes with the older adult's perception to void (e.g., medications, depression, limited fluid intake, neurologic impairments) or delays his or her ability to reach the toilet can cause incontinence.
5. Other physiologic components of aging that contribute to incontinence are the diminished ability of kidneys to concentrate urine, decreasing muscle tone of the pelvic floor muscles, and the ability to postpone urination.
6. Frequent voiding out of habit or limiting fluids may contribute to urgency by impairing the neurologic mechanisms that signal the need to void, because the bladder is rarely fully expanded.
7. The diminished vision, impaired mobility, and decreased energy level that may accompany aging mean that increased time is needed to locate the toilet, which also requires the person to be able to delay urination.
8. In one study, incontinent elderly women reported a history of vaginal deliveries, bacteriuria, and a greater number of functional impairments (Ouslander, Morishita, Blaustein, Orzeck, Dunne, & Sayre, 1987).

9. Older adults experience urgency owing to the bladder's limited capacity and their decreased ability to inhibit bladder contractions.

Focus Assessment Criteria

Subjective Data

A. Assess for defining characteristics

1. "Do you have a problem with controlling your urine (or going to the bathroom)?"
2. History of symptoms
   a. Complaints of

Lack of control	Pain or discomfort
Dribbling	Burning
Hesitancy	Change in voiding pattern
Urgency	Retention
Frequency	

   b. Onset and duration
   c. Description
   d. Frequency
   e. Precipitated by what?
   f. Relieved by what?
   g. Aggravated by what?
   h. Restrictions on life-style

Social	Sexual
Occupational	Role responsibilities

3. Incontinence (adult)
   a. History of continence

Is degree of continence acceptable?	History of "weak" bladder?
Age of attainment of continence?	Family history of incontinence?
Previous history of enuresis?	

   b. Onset and duration (day, night, just certain times)
   c. Factors that increase incidence (Newman, Lynch, Smith, & Cell, 1991; Ruff & Reaves, 1989):

Coughing	Delay in getting to bathroom
Laughing	When excited
Standing	Leaving bathroom
Turning in bed	Running

   d. Perception of need to void

Present	Absent
Diminished	

   e. Ability to delay urination after urge
   Present (how long)?
   Absent
   f. Sensations occurring before or during micturition

Difficulty starting stream	Need to force urine out
Difficulty stopping stream	Lack of sensation to void
Painful straining (tenesmus)	

   g. Relief after voiding
   Complete
   Continued desire to void after bladder is emptied
   h. Use of catheters, diapers, bed pads
4. Enuresis (child)
   a. Onset and pattern (day, night)
   b. Toilet training history
   c. Family history of bed-wetting
   d. Response of others to child (parents, siblings, peers)

B. Assess for related factors
　　1. Presence of risk factors
　　　　a. Physiologic
　　　　　　Fluid intake pattern (type and amount especially before bedtime)
　　　　　　Dehydration (self-imposed, overuse of diuretics, caffeine, alcohol)
　　　　　　Prostatic hypertrophy
　　　　　　Bladder, vaginal infections
　　　　　　Chronic illnesses (*e.g.*, diabetes, alcoholism, Parkinson's disease, Alzheimer's
　　　　　　　　disease, multiple sclerosis, cerebrovascular accident, vitamin B_{12} defi-
　　　　　　　　ciency)
　　　　　　Metabolic disturbances (*e.g.*, hypokalemia, hypercalcemia)
　　　　　　Fecal impaction/severe constipation
　　　　　　Certain medications (diuretics, anticholinergics, antihistamines, sedatives,
　　　　　　　　acetaminophen, amitriptyline, aspirin, barbiturates, chlorpropamide, clofi-
　　　　　　　　brate, fluphenazine, haloperidol, narcotics)
　　　　　　Multiple or difficult deliveries
　　　　　　Pelvic, bladder, or uterine surgery, disorders
　　　　b. Functional ability
　　　　　　Perception of bladder cues　　　　　　　　Ability to reach toilet in time
　　　　　　Walking, balance, manual dexterity
　　　　c. Environmental barriers
　　　　　　Location of bathroom within 40 feet
　　　　　　Stairs, narrow doorways
　　　　　　Dim lighting
　　　　　　Ability to locate bathroom in social settings

Objective Data

A. Assess for defining characteristics
　　1. Urination stream
　　　　Slow　　　　　　Sprays
　　　　Small　　　　　Starts and stops
　　　　Drops　　　　　Slow or hard to start
　　　　Dribble
　　2. Urine
　　　　a. Color
　　　　　　Yellow　　　　　　Yellow-brown
　　　　　　Amber　　　　　　Green-brown
　　　　　　Straw color　　　　Dark brown
　　　　　　Red-brown　　　　Black
　　　　b. Odor
　　　　　　Faint　　　　　　Offensive
　　　　　　Ammoniac　　　Acetonic
　　　　c. Appearance
　　　　　　Clear
　　　　　　Cloudy
　　　　d. Reaction (normal, pH 4.6–7.5, or alkaline, over 7.5)
　　　　　　Specific gravity
　　　　　　Dilute ($<$1.003)
　　　　　　Concentrated ($>$1.025)
　　　　　　Normal (1.003–1.025)
　　　　f. Negative or positive for
　　　　　　Glucose　　　　Bacteria
　　　　　　Protein　　　　Red blood cells
　　　　　　Ketone

B. Assess for related factors
   1. Voiding and fluid intake patterns (record for 2–4 days to establish a baseline)
      a. What is daily fluid intake?
      b. When does incontinence occur?
   2. Muscle tone
      a. Abdomen firm, or soft and pendulous?
      b. History of recent significant weight loss or gain?
   3. Reflexes
      a. Presence or absence of cauda equina reflexes
            Anal
            Bulbocavernosus
   4. Bladder
      a. Distention (palpable)
      b. Can it be emptied by external stimuli? (Credé's method, gentle suprapubic tapping, or warm water over the perineum, Valsalva maneuver, pulling of pubic hair, anal stretch)
      c. Capacity (at least 400–500 mL)
      d. Residual urine
            None
            Present in what amount?
   5. Functional ability
      a. Get in/out of chair
      b. Walk alone to bathroom
      c. Maintain balance
      d. Manipulate clothing
   6. Cognitive ability
      a. Asks to go to bathroom
      b. Initiates toileting with reminders
      c. Aware of incontinence
      d. Expects to be incontinent
   7. Assess for presence of
Constipation	Depression
Fecal impaction	Mobility disorders
Dehydration	Sensory disorders

Maturational Enuresis*

DEFINITION
Maturational Enuresis: The state in which a child experiences involuntary voiding during sleep that is not pathophysiologic in origin.

DEFINING CHARACTERISTICS
Major (Must Be Present)
Reports or demonstrates episodes of involuntary voiding during sleep

* This diagnosis is not currently on the NANDA list but has been included for clarity or usefulness.

RELATED FACTORS
Situational (Personal, Environmental)
Related to stressors (school, siblings)
Related to inattention to bladder cues
Related to unfamiliar surroundings

Maturational
Child
Related to small bladder capacity
Related to lack of motivation
Related to attention-seeking behavior

Author's Note

Enuresis can be due to physiologic or maturational factors. Certain etiologies, such as strictures, urinary tract infection, constipation, nocturnal epilepsy, and diabetes, should be ruled out when enuresis is present. These situations do not represent nursing diagnoses.

When enuresis results from small bladder capacity, failure to perceive cues because of deep sleep, or inattention to bladder cues, or is associated with a maturational issue (*e.g.*, new sibling, school pressures), the nursing diagnosis *Maturational Enuresis* is appropriate. Psychological problems usually are not the cause of enuresis, but may result from lack of understanding or insensitivity to the problem. Interventions that punish or shame the child must be avoided.

Errors in Diagnostic Statements

Maturational Enuresis related to stressors and conflicts

Rather than focus on etiology for maturational enuresis, the nurse should focus on teaching the child and parents management strategies. The nurse also should encourage parents to share their concerns and direct them away from punishing behaviors. Given this nursing focus, the diagnosis could be restated as *Maturational Enuresis related to unknown etiology, as evidenced by reported episodes of bed-wetting.*

Key Concepts

1. The newborn may void up to 20 times per day because of small bladder capacity (Wong, 1995). As the child grows, bladder capacity increases and frequency of urination decreases (Chow, Durand, Feldman, & Mills, 1984).
2. Most children by age 4–5 years have complete neuromuscular control of urination (Chow et al., 1984).
3. Foye and Sulkes (1990) define enuresis as urinary incontinence at any age when urinary control would be expected.
4. The etiology of enuresis is complex and not well understood. The following factors have been implicated:
   a. Developmental/maturational delay (*e.g.*, small functional bladder capacity, deep sleep, or mental retardation)
   b. Organic factors (*e.g.*, infection, sickle cell anemia, diabetes, and neuromuscular disorders)
   c. Psychological/emotional factors (*e.g.*, stressors such as birth of sibling, hospitalization, or divorce of parents) (Chow et al., 1984; Van Cleve & Baldwin, 1989)
5. Children at risk for urinary retention include those who
   a. Have congenital anomalies of the urinary tract
   b. Are neurologically impaired (Wong, 1995)
   c. Have undergone surgery (Hunsberger, 1989)

6. Enuresis is primarily a maturational problem and usually ceases between the ages of 6 and 8 years. It is more common in boys (Warrady, 1991). Ninety-nine percent become continent by adolescence.
7. There is a high frequency of bed-wetting in children whose parents or other near relatives were bed-wetters (Warrady, 1991).
8. High anxiety can impede the child's ability to master the necessary skills for the maintenance of continence (Carpenter, 1994).
9. Most children with nocturnal enuresis have neither a psychiatric nor an organic illness (Carpenter, 1994; Warrady, 1991).

Focus Assessment Criteria

Subjective Data
A. Assess for defining characteristics
1. Onset
2. Pattern (day, night)
3. Number of episodes in month

B. Assess for related factors
1. Toilet training history
2. Family history of bed-wetting
3. Response of others (parents, peers, siblings)
4. Recent change or stressor

School	Relocation
Peers	Family problems
New sibling	

5. Inattention to bladder cues

Outcome Criteria

- The child will remain dry during the sleep cycle
- The child or family will be able to state the nature and causes of enuresis

---

Interventions
A. Assess for contributing factors
1. Small bladder capacity
2. Sound sleeper
3. Response to stress (at school or at home, *e.g.*, new sibling)

B. Promote a positive parent–child relationship
1. Explain the nature of enuresis to parents and child as developmental, and that it usually resolves with time.
2. Explain to parents that disapproval (shaming, punishing) is useless in stopping enuresis, but can make child shy, ashamed, and afraid.
3. Offer reassurance to child that other children wet the bed at night and that he is not bad or sinful.

C. Reduce contributing factors, if possible
1. Small bladder capacity: After child drinks fluids, encourage him to postpone voiding to help stretch the bladder.

2. Sound sleeper
   a. Have child void before retiring.
   b. Restrict fluids at bedtime.
   c. If child is awakened later (about 11 P.M.) to void, attempt to awaken child fully for positive reinforcement.
3. Too busy to sense a full bladder (if daytime wetting occurs)
   a. Teach child awareness of sensations that occur when it is time to void.
   b. Teach child ability to control urination (have him start and stop the stream; have him "hold" the urine during the day, even if for only a short time).
   c. Have child keep a record of how he is doing; emphasize dry days or nights (*e.g.*, stars on a calendar).
   d. If child wets, have him explain or write down, if he can, why he thinks it happened.

D. Initiate health teaching and referrals, as indicated
   1. For children with enuresis
      a. Teach child and parents the facts about enuresis.
      b. Teach child and family techniques to control the adverse effects of enuresis (*e.g.*, use of plastic mattress covers, use of child's own sleeping bag [machine washable] when staying overnight away from home).
   2. Seek out opportunities to teach the public about enuresis and incontinence (*e.g.*, school and parent organizations, self-help groups).

Rationale

- Anger, punishment, and rejection by parents and peers contribute to feelings of shame, embarrassment, and low self-esteem (Carpenter, 1994).
- Explaining that enuresis is developmental reduces blaming of child and parent frustration (Carpenter, 1994).
- Behavioral reward system can enhance parent–child interactions related to toileting and decrease episodes of incontinence (Carpenter, 1994).

Functional Incontinence

DEFINITION

Functional Incontinence: The state in which an individual experiences incontinence because of a difficulty or inability to reach the toilet in time.

DEFINING CHARACTERISTICS
Major (Must Be Present)

Incontinence before or during an attempt to reach the toilet

RELATED FACTORS
Pathophysiologic

Related to diminished bladder cues and impaired ability to recognize bladder cues secondary to:

Brain injury/tumor/infection	Alcoholic neuropathy
Cerebrovascular accident	Parkinsonism

Demyelinating diseases   Progressive dementia
Multiple sclerosis

Treatment-Related

Related to decreased bladder tone secondary to:

Antihistamines	Immunosuppressant therapy
Epinephrine	Diuretics
Anticholinergics	Tranquilizers
Sedatives	Muscle relaxants

Situational (Personal, Environmental)

Related to impaired mobility
Related to decreased attention to bladder cues

     Depression   Intentional suppression (self-induced deconditioning)
     Confusion

Related to environmental barriers to bathroom

Distant toilets	Bed too high
Poor lighting	Side rails
Unfamiliar surroundings	

Maturational

Older Adult

     Related to motor and sensory losses

Key Concepts

1. Functional incontinence is the inability or unwillingness of the person with a normal bladder and sphincter to reach the toilet in sufficient time.
2. Functional incontinence may be caused by conditions affecting the individual's physical and emotional ability to manage the act of urination.
3. Underlying psychological problems can be a functional etiology of incontinence.
4. Approximately 45% of all nursing home residents are incontinent. Of those with bladder incontinence, 82% are mobility limited.

Focus Assessment Criteria

See *Altered Patterns of Urinary Elimination*

Outcome Criteria

The person will
- Remove or minimize environmental barriers from home
- Use proper adaptive equipment to assist with voiding, transfers, and dressing
- Describe causative factors for incontinence

Interventions

A. Assess causative or contributing factors

     1. Assess for

       a. Obstacles to toilet

         Poor lighting, slippery floor, misplaced furniture and rugs, inadequate footwear, toilet too far, bed too high, side rails up

         Inadequate toilet

           Too small for walkers, wheelchair, seat too low/high, no grab bars

         Inadequate signal system for requesting help

         Lack of privacy

b. Sensory/cognitive deficits
   Visual deficits (blindness, field cuts, poor depth perception)
   Cognitive deficits due to aging, trauma, stroke, tumor, infection
c. Motor/mobility deficits
   Limited upper and/or lower extremity movement/strength (inability to remove clothing)
   Barriers to ambulation (*e.g.*, vertigo, fatigue, altered gait, hypertension)

B. Reduce or eliminate contributing factors, if possible
   1. Environmental barriers
      a. Assess path to bathroom for obstacles, lighting, and distance.
      b. Assess adequacy of toilet height and need for grab bars.
      c. Assess adequacy of room size.
      d. Provide a commode between bathroom and bed, if necessary.
   2. Sensory/cognitive deficits
      a. For an individual with diminished vision
         Ensure adequate lighting.
         Encourage person to wear prescribed corrective lens.
         Provide clear, safe pathway to bathroom.
         Keep call bell easily accessible.
         If bedpan or urinal is used, make sure it is within easy reach in the same location at all times.
         Assess person for safety in bathroom.
         Assess person's ability to provide self-hygiene.
      b. For an individual with cognitive deficits
         Offer toileting reminders every 2 hours, after meals, and before bedtime.
         Establish appropriate means to communicate need to void.
         Answer call bell immediately.
         Encourage wearing ordinary clothes.
         Provide a normal environment for elimination (use bathroom if possible).
         Allow for privacy while maintaining safety.
         Allow sufficient time for task.
         Reorient individual to where he is and what task he is doing.
         Be consistent in your approach to person.
         Give simple step-by-step instructions; use verbal and nonverbal cues.
         Give positive reinforcement for success.
         Assess person for safety in bathroom.
         Assess need for adaptive devices on clothing to make dressing and undressing easier.
         Assess person's ability to provide self-hygiene.
   3. Motor/mobility deficits
      a. For people with limited hand function
         Assess person's ability to remove and replace clothing.
         Clothing that is loose is easier to manipulate.
         Provide dressing aids as necessary (*e.g.*, Velcro closures in seams for wheelchair patients, zipper pulls; all garments with fasteners may be adapted with Velcro closures).

C. Provide for factors that promote continence
   1. Maintain optimal hydration.
      a. Increase fluid intake to 2000–3000 mL/day, unless contraindicated.
      b. Teach older adults not to depend on thirst sensations but to drink liquids even when not thirsty.
      c. Space fluids every 2 hours.
      d. Decrease fluid intake after 7 P.M. and provide only minimal fluids during the night.
      e. Reduce intake of coffee, tea, dark colas, alcohol, and grapefruit juice because of their diuretic effect.

    f. Avoid large amounts of tomato and orange juice because they tend to make the urine more alkaline.

    g. Encourage cranberry juice to acidify urine.

2. Maintain adequate nutrition to ensure bowel elimination at least once every 3 days.

    a. Monitor elimination pattern; check for fecal impaction if indicated.

    b. Assess daily dietary intake for daily requirements of roughage, basic five food groups, and adequate fluids.

    c. See *Altered Nutrition* and *Constipation* for additional interventions.

3. Promote micturition.

    a. Ensure privacy and comfort.

    b. Use toilet facilities, if possible, instead of bedpans.

    c. Provide man with opportunity to stand, if possible.

    d. Assist person on bedpan to flex knees and support back.

    e. Teach postural evacuation (bend forward while sitting on toilet).

    f. Ensure safe access to facilities.

        Provide person with access to urinal or bedpan.

        Provide person with call light.

        Reduce obstacles to toilet facilities (path that is well lighted and free of obstacles, bed at lowest level).

        Modify path to bathroom with rails.

        Modify bathroom with grab rails, elevated seats.

    g. Stimulate the cutaneous surface to trigger the voiding reflex.

        Have person brush or stroke inner thigh or abdomen.

        Pour warm water over perineum.

        Give glass of water to drink while sitting on the toilet.

4. Promote personal integrity and provide motivation to increase bladder control.

    a. Encourage person to share his feelings about incontinence and determine its effect on his social patterns.

    b. Convey to him that incontinence can be cured or at least controlled to maintain dignity.

    c. Expect him to be continent, not incontinent (*e.g.*, encourage street clothes, discourage use of bedpans).

    d. Use protective pads or garments only after conscientious reconditioning efforts have been completely unsuccessful after 6 weeks.

    e. Work to achieve daytime continence before expecting nighttime continence.

    f. Encourage socialization.

        Encourage and assist person to groom self.

        If hospitalized, provide opportunities to eat meals outside bedroom (day room, lounge).

        If fear or embarrassment is preventing socialization, instruct person to use sanitary pads or briefs temporarily until control is established.

        Change clothes as soon as possible when wet to avoid indirectly sanctioning wetness.

        Advise the oral use of chlorophyll tablets to deodorize urine and feces.

        See *Social Isolation* and *Ineffective Individual Coping* for additional interventions, if indicated.

5. Promote skin integrity.

    a. Identify individuals at risk for development of pressure ulcers.

    b. Wash area, rinse, and dry well after incontinent episode.

    c. Use a protective ointment if needed (for area burns, use hydrocortisone cream; for fungal irritations, use antifungal ointment).

    d. See *Risk for Impaired Skin Integrity* for additional information.

6. Promote personal hygiene

    a. Take showers rather than baths to prevent bacteria from entering urethra.

    b. Instruct women to cleanse the perineum and urethra from front to back after each bowel movement.

D. Teach prevention of urinary tract infections (UTI)
1. Encourage regular, complete emptying of the bladder.
2. Ensure adequate fluid intake.
3. Keep urine acidic; avoid citrus juices, dark colas, and coffee.
4. Monitor urine pH.
5. Teach individual to recognize abnormal changes in urine properties.
   a. Increase in mucus and sediment
   b. Blood in urine (hematuria)
   c. Change in color (from normal straw-colored) or odor
6. Teach individual to monitor for signs and symptoms of UTI.
   a. Elevated temperature, chills, and shaking
   b. Changes in urine properties
   c. Suprapubic pain
   d. Painful urination
   e. Urgency
   f. Frequent small voids or frequent small incontinences
   g. Increased spasticity in spinal cord-injured individuals
   h. Increase in urine pH
   i. Nausea/vomiting
   j. Lower back and/or flank pain

E. Explain age-related effects on bladder function and that urgency and nocturia do not necessarily lead to incontinence

F. Initiate health teaching referral, when indicated
1. Referral to visiting nurse (occupational therapy department) for assessment of bathroom facilities at home

Rationale

- Barriers can delay access to the toilet and cause incontinence if the client cannot delay urination.
- A few seconds' delay in reaching the bathroom can make the difference between continence and incontinence.
- Wearing normal clothing or nightwear helps simulate the home environment, where incontinence may not occur. A hospital gown may reinforce incontinence.
- A client with a cognitive deficit needs constant verbal cues and reminders to establish a routine and reduce incontinence (Urinary Incontinence Guideline Panel, 1992).
- Dehydration can prevent the sensation of a full bladder and can contribute to loss of bladder tone. Spacing fluids helps promote regular bladder filling and emptying.
- Coffee, tea, colas, and grapefruit juice act as diuretics, which can cause urgency.
- Dilute urine helps prevent infection and bladder irritation.
- Bacteria multiply rapidly in stagnant urine retained in the bladder. Moreover, overdistention hinders blood flow to the bladder wall, increasing the susceptibility to infection from bacterial growth. Regular, complete bladder emptying greatly reduces the risk of infection.
- Acidic urine deters the growth of most bacteria implicated in cystitis.

Interventions—*Older Adult Focus*

1. Emphasize that incontinence is not an inevitable age-related event.
2. Explain not to restrict fluid intake for fear of incontinence.
3. Explain not to rely on thirst as a signal to drink fluids.
4. Teach the need to have easy access to bathroom at night. If needed, consider commode chair or urinal.

Rationale

- Explaining the cause can motivate the person to participate.
- Dehydration can cause incontinence by eliminating the sensation of a full bladder (the signal to urinate) and also by reducing the person's alertness to the sensation.
- The older adult has an age-related decrease in thirst (Miller, 1995).

Reflex Incontinence

DEFINITION

Reflex Incontinence: The state in which the individual experiences predictable involuntary loss of urine with no sensation of urge, voiding, or bladder fullness.

DEFINING CHARACTERISTICS
Major (Must Be Present)

Uninhibited bladder contractions
Involuntary reflexes producing spontaneous voiding
Partial or complete loss of sensation of bladder fullness or urge to void

RELATED FACTORS
Pathophysiologic

Related to impaired conduction of impulses above the reflex arc level secondary to:
Cord injury/tumor/infection

Key Concepts

1. A lesion above the sacral cord segments (above T12) involving both motor and sensory tracts of the spinal cord results in a reflex bladder. Other common names for this type of bladder dysfunction are spastic, supraspinal, hypertonic, automatic, and upper motor neuron bladder.
2. A lesion that does not completely transect the spinal cord can produce variable findings.
3. Control from higher cerebral centers is removed in the reflex neurogenic bladder. Therefore, micturition cannot be started or stopped in a voluntary manner.
4. The simple spinal reflex arc takes over the control of micturition.
5. A positive bulbocavernosus reflex suggests that the voiding reflex (spinal reflex arc) is intact.
6. If the opening of the urinary sphincter and the relaxation of the striated muscle surrounding the urinary sphincter are uncoordinated, there is a potential for large residual urine volumes after triggered voiding.
7. Autonomic dysreflexia is an abnormal hyperactive reflex activity that occurs only in spinal cord–injured individuals with a lesion above T8. Most often, these individuals have an upper motor neuron bladder (reflex incontinence). This is a life-threatening situation in which the blood pressure rises to lethal levels. Autonomic hyperreflexia is most often set off by stimuli resulting from an overstretched bladder or bowel.

Outcome Criteria

The person will
- Report a state of dryness that is personally satisfactory
- Have a residual urine volume of less than 50 mL
- Use triggering mechanisms to initiate reflex voiding

Interventions

A. Assess for causative and contributing conditions
   1. Spinal cord lesion above T12
   2. Traumatic injury
   3. Infection
   4. Tumor
   5. Syringomyelia
   6. Multiple sclerosis
   7. Brown-Séquard syndrome
   8. Transverse myelitis
   9. Pernicious anemia

B. Explain to person rationale for treatment

C. Develop a bladder retraining or reconditioning program (see Interventions under *Total Incontinence*)

D. Teach techniques to stimulate reflex voiding
   1. Cutaneous triggering mechanisms
      a. Repeated deep, sharp suprapubic tapping (most effective)
      b. Instruct individual to:
         Position self in a half-sitting position.
         Tapping is aimed directly at bladder wall with a rate of seven to eight times for 5 seconds (50 single blows).
         Use only one hand.
         Shift site of stimulation over bladder to find most successful site.
         Continue stimulation until a good stream starts.
         Wait approximately 1 minute, repeat stimulation until bladder is empty.
         One or two series of stimulations without response signifies that nothing more will be expelled.
      c. If the preceding measures are ineffective, instruct to perform each of the following for 2–3 minutes each, waiting 1 minute between facilitation attempts.
         Stroking glans penis
         Punching abdomen above inguinal ligaments (lightly)
         Stroking inner thigh
      d. Encourage person to void or trigger at least every 3 hours.
      e. Indicate on intake and output sheet which mechanism was used to induce voiding.
      f. People with abdominal muscle control should use the Valsalva maneuver during triggered voiding.
      g. Teach person that if he increases his fluid intake he also needs to increase the frequency of triggering to prevent overdistention.
      h. Schedule intermittent catheterization program (see *Total Incontinence*).

E. Initiate health teaching, as indicated
   1. Teach bladder reconditioning program (see *Total Incontinence*).
   2. Teach intermittent catheterization (see *Total Incontinence*).

3. Teach prevention of urinary tract infections (see *Total Incontinence*).

4. If at high risk for dysreflexia, see *Dysreflexia*.

Rationale

- Because the voiding reflex located in the sacral cord segments is spared, micturition can occur automatically after external cutaneous stimulation (manual triggering).
- Stimulating the reflex arc replaces the internal sphincter of the bladder, allowing urination. The reflex arc can be triggered by stimulating the bladder wall or cutaneous sites (*e.g.*, suprapubic and pubic).
- Individuals with reflex neurogenic bladders can learn methods for stimulating the reflex arc to stimulate bladder emptying.
- Preferred cutaneous triggering methods are light, rapid suprapubic tapping, light pulling of pubic hairs, massage of the abdomen, and digital rectal stimulation.
- Avoid the use of Credé's maneuver with a reflex bladder because the urethra may be damaged or vesicoureteral reflux may occur if the external sphincter is contracted.
- Contraction of abdominal muscles compresses the bladder to empty it.
- A regular voiding pattern can prevent incontinent episodes.

Stress Incontinence

DEFINITION

Stress Incontinence: The state in which an individual experiences an immediate involuntary loss of urine with an increase in intra-abdominal pressure.

DEFINING CHARACTERISTICS
Major (Must Be Present)

The individual reports loss of urine (usually less than 50 mL) occurring with increased abdominal pressure from standing, sneezing, coughing, running, or lifting heavy objects.

RELATED FACTORS
Pathophysiologic

Related to incompetent bladder outlet secondary to congenital urinary tract anomalies

Related to degenerative changes in pelvic muscles and structural supports secondary to estrogen deficiency

Situational (Personal, Environmental)

Related to high intraabdominal pressure and weak pelvic muscles secondary to:

Obesity	Sex
Pregnancy	Poor personal hygiene

Related to weak pelvic muscles and structural supports secondary to:

Recent substantial weight loss   Childbirth

Maturational

Older Adult

Related to loss of muscle tone

Key Concepts

1. Urinary continence is maintained by the junction of the bladder and the urethra, by support from the perineal floor, and by the muscle around the urethra.
2. Stress incontinence is the leakage of small amounts of urine when the urethral outlet is unable to control passage of urine in the presence of increased intra-abdominal pressure.
3. Stress incontinence is usually made worse by the menopausal decrease in elasticity.
4. A trial of vaginal estrogen cream in the postmenopausal woman who exhibits a pale, atrophic vaginal vault may be helpful in reducing the incidence of incontinence.
5. A stress test is used to help diagnose stress incontinence. It involves observation of the urethral meatus of a client with a full bladder in the standing position while she coughs or strains. Short spurts of urine escaping simultaneously with cough or strain suggest a probable diagnosis of stress incontinence.
6. The client with pure stress incontinence has a normal cystometrogram.
7. The degrees of stress incontinence are designated as:
   a. Grade 1—Loss of urine with sudden increase in abdominal pressure, but never at night.
   b. Grade 2—Lesser degrees of physical stress, such as walking, standing erect from a sitting position, or sitting up in bed, produce incontinence.
   c. Grade 3—In this stage, there is total incontinence, and urine is lost without any relation to physical activity or to position.

Key Concepts—Maternal

1. Pressure of the uterus can cause stress incontinence, which can be misinterpreted as amniotic fluid.

Focus Assessment Criteria

See *Altered Patterns of Urinary Elimination*

Outcome Criteria

The person will
• Report a reduction or elimination of stress incontinence
• Be able to explain the cause of incontinence and rationale for treatment

---

Interventions

A. Assess for contributing factors
   1. Loss of tissue or muscle tone due to:
      a. Childbirth
      b. Obesity
      c. Aging
      d. Recent weight loss
      e. Cystocele
      f. Rectocele
      g. Prolapsed uterus
      h. Atrophic vaginitis or urethritis
   2. History of surgery of the bladder and urethra with adhesions to the vaginal wall
   3. Increased intra-abdominal pressure from:
      a. Pregnancy
      b. Overdistention between voidings
      c. Obesity

B. Assess pattern of voiding/incontinence and fluid intake

1. Promote optimal hydration (see *Total Incontinence*).
2. Assess voiding (see *Total Incontinence*).
3. Instruct person to avoid fluids such as coffee, tea, dark colas, and alcohol, which act as diuretics and irritants.

C. Reduce or eliminate causative or contributing factors

1. Loss of tissue and muscle tone
   a. Explain the effect of incompetent floor muscles on continence (see Key Concepts).
   b. Teach to identify her pelvic floor muscles and strengthen them with exercise (Kegel exercises: 25 times, 4–6 sets a day); provide the following instructions (Urinary Incontinence Guideline Panel, 1992):

      "For posterior pelvic floor muscles, imagine you are trying to stop the passage of stool and tighten your anal muscles for 10 seconds without tightening your legs or your abdominal muscles."

      "For anterior pelvic floor muscles, imagine you are trying to stop the passage of urine, tighten the muscles (back and front) for 10 seconds and then release them; repeat ten times, four times a day." (Can be increased to four times an hour if indicated)

      Stop and start the urine stream several times during voiding.
2. Increased abdominal pressure with obesity
   a. Instruct person to void every 2 hours.
   b. Avoid prolonged periods of standing.
   c. Explain the relation between obesity and stress incontinence.
   d. Teach Kegel exercises.
   e. If person desires to lose weight, refer to *Altered Health Maintenance*.

D. Initiate health teaching for people who continue to remain incontinent after attempts at bladder reconditioning or muscle retraining

1. Promote personal integrity (see *Total Incontinence*).
2. Promote skin integrity (see *Total Incontinence*).
3. Schedule intermittent catheterization program, if appropriate (see *Total Incontinence*).
4. Discuss use of incontinence briefs to contain incontinence.

Rationale

- In stress incontinence, the pelvic floor muscles (pubococcygeus) and levator ani muscles have been weakened or stretched by childbirth, trauma, menopausal atrophy, or obesity.
- Kegel exercises, or pelvic muscle exercises, strengthen and tone the muscles of the pelvic floor. They may provide enough augmentation or urethral pressure to prevent mild stress incontinence. They should be taught to all women as a preventive measure. Studies have shown that pelvic muscle exercises improve or completely control stress incontinence (Urinary Incontinence Guideline Panel, 1992).

Interventions—*Maternal Focus*

1. For increased abdominal pressure during pregnancy
   a. Teach to avoid prolonged periods of standing.
   b. Teach the benefit of frequent voidings at least every 2 hours.
   c. Teach Kegel exercises.

Rationale

- Pressure of the uterus on the bladder can cause involuntary loss of urine.

Total Incontinence

DEFINITION

Total Incontinence: The state in which an individual experiences continuous, unpredictable loss of urine without distention or awareness of bladder fullness.

DEFINING CHARACTERISTICS
Major (Must Be Present)

Constant flow of urine without distention
Nocturia more than two times during sleep time
Incontinence refractory to other treatments

Minor (May Be Present)

Unaware of bladder cues to void
Unaware of incontinence

RELATED FACTORS

Refer to *Altered Patterns of Urinary Elimination*

Key Concepts

See *Altered Patterns of Urinary Elimination*

Focus Assessment Criteria

See *Altered Patterns of Urinary Elimination*

Outcome Criteria

The person will
- Be continent (specify during day, night, 24 hours)
- Be able to identify the cause of incontinence and rationale for treatment

---

Interventions

A. Develop a bladder retraining or reconditioning program to include communication, assessment of voiding pattern, scheduled fluid intake, and scheduled voiding times

   1. Promote communication among all staff members and among individual, family, and staff.
      a. Provide all staff with sufficient knowledge concerning the program planned.
      b. Assess staff's response to program.
   2. Assess the person's potential for participation in a bladder retraining program.
      a. Cognition
      b. Desire to change behavior
      c. Ability to cooperate
      d. Willingness to participate

3. Provide individual with rationale for plan and acquire his informed consent.
4. Encourage individual to continue program by providing accurate information concerning reasons for success or failure.
5. Assess voiding pattern (Fig. II-7).
   a. Monitor and record intake and output.
   b. Time and amount of fluid intake
   c. Type of fluid
   d. Amount of incontinence; measure if possible or estimate amount as small, moderate, or large
   e. Amount of void, whether it was voluntary or involuntary
   f. Presence of sensation of need to void
   g. Amount of retention (retention is the amount of urine left in the bladder after an unsuccessful attempt at manual triggering or voiding)
   h. Amount of residual (residual is the amount of urine left in the bladder after either a voluntary or manual triggered voiding; also called a postvoid residual)
   i. Amount of triggered urine (triggered voiding is urine that is expelled after manual triggering [*e.g.*, tapping, Credé's method])
   j. Identify certain activities that precede voiding (*e.g.*, restlessness, yelling, exercise).
   k. Record in appropriate column.

	Intake	Output					
Time	Type of Fluids	Incontinence	Void	Manual Trigger	Retention	Residual	Behavior/ Activity
12M							
01							
02							
03							
04							
05							
06							
07							
08							
09							
10							
11							
12N							
1							
2							
3							
4							
5							
6							
7							
8							
9							
10							
11							
Totals							

Fig. II-7   Chart used for the assessment of voiding patterns.

6. Schedule fluid intake and voiding times.
   a. Provide for fluid intake of 2000 mL each day unless contraindicated.
   b. Discourage fluids after 7 P.M.
   c. Initially, bladder emptying is done at least every 2 hours and at least twice during the night; goal is 2- to 4-hour intervals.
   d. If the person is incontinent before scheduled voids, shorten the time between voids.
   e. If the person has a postvoid residual greater than 100–150 mL, schedule intermittent catheterization.

B. Schedule intermittent catheterization program (ICP), if indicated
   1. Monitor intake and output.
   2. Fluid intake should be at least 2000 mL/day.
   3. Use sterile catheterization technique in the hospital, clean technique at home.
   4. Desired catheter volumes are less than 500 mL.
   5. Increase or decrease the interval between catheterization to obtain the desired catheter volumes.
   6. Usual catheterization times are every 4–6 hours.
   7. Urine volumes may increase at night; thus, it may be necessary to catheterize more frequently at night.
   8. Encourage the individual to attempt to void before scheduled catheterization time.
   9. Initially obtain postvoid residuals at least every 6 hours.
   10. Terminate ICP when the bladder is consistently emptied voluntarily or by triggering with less than a 50-mL residual urine after each void.

C. Teach intermittent catheterization to person and family for long-term management of bladder (see Key Concepts)
   1. Explain the reasons for the catheterization program.
   2. Explain the relation of fluid intake and the frequency of catheterization.
   3. Explain the importance of emptying the bladder at the prescribed time, regardless of circumstances, because of the hazards of an overdistended bladder (*e.g.*, circulation contributes to infection, and stasis of urine contributes to bacterial growth).

D. Teach the individual about his bladder reconditioning program
   1. Explain rationale and treatments of bladder reconditioning program (see Key Concepts).
   2. Explain the schedule of fluid intake, voiding attempts, manual triggering, and catheterization to control incontinence.
   3. Teach person and family the importance of positive reinforcement and adherence to program for best results.
   4. Refer to community nurses for assistance in bladder reconditioning if indicated.

E. If bladder retraining fails, consider use of an indwelling catheter
   1. For men, a catheter no larger than 16 Fr.
   2. For women, up to a 18 Fr for routine use
   3. Teach care of indwelling catheter.
      a. Maintain 3000-mL fluid intake every day.
      b. Keep urine acidic.
      c. Change catheter at least every 2 weeks or when it does not drain properly.
      d. Tape catheter to prevent pulling.
         Men—to suprapubic abdominal area
         Women—to inner aspect of thighs
      e. Perform thorough cleaning of the meatus, distal catheter, and perineum at least twice a day.
      f. Maintain sterile drainage system at all times in the hospital; at home may use clean system.
      g. Know that the urine collection system should drain by gravity.

    h. Do not lift collection bag above the level of the bladder without pinching off the tubing to prevent backflow.

    i. Connect the catheter to a leg bag drainage system during the day.

F. Initiate health teaching

    1. If appropriate, teach intermittent catheterization.

    2. Instruct person in prevention of urinary tract infection.

    3. Teach person how to change indwelling catheter.

    4. For people living in the community, initiate a referral to the visiting nurse for follow-up and/or regular indwelling catheter changes.

Rationale

- Continence training programs are either self-directed or caregiver directed. Self-directed programs of bladder training, retraining, and exercises are for motivated, cognitively intact individuals. Caregiver-directed programs of scheduled toileting or habit training are appropriate for motivated caregivers of cognitively impaired people (Miller, 1995).
- The essential components of any continence training program (self-directed or caregiver directed) include motivation, assessment of voiding and incontinent patterns, a regular fluid intake of 2000–3000 mL/day, timed voiding of 2- to 4-hour intervals in an appropriate place, and ongoing assessment (Miller, 1995).
- Obstruction of the bladder neck that progresses to bladder distention and overflow (incontinence) can be caused by fecal impaction and enlarged prostate gland.
- Dehydration can cause incontinence by eliminating the sensation of a full bladder (the signal to urinate) and also by reducing the person's alertness to the sensation.
- Intermittent self-catheterization, periodic drainage of urine by the individual by the use of a catheter in the bladder, is indicated when a neurologic impairment impairs bladder emptying.
- Intermittent catheterization, when performed in a health care facility, should follow aseptic technique because the organisms present in such a facility are more virulent and resistant to drugs than organisms found outside. People at home can practice clean technique because of the lack of virulent organisms in the home environment.
- An overdistended bladder reduces blood flow to the bladder wall, making it more susceptible to infection from bacterial growth.
- Intermittent catheterization provides for a decrease in morbidity associated with long-term use of indwelling catheters, increased independence, a more positive self-concept, and more normal sexual relations.

Urge Incontinence

DEFINITION

Urge Incontinence: The state in which an individual experiences an involuntary loss of urine associated with a strong, sudden desire to void.

DEFINING CHARACTERISTICS
Major (Must Be Present)

Urgency followed by incontinence

Related Factors

Pathophysiologic

Related to decreased bladder capacity secondary to:

Infection

Trauma

Urethritis

Neurogenic disorders or injury

Brain injury/tumor/infection

Cerebrovascular accident

Demyelinating diseases

Diabetic neuropathy

Alcoholic neuropathy

Parkinsonism

Treatment-Related

Related to decreased bladder capacity secondary to:

Abdominal surgery

Post-indwelling catheters

Situational (Personal, Environmental)

Related to irritation of bladder stretch receptors secondary to:

Alcohol

Caffeine

Excess fluid intake

Related to decreased bladder capacity secondary to frequent voiding

Maturational

Child: Related to small bladder capacity

Older Adult: Related to decreased bladder capacity

Key Concepts

1. Urge incontinence is an involuntary loss of urine associated with a strong desire to void. This is characterized by loss of large volumes of urine and may be triggered by emotional factors, body position changes, or the sight and sound of running water. This type of urge incontinence is commonly called bladder detrusor instability or vesical instability.
2. Detrusor instability is characterized by the presence of uninhibited detrusor contractions sufficient to cause urinary incontinence. Common causes include central nervous system disease, hyperexcitability of the afferent pathways, and deconditioned voiding reflexes.
3. A person with an uninhibited neurogenic bladder has damage to the cerebral cortex (*e.g.*, cerebrovascular accident, Parkinson's disease, brain injury/tumor) affecting the ability to inhibit urination. Sensation of bladder fullness is also limited; this is manifested by urgency. There is little time between the sensation to void and the uninhibited contraction.
4. Warning time is the amount of time the individual can delay urination after the urge to void is felt.
5. Diminished warning time can cause incontinence if the individual is unable to reach a toilet in time.

Focus Assessment Criteria

See *Altered Patterns of Urinary Elimination*

Outcome Criteria

The person will
- Report an absence or decreased episodes of incontinence (specify)
- Explain causes of incontinence

Interventions

A. Assess for causative or contributing factors
   1. Bladder irritants
      a. Infection
      b. Inflammation
      c. Alcohol, caffeine, or dark cola ingestion
      d. Concentrated urine
   2. Diminished bladder capacity
      a. Self-induced deconditioning (frequent small voids)
      b. Post-indwelling catheterization
   3. Overdistended bladder
      a. Increased urine production (diabetes mellitus, diuretics)
      b. Intake of alcohol and/or large quantities of fluids
   4. Uninhibited bladder contractions due to neurologic disorder
      a. Cerebrovascular accident
      b. Brain tumor/trauma/infection
      c. Parkinson's disease

B. Assess pattern of voiding/incontinence and fluid intake
   1. Maintain optimal hydration (see *Total Incontinence*).
   2. Assess voiding pattern (see *Total Incontinence*).

C. Reduce or eliminate causative and contributing factors, when possible
   1. Bladder irritants
      a. Infection/inflammation
         Refer to physician for diagnosis and treatment.
         Initiate bladder reconditioning program (see *Total Incontinence*).
         Explain the relation between incontinence and intake of alcohol, caffeine, and dark colas (irritants).
      b. Explain the risk of insufficient fluid intake and its relation to infection and concentrated urine.
   2. Diminished bladder capacity
      a. Determine amount of time between urge to void and need to void (record how long person can hold off urination).
      b. For a person with difficulty prolonging waiting time, communicate to personnel the need to respond rapidly to his request for assistance for toileting (note on care plan).
      c. Teach person to increase waiting time by increasing bladder capacity.
         Determine volume of each void.
         Ask person to "hold off" urinating as long as possible.
         Give positive reinforcement.
         Discourage frequent voiding that is result of habit, not need.
         Develop bladder reconditioning program (see *Total Incontinence*).
   3. Overdistended bladder
      a. Explain that diuretics are given to help reduce the amount of water in the body; they work by acting on the kidneys to increase the flow of urine.
      b. Explain that in diabetes mellitus, insulin deficiency causes high levels of blood sugar. The high level of blood sugar pulls fluid from body tissues, causing osmotic diuresis and increased urination (polyuria).
      c. Explain that because of the increased urine flow, regular voiding is needed to prevent overdistention of the bladder. Explain that overdistention can result in loss of bladder sensation, which increases incontinent episodes (diabetic neuropathy).
      d. Assess voiding pattern (see *Total Incontinence*).
      e. Check postvoid residual; if greater than 100 mL, include intermittent catheterization in bladder reconditioning program.
      f. Initiate bladder reconditioning program (see *Total Incontinence*).

4. Uninhibited bladder contractions
   a. Assess voiding pattern (see *Total Incontinence*).
   b. Establish method to communicate urge to void (document on care plan).
   c. Communicate to personnel the need to respond rapidly to a request to void.
   d. Establish a planned-voiding pattern.

      Provide an opportunity to void on awakening; after meals, physical exercise, bathing, and drinking coffee or tea; and before going to sleep.

      Begin by offering bedpan, commode, or toilet every half-hour initially, and gradually lengthen the time to at least every 2 hours.

      If person has incontinent episode, reduce the time between scheduled voidings.

      Document behavior/activity that occurs with void or incontinence (see Assessment of voiding pattern in *Total Incontinence*).

      Encourage person to try to "hold" urine until voiding time, if possible.

      Refer to *Total Incontinence* for additional information on developing a bladder reconditioning program.

D. Initiate health teaching

   1. Instruct person on prevention of urinary tract infections (see *Functional Incontinence*).

Rationale

- The essential components of any continence training program (self-directed or caregiver directed) include motivation, assessment of voiding and incontinent patterns, a regular fluid intake of 2000–3000 mL/day, timed voiding of 2- to 4-hour intervals in an appropriate place, and ongoing assessment (Miller, 1995).
- Deconditioning of the voiding reflex can result in incontinence through self-induced or iatrogenic causes. Frequent toileting (more than every 2 hours) causes chronic low-volume voiding, which reduces bladder capacity and increases detrusor tone and bladder wall thickness, which in turn potentiate incontinent episodes.
- Iatrogenic causes include placing a person on the toilet after the incontinent episode or using uncomfortable equipment to make him continent.
- Factors that contribute to urgency include acute urinary tract infection, neurologic impairments, diuretics, diabetes mellitus, inadequate fluid intake, and habitual frequent voiding.
- Optimal hydration is needed to prevent urinary tract infection and renal calculi.

Urinary Retention

DEFINITION

Urinary Retention: The state in which an individual experiences a chronic inability to void followed by involuntary voiding (overflow incontinence).

DEFINING CHARACTERISTICS
Major (Must Be Present)

Bladder distention (not related to acute reversible etiology) or
Bladder distention with small, frequent voids or dribbling (overflow incontinence)
100 mL or more residual urine

Minor (May Be Present)

Report that it feels like the bladder is not emptying after voiding.

RELATED FACTORS
Pathophysiologic

Related to sphincter blockage secondary to:
   Strictures
   Ureterocele
   Bladder-neck contractures
   Prostatic enlargement
   Perineal swelling
Related to impaired afferent pathways or inadequacy secondary to:
   Cord injury/tumor/infection
   Brain injury/tumor/infection
   Cerebrovascular accident
   Demyelinating diseases
   Multiple sclerosis
   Diabetic neuropathy
   Alcoholic neuropathy
   Tabes dorsalis

Treatment-Related

Related to bladder outlet obstruction or impaired afferent pathways secondary to drug
   therapy (iatrogenic)
   Antihistamines   Theophylline
   Epinephrine   Isoproterenol
   Anticholinergics

Situational (Personal, Environmental)

Related to bladder outlet obstruction secondary to fecal impaction
Related to detrusor inadequacy secondary to:
   Deconditioned voiding
   Association with stress or discomfort

Key Concepts

1. Urinary retention can be caused by three different entities: bladder outlet obstruction, detrusor inadequacy, and impaired afferent pathways.
2. Detrusor inadequacy is characterized by the pressure of uninhibited detrusor contractions sufficient to cause urinary incontinence. One cause of detrusor inadequacy is deconditioned voiding reflexes characterized by anxiety or discomfort associated with voiding. Another cause is central nervous system diseases.
3. Impaired afferent pathways occur when both the sensory and motor branches of the simple reflex arc are damaged. Therefore, there are no sensations to tell the individual the bladder is full or no motor impulses for emptying the bladder. Thus, the individual develops a neurogenic bladder (autonomous).
4. With this type of neurogenic bladder, the individual is likely to dribble urine when the pressure in the bladder rises because of the bladder filling beyond its normal capacity or because of coughing, straining, or exercising.
5. Other common names for this type of bladder are lower motor neuron, hypotonic, flaccid, cord, tabetic, and atonic bladder.
6. External manual compression and/or abdominal straining are the most effective methods to empty a neurogenic bladder.

Focus Assessment Criteria

See *Altered Patterns of Urinary Elimination*

Outcome Criteria

The person will
- Empty the bladder using the Créde and/or Valsalva maneuvers with a residual urine of less than 50 mL if indicated
- Void voluntarily
- Achieve a state of dryness that is personally satisfactory

Interventions

A. Assess for causative or contributing factors

   1. Factors that cause impaired afferent pathways
     a. Cerebrovascular accidents
     b. Demyelinating diseases
     c. Spinal cord injury/trauma/infection
     d. Peripheral nerve damage
        Diabetic neuropathy   Pelvic fractures/extensive surgery
        Alcoholic neuropathy
   2. Loss of bladder tone (detrusor weakness)
     a. Benign prostatic hypertrophy (postoperative)
     b. Spinal cord injury/tumor/infection
     c. Cerebrovascular accident
     d. Brain injury/tumor/infection
     e. Medications
        Anticholinergics
        α-Adrenergics
   3. Conditions contributing to bladder neck obstruction
     a. Strictures/contracture/spasms
     b. Edema (postsurgical, postpartum, vaginal or rectal packing)
     c. Prostatic hypertrophy
     d. Fecal impaction
     e. Tumor
     f. Congenital abnormalities
   4. Conditions that inhibit micturition
     a. Poor fluid intake
     b. Anxiety

B. Explain rationale for treatment

C. Develop a bladder retraining or reconditioning program (see *Total Incontinence*)

D. Instruct on methods to empty bladder

   1. Assist person to a sitting position.
     a. Teach abdominal strain and Valsalva maneuver; instruct person to:
        Lean forward on thighs.
        Contract abdominal muscles if possible and strain or "bear down"; hold breath while straining (Valsalva maneuver).
        Hold strain or breath until urine flow stops; wait 1 minute, and strain again as long as possible.
        Continue until no more urine is expelled.
     b. Teach Créde's maneuver; instruct person to:
        Place hands flat (or place fist) just below umbilical area.
        Place one hand on top of the other.

Press firmly down and in toward the pelvic arch.

Repeat six or seven times until no more urine can be expelled.

Wait a few minutes and repeat to ensure complete emptying.

c. Teach anal stretch maneuver; instruct person to:

Sit on commode or toilet.

Lean forward on thighs.

Place one gloved hand behind buttocks.

Insert one to two lubricated fingers into the anus to the anal sphincter.

Spread fingers apart or pull to posterior direction.

Gently stretch the anal sphincter and hold it distended.

Bear down and void.

Take a deep breath and hold it while straining (Valsalva maneuver).

Relax and repeat the procedure until the bladder is empty.

2. Instruct individual to try all three techniques or a combination of techniques to determine which is most effective in emptying the bladder.

3. Indicate on the intake and output record which technique was used to induce voiding.

4. Obtain postvoid residuals after attempts at emptying bladder; if residual urine volumes are greater than 100 mL, schedule intermittent catheterization program (see Interventions).

E. Initiate health teaching

1. Teach bladder reconditioning program (see *Total Incontinence*).
2. Teach intermittent catheterization (see *Total Incontinence*).
3. Instruct person on prevention of urinary tract infections (see *Total Incontinence*).

Rationale

- Dribbling of urine often can be reduced by reducing the pressure in the bladder and abdomen and strengthening the periurethral tissue.
- To increase comfort associated with voiding, the client must condition the voiding reflex by ingesting adequate fluids and inhibiting bladder contractions. Frequent toileting causes chronic low-volume voiding and increase detrusor activity. Resisting the urge to void may increase voiding intervals and reduce detrusor muscle activity.
- In many clients, Credé's maneuver can help empty the bladder. This maneuver is inappropriate, however, if the urinary sphincters are chronically contracted. In this case, pressing the bladder can force urine up the ureters as well as through the urethra. Reflux of urine into the renal pelvis may result in renal infection.
- External cutaneous stimulation can stimulate the voiding reflex.
- Valsalva maneuver contracts the abdominal muscles, which manually compresses the bladder.
- Anal sphincter stimulation can stimulate the voiding reflex.
- Clean intermittent self-catheterization (CISC) prevents overdistention, helps maintain detrusor muscle tone, and ensures complete bladder emptying. CISC may be used initially to determine residual urine following Credé's maneuver or tapping. As residual urine decreases, catheterization may be tapered. CISC may recondition the voiding reflex in some clients.
- If bladder emptying techniques are unsuccessful, other methods of managing incontinence are necessary.

References/Bibliography

Carpenter, R. O. (1994). Disorders of elimination. In F. Oski (Ed.). *Principles and practice of pediatrics* (2nd ed.). Philadelphia: J. B. Lippincott.

Cella, M. (1988). The nursing costs of urinary incontinence in nursing home population. *Nursing Clinics of North America, 23,* 159–168.

Chow, M. P., Durand, B. A., Feldman, M. N., & Mills, M. A. (1984). *Handbook of pediatric primary care* (2nd ed.). New York: John Wiley & Sons.

Foye, H., & Sulkes, S. (1990). Developmental and behavioral pediatrics. In R. E. Behrman & R. Kliegman (Eds.). *Nelson essentials of pediatrics*. Philadelphia: W. B. Saunders.

Hunsberger, M. (1989). Principles and skills adapted to the care of children. In R. L. Foster, M. M. Hunsberger, & J. J. T. Anderson (Eds.). *Family-centered nursing care of children*. Philadelphia: W. B. Saunders.

Miller, C. A. (1995). *Nursing care of older adults* (2nd ed.). Glenview, IL: Scott, Foresman.

Newman, D. K., Lynch, K., Smith, D. A., & Cell, P. (1991). Restoring urinary continence. *American Journal of Nursing, 91*, 28–36.

Ouslander, J. G., Morishita, L., Blaustein, J., Orzeck, S., Dunn, S., & Sayre, J. (1987). Clinical, functional and psychosocial characteristics of an incontinent nursing home population. *Journal of Gerontology, 42*, 631–637.

Porth, C. M. (1994). *Pathophysiology: Concepts of altered health states* (4th ed.). Philadelphia: J. B. Lippincott.

Resnick, N., & Yalla, S. (1985). Management of urinary incontinence in the elderly. *New England Journal of Medicine, 5*(13), 800–805.

Smith, D., & Newmen, D. K. (1991). Nursing management of urinary incontinence associated with Alzheimer's disease. *Journal of Home Health Care Practice, 3*(4), 25–32.

Urinary Incontinence Guideline Panel. (1992, March). *Urinary incontinence in adults: Clinical practice guideline*. AHCPR Pub. No. 92-0038. Rockville, MD: Agency for Health Care Policy and Research, Public Health Service, U.S. Department of Health and Human Services.

Van Cleve, S. N., & Baldwin, S. E. (1989). Nursing strategies: Altered genitourinary function. In R. L. Foster, M. M. Hunsberger, & J. J. T. Anderson (Eds.). *Family-centered nursing care of children*. Philadelphia: W. B. Saunders.

Warrady, B. A. (1991). Primary nocturnal enuresis: Current concepts about an old problem. *Pediatric Annals, 20*, 246–251.

Wong, D. L. (1995). *Nursing care of infants and children* (5th ed.). St. Louis: Mosby–Year Book.

Wyman, J. F. (1988). Nursing assessment of the incontinent geriatric outpatient population. *Nursing Clinics of North America, 23*, 169–179.

Violence, Risk for

DEFINITION

Risk for Violence: A state in which an individual has been, or is at risk to be, assaultive toward others or the environment.

RISK FACTORS
Major (Must Be Present)
Presence of risk factors (see Related Factors)

RELATED FACTORS
Pathophysiologic

Related to history of aggressive acts and perception of environment as threatening secondary to:

or

Related to history of aggressive acts and delusional thinking secondary to:

or

Related to history of aggressive acts and manic excitement secondary to:

or

Related to history of aggressive acts and inability to verbalize feelings secondary to:

or

Related to history of aggressive acts and psychic overload secondary to:
    Temporal lobe epilepsy
    Head injury
    Progressive central nervous system deterioration (brain tumor)
    Hormonal imbalance
    Viral encephalopathy
    Mental retardation
    Minimal brain dysfunction
Related to toxic response to alcohol or drugs
Related to organic brain syndrome

Treatment-Related

Related to toxic reaction to medication

Situational (Personal, Environmental)

Related to history of overt aggressive acts
Related to increase in stressors within a short period
Related to acute agitation
Related to suspiciousness
Related to persecutory delusions
Related to verbal threats of physical assault
Related to low frustration tolerance
Related to poor impulse control
Related to fear of the unknown
Related to response to catastrophic event
Related to response to dysfunctional family throughout developmental stages
Related to dysfunctional communication patterns
Related to drug or alcohol abuse

Author's Note

The diagnosis *Risk for Violence* describes a person who has been assaultive or because of certain factors (*e.g.*, toxic response to alcohol or drugs, hallucinations or delusions, brain dysfunction) is at high risk for assaulting others. In such a situation, the nursing focus is on decreasing violent episodes and protecting the person and others.

    The nurse should not use this diagnosis to address underlying problems such as anxiety or poor self-esteem, but instead should refer to the diagnoses of *Anxiety* and/or *Ineffective Individual Coping* for a focus on the sources of the violence (spouse, child, elder). When domestic violence is present or suspected, the nurse should explore the diagnosis *Ineffective Family Coping: Disabling*. A person at risk for suicide would warrant the diagnosis *Risk for Suicide*.

Errors in Diagnostic Statements

Risk for Violence related to reports of abuse by wife

    Reports of abuse by a spouse represents a family dysfunction, which is not a situation covered by *Risk for Violence*. Spouse abuse is a complex situation necessitating individual and family therapy. The nursing diagnoses *Ineffective Family Coping: Disabling* and *Ineffective Individual Coping* for the abuser and the victim would be more clinically useful.

    Risk for Violence related to poor management of agitation by staff

    This diagnostic statement is legally problematic and does not offer constructive strategies. In a situation in which staff inappropriately manage an agitated client, the nurse must treat this as a staff management problem, not a client problem. If the staff increased the client's agitation because of their lack of knowledge, the nurse must outline specific dos and don'ts in the nursing care plan. In addition, an inservice program on identifying precursors to violence and agitation reduction strategies should be held for the staff. For the client, the nurse could rewrite the diagnosis as *Risk for Violence related to mental dysfunction and persecutory delusions*.

Key Concepts

1. A central theme in violent individuals is helplessness. Assaultive behavior is a defense against passivity and helplessness (Turnbull, Aitken, Black, & Patterson, 1990).
2. Aggressive behavior is a defense against anxiety. This coping mechanism is reinforced because it reduces anxiety by increasing the individual's sense of power and control. (Refer to Key Concepts, *Anxiety* for further discussion of anger.) Interventions that encourage "acting out of anger" reinforce assaultiveness, and thus are to be avoided.
3. Violence is usually preceded by a predictable sequence of events (*e.g.*, a stressor or a series of stressors) (Munns & Nolan, 1991).
4. When brain dysfunction is a prime or contributing factor in violent behavior, social and environmental variables still need to be evaluated. Organic impairment may interfere with an individual's ability to handle certain stresses. A person's normal behavior can be altered by exposure to or ingestion of toxic chemicals, such as lead and pesticides. Examples of violent behavior in brain dysfunction are biting, scratching, temper outbursts, and mood lability (Bauer & Hill, 1994).
5. Fear and anxiety can distort an individual's perception of the environment. Suspicious, delusional people often misinterpret stimuli. Alcohol and drugs also impair judgment and decrease internal controls over behavior.
6. Individuals who had a history of emotional deprivation in childhood are particularly vulnerable to attacks on their self-esteem.
7. Even though the individual may identify the person with whom he is angry, this may not be the real object of his aggression. Individuals often cannot allow themselves to express anger toward a person on whom they are dependent.
8. Staff frequently respond to violent individuals with actual fear or overreactions. This can lead to punitive sanctions such as heavier medication, seclusion, or attempts to cope by avoidance and withdrawal from the individual (Maier, Stava, Morrow, Van Rybroek, & Bauman, 1987). Staff must identify their own reactions to violent individuals so that they can more effectively manage the situation. Staff should trust an intuition that the person is potentially violent.
9. In studies of client's perception of seclusion, the sense of powerlessness seemed to be the worst feeling. It was followed by fear, humiliation, loneliness, and shame (Norris & Kennedy, 1992).
10. Physical aggression in long-term care, such as swearing, biting, kicking, spitting, and grabbing, may be in response to a loss of control over life. The more importance the individual attaches to freedom and choice, the more forcefully he or she is likely to respond (Meddaugh, 1990).

Key Concepts—Child

1. Violence, including homicide, child abuse and neglect, and assault by peers and others, causes more than 2000 deaths a year to U.S. children older than 0–19 years (Christoffel, 1990).
2. Homicide is a leading cause of death for U.S. children and adolescents, and therefore a major cause of years of potential lost life (Christoffel, 1990).
3. Recent research findings indicate that the shaking of infants, by itself, is sufficient to cause severe or fatal intracranial injury (Alexander, 1990).

Focus Assessment Criteria

(Refer also to Focus Assessment Criteria for *Ineffective Individual Coping, Ineffective Family Coping, Altered Thought Processes, Anxiety*)

Subjective Data

A. Assess for risk factors

1. Medical history

Epilepsy	Hormonal imbalance
Head injury	Present medication
Brain disease	Drug abuse (amphetamines, PCP, marijuana)

2. Psychiatric history
      Previous hospitalizations   Outpatient therapy
3. History of emotional difficulties in individual and/or family
      Alcoholism   Parental brutality
      Cruelty to animals   Pyromania
4. Interaction patterns (note changes)
      Family   Coworkers
      Friends   Others
5. Coping patterns (past and present)
6. Sources of stress in current environment
7. Work/school history
      How does he function under stress?   Employment
      Level of education attained   Stable
      Learning disabilities   Frequency of job changes
      Fights in school   Periods of unemployment
8. Legal history
      Arrests and convictions for violent crimes
      Juvenile offenses for violent behavior
9. History of violence
      Assess recency, severity, and frequency
         "What is the most violent thing you have ever done?"
         "What is the closest you have ever come to striking someone?"
         "In what kinds of situations have you hit someone or destroyed property?"
         "When was the last time this happened?"
         "How often does this occur?"
         "Were you using drugs or alcohol when these episodes occurred?"
10. Present thoughts about violence
      Identify possible victim and weapon
         "How do you feel after an incident?"
         "Are you currently having thoughts about harming someone?"
         "Is there anyone in particular you think about harming?" (Identify the victim
            and the person's access to victim.)
         "Do you have a specific plan for how you might accomplish this?" (Identify plan,
            type of weapon, and availability of weapon.)
11. Thought content
      Helplessness
      Suspiciousness or hostility
      Perceived intention (*e.g.*, "He meant to hit me" in response to a slight bump)
      Fear of loss of control
      Persecutory delusions
      Disorientation

Objective Data

A. Assess for risk factors
   1. Body language
         Posture (relaxed, rigid)   Hands (relaxed, rigid, clenched)
         Facial expression (calm, annoyed, tense)
   2. Motor activity
         Within normal limits   Pacing
         Immobile   Agitation
         Increased
   3. Affect
         Within normal limits   Flat
         Labile   Inappropriate
         Controlled

Outcome Criteria

The person will
- Demonstrate control of behavior with assistance from others
- Have a decreased number of violent responses
- Describe causation and possible preventive measures
- Explain rationale for interventions

Interventions

The nursing interventions for the diagnosis *Risk for Violence* apply to any individual who is potentially violent, regardless of related factors.

A. Promote interactions that increase the individual's sense of trust
   1. Acknowledge the individual's feelings (*e.g.*, "You are having a rough time.").
       a. Be genuine and empathetic.
       b. Tell individual that you will help him control his behavior and not let him do anything destructive.
       c. Be direct and frank ("I can see you are angry.").
       d. Be consistent and firm.
   2. Set limits when individual presents a risk to others. Refer to *Anxiety* for further interventions on limit-setting.
   3. Offer the individual choices and options. At times, it is necessary to give in on some demands to avoid a power struggle.
   4. Encourage individual to express anger and hostility verbally instead of "acting out."
   5. Encourage walking or exercise as activities that may diffuse aggression.
   6. Maintain person's personal space.
       a. Do not touch the individual.
       b. Avoid feelings of physical entrapment of individual or staff.
   7. Be aware of your own feelings and reactions.
       a. Do not take verbal abuse personally.
       b. Remain calm if you are becoming upset; leave the situation in the hands of others, if possible.
       c. After a threatening situation, ventilate your feelings with other staff.

B. Initiate immediate management of high-risk person
   1. Allow the acutely agitated individual space that is five times greater than that for an individual who is in control. Do not touch the person unless you have a trusting relationship. Avoid physical entrapment of individual or staff.
   2. Convey empathy by acknowledging the individual's feelings. Let him know you will not let him lose control. Remind of previous successes at self-control.
   3. Do not approach a violent individual alone. Often the presence of three to four staff members will be enough to reassure the individual that you will not let him lose control. Use a positive tone; do not demand or cajole.
   4. Give the individual control by offering him alternatives (*e.g.*, walking, talking).
   5. Set limits on actions, not feelings. Use concise, easily understood statements.
   6. Maintain eye contact, but do not stare. Stand at a friendly angle (45 degrees); keep an open posture if person is standing, sit when the person sits.
   7. Do not make promises you cannot keep.
   8. Avoid using "always" and "never."
   9. When assault is imminent, quick, coordinated action is essential.
   10. Approach individual in a calm, self-assured manner so as not to communicate your anxiety or fear.

11. Avoid using force in giving intramuscular injections, when possible, because it increases the person's sense of powerlessness. Use only when a clear danger to others or self exists.

12. If the person has a weapon, do not attempt to grab it. Instruct the person to put it down. Attempt to calm the person without risking bodily harm to yourself.

C. Establish an environment that reduces agitation

1. Decrease noise level.
2. Give short, concise explanations.
3. Control the number of persons present at one time.
4. Provide single or semiprivate room.
5. Allow individual to arrange personal possessions.
6. Be aware that darkness can increase disorientation and enhance suspiciousness.
7. Decrease situations in which the individual is frustrated.
8. Provide music if individual is receptive.

D. Assist the individual in maintaining control over his behavior (Bauer & Hill, 1994)

1. Establish the expectation that he can control his behavior, and continue to reinforce the expectation. Explain exactly which behavior is inappropriate and why.
2. Give three options: two offer a choice, the third is the consequence of violent behavior.
3. Allow time for person to make choice.
4. Provide positive feedback when person is able to exercise restraint.
5. Enforce consequences when indicated.
6. Reassure individual that you will provide control if he cannot ("I am concerned about you, I will get [more staff, medications] to keep you from doing anything impulsive.").
7. Set firm, clear limits when individual presents a danger to self or others. ("Put the chair down.").
8. Call person by name in a calm, quiet respectful manner.
9. Avoid threats; refer to yourself, not policies, rules, or supervisors.
10. Allow appropriate verbal expressions of anger. Give positive feedback.
11. Set limits on verbal abuse. Do not take insults personally. Support others (clients, staff) who may be targets of abuse.
12. Do not give attention to person who is being verbally abusive. Tell the person what you are doing and why.
13. Assist with external controls, as necessary.
    a. Maintain observation every 15–30 minutes.
    b. Remove items that could be used as weapons (*e.g.*, glass, sharp objects).
    c. Assess ability to tolerate off-unit procedures.
    d. If person is acutely agitated, be cautious with items such as hot coffee.

E. Plan for unpredictable violence

1. Monitor for signs of escalating aggression (Munns & Nolan, 1991).
    a. Hostile body language (*e.g.*, rigid, clenched fists, glaring eyes)
    b. Threats, boasting of prior aggressive acts
    c. Pacing, irritability
    d. Passive–aggressive behavior (*e.g.*, derogatory jokes)
    e. Repetitive complaints, requests, or demands
    f. Argumentative, hypersensitive
    g. Fearful of others
    h. Aggression toward objects (*e.g.*, slamming doors, damaging property)
2. Ensure availability of staff before potential violent behavior (never try to assist person alone when physical restraint is necessary).
3. Determine who will be in charge of directing personnel to intervene in violent behavior if it occurs.
4. Ensure protection for oneself (door nearby for withdrawal, pillow to protect face).

F. Use seclusion and/or restraint, if indicated

   1. Remove individual from situation if environment is contributing to aggressive behavior, using the least amount of control needed (*e.g.*, ask others to leave, and take individual to quiet room).

   2. Reinforce that you are going to help him control himself.

   3. Repeatedly tell the person what is going to happen before external control is begun.

   4. Protect individual from injuring self or others through use of restraints or seclusion.*

   5. When using seclusion, institutional policy provides specific guidelines; the following are general.

     a. Observe individual at least every 15 minutes.

     b. Search the individual before secluding to remove harmful objects.

     c. Check seclusion room to see that safety is maintained.

     d. Offer fluids and food periodically (in nonbreakable containers).

     e. When approaching an individual to be secluded, have sufficient staff present.

     f. Explain concisely what is going to happen ("You will be placed in a room by yourself until you can better control your behavior.") and give person a chance to cooperate.

     g. Assist person in toileting and personal hygiene (assess his ability to be out of seclusion; a urinal or commode may need to be used).

     h. If person is taken out of seclusion, someone must be present continually.

     i. Maintain verbal interaction during seclusion (provides information necessary to assess person's degree of control).

     j. When person is allowed out of seclusion, a staff member needs to be in constant attendance to determine whether person can handle additional stimulation.

   6. When using restraint, institutional policy provides specifics. The following are general measures.

     a. A person in a four-point or two-point restraint must be in seclusion or with one-on-one nursing care for protection. Seclusion guidelines should be followed.

     b. Restraints must be loosened every hour (one limb at a time).

     c. Waist restraints must allow enough arm movement to enable eating/smoking and self-protection from falling.

     d. Restraints should be padded.

     e. Restraints never should be attached to side rails, but rather to the bed frame.

   7. Provide an opportunity to clarify the rationale for seclusion and to discuss the person's reactions after the seclusion period is ended.

G. Convene a group discussion after a violent episode on an inpatient unit (Wilson & Kneisl, 1996)

   1. Include all those who witnessed the episode (client, staff).

   2. Include individual(s) exhibiting the violent behavior, if possible.

   3. Discuss what happened, the consequences, and the feelings of the community.

H. If the client has assaulted another client or staff member, reintegrate the client with the assaulted individual when control has been regained, but before release from seclusion (Wilson & Kneisl, 1996)

I. Assist individual in developing alternative coping strategies when crisis has passed and learning can occur

   1. Explore what precipitates the person's loss of control ("What was happening before you began to feel like hitting her?").

   2. Assist the person in recalling the physical symptoms associated with anger.

   3. Help person evaluate where in the chain of events change was possible.

     a. Use role playing to practice communication techniques.

* May require a primary care professional's order.

b. Discuss how issues of control interfere with communication.

c. Help the person recognize negative thinking patterns associated with low self-esteem.

4. Practice negotiation skills with significant others and people in authority.

5. Encourage an increase in recreational activities.

6. Use group therapy to decrease sense of aloneness and increase communication skills.

a. Instruct or refer for assertiveness training.

b. Instruct or refer for negotiation skills development.

Rationale

- The client is in an agitated/mentally compromised state, and environmental stimuli unnecessarily increase this state and send client "over the edge."
- There can be a pattern to violence. Detecting and changing the pattern can eliminate the violence.
- The presence of four to five staff members reassures the individual that you will not let him lose control.
- Assaultive behavior tends to occur when conditions are crowded, are without structure, and involve staff-"demanded" activity (Harris & Varnly, 1986).
- Staff activities may be counterproductive in managing aggressive behavior. Recognition and replacement of attitudes such as "I must be calm and relaxed at all times" with "No matter how anxious I feel, I will keep thinking and decide on the best approach" often prevent escalation of aggression (Davies, 1989).
- Although individuals may verbalize hostile threats and take a defensive stance, most are fearful of losing control and want assistance in maintaining their control (Bauer & Hill, 1994; Lion, 1972).
- A habitually violent person exhibits a wider-than-average body buffer zone (Davies, 1989).
- Eye contact can increase arousal and be misinterpreted as hostility; the best approach is to maintain short periods of eye contact with no staring (Davies, 1989).
- Maintain the same physical level (*e.g.*, both people either sitting or standing prevents feelings of intimidation) (Bauer & Hill, 1994). The least aggressive stance is at a 45 degree angle to the person, rather than face-to-face (Davies, 1989).
- Crisis management techniques can help prevent escalation of aggression and help the person achieve self-control. The least restrictive safe and effective measure should be used (Bauer & Hill, 1994).
- Seclusion and restraint are options for a person exhibiting serious, persistent aggression. The person's safety must be protected at all times. Use of the least restrictive measures allows the person the most opportunity to regain self-control (Ropor, Coutts, Sather, & Taylor, 1985). Use of ambulatory waist restraints offers a less restrictive alternative to seclusion and restraint (Maier et al., 1987).
- After a violent act occurs, leading a group discussion of the event, outcome, and feelings can decrease anxiety and increase understanding of violence (Wilson & Kneisl, 1996).
- Setting the limits clarifies rules, guidelines, and standards of acceptable behavior and establishes the consequences of violating the rules (Bauer & Hill, 1994).
- Physical activity can help reduce muscle tension (Bauer & Hill, 1994).
- Diversions that requires a short attention span are useful because high anxiety causes scattered thinking (Bauer & Hill, 1994).

References/Bibliography

Alexander, R. (1990). Incidence of impact trauma with cranial injuries ascribed to shaking. *American Journal of Diseases of Children, 144*, 724–726.

Bauer, B.,& Hill, S. (1994). People who defend against anxiety through aggression towards others. In E. M. Varcarolis (Ed.). *Foundations of psychiatric–mental health nursing* (2nd ed.). Philadelphia: W. B. Saunders.

Christoffel, K. K. (1990). Violent death and injury in U.S. children and adolescents. *American Journal of Diseases of Children, 144*, 697–706.

Davies, W. (1989). The prevention of assault of professional helpers. In K. Howells & C. Hallin

(Eds.). *Clinical approaches to violence.* New York: John Wiley & Sons.

Harris, G. T., & Varnly, G. W. (1986). Assaults and assaulters in maximum security. *Research Reports, 3*(2), Mental Health Center, Penetanguishene, Ontario.

Hunter, D. S. (1989). The use of physical restraint in managing out-of-control behavior in youth: A frontline perspective. *Child and Youth Care Quarterly, 18,* 141–154.

Lion, J. (1972). *Evaluation and management of the violent patient.* Springfield, IL: Charles C Thomas.

Maier, G., Stava, L., Morrow, B., Van Rybroek, G., & Bauman, K. (1987). A model for understanding and managing cycles of aggression among psychiatric inpatients. *Hospital and Community Psychiatry, 38,* 520–524.

Meddaugh, D. (1990). Reactance: Understanding aggressive behavior in long-term care. *Journal of Psychosocial Nursing, 28*(2), 28–32.

Munns, D., & Nolan L. (1991). Potential for violence. In Mass, M., Buckwalter, K., & Hardy, M. (Eds.). *Nursing diagnoses and interventions for the elderly.* Redwood City, CA: Addison-Wesley Nursing.

Norris, M., & Kennedy, C. (1992). How patients perceive the seclusion process. *Journal of Psychosocial Nursing, 30*(6), 7–13.

Ropor, J., Coutts, A., Sather, J., & Taylor, R. (1985). Restraint and seclusion. *Journal of Psychosocial Nursing, 23*(6), 18–23.

Turnbull, J., Aitken, I., Black, L., & Patterson, B. (1990). Turn it around: Short term management for aggression and anger. *Journal of Psychosocial Nursing, 28,* 7–10.

Wilson, H. S., & Kneisl, C. R. (1996). *Psychiatric nursing* (5th ed.). Redwood City, CA: Addison-Wesley Nursing.

Section III

Manual of Collaborative Problems

Introduction

This Manual of Collaborative Problems presents 52 specific collaborative problems grouped under 9 generic collaborative problem categories. These problems have been selected because of their high incidence or morbidity. Appendix XI provides a more comprehensive list. Information on each generic collaborative problem is presented under the following subheads:

- Physiologic Overview
- Definition
- Author's Note: Discussion of the problem to clarify its clinical use
- Focus Assessment Criteria: Subjective and objective, guiding the nurse in data collection for client monitoring
- Significant Laboratory/Diagnostic Assessment Criteria: Laboratory findings useful in monitoring

Discussions of the 52 specific collaborative problems cover the following information:
- Definition
- High-Risk Populations
- Nursing Goals: A statement specifying the nursing accountability for the collaborative problem
- Generic Interventions: These specifically direct the nurse to:
  Monitor for onset or early changes in status
  Initiate physician-prescribed interventions as indicated
  Initiate nurse-prescribed interventions as indicated
  Evaluate the effectiveness of these interventions
- Rationale: A statement in parentheses explaining why a sign or symptom is present or giving the scientific explanation for why an intervention produces the desired response

Keep in mind that for many of the collaborative problems in Section III, associated nursing diagnoses also can be predicted to be present. For example, a client with diabetes mellitus would receive care under the collaborative problem *PC: Hypo/Hyperglycemia* along with the nursing diagnosis *Risk for Altered Health Maintenance related to insufficient knowledge of (specify)*; a client with renal calculi would be under the collaborative problem *PC: Renal Calculi* and also the nursing diagnosis *Risk for Ineffective Management of Therapeutic Regimen related to insufficient knowledge of prevention of recurrence, dietary restrictions, and fluid requirements.*

Potential Complication: Cardiac/Vascular

PC: Decreased Cardiac Output

PC: Dysrhythmias

PC: Pulmonary Edema

PC: Deep Vein Thrombosis

PC: Hypovolemia

PC: Compartmental Syndrome

PC: Pulmonary Embolism

Cardiovascular System Overview

The cardiovascular system consists of the heart, arteries, arterioles, veins, venules, capillaries, and lymphatic vessels. The hollow, muscular heart pumps blood to tissues; blood supplies oxygen and other nutrients and carries away tissue waste products such as carbon dioxide back to the lungs. The liters per minute of blood pumped by the heart's ventricles during a given period—*cardiac output*—is affected by the amount of blood ejected with each heartbeat—*stroke volume*. The cardiac index is the cardiac output divided by body surface area. Cardiac index reflects the heart's ability to meet body tissue demands. Any change in circulatory blood volume and/or in heart rate affects cardiac index. The contractility or pumping action of the myocardium results from the stimulation of sympathetic and parasympathetic fibers supplying the heart. In addition, the cardiac conduction system generates and sends electrical impulses throughout the myocardium. Problems that can alter these electrical impulses, leading to altered cardiac output, include cardiac muscle cell damage, tissue hypoxia, medications, and abnormal serum calcium or potassium levels. Disorders of the heart or circulatory system can cause serious, even fatal, hypoxic states.

Considered part of the circulatory system, the lymphatic system consists of capillaries, vessels, and nodes. This system contains and maintains the immune system, transports fluids and proteins from interstitial spaces back to the veins, and reabsorbs fats (chyme) from the small intestine.

Potential Complication: Cardiac/Vascular

DEFINITION

PC: Cardiac/Vascular: Describes a person experiencing or at high risk to experience various cardiac and/or vascular dysfunctions.

Author's Note

The nurse can use this generic collaborative problem to describe a person at risk for several types of cardiovascular problems. For example, for a client in a critical care unit vulnerable to cardiovascular dysfunction, using *PC: Cardiac/Vascular* would direct nurses to monitor cardiovascular status for various problems, based on focus assessment findings. Nursing interventions for this client would focus on detecting and diagnosing abnormal functioning.

For a client with a specific cardiovascular complication, the nurse would add the applicable collaborative problem to the client's problem list, along with specific nursing interventions for that problem. For example, a Standard of Care for a client postmyocardial infarction could contain the collaborative problem *PC: Cardiac/Vascular*, directing nurses to monitor cardiovascular status. If this client later experienced a dysrhythmia, the nurse would add *PC: Dysrhythmia* to the problem list, along with specific nursing management information (*e.g., PC: Dysrhythmia related to myocardial infarction*). When the risk factors or etiology are not directly related to the primary medical diagnosis, the nurse still should add them, if known (*e.g., PC: Hypo/Hyperglycemia related to diabetes mellitus* in a client who has sustained myocardial infarction).

Focus Assessment Criteria

Subjective Data

1. Discomfort (pain, burning, squeezing, pressure, tightness, and/or aching)
    a. Location (chest, jaw, neck, scapula)
    b. Description (location, radiation, character, duration, severity, onset)
    c. Precipitating/aggravating factors (*e.g.*, activity, eating)
    d. Alleviating measures (*e.g.*, rest, medications)
    e. Associated symptoms (*e.g.*, nausea, vomiting, vertigo, diaphoresis)
2. Perception of heart rate (*e.g.*, too fast, skipping beats)
3. Complaints of
    a. Shortness of breath
    b. Lightheadedness
    c. Fatigue
    d. Nausea

Objective Data

1. Apical pulse
    a. Rate (normal, above 100 beats/min, below 60 beats/min)
    b. Rhythm (regular, irregular, pulse deficits)
    c. Apical–radial pulse deficit
    d. Heart sounds (normal, S_3, S_4, murmurs, friction rubs)
2. Jugular veins, at a 45-degree angle (nondistended or distended)

3. Blood pressure and pulse pressure, any postural changes (compare readings between arms)
4. Bilateral pulses (radial, posterior tibial, dorsalis pedis, brachial, popliteal)
   a. Rate and rhythm
   b. Volume
       0 = Absent, nonpalpable
       +1 = Thready, weak, fades in and out
       +2 = Present but diminished
       +3 = Normal, easily palpable
       +4 = Bounding
5. Skin
   a. Temperature (cool, warm)
   b. Color (pale, dependent rubor, flushed, cyanotic, mottled, brown discolorations)
   c. Ulcerations (size, location, description of surrounding tissue)
6. Edema (location, pitting or nonpitting)
7. Capillary refill time (normal, less than 3 seconds)
8. Motor ability (normal or compromised)
9. Urine output
10. Level of orientation, anxiety, confusion
11. Mucous membranes
12. Electrocardiogram (ECG) (S-T segment changes, PR, QRS, or QT interval changes, rate or rhythm changes)
13. Hemodynamic monitoring parameters
14. Oxygen saturation obtained with pulse oximetry

Significant Laboratory/Diagnostic Assessment Criteria

1. Cardiac enzymes (elevated with cardiac tissue damage, *e.g.*, in myocardial infarction)
   a. Creatinine phosphokinase, isoenzymes
   b. Lactic dehydrogenase (LDH), isoenzymes
2. Serum potassium (fluctuates with diuretic therapy, parenteral fluid replacement)
3. Serum calcium, magnesium, phosphate
4. White blood cell count (elevated with inflammation)
5. Erythrocyte sedimentation rate (elevated with inflammation, tissue injury)
6. Arterial blood gas (ABG) values (lowered SaO_2 indicates hypoxemia; elevated pH, alkalosis; lowered pH, acidosis)
7. Coagulation studies (elevated with anticoagulant and/or thrombolytic therapy or coagulopathies)
8. Hemoglobin and hematocrit (elevated with polycythemia, lowered with anemia)
9. Doppler ultrasonic flowmeter
10. Cardiac catheterization
11. Stress test

PC: Decreased Cardiac Output

DEFINITION

PC: Decreased Cardiac Output: Describes a person experiencing or at high risk to experience inadequate blood supply for tissue needs because of insufficient blood pumping by the heart.

High-Risk Populations

- Acute myocardial infarction
- Aortic or mitral valve disease
- Cardiomyopathy
- Cardiac tamponade
- Hypothermia
- Septic shock
- Coarctation of the aorta
- Chronic obstructive pulmonary disease (COPD)
- Congenital heart disease
- Hypovolemia (*e.g.*, due to severe bleeding or burns)
- Bradycardia
- Tachycardia
- Congestive heart failure
- Cardiogenic shock
- Hypertension
- Angina

Nursing Goals

The nurse will monitor and manage episodes of decreased cardiac output.

Interventions

1. Monitor for signs and symptoms of decreased cardiac output/index:
   a. Decreased and/or irregular pulse rate
   b. Increased respiratory rate
   c. Decreased blood pressure
   d. Abnormal heart sounds
   e. Abnormal lung sounds (crackles)
   f. Decreased urine output (less than 30 mL/hour)
   g. Changes in mentation
   h. Cool, moist, cyanotic, mottled skin
   i. Delayed capillary refill time
   j. Neck vein distention
   k. Weak peripheral pulses
   l. Abnormal pulmonary artery pressures
   m. Decreased mixed venous oxygen saturation
   n. ECG changes
   o. Dysrhythmias
   p. Decreased SaO_2
   q. Decreased SvO_2

(Decreased cardiac output/index leads to an insufficient supply of oxygenated blood to meet the metabolic needs of tissues. Decreased circulating volume can result in hypoperfusion of the kidneys and decreased tissue perfusion with a compensatory response of decreased circulation to extremities and increased pulse and respiratory rates. Changes in mentation may result from cerebral hypoperfusion. Vasoconstriction and venous congestion in dependent areas [*e.g.*, limbs] produce changes in skin and pulses.)

2. Initiate appropriate protocols or standing orders, depending on the underlying etiology of the problem affecting the function of the ventricles.
   (Nursing management differs based on etiology, *e.g.*, measures to help increase preload for hypovolemia and to decrease preload for impaired ventricular contractility.)

3. Position the client with the legs elevated, unless ventricular function is impaired.
   (This position can help increase preload and enhance cardiac output.)

4. During acute episodes, maintain absolute bed rest and minimize all controllable stressors. Administer IV morphine PRN according to protocol. Use with caution if hypotensive.
   (These measures decrease metabolic demands.)

5. Assist the client with measures to conserve strength, such as resting before and after activities (*e.g.*, meals, baths).
   (Adequate rest reduces oxygen consumption and decreases the risk of hypoxia.)

6. In a client with impaired ventricular function, cautiously administer IV fluids. Consult with the physician if the ordered rate exceeds 125 mL/hour. Be sure to include any additional IV fluids (*e.g.*, antibiotics) when calculating the hourly allocation.
   (A client with poorly functioning ventricles may not tolerate increased blood volumes.)

7. If decreased cardiac output results from hypovolemia, septic shock, or dysrhythmia, refer to the specific collaborative problem in this section.

8. Administer inotropic and vasoactive agents as prescribed to improve contractility (*e.g.*, digoxin, dopamine, dobutamine).

9. Assist with insertion and/or maintenance of mechanical cardiac assist devices as indicated (intra-aortic balloon pump, hemapump, ventricular assist devices).

PC: Dysrhythmias

DEFINITION

PC: Dysrhythmias: Describes a person experiencing or at high risk to experience a disorder of the heart's conduction system that results in an abnormal heart rate, abnormal rhythm, or a combination of both.

High-Risk Populations

- Myocardial infarction
- Congestive heart failure
- Hypoendocrine or hyperendocrine status
- Increased intracranial pressure
- Electrolyte imbalance (calcium, potassium, magnesium, phosphorus)
- Atherosclerotic heart disease
- Medication side effects (*e.g.*, aminophylline, dopamine, stimulants, digoxin, β blockers, dobutamine, lidocaine, procainamide, quinidine, diuretics)

- COPD
- Cardiomyopathy, valvular heart disease
- Anemia
- Postoperative cardiac surgery

Nursing Goals

The nurse will manage and minimize dysrhythmic episodes.

Generic Interventions

1. Monitor for signs and symptoms of dysrhythmias.
    a. Abnormal rate, rhythm
    b. Palpitations, chest pain, syncope
    c. Decreased SaO_2
    d. ECG changes
    e. Hypotension
    (Ischemic tissue is electrically unstable, causing dysrhythmias. Certain congenital cardiac conditions, electrolyte imbalances, and medications can also cause disturbances in cardiac conduction.)
2. Initiate appropriate protocols depending on the type of dysrhythmia; this may include
    a. Supraventricular tachycardia: vagal stimulation (direct or indirect), IV calcium channel blockers, digoxin (IV), adenosine, synchronized cardioversion, overdrive pacing
    b. Atrial fibrillation: digitalization, electrical cardioversion
    c. Premature ventricular contractions, ventricular tachycardia: IV lidocaine, IV procainamide, IV bretylium, oxygen
    d. Ventricular tachycardia: oxygen, lidocaine, procainamide, bretylium, synchronized cardioversion, precardial thump if witnessed
    e. Bradycardia or heart blocks: atropine, pacing, dopamine infusion, epinephrine infusion
    f. Ventricular fibrillation: cardiopulmonary resuscitation (CPR) defibrillation, epinephrine, lidocaine, bretylium
    g. Pulseless electrical activity: CPR, epinephrine, (diagnose and treat the cause)
    h. Asystole: CPR, epinephrine, atropine, pacing
3. Administer supplemental oxygen, if indicated.
    (Supplemental oxygen therapy increases circulating oxygen levels.)
4. Monitor oxygen saturation (SaO_2) with pulse oximetry and ABGs as necessary.
5. Monitor serum electrolyte levels (*e.g.*, sodium, potassium, calcium, magnesium; high or low electrolyte levels may exacerbate a dysrhythmia.)
6. Monitor pacemaker and automatic implantable cardioverter defibrillator therapy.

PC: Pulmonary Edema

DEFINITION

PC: Pulmonary Edema: Describes a person experiencing or at high risk to experience insufficient gas exchange because of accumulation of fluid related to left-sided heart failure.

High-Risk Populations

- Hypertension
- Dysrhythmias
- Myocardial infarction
- Congestive heart failure
- Cardiomyopathy
- Coronary artery disease
- Aortic or mitral cardiac valve disease
- Diabetes mellitus
- Inhalation of toxins
- Drug overdose
- Smoking

Nursing Goals

The nurse will manage and minimize episodes of pulmonary edema.

Interventions

1. Monitor for signs and symptoms of pulmonary edema
   a. Dyspnea, cyanosis
   b. Tachypnea
   c. Adventitious breath sounds, crackles
   d. Persistent cough or productive cough with frothy, pink-tinged sputum
   e. Abnormal ABGs
   f. Decreased O_2 saturation by pulse oximetry
   g. Decreased cardiac output/cardiac index
   h. Elevated pulmonary artery pressure
   i. Tachycardia
   j. Abnormal heart sounds (S_3)
   (Impaired pumping of left ventricle accompanied by a decreased cardiac output and increased pulmonary venous pressure and pulmonary artery pressure produces pulmonary edema.)
2. If indicated, administer oxygen as prescribed.
3. Initiate appropriate treatments according to protocol, which may include
   a. Diuretics (to decrease preload)
   b. Vasodilators (to decrease afterload)
   c. Positive inotropics (*e.g.*, digitalis) (to enhance ventricular contractions)
   d. Morphine (to decrease anxiety, decrease preload and afterload, and lower metabolic demands)
4. Monitor urine hemodynamic parameters, specific gravity, intake/output, weight, and serum osmolality values.
   (These values can help evaluate hydration.)
5. Take steps to maintain adequate hydration while avoiding overhydration.
   (Adequate hydration helps liquefy pulmonary secretions; overhydration can increase preload and worsen pulmonary edema.)
6. Change the client's position every 2 hours. Determine which position provides optimum oxygenation by analyzing PaO_2 from pulse oximetry and/or ABG values with the client in various positions.
   (Limiting time the client spends in positions that compromise oxygenation improves PaO_2.)
7. Place the client in high Fowler's position with legs dependent if severely dyspneic.
   (This positioning helps decrease venous return, increase venous pooling, and decrease preload.)

8. Minimize controllable stressors (*e.g.*, noise, long series of tests and procedures) and explain all procedures and treatments.
   (These measures may reduce anxiety, which can help decrease metabolic demands.)
9. Continue monitoring cardiovascular status—vital signs, ABG values, cardiac output, fluid balance, weight.
   (This monitoring helps evaluate the client's response to treatment.)

PC: Deep Vein Thrombosis

DEFINITION

PC: Deep Vein Thrombosis: Describes a person experiencing venous clot formation because of blood stasis, vessel wall injury, or altered coagulation.

High-Risk Populations

- Immobility
- Extremity paralysis
- Fractures
- Chemical irritation of vein
- Blood dyscrasias
- Orthopedic, urologic, or gynecologic surgery
- History of venous insufficiency
- Obesity
- Oral contraceptive use
- Malignancy
- Heart failure

Nursing Goals

The nurse will manage and minimize complications of deep vein thrombosis.

Interventions

1. Monitor the status of venous thrombosis, noting
   a. Diminished or absent peripheral pulses
      (Insufficient circulation causes pain and diminished peripheral pulses.)
   b. Unusual warmth and redness or coolness and cyanosis
      (Unusual warmth and redness point to inflammation; coolness and cyanosis indicate vascular obstruction.)
   c. Increasing leg pain
      (Leg pain results from tissue hypoxia.)
   d. Sudden, severe chest pain, increased dyspnea, tachypnea
      (May indicate mobilization of thrombi to the lungs.)
   e. Positive Homans' sign
      (In a positive Homans' sign, dorsiflexion of the foot causes pain because of insufficient circulation.)

2. Consult physician for use of antiembolic stockings or sequential pressure devices, low-dose Dextran, or anticoagulant therapy for high-risk clients. (These assist in the reduction of venous stasis.) High-risk people are those older than 40 years of age, obese with multiple trauma or history of circulation deficits; on estrogen therapy; with systemic infection; and/or are cigarette smokers (Carroll, 1993).

3. Evaluate hydration status based on urine specific gravity, intake/output weights, and serum osmolality. Take steps to ensure adequate hydration.
   (Increased blood viscosity and coagulability and decreased cardiac output may contribute to thrombus formation.)

4. Encourage the client to perform isotonic leg exercises.
   (Isotonic leg exercises promote venous return.)

5. Ambulate as soon as possible with at least 5 minutes of walking each waking hour. Avoid prolonged chair sitting with legs dependent.
   (Walking contracts leg muscles, stimulates the venous pump, and reduces stasis [Carroll, 1993].)

6. Elevate the affected extremity above the level of the heart.
   (This positioning can help reduce interstitial swelling by promoting venous return.)

7. Discourage the person from smoking.
   (Nicotine can cause vasospasms.)

8. Administer anticoagulant therapy as the physician prescribes, and monitor blood coagulation results daily.
   (Anticoagulant therapy prevents extension of a thrombosis by delaying the clotting time of blood.)

9. For a client receiving anticoagulant therapy, monitor for early signs of abnormal bleeding (*e.g.*, hematuria, bleeding gums, ecchymoses, petechiae, epistaxis).
   (Prolonged clotting time can increase the risk of bleeding.)

10. Administer analgesics for leg pain as prescribed.

11. Explain the importance of antiembolic stockings (These stockings reduce venous stasis by applying a graded degree of compression to the ankle and the calf) (Carroll, 1993).

PC: Hypovolemia

DEFINITION

PC: Hypovolemia: Describes a person experiencing or at high risk to experience inadequate cellular oxygenation and inability to excrete waste products of metabolism secondary to decreased fluid volume (*e.g.*, from bleeding, plasma loss, prolonged vomiting, or diarrhea).

High-Risk Populations

- Intraoperative status
- Postoperative status
- Anaphylactic shock
- Trauma
- Bleeding
- Diabetic ketoacidosis
- Prolonged vomiting or diarrhea

- Infants, children, elderly
- Acute pancreatitis
- Major burns
- Disseminated intravascular coagulation
- Rupture of esophageal varices
- Dissecting aneurysms
- Prolonged pregnancy
- Trauma in pregnancy

Nursing Goals

The nurse will manage and minimize hypovolemic episodes.

Interventions

1. Monitor fluid status; evaluate
   a. Intake (parenteral and oral)
   b. Output and other losses (urine, drainage, and vomiting)
      (Early detection of fluid deficit enables interventions to prevent shock.)
2. Monitor the surgical site for bleeding, dehiscence, and evisceration.
   (Careful monitoring allows early detection of complications.)
3. Teach the client to splint the surgical wound with a pillow when coughing, sneezing, or vomiting.
   (Splinting reduces stress on the suture line by equalizing pressure across the wound.)
4. Monitor for signs and symptoms of shock:
   a. Increased pulse rate with normal or slightly decreased blood pressure
   b. Urine output less than 30 mL/hour
   c. Restlessness, agitation, decreased mentation
   d. Increased respiratory rate, thirst
   e. Diminished peripheral pulses
   f. Cool, pale, moist, or cyanotic skin
   g. Decreased oxygenation saturation (SaO_2, SvO_2), pulmonary artery pressures
   h. Decreased hemoglobin/hematocrit, decreased cardiac output/index
   (The compensatory response to decreased circulatory volume aims to increase oxygen delivery through increased heart and respiratory rates and decreased peripheral circulation [manifested by diminished peripheral pulses and cool skin]. Decreased oxygen to the brain results in altered mentation. Decreased circulation to the kidneys leads to decreased urine output. Hemoglobin and hematocrit values decline if significant bleeding occurs.)
5. If shock occurs, place the client in the supine position unless contraindicated (*e.g.*, if he has a head injury).
   (This position increases blood return [preload] to the heart.)
6. Insert an IV line; use a large-bore catheter if blood replacement is anticipated. Initiate appropriate protocols for shock (*e.g.*, vasopressor therapy). Refer also to *PC: Acidosis* or *PC: Alkalosis*, if indicated, for more information.
   (Protocols aim to increase peripheral resistance and elevate blood pressure.)
7. Collaborate with the physician to replace fluid losses at a rate sufficient to maintain urine output greater than 0.5 mL/kg/hour.
   (This measure promotes optimal renal tissue perfusion.)
8. Restrict the client's movement and activity.
   (This helps decrease tissue demands for oxygen.)
9. Provide reassurance, simple explanations, and emotional support to help reduce anxiety.
   (High anxiety increases metabolic demands for oxygen.)

PC: Compartmental Syndrome

DEFINITION

PC: Compartmental Syndrome: Describes a person experiencing increased pressure in a limited space, such as a fascial envelope, which compromises circulation and function, usually in the forearm or leg (Slye, 1991).

High-Risk Populations

- Fractures
- Musculoskeletal surgery
- Injuries (crush, electrical, vascular)
- Allergic response (snake, insect bites)
- Excessive edema
- Thermal injuries
- Vascular obstruction
- Intramuscular bleeding
- External constriction (casts, inflatable splints, antishock garment, traction)

Nursing Goals

The nurse will manage and minimize compartmental syndrome.

Interventions

1. Refer to nursing diagnosis *Risk for Peripheral Neurovascular Dysfunction* for specific extremity assessment techniques and prevention of compartmental syndrome.
2. Monitor for signs of compartmental syndrome:
   a. Early signs
      Unrelieved or increasing pain
      Pain with passive stretch movement of toes or fingers
      Mottled or cyanotic skin
      Excessive swelling
      Delay in capillary refill
      Paresthesia
      Inability to move toes or fingers
   (Pain and paresthesia indicate compression of nerves and increasing pressure within muscle compartment. Passive stretching of muscles decreases muscle compartment, thus increasing pain. Delayed capillary refill or mottled or cyanotic skin indicates obstructed capillary blood flow.)
   b. Late signs
      Pallor
      Diminished or absent pulse
      Cold skin
   (Arterial occlusion produces these late signs.)
3. Assess peripheral nerve function at least every hour for first 24 hours.
   (Peripheral neurovascular compromise may be the first sign [Ross, 1991].)
4. Instruct to report unusual, new, or different sensations (*e.g.*, tingling, numbness, and/or decreased ability to move toes or fingers).
   (Early detection of compromise can prevent serious impairment [Ross, 1991].)

5. If signs of compartmental syndrome occur, notify physician and
   a. Discontinue elevation and ice applications.
   b. Loosen circumferential dressings, splints, casts per protocol,
6. If invasive compartmental monitoring system is used, follow procedure for use.
7. Monitor and document compartmental pressures according to protocol. Report elevated pressures promptly.
8. Carefully maintain hydration.
(Hypovolemia can result from fluid volume shift.)
9. Evaluate cardiovascular and renal status:
     Pulse, respiration
     Blood pressure
     Urine output
(Eight liters of fluid can extravasate into a limb, causing hypovolemia, decreased renal function, and shock [Lucas, 1985].)
10. Notify the physician of any early signs and symptoms of neurovascular compromise.
(The physician will evaluate the cause and determine the necessary treatment, *e.g.*, cast-splitting, removal of medical antishock trousers [MAST], removal of intra-aortic balloon pump, surgery [*e.g.*, fasciotomy].)

PC: Pulmonary Embolism

DEFINITION

PC: Pulmonary Embolism: Describes a person experiencing or at high risk to experience obstruction of one or more pulmonary arteries from a blood clot or air or fat embolus.

High-Risk Populations

- Prolonged immobilization
- Prolonged sitting/traveling
- Varicose veins
- Vascular injury
- Tumor
- Increased platelet count (*e.g.*, from polycythemia, splenectomy)
- Thrombophlebitis
- Vascular disease
- Presence of foreign bodies (*e.g.*, IV or central venous catheters)
- Heart disease (especially congestive heart failure)
- Surgery or trauma (especially of hip, pelvis, spine, lower extremities)
- Postoperative state
- Pregnancy
- Postpartum state
- Diabetes
- COPD
- History of previous pulmonary embolism or thrombophlebitis
- Obesity
- Oral contraceptive use, estrogen therapy

- Acute spinal cord injury
- Thrombus formation in heart from cardioversion, bacterial endocarditis, atrial fibrillation, or myocardial infarction

For air embolism
- Central line insertion or removal
- Central line tubing changes

Nursing Goals

The nurse will manage and minimize complications of pulmonary embolism.

Interventions

1. Consult with the physician for low-dose heparin therapy for a high-risk client until ambulatory.
   (Heparin therapy decreases blood viscosity and platelet adhesiveness, reducing the risk of embolism.)
2. Refer to the nursing diagnosis *Risk for Altered Peripheral Tissue Perfusion* in Section II for information on preventing deep vein thrombosis.
3. Monitor for signs and symptoms of pulmonary embolism:
   a. Acute, sharp chest pain
   b. Dyspnea, restlessness, cyanosis
   c. Decreased oxygen saturation (SaO_2, SvO_2)
   d. Tachycardia
   e. Neck vein distention
   f. Hypotension
   g. Acute right ventricular dilation without parenchymal disease (on chest x-ray)
   h. Confusion
   i. Cardiac dysrhythmias
   (Occlusion of pulmonary arteries impedes blood flow to the distal lung, producing a hypoxic state.)
4. If these manifestations occur, promptly initiate protocols for shock.
   a. Establish an IV line (for medication and fluid administration).
   b. Administer fluid replacement therapy according to protocol.
   c. Insert an indwelling urinary (Foley) catheter (to monitor circulatory volume through urine output).
   d. Initiate ECG monitoring and invasive hemodynamic monitoring (to detect dysrhythmias and guide therapy).
   e. Administer vasopressors to increase peripheral resistance and raise blood pressure.
   f. Administer sodium bicarbonate as indicated (to correct metabolic acidosis).
   g. Administer digitalis glycosides and IV diuretics and antiarrhythmic agents, as indicated.
   h. Administer small IV doses of morphine (to reduce anxiety and decrease metabolic demands).
   i. Refer to *PC: Hypovolemic Shock* for additional interventions.
   j. Prepare for angiography and/or perfusion lung scans (to confirm diagnosis and detect the extent of atelectasis).
   (Because death from massive pulmonary embolism commonly occurs in the first 2 hours after onset, prompt intervention is crucial.)
5. Initiate oxygen therapy through nasal cannula; monitor oxygen saturation.
   (This measure rapidly increases circulating oxygen levels.)
6. Monitor serum electrolyte levels, ABG values, blood urea nitrogen, and complete blood count results.
   (These laboratory tests help determine perfusion and volume status.)

7. Initiate thrombolytic therapy (*e.g.*, urokinase, streptokinase) per physician's orders.
   (Thrombolytics can cause lysis of emboli and increase pulmonary capillary perfusion.)
8. When prescribed after thrombolytic infusion, initiate heparin therapy (continuous IV infusion or intermittent). Monitor clotting times during heparin therapy.
   (Heparin can slow or halt the underlying thrombotic process, helping prevent clot extension or recurrence.)
9. For a client receiving thrombolytics and/or anticoagulant therapy, monitor for signs of abnormal bleeding (*e.g.*, hematuria, bleeding gums, ecchymosis, petechiae, epistaxis).

For PC: Air Embolism
1. Before central line catheter insertion and tubing changes, place the client in Trendelenburg's position and instruct him to perform Valsalva maneuver during the procedure.
   (These measures increase intrathoracic pressure and help prevent air from entering the catheter.)
2. Secure the proximal catheter connection with a Luer-Lok IV set, and tape all connections securely.
   (These measures help prevent accidental tubing disconnection, the most common cause of air embolism.)
3. Tape a loop of IV tubing to the client's chest (Thielen, 1990).
   (This measure eliminates traction on the catheter, which can enlarge the insertion site and increase the risk of air entry.)
4. Use only clamps designed for central lines. If tubing is difficult to disconnect during changes, *do not* use hemostats—instead, try using a rubber tourniquet with ends wrapped around the tubing to improve your grip.
   (These measures can help prevent damage to the tubing and resultant air leaks.)
5. Explain the potential problems associated with tubing disconnection, and instruct the client to crimp the tubing near the entry site if separation occurs.
   (Immediate action can prevent air embolism.)
6. Before IV catheter removal, place the client in Trendelenburg's position and instruct him to perform Valsalva maneuver or at least hold his breath during the procedure. After removal, immediately apply direct pressure to the catheterization site, then apply a sterile nonpermeable dressing. Leave the dressing in place for 24–48 hours.
   (These measures help prevent air entry.)
7. Monitor for signs and symptoms of air embolism during dressing and IV tubing changes and after any accidental separation of IV connections:
   a. Sucking sound on insertion
   b. Dyspnea
   c. Tachypnea
   d. Wheezing
   e. Substernal chest pain
   f. Anxiety
   (Air embolism can occur with IV tubing changes, with accidental tubing separation, and during catheter insertion and disconnection. [For example, a client can aspirate as much as 200 mL of air from a deep breath during subclavian line disconnection.] Entry of air into the pulmonary arterial system can obstruct blood flow, causing bronchoconstriction of the affected lung area.)
8. If air embolism is suspected
   a. Place the client in steep Trendelenburg's position on the left side.
      (This position allows air to be displaced away from the pulmonary valve and prevents more air from entering [Thielen, 1990].)
   b. Administer oxygen through face mask according to protocol.
      (This promotes diffusion of nitrogen, which compresses an air embolism in about 80% of cases.)
   c. Initiate protocols for respiratory or cardiac arrest if indicated.

For PC: Fat Embolism

1. Monitor for sign and symptoms of fat embolism:
   a. Tachypnea >30/minute
   b. Sudden onset of chest pain or dyspnea
   c. Restlessness, apprehension
   d. Confusion
   e. Elevated temperature >103°F
   f. Increased pulse rate >140/minute
   g. Petechial skin rash (12–96 hours postoperative)

   (These changes are the result of hypoxemia. Fatty acids attack red blood cells and platelets to form microaggregates, which impair circulation to vital organs, such as the brain. Fatty globules passing through the pulmonary vasculature cause a chemical reaction that decreases lung compliance and ventilation/perfusion ratio and raises body temperature. The rash is the result of capillary fragility. Common sites are conjunctiva, axilla, chest, and neck [Slye, 1991].)

2. Minimize movement of a fractured extremity for the first 3 days after the injury.
   (Immobilization minimizes further tissue trauma and reduces the risk of embolism dislodgement [Slye, 1991].)

3. Ensure adequate hydration.
   (Optimal hydration dilutes the irritating fatty acids through the system [Slye, 1991].)

4. Monitor intake/output, urine color, and specific gravity.
   (These data reflect hydration status.)

References/Bibliography

American Heart Association. (1994). *Advanced cardiac life support*. Dallas: Author.

Bousquet, G. L. (1990). Congestive heart failure: A review of nonpharmacologic therapies. *Journal of Cardiovascular Nursing, 4*(3), 35–46.

Braunwald, E., Mark, D. B., & Jones, R. H. (1994). *Unstable angina: Diagnosis and management, clinical practice guideline number 10*. Rockville, MD: AHCPR and NHLBI.

Carroll, P. (1993). Deep venous thrombosis: Implications for orthopedic nursing. *Orthopedic Nursing, 12*(3), 33–41.

Caswell, D. (1993). Thromboembolic phenomena. *Critical Care Nursing Clinics of North America, 5*, 489–497.

Curie, D. (1990). Pulmonary embolism: Diagnosis and management. *Critical Care Nursing Quarterly, 13*(2), 41–49.

Guzzetta, C. E., & Dossey, B. M. (1992). *Cardiovascular nursing: Holistic practice*. St. Louis: Mosby–Year Book.

Kinney, M. R., Packa, D. R., & Dunbar, S. B. (1993). *AACN clinical reference for critical-care nursing* (3rd ed.). New York: McGraw-Hill.

Kleven, M. (1988). Comparison of thrombolytic agents: Mechanism of action, efficacy, and safety. *Heart and Lung, 17*(Suppl), 750–755.

Ley, J. (1993). Myocardial depression after cardiac surgery: Pharmacologic and mechanical support. *AACN Clinical Issues in Critical Care Nursing, 4*, 293–308.

Lucas, C. (1985). Answers to questions on crush injury. *Hospital Medicine, 21*(5), 100–112.

Morton, P. (1994). Update on new antiarrhythmic drugs. *Critical Care Nursing Clinics of North America, 6*, 69–83.

Norris, S. O. (1993). Managing low cardiac output states: Maintaining volume after cardiac surgery. *AACN Clinical Issues in Critical Care Nursing, 4*, 309–319.

Peck, S. (1990). Crush syndrome. *Orthopedic Nursing, 9*(3), 33–40.

Rice, V. (1991). Shock, a clinical syndrome: An update, Part 4. Nursing care of the shock patient. *Critical Care Nurse, 11*(7), 28–40.

Ross, D. (1991). Acute compartmental syndrome. *Orthopedic Nursing, 10*(2), 33–38.

Slye, D. A. (1991). Orthopedic complications. *Nursing Clinics of North America, 26*, 113–132.

Stanley, R. (1990). Drug therapy in heart failure. *Journal of Cardiovascular Nursing, 4*, 17–34.

Thelan, L., Davie, J., & Urden, L. (1990). *Textbook of critical care nursing*. St. Louis: C. V. Mosby.

Thielen, J. B. (1990). Air emboli: A potentially lethal complication of central venous lines. *Focus on Critical Care, 17*, 374–383.

Underhill, S. L., Woods, S. L., Sivarajan, E. S., & Halpenny, C. J. (1994). *Cardiac nursing* (3rd ed.). Philadelphia: J. B. Lippincott.

Potential Complication: Respiratory

PC: Hypoxemia

PC: Atelectasis/Pneumonia

PC: Tracheobronchial Constriction

PC: Pneumothorax

Respiratory System Overview

Respiratory functioning primarily depends on two systems: the conducting system and the respiratory center in the brain stem. Consisting of the upper airway (nose, nasal mucosa, pharynx, larynx, epiglottis) and lower airway (trachea, bronchi, bronchioles, alveolar ducts), the conducting system conducts and filters air, traps foreign bodies to be expectorated or swallowed, and warms and humidifies inspired air. The lungs consist of three lobes on the right side and two lobes on the left side. Oxygen (O_2) is exchanged for carbon dioxide (CO_2) across the alveolar capillary membrane by simple diffusion, and wastes are removed by alveolar macrophages. Surfactant, a phospholipid secreted by the alveoli, prevents lung collapse by reducing surface tension of the lungs. Blood supply to the lungs consists of pulmonary circulation and bronchial circulation.

Located in the medulla oblongata in the brain stem, the respiratory center increases or decreases respiratory rate in response to CO_2 and hydrogen ion (H^+) concentrations in the cerebrospinal fluid.

The diaphragm is the major muscle of respiration. Additional respiratory muscles are the external intercostals, the scaleni, and the sternocleidomastoid. Normally, expiration is passive. Diaphragmatic movement during inspiration and expiration changes the space in the thoracic cavity, allowing the lungs to expand and deflate.

The right and left pulmonary arteries transport deoxygenated blood from the right side of the heart to the lungs. The pulmonary veins transport oxygenated blood to the left side of the heart to be pumped through the body. The bronchial circulation supplies the lungs with oxygenated blood for nutrition of the pulmonary nerves and ganglia, arteries and veins, pleura, and connective tissue.

The mechanics of respiration can be adversely affected by various factors, including foreign body obstruction, excessive or thickened secretions, edema, and poor positioning. Respiratory muscle movements may be impeded because of fatigue, mechanical ventilation, or depression of the respiratory center. Perfusion at the alveolar level can be impaired by compromised cardiac functioning, inadequate blood supply, inadequate oxyhemoglobin levels, or abnormalities in the alveoli (*e.g.*, excessive mucus, tumor).

Potential Complication: Respiratory

DEFINITION

PC: Respiratory: Describes a person experiencing or at high risk to experience various respiratory problems.

Author's Note

The nurse uses the generic collaborative problem *PC: Respiratory* to describe a person at risk for several types of respiratory problems and to identify the nursing focus—monitoring respiratory status for detection and diagnosis of abnormal functioning. Nursing management of a specific respiratory complication is then described under the appropriate collaborative problem for that complication. For example, a nurse using *PC: Respiratory* for a client in whom hypoxemia later develops would then add *PC: Hypoxemia* to the client's problem list. If the risk factors or etiology were not directly related to the primary medical diagnosis, the nurse would add this information to the diagnostic statement (*e.g., PC: Hypoxemia related to COPD* in a client with COPD [chronic obstructive pulmonary disease] who experiences respiratory problems after gastric surgery).

For a person vulnerable to respiratory problems due to immobility or excessive tenacious secretions, the nurse should apply the nursing diagnosis *Risk for Altered Respiratory Function related to immobility* rather than *PC: Respiratory*.

Focus Assessment Criteria

Subjective Data

1. History of
   a. Allergies
   b. Bronchitis
   c. Asthma
   d. Emphysema
   e. Tuberculosis (drug-resistant TB)
   f. Respiratory infection
   g. Heart disease
   h. Sarcoidosis
   i. Exposure to environmental inhalants (chemical dusts, fumes, asbestos)
   j. Exposure to respiratory infections
   k. Immune system compromise
2. Medication use (prescribed and over-the-counter, immunizations)
3. Tobacco use (type, amount, length of time)
4. Complaints of
   a. Shortness of breath (related to activity, during sleep)
   b. Weight loss
   c. Fatigue
   d. Fever and chills
   e. Anorexia (decreased appetite)
   f. Cough (dry or productive, sputum, frequency)
   g. Chest pain

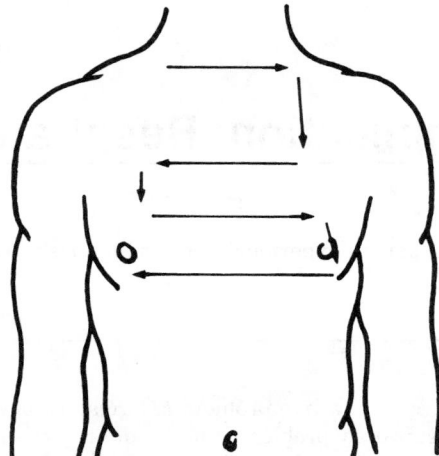

Fig. III-1   Sequence for chest auscultation.

Objective Data

1. Thoracic expansion (symmetric or asymmetric)
2. Diaphragmatic excursion (normal: descends 3–6 cm; abnormal: descends less than 3 or more than 6 cm, equal bilaterally vesicular/bronchial)
3. Breath sounds in all lung fields (Fig. III-1) (normal [vascular], rales, rhonchi, wheezes, pleural friction rub)
4. Ability to cough (effective or ineffective)
5. Effect of coughing on rhonchi

Significant Laboratory/Diagnostic Assessment Criteria

1. Blood pH (elevated in alkalosis, lowered in acidosis)
2. Arterial blood gas (ABG) values
   a. pH (elevated in alkalemia, lowered in acidemia)
   b. PCO_2 (elevated in pulmonary disease, lowered in hyperventilation)
   c. PO_2 (lowered in pulmonary disease)
   d. CO_2 content (elevated in COPD, lowered in hyperventilation)
3. Sputum stain and culture
4. Chest x-ray
5. Ventilation perfusion scanning

PC: Hypoxemia

DEFINITION

PC: Hypoxemia: Describes a person experiencing or at high risk to experience insufficient plasma oxygen saturation (PO_2 less than normal for age) because of alveolar hypoventilation, pulmonary shunting, or ventilation–perfusion inequality.

High-Risk Populations

- COPD
- Pneumonia
- Atelectasis
- Pulmonary edema
- Adult respiratory distress syndrome
- Central nervous system depression
- Medulla or spinal cord disorders
- Guillain-Barré syndrome
- Myasthenia gravis
- Muscular dystrophy
- Obesity
- Compromised chest wall movement (*e.g.*, trauma)
- Drug overdose
- Head injury
- Near-drowning
- Multiple trauma

Nursing Goals

The nurse will manage and minimize complications of hypoxemia.

Interventions

1. Monitor for signs of acid–base imbalance:
   a. ABG analysis: pH less than 7.35, $PaCO_2$ greater than 48 mm Hg
      (ABG analysis helps evaluate gas exchange in the lungs. In mild to moderate COPD, the client may have a normal $PaCO_2$ level as chemoreceptors in the medulla respond to increased $PaCO_2$ by increasing ventilation. In severe COPD, however, the client cannot sustain this increased ventilation, and the $PaCO_2$ value gradually increases.)
   b. Increased and irregular pulse, and increased respiratory rate initially, followed by decreased rate
      (Respiratory acidosis develops as a result of excessive CO_2 retention. A client with respiratory acidosis from chronic disease at first experiences increased heart rate and respirations in an attempt to compensate for decreased oxygenation. After a while, the client breathes more slowly and with prolonged expiration. Eventually, his respiratory center may stop responding to the higher CO_2 levels, and breathing may stop abruptly.)
   c. Changes in mentation (somnolence, confusion, irritability)
      (Changes in mentation result from cerebral tissue hypoxia.)
   d. Decreased urine output (less than 30 mL/hour); cool, pale, or cyanotic skin.
      (The compensatory response to decreased circulatory oxygen aims to increase blood oxygen by increasing heart and respiratory rates and to decrease circulation to the kidneys and to the extremities [marked by decreased pulses and skin changes].)
2. Administer low-flow (2 L/minute) oxygen as needed through a mask or nasal cannula, if indicated.
   (Oxygen therapy increases circulating oxygen levels. High flow rates increase CO_2 retention in people with COPD. Using a cannula rather than a mask may help reduce the client's fears of suffocation.)
3. Evaluate the effects of positioning on oxygenation, using ABG values as a guide. Change the client's position every 2 hours, avoiding those positions that compromise oxygenation. (This measure promotes optimal ventilation.)
4. Ensure adequate hydration. Teach the client to avoid dehydrating beverages (*e.g.*, caffeinated drinks, grapefruit juice).
   (Optimal hydration helps liquefy secretions.)

5. Teach the client effective coughing technique.
   (Effective coughing moves mucus from the lower airways to the trachea for expectoration.)

6. If the client cannot expectorate secretions, use coughing and/or chest physiotherapy to move secretions up from the trachea for suctioning.
   (Suctioning is effective only at the tracheal level.)

7. Administer supplemental oxygen before and after suctioning.
   (This measure helps prevent a decrease in PO_2 due to suctioning.)

8. Obtain a sputum sample for culture and sensitivity and Gram stain testing.
   (Sputum culture and sensitivity determine whether an infection is contributing to symptoms.)

9. Eliminate smoke and strong odors from the client's room.
   (Irritation of the respiratory tract can exacerbate symptoms.)

10. Monitor the electrocardiogram for dysrhythmias secondary to altered oxygenation.
    (Hypoxemia may precipitate cardiac dysrhythmias.)

11. Monitor for signs of right-sided congestive heart failure
    a. Elevated diastolic pressure
    b. Distended neck veins
    c. Peripheral edema
    d. Elevated central venous pressure
       (The combination of arterial hypoxemia and respiratory acidosis acts locally as a strong vasoconstrictor of pulmonary vessels. This leads to pulmonary arterial hypertension, increased right ventricular systolic pressure, and, eventually, right ventricular hypertrophy and failure.)

12. Refer to the nursing diagnosis *Activity Intolerance* in Section II for specific adaptive techniques to teach a client with chronic pulmonary insufficiency.

PC: Atelectasis, Pneumonia

DEFINITION

PC: Atelectasis, Pneumonia: Describes a person experiencing impaired respiratory functioning because of alveolar collapse, which can result in pneumonia.*

High-Risk Populations

- Postoperative status (abdominal or thoracic surgery)
- Immobilization
- Decreased level of consciousness
- Nasogastric feedings
- Chronic lung disease
- Debilitation
- Decreased surfactant production

* The nurse should use the nursing diagnosis *Risk for Altered Respiratory Function* for people at high risk for atelectasis and pneumonia, to focus on prevention. The collaborative problem *PC: Atelectasis, Pneumonia* is applicable only if the condition occurs.

- Compression of lung tissue (*e.g.*, from cancer, abdominal distention, obesity, pneumothorax)
- Airway obstruction

Nursing Goals

The nurse will manage and minimize complications of atelectasis or pneumonia.

Interventions

1. Monitor respiratory status and assess for signs and symptoms of inflammation:
   a. Increased respiratory rate
   b. Fever and chills (sudden or insidious)
   c. Productive cough
   d. Diminished or absent breath sounds
   e. Pleuritic chest pain
   f. Tachycardia
   g. Marked dyspnea
   h. Cyanosis
      (Tracheobronchial inflammation, impaired alveolar capillary membrane function, edema, fever, and increased sputum production disrupt respiratory function and compromise the blood's oxygen-carrying capacity. Reduced chest wall compliance in older adults affects the quality of respiratory effort. In the elderly, tachypnea, at over 26 respirations per minute, is one of the earliest signs of pneumonia, often occurring 3–4 days before a confirmed diagnosis. Delirium or mental status changes are often seen early in pneumonia in the elderly [Brown, 1993].)
   i. Lethargy
2. Monitor for signs and symptoms of infection:
   a. Fever of 101°F (39.4°C) or higher
   b. Chills
   c. Tachycardia
   d. Manifestations of shock: restlessness or lethargy, confusion, decreased systolic blood pressure
      (Endogenous pyrogens are released and reset the hypothalamic set point to febrile levels. The body temperature is sensed as "too cool"; shivering and vasoconstriction result to generate and consume heat. Core temperature rises to the new level of the set point, resulting in fever. White blood cells are released to destroy some pathogens. The impaired respiratory system cannot compensate; tissue hypoxia results [Holtzclaw, 1990].)
3. If fever occurs, provide cooling measures (*e.g.*, reduced clothing and bed linen, tepid baths, increased fluids, hypothermia blanket).
   (Reducing body temperature is necessary to lower metabolic rate and reduce oxygen consumption.)
4. Monitor for signs and symptoms of septic shock:
   a. Altered body temperature (>38°C or <36°C)
   b. Hypotension
   c. Decreased level of consciousness
   d. Weak, rapid pulse
   e. Rapid, shallow respirations or $CO_2 < 32$
   f. Cold, clammy skin
   g. Oliguria
      (Septic shock is a systemic inflammatory response syndrome [SIRS] associated with infection due to microorganisms or their other products associated with hypotension and perfusion abnormalities despite fluid resuscitation or vasopressors.)

5. Evaluate the effectiveness of cough suppressants and expectorants.
   (A dry, hacking cough interferes with sleep and affects energy. Cough suppressants should be used judiciously, however, because complete depression of the cough reflex can lead to atelectasis by hindering movement of tracheobronchial secretions.)
6. Maintain oxygen therapy, as prescribed, and monitor its effectiveness.
   (Oxygen therapy may help prevent dyspnea and also reduce the risk of pulmonary edema.)
7. Provide respiratory physiotherapy (*e.g.*, chest percussion, postural drainage) to move thick, tenacious secretions along the tracheobronchial tree.
   (Exudate in the alveoli and bronchospasms linked to increased bronchopulmonary secretions can decrease ventilatory effort and impair gas exchange.)
8. Teach the client how to do diaphragmatic breathing.
   (This technique increases tidal volume by maximizing diaphragmatic descent.)
9. Refer to *PC: Hypoxemia* for additional interventions.

PC: Tracheobronchial Constriction

DEFINITION

PC: Tracheobronchial Constriction: Describes a person experiencing or at high risk to experience airflow limitations through the tracheobronchial tree because of asthma, bronchitis, emphysema, and/or allergic reaction.

High-Risk Populations

- COPD
- Allergies
- Asthma
- Chronic bronchitis
- Viral infections (<6 months of age)

Nursing Goals

The nurse will manage and minimize episodes of tracheobronchial constriction.

Interventions

1. Monitor respiratory status continuously during acute exacerbation; evaluate
   a. Use of accessory muscles
   b. Respiratory rate, pulse rate, blood pressure
   c. Breath sounds (*e.g.*, wheezing)
   d. ABG values
   e. Peripheral perfusion (skin color, pulses)
   f. Level of consciousness
   (A client's respiratory status can change rapidly, with specific changes depending on response to treatments, level of fatigue, and severity of the episode.)

2. Administer oxygen through nasal cannula at a rate of 2–3 L/minute.
   (Oxygen therapy reduces hypoxemic effects; using a cannula rather than a mask may help minimize feelings of suffocation.)
3. Ensure adequate hydration either orally or intravenously.
   (Good hydration status helps prevent tenacious, impacted mucus.)
4. During acute episodes, stay with the client and have him breathe using pursed-lip or diaphragmatic breathing.
   (A panicky, dyspneic client needs a nurse's constant presence to help him gain control over his breathing.)
5. Maintain the client in an upright position.
   (The upright position promotes optimal lung expansion.)
6. Initiate physician-prescribed interventions, which may include anti-inflammatory agents, β_2-agonists, theophylline preparations, or corticosteroids (systemic or inhaled).
7. Avoid administering narcotics and sedatives.
   (Sedation depresses respiratory drive.)
8. Monitor for medication side effects (*e.g.*, dysrhythmias, hypotension, hypertension, vomiting, theophylline blood levels).
   (Early detection of side effects enables prompt intervention to minimize their seriousness.)
9. Monitor for early signs of status asthmaticus:
   a. Previous severe asthma attack
   b. Little or no response to bronchodilator therapy after 1 hour
   c. Altered level of consciousness
   (Status asthmaticus is not relieved by usual treatment for an acute asthmatic episode and requires IV corticosteroids.)
10. Consult with the physician for possible intubation if the work of breathing becomes increasingly difficult for the client.
    (Exhaustion brought on by excessive respiratory effort can lead to pulmonary arrest.)
11. When indicated, initiate health teaching, using the nursing diagnosis *Risk for Altered Health Maintenance related to insufficient knowledge of (specify)*.

🕭 Interventions—*Child Focus*

1. Refer also to Interventions.
2. Monitor respiratory status.
   a. Pulse rate, respiratory rate
   b. Use of accessory respiratory muscles, retractions, nasal flaring
   c. Diaphoresis, cyanosis
   d. Wheezing, cough
   (Pulse and respiratory rate increases indicate hypoxia. Asthma can often manifest as a cough rather than wheezing.)
3. Assess for signs of dehydration.
   (Children with dyspnea may refuse fluids.)
4. Ensure adequate hydration.
   (Good hydration status helps prevent tenacious, impacted mucus.)
5. Evaluate child's and parents' understanding of condition, triggers, monitoring, and treatment.
6. Ask child and/or parent to demonstrate use of inhaler, spacer, or nebulizer.
   (Many drug failures are the result of improper use of equipment.)
7. Teach how to monitor peak expiratory flow rates (PEFR) twice daily, before and after treatments, in a diary.
   a. Determine the child's personal-best values.
   b. Instruct to increase medications if PEFR falls below 50%–80% of personal best.
   c. Instruct to use bronchodilator immediately if rate is below 50%, and seek emergency treatment if not improved immediately.
   (PEFR monitoring is critical to effective prevention of acute exacerbations in children with moderate or severe asthma.)

PC: Pneumothorax

DEFINITION

PC: Pneumothorax: Describes a person experiencing or at high risk to experience accumulation of air in the pleural space because of lung injury.

High-Risk Populations

- Severe blunt or penetrating chest injury
- Postoperative status (cardiac or thoracic surgery)
- Mechanically ventilated with positive end-expiratory pressure

Nursing Goals

The nurse will manage and minimize complications of pneumothorax.

Interventions

1. Monitor for signs and symptoms of pneumothorax:
   a. Acute pleuritic chest pain
   b. Dyspnea, tachypnea, tachycardia
   c. Hyperresonant percussion sounds with loss of breath sounds over the affected side
   d. Shifting of trachea
   (Early detection and prompt intervention are necessary to prevent serious complications.)
2. Administer oxygen, if indicated. If chronic CO_2 retention occurs, limit the flow rate to no more than 2 L/min.
   (Higher flow rates can depress ventilatory drive.)
3. Prepare for stat chest x-ray.
4. Evaluate the need for analgesics to manage thoracic pain.
   (Pain interferes with lung expansion on inspiration, compromising oxygenation.)
5. Position the client with the head of the bed elevated, unless contraindicated.
   (This position helps maximize lung expansion.)
6. Reposition the client every 2 hours, keeping the unaffected lung in the dependent position.
   (This position limits pain and improves oxygenation by better equalizing ventilation and perfusion [Thelan, Davie, & Urden, 1990].)
7. Explain and supervise deep breathing with sustained maximum inspiration.
   (Deep breathing expands the lungs and evacuates air from the pleural space into the chest drainage system [if present].)
8. Instruct the person to avoid coughing except when necessary to clear secretions.
   (Coughing increases pain.)
9. Minimize environmental stimuli, provide emotional support, and offer simple explanations for all procedures.
   (These measures may help reduce anxiety, which increases respiratory rate.)
10. If use of a chest drainage system is indicated, follow institutional protocols for set-up, assessment, and maintenance.

References/Bibliography

Brown, L. H. (1990). Pulmonary oxygen toxicity. *Focus on Critical Care, 17*, 68–75.

Brown, R. (1993). Community-acquired pneumonia: Diagnosis and therapy of older adults. *Geriatrics, 48*(2), 43–44, 46–50.

Case, S., & Sabo, C. (1992). Adult respiratory distress syndrome: A deadly complication of trauma. *Focus on Critical Care, 19*, 116–121.

Ely, E., & Haponik, E. (1991). Pneumonia in the elderly. *Journal of Thoracic Imaging, 6*(3), 45–61.

Fontaine, D. K. (1989). Positioning as a nursing therapy in trauma care. *Critical Care Nursing Clinics of North America, 9*, 105–121.

Holtzclaw, B. J. (1990). Temperature problems in the postoperative period. *Critical Care Nursing Clinics of North America, 2*, 589–597.

Hudak, C., Gallo, B., & Benz, J. (1990). *Critical care nursing* (5th ed.). Philadelphia: J. B. Lippincott.

Marrie, T. (1992). Pneumonia. *Clinics in Geriatric Medicine, 8*, 721–734.

Mims, B. C. (1989). Fat embolism syndrome, a variant of ARDS. *Orthopedic Nursing, 8*(3), 22–27.

Pfister, S. M. (1989). Arterial blood gas evaluation: Metabolic acidemia. *Critical Care Nurse, 9*(1), 70–72.

Thelan, L., Davie, J., & Urden, L. (1990). *Textbook of critical care nursing*. St. Louis: C. V. Mosby.

Potential Complication: Metabolic/Immune/Hematopoietic

PC: Hypo/Hyperglycemia

PC: Negative Nitrogen Balance

PC: Electrolyte Imbalances

PC: Sepsis

PC: Acidosis (Metabolic, Respiratory)

PC: Alkalosis (Metabolic, Respiratory)

PC: Allergic Reaction

PC: Thrombocytopenia

PC: Opportunistic Infections

PC: Sickling Crisis

Metabolic/Immune/Hematopoietic System Overview

Metabolic functioning influences all physical and chemical changes occurring within the body. *Catabolism* refers to the breakdown of ingested substances into simpler substances (*e.g.*, food); *anabolism* refers to the conversion of ingested substances to protoplasm for cellular activities and tissue growth and repair.

For proper metabolic functioning, adequate amounts of carbohydrates, protein, fats, vitamins, electrolytes, minerals, and trace elements are needed. These nutrients are digested and absorbed into circulating blood and lymph.

Carbohydrates provide the preferred source of energy for cellular activity and are broken down into glucose, fructose, and galactose. Serum glucose levels are controlled primarily by the pancreatic hormones insulin and glucagon. Insulin facilitates glucose transport into cells. Glucagon, which stimulates the conversion of liver glycogen to glucose, is available for release when the blood glucose level falls below normal.

Proteins provide the structural basis of all lean body mass and are required for visceral functions, initiation of chemical reactions, transportation of apoproteins, preservation of immune function, and maintenance of osmotic pressure and blood neutrality (Thelan, Davie, & Urden, 1990). Proteins are broken down by gastric and pancreatic digestion into amino acids. About half the amino acids digested comes from ingested foods (essential); the other half is derived from enzymes secreted into the intestine and from desquamated mucosal cells (nonessential). Nonessential amino acids cannot be manufactured if the supply of essential amino acids is inadequate. Nitrogen remains after protein is metabolized and must be excreted by the kidneys.

Lipids or fats (fatty acids, triglycerides, phospholipids, cholesterol, cholesterol esters) are responsible for insulation, structure and temperature control, and the manufacture of prostaglandins, and serve as carriers of fat-soluble vitamins. Lipids also are a stored source of energy when glucose supply is low (*e.g.*, an overnight fast).

Dietary fats are hydrolyzed in the small intestine to form short-chain and long-chain fatty acids. Bile from the gallbladder emulsifies the fat so that pancreatic lipase can break down the fat more effectively. Short-chain fatty acids are absorbed and transported to the liver; long-chain fatty acids are transported by the lymphatic system to the liver and other tissues. When fatty acids are used for energy, ketones are produced. Large amounts of circulating ketones can cause metabolic acidosis.

Endocrine glands—the pituitary, adrenals, thyroid, parathyroids, and parts of the pancreas—secrete various hormones into the bloodstream. These hormones control metabolic functions such as rate of chemical reaction in cells, transport of substances across cell membranes, and growth and secretion. Chemical and neurologic stimuli regulate the release of hormones. Chemical control is accomplished by negative feedback (*e.g.*, a rise or fall of the blood level of one hormone causes a corresponding rise or fall of the blood level of another hormone).

Neurologic stimuli are controlled by the autonomic and central nervous systems (CNS). For example, the autonomic system regulates blood pressure through glandular secretions and release of renin. In response to stimuli, the CNS activates the hypothalamus, which in turn activates the pituitary. Depending on the problem, the pituitary can then activate various other glands. Altered endocrine functions include hypofunction, hyperfunction, secondary failure, functional disorders, end-stage organ failure, abnormal hormone production, inborn errors of metabolism, ectopic hormone secretion, and organ-induced endocrine dysfunction.

The hematopoietic system encompasses the functions of blood and blood-forming processes. A type of connective tissue, blood contains plasma and cellular components. Plasma is composed of ions, proteins (*e.g.*, albumin, globulins), nonprotein nitrogen, glucose, and electrolytes. Albumin maintains an osmotic force that keeps fluid within the vascular space. Globulins are varied and have distinct purposes (*e.g.*, gamma globulins are antibodies). Cellular components of blood include erythrocytes, leukocytes, platelets, and fat droplets (chylomicrons). In the interior of spongy bones and the central cavity of long bones, red bone marrow produces blood cells.

The primary functions of the hematopoietic system include blood cell production (bone marrow); oxygen transport to tissues (erythrocytes); clot formation (platelets); defense against bacterial, viral (*e.g.*, lymphocyte B cell), fungal, and parasitic infections, cancer, and foreign tissue invasion (lymphocyte, T cell); and providing anticoagulation (basophils).

Potential Complication: Metabolic/Immune/Hematopoietic

DEFINITION

PC: Metabolic/Immune/Hematopoietic: Describes a person experiencing or at high risk to experience various endocrine, immune, or metabolic dysfunctions.

Author's Note

The nurse can use this generic collaborative problem to describe a person at risk for several types of metabolic and immune system problems. For example, for a client with pituitary dysfunction, who is at risk for various metabolic problems, using *PC: Metabolic* directs nurses to monitor endocrine system function for specific problems, based on focus assessment findings. Under this collaborative problem, nursing interventions would focus on monitoring metabolic status to detect and diagnose abnormal functioning. If a specific complication developed in the client, the nurse would add the appropriate specific collaborative problem, along with nursing management information, to the client's problem list. For a client with diabetes mellitus, the nurse would add the diagnostic statement *PC: Hypo/Hyperglycemia*. For a client receiving chemotherapy, the nurse would use *PC: Immunodeficiency*, a collaborative problem that encompasses leukopenia, thrombocytopenia, and erythrocytopenia. If thrombocytopenia were an isolated problem, it would warrant a separate diagnostic statement (*i.e., PC: Thrombocytopenia*).

For a client with a condition or undergoing a treatment that produces immunosuppression (*e.g.*, acquired immunodeficiency syndrome [AIDS], graft-versus-host disease, immunosuppressant therapy), the collaborative problem *PC: Immunosuppression* would be appropriate. When conditions have or possibly could have affected coagulation (*e.g.*, chronic renal failure, alcohol abuse, anticoagulant therapy), a collaborative problem such as *PC: Hemolysis* or *PC: Erythrocytopenia* would be indicated. If the risk factors or etiology were not directly related to the primary medical diagnosis, they could be added (*e.g.*, *PC: Immunosuppression related to chronic corticosteroid therapy* in a client who has sustained a myocardial infarction).

Focus Assessment Criteria

Subjective Data

1. Complaints of change in appearance of face, hair (distribution, growth, texture), skin (pigmentation, dryness), eyesight, weight (gain or loss)
2. Complaints of headaches, change in libido and/or menses, excessive sweating, easy bruising, poor wound healing, sensitivity to cold or heat, nausea, anorexia, excessive urination, excessive thirst, excessive appetite, diarrhea, constipation, easy fatigability, frequent infections

Objective Data

1. Temperature
2. Pulse, respiration
3. Blood pressure
4. Urine: ketones, specific gravity
5. Weight for height
6. Ability to eat
7. Diet: calories and protein adequate to meet metabolic demands

Significant Laboratory/Diagnostic Assessment Criteria

1. Serum amylase (elevated in acute pancreatitis, lowered in chronic pancreatitis)
2. Serum albumin (lowered in malnutrition)
3. Lymphocyte count (lowered in malnutrition)
4. Serum calcium (elevated in hyperparathyroidism, certain cancers, and acute pancreatitis, lowered in hypoparathyroidism)
5. Blood pH (elevated in alkalosis, lowered in acidosis)
6. Serum glucose (elevated in diabetes mellitus and pancreatic insufficiency, lowered in pancreatic islet cell tumors)
7. Serum glycosylated hemoglobin (reflects mean glucose levels for preceding 2–3 months)
8. Urine acetone, urine glucose (present in diabetes mellitus)
9. Urine ketone bodies (present in uncontrolled diabetes)
10. Platelets (elevated in polycythemia and chronic granulocytic leukemia, lowered in anemia and acute leukemia)
11. Immunoglobins (elevated in autoimmune disease)
12. Coagulation tests (elevated in thrombocytopenia, purpura, and hemophilia)
13. Prothrombin time (elevated in anticoagulant therapy, cirrhosis, and hepatitis)
14. Red blood cell (RBC) count (lowered in anemia, leukemia, and renal failure)

PC: Hypo/Hyperglycemia

DEFINITION

PC: Hypo/Hyperglycemia: Describes a person experiencing or at high risk to experience a blood glucose level that is too low or too high for metabolic function.*

High-Risk Populations

- Diabetes mellitus
- Parenteral nutrition
- Sepsis
- Enteral feedings
- Corticosteroid therapy
- Neonate of diabetic mother
- Small-for-gestational-age neonate
- Neonate of narcotic-addicted mother
- Thermal injuries (severe)
- Pancreatitis (hyperglycemia), cancer of pancreas
- Addison's disease (hypoglycemia)
- Adrenal gland hyperfunction
- Liver disease (hypoglycemia)

Nursing Goals

The nurse will manage and minimize episodes of hypoglycemia or hyperglycemia.

Interventions

For Hypoglycemia

1. Monitor serum glucose level at the bedside before administering hypoglycemic agents and/or before meals and hour of sleep.
   (Serum glucose is a more accurate parameter than urine glucose, which is affected by renal threshold and renal function.)
2. Monitor for signs and symptoms of hypoglycemia:
   a. Blood glucose level below 70 mg/dL
   b. Pale, moist, cool skin
   c. Tachycardia, diaphoresis
   d. Jitteriness, irritability
   e. Hypoglycemia unawareness
   f. Incoordination
   g. Drowsiness, confusion
   (Hypoglycemia [insufficient glucose levels] can result from excessive insulin, insufficient food intake, or excessive physical activity. A rapid drop in blood glucose level stimulates the sympathetic system to produce adrenaline, which causes diaphoresis, cool skin, tachycardia, and jitteriness [American Diabetes Association, 1989; Hass, 1993].)

* If the person is not at risk for both, the diagnosis should specify the problem (*e.g.*, PC: Hyperglycemia related to corticosteroid therapy).

3. If the client can swallow, give him ½ cup of orange juice, cola, or ginger ale every 15 minutes until his blood glucose level reaches above 69 mg/dL.
(Simple carbohydrates are metabolized quickly.)

4. If the client cannot swallow, administer glucagon hydrochloride subcutaneously or 50 mL of 50% glucose in water IV, according to protocol.
(Glucagon causes glycogenolysis in the liver in the presence of adequate glycogen stores. In a client in critical condition who has been in a coma for some time, glycogen stores likely have already been used up, and IV glucose is the only effective treatment.)

5. Recheck blood glucose level 1 hour after an initial blood glucose reading of greater than 69 mg/dL.
(Regular monitoring detects early signs of high or low levels.)

6. If indicated, consult with a dietitian to provide a complex carbohydrate snack at bedtime.
(This measure can help prevent hypoglycemia during the night.)

For Hyperglycemia

1. Monitor for signs and symptoms of diabetic ketoacidosis:
   a. Blood glucose level greater than 300 mg/dL
   b. Positive plasma ketone, acetone breath
   c. Headache
   d. Kussmaul's respirations
   e. Anorexia, nausea, vomiting
   f. Tachycardia
   g. Decreased blood pressure
   h. Polyuria, polydipsia
   i. Decreased serum sodium, potassium, and phosphate levels
   (When insulin is not available, blood glucose levels rise and the body metabolizes fat for energy-producing ketone bodies. Excessive ketone bodies cause headaches, nausea, vomiting, and abdominal pain. Respiratory rate and depth increase to help increase CO_2 excretion and reduce acidosis. Glucose inhibits water reabsorption in the renal glomerulus, leading to osmotic diuresis with severe loss of water, sodium, potassium, and phosphates. Diabetic ketoacidosis occurs in type I diabetes [Davidson, 1991].)

2. If ketoacidosis occurs, initiate appropriate protocols to reverse dehydration, restore the insulin–glucagon ratio, and treat circulatory collapse, ketoacidosis, and electrolyte imbalance (Thelan et al., 1990):
   a. IV infusion of physiologic saline or half-strength sodium chloride
      (Infusion rate is adjusted according to urinary output to achieve rapid hydration.)
   b. IV infusion of 5% dextrose in ½ normal saline when serum glucose is 250–300 mg/dL
      (This replenishes glucose stores and prevents cerebral edema.)
   c. Insulin in IV fluids (approximately 6–10 U/hour)
      (Insulin is needed to facilitate entry of glucose in cells.)
   d. IV potassium and phosphate supplements
      (Deficits may occur as potassium and phosphate return to the cells because of insulin.)
   e. IV bicarbonate
      (For severe acidosis [pH >7], bicarbonate levels should be above 5 mEq/L.)
   f. Identify the etiology of diabetic ketoacidosis

3. Continue to monitor hydration status every ½ hour, assess skin moisture and turgor, urine output and specific gravity, and fluid intake.
(Accurate assessments are needed during the acute stage [first 10–12 hours] to prevent overhydration or underhydration.)

4. Continue to monitor blood glucose levels every ½ hour until stable.
(Careful monitoring enables early detection of medication-induced hypoglycemia or continued hyperglycemia.)

5. Monitor serum potassium, sodium, and phosphate levels.
(Acidosis causes hyperkalemia and hyponatremia. Insulin therapy promotes potassium and phosphate return to the cells, causing serum hypokalemia and hypophosphatemia).

6. Monitor neurologic status every hour.
   (Fluctuating glucose levels, acidosis, and fluid shifts can affect neurologic functioning.)
7. Carefully protect the client's skin from microorganism invasion, injury, and shearing force; reposition every 1–2 hours.
   (Dehydration and tissue hypoxia increase the skin's vulnerability to injury.)
8. Do not allow a recovering client to drink large quantities of water. Give a conscious client ice chips to quench thirst.
   (Excessive fluid intake can cause abdominal distention and vomiting.)
9. Monitor for signs and symptoms of hyperosmolar hyperglycemic nonketotic (HHNK) coma:
   a. Blood glucose 600–2000 mg/dL
   b. Serum sodium, potassium normal or elevated
   c. Elevated hematocrit, BUN
   d. Nausea, vomiting
   e. Hypotension, tachycardia
   f. Dehydration, weight loss, poor skin turgor
   g. Lethargy, stupor, coma
   h. Elevated urine glucose ($>2^+$)
   i. Urine ketones negative or $<2^+$
   j. Polyuria
   (HHNK occurs as a result of relative insulin deficiency. Hyperglycemia and hyperosmolality are present, but these are an absence of significant ketones. HHNK coma can occur in response to acute stress [*e.g.*, from myocardial infarction, burns, severe infection, dialysis, or hyperalimentation]. People with type II insulin-resistant diabetes who experience marked dehydration are especially at risk. Glucose inhibits water reabsorption in the renal glomerulus, leading to osmotic diuresis with loss of water, sodium, potassium, and phosphates. Cerebral impairment results from intracellular dehydration in the brain.)
10. Monitor cardiac function and circulatory status; evaluate
    a. Rate, rhythm (cardiac, respiratory)
    b. Skin color
    c. Capillary refill time, central venous pressure
    d. Peripheral pulses
    e. Serum potassium
    (Severe dehydration can cause reduced cardiac output and compensatory vasoconstriction. Cardiac dysrhythmias can result from potassium imbalances.)
11. Follow protocols for ketoacidosis, as indicated.
12. Investigate for causes of ketoacidosis or hypoglycemia, and teach prevention and early management, using the nursing diagnosis *Risk for Ineffective Management of Therapeutic Regimen related to insufficient knowledge of (specify)* (see Section II).

🌀 Interventions—*Child Focus*

1. Refer also to Interventions.
2. Consult with dietitian for nutritional management.
   (The goal is a consistent, well-balanced diet to ensure normal growth and development.)
3. Evaluate child's growth and development.
   (Poor control of glucose levels affects growth.)
4. Teach about condition, insulin therapy, self-monitoring of glucose, nutrition, exercise, and prevention of complications.
5. Consult with school nurse for management at school.
   (Effective management is a team effort.)

PC: Negative Nitrogen Balance

DEFINITION

PC: Negative Nitrogen Balance: Describes a person experiencing or at risk to experience catabolism, when more nitrogen is excreted from tissue breakdown than is replaced by intake.

High-Risk Populations

- Severe malnutrition
- Prolonged NPO state
- Elderly with chronic disease
- Uncontrolled diabetes
- Digestive disorders
- Prolonged use of glucose or saline IV therapy
- Inadequate enteral replacement
- Excessive catabolism (*e.g.*, due to cancer, infection, burns, surgery, excess stress)
- Anorexia nervosa, bulimia
- Critical illness
- Chemotherapy
- Sepsis

Nursing Goals

The nurse will manage and minimize negative nitrogen balance.

Interventions

1. Establish the client's optimum weight for height.
   (This establishes baseline goals.)
2. Weigh the client daily at the same time, wearing same amount of clothes, same scale, and same bedding.
   (Monitoring weight helps detect excessive catabolism.)
3. Monitor for signs of negative nitrogen balance.
   a. Weight loss
   b. 24-Hour urine nitrogen balance below zero
   (Cachexia results from the increased metabolic demands, insufficient replacement, and anorexia. Impaired carbohydrate metabolism causes increased metabolism of fats and protein, which—especially in the presence of metabolic acidosis—can lead to negative nitrogen balance and weight loss.)
4. Monitor for signs and symptoms of hypoalbuminemia, which can have a rapid or insidious onset:
   a. Emotional depression, fatigue
   (These effects result from decreased energy supplies.)
   b. Muscle wasting
   (This results from insufficient protein available for tissue repair.)
   c. Poorly healing wounds
   (This results from insufficient protein available for tissue repair.)
   d. Edema
   (Edema results from a plasma-to-interstitial fluid shift due to insufficient vascular osmotic pressure.)
5. Monitor laboratory values:
   a. Serum prealbumin and transferrin

(These values evaluate visceral protein. Prealbumin is a precursor to albumin and a much more sensitive measure of visceral protein [Ackerman, Evans, & Ecklund, 1994].)

   b. Blood urea nitrogen

(This value measures kidney clearance ability.)

   c. 24-Hour urine nitrogen

(Because the glomerulus of the kidney reabsorbs 99% of what is filtered, measurement of urea nitrogen, a waste product of protein metabolism, gives data to calculate the nitrogen balance [Ackerman et al., 1994].)

   d. Electrolytes, osmolality

(These values help assess kidney function.)

   e. Total lymphocyte count

(Lymphocyte production requires protein.)

6. Continually reevaluate the client's energy/protein requirements. Consult with a registered dietitian for evaluation (*e.g.*, indirect calorimetry test, anthropometric measures). (The person's calorie/protein requirements will change depending on metabolic demands, *e.g.*, from stress, fever, or infection.)

7. Administer total parenteral solutions, intralipid fat emulsions, and/or enteral formulas as prescribed by the physician and in accordance with appropriate procedures and protocols. (This client's increased caloric requirements for tissue repair cannot be met with routine IV therapy.)

8. For specific nursing interventions to increase oral nutrient intake, refer to the nursing diagnosis *Altered Nutrition: Less Than Body Requirements* (see Section II).

PC: Electrolyte Imbalances*

- *Related to* **Hypokalemia**
- *Related to* **Hyperkalemia**
- *Related to* **Hyponatremia**
- *Related to* **Hypernatremia**
- *Related to* **Hypocalcemia**
- *Related to* **Hypercalcemia**
- *Related to* **Hypophosphatemia**
- *Related to* **Hyperphosphatemia**
- *Related to* **Hypomagnesemia**
- *Related to* **Hypermagnesemia**
- *Related to* **Hypochloremia**
- *Related to* **Hyperchloremia**

DEFINITION

PC: Electrolyte Imbalances: Describes a person experiencing or at risk to experience a deficit or excess of one or more electrolytes.

* For a person experiencing or at high risk to experience a deficit or excess in a single electrolyte, the diagnostic statement should specify the problem (*e.g., PC: Hypokalemia related to diuretic therapy*).

High-Risk Populations

For Hypokalemia
- Crash dieting (diabetic ketoacidosis [DKA])
- Metabolic or respiratory alkalosis
- Excessive intake of licorice
- Diuretic therapy
- Loss of gastrointestinal (GI) fluids (through excessive nasogastric suctioning, nausea, vomiting, or diarrhea)
- Steroid use
- Estrogen use
- Hyperaldosteronism
- Severe burns
- Decreased potassium intake
- Liver disease with ascites
- Renal tubular acidosis
- Malabsorption
- Severe catabolism
- Salt depletion
- Hemolysis
- Hypoaldosteronism
- Rhabdomyolysis

For Hyperkalemia
- Renal failure
- Excessive potassium intake (oral or IV)
- Cell damage (*e.g.*, from burns, trauma, surgery)
- Crushing injuries
- Potassium-sparing diuretic use
- Adrenal insufficiency
- Lupus
- Sickle cell disease
- Post transplant
- Chemotherapy
- Metabolic acidosis
- Transfusion of old blood
- Internal hemorrhage

For Hyponatremia
- Water intoxication (oral or IV)
- Renal failure
- Gastric suctioning
- Vomiting, diarrhea
- Burns
- Potent diuretic use
- Excessive diaphoresis
- Excessive wound drainage
- Congestive heart failure
- Hyperglycemia
- Malabsorption syndrome
- Cystic fibrosis
- Addison's disease
- Psychogenic polydipsia
- Oxytocin administration
- Syndrome of inappropriate antidiuretic hormone (resulting from CNS disorders, major trauma, malignancies, or endocrine disorders)

For Hypernatremia
- Elderly, infants
- Inadequate fluid intake
- Heat stroke
- Diarrhea
- Severe insensible fluid loss (*e.g.*, through hyperventilation or sweating)
- Diabetes insipidus
- Excessive sodium intake (oral, IV, medications)
- Hypertonic tube feeding
- Coma

For Hypocalcemia
- Renal failure ($\uparrow$ phosphorus)
- Protein malnutrition (*e.g.*, due to malabsorption)
- Inadequate calcium intake
- Diarrhea
- Burns
- Malignancy
- Hypoparathyroidism
- Vitamin D deficiency
- Excessive antacid use
- Osteoblastic tumors

For Hypercalcemia
- Chronic renal failure
- Sarcoidosis and granulomatous disease
- Excessive vitamin D intake
- Hyperparathyroidism
- Decreased hypophosphatemia
- Bone tumors
- Cancers (Hodgkin's disease, myeloma, leukemia, neoplastic bone disease)
- Prolonged use of thiazide diuretics
- Paget's disease
- Parathyroid hormone-secreting tumors (*e.g.*, lung, kidney)
- Hemodialysis
- Multiple fractures
- Prolonged immobilization

For Hypophosphatemia
- Diabetic ketoacidosis
- Prolonged use of IV dextrose solutions
- Malabsorption disorders
- Renal wasting of phosphorus
- Low-phosphate diet (oral, total parenteral nutrition)
- Rickets
- Excessive use of phosphate binders
- Osteomalacia
- Alcoholism

For Hyperphosphatemia
- Excessive vitamin D intake
- Renal failure
- Healing fractures
- Bone tumors
- Hypoparathyroidism
- Hypocalcemia
- Phosphate laxatives
- Excessive IV or PO phosphate

- Chemotherapy
- Catabolism
- Lactic acidosis

For Hypomagnesemia
- Malnutrition
- Prolonged diuretic use
- Chronic alcoholism
- Excessive lactation
- Severe diarrhea, nasogastric suctioning
- Cirrhosis
- Severe dehydration
- Ulcerative colitis
- Toxemia
- Burns
- Cisplatinum use
- Hyperthryroidism/Cushing's disease
- Prolonged IV therapy without magnesium

For Hypermagnesemia
- Addison's disease
- Renal failure
- Severe dehydration with oliguria
- Excessive intake of magnesium-containing antacids, laxatives
- Thiazide use

For Hypochloremia
- Loss of GI fluids (*e.g.*, through vomiting, diarrhea, suctioning)
- Metabolic alkalosis
- Diabetic acidosis
- Prolonged use of IV dextrose
- Excessive diaphoresis
- Excessive diuretic use
- Ulcerative colitis
- Fever
- Acute infections
- Severe burns

For Hyperchloremia
- Metabolic acidosis
- Severe diarrhea
- Excessive parenteral isotonic saline solution infusion
- Urinary diversion
- Renal failure
- Cushing's syndrome
- Hyperventilation
- Eclampsia
- Anemia
- Cardiac decompensation

Nursing Goals

The nurse will manage and minimize episodes of electrolyte imbalance(s).

Interventions

Identify the electrolyte imbalance(s) for which the client is vulnerable, and intervene as follows. (Refer to High-Risk Populations under the specific imbalance.)

PC: Hypo/Hyperkalemia

1. Monitor for signs and symptoms of hyperkalemia:
   a. Weakness to flaccid paralysis
   b. Muscle irritability
   c. Paresthesias
   d. Nausea, abdominal cramping, or diarrhea
   e. Oliguria
   f. Electrocardiogram (ECG) changes: tall, tented T-waves, ST segment depression, prolonged PR interval (greater than 0.2 second), first-degree heart block, bradycardia, broadening of the QRS complex, eventual ventricular fibrillation, and cardiac standstill (Baer & Lancaster, 1992)

   (Hyperkalemia can result from the kidney's decreased ability to excrete potassium or from excessive potassium intake. Acidosis increases the release of potassium from cells. Fluctuations in potassium level affect neuromuscular transmission, producing cardiac dysrhythmias, and reducing action of GI smooth muscle.)

2. For a client with hyperkalemia
   a. Restrict potassium-rich foods, fluids, and IV solutions with potassium.
      (High potassium levels necessitate a reduction in potassium intake.)
   b. Provide range-of-motion (ROM) exercises to extremities.
      (ROM improves muscle tone and reduces cramps.)
   c. Per physician orders or protocols give medications to reduce serum potassium levels, such as

      IV calcium
      (To block effects on the heart muscle temporarily)
      Sodium bicarbonate, glucose, insulin
      (To force potassium back into cells)
      Cation-exchange resins (*e.g.*, kayexalate, hemodialysis)
      (To force excretion of potassium)

3. Monitor for signs and symptoms of hypokalemia:
   a. Weakness or flaccid paralysis
   b. Decreased or absent deep tendon reflexes
   c. Hypoventilation, change in consciousness
   d. Polyuria
   e. Hypotension
   f. Paralytic ileus
   g. ECG changes: U wave, low-voltage or inverted T wave, dysrhythmias, and prolonged QT interval
   h. Nausea, vomiting, anorexia

   (Hypokalemia results from losses associated with vomiting, diarrhea, or diuretic therapy, or from insufficient potassium intake. Hypokalemia impairs neuromuscular transmission and reduces the efficiency of respiratory muscles. Kidneys are less sensitive to antidiuretic hormone and thus excrete large quantities of dilute urine. GI smooth muscle action also is reduced. Abnormally low potassium levels also impair electrical conduction of the heart. [Baer & Lancaster, 1992].)

4. For a client with hypokalemia
   a. Encourage increased intake of potassium-rich foods.
      (An increase in dietary potassium intake helps ensure potassium replacement.)
   b. If parenteral potassium replacement (always diluted) is instituted, do not exceed 20 mEq/hour in adults. Monitor serum potassium levels during replacement.
      (Excessive levels can cause cardiac dysrhythmias.)
   c. Observe the IV site for infiltration.
      (Potassium is very caustic to tissues.)

PC: Hypo/Hypernatremia

1. Monitor for signs and symptoms of hyponatremia:
   a. CNS effects ranging from lethargy to coma, headache

    b. Weakness

    c. Abdominal pain

    d. Muscle twitching or convulsions

    e. Nausea, vomiting, diarrhea

    f. Apprehension

(Hyponatremia results from sodium loss through vomiting, diarrhea, or diuretic therapy; excessive fluid intake; or insufficient dietary sodium intake. Cellular edema, caused by osmosis, produces cerebral edema, weakness, and muscle cramps.)

2. For a client with hyponatremia, initiate IV sodium chloride solutions and discontinue diuretic therapy, as ordered.

(These interventions prevent further sodium losses.)

3. Monitor for signs and symptoms of hypernatremia with fluid overload:

    a. Thirst, decreased urine output

    b. CNS effects ranging from agitation to convulsions

    c. Elevated serum osmolality

    d. Weight gain, edema

    e. Elevated blood pressure

    f. Tachycardia

(Hypernatremia results from excessive sodium intake or increased aldosterone output. Water is pulled from the cells, causing cellular dehydration and producing CNS symptoms. Thirst is a compensatory response to dilute sodium.)

4. For a client with hypernatremia

    a. Initiate fluid replacement in response to serum osmolality levels, as ordered.

      (Rapid reduction in serum osmolality can cause cerebral edema and seizures.)

    b. Monitor for seizures.

      (Sodium excess causes cerebral edema.)

5. Monitor intake and output, weight

(This evaluates fluid balance.)

PC: Hypo/Hypercalcemia

1. Monitor for signs and symptoms of hypocalcemia:

    a. Altered mental status

    b. Numbness or tingling in fingers and toes

    c. Muscle cramps

    d. Seizures

    e. ECG changes: prolonged QT interval, prolonged ST segment, and dysrhythmias

    f. Chvostek's or Trousseau's sign

    g. Tetany

(Hypocalcemia can result from the kidney's inability to metabolize vitamin D [needed for calcium absorption]. Retention of phosphorus causes a reciprocal drop in serum calcium level. A low serum calcium level produces increased neural excitability, resulting in muscle spasms [cardiac, facial, extremities] and CNS irritability [seizures]. It also causes cardiac muscle hyperactivity, as evidenced by ECG changes.)

2. For a client with hypocalcemia

    a. Per physician orders for acute hypocalcemia, administer calcium via IV bolus infusion.

    b. Consult with the dietitian for a high-calcium, low-phosphorus diet.

      (Lower serum calcium level necessitates dietary replacement.)

    c. Assess for hyperphosphatemia or hypomagnesemia.

      (Hyperphosphatemia inhibits calcium absorption; in hypomagnesemia, the kidneys will excrete calcium to retain magnesium.)

    d. Monitor for ECG changes: prolonged QT interval, irritable dysrhythmias, and atrioventricular conduction defects.

      (Calcium imbalances can cause cardiac muscle hyperactivity.)

3. Monitor for signs and symptoms of hypercalcemia:

    a. Altered mental status

    b. Anorexia, nausea, vomiting, constipation

    c. Numbness or tingling in fingers and toes
    d. Muscle cramps, hypotoxicity
    e. Deep bone pain
    f. AV blocks (ECG)
  (Insufficient calcium level reduces neuromuscular excitability, resulting in decreased muscle tone, numbness, anorexia, and mental lethargy.)
4. For a client with hypercalcemia
    a. Initiate normal saline IV therapy and loop diuretics, as ordered; avoid thiazide diuretics.
    (IV fluids dilute serum calcium. Loop diuretics enhance calcium excretion; thiazide diuretics inhibit calcium excretion.)
    b. Per physician's order, administer phosphorus preparations and mithramycin (contraindicated in clients with renal failure.)
    (These increase bone deposition of calcium.)
    c. Monitor for renal calculi (see *PC: Renal Calculi*).

PC: Hypo/Hyperphosphatemia

1. Monitor for signs and symptoms of hypophosphatemia:
    a. Muscle weakness, pain
    b. Bleeding
    c. Depressed white cell function
    d. Confusion
    e. Anorexia
  (Phosphorus deficiency impairs cellular energy resources and oxygen delivery to tissues and also causes decreased platelet aggregation.)
2. For a client with hypophosphatemia, per physician order replace phosphorus stores slowly by oral supplements, and discontinue phosphate binders.
  (This helps prevent precipitation with calcium.)
3. Monitor for signs and symptoms of hyperphosphatemia:
    a. Tetany
    b. Numbness or tingling in fingers and toes
    c. Soft tissue calcification
    d. Chvostek's and Trousseau's signs
    e. Coarse, dry skin
  (Hyperphosphatemia can result from the kidneys' decreased ability to excrete phosphorus. Elevated phosphorus does not cause symptoms in itself, but contributes to tetany and other neuromuscular symptoms in the short term and to soft tissue calcification in the long term.)
4. For a client with hyperphosphatemia
    a. Administer phosphorus-binding antacids, calcium supplements, or vitamin D, and restrict phosphorus-rich foods.
  (Supplements are needed to overcome vitamin D deficiency and to compensate for a calcium-poor diet. High phosphate decreases calcium, which increases parathyroid hormone [PTH]. PTH is ineffective in removing phosphates due to renal failure, but causes calcium reabsorption from bone and decreases tubular reabsorption of phosphate.)

PC: Hypo/Hypermagnesemia

1. Monitor for hypomagnesemia:
    a. Dysphagia, nausea, anorexia
    b. Muscle weakness
    c. Facial tics
    d. Athetoid movements (slow, involuntary twisting movements)
    e. Cardiac dysrhythmias, flat or inverted T waves, prolonged QT intervals, tachycardia, depressed ST segment
    f. Confusion
  (Magnesium deficit causes neuromuscular changes and hyperexcitability.)

2. For a client with hypomagnesemia, initiate magnesium sulfate replacement (dietary for mild deficiency, parenteral for severe deficiency), as ordered.
3. Initiate seizure precautions.
   (This protects from injury.)
4. Monitor for hypermagnesemia:
   a. Decreased blood pressure, bradycardia, decreased respirations
   b. Flushing
   c. Lethargy, muscle weakness
   d. Peaked T waves
   (Magnesium excess causes depression of central and peripheral neuromuscular function, producing vasodilation.)
5. If respiratory depression occurs, consult with the physician for possible hemodialysis.
   (Magnesium-free dialysate causes excretion.)

PC: Hypo/Hyperchloremia

1. Monitor for hypochloremia:
   a. Hyperirritability
   b. Slow respirations
   c. Decreased blood pressure
   (Hypochloremia occurs with metabolic alkalosis, resulting in loss of calcium and potassium, which produces the symptoms.)
2. For a client with hypochloremia, see *PC: Alkalosis* for interventions.
3. Monitor for hyperchloremia:
   a. Weakness
   b. Lethargy
   c. Deep, rapid breathing
   (Metabolic acidosis causes loss of chloride ions.)
4. For a client with hyperchloremia, see *PC: Acidosis* for interventions.

PC: Sepsis

DEFINITION

PC: Sepsis: Describes a person experiencing or at high risk to experience a systemic response to the presence of pathogenic bacteria, viruses, fungi, or their toxins. The microorganisms may or may not be present in the bloodstream (Ackerman, 1994).

High-Risk Populations

- Extreme age
- Drug dependency, alcoholism
- Burns, multiple trauma
- Infection (urinary, respiratory, wound)
- Immunosuppression
- Invasive lines (urinary, arterial, or central venous catheter)
- AIDS

- Disseminated intravascular coagulation
- Pressure ulcers
- Extensive slow-healing wounds
- Surgical procedures (GI, thoracic, cardiac)
- Diabetes mellitus
- Malnutrition
- Cancer
- Cirrhosis, pancreatitis
- Transplants

Infants/Children
- Viral upper respiratory infection
- Bacterial enteritis
- Burns
- Urinary tract infections
- Bite wounds (*e.g.*, dog, human)
- Craniofacial surgery
- Compromised host defenses

Nursing Goals

The nurse will manage and monitor the complications of sepsis.

Interventions

1. Monitor for signs and symptoms of sepsis (AACP/SCCM Consensus Conference Committee, 1992):
   a. Temperature >38°C or <36°C
   b. Heart rate >90 beats/minute
   c. Respiratory rate >20 breaths+/minute or $PaCO_2$ <32 torr (<4.3 kPa)
   d. White blood cell (WBC) count >12,000 cells/mm^3, <4000 cells/mm^3, or >10% immature (band) forms
2. Monitor the elderly for changes in mentation; weakness, malaise; normothermia or hypothermia; and anorexia.
   (The elderly do not exhibit the typical signs of infection. Usual presenting findings—fever, chills, tachypnea, tachycardia, and leukocytosis—frequently are absent in the elderly with significant infection [Stegle & Dries, 1994].)
3. Per physician orders, initiate anti-infectives, monitoring and management of oxygen consumption and delivery, immunomodulation, and nutritional support.
   (These four areas in the management of septic clients show promise in reducing morbidity and mortality [Ackerman, 1994].)
4. If indicated, refer to *PC: Hypovolemic Shock* for more information.

🌀 Interventions—*Child Focus*

1. Monitor temperature (temperature >41°C [105.8°F] implies bacteremia). Very young infants can be hypothermic (Boyer & Hayden, 1994).
2. Monitor for behavior changes (Boyer & Hayden, 1994).
   a. Quality of cry
   b. Response to parent stimulation
   c. State variation
   d. Response to social stimulation
   (These changes reflect compromised cerebral circulation.)
3. Monitor respiratory pattern
   (Tachypnea and acrocyanosis may reflect poor peripheral perfusion.)
4. Monitor blood pressure, peripheral pulses, and capillary refill times.

(Circulatory inadequacy can be present even with normal blood pressures [Boyer & Hayden, 1994]).

5. Monitor for cutaneous changes.
   (Petechiae, ecchymoses of distal extremities, and diffuse erythroderma can manifest with sepsis.)
6. Monitor oxygen saturation.
   (Pulse oximetry measures oxygen levels.)
7. See #3 under Interventions.

PC: Acidosis (Metabolic, Respiratory)*

DEFINITION

PC: Acidosis: Describes a person experiencing or at high risk for experiencing an acid–base imbalance due to increased production of acids or excessive loss of base.

High-Risk Populations

For Respiratory Acidosis
- Hypoventilation
- Acute pulmonary edema
- Airway obstruction
- Pneumothorax
- Sedative overdose
- Severe pneumonia
- Chronic obstructive pulmonary disease
- Asthma
- Central nervous system lesions
- Disorders of respiratory system, muscle and chest wall (myasthenia gravis, amyotrophic lateral sclerosis, Guillain-Barré syndrome)

For Metabolic Acidosis
- Diabetes mellitus
- Lactic acidosis
- Late-phase salicylate poisoning
- Uremia
- Methanol or ethylene glycol ingestion
- Diarrhea
- Intestinal fistulas
- Intake of large quantities of isotonic saline or ammonium chloride
- Renal failure (acute or chronic)

---

* When indicated, the nurse should specify the diagnosis as either *PC: Metabolic Acidosis* or *PC: Respiratory Acidosis*.

Nursing Goals

The nurse will manage and minimize complications of acidosis.

Interventions

For Metabolic Acidosis
1. Monitor for signs and symptoms of metabolic acidosis:
    a. Rapid, shallow respirations
    b. Headache, lethargy, coma
    c. Nausea and vomiting
    d. Low plasma bicarbonate and pH of arterial blood
    e. Behavior changes, drowsiness
    f. Increased serum potassium
    g. Increased serum chloride
    h. PCO_2 less than 35–40 mm Hg
    i. Decreased HCO_3
    (Metabolic acidosis results from the kidney's inability to excrete hydrogen ions, phosphates, sulfates, and ketone bodies. Bicarbonate loss results when the kidney reduces its reabsorption. Metabolic acidosis is aggravated by hyperkalemia, hyperphosphatemia, and decreased bicarbonate levels. Excessive ketone bodies cause headaches, nausea, vomiting, and abdominal pain. Respiratory rate and depth increase to increase CO_2 excretion and reduce acidosis. Acidosis affects the CNS and can increase neuromuscular irritability because of the cellular exchange of hydrogen and potassium.)
2. For a client with metabolic acidosis
    a. Initiate IV fluid replacement as ordered, depending on the underlying etiology.
       (Dehydration may result from gastric and urinary fluid losses.)
    b. If the etiology is diabetes mellitus, refer to *PC: Hypo/Hyperglycemia* for interventions.
    c. Assess for signs and symptoms of hypocalcemia, hypokalemia, and alkalosis as acidosis is corrected.
       (Rapid correction of acidosis may cause rapid excretion of calcium and potassium and rebound alkalosis.)
    d. Correct, per physician orders, any electrolyte imbalances. Refer to *PC: Electrolyte Imbalances* for specific interventions for each type of electrolyte imbalance.
    e. Monitor arterial blood gas (ABG) values, urine pH.
       (These values help evaluate the effectiveness of therapy.)

For Respiratory Acidosis
1. Monitor for signs and symptoms of respiratory acidosis:
    a. Tachycardia, dysrhythmias
    b. Blurred vision
    c. Diaphoresis
    d. Nausea and/or vomiting
    e. Restlessness, headaches
    f. Dyspnea, hypoventilation
    g. Increased respiratory effort
    h. Decreased respiratory rate
    i. Increased PCO_2
    j. Normal or decreased PO_2
    k. Increased serum calcium
    l. Decreased sodium chloride
    (Respiratory acidosis can occur when an impaired respiratory system is unable to remove CO_2, or when compensatory mechanisms that stimulate increased cardiac and respiratory efforts to remove excess CO_2 are overtaxed. An elevated $PaCO_2$ is the chief criterion. Elevated $PaCO_2$ increases cerebral blood flow, which decreases perfusion to heart, kidneys, and GI tract.)
2. For a client with respiratory acidosis

  a. Improve ventilation by
       Positioning with head of bed up
     (To promote diaphragmatic descent)
       Coaching in deep-breathing with prolonged expiration
     (To increase exhalation of CO_2)
       Aiding expectoration of mucus followed by suctioning, if needed
     (To improve ventilation–perfusion)
  b. Consult with the physician for possible use of mechanical ventilation if improvement does not occur after the preceding interventions.
  c. Administer oxygen after the client is breathing better.
     (Use of oxygen is of no value if the client is not breathing effectively [Thelan et al., 1990].)
  d. Promote optimal hydration.
     (This helps liquefy secretions and prevent mucous plugs.)
  e. Limit use of sedatives and tranquilizers.
     (Both can cause respiratory depression.)
  f. Initiate Interventions 2a–2e to correct metabolic acidosis.

PC: Alkalosis (Metabolic, Respiratory)*

DEFINITION

PC: Alkalosis: Describes a person experiencing or at high risk for experiencing an acid–base imbalance due to excessive bicarbonate or loss of hydrogen ions.

High-Risk Populations

For Respiratory Alkalosis
- Pulmonary disease
- Central nervous system disorders/lesions
- Hyperventilation
- Severe infection, fever
- Asthma
- Overly vigorous mechanical ventilation
- Restricted diaphragmatic movement (*e.g.*, due to obesity, pregnancy)
- Inadequate oxygen in inspired air
- Congestive heart failure
- Alcohol intoxication
- Cirrhosis
- Thyrotoxicosis
- Paraldehyde, epinephrine, early salicylate overdose
- Overrapid correction of metabolic acidosis

For Metabolic Alkalosis
- Prolonged vomiting, gastric suctioning, diarrhea
- Use of potent diuretics (*e.g.*, thiazides), with resultant hydrogen and potassium loss
- Corticosteroid therapy
- IV replacement with potassium-free IV solutions

* When indicated, the nurse should specify the diagnosis as either *PC: Metabolic Acidosis* or *PC: Respiratory Acidosis*.

- Primary and secondary hyperaldosteronism
- Adrenocortical hormone disease
- Prolonged hypercalcemia or hypokalemia
- Excessive correction of metabolic acidosis

Nursing Goals

The nurse will manage and minimize complications of alkalosis.

Interventions

For Metabolic Alkalosis
1. Monitor for early signs and symptoms of metabolic alkalosis:
   a. Tingling of fingers, dizziness
   b. Hypertonic muscles (tremors)
   c. Hypoventilation (to conserve carbonic acid)
   d. Increased HCO_3
   e. Slightly increased PCO_2
   f. Decreased serum chloride, serum potassium, serum calcium
   g. Hypoventilation
   h. Polydipsia
   (A decrease in ionized calcium produces most symptoms.)
2. For a client with metabolic alkalosis
   a. Initiate physician order for parenteral fluids.
      (To correct sodium, water, chloride deficits)
   b. Monitor carefully the administration of ammonium chloride if ordered.
      (Ammonium chloride increases the amount of circulating hydrogen ions, which results in a decrease in pH. Treatment can cause too-rapid decrease in pH and hemolysis of RBCs.)
   c. Evaluate renal and hepatic function before administration of ammonium chloride.
      (Impaired renal or hepatic function cannot accommodate increased hemolysis.)
   d. Administer sedatives and tranquilizers cautiously, if ordered.
      (Both depress respiratory function.)
   e. Monitor ABG values, urine pH, serum electrolyte levels, and blood urea nitrogen.
      (These values help evaluate response to treatment and detect rebound metabolic acidosis resulting from too-rapid correction.)

For Respiratory Alkalosis
1. Monitor for respiratory alkalosis:
   a. Lightheadedness
   b. Numbness, tingling
   c. Carpopedal spasm
   d. Muscle weakness
   e. Normal or decreased HCO_3
   f. Decreased PCO_2
   g. Decreased serum potassium
   h. Increased serum chloride
   i. Decreased serum calcium
   (Decrease in plasma carbonic acid content causes vasoconstriction, decreased cerebral blood flow, and decreased ionized calcium.)
2. For a client with respiratory alkalosis
   a. Determine the cause of hyperventilation.
      (Different etiologies warrant different interventions, *e.g.*, anxiety versus incorrect mechanical ventilation.)
   b. Calm the anxious person by maintaining eye contact and remaining with him or her.
      (Anxiety increases respiratory rate and CO_2 retention.)

c. Instruct the person to breathe slowly with you.
(This increases CO_2 retention.)

d. Alternatively, have the anxious person breathe into a paper bag and rebreathe from the bag.
(This increases $PaCO_2$ as the person rebreathes his own exhaled CO_2.)

e. If anxiety is causative, refer to the nursing diagnoses *Anxiety* and *Ineffective Breathing Patterns* in Section II for additional interventions.

f. Consult with the physician for use of sedation as necessary.
(Sedation can help reduce respiratory rate and anxiety.)

g. Monitor ABG values and electrolyte levels (*e.g.*, potassium, calcium).
(Monitoring these values helps evaluate the client's response to treatment.)

h. As necessary, refer to *PC: Electrolyte Imbalances* for specific management of electrolyte imbalance.

PC: Allergic Reaction

DEFINITION

PC: Allergic Reaction: Describes a person experiencing or at high risk to experience hypersensitivity and release of mediators to specific substances (antigens).

High-Risk Populations

- History of allergies
- Asthma
- Immunotherapy
- Individuals exposed to high-risk antigens:
  - Insect stings (*e.g.*, bee, wasp, hornet, ant)
  - Animal bites/stings (*e.g.*, stingray, snake, jellyfish)
  - Radiologic iodinated contrast media (*e.g.*, used in arteriography, intravenous pyelography)
  - Transfusion of blood and blood products
- High-risk individuals exposed to
  - High-risk medications (*e.g.*, aspirin, antibiotics, tetanus, opiates, local anesthetics, animal insulin, chymopapain)
  - High-risk foods (*e.g.*, peanuts, chocolate, eggs, seafood, shellfish, strawberries, milk)
  - Chemicals (*e.g.*, floor waxes, paint, soaps, perfume, new carpets)

Nursing Goals

The nurse will manage and minimize complications of allergic reactions.

Interventions

1. Carefully assess for history of allergic responses (*e.g.*, rashes, difficulty breathing).
(Identifying a high-risk client allows precautions to prevent anaphylaxis.)

2. If the client has a history of allergic response, consult with the physician regarding skin tests, if indicated.
   (Skin testing can confirm hypersensitivity.)
3. Monitor for signs and symptoms of localized allergic reaction:
   a. Wheals, flares (due to histamine release)
   b. Itching
   c. Nontraumatic edema (perioral, periorbital)
   (These early manifestations can indicate the beginning of a continuum of localized reaction to systemic reaction to anaphylactic shock.)
4. At the first sign of hypersensitivity, consult with the physician for pharmacologic intervention, such as antihistamines.
   (Antihistamines are commonly used to treat mild localized reactions by inhibiting histamine release.)
5. Monitor for signs and symptoms of systemic allergic reaction and anaphylaxis:
   a. Lightheadedness, skin flushing, and slight hypotension (resulting from histamine-induced vasodilation)
   b. Throat or palate tightness, wheezing, hoarseness, dyspnea, and chest tightness (due to smooth muscle contraction from prostaglandin release)
   c. Irregular, increased pulse and decreased blood pressure (due to leukotriene release, which constricts airways and coronary vessels)
   d. Decreased level of consciousness, respiratory distress, and shock (resulting from severe hypotension, respiratory insufficiency, and tissue hypoxia)
   (Within minutes, such reactions can progress to severe hypotension, decreased level of consciousness, and respiratory distress, and can prove rapidly fatal.)
6. Promptly initiate emergency protocol for anaphylaxis and/or stat page physician.
   a. Start an IV line.
      (For rapid medication administration)
   b. Administer epinephrine IV or endotracheally.
      (To produce peripheral vasoconstriction, which raises blood pressure and acts as a β agonist to promote bronchial smooth muscle relaxation, and to enhance inotropic and chronotropic cardiac activity)
   c. Administer oxygen, establish a patent airway if indicated. Oropharyngeal intubation may be required.
      (Laryngeal edema interferes with breathing.)
7. Administer other medications, as ordered, which may include:
   a. Corticosteroids
      (To inhibit enzyme and WBC response to reduce bronchoconstriction)
   b. Aminophylline
      (To produce bronchodilation)
   c. Vasopressins
      (To counter profound hypotension)
   d. Diphenhydramine
      (To prevent further antigen–antibody reaction)
8. Frequently evaluate response to therapy; assess
   a. Vital signs
   b. Level of consciousness
   c. Lung sounds, peak flows
   d. Cardiac function
   e. Intake and output
   f. ABG values
   (Careful monitoring is necessary to detect complications of shock and identify the need for additional interventions.)
9. After recovery, discuss with the client and family preventive measures for anaphylaxis and the need to carry an anaphylaxis kit, which contains injectable epinephrine and oral histamines for use in self-treating allergic reaction.

PC: Thrombocytopenia

DEFINITION

PC: Thrombocytopenia: Describes a person experiencing or at high risk to experience insufficient circulating platelets. This decrease can be caused by a reduction in platelet production, a change in platelet distribution, platelet destruction, or vascular dilution (Goebel, 1993).

High-Risk Populations

Decreased Platelet Production due to

- Chemotherapy
- Radiation therapy
- Bone marrow invasion by tumor
- Leukemia
- Heparin therapy
- Toxins
- Severe infection
- Alcoholism
- Aplastic anemia

Increased Platelet Destruction due to

- Antibodies
- Aspirin
- Alcohol
- Quinine, quinidine
- Digoxin
- Sulfonamides
- Entrapment in large spleen
- Infections (bacteremia, postviral infections)
- Renal disease
- Post-transfusion status

Increased Platelet Utilization due to

- Disseminated intravascular coagulation
- Thrombotic thrombocytopenic purpura
- Liver disease
- Administration of several units of non–platelet-containing fluids

Nursing Goals

The nurse will manage and minimize complications of decreased platelets.

Interventions

1. Monitor complete blood count (CBC), hemoglobin, coagulation tests, and platelet counts. (These values help evaluate response to treatment and risk for bleeding. Platelet count $<20,000/mm^3$ indicates a high risk for intracranial bleeding.)
2. Assess for other factors that may lower platelet count in addition to the primary cause, such as
   a. Abnormal hepatic function
   b. Abnormal renal function

    c. Infection, fever

    d. Anticoagulant use

    e. Alcohol use

    f. Aspirin use

    g. Administration of several units of non–platelet-containing fluids (*e.g.*, packed RBCs)

  (Assessment may identify factors that could be controllable [McNally, Stair, & Smernilly, 1985].)

3. Monitor for signs and symptoms of spontaneous or excessive bleeding:

    a. Spontaneous petechiae, ecchymoses, hematomas

    b. Bleeding from nose or gums

    c. Prolonged bleeding from invasive procedures such as venipunctures or bone marrow aspiration

    d. Hematemesis or coffee-ground emesis

    e. Hemoptysis

    f. Hematuria

    g. Vaginal bleeding

    h. Rectal bleeding

    i. Gross blood in stools

    j. Black, tarry stools

    k. Change in vital signs

    l. Change in neurologic status (blurred vision, headache, disorientation)

    m. Urine, feces, and emesis positive for occult blood

    n. High pad count for menstruating women

  (Constant monitoring is needed to ensure early detection of bleeding episodes [McNally et al., 1985].)

4. Assess for systemic signs of bleeding and hypovolemia:

    a. ↑ Pulse, ↑ respirations, ↓ blood pressure

    b. Changes in neurologic status (*e.g.*, subtle mental status changes, blurred vision, headache, disorientation)

  (Changes in circulatory oxygen levels produce changes in cardiac, vascular, and neurologic functioning.)

5. If hemorrhage is suspected, refer to *PC: Hypovolemic Shock* for specific interventions. Anticipate platelet transfusion.

6. Apply direct pressure for 5–10 minutes, then a pressure dressing, to all venipuncture sites. Monitor carefully for 24 hours.

  (These measures promote clotting and reduce blood loss.)

7. Treat nausea aggressively to prevent vomiting.

  (Severe vomiting can cause GI bleeding.)

8. Minimize rectal probing.

  (This avoids injury to rectal tissue and bleeding.)

9. Using the nursing diagnosis *Risk for Injury related to bleeding tendency* (see Section II), implement nursing interventions and teaching to reduce the risk of trauma.

PC: Opportunistic Infections

DEFINITION

PC: Opportunistic Infections: Describes a person experiencing or at high risk to experience an infection by an organism capable of causing disease only when immune system dysfunction is present.

High-Risk Populations

- Immunosuppressive therapy (chemotherapy, antibiotics)
- Malignancy
- Sepsis
- AIDS
- Nutritional deficits
- Burns
- Trauma
- Extensive pressure ulcers
- Radiation therapy (long bones, skull, sternum)
- Elderly with chronic illness
- Drug/alcohol addiction

Nursing Goals

The nurse will manage and minimize complications of immunodeficiency.

Interventions

1. Monitor CBC, WBC differential (neutrophils, lymphocytes), and absolute neutrophil count (WBC × neutrophil).
   (These values help evaluate response to treatment.)
2. Monitor for signs and symptoms of primary or secondary infection:
   a. Slightly increased temperature
   b. Chills
   c. Adventitious breath sounds
   d. Cloudy or foul-smelling urine
   e. Complaints of urinary frequency, urgency, or dysuria
   f. Presence of WBCs and bacteria in urine
   g. Redness, change in skin temperature, swelling or unusual drainage in any area of disrupted skin integrity, including previous and current puncture sites
   h. Irritation or ulceration of oral mucous membrane
   i. Complaints of perineal or rectal pain and any unusual vaginal or rectal discharge
   j. Increased hemorrhoidal pain, redness, or bleeding
   k. Painful, pruritic skin lesions (herpes zoster), particularly in cervical or thoracic area
   l. Change in WBC count, especially an increase in immature neutrophils
   (In a client with severe neutropenia, the usual inflammatory responses may be decreased or absent.)
3. Obtain culture specimens (*e.g.,* urine, vaginal, rectal, mouth, sputum, stool, blood, skin lesions) as ordered.
   (Testing determines the type of causative organism and guides treatment.)

4. Monitor for signs and symptoms of septicemia.
   (Gram-positive and gram-negative organisms can invade open wounds, causing septicemia. A debilitated client is at increased risk. Sepsis produces massive vasodilation, resulting in hypovolemia and subsequent tissue hypoxia. Hypoxia leads to decreased renal function and cardiac output, triggering a compensatory response of increased respirations and heart rate in an attempt to correct hypoxia and acidosis. Bacteria in urine or blood indicates infection.)
5. Monitor for therapeutic and nontherapeutic effects of antibiotics.
6. Monitor for signs and symptoms of opportunistic protozoal infections:
   a. *Pneumocystis carinii* pneumonia: dry, nonproductive cough, fever, gradual to severe dyspnea
   b. *Toxoplasma gondii* encephalitis: headache, lethargy, seizures
   c. *Cryptosporidium* enteritis: watery diarrhea, nausea, abdominal cramps, malaise
   (Immunodeficient clients are at risk for secondary diseases of opportunistic infections; protozoal infections are the most common and serious.)
7. Monitor for signs and symptoms of opportunistic viral infections:
   a. Herpes simplex oral or perirectal abscesses: severe pain, bleeding, rectal discharge
   b. Cytomegalovirus retinitis, colitis, pneumonitis, encephalitis, or other organ disease
   c. Progressive multifocal leukoencephalopathy: headache, decreased mentation
   d. Varicella zoster, disseminated (shingles)
8. Monitor for signs and symptoms of opportunistic fungal infections:
   a. *Candida albicans* stomatitis and esophagitis: exudate, complaints of unusual taste in mouth
   b. *Cryptococcus neoformans* meningitis: fever, headaches, blurred vision, stiff neck, confusion
9. Monitor for signs and symptoms of opportunistic bacterial infections, which commonly affect the pulmonary system:
   a. *Mycobacterium avium* (intracellular disseminated)
   b. *Mycobacterium tuberculosis* (extrapulmonary and pulmonary)
10. Emphasize the need to report symptoms promptly.
    (Early treatment of adverse manifestations often can prevent serious complications [*e.g.*, septicemia] and also increases the likelihood of a favorable response to treatment.)
11. Explain the need to balance activity and rest and to consume a nutritious diet.
    (Rest and a nutritious diet provide the client with energy to heal and to enhance the body's defense system.)
12. Avoid or minimize invasive procedures (*e.g.*, urinary catheterization, arterial or venous punctures, injections, rectal tubes, suppositories).
    (This precaution helps prevent introduction of microorganisms.)
13. Refer to the nursing diagnosis *Risk for Infection* in Section II for interventions to prevent introduction of microorganisms and to increase resistance.

PC: Sickling Crisis

DEFINITION

PC: Sickling Crisis: Describes a person with sickle cell disease experiencing vascular occlusion by the sickled cells and the hemolytic anemia (Bunn, 1991).

High-Risk Populations

People With Sickle Cell Disease With Precipitating Factors, e.g.:

- High altitude (>7000 feet above sea level)
- Unpressurized aircraft
- Dehydration (*e.g.*, diaphoresis, diarrhea, vomiting)
- Strenuous physical activity
- Cold temperatures (*e.g.*, iced liquids)
- Infection (*e.g.*, respiratory, urinary, vaginal)
- Ingestion of alcohol
- Cigarette smoking

Nursing Goals

The nurse will manage and minimize the sickling crisis.

Interventions

1. Monitor for signs and symptoms of anemia:
   a. Lethargy
   b. Weakness
   c. Fatigue
   d. Increased pallor
   e. Dyspnea on exertion
   (Because anemia is common with most of these clients, and low hemoglobins are relatively tolerated, changes should be described in reference to person's baseline or acute symptoms [Bunn, 1991].)
2. Monitor laboratory values, including CBC with reticulocyte count.
   (Reticulocyte [normal level about 1%] elevation represents active erythropoiesis. Lack of elevation in the presence of anemia may represent a problem [Eckman & Platt, 1991].)
3. Monitor for signs and symptoms of acute chest syndrome:
   a. Fever
   b. Acute chest pain
   (Acute chest syndrome is the term used to represent the group of symptoms—acute pleuritic chest pain, fever, leukocytosis, and infiltrates on chest x-ray—seen in sickle cell disease [Eckman & Platt, 1991]. This represents a medical emergency and may be caused by "sickling" leading to pulmonary infarction.)
4. Monitor for signs and symptoms of infection:
   a. Fever
   b. Pain
   c. Chills
   d. Increased WBCs
   (Bacterial infection is one of the major causes of morbidity and mortality. Decreased functioning of the spleen [asplenia] results from sickle cell anemia. The loss of the spleen's ability to filter and destroy various infectious organisms increases the risk of infection [Bunn, 1991].)
5. Monitor for changes in neurologic function:
   a. Speech disturbances
   b. Sudden headache
   c. Numbness, tingling
   (Cerebral infarction and intracranial hemorrhage are complications of sickle cell disease. Occlusion of nutrient arteries to major cerebral arteries causes progressive wall damage and eventual occlusion of the major vessel. Intracerebral hemorrhage may be secondary to hypoxic necrosis of vessel walls [Dahl, 1983].)

6. Monitor for splenic dysfunction.

(The spleen is responsible for filtering blood to remove old bacteria. Sluggish circulation and increased viscosity of sickled cells causes splenic blockage. The normal acidotic and anoxic environment of the spleen stimulates sickling, which increases blood flow obstruction [Bushanon, 1983].)

7. Monitor for splenic sequestration crisis:
   a. Sudden onset of lassitude
   b. Very pale, listless
   c. Rapid pulse
   d. Shallow respirations
   e. Low blood pressure

(Increased obstruction of blood from the spleen together with rapid sickling can cause sudden pooling of blood into the spleen. This causes intravascular hypovolemia and hypoxia, progressing to shock [Bushanon, 1983].)

8. Instruct to report the following:
   a. Any acute illness
   b. Severe joint or bone pain
   c. Chest pain
   d. Abdominal pain
   e. Headaches, dizziness
   f. Gastric distress

(These symptoms may indicate vaso-occlusion in varied sites due to sickling. Some illnesses may predispose the client to dehydration [Bunn, 1991].)

9. Initiate therapy per physician prescription (*e.g.*, antisickling agents, analgesics, transfusions).

10. Refer to the nursing diagnosis *Acute Pain* (see Section II) for interventions to manage the pain associated with a sickling crisis.

References/Bibliography

ACCP-SCCM Consensus Conference Committee. (1992). American College of Chest Physicians/Society of Critical Care Medicine Consensus Conference: Definitions for sepsis and organ failure and guidelines for the use of innovative therapies in sepsis. *Critical Care Medicines, 20*, 6.

Ackerman, M. (1994). The systemic inflammatory response, sepsis, and multiple organ dysfunction: New definitions for an old problem. *Critical Care Nursing Clinics of North America, 6*, 243–250.

Ackerman, M., Evans, N., & Ecklund, M. (1994). Systemic inflammatory response, sepsis and nutritional support. *Critical Care Nursing Clinics of North America, 6*, 321–340.

American Diabetes Association. (1989). *The physician's guide to non–insulin-dependent (type II) diabetes: Diagnosis and treatment* (2nd ed.). Reston, VA: Author.

Baer, C., & Lancaster, L. (1992). Acute renal failure. *Critical Care Nursing Quarterly, 14*(4), 1–21.

Boyer, K. M., & Hayden, W. (1994). Sepsis and septic shock. In F. Oski (Ed.). *Principles and practice of pediatrics* (2nd ed.). Philadelphia: J. B. Lippincott.

Bunn, I. H. (1991). Disorders of hemoglobin. In D. Wilson (Ed.). *Harrison's principles of internal medicine* (12th ed.). New York: McGraw-Hill.

Bushanon, I. (1983). Splenic sequestration crisis in complication of sickle cell anemia. *Nursing Clinics of North America, 18*, 145–149.

Champagne, M., & Ashley, M. (1989). Nutritional support in the critically ill elderly patient. *Critical Care Nursing Quarterly, 12*(1), 15–25.

Cohen, F. (1989). Immunologic impairment, infection and AIDS in the aging patient. *Critical Care Nursing Quarterly, 12*(1), 38–45.

Dahl, J. (1983). Cerebral vascular accidents in sickle cell disease in complication of sickle cell anemia. *Nursing Clinics of North America, 18*, 145–149.

Davidson, J. K. (1991). *Clinical diabetes mellitus: A problem-oriented approach* (2nd ed.). New York: Thieme.

Eckman, J., & Platt, A. (1991). *Problem oriented management of sickle syndromes*. Atlanta: Grady Memorial Hospital.

Goebel, B. H. (1983). Bleeding disorders. In S. Groenwald, M. Frogge, M. Goodman, & C. Yarbo (Eds.). *Cancer nursing: Principles and practice*. Boston: Jones and Bartlett.

Hass, L. B. (1993). Chronic complications of diabetes mellitus. *Nursing Clinics of North America, 28*, 71–85.

Hudak, C., Gallo, B., & Benz, J. (1990). *Critical care nursing* (5th ed.). Philadelphia: J. B. Lippincott.

Isley, W., & Hamburger, S. (Eds.). (1990). Endocrine/metabolic disorders. *Critical Care Nursing Quarterly, 13*(3), 1–88.

Mahoney, E., & Flynn, J. (1986). *Handbook of medical–surgical nursing.* New York: John Wiley & Sons.

McNally, J., Stair, J. C., & Smernilly, E. (1985). *Guidelines for cancer nursing practice.* Orlando, FL: Grune & Stratton.

Porth, C. (1994). *Pathophysiology: Concepts of altered health states* (4th ed.). Philadelphia: J. B. Lippincott.

Sabo, C. E. (1989). Diabetic ketoacidosis: Pathophysiology, nursing diagnoses, and nursing interventions. *Focus on Critical Care, 16*(1), 21–28.

Schneiderman, E. (1990). Thrombocytopenia in the critically ill patient. *Critical Care Nursing Quarterly, 13*(2), 1–6.

Stegle, J., & Dries, D. (1994). Sepsis in the elderly. *Critical Care Nursing Clinics of North America, 6*, 421–428.

Thelan, L., Davie, J., & Urden, L. (1990). *Textbook of critical care nursing.* St. Louis: C. V. Mosby.

Tribett, D. (Ed.). (1989). The immunocompromised patient. *Critical Care Nursing Clinics of North America, 1*, 723–724.

U.S. Department of Health and Human Services. (1992). *Management and therapy of sickle cell disease.* U.S. Department of Health and Human Services, NIH Publication No. 92-2117. Washington, DC: U.S. Health Service.

Potential Complication: Renal/Urinary

Acute Urinary Retention

PC: Renal Insufficiency

PC: Renal Calculi

Renal and Urinary System Overview

The kidneys and urinary system have related functions but also very distinct purposes. The kidneys regulate fluid and electrolyte balance, acid–base balance, and excretion of metabolic waste products. They also regulate arterial blood pressure, erythropoiesis, and vitamin D metabolism. Highly vascular, the kidneys receive the entire circulatory volume 20 times each hour to regulate body fluid composition. Factors affecting renal clearance include age, fluid volume, renal blood flow, glomerular membrane permeability, blood pressure, and cardiac output.

The urinary system (ureters, bladder, urethra) serves as a reservoir and conduit for urine from the kidney to elimination through urination. Factors that can affect this function are infections, prostate enlargement, neurogenic bladder, and tumors.

Potential Complication: Renal/Urinary

DEFINITION

PC: Renal/Urinary: Describes a person experiencing or at high risk to experience various renal or urinary tract dysfunctions.

Author's Note

The nurse can use this generic collaborative problem to describe a person at risk for several types of renal or urinary problems. For such a client (*e.g.*, a client in a critical care unit, who is vulnerable to a variety of renal/urinary problems), using *PC: Renal/Urinary* directs nurses to monitor renal and urinary status, based on the focus assessment, to detect and diagnose abnormal functioning. Nursing management of a specific renal or urinary complication would be addressed under the collaborative problem applying to the specific complication. For example, a standard of care for a client recovering from coronary bypass surgery could contain the collaborative problem *PC: Renal/Urinary*, directing the nurse to monitor renal and urinary status. If urinary retention developed in this client, the nurse would add *PC: Urinary Retention* to the problem list, along with specific nursing interventions to manage this problem. If the risk factors or etiology were not directly related to the primary medical diagnosis, the nurse still would specify them in the diagnostic statement (*e.g.*, *PC: Renal Insufficiency related to chronic renal failure* in a client who has sustained a myocardial infarction).

Keep in mind that the nurse must differentiate those problems in bladder function that can be treated primarily by nurses as nursing diagnoses (*e.g.*, incontinence, chronic urinary retention) from those that nurses manage using both nurse-prescribed and physician-prescribed interventions (*e.g.*, acute urinary retention).

Focus Assessment Criteria

Subjective Data

1. History of symptoms
   a. Onset and duration
   b. Description
   c. Frequency
   d. Precipitating factors
   e. Alleviating factors
2. Weight (gain, loss, fluctuations)
3. Complaints of
   a. Pain, aching (costovertebral angle, urethral, bladder, scrotum/vulva, constant, with voiding)
   b. Dry, scaly skin
   c. Fatigue
   d. Inability to concentrate
   e. Fever
   f. Edema
4. History of
   a. Recent trauma
   b. Renal trauma (can have residual effects years later)
   c. Renal disease (family history)
   d. Hypertension
   e. Diabetes mellitus
   f. Lupus erythematosus
   g. Renal calculi
5. Medication use (prescribed and over-the-counter)

Objective Data

1. Urine characteristics
   a. Color
   b. Odor
   c. Appearance
   d. Specific gravity
   e. Presence of glucose, protein, ketones, red blood cells, myoglobin

Significant Laboratory/Diagnostic Assessment Criteria

1. Blood
   a. Prealbumin, albumin (lowered in renal disease)
   b. Amylase (elevated with renal insufficiency)
   c. pH, base excess, bicarbonate (lowered in metabolic acidosis, elevated in metabolic alkalosis)
   d. Calcium (lowered in uremic acidosis)
   e. Chloride (elevated with renal tubular acidosis)

    f. Creatinine (elevated with kidney disease)

    g. Magnesium (lowered in chronic nephritis)

    h. Phosphorus (elevated with chronic glomerular disease, lowered with renal tubular acidosis)

    i. Potassium (elevated in renal failure, lowered with chronic diuretic therapy, renal tubular acidosis)

    j. Proteins (total, albumin, globulin) (lowered in nephritic syndrome)

    k. Sodium (elevated with nephritis, lowered with chronic renal insufficiency)

    l. Blood urea nitrogen (BUN) (elevated in acute or chronic renal failure)

    m. Uric acid (elevated with chronic renal failure)

    n. White blood cell (WBC) count (elevated, lowered with acute and chronic infections)

2. Urine

    a. Blood (present with hemorrhagic cystitis, renal calculi, renal, bladder tumors)

    b. Creatinine (elevated in acute/chronic glomerulonephritis, nephritis, lowered in advanced degeneration of kidneys)

    c. pH (elevated with metabolic acidosis, lowered with metabolic alkalosis)

    d. Specific gravity (elevated with dehydration, lowered with overhydration, renal tubular disease)

    e. WBC count (elevated with urinary tract infections)

    f. Myoglobin

3. Renal ultrasound

4. Kidneys, ureters, bladder x-ray.

PC: Acute Urinary Retention

DEFINITION

PC: Acute Urinary Retention: Describes a person experiencing or at high risk to experience an acute abnormal accumulation of urine in the bladder and the inability to void due to a temporary situation (*e.g.*, postoperative status) or to a condition reversible with surgery (*e.g.*, prostatectomy) or medications.

High-Risk Populations

- Postoperative status (*e.g.*, surgery of the perineal area, lower abdomen)
- Postpartum status
- Anxiety
- Prostate enlargement, prostatitis
- Medication side effects (*e.g.*, atropine, antidepressants, antihistamines)
- Postarteriography status
- Bladder outlet obstruction (infection, tumor)
- Impaired detrusor contractility

Nursing Goals

The nurse will manage and minimize acute urinary retention episodes.

Interventions

1. Monitor a postoperative client for urinary retention.
   (Trauma to the detrusor muscle and injury to the pelvic nerves during surgery can inhibit bladder function. Anxiety and pain can cause spasms of the reflex sphincters. Bladder neck edema can also cause retention. Sedatives and narcotics can affect the central nervous system and the effectiveness of smooth muscles [Kemp & Tabalea, 1990].)
2. Observe for
   a. Bladder distention
   b. Urine overflow (30–60 mL of urine every 15–30 minutes)
   (Overdistention of the bladder can aggravate one's ability to empty the bladder [Kemp & Tabalea, 1990].)
3. Instruct the client to report bladder discomfort or inability to void.
   (Bladder discomfort and failure to void may be early signs of urinary retention.)
4. Monitor for urinary retention in postpartum women.
   (Labor and delivery can temporarily slacken the tone of the bladder wall, causing urinary retention.)
5. Encourage the client to void within 6 to 8 hours after delivery.
   (The desire to void may be diminished because of an increased bladder capacity related to reduced intraabdominal pressure after delivery.)
6. In a postpartum client, differentiate between bladder distention and uterine enlargement; keep in mind that
   a. A distended bladder protrudes above the symphysis pubis.
   b. When the nurse massages the uterus to return it to its midline position, the bladder protrudes further.
   c. Percussion and palpation can distinguish between a rebounding bladder (due to fluid) and a firm uterus.
   (A distended bladder can push the uterus upward and to the side and can cause uterine relaxation.)
7. If the client does not void within 8 to 10 hours after surgery or complains of bladder discomfort, take the following steps:
   a. Warm the bedpan.
   b. Encourage the client to get out of bed to use the bathroom, if possible.
   c. Instruct a man to stand when urinating, if possible.
   d. Run water in the sink as the client attempts to void.
   e. Pour warm water over the client's perineum.
   (These measures may help promote relaxation of the urinary sphincter and facilitate voiding.)
8. After the first voiding postdelivery or postsurgery, continue to monitor and encourage the client to void again in an hour or so.
   (This first voiding usually does not empty the bladder completely.)
9. If the client still cannot void after 10 hours, follow protocols for straight catheterization, as ordered by the physician.
   (Straight catheterization is preferable to indwelling catheterization because it carries less risk of urinary tract infection from ascending pathogens.)
10. For a client with chronic urinary retention, refer to the nursing diagnosis *Urinary Retention* in Section II.

PC: Renal Insufficiency

DEFINITION

PC: Renal Insufficiency: Describes a person experiencing or at high risk to experience a decrease in glomerular filtration rate that results in oliguria or anuria.

High-Risk Populations

- Renal tubular necrosis due to ischemic causes
  - Excessive diuretic use
  - Pulmonary embolism
  - Burns
  - Intrarenal thrombosis
  - Renal infections
  - Renal artery stenosis/thrombosis
  - Peritonitis
  - Sepsis
  - Hypovolemia
  - Hypotension
  - Congestive heart failure
  - Myocardial infarction
- Renal tubular necrosis due to toxicity (Thelan, Davie, & Urden, 1990)
  - Nonsteroidal antiinflammatory drugs
  - Gout
  - Hypercalcemia
  - Certain street drugs (*e.g.*, PCP)
  - Gram-negative infection
  - Radiocontrast media
  - Aminoglycoside antibiotics
  - Antineoplastic agents
  - Methanol
  - Rhabdomyolysis
  - Carbon tetrachloride
  - Phenacetin-type analgesics
  - Heavy metals
  - Insecticides
  - Aminoglycosides
- Diabetes mellitus
- Primary hypertensive disease
- Hemolysis (*e.g.*, from transfusion reaction)

Nursing Goals

The nurse will manage and minimize complications of renal insufficiency.

Interventions

1. Monitor for early signs and symptoms of renal insufficiency:
   a. Sustained elevated urine specific gravity, elevated urine sodium levels
   b. Sustained insufficient urine output (less than 30 mL/hour), elevated blood pressure

    c. Elevated BUN, serum creatinine, potassium, phosphorus, and ammonia; decreased creatinine clearance

    d. Dependent edema (periorbital, pedal, pretibial, sacral)

    e. Nocturia

    f. Lethargy

    g. Itching

    h. Nausea/vomiting

(Hypovolemia and hypotension activate the renin–angiotensin system, resulting in increased renal vasculature resistance, which decreases renal plasma flow and glomerular filtration rate [Krumberger, 1993]. Decreased glomerular filtration rate eventually causes insufficient urine output and stimulates renin production, resulting in elevated blood pressure in an attempt to increase blood flow to the kidney. Decreased excretion of urea and creatinine in the urine elevates BUN and creatinine levels. Dependent edema results from increased plasma hydrostatic pressure, salt and water retention, and/or decreased colloid osmotic pressure due to plasma protein losses.)

2. Weigh the client daily at a minimum; more often, if indicated. Ensure accurate findings by weighing at the same time each day, on the same scale, and with the client wearing the same amount of clothing.
(Daily weights and intake and output records help evaluate fluid balance and guide fluid intake recommendations.)

3. Maintain strict intake and output records: determine the net fluid balance and compare with daily weight loss or gain for correlation. (A 1-kg [2.2-lb] weight gain correlates with excess intake of 1 L.)

4. Explain prescribed fluid management goals.
(The client's and family's understanding may enhance cooperation.)

5. Adjust the client's daily fluid intake so it approximates fluid loss plus 300–500 mL/day.
(Careful replacement therapy is necessary to prevent fluid overload.)

6. Distribute fluid intake fairly evenly throughout the entire day and night. It may be necessary to match fluid intake with loss every 8 hours or even every hour if the client is critically imbalanced.
(Maintaining a constant fluid balance, without major fluctuations, is essential. Allowing toxins to accumulate because of poor hydration can cause complications such as nausea and sensorium changes.)

7. Encourage the client to express feelings and frustrations; give positive feedback.
(Fluid and diet restrictions can be extremely frustrating. Emotional support can help reduce anxiety and may improve compliance with the treatment regimen.)

8. Consult with a dietitian regarding the fluid and diet plan.
(Important considerations in fluid management, requiring a specialist's attention, include the fluid content of nonliquid food, appropriate amount and type of liquids, liquid preferences, and sodium content.)

9. Administer oral medications with meals whenever possible. If medications must be administered between meals, give with the smallest amount of fluid necessary.
(This measure avoids using parts of the fluid allowance unnecessarily.)

10. Avoid continuous IV fluid infusion whenever possible. Dilute all necessary IV drugs in the smallest amount of fluid that is safe for IV administration. Use small IV bags and an IV controller or pump, if possible, to prevent accidental infusion of a large volume of fluid.
(Extremely accurate fluid infusion is necessary to prevent fluid overload.)

11. Monitor for signs and symptoms of metabolic acidosis:
    a. Rapid, shallow respirations

    b. Headaches

    c. Nausea and vomiting

    d. Low plasma pH

    e. Behavioral changes, drowsiness, lethargy

(Acidosis results from the kidney's inability to excrete hydrogen ions, phosphates, sulfates, and ketone bodies. Bicarbonate loss results from decreased renal reabsorption. Metabolic acidosis is aggravated by hyperkalemia, hyperphosphatemia, and decreased bicarbonate levels. Excessive ketone bodies cause headaches, nausea, vomiting, and abdominal pain. Respiratory rate and depth increase in an attempt to increase CO_2 excretion and thus reduce acidosis. Acidosis affects the central nervous system [CNS] and can increase neuromuscular irritability because of the cellular exchange of hydrogen and potassium [Baer & Lancaster, 1992].)

12. For a client with metabolic acidosis, ensure adequate caloric intake while limiting fat and protein intake. Consult with a dietitian for an appropriate diet.
 (Restricting fats and protein helps prevent accumulation of acidic end products.)

13. Assess for signs and symptoms of hypocalcemia, hypokalemia, and alkalosis as acidosis is corrected.
 (Rapid correction of acidosis may cause rapid excretion of calcium and potassium and result in rebound alkalosis.)

14. Consult with the physician to initiate bicarbonate/acetate dialysis if the preceding measures do not correct metabolic acidosis:
 a. Bicarbonate dialysis for severe acidosis: dialysate − $NaHCO_3$ = 100 mEq/L
 b. Bicarbonate dialysis for moderate acidosis: dialysate − $NaHCO_3$ = 60 mEq/L
 (The acetate anion, converted by the liver to bicarbonate, is used in dialysate to combat metabolic acidosis. Bicarbonate dialysis is indicated for clients with liver impairment, lactic acidosis, or severe acid–base imbalance.)

15. Monitor for signs and symptoms of hypernatremia with fluid overload:
 a. Extreme thirst
 b. CNS effects ranging from agitation to convulsion
 (Hypernatremia results from excessive sodium intake or from increased aldosterone output. Water is pulled from the cells, causing cellular dehydration and producing CNS symptoms. Thirst is a compensatory response aimed at diluting sodium.)

16. Maintain prescribed sodium restrictions.
 (Hypernatremia must be corrected slowly to minimize CNS deterioration.)

17. Monitor for electrolyte imbalances:
 a. Potassium
 b. Calcium
 c. Phosphorus
 d. Sodium
 e. Magnesium
 (Refer to *PC: Electrolyte Imbalance* for specific signs and symptoms and interventions.)
 (Renal dysfunction can result in hyperkalemia, hypernatremia, hypocalcemia, hypermagnesemia, or hyperphosphatemia. Diuretic therapy can cause hypokalemia or hyponatremia.)

18. Monitor for gastrointestinal (GI) bleeding. (Refer to *PC: GI Bleeding* for more information and specific interventions.)
 (Bleeding may be aggravated by the poor platelet aggregation and capillary fragility associated with high serum levels of nitrogenous wastes. Heparinization required during dialysis in the presence of gastric ulcer disease also may precipitate GI bleeding.)

19. Monitor for manifestations of anemia:
 a. Dyspnea
 b. Fatigue
 c. Tachycardia, palpitations
 d. Pallor of nail beds and mucous membranes
 e. Low hemoglobin and hematocrit levels
 f. Easy bruising
 (Chronic renal failure results in decreased red blood cell production and survival time because of elevated uremic toxins.)

20. Avoid unnecessary collection of blood specimens.
 (Some blood loss occurs with every blood collection.)

21. Instruct the client to use a soft toothbrush and avoid vigorous nose blowing, constipation, and contact sports.
 (Trauma should be avoided to reduce the risk of bleeding and infection.)

22. Demonstrate the pressure method to control bleeding should it occur.
    (Applying direct, constant pressure on a bleeding site can help prevent excessive blood loss.)
23. Monitor for manifestations of hypoalbuminemia:
    a. Serum albumin level less than 3.5 g/dL; proteinuria (<100–150 mg protein/24 hours)
    b. Edema formation: pedal, facial, sacral
    c. Hypovolemia
    d. Increased hematocrit and hemoglobin levels.
    (Refer to *PC: Negative Nitrogen Balance* for more information and interventions.)
    (When albumin leaks into the urine because of changes in the glomerular electrostatic barrier or because of peritoneal dialysis, the liver responds by increasing production of plasma proteins. However, when the loss is great, the liver cannot compensate, and hypoalbuminemia results.)
24. Monitor for hypervolemia. Evaluate daily
    a. Weight
    b. Fluid intake and output records
    c. Circumference of the edematous parts
    d. Laboratory data: hematocrit, serum sodium, and plasma protein in specific serum albumin
    (As glomerular filtration rate decreases and the functioning nephron mass continues to diminish, the kidneys lose the ability to concentrate urine and to excrete sodium and water, resulting in hypervolemia.)
25. Monitor for signs and symptoms of congestive heart failure and decreased cardiac output:
    a. Gradual increase in heart rate
    b. Increasing dyspnea
    c. Diminished breath sounds, rales
    d. Decreased systolic blood pressure
    e. Presence of or increase in S_3 and/or S_4 heart sounds
    f. Gallop rhythm
    g. Peripheral edema
    h. Distended neck veins
    (Congestive heart failure can occur as a result of increased cardiac output, hypervolemia, dysrhythmias, and hypertension, resulting in reduced ability of the left ventricle to eject blood and consequent decreased cardiac output and increased pulmonary vascular congestion.)
26. Encourage adherence to strict fluid restrictions: 800–1000 mL/24 hours, or 24-hour urine output plus 500 mL.
    (Fluid restrictions are based on urine output. In an anuric client, restriction usually is 800 mL/day, which accounts for insensible losses from metabolism, the GI tract, perspiration, and respiration.)
27. Collaborate with the physician or dietitian in planning an appropriate diet. Encourage adherence to a low-sodium diet (2–4 g/day).
    (Sodium restrictions should be adjusted based on urine sodium excretion.)
28. If hemodialysis or peritoneal dialysis is initiated, follow institutional protocols.

🙋 Interventions—*Child Focus*

1. Assess for signs and symptoms unique to children with renal failure (Kohaut, 1994).
   a. Growth failure
   b. Bone deformities
   c. Abnormal tooth development
   d. Unexplained dehydration
   e. Salt craving
   (Children with renal insufficiency present differently from adults.)
2. Explore with parents child's response to exercise.
   (Lethargy and reduced exercise tolerance are two early signs of renal insufficiency [Kohaut, 1994].)

3. Per physician orders, initiate treatment for anemia, hypertension, acidosis, and renal osteodystrophy.

(These represent the key nondialytic therapy goals.)

4. Consult with dietitian.

(Children with renal dysfunction present a challenge for obtaining adequate protein for growth and development and to prevent worsening of renal function [Kohaut, 1994].)

PC: Renal Calculi

DEFINITION

PC: Renal Calculi: Describes a person with or at high risk for development of a solid concentration of mineral salts in the urinary tract.

High-Risk Populations

- History of renal calculi
- Urinary infection
- Urinary stasis
- Immobility
- Hypercalcemia (dietary)
- Conditions that cause hypercalcemia
  - Hyperparathyroidism
  - Renal tubular acidosis
  - Myeloproliferative disease (leukemia, polycythemia vera, multiple myeloma)
- Excessive excretion of uric acid
- Inflammatory bowel disease

Nursing Goals

The nurse will manage and minimize complications of renal calculi.

Interventions

1. Monitor for signs and symptoms of calculi:
   a. Increased or decreased urine output
   b. Sediment in urine
   c. Flank or loin pain
   d. Hematuria
   e. Abdominal pain, distention, nausea, diarrhea

   (Stones in the urinary tract can produce obstruction, infection, and edema, manifested by loin or flank pain, hematuria, and dysuria. Calculi in the renal pelvis may increase urine production. GI symptoms can result from calculi stimulating renointestinal reflexes [Smith, 1990].)

2. Strain urine to obtain a stone sample; send samples to the laboratory for analysis.

   (Acquiring a stone sample confirms stone formation and enables analysis of stone constituents.)

3. If the client complains of pain, consult with the physician for aggressive therapy (*e.g.*, narcotics, antispasmodics).
   (Calculi can produce severe pain from spasms and proximity of the nerve plexus.)
4. Track the pain by documenting location, any radiation, duration, and intensity (using a rating scale of 0–10).
   (This measure helps evaluate movement of calculi [Smith, 1990].)
5. Instruct the client to increase fluid intake, if not contraindicated.
   (Increased fluid intake promotes increased urination, which can help facilitate stone passage and flush bacteria and blood from the urinary tract.)
6. Monitor for signs and symptoms of pyelonephritis:
   a. Fever, chills
   b. Costovertebral angle pain (a dull, constant backache below the 12th rib)
   c. Leukocytosis
   d. Bacteria, blood, and pus in urine
   e. Dysuria, frequency
   (Urinary tract infections can be caused by urinary stasis or irritation of tissue by calculi. Signs and symptoms reflect various mechanisms. Bacteria can act as pyrogens by raising the hypothalamic thermostat through the production of endogenous pyrogen, which may be mediated through prostaglandins. Chills can occur when the temperature set-point of the hypothalamus changes rapidly. Costovertebral angle pain results from distention of the renal capsule. Leukocytosis reflects an increase in leukocytes to fight infection through phagocytosis. Bacteria and pus in urine indicate a urinary tract infection. Bacteria can irritate bladder tissue, causing spasms and frequency.)
7. Monitor for early signs and symptoms of renal insufficiency. (Refer to *PC: Renal Insufficiency.*)

References/Bibliography

Baer, C., & Lancaster, L. (1992). Acute renal failure. *Critical Care Nursing Quarterly, 14*(4), 1–21.

Hudak, C., Gallo, B., & Benz, J. (1990). *Critical care nursing* (5th ed.). Philadelphia: J. B. Lippincott.

Kaye, D. (1991). Urinary tract infection. *Medical Clinics of North America, 75*, 241–513.

Kemp, D., & Tabalea, N. (1990). Postoperative urinary retention. *Journal of Post Anesthesia Nursing, 5*, 338–341.

Kohaut, E. C. (1994). Chronic renal failure. In F. Oski (Ed.). *Principles and practice of pediatrics* (2nd ed.). Philadelphia: J. B. Lippincott.

Krumberger, J. (1993). Acute pancreatitis. *Critical Care Nursing Clinics of North America, 5*, 185–202.

Smith, L. H. (1990). The pathophysiology and medical treatment of urolithiasis. *Seminars in Nephrology, 10*, 31–52.

Thelan, L., Davie, J., & Urden, L. (1990). *Textbook of critical care nursing*. St. Louis: C. V. Mosby.

Potential Complication: Neurologic/Sensory

PC: Increased Intracranial Pressure

PC: Seizures

PC: Increased Intraocular Pressure

PC: Neuroleptic Malignant Syndrome

PC: Alcohol Withdrawal

Neurologic/Sensory System Overview

The neurologic system, in conjunction with the endocrine system, controls all body functions. Composed of the brain and spinal cord, the *central nervous system* (CNS) is divided into three major functional units: the spinal cord, the lower brain level, and the higher brain level or cortical function.

The brain contains four major structures. The *cerebrum* is divided into two hemispheres with four lobes in each (frontal, parietal, temporal, and occipital). Its functions include maintaining consciousness and controlling memory, mental processes, sensations, emotions, and voluntary movements. Included in these functions are speech, auditory recognition of written and spoken language, and vision. Located under the occipital lobe, the *cerebellum* controls balance and coordination. The *diencephalon* consists of the right and left thalamus, which function as conducting pathways for sensory impulses to the cerebral cortex, and the hypothalamus, which controls the autonomic nervous system, body temperature, and water balance and influences appetite and wakefulness.

Brain stem structures include the midbrain, pons, and medulla. The midbrain serves as a nerve pathway of the cerebral hemispheres and the lower brain. All but two of the cranial nerves originate from the brain stem. Cranial nerves III and IV originate from the midbrain; V, VI, VII, and VIII originate from the pons; and IX, X, XI, and XII originate from the medulla. The medulla contains the vasomotor center controlling heart rate and blood pressure. Respiratory centers are located throughout the brain stem (Hickey, 1992).

Consisting of 31 segments, the *spinal cord* provides conduction pathways to and from the brain and serves as the center for reflex actions.

In the *peripheral nervous system*, cranial and spinal nerves and ganglia control movements (descending pathways) and sensations (ascending pathways). The *autonomic nervous system* controls involuntary functions through the sympathetic and parasympathetic nervous systems. Sympathetic system responses include increased cardiovascular response, vasodilation, pupillary dilatation, decreased peristalsis, temperature regulation, blood glucose increases, rectal and bladder sphincter contraction, and increased secretion of sweat glands and thick saliva. The parasympathetic nervous system acts to constrict blood vessels, constrict pupils, slow heart rate, increase peristalsis, increase secretion of thin saliva, and relax rectal and bladder sphincters.

The sensory system comprises vision, hearing, olfaction, taste, and proprioception.

The eye consists of external structures, extraocular muscles, internal structures, refractory structures, and an anterior chamber. The external structures (orbit, eyelid, glands of eyelid, conjunctiva, lacrimal gland, and duct) protect and lubricate the eye. The sclera, an internal structure, provides rigid structure. The cornea allows passage of images to the retina, another internal structure. The uveal tract (choroid, ciliary body, and iris) prevents internal reflection of light, changes the shape of the lens for focusing, and controls the amount of light reaching the retina. The retina consists of the macula, retinal periphery, and optic disc. The macula provides color vision and differentiates fine details; the retinal periphery detects moving objects; and the optic disc carries impulses to the brain through the optic nerve. The refractory structures are the cornea, aqueous humor, lens, and vitreous humor. The cornea allows passages of images to the retina, and the lens performs the function of accommodation. The aqueous humor refracts light, supplies nutrients to the refractory structures, and maintains internal pressure. The vitreous humor also refracts light and maintains the spherical shape of the eyeball. The anterior chamber produces an aqueous fluid and regulates its flow, thus maintaining intraocular pressure.

The ear consists of three components: the external, middle, and inner ear. The external ear receives sound waves and directs them to the middle ear. The middle ear amplifies the waves and transmits sound to the inner ear; it also equalizes pressure. The inner ear is the receptor end organ of hearing and equilibrium; it also contains the acoustic nerve, which connects the inner ear with the brain.

The senses of olfaction and taste are discussed under the nursing diagnosis of *Altered Nutrition*. Proprioception is discussed under *Risk for Injury*.

Potential Complication: Neurologic/Sensory

DEFINITION

PC: Neurologic/Sensory: Describes a person experiencing or at high risk to experience various neurologic or sensory dysfunctions.

Author's Note

The nurse can use this generic collaborative problem to describe a person at risk for several types of neurologic or sensory problems (*e.g.*, a client recovering from cranial surgery or one who has sustained multiple trauma). For such a person, using *PC: Neurologic/Sensory* directs nurses to monitor neurologic and sensory function based on focus assessment findings. Should a complication occur, the nurse would add the applicable specific collaborative problem (*e.g.*, *PC: Increased Intracranial Pressure*) to the client's problem list to describe nursing management of the complication. If the risk factors or etiology were not directly related to the primary medical diagnosis or treatment, the nurse could add this information to the diagnostic statement. For example, for a client with a seizure disorder admitted for abdominal surgery, the nurse would add *PC: Seizures related to epilepsy* to the problem list.

In addition to the collaborative problem, the nurse should assess for other actual or potential responses that can compromise functioning. Some of these responses may represent nursing diagnoses (*e.g., Risk for Injury related to poor awareness of environmental hazards secondary to decreased sensorium*).

Focus Assessment Criteria

Subjective Data

1. Complaints of
   a. Headaches (precipitating factors, location, duration, frequency, relieving factors)

b. Vision problems (loss, double, blurred)
c. Eye pain
d. Numbness, tingling, paralysis
e. Swallowing problems (liquids or solids)
f. Speech problems (initiating, expressing)
g. Memory problems (remote, recent)
h. Inability to comprehend
i. Changes in taste, smell, hearing
j. Inability to sense hot, cold with hands, feet
k. Unstable gait
2. History of seizures (type, precipitating factors, duration, progression of symptoms)
3. History of drinking pattern (Kappas-Larson, 1993):
a. What was the day of last drink?
b. How much was consumed on that day?
c. On how many days of last 30 was alcohol consumed?
d. What was the average intake?
e. What was the most you drank?
4. Attitude toward drinking (CAGE questions):
a. Have you ever thought you should *Cut* down your drinking?
b. Have you ever been *Annoyed* by criticism of your drinking?
c. Have you ever felt *Guilty* about your drinking?
d. Do you drink in the morning (*i.e.*, *Eyeopener*) (Ewing, 1984)?

Objective Data
1. Mental status
a. Alert
b. Receptive aphasia
c. Poor memory
d. Oriented to person, place, and time
e. Confused
f. Combative
g. Unresponsive
2. Speech
a. Normal
b. Slurred
c. Garbled
d. Expressive aphasia
e. Language barrier
3. Pupils
a. Equal or unequal size
b. Reactive to light (left, right, yes, no/specify)
4. Eyes
a. Clear
b. Draining
c. Reddened
d. Other
5. Glasgow Coma Scale
a. Eyes open: spontaneously, to speech, to pain, not at all
b. Best verbal response: oriented, confused, inappropriate words, incomprehensible sounds, no response
c. Best motor response: obeys verbal commands, localizes pain, abnormal flexion withdrawal to pain, abnormal extension to pain, no response
6. Balance and gait
a. Steady
b. Unsteady
c. Description

7. Hand grasp
   a. Bilateral equality
   b. Strength
   c. Weakness/paralysis
8. Leg muscles
   a. Bilateral equality
   b. Strength
   c. Weakness/paralysis
9. Sensory acuity
   a. Visual
   b. Auditory
   c. Tactile
   d. Olfactory/gustatory
10. Cranial nerve function
    a. I (olfactory): ability to smell with each nostril
    b. II (optic): visual acuity
    c. III (oculomotor): pupillary constriction, accommodation, extraocular movements, and elevation of eyelids
    d. IV (trochlear): extraocular movements
    e. V (trigeminal): facial sensation
    f. VI (abducens): extraocular movements
    g. VII (facial): voluntary facial movements, symmetry, taste on anterior two thirds of tongue
    h. VIII (acoustic): hearing acuity
    i. IX (glossopharyngeal): pharynx, speech quality
    j. X (vagus): pharynx, speech quality
    k. XI (spinal accessory): shoulder movement, sternocleidomastoid
    l. XII (hypoglossal): voluntary tongue movements, symmetry

Significant Laboratory/Diagnostic Assessment Criteria

1. Cerebrospinal fluid
   a. Protein (increased in meningitis)
   b. White blood cell (WBC) count (increased in meningitis)
   c. Albumin (elevated with brain tumors)
   d. Glucose (decreased with bacterial meningitis)
2. Blood
   a. WBC count (elevated with bacterial infection, decreased in viral infection)
   b. Alcohol level

PC: Increased Intracranial Pressure

DEFINITION

PC: Increased Intracranial Pressure: Describes a person experiencing or at high risk to experience increased pressure (greater than 15 mm Hg) exerted by cerebrospinal fluid within the brain's ventricles or the subarachnoid space.

High-Risk Populations

- Intracerebral mass (lesions, hematomas, tumors, abscesses)
- Blood clots
- Blockage of venous outflow
- Head injuries
- Reye's syndrome
- Meningitis
- Premature birth
- Cranial surgery

Nursing Goals

The nurse will manage and minimize episodes of increased intracranial pressure (ICP).

Interventions

1. Monitor for signs and symptoms of increased ICP.
   a. Assess the following:
      Best eye opening response: spontaneously, to auditory stimuli, to painful stimuli, or no response
      Best motor response: obeys verbal commands, localizes pain, flexion–withdrawal, flexion–decorticate, extension–decerebrate, or no response
      Best verbal response: oriented to person, place, and time; confused conversation; inappropriate speech; incomprehensible sounds; or no response
   (Cerebral tissue is compromised by deficiencies of cerebral blood supply caused by hemorrhage, hematoma, cerebral edema, thrombus, or emboli. These responses evaluate the client's ability to integrate commands with conscious and involuntary movement. Cortical function can be assessed by evaluating eye opening and motor response. No response may indicate damage to the midbrain.)
   b. Assess for changes in vital signs:
      Pulse changes: slowing rate to 60 beats/minute or lower or increasing rate to 100 beats/minute or higher
   (Bradycardia is a late sign of brain stem ischemia. Tachycardia may indicate hypothalamic ischemia and sympathetic discharge.)
      Respiratory irregularities: slowing rate with lengthening apneic periods
   (Respiratory patterns vary depending on the site of impairment. Cheyne-Stokes breathing [a gradual increase followed by a gradual decrease, then a period of apnea] points to damage in both cerebral hemispheres, midbrain, and upper pons. Central neurogenic hyperventilation occurs with midbrain and upper pontine lesions. Ataxic breathing [irregular with random sequence of deep and shallow breaths] indicates pontine dysfunction. Hypoventilation and apnea occur with medullary lesions.)
      Rising blood pressure and/or widening pulse pressure
      Cushing's triad: bradycardia, increased systolic blood pressure, and increased pulse pressure
   (These are late signs of brain stem ischemia leading to cerebral herniation.)
   c. Assess pupillary responses:
      (Pupillary changes indicate pressure on oculomotor or optic nerves.)
      Inspect the pupils with a bright pinpoint light to evaluate size, configuration, and reaction to light. Compare both eyes for similarities and differences.
      (Pupil reactions are regulated by the oculomotor nerve [cranial nerve III] in the brain stem.)
      Evaluate gaze to determine whether it is conjugate (paired, working together) or if eye movements are abnormal.
      (Conjugate eye movements are regulated from parts of the cortex and brain stem.)
      Evaluate the ability of the eyes to adduct and abduct.

(Cranial nerve VI, or the abducens nerve, regulates abduction and adduction of the eyes. Cranial nerve IV, or the trochlear nerve, also regulates eye movement.)

   d. Note any other signs and symptoms:

      Vomiting

(Vomiting results from pressure on the medulla, which stimulates the brain's vomiting center.)

        Headache (constant, increasing in intensity, or aggravated by movement or straining)

(Compression of neural tissue increases ICP and causes pain.)

        Subtle changes (*e.g.*, lethargy, restlessness, forced breathing, purposeless movements, changes in mentation)

(These signs may be the earliest indicators of cranial pressure changes.)

2. Elevate the head of the bed 30 to 45 degrees unless contraindicated.

(Slight head elevation can aid venous drainage to reduce cerebrovascular congestion, thereby decreasing ICP.)

3. Avoid the following situations or maneuvers, which can increase ICP (Lee, 1989):

   a. Carotid massage

(This slows the heart rate and reduces systemic circulation, which is followed by a sudden increase in circulation.)

   b. Neck flexion or extreme rotation

(This inhibits jugular venous drainage, which increases cerebrovascular congestion and ICP.)

   c. Digital anal stimulation, breath-holding, straining

(These can initiate the Valsalva maneuver, which impairs venous return by constricting the jugular veins, thus increasing ICP.)

   d. Extreme flexion of the hips and knees

(Flexion increases intrathoracic pressure, which inhibits jugular venous drainage, increasing cerebrovascular congestion and, thus, ICP.)

   e. Rapid position changes

4. Teach the client to exhale during position changes.

(This helps prevent the Valsalva maneuver.)

5. Consult with the physician for stool softeners, if needed.

(Stool softeners prevent constipation and straining during defecation, which can trigger the Valsalva maneuver.)

6. Maintain a quiet, calm, softly lit environment. Schedule several lengthy periods of uninterrupted rest daily. Cluster necessary procedures and activities to minimize interruptions.

(These measures promote rest and decrease stimulation, both of which can help decrease ICP.)

7. Avoid sequential performance of activities that increase ICP (*e.g.*, coughing, suctioning, repositioning, bathing).

(Research has validated that such sequential activities can cause a cumulative increase in ICP [Mitchell, 1986].)

8. Monitor temperature. As indicated, initiate external hypothermia or hyperthermia measures according to the physician's orders and institutional protocol.

(Impaired hypothalamic function can interfere with temperature regulation, necessitating intervention. Hypothermia may reduce ICP, whereas hyperthermia may increase it.)

9. Limit suctioning time to 10 seconds at a time; hyperoxygenate and hyperventilate the client both before and after suctioning.

(These measures help prevent hypercapnia, which can increase cerebral vasodilation and raise ICP and prevent hypoxia, which may increase cerebral ischemia.)

10. Consult with the physician about administering prophylactic lidocaine before suctioning.

(This measure may help prevent acute intracranial hypertension [Thelan, Davie, & Urden, 1990].)

11. Maintain optimal ventilation through proper positioning and regular suctioning.

(These measures help prevent hypoxemia and hypercapnia.)

12. Monitor arterial blood gas values.
    (Arterial blood gas values help evaluate gas exchange in the lungs and determine the circulating oxygen level and arterial CO_2. It is recommended that arterial O_2 be in the range of 90–100 torr, and that arterial CO_2 be in the range of 25–30 mmHg, to prevent cerebral ischemia and cerebrovascular congestion, which increase ICP.)
13. If indicated, initiate protocols or collaborate with the physician for drug therapy, which may include the following (Thelan et al., 1990):
    a. Sedation, barbiturates
       (These drugs reduce cerebral metabolic rate, contributing to decreased ICP.)
    b. Anticonvulsants
       (These agents help prevent seizures, which increase cerebral metabolic rate.)
    c. Osmotic diuretics
       (These agents draw water from brain tissue to the plasma to reduce cerebral edema.)
    d. Nonosmotic diuretics
       (These agents draw sodium and water from edematous areas to reduce cerebral edema.)
    e. Steroids
       (These drugs can reduce capillary permeability, limiting cerebral edema.)
14. Carefully monitor hydration status; evaluate fluid intake and output, serum osmolality, and urine specific gravity and osmolality.
    (Dehydration from diuretic therapy can cause hypotension and decreased cardiac output.)
15. If IV fluid therapy is prescribed, carefully administer IV fluids with an infusion pump.
    (Careful IV fluid administration is necessary to prevent overhydration, which increases ICP.)
16. If using an ICP monitoring device, refer to the procedures manual for guidelines.

PC: Seizures

DEFINITION

PC: Seizures: Describes a person experiencing or at high risk to experience paroxysmal episodes of involuntary muscular contraction (tonus) and relaxation (clonus).

High-Risk Populations

- Family history of seizure disorder
- Cerebral cortex lesions
- Head injury
- Infectious disorder (*e.g.*, meningitis)
- Cerebral circulatory disturbance (*e.g.*, cerebral palsy, stroke)
- Brain tumor
- Alcohol overdose or withdrawal (*e.g.*, theophylline)
- Drug overdose or withdrawal
- Electrolyte imbalances
- Hypoglycemia
- High fever
- Eclampsia
- Metabolic abnormalities (renal, hepatic, electrolyte)

Nursing Goals

The nurse will manage and minimize seizure episodes.

Interventions

1. Determine whether the client senses an aura before onset of seizure activity. If so, reinforce safety measures to take when an aura is felt (*e.g.*, lie down, pull car over to roadside and shut off ignition).
2. If seizure activity occurs, observe and document the following (Hickey, 1992):
   a. Where seizure began
   b. Type of movements, parts of body involved
   c. Changes in pupil size or position
   d. Urinary or bowel incontinence
   e. Duration
   f. Unconsciousness (duration)
   g. Behavior postseizure
   h. Weakness, paralysis postseizure
   i. Sleep postseizure (postictal period)
   (Progression of seizure activity may assist in identifying the anatomic focus of the seizure.)
3. Provide privacy during and after seizure activity.
   (To protect the client from embarrassment)
4. During seizure activity, take measures to ensure adequate ventilation (*e.g.*, loosen clothing). *Do not* try to force an airway or tongue blade through clenched teeth, however.
   (Strong clonic/tonic movements can cause airway occlusion. Forced airway insertion can cause injury.)
5. During seizure activity, gently guide movements to prevent injury. Do not attempt to restrict movements.
   (Physical restraint could result in musculoskeletal injury.)
6. If the client is sitting when seizure activity occurs, ease him to the floor and place something soft under his head.
   (These measures help prevent injury.)
7. After seizure activity subsides, position the client on his side.
   (This position helps prevent aspiration of secretions.)
8. Allow the person to sleep after seizure activity; reorient on awakening.
   (The person may experience amnesia; reorientation can help him regain a sense of control and can help reduce anxiety.)
9. If person continues to have generalized convulsions, notify physician and initiate protocol:
   a. Establish airway.
   b. Suction PRN.
   c. Administer oxygen through nasal catheter.
   d. Initiate an intravenous line.
   (Status epilepticus is a medical emergency. Impaired respiration can cause systemic and cerebral hypoxia. Intravenous administration of a rapid-acting anticonvulsant [*e.g.*, diazepam] is indicated [Hickey, 1992].)
10. Keep the bed in a low position with the side rails up, and pad the side rails with blankets.
    (These precautions help prevent injury from fall or trauma.)
11. If the client's condition is chronic, evaluate the need for teaching self-management techniques. Use the nursing diagnosis *Risk for Ineffective Management of Therapeutic Regimen related to insufficient knowledge of condition, medication regimen, safety measures, and community resources* (see Section II).

PC: Increased Intraocular Pressure

DEFINITION

PC: Increased Intraocular Pressure: Describes a person experiencing or at high risk to experience increased aqueous humor production or resistance to outflow, which can cause compression of nerve fibers and blood vessels in the optic disc.

High-Risk Population

- Glaucoma
- Corneal transplant
- Radiation therapy
- Eye trauma
- Ophthalmic surgery

Nursing Goals

The nurse will manage and minimize increased intraocular pressure.

Interventions

1. Reinforce prescribed postoperative activity restrictions, which may include avoiding the following:
   a. Bending at the waist
   b. Making sudden head movements
   c. Valsalva maneuver (*e.g.*, straining during bowel movements)
   (These activities can increase intraocular pressure.)
2. Reinforce the need to wear eye protection (patch and shield).
   (These protect the eye from trauma.)
3. Monitor for bleeding, dehiscence, and evisceration.
   (Ocular tissue is vulnerable to these problems because of its high vascularity and fragile vessels.)
4. Monitor for signs and symptoms of increased intraocular pressure:
   a. Eyebrow pain
   b. Nausea
   c. Halos around lights
   (Intraocular pressure may increase in response to surgery or owing to medications, such as steroid eye drops [Schremp, 1995b].)
5. Administer an antiemetic if nausea develops.
   (Vomiting increases intraocular pressure and must be avoided.)
6. Monitor visual acuity and note any changes (*e.g.*, halos around lights).
   (Factors that can alter vision include blood in the vitreous or from the incision, infection, dislocation of the lens implant, redetachment of the retina, and increased intraocular pressure.)
7. Position the client on his back with the head elevated; turn on the unaffected side.
   (This positioning can help reduce pressure in the affected eye.)
8. Maintain a quiet environment; limit external stimuli and activities.
   (These measures can help reduce stress and may promote a decrease in intraocular pressure.)

PC: Neuroleptic Malignant Syndrome

DEFINITION

PC: Neuroleptic Malignant Syndrome (NMS): Describes a person experiencing or at high risk to experience an acute, life-threatening reaction to neuroleptic medication. The pathophysiology of NMS is poorly understood, but like other forms of extrapyramidal symptoms, there appears to be neuroleptic-induced dopaminergic blockade and dopamine depletion in the CNS, particularly in the basal ganglia and hypothalamus, which causes the various symptoms. It is most often characterized by the rapid onset of severe muscular rigidity, autonomic instability, hyperthermia, and deteriorating mental state. It occurs in 10% of patients receiving neuroleptic agents.

High-Risk Populations

- Use of neuroleptic, especially the higher-potency drugs haloperidol, fluphenazine, and chlorpromazine
- Use of long-acting depot neuroleptics
- Use of neuroleptic medications in combination with:
  - Concurrent lithium therapy
  - Physiologic stress
  - Nutritional deficiencies
  - Concurrent organic brain syndrome
  - Physical exhaustion
  - Dehydration
  - Acquired immunodeficiency syndrome
  - Restraints
  - Anticholinergic drugs
  - Agitation
  - Mood Disorders
  - High room temperature
- High doses of neuroleptic
- Concurrent use of two or more neuroleptics
- Previous history of NMS
- Male gender, younger than 40 years of age (80% of cases)
- Undergoing "rapid neuroleptization," especially if administered by injections
- Initial 2 weeks of therapy (however, it can occur at any point in neuroleptic therapy)
- Discontinuation of antiparkinsonian drugs

Nursing Goals

The nurse will manage and minimize NMS episodes.

Interventions

1. Hold doses of all neuroleptic drugs and drugs with anticholinergic properties, and notify physician.
2. Maintain airway.
   (Any patient with altered level of consciousness is at risk for airway compromise and hypoventilation. Chest wall muscle rigidity also contributes to this.)
3. Prompt recognition and treatment of cardiac dysrhythmias and blood pressure instabilities is necessary.

4. Monitor for signs and symptoms.
   a. Severe extrapyramidal symptoms
      Muscular rigidity
      Dysarthria
      Dysphagia (difficulty swallowing)
      Excess salivation
      Myoglobinuria (urine turning red)
      Akinesis
      Cogwheel rigidity
      Muteness
      Waxy flexibility
      Exaggerated deep tendon reflexes
   b. Autonomic dysfunction
      Tachycardia
      Diaphoresis
      Urinary incontinence
      Labile or sustained hypertension
      Hypotension (abnormal blood pressure)
      Dyspnea
      Tachypnea
      Pallor
      Cardiac dysrhythmias
   c. Fever above 100°F
   d. Behavioral changes or fluctuations (*e.g.*, confusion, delirium, agitation, coma, cata-
      tonic-like posturing, combativeness)
   (The underlying pathophysiology is not well understood but appears to be related to the
   blockage or depletion of the CNS neurotransmitter dopamine. Signs and symptoms of
   NMS appear to be related to the degree and sites of involvement of dopamine blockade.
   For example, muscular rigidity appears to be caused by dopamine blockade in the nigro-
   striatal pathway: fever appears to be caused by dopamine impairment in the preoptic
   anterior hypothalamus, which regulates temperature; autonomic dysfunction may be
   caused by dopamine disturbance in the spinal cord [Lazarus, 1989].)
5. Monitor for abnormal laboratory findings
      Elevated creatine phosphokinase
      Elevated WBC count
      Elevated liver functions
      Arterial blood gas
      Electrolytes
   (As the body reacts to dopamine depletion, WBC count rises, creatine phosphokinase is
   elevated because of micronecrosis of the skeletal muscles, and hepatic enzymes are elevated. Blood gas determinations measure the degree of autonomic instability. Electrolytes
   measure the effect the autonomic instability and micronecrosis have on the body systems.)
6. Assess vital signs frequently (blood pressure; temperature, pulse, respiration; and electrocardiogram) for signs of respiratory and cardiovascular decompensation.
7. Monitor degree of rigidity through deep tendon reflexes. If rigidity is worsening, further
   measures must be taken because it can affect the muscles of the vital organs.
   (Deep tendon reflexes indicate objectively whether the rigidity is worsening or improving.)
8. Monitor fluid intake and output and for signs of renal decompensation.
   (Excessive muscle breakdown [micronecrosis] can cause myoglobinuria and renal failure.)
9. Auscultate and evaluate lungs for pulmonary stasis and embolus.
   (Dysphagia can lead to aspiration pneumonia. Immobility places a person at risk for pulmonary stasis or embolus).
10. If physician orders dantrolene to help decrease muscle rigidity, remain alert for:
   a. Liver toxicity
   b. Phlebitis and tissue damage (if administered intravenously)
   (Dantrolene, a skeletal muscle relaxant, acts at the level of the sarcoplasmic reticulum,
   complementing the effects of a dopaminergic agent.)

11. Apply cooling blankets, antipyretic medications, and cool sponge baths.
    (To control fever)
12. If dysphagia is present
       Monitor food intake closely.
       Provide soft or liquid diet.
       Tube feedings or total parenteral nutrition may be needed if nutritional status continues to decline.
       Refer also to *Impaired Swallowing*.
13. Refer to *Risk for Impaired Skin Integrity* to prevent pressure ulcers.
    (Profuse diaphoresis, dehydration, urinary incontinence, and contracted limbs set the stage for skin breakdown.)
14. Provide mouth care and suctioning as needed.
    (Dysphagia can cause increased salivation.)
15. Apply eye patches and lubricants as needed.
    (These prevent exposure keratitis secondary to inadequate blinking.)
16. After recovery
       Teach client and significant others the importance of maintaining proper nutrition, sleep, exercise.
    (Physiologic depletion predisposes the person to NMS.)
       Review manifestations of NMS and teach client and significant others that if stiffness, fever, excess sweating, and racing pulse occur, immediate medical help should be sought.
(Early detection can prevent serious complications; NMS has a 11.6% mortality rate [Teglia, Hopkins, & Cunha, 1991].)

PC: Alcohol Withdrawal

DEFINITION

PC: Alcohol Withdrawal: Describes a person experiencing or at high risk to experience the complications of alcohol withdrawal (*e.g.*, delirium tremens, autonomic hyperactivity, seizures, alcohol hallucinosis, and hypertension).

High-Risk Populations

- Alcoholics

Nursing Goals

The nurse will manage and minimize alcohol withdrawal complications.

Interventions

1. Carefully attempt to determine if the client abuses alcohol. Consult with the family regarding their perception of alcohol consumption. Explain why accurate information is necessary.
   (It is critical that high-risk people be identified so that potentially fatal withdrawal symptoms can be prevented [Lerner, Marx, & Mathews, 1988].)

2. Obtain history of previous withdrawals.
   a. Delirium tremens
      Time of onset
      Manifestation
   b. Seizures
      Time of onset
      Type
   (Withdrawal occurs between 6 to 96 hours after the cessation of drinking. Withdrawal can occur in individuals who are considered "social drinkers" [6 oz of alcohol daily for a period of 3–4 weeks]. Withdrawal patterns may resemble those of previous episodes. If seizure patterns are unlike previous episodes, it may indicate another underlying pathology [Lerner et al., 1988].)
3. Obtain a complete history of prescription and nonprescription drugs taken.
   (Benzodiazepine or barbiturate withdrawal may mimic alcohol withdrawal and complicate the picture [Lerner et al., 1988].)
4. Consult with the primary physician regarding the risk of the client and initiation of benzodiazepine therapy with dosage determined by assessment findings.
   (Benzodiazepine requirements in alcohol withdrawal are highly variable and client specific. Fixed schedules may oversedate or undersedate [Lerner et al., 1988].)
5. Observe for the desired effects of benzodiazepine therapy:
   a. Relief from withdrawal symptoms
   b. Peaceful sleep but rousable
   (Benzodiazepine is the drug of choice in controlling withdrawal symptoms. Neuroleptics cause hypotension and lower seizure threshold. Barbiturates may effectively control symptoms of withdrawal but have no advantages over benzodiazepines [Lerner et al., 1988].)
6. Monitor for indicators of a drop in blood alcohol level and determine the time of onset:
   a. Anxiety
   b. Insomnia
   c. Mild tachycardia
   d. Tremors
   e. Sensory hyperacuity
   f. Low-grade fever
   g. Disorientation
   h. Dehydration
   (Once a level drops $\leq$ 100 mg/dL below the person's normal level, he or she typically manifests withdrawal. These symptoms can last up to 5 days. Withdrawal results in a hypermetabolic state due to adrenergic excess and possible alteration of prostaglandin E_1 levels [Lenzer, 1988].)
7. Monitor for withdrawal seizures.
   a. Determine time of onset.
   b. Refer also to *PC: Seizures.*
   (Withdrawal seizures can occur between 6 to 96 hours after cessation of drinking. Seizures are usually nonfocal and grand mal, last for minutes or less, and occur singly or in clusters of two to six [Lerner et al., 1988].)
8. Monitor for and intervene promptly in cases of status epilepticus.
   a. Follow institution's emergency protocol.
   (Status epilepticus is life threatening if not controlled immediately with IV diazepam.)
9. Monitor for delirium tremens:
   a. Delirium component (vivid hallucinations, confusion, extreme disorientation, and fluctuating levels of awareness)
   b. Extreme hyperadrenergic stimulation (tachycardia, hypertension or hypotension, extreme tremor, agitation, diaphoresis, and fever)
   (Delirium tremens appears on either the fourth or fifth day after cessation of drinking and resolves within 5 days [Lerner et al., 1988].)

10. Monitor and determine onset of alcohol hallucinosis.
    a. Visual, auditory, and tactile hallucinations (however, the person senses that the hallucinations are not real and is aware of his or her surroundings)
    (Alcohol hallucinosis occurs between 6 to 96 hours after abstinence and can last up to 3 days [Lerner et al., 1988].)
11. Monitor vital signs every 2 hours:
    a. Temperature, pulse, and respiration
    b. Blood pressure
    (Patients in withdrawal have elevated heart rate, respirations, and fever [Lerner et al., 1988]. Patients experiencing delirium tremens can be expected to have a low-grade fever. However, a rectal temperature greater than 37.7°C (99.9°F) is a clue to possible infection [Lenzer, 1988].)
12. Maintain the client's IV running continuously.
    (This is necessary for fluid replacement, dextrose, thiamine bolus, benzodiazepine, and magnesium sulfate administrations. Chlordiazepoxide and diazepam should not be given IM because of unpredictable absorption [Lerner et al., 1988].)
13. Refer to the nursing diagnosis *Ineffective Denial* for interventions for substance abuse.

References/Bibliography

Bolin, A. (1994). Drug watch: Neuroleptic malignant syndrome. *Emergency, 26*(11), 18–25.

Byrd, C. (1993). Neuroleptic malignant syndrome: A dangerous complication of neuroleptic therapy. *Journal of Neuroscience Nursing, 25*(1), 61–65.

Cahaill, C., & Arana, G. W. (1986). Navigating neuroleptic malignant syndrome. *American Journal of Nursing, 86*, 670–673.

Dauner, A., & Blair, D. T. (1994). Neuroleptic malignant syndrome: An unrecognized killer. *Nurse Practitioner, 19*(2), 11–16.

Drummond, B. (1990). Preventing increased intracranial pressure. *Focus on Critical Care, 17*(21), 116–122.

Ewing, J. A. (1984). Detecting alcoholism: The CAGE questionnaire. *Journal of the American Medical Association, 252*, 1905–1907.

Foley, J. (1993). Recognition and treatment of neuroleptic malignant syndrome. *Journal of Emergency Nursing, 19*(2), 139–141.

Hickey, J. V. (1992). *The clinical practice of neurological and neurosurgical nursing* (2nd ed.). Philadelphia: J. B. Lippincott.

Hudak, C., Gallo, B., & Benz, J. (1990). *Critical care nursing* (5th ed.). Philadelphia: J. B. Lippincott.

Kappas-Larson, P. (1993). Early detection and intervention for hazardous ethanol use. *Nurse Practitioner, 18*(7), 50–55.

Lazarus, A. (1989). Neuroleptic malignant syndrome. *Hospital and Community Psychiatry, 40*(12), 1229–1230.

Lee, S. (1989). Intracranial pressure changes during positioning of patients with severe head injury. *Heart and Lung, 18*, 411–414.

Lenzer, J. (1988). Infection and immune deficits in the alcoholic patient. *Physician Assistant, 7*(4), 140–151.

Lerner, W. D., Marx, J. A., & Mathews, J. J. (1988). Alcohol emergencies. *Patient Care, 30*, 112–136.

Mitchell, P. H. (1986). Intracranial hypertension: Influence of nursing care activities. *Nursing Clinics of North America, 21*, 563–567.

Rosebush, P. (1994). What is neuroleptic malignant syndrome and how it is treated? *Harvard Mental Health Letter, 11*(6), 8.

Schremp, P. (1995a). Assessment of the eye and vision. In D. Ignatavicius, M. Workman, & M. Mishler (Eds.). *Medical–surgical nursing: A nursing process approach* (2nd ed.). Philadelphia: W. B. Saunders.

Schremp, P. (1995b). Interventions for clients with eye and vision problems. In D. Ignatavicius, M. Workman, & M. Mishler (Eds.). *Medical–surgical nursing: A nursing process approach* (2nd ed.). Philadelphia: W. B. Saunders.

Staab, W. (1994). Neuroleptic malignant syndrome: Critical factors. *Critical Care Nurse, 14*(6), 77–81.

Stewart, K. (1995). What's wrong with this patient? . . . Neuroleptic malignant syndrome. *RN, 58*(2), 45–46.

Teglia, M., Hopkins, T., & Cunha, B. (1991). Neuroleptic malignant syndrome. *Heart and Lung, 20*, 202–205.

Thelan, L., Davie, J., & Urden, L. (1990). *Textbook of critical care nursing*. St. Louis: C. V. Mosby.

Potential Complication: Gastrointestinal/Hepatic/Biliary

PC: Paralytic Ileus

PC: GI Bleeding

PC: Hepatic Dysfunction

PC: Hyperbilirubinemia

Gastrointestinal, Hepatic, and Biliary Systems Overview

A tube extending from the mouth to anus, the gastrointestinal (GI) system also includes the esophagus, stomach, and small and large intestines. Its functions include ingesting and breaking down food particles into small molecules for digestion, absorbing the small molecules into the bloodstream, and eliminating undigested and unabsorbed foodstuffs and other body wastes. Specific hormones (*e.g.*, gastrin, secretin) and enzymes (*e.g.*, pepsin, hydrochloric acid), as well as large volumes of fluid, are needed for digestion, absorption, and elimination. Blood supply to the GI tract, through the thoracic and abdominal arteries, comprises about 20% of the total cardiac output—more after eating.

The body's largest gland, the liver, performs various regulatory, digestive, and other biochemical functions. Important functions include carbohydrate metabolism, fat metabolism, protein metabolism, phagocytosis (Kupffer cells), bile formation, vitamin storage (A, D, B complex), iron storage, and formulation of coagulation factors (fibrinogen, prothrombin, acceleration globulin, and factor VII). About 75% of the blood that perfuses the liver comes from the portal vein; this blood is rich with nutrients from the GI tract. The remaining hepatic blood supply comes from the hepatic artery and is oxygen rich. The hepatic vein provides the only exit pathway. Hepatic dysfunction can involve local enlargement and portal hypertension, as well as systemic effects such as altered blood coagulation and nutritional and metabolic problems.

A small, pear-shaped organ attached to the liver's inferior surface, the gallbladder stores bile for release into the intestines, where it acts in fat emulsification. The hepatic duct from the liver and the cystic duct from the gallbladder join to form the common bile duct to the duodenum.

Potential Complication: Gastrointestinal/Hepatic/Biliary

DEFINITION

PC: Gastrointestinal/Hepatic/Biliary: Describes a person experiencing or at high risk to experience compromised function in the GI, hepatic, or biliary systems. (Note: These three systems are grouped together for classification purposes. In a clinical situation, the nurse would use either *PC: Gastrointestinal, PC: Hepatic*, or *PC: Biliary* to specify the applicable system.)

Author's Note

The nurse can use these generic collaborative problems to describe a person at risk for various problems affecting the GI, hepatic, or biliary systems. Doing so focuses nursing interventions on monitoring GI, hepatic, or biliary status to detect and diagnose abnormal functioning. Should a complication develop, the nurse would add the applicable specific collaborative problem (*e.g., PC: GI Bleeding, PC: Hepatic Dysfunction*) to the problem list, specifying appropriate nursing management.

In most cases, along with these collaborative problems, the nurse treats other associated responses, using nursing diagnoses (*e.g., Altered Comfort related to accumulation of bilirubin pigment and bile salts*).

Focus Assessment Criteria

Subjective Data

1. Alcohol use (past and present)
2. IV drug use (past and present)
3. Exposure to toxins (environmental, travel, occupational)
4. History of
    a. Hepatitis
    b. Cirrhosis
    c. Peptic ulcer
    d. Renal failure
5. Complaints of
    a. Anorexia, indigestion
    b. Pruritus, jaundice
    c. Nausea, vomiting
    d. Constipation, diarrhea
    e. Edema
    f. Bleeding, easy bruising
    g. Tarry or clay-colored stools
    h. Abdominal distention
    i. Tea-colored urine

Objective Data

1. Height and weight, general nutritional status
2. Bowel sounds
3. Stool color, presence of occult blood
4. Presence of jaundice (yellowed skin, sclera)
5. Presence of spider nevi
6. Central nervous system changes

Significant Laboratory/Diagnostic Assessment Criteria

1. Serum albumin (lowered in chronic liver disease)
2. Serum amylase (elevated in biliary tract disease)
3. Bilirubin (elevated in hepatic disease, newborn hyperbilirubinemia)
4. Potassium (lowered in liver disease with ascites, vomiting, diarrhea)
5. Blood urea nitrogen (BUN; increased in hepatic failure)
6. Prothrombin time (elevated in cirrhosis, hepatitis)
7. Hemoglobin, hematocrit (decreased with bleeding)
8. Sodium (decreased with dehydration)
9. Platelets (decreased with liver disease or bleeding)
10. Abdominal x-ray
11. Urinalysis
12. Colonoscopy, barium enema
13. Endoscopy, upper GI series

PC: Paralytic Ileus

DEFINITION

PC: Paralytic Ileus: Describes a person experiencing or at high risk to experience neurogenic or functional bowel obstruction.

High-Risk Populations

- Postoperative status (bowel, retroperitoneal, or spinal cord surgery)
- Hypokalemia
- Postshock status
- Hypovolemia
- Post-trauma (*e.g.*, spinal cord)

Nursing Goals

The nurse will manage and minimize complications of paralytic ileus.

Interventions

1. In a postoperative client, monitor bowel function, looking for
   a. Bowel sounds in all quadrants returning within 24 to 48 hours of surgery
   b. Flatus and defecation resuming by the second or third postoperative day
   (Surgery and anesthesia decrease innervation of the bowels, reducing peristalsis and possibly leading to transient paralytic ileus.)
2. Do not allow the client any fluids until bowel sounds are present. When indicated, begin with small amounts. Monitor the client's response to resumption of fluid and food intake, and note the nature and amount of any emesis or stools.
   (The client will not tolerate fluids until bowel sounds resume.)

3. Monitor for signs of paralytic ileus—primarily pain, typically localized, sharp, and intermittent.
   (Intraoperative manipulation of abdominal organs and the depressive effects of narcotics and anesthetics on peristalsis can cause paralytic ileus, typically developing between the third and fifth postoperative day.)
4. If paralytic ileus is related to hypovolemia, refer to *PC: Hypovolemia* for more information and specific interventions.

PC: GI Bleeding

DEFINITION

PC: GI Bleeding: Describes a person experiencing or at high risk to experience GI bleeding.

High-Risk Populations

- Disorders of GI, hepatic, and biliary systems
- Transfusion of 5 U (or more) of blood
- Recent stress (*e.g.*, trauma, sepsis), prolonged mechanical ventilation
- Esophageal varices
- Peptic ulcer
- Colon cancer
- Platelet deficiency
- Coagulopathy
- Shock, hypotension
- Major surgery (>3 hours)
- Head injury
- Severe vascular disease
- Burns (>35% of body)

Infants/Children (Brown, 1994)
- Neonate (*swallowed maternal blood, *hemorrhagic disease, anal fissure, stress ulcers, enterocolitis, vascular malformations)
- 6 months (same as above except [*], intussusception, lymphonodular hyperplasia)
- 6 months–5 years (same as above, epistaxis, esophagitis, varices, gastritis, Meckel's diverticulum, Henoch-Schönlein purpura, polyps)
- 5–18 years (same as above, Mallory-Weiss tear, peptic ulcer, chronic ulcerative colitis, Crohn's disease, hemorrhoids)

Nursing Goals

The nurse will manage and minimize complications of GI bleeding.

Interventions

1. Monitor for signs and symptoms of GI bleeding:
   a. Nausea
   b. Hematemesis

   c. Blood in stool

   d. Decreased hematocrit or hemoglobin

   e. Hypotension, tachycardia

   f. Diarrhea or constipation

   g. Anorexia

(Clinical manifestations depend on the amount and duration of GI bleeding. Early detection enables prompt intervention to minimize complications.)

2. Monitor for occult blood in gastric aspirates and bowel movements.

3. Monitor gastric pH every 2–4 hours (Prevost & Oberle, 1993).

(Maintenance of gastric pH below 5 has decreased bleeding complications by 89% [Eisenberg, 1990].)

   a. Use pH paper that has a range from 0–7.5. Use good light to interpret the color on the pH paper.

   b. Position the client on the left side lying down.

   (The left side down position allows the tip of the nasogastric or gastrostomy tube to move into the greater curvature of the stomach and usually below the level of gastric fluid [Eisenberg, 1990].)

   c. Use two syringes (>30 mL) to obtain the aspirate. Aspirate a gastric sample and discard. Use aspirate in the second syringe for testing.

   (The first aspirate clears the tube of antacids and other substances that can alter the pH of the sample [Prevost & Oberle, 1993].)

4. Evaluate for other factors that affect the pH reading.

   a. Medications (*e.g.*, cimetidine)

   b. Tube feeding

   c. Irrigations

(False-positive and false-negative findings can result when aspirate contains certain substances.)

5. Consult with the physician for the specific prescription for titration ranges of pH and antacid administration.

(Most investigators recommend a range of 3.5–5.0 [Eisenberg, 1990].)

6. Monitor vital signs often, particularly blood pressure and pulse.

(Careful monitoring can detect early changes in blood volume.)

7. If nasogastric intubation is prescribed, use a large-bore (18-gauge) tube and follow protocols for insertion and client care.

(A nasogastric tube can remove irritating gastric secretions, blood, and clots and can reduce abdominal distention.)

8. Follow the protocol for gastric lavage, if ordered.

(Lavage provides local vasoconstriction and may help control GI bleeding.)

9. Monitor hemoglobin, hematocrit, red blood cell count, platelets, prothrombin time, partial thromboplastin time, and BUN values.

(These values reflect the effectiveness of therapy.)

10. If hypovolemia occurs, refer to *PC: Hypovolemia* for more information and specific interventions.

11. Prepare for transfusion per physician order.

(To re-establish volume status)

PC: Hepatic Dysfunction

DEFINITION

PC: Hepatic Dysfunction: Describes a person experiencing or at high risk to experience progressive liver dysfunction.

High-Risk Populations

- Cirrhosis, alcoholism
- Renal failure
- Hepatitis
- Nutritional deficiencies
- Drug or chemical toxicity (*e.g.*, ethanol, carbon tetrachloride, chloroform, phosphorus, arsenicals)
- Hyperbilirubinemia
- Cystic fibrosis
- Thalassemia
- Rh incompatibility
- Ingestion of raw fish

Nursing Goals

The nurse will manage and minimize the complications of hepatic dysfunction.

Interventions

1. Monitor for signs and symptoms of hepatic dysfunction:
   a. Anorexia, indigestion
      (GI effects result from circulating toxins.)
   b. Jaundice
      (Yellowed skin and sclera result from excessive bilirubin production.)
   c. Petechiae, ecchymoses
      (These skin changes reflect impaired synthesis of clotting factors.)
   d. Clay-colored stools
      (This can result from decreased bile in stools.)
   e. Elevated liver function tests (*e.g.*, serum bilirubin, serum transaminase)
      (Elevated values indicate extensive liver damage.)
   f. Prolonged prothrombin time
      (This reflects reduced production of clotting factors.)
2. With hepatic dysfunction, monitor for hemorrhage.
   (The liver has a central role in hemostasis. Decreased platelet count results from impaired production of new platelets from the bone marrow. Decreased clearance of old platelets by the reticuloendothelial system also results. In addition, the synthesis of coagulation factors [II, V, VII, IX, and X] is impaired, resulting in bleeding. The most frequent site is the upper GI tract. Other sites include the nasopharynx, lungs, retroperitoneum, kidneys, and intracranial, and skin puncture sites [Kucharski, 1993].)
3. Teach the client to report any unusual bleeding (*e.g.*, in the mouth after brushing teeth).
   (Mucous membranes are prone to injury because of their high surface vascularity.)
4. Monitor for portal systemic encephalopathy by assessing
   a. General appearance and behavior
   b. Orientation

    c. Speech patterns

    d. Laboratory values: blood pH and ammonia level

(Profound liver failure results in accumulation of ammonia and other toxic metabolites in the blood. The blood–brain barrier permeability increases, and both toxins and plasma proteins leak from capillaries to the extracellular space, causing cerebral edema [Kucharski, 1993].)

5. Monitor for signs and symptoms of (refer to the index under each electrolyte for specific signs and symptoms):

    a. Hypoglycemia

    (Hypoglycemia is caused by loss of glycogen stores in the liver from damaged cells and decreased serum concentrations of glucose, insulin, and growth hormones [Kucharski, 1993].)

    b. Hypokalemia

    (Potassium losses occur from vomiting, nasogastric suctioning, diuretics, or excessive renal losses [Kucharski, 1993].)

    c. Hypophosphatemia

    (The loss of potassium ions causes the proportional loss of magnesium ions [Kucharski, 1993].)

    d. Hypophosphatemia

    (Increased phosphate loss, transcellular shifts, and decreased phosphate intake contribute to hypophosphatemia [Kucharski, 1993].)

6. Monitor for acid–base disturbances.

    a. Hepatocellular necrosis can result in accumulation of organic anions, resulting in metabolic acidosis. (People with ascites often have metabolic alkalosis from increased bicarbonate levels resulting from increased sodium/hydrogen exchange in the distal tubule [Kucharski, 1993].)

7. Assess for side effects of medications. Avoid administering narcotics, sedatives, and tranquilizers and exposing the client to ammonia products.

(Liver dysfunction results in decreased metabolism of certain medications [*e.g.*, opiates, sedatives, tranquilizers], increasing the risk of toxicity from high drug blood levels. Ammonia products should be avoided because of the client's already high serum ammonia level.)

8. Monitor for signs and symptoms of renal failure. (Refer to *PC: Renal Failure* for more information.)

(Obstructed hepatic blood flow results in decreased blood to the kidneys, impairing glomerular filtration and leading to fluid retention and decreased urinary output.)

9. Monitor for hypertension.

(Fluid retention and overload can cause hypertension.)

10. Teach the client and family to report signs and symptoms of complications, such as

    a. Increased abdominal girth

    (Increased abdominal girth may indicate worsening portal hypertension.)

    b. Rapid weight loss or gain

    (Rapid weight loss points to negative nitrogen balance; weight gain, to fluid retention.)

    c. Bleeding

    (Unusual bleeding indicates decreased prothrombin time and clotting factors.)

    d. Tremors

    (Tremors can result from impaired neurotransmission due to failure of the liver to detoxify enzymes that act as false neurotransmitters.)

    e. Confusion

    (Confusion can result from cerebral hypoxia caused by high serum ammonia levels due to the liver's impaired ability to convert ammonia to urea.)

PC: Hyperbilirubinemia

DEFINITION

PC: Hyperbilirubinemia: Describes a neonate with or at high risk for development of excessive serum bilirubin levels (greater than 0.15 mg/dL).

High-Risk Neonates

- ABO incompatibility
- Rh-negative mother
- Polycythemia
- Small for gestational age
- Preterm status
- Large for gestational age
- Diabetic mother

Nursing Goals

The nurse will manage and minimize complications of hyperbilirubinemia.

Interventions

1. Prevent cold stress.
   (Metabolism of brown adipose tissue releases nonesterified free fatty acids, which compete with bilirubin for albumin-binding sites.)
2. Ensure adequate hydration and intake.
   (Optimal fluid and feedings facilitates bilirubin excretion.)
3. Monitor for signs of hyperbilirubinemia:
   a. Jaundice
      (Yellowed skin and sclera reflect excessive bilirubin production.)
   b. Manifestations of central nervous system depression (*e.g.*, lethargy, absent Moro reflex, poor sucking reflex) or excitation (*e.g.*, tremors, twitching, high-pitched cry).
      (Central nervous system effects result from deposition of unconjugated bilirubin in brain cells.)
4. Initiate phototherapy according to protocol, if indicated.
   (Phototherapy breaks down bilirubin into water-soluble products that can be excreted.)
5. If phototherapy is performed, ensure optimal hydration. Weigh the infant daily to assess fluid status.
   (Phototherapy increases fluid loss through diaphoresis.)
6. Protect the infant's eyes during phototherapy treatment. Use Plexiglas shields; ensure that lids are closed before applying shields. Provide periods out of light with eye shields removed.
   (These precautions help ensure safe treatment.)
7. Monitor for eye discharge, excessive pressure on lids, and corneal irritation.
   (These complications may result from use of eye shields.)
8. Turn the infant frequently during phototherapy.
   (Any areas not exposed to the light will remain jaundiced.)
9. Monitor temperature, checking it at least every 4 hours.
   (A nude infant is vulnerable to hypothermia; use of radiant warmers increases the risk of hyperthermia.)

References/Bibliography

Brown M. (1994). Gastrointestinal bleeding. In F. Oski (Ed.). *Principles and practice of pediatrics* (2nd ed.). Philadelphia: J. B. Lippincott.

Clochesy, J. M., Breu, C., Cardin, S., Rudy, E. B., & Whittaker, A. A. (1993). *Critical care nursing*. Philadelphia: W. B. Saunders.

Eisenberg, P. (1990). Monitoring gastric pH to prevent stress ulcer syndrome. *Focus on Critical Care, 17*, 316–322.

Hudak, C., Gallo, B., & Benz, J. (1990). *Critical care nursing* (5th ed.). Philadelphia: J. B. Lippincott.

Groenwald, S., Frogge, M., Goodman, M., & Yarbro, C. (1993). *Cancer nursing: Principles and practice* (3rd ed.). Boston: Jones & Bartlett.

Kucharski, S. (1993). Fulminant hepatic failure. *Critical Care Nursing Clinics of North America, 5*, 141–151.

Littleton, M. T. (1989). Complications of multiple trauma. *Critical Care Nursing Clinics of North America, 1*, 75–84.

Porth, C. (1994). *Pathophysiology: Concepts of altered health states* (4th ed.). Philadelphia: J. B. Lippincott.

Prevost, S., & Oberle, A. (1993). Stress ulceration in the critically ill patient. *Critical Care Nursing Clinics of North America, 5*, 163–169.

Yamada, T. (Ed.). (1995). *Textbook of gastroenterology* (2nd ed.). Philadelphia: J. B. Lippincott.

Potential Complication: Muscular/Skeletal

PC: Pathologic Fractures

PC: Joint Dislocation

Musculoskeletal System Overview

Providing the support structure for the body and housing all body systems, the skeletal system contains 206 bones, as well as ligaments (which provide stability to joints) and tendons (which connect bone to muscle). Besides their structural function, bones also provide a site for red blood cell production and mineral—especially calcium—storage. Joints, the unions between two or more bones, are classified as fibrous (*e.g.*, distal tibiofibular junction), cartilaginous (*e.g.*, symphysis pubis), or synovial (*e.g.*, wrist bones). Cartilage, a connective tissue, provides support and facilitates movement in joints, while also absorbing shock.

Skeletal muscles serve important functions in movement, posture, and heat production. Each skeletal muscle is composed of many elongated multinucleated muscle fibers, through which run slender protein threads known as myofibrils. Motor impulses transmitted from the brain through peripheral motor nerves trigger neurochemical mechanisms—acetylcholine release, calcium release, adenosine triphosphate release—that in turn control muscle contraction and relaxation.

Musculoskeletal injuries are common and range from mild to severe. Although not usually life threatening, disorders of this system—especially when chronic—can adversely affect a person's ability to perform all activities of daily living.

Potential Complication: Muscular/Skeletal

DEFINITION

PC: Muscular/Skeletal: Describes a person experiencing or at high risk to experience various musculoskeletal problems.

Author's Note

The nurse can use this generic collaborative problem to describe people at risk for several types of musculoskeletal problems (*e.g.*, all clients who have sustained multiple trauma). This collaborative problem focuses nursing management on assessing musculoskeletal status to detect and diagnose abnormalities.

For a client exhibiting a specific musculoskeletal problem, the nurse would add the applicable collaborative problem (*e.g.*, PC: *Pathologic Fractures*) to the problem list. If the risk factors or etiology were not directly related to the primary medical diagnoses, this information would be added to the diagnostic statement (*e.g.*, PC: *Pathologic Fractures related to osteoporosis*).

Because musculoskeletal problems typically affect daily functioning, the nurse must assess the client's functional patterns for evidence of impairment. Findings may have significant implications—for instance, a casted leg that prevents a woman from assuming her favorite sleeping position and impairs her ability to perform housework. After identifying any such problems, the nurse should use nursing diagnoses to address specific responses of actual or potential altered functioning.

Focus Assessment Criteria

Subjective Data

1. Complaints of
   a. Pain, tenderness (site, precipitating factors, relieving factors)
   b. Change in shape and/or size of extremity
   c. Paresthesias, paralysis
   d. Swelling, stiffness (site, precipitating factors, alleviating factors)
   e. Fatigue (pattern, alleviating factors)
   f. Difficulty moving (pattern)
2. History of
   a. Osteoporosis
   b. Joint disease
   c. Fractures
   d. Orthopedic surgery
   e. Tick bite (possibility of Lyme disease)
3. Medication use (prescribed and over-the-counter)

Objective Data

1. Balance and gait
2. Restrictive devices (*e.g.*, cast, brace)
3. Range of motion (flexion, extension, adduction, abduction, external rotation, internal rotation) in
   a. Neck
   b. Shoulders
   c. Elbows, wrists, hands, and fingers
   d. Hips
   e. Knees, ankles, feet, and toes
4. In all extremities
   a. Pulses
   b. Color and temperature
   c. Thermal sensation
   d. Sensitivity (light touch, two-point discrimination)
   e. Strength
   f. Presence of edema, atrophy

Significant Laboratory/Diagnostic Assessment Criteria

1. Laboratory
   Serum calcium (decreased in osteoporosis)
   Serum phosphorus (decreased in osteoporosis)
   Sedimentation rate (increased in inflammatory disorders)
2. Diagnostic
   X-ray   Computed tomography scan
   Magnetic resonance imaging   Bone scan
   Aspiration

PC: Pathologic Fractures

DEFINITION

PC: Pathologic Fractures: Describes a person experiencing or at high risk to experience a fracture unrelated to trauma because of defects in bone structure

High-Risk Populations

- Osteoporosis
- Cushing's syndrome
- Malnutrition
- Long-term corticosteroid therapy
- Osteogenesis imperfecta
- Bone tumors (primary or metastatic)
- Paget's disease
- Prolonged immobility

Nursing Goals

The nurse will manage and minimize complications of pathologic fractures.

Interventions

1. Monitor for signs and symptoms of pathologic fractures:
   a. Localized pain that is continuous and unrelenting (back, neck, or extremities)
   b. Visible bone deformity
   c. Crepitation on movement
   d. Loss of movement or use
   e. Localized soft tissue edema
   f. Skin discoloration
   (Detection of pathologic fractures enables prompt intervention to prevent or minimize further complications.)
2. In a client with osteoporosis, monitor for signs and symptoms of vertebral, hip, and wrist fractures, such as
   a. Pain in the lower back, neck, or wrist
   b. Localized tenderness
   c. Pain radiating to abdomen and flank
   d. Spasm of paravertebral muscles
   (Bones with high amounts of trabecular tissue [*e.g.*, hip, vertebrae, wrist] are more readily affected by progressive osteoporosis.)
3. Promote weight-bearing activities as soon as possible.
   (Weight-bearing prevents bone demineralization.)
4. Teach measures to help prevent injury and promote weight bearing, such as
   a. Using smooth movements to avoid pulling or pushing on limbs
   b. Supporting the extremities when turning in bed
   c. Lifting the buttocks up slightly when sitting to provide weight bearing to the legs and arms
5. Monitor x-ray results and serum calcium levels.
   (These diagnostic findings help evaluate the client's risk for fractures.)

6. If a fracture is suspected, maintain proper alignment and immobilize the site using pillows or a splint; notify the physician promptly.
   (Timely, appropriate intervention can prevent or minimize soft tissue damage.)
7. Teach the client and family measures to prevent or delay bone demineralization, using the nursing diagnosis *Health-Seeking Behaviors: Management of osteoporosis.*

PC: Joint Dislocation

DEFINITION
PC: Joint Dislocation: Describes a person experiencing or at high risk to experience displacement of a bone from its position in a joint.

High-Risk Populations

- Total hip replacement
- Total knee replacement
- Fractured hip, knee, shoulder

For Infants/Children
- Birth trauma (*e.g.*, breech, first born)
- Sports
- Cerebral palsy (hip)

Nursing Goals

The nurse will manage and minimize complications of joint dislocation.

Interventions

1. Maintain correct positioning:
   a. Hip: Maintain the hip in abduction, neutral rotation, or slight external rotation.
   b. Hip: Avoid hip flexion over 60 degrees.
   c. Knee: Slightly elevated from hip; avoid using bed knee gatch or placing pillows under the knee (to prevent flexion contractures). Pillows should be placed under the calf.
   (Specific positions are used to prevent prosthesis dislocation.)
2. Assess for signs of joint (hip, knee) dislocation:
   a. Hip
      Acute groin pain in operative hip
      Shortening of leg and in external rotation
   b. Hip, knee, shoulder
      "Popping" sound heard by the client   Bulge at the surgical site
      Inability to move   Pain with mobility
   (Until the surrounding muscles and joint capsule heal, joint dislocation may occur if positioning exceeds the limits of the prosthesis, as in flexing or hyperextending the knee or abducting the hip more than 45 degrees.)

3. Maintain bed rest as ordered. Keep the affected joint in a neutral position with rolls, pillows, or specified devices.

    (Bed rest typically is ordered for 1–3 days after surgery to allow stabilization of the prosthesis.)

4. The client may be turned toward either side unless contraindicated by the physician. Always maintain an abduction pillow when turning; limit the use of Fowler's position.

    (If proper positioning is maintained, including the abduction pillow, clients may safely be turned toward the operative and nonoperative side. This promotes circulation and decreases the potential for pressure ulcer formation as a result of immobility. A prolonged Fowler's position can dislocate the prosthesis [Johnson, 1993].)

5. Monitor for shoulder joint dislocation/subluxation.

    (Total shoulder arthroplasty has a higher risk of joint dislocation/subluxation because the shoulder is capable of movement in three planes [flexion/extension, abduction/adduction, internal/external rotation] [Johnson, 1993].)

Interventions—*Child Focus*

1. Evaluate neonate for developmental dysplasia of the hip (Sponsellar, 1994).
    a. "Clunk" sound of subluxation or dislocation (Barlow test)
    b. Abducting and lifting hip back in place (Ortolani test).
    (These maneuvers test for instability.)
2. For infants older than 6 months, assess for (Sponsellar, 1994)
    a. Asymmetry
    b. Abduction and full extension limitations
    c. Shortened flexed thigh length on dysplasic side
    (After 6 months, the Barlow and Ortolani tests are often falsely negative because of diminished laxity.)

References/Bibliography

Groenwald, S., Frogge, M., Goodman, M., & Yarbro, C. (Eds.). (1995). *Cancer nursing: Principles and practice* (3rd ed.). Boston: Jones & Bartlett.

Johnson, R. (1993). Total shoulder arthroplasty. *Orthopedic Nursing, 12*(1), 14–22.

National Association of Orthopaedic Nurses. (1991). *Core curriculum for orthopaedic nursing* (2nd ed.). Pitman, NJ: Anthony J. Jannetti.

Orr, P. M. (1990). An educational program for total hip and knee replacement patients as part of a total arthritis center program. *Orthopaedic Nursing, 9*(15), 61–69.

Sponsellar, P. (1994). Bone, joint and muscle problems. In F. Oski (Ed.). *Principles and practice of pediatrics* (2nd ed.). Philadelphia: J. B. Lippincott.

Thelan, L., Davie, J., & Urden, L. (1990). *Textbook of critical care nursing*. St. Louis: C. V. Mosby.

Potential Complication: Reproductive

PC: Prenatal Bleeding

PC: Preterm Labor

PC: Pregnancy-Associated Hypertension

PC: Fetal Distress

PC: Postpartum Hemorrhage

Reproductive System Overview

The female reproductive system is composed of external genitalia (mons pubis, labia majora, labia minora, clitoris, vestibule) and internal genitalia (ovaries, fallopian tubes, uterus, vagina). Neuroendocrine interactions control the reproductive cycle. In this cycle, the ovarian follicle grows into the graafian follicle in response to secretion of follicle-stimulating hormone (FSH) and luteinizing hormone (LH) by the anterior pituitary. The preovulatory phase involves the maturation of graafian follicle and rising estrogen production. Anterior pituitary secretion of LH then stimulates ovulation. The graafian follicles release the ovum, then form the corpus luteum, which secretes increased amounts of estrogen and progesterone to stimulate endometrial growth. If the ovum is not fertilized, the corpus luteum regresses and decreases secretion of estrogen and progesterone, and menstruation—uterine discharge of blood, epithelial cells, fluid, and mucus—occurs.

The male reproductive system also consists of external genitalia (scrotum, testes, penis, epididymis) and internal genitalia (vas deferens, spermatic cord, inguinal canal, ejaculatory ducts, urethra). Accessory glands—seminal vesicles, prostate gland, and Cowper's glands—secrete substances that contribute to semen volume.

Androgens, especially testosterone, control differentiation of fetal external genitalia, development of secondary male sex characteristics, maturation of sperm, and growth and development of male sex organs. The anterior pituitary secretes FSH, which stimulates production of spermatogenesis, and interstitial cell–stimulating hormone, which stimulates production of spermatogenesis and activates cells of Leydig to produce testosterone.

Factors that can cause problems with male or female reproductive system function include hormone imbalances, trauma, tumors, vascular and structural defects, and bacterial and viral infections.

Potential Complication: Reproductive

DEFINITION

PC: Reproductive: Describes a person experiencing or at high risk to experience a problem in reproductive system functioning.

> ### Author's Note
>
> This generic collaborative problem provides a category under which to classify more specific collaborative problems affecting the reproductive system. Unlike the other generic collaborative problems (*e.g., PC: Respiratory, PC: Cardiac*), it is of little clinical use by itself. So instead of adding this generic collaborative problem to a client's problem list, the nurse should use the appropriate specific collaborative problem, such as *PC: Fetal Distress* or *PC: Postpartum Hemorrhage.*

Focus Assessment Criteria

Subjective Data

1. Menses (usual, change, midcycle, bleeding)
2. Pregnancy history
3. Contraceptive history
4. If pregnant, date of last menstrual period, presence of cramping, bleeding, or spotting
5. Complaints of
   a. Discomfort or pain with intercourse and/or urination
   b. Penile or vaginal discharge
   c. Breast discharge, lumps, other changes
   d. Stress incontinence
   e. Rectal pain or itching
   f. Difficulty starting or stopping urinary stream
   g. Genital rashes, lesions, or growths
   h. Testicular swelling, pain
   i. Excess warmth or hot flushes
   j. Sleep disturbances
6. Does client or family have special practices or remedies during menses? During pregnancy?

Objective Data

1. Vital signs (fetal heart rate, rhythm)
2. Presence of edema (peripheral, facial)
3. Presence of discharge
4. Breast examination findings
5. Female genital examination findings
6. Male genital examination findings
7. Postpartum monitoring
   a. Vital signs
   b. Urine output
   c. Uterine fundus (height, size, tone)

    d. Perineum
    e. Lochia
    f. Breast assessment

Significant Laboratory/Diagnostic Assessment Criteria

1. Gram stain for diplococci (positive in gonorrhea)
2. Venereal Disease Research Laboratory (VDRL) test (positive in syphilis)
3. Cervical, urethral smears (positive in infections)
4. Pap smear (positive in dysplasia, carcinoma)
5. Fetal pH (lowered in hypoxia)

PC: Prenatal Bleeding

DEFINITION

PC: Prenatal Bleeding: Describes a woman experiencing or at high risk to experience bleeding during pregnancy.

High-Risk Populations

- Spontaneous therapeutic abortion
- Ectopic pregnancy
- Gestational trophoblastic disease (hydatidiform mole)

For Placenta Previa
- Multiparity
- Previous placenta previa
- Uterine abnormalities
- Increased maternal age
- Multiple gestation
- Previous cesarean section
- Endometritis

For Abruptio Placentae
- Shortened umbilical cord
- Trauma
- Precipitous labor
- Uterine abnormalities
- Hypertension
- Folic acid deficiency
- Compression of vena cava
- History of abruption
- High multiparity
- Oxytocin induction
- Second born of multiple births (*e.g.*, twins, triplets)
- Increased maternal age
- Cocaine/amphetamine use

- Cigarette smoking
- Excessive alcohol consumption

Nursing Goals

The nurse will manage and minimize complications of prenatal bleeding.

Interventions

1. Teach the client to report unusual bleeding immediately.
2. If bleeding occurs, notify physician and monitor
    a. Amount
    b. Presence of cramps, contractions, pain, or tenderness
    c. Vital signs
    d. Urine output
3. Monitor fetal heart tones (refer to *PC: Fetal Distress* for specific guidelines).
4. Do not perform vaginal or rectal examinations if placenta previa is suspected. (These procedures can tear the placenta, causing life-threatening hemorrhage.)
5. Maintain the client in a supine position. (This position reduces compression on the vena cava, which increases perfusion to the fetus.)
6. Administer oxygen by face mask at a rate of 8 L/minute, as indicated. (Supplemental oxygen therapy increases maternal circulating oxygen to the fetus.)
7. If signs of shock occur, refer to *PC: Hypovolemic shock* for more information on nursing management.
8. Refer to the nursing diagnosis *Grieving* for interventions to provide support.

PC: Preterm Labor

DEFINITION

PC: Preterm Labor: Describes a woman experiencing or at high risk to experience expulsion of a viable fetus before the 38th week of gestation.

High-Risk Population

- Age (younger than 19 years or older than 40 years)
- Low socioeconomic status
- Maternal medical conditions (*e.g.*, infection, renal disease, hypertension)
- Premature membrane rupture
- Multifetal gestation
- Previous premature birth
- Previous second trimester abortion
- Uterine anomalies
- Cervical incompetency
- Closely spaced pregnancies
- Low-weight, small-stature mother

- Heavy work outside home
- Hydramnios
- Poor weight gain
- Tobacco use
- Substance abuse
- Premature bleeding
- Reproductive tract infection
- Cervical dilation >2 cm by 32 weeks
- Diethylstilbestrol exposure in utero

Nursing Goals

The nurse will manage and minimize complications of premature labor.

Interventions

1. Teach the client to watch for and report (May & Mahlmeister, 1994)
   a. Menstrual-like cramps, abdominal tightening
   b. Low backache
   c. Pelvic pressure
   d. Change in character of vaginal secretions
   e. Diarrhea
   f. Vaginal spotting or bleeding
   g. Urinary tract infection
   (Early detection of impending premature labor enables interventions to ensure successful delivery and decrease the risk of complications.)
2. Once labor begins, stay with the client and provide emotional support.
   (Reassurance and support can help the client prepare for and cope with premature birth.)
3. Maintain constant bed rest.
   (Bed rest is thought to reduce pressure of the fetal presenting part on the cervix, thus improving uterine blood flow [May & Mahlmeister, 1994].)
4. Ensure optimal hydration (oral and/or IV).
   (Studies indicate that hydration inhibits the antidiuretic hormone and suppresses uterine activity [Armson, Samuels, & Miller, 1992].)
5. Monitor fetal heart rate and rhythm.
6. If intravenous tocolytic therapy (*e.g.*, magnesium sulfate, ritodrine, nifedipine, indomethacin) is prescribed, refer to protocol for preparation (*e.g.*, baseline laboratory tests, electrocardiogram [ECG]) and administration.
7. During intravenous tocolytic therapy (Mandeville & Troiano, 1992)
   a. Establish a baseline and then assess pulse, respirations, blood pressure, breath sounds.
      Every 15 minutes during loading doses, with dosage increases, or with unstable vital signs
      Every 1 hour during maintenance
      (Cardiopulmonary complications of tocolytic therapy can be fatal; close monitoring is essential.)
   b. With magnesium sulfate
      Assess deep tendon reflexes and level of consciousness every 1 hour.
      (Hypermagnesemia can cause central nervous system [CNS] depression.)
      Ensure antidote calcium gluconate is available at bedside.
   c. Evaluate uterine activity every 1 hour.
      (This information is necessary to evaluate the effectiveness of the therapy.)
   d. With ritodrine
      Assess urine for ketones hourly or with every void.
      Auscultate breath sounds and assess for cough, chest pain, or shortness of breath every 2 hours.

   e. Maintain NPO status and hourly intake and output during infusion.
   f. Maintain bed rest in lateral recumbent position.
     (Uterine perfusion is increased in this position.)
   g. Notify physician if the following occur:
        Respiratory rate less than 12/minute or more than 24/minute
        Abnormal breath sounds, signs and symptoms of dyspnea, or mild coughing
        Pulse rate greater than 120 beats/minute, systolic pressure less than 90 mm Hg or
           diastolic pressure less than 40 mm Hg
        Decreasing deep tendon reflexes or level of consciousness
        Fetal heart rate above 160 beats/minute or nonreassuring
        Six or more uterine contractions per minute
        ECG changes

PC: Pregnancy-Associated Hypertension

DEFINITION

PC: Pregnancy-Associated Hypertension: Describes a woman experiencing or at high risk to experience a multisystem disease with vasoconstriction, hypertension (systolic pressure 140 mm Hg or higher or a diastolic pressure 90 mm Hg or higher), proteinuria, and edema during pregnancy.

High-Risk Populations

- Younger than 21 years of age
- Older than 35 years of age
- Preexisting renal disease
- Diabetes mellitus
- Vascular disease
- Multifetal pregnancy
- Hydatidiform mole
- Chronic hypertensive disease
- History of pregnancy-associated hypertension

Nursing Goals

The nurse will manage and minimize complications of hypertension.

Interventions

1. Monitor blood pressure and compare readings to those taken earlier in the pregnancy.
   (Midway through pregnancy, blood pressure commonly is lower than the woman's usual reading; thus, any elevation—even if readings still are within normal limits—may be significant [May & Mahlmeister, 1994].)
2. Monitor daily weights.
   (Sudden weight gain of 2 lb or more can indicate tissue or occult edema.)

3. Monitor for edema, particularly in the ankles, fingers, and face.
   (Edema results from sodium retention related to decreased glomerular filtration.)
4. Monitor laboratory results for proteinuria.
   (Peripheral arterial vasoconstriction leads to decreased glomerular filtration.)
5. Assess for and teach to report (Mandeville & Troiano, 1992)
   > Edema
   > Visual disturbances
   > Dyspnea
   > Decreased urine output
   > Headache
   > Blurred vision
   > Nausea and vomiting
   > Change in level of consciousness
   > Epigastric pain

   (These are indicators of cerebral edema, pulmonary edema, and GI, renal, or hepatic impairments.)
6. Teach a client exhibiting mild hypertension with minimal or no edema or proteinuria to
   a. Restrict activities and rest in bed most of the day.
   b. Increase dietary protein intake to compensate for losses in urine.
   c. Measure and record intake, output, and weight daily.
7. For a client with progressive or severe hypertension and/or proteinuria, hospitalization may be indicated with
   a. Complete bed rest in left lateral position
   b. Daily weight, intake, and output monitoring
   c. Daily urinalysis for protein and casts
   d. Sedation
   e. Magnesium sulfate therapy
8. Ensure that the client gets as much undisturbed rest as possible.
   (Adequate rest promotes relaxation and may help reduce hypertension and decrease the risk of seizure activity.)
9. Assess deep tendon reflexes of biceps and quadriceps and compare responses on each side (May & Mahlmeister, 1994).
   (CNS irritability increases the reflex response.)
10. Assess for signs and symptoms of impending convulsion (May & Mahlmeister, 1994):
    a. Epigastric or right upper quadrant pain
    b. Increasing hyperreflexia
    c. Development or worsening of clonus (alternating contraction and relaxation, *e.g.*, twitching)
    (Convulsions are a sign of cerebral hemorrhage.)
11. Assess fetal heart tones for incidence of late decelerations, absent long-term variability, or bradycardia.
    (Decreased placental perfusion causes late deceleration; hypoxia causes bradycardia [May & Mahlmeister, 1994].)
12. Consult with physician regarding low-dose aspirin therapy or calcium supplements for high-risk women during pregnancy.
    (Studies have shown a reduction of pregnancy-associated hypertension in high-risk women from these therapies [May & Mahlmeister, 1994].)
13. If seizures occur, refer to *PC: Seizures* for nursing interventions.
14. Refer to *PC: Preterm Labor* for nursing interventions with magnesium sulfate therapy.

PC: Fetal Distress

DEFINITION

PC: Fetal Distress: Describes a fetus experiencing or at high risk to experience a disruption of the physiologic exchange of nutrients, oxygen, and metabolites.

High-Risk Populations

Fetal Factors
- Prematurity
- Intrauterine growth retardation
- Atresia of umbilical cord
- Cord compression
- Placental insufficiency
- Infection
- Multiple gestation
- Congenital anomalies
- Dysmaturity
- Acute hemolytic crisis
- Prolonged labor
- Prolonged rupture of membranes
- Rh disease

Maternal Factors
- Chronic hypertension
- Pregnancy-associated hypertension
- Diabetes mellitus
- Third trimester bleeding
- Maternal hypoxia (*e.g.*, respiratory insufficiency)
- Seizures, hypotension
- Prolonged uterine activity
- Abruptio placentae
- Cardiovascular disease
- Substance abuse
- Malnutrition

Nursing Goals

The nurse will manage and minimize episodes of fetal distress.

Interventions

1. Determine baseline fetal heart tones and evaluate as reassuring if:
   a. Rate of 120–160 beats/minute
   b. Presence of beat-to-beat variation (normal fetal rate has a fine irregularity of more than 5–10 beats/minute)
   c. Early decelerations (transient slowing of fetal heart rate with compression of the contraction causing parasympathetic stimulation)
2. Monitor for nonreassuring fetal heart rate or rhythm, including:
   a. Decreased variability (<6 beats/minute)
   b. Tachycardia (>160 beats/minute)

  c. Bradycardia (<110 beats/minute)
  d. Late decelerations (a drop in fetal heart rate of 15–45 beats/minute after the contraction)
  e. Variable decelerations, caused by compression of the umbilical cord
  f. Sinusoidal pattern (repetitive undulation of baseline)
  (Changes in fetal heart rate can be caused by fetal hypoxia, maternal drugs, maternal anemia, or dysrhythmias [May & Mahlmeister, 1994].)
3. If tachycardia occurs, assess
  a. Maternal temperature
    (Fetal tachycardia occurs when maternal core temperature rises. It may increase before the mother's temperature can be measured orally or rectally.)
  b. Maternal intake, output, and urine specific gravity
    (Maternal dehydration can cause fetal tachycardia.)
  c. Maternal anxiety level
    (Severe anxiety can increase fetal heart rate.)
  d. Maternal medication use
    (Certain medications used by the mother can cause increased fetal heart rate, *e.g.*, atropine, ritodrine hydrochloride, scopolamine.)
4. Increase maternal hydration.
  (Maternal dehydration can cause fetal tachycardia.)
5. Notify the physician of the situation and your assessment findings.
6. Position the mother on her left side.
  (This position decreases occlusion of the inferior vena cava by the uterus, promoting venous return to the heart.)
7. If decreased variability occurs, evaluate possible causes, which can include:
  a. Sleeping fetus
  b. Effects of narcotics or sedatives
  c. Fetal hypoxia
  d. Maternal position
8. If nonreassuring fetal heart patterns continue, notify the physician and take the following steps:
  a. Keep the mother in a left side-lying position.
    (See Intervention 6, above.)
  b. Administer oxygen by face mask at a flow rate of 8 L/minute, according to protocol.
    (This increases oxygen delivery to the fetus.)
  c. Acquire a fetal scalp blood sample according to protocol.
    (To evaluate fetal pH and metabolic status)
  d. If fetal scalp monitoring is not immediately available, perform fetal scalp stimulation with a gloved finger.
    (Immediate fetal heart rate accelerations indicate a well-oxygenated brain and fetal reserve [May & Mahlmeister, 1994].)
  e. Discontinue oxytocin infusion, if indicated, according to protocol.
9. Initiate electronic fetal monitoring according to protocol, if indicated.
10. Remain with the mother and partner, provide information, and give them opportunities to share concerns and fears.
  (This ensures constant monitoring and also may help reduce the mother's anxiety.)
11. If the mother's condition worsens or if fetal pH is 7.2 or below, anticipate a cesarean section and assist as indicated.
12. If mild variable decelerations occur, change the mother's position from supine to lateral or from one side to the other. If fetal heart rate does not improve, see Intervention 13.
  (Position shifts may relieve cord compression.)
13. If severe variable decelerations occur, take the following steps.
  a. Notify the physician.
  b. Discontinue oxytocin infusion per protocol.
  c. Perform a vaginal examination to assess for cord prolapse.

    d. Shift the mother's position to left side lying and evaluate fetal heart rate; if not improved, turn the mother on her right side.

    e. If these position changes do not improve fetal heart rate, or if cord is prolapsed, help the mother assume a knee–chest position.
(This reduces pressure on the cord and increases perfusion to the fetus.)

    f. Administer oxygen by face mask at a rate of 8–12 L/minute, according to protocol.
(This increases oxygen delivery to the fetus.)

    g. Assess for improvement in fetal heart rate within 1 minute.

14. Anticipate an emergency vaginal delivery or cesarean section if the mother's condition worsens, if cord prolapse occurs, and/or if fetal pH is 7.2 or lower.

PC: Postpartum Hemorrhage

DEFINITION

PC: Postpartum Hemorrhage: Describes a woman who is experiencing or is at high risk to experience acute blood loss greater than 500 mL within the first 24 hours postpartum or occurring after 24 hours and before the sixth week postpartum.

High-Risk Populations

- Problematic third stage of labor
- Overdistended uterus (*e.g.*, due to hydramnios, large fetus, multiple gestation)
- Prolonged labor
- Precipitous labor
- Oxytocin induction
- Multiparity
- Maternal exhaustion
- Instrument delivery
- History of uterine atony
- History of blood dyscrasias
- Excessive analgesic use
- Pregnancy-associated hypertension
- Retained placental fragments

Nursing Goals

The nurse will manage and minimize postpartum bleeding.

Interventions

1. Assess the uterine fundus every 5 minutes for the first hour postpartum and PRN thereafter for the first 24 hours; evaluate
   a. Height (normally should be at the level of the umbilicus after delivery)
   b. Size (when contracted, should be about the size of an apple)
   c. Consistency (should feel firm)
   (A boggy or relaxed uterus will not control bleeding by compression of the uterine muscle fibers.)

2. If the uterus is relaxed or relaxing, massage it with firm but gentle circular strokes until it contracts.
   (Massage stimulates the uterine muscle to contract.)
3. Avoid routine massage or overmassaging the uterus.
   (Unnecessary massage can cause pain and muscle fatigue, with subsequent uterine relaxation.)
4. Monitor blood pressure and pulse every 15 minutes for 1 hour, then every 30 minutes for the next hour, and then once every hour until the mother's condition stabilizes.
   (Careful vital sign monitoring provides accurate evaluation of hemodynamic status.)
5. Monitor perineal blood loss. Keep a record of the number of pads used and the amount of saturation.
   (Continuous seepage of blood with a firm uterus can indicate cervical or vaginal lacerations. Bleeding after the first 24 hours can indicate retained placental fragments or subinvolution.)
6. Obtain hemoglobin and hematocrit levels. Report a decrease to the physician or midwife.
   (A decrease in the hemoglobin value of 1.0–1.5 g/dL and a four-point drop in hematocrit indicate a blood loss of 450–500 mL [May & Mahlmeister, 1994].)
7. Monitor bladder size and urine output with the same frequency as for vital signs (see Intervention 4, above).
   (A distended bladder can displace the uterus and increase uterine atony.)
8. If bleeding becomes excessive, if the uterus fails to contract, or if vital sign changes occur, notify the physician.
9. If the woman exhibits signs of shock, refer to *PC: Hypovolemic Shock* for nursing interventions.

References/Bibliography

Armson, A., Samuels, P., & Miller, F. (1992). Evaluation of maternal fluid dynamics during tocolytic therapy with ritodrine hydrochloride and magnesium sulfate. *American Journal of Obstetrics and Gynecology, 167*, 758.

Bennett, N., & Bott, J. (1989). New strategies for preterm labor. *Nurse Practitioner, 14*(4), 27–38.

Groenwald, S., Frogge, M., Goodman, M., & Yarbro, C. (Eds.). (1993). *Cancer nursing: Principles and practice* (3rd ed.). Boston: Jones & Bartlett.

Haubrich, K. L. (1990). Amnioinfusion: A technique for the relief of variable deceleration. *Journal of Obstetric, Gynecologic, and Neonatal Nursing, 19*, 299–303.

Hudak, C., Gallo, B., & Benz, J. (1994). *Critical care nursing* (6th ed.). Philadelphia: J. B. Lippincott.

Mandeville, L., & Troiano, N. (1992). *High risk intrapartum nursing*. Philadelphia: J. B. Lippincott.

May, K., & Mahlmeister, L. (1994). *Maternal and neonatal nursing: Family-centered care* (3rd ed.). Philadelphia: J. B. Lippincott.

Sala, D. J., & Moise, K. (1990). The treatment of preterm labor using a portable subcutaneous terbutaline pump. *Journal of Obstetric, Gynecologic, and Neonatal Nursing, 19*, 108–115.

Scott, J., Disaia, P., Hammond, C., & Spellacy, W. (1994). *Obstetrics and gynecology* (7th ed.). Philadelphia: J. B. Lippincott.

Thelan, L., Davie, J., & Urden, L. (1990). *Textbook of critical care nursing*. St. Louis: C. V. Mosby.

Potential Complication: Medication Therapy Adverse Effects

PC: Anticoagulant Therapy Adverse Effects

PC: Antianxiety Therapy Adverse Effects

PC: Adrenocorticosteroid Therapy Adverse Effects

PC: Antineoplastic Therapy Adverse Effects

PC: Anticonvulsant Therapy Adverse Effects

PC: Antidepressant Therapy Adverse Effects

PC: Antiarrhythmic Therapy Adverse Effects

PC: Antipsychotic Therapy Adverse Effects

PC: Antihypertensive Therapy Adverse Effects

Potential Complication: Medication Therapy Adverse Effects*

DEFINITION

PC: Medication Therapy Adverse Effects: Describes a client experiencing or at high risk to experience potentially serious effects or reactions related to medication therapy.

Author's Note

The nurse can use these collaborative problems to describe a client who has experienced or who is at risk for adverse effects of medication therapy. In contrast to side effects, which are troublesome and annoying but rarely serious, adverse effects are unusual, unexpected, and potentially serious reactions (Malseed, 1990). Examples of adverse effects

* This section is intended as an overview of the nursing accountability for adverse effects of medication therapy. It is not intended to provide the reader with complete information on individual drugs, which can be found in pharmacology texts or manuals.

include dysrhythmias, gastric ulcers, blood dyscrasias, and anaphylactic reactions; examples of side effects include drowsiness, dry mouth, nausea, and weakness. Side effects usually can be managed by changing the dose, form, route of administration, or diet, or by using preventive measures with continuation of the medication (Malseed, 1990). Adverse effects may require discontinuation of the medication. A care plan will not contain a collaborative problem for every medication that the client is taking. Nurses routinely teach clients about side effects of medications and monitor for side effects as part of the standard of care for every client. These collaborative problems are indicated for clients who are at high risk for adverse effects or reactions because of the duration of the therapy, high predictability of their occurrence, the potential seriousness if they occur, and previous history of an adverse response. Students may add these collaborative problems to care plans. Practicing nurses should have access to standardized plans for *Medication Therapy Adverse Effects* for major medications.

High-Risk Populations

- Prolonged medication therapy
- History of hypersensitivity
- History of adverse reactions
- High single or daily doses
- Multiple medication therapy
- Mental instability
- Hepatic insufficiency
- Renal insufficiency
- Disease or condition that increases the risk of a specific adverse response (*e.g.*, history of gastric ulcer)

PC: Anticoagulant Therapy Adverse Effects

High-Risk Populations

- Diabetes mellitus
- Hypothyroidism
- Gastrointestinal bleeding
- X-ray therapy
- Bleeding tendency
- Hyperlipidemia
- Elderly women
- Vitamin K deficiency
- Debilitation
- Congestive heart failure
- Children

- Mild hepatic or renal dysfunction
- Indwelling catheterization
- Tuberculosis
- Menstruation
- Pregnancy
- Immediately postpartum

Nursing Goals

The nurse will manage or assist the client and family to manage and minimize adverse effects.

Interventions

Refer also to a pharmacology text for specific information on the individual drug.
1. Assess for contraindications to anticoagulant therapy:
   a. History of hypersensitivity
   b. Wounds
   c. Presence of active bleeding
   d. Blood dyscrasias
   e. Anticipated or recent surgery
   f. Gastrointestinal ulcers
   g. Subacute bacterial endocarditis
   h. Pericarditis
   i. Severe hypertension
   j. Impaired renal function
   k. Impaired hepatic function
   l. Hemorrhagic cerebrovascular accident
   m. Use of drugs that affect platelet formation (*e.g.*, salicylates, dipyridamole, nonsteroidal anti-inflammatory drugs)
   n. Presence of drainage tubes
   o. Eclampsia
   p. Hemorrhagic tendencies
   q. Threatened abortion
   r. Ascorbic acid deficiency
   s. Spinal puncture
   t. Regional anesthesia
2. Explain possible adverse effects:
   a. Systemic
         Hypersensitivity (fever, chills, runny nose, headache, nausea, vomiting, rash, itching, tearing)
         Bleeding, hemorrhage
   b. Gastrointestinal
         Vomiting
         Diarrhea
   c. Cardiovascular
         Hypertension
         Chest pain
   d. Renal
         Impaired renal function
3. Monitor for and reduce the severity of adverse effects.
   a. Establish baseline prothrombin time (PT) and partial thromboplastin time (PTT) levels.
   b. Report PTT below or above the therapeutic range (usually 1.5 to 2 times the normal value).

    c. Monitor for signs of bleeding (*e.g.*, bleeding gums, skin bruises, tarry stools, hematuria, epistaxis).

    d. For a client receiving heparin therapy, have protamine sulfate available during administration.
(Protamine sulfate is the antidote to reverse the effects of heparin.)

    e. Consult with the pharmacist about medications that can potentiate (*e.g.*, antibiotics, cimetidine, salicylates) or inhibit (*e.g.*, antacids, barbiturates, oral contraceptives) anticoagulant action.

4. Reduce hematomas and bleeding at injection sites.

    a. Use small-gauge needles.

    b. Do not massage sites.

    c. Rotate sites.

    d. Use subcutaneous route.

    e. Apply steady pressure for 1–2 minutes.

  (These techniques reduce the trauma to tissues and avoid highly vascular areas [*e.g.*, muscles].)

5. Teach the client and family how to prevent or reduce the severity of adverse effects.

    a. Instruct them to monitor for and report signs of bleeding.

    b. Tell them to inform physicians, dentists, and other health care providers of anticoagulant therapy before invasive procedures.
(Precautions may be needed to prevent bleeding.)

    c. Instruct them to contact the physician immediately after the onset of a fever or rash.
(Can indicate an infection or allergic response)

    d. Tell them that it takes 2–10 days for PT levels to return to normal after warfarin (Coumadin) is stopped.

    e. Explain that certain medications can inhibit or potentiate anticoagulant effect, and advise them to consult with a pharmacist before taking any prescribed or over-the-counter drug.

    f. Teach them to avoid foods high in vitamin K; such foods include turnip greens, asparagus, broccoli, watercress, cabbage, beef liver, lettuce, and green tea.
(Vitamin K decreases anticoagulant action.)

    g. Instruct the client to wear MedicAlert identification.

    h. Stress the importance of regular follow-up care.

6. Instruct the client and family to report the following signs and symptoms:

    a. Bleeding

    b. Tarry stools

    c. Fever

    d. Chills

    e. Sore throat

    f. Itching

    g. Dark urine

    h. Jaundice

    i. Mouth sores

PC: Antianxiety Therapy Adverse Effects

High-Risk Populations

- Children
- Older adult
- Impaired liver or kidney function
- Psychosis
- Depression
- Pregnancy or breast-feeding
- Severe muscle weakness
- Limited pulmonary reserves

Nursing Goals

The nurse will manage or assist the client and family to manage and minimize adverse effects.

Interventions

Refer also to a pharmacology text for specific information on the individual drug.
1. Assess for contraindications to antianxiety therapy:
   a. Hypersensitivity
   b. Impaired consciousness
   c. Compromised respiratory function
   d. Shock
   e. Porphyria
   f. History of drug abuse
   g. Undiagnosed neurologic disorders
   h. Glaucoma, paralytic ileus, prostatic hypertrophy (for benzodiazepines)
   i. Pregnancy or breast-feeding
2. Explain possible adverse effects:
   a. Systemic
        Hypersensitivity (pruritus, rash, hypotension)
        Drug dependency
        Sleep disturbances
   b. Cardiovascular
        Decreased heart rate, blood pressure
        Transient tachycardia, bradycardia
        Edema
   c. Central nervous system
        Impaired judgment   Paradoxical excitement
        Excessive drowsiness   Tremors
        Dizziness   Slurred speech
        Confusion   Dysphagia
   d. Respiratory
        Respiratory depression
   e. Hematologic
        Leukopenia

    f. Ophthalmic
       Blurred vision
    g. Genitourinary
       Urine retention
    h. Hepatic
       Jaundice

3. Monitor for and reduce the severity of adverse effects.
   a. Evaluate the client's mental status before drug administration. Consult the physician if the client exhibits confusion or excessive drowsiness.
   b. Evaluate the client's risk for injury; see *Risk for Injury* for more information.
   c. Monitor for signs of overdose (*e.g.*, slurred speech, continued somnolence, respiratory depression, confusion).
   d. Monitor for signs of tolerance (*e.g.*, increased anxiety, wakefulness).

4. Teach the client and family how to prevent or reduce the severity of adverse effects.
   a. Instruct the client never to discontinue taking the medication abruptly after long-term use.
      (Abrupt cessation can cause vomiting, tremors, and convulsions.)
   b. Teach the family or significant others the signs of overdose (*e.g.*, slurred speech, continued somnolence, respiratory depression, confusion).
   c. Remind the client and family that alcohol and other sedatives potentiate the action of the medication.
   d. Instruct client to avoid driving and other hazardous activities when drowsy.
   e. Discuss the possibility of drug tolerance and dependence with long-term use.

5. Instruct the client and family to report the following signs or symptoms:
   a. Slurred speech
   b. Continued somnolence
   c. Confusion
   d. Respiratory insufficiency
   e. Hostility, rage
   f. Muscle spasms
   g. Vivid dreams
   h. Euphoria
   i. Hallucinations
   j. Sore throat
   k. Fever
   l. Mouth ulcers

PC: Adrenocorticosteroid Therapy Adverse Effects

High-Risk Populations

- Acquired immunodeficiency syndrome
- Thrombophlebitis
- Congestive heart failure

- Diabetes mellitus
- Hypothyroidism
- Glaucoma
- Osteoporosis
- Myasthenia gravis
- Bleeding ulcers
- Seizure disorders or mental illness
- Older adult
- Pregnancy or breast-feeding
- Severe stress, trauma, or illness

Nursing Goals

The nurse will manage or assist the client and family to manage and minimize adverse effects.

Interventions

Refer also to a pharmacology text for specific information on the individual drug.
1. Assess for contraindications to steroid therapy:
    a. History of hypersensitivity
    b. Active peptic ulcer disease
    c. Active tuberculosis
    d. Active fungus infection
    e. Herpes
    f. Cardiac disease
    g. Hypertension
2. Explain possible adverse effects:
    a. Systemic
        Hypersensitivity (rash, hives, hypotension, respiratory distress, anaphylaxis)
        Increased susceptibility to infection
        Acute adrenal insufficiency (response to withdrawal)
        Hypokalemia
        Delayed wound healing
    b. Central nervous system
        Hallucinations   Psychosis
        Headaches   Papilledema
        Depression
    c. Ophthalmic
        Glaucoma
        Cataracts
    d. Cardiovascular
        Thrombophlebitis   Hypertension
        Embolism   Edema
        Dysrhythmias
    e. Gastrointestinal
        Bleeding   Pancreatitis
        Ulcers
    f. Musculoskeletal
        Osteoporosis   Growth retardation in children
        Muscle wasting
3. Monitor for adverse effects.
    a. Establish baseline assessment data.
        Weight   Serum potassium
        Complete blood count (CBC) Blood glucose
        Blood pressure   Serum sodium

    b. Monitor:

Weight	Blood glucose
CBC	Serum sodium
Blood pressure	Stool for guaiac
Serum potassium	

    c. Report changes in monitored data.

4. Teach the client and family how to prevent or reduce the severity of adverse effects.

    a. Instruct to take the medication with food or milk.
      (This reduces gastric distress.)

    b. Advise to weigh self daily at the same time and wearing the same clothes each time.
      (Weight gain may indicate fluid retention.)

    c. Instruct to avoid people with infections.
      (The client's compromised immune system increases his vulnerability to infection.)

    d. Advise to consult with a physician or pharmacist before taking any over-the-counter drugs.
      (Serious drug interactions can occur.)

    e. Instruct to inform physicians, dentists, and other health care providers of therapy before any invasive procedure.
      (Precautions should be taken to prevent bleeding.)

    f. Instruct to contact the physician if signs of infection occur.

    g. Teach to take anticoagulant medication in the morning.
      (This can help reduce adrenal suppression.)

    h. Instruct to wear MedicAlert identification.
      (He may need more medication in an emergency.)

    i. Warn never to discontinue the medication without consulting the physician about side effects.
      (Adrenal function needs a gradual return time.)

    j. Discuss the possible problems of weight gain and sodium retention (refer to *Altered Nutrition: More than Body Requirements* and *Fluid Volume Excess* for more information).

    k. Explain possible drug-induced appearance changes (*e.g.*, moon face, hirsutism, abnormal fat distribution).

    l. Encourage to establish a system to prevent dosage omission or double dosage (*e.g.*, check sheet, prefilled daily dose containers).

    m. Explain the risk for hyperglycemia.
      (Steroids interfere with glucose metabolism.)

5. Instruct the client and family to report the following signs and symptoms:

    a. Gastric pain

    b. Darkened stool color

    c. Unusual weight gain

    d. Vomiting

    e. Sore throat, fever

    f. Adrenal insufficiency (fatigue, anorexia, palpitations, nausea, vomiting, diarrhea, weight loss, mood swings)

    g. Menstrual irregularities

    h. Change in vision, eye pain

    i. Persistent, severe headache

    j. Leg pain, cramps

    k. Excessive thirst, hunger, urination

PC: Antineoplastic Therapy Adverse Effects

High-Risk Populations

- Debilitation
- Bone marrow depression
- Malignant infiltration of kidney
- Malignant infiltration of bone marrow
- Liver dysfunction
- Renal insufficiency
- Older adult
- Children

Nursing Goals

The nurse will manage or assist the client and family to manage and minimize adverse effects.

Interventions

Refer also to a pharmacology text for specific information on the individual drug.

1. Assess for contraindications to antineoplastic therapy:
   a. Hypersensitivity to the drug
   b. Radiation therapy within the previous 4 weeks
   c. Severe bone marrow depression
   d. Breast-feeding
   e. First trimester of pregnancy
2. Explain possible adverse effects:
   a. Systemic
      Hypersensitivity (pruritus, rash, chills, fever, difficulty breathing, anaphylaxis)
      Immunosuppression
      Alopecia
      Fever
   b. Cardiovascular
      Congestive heart failure
      Dysrhythmias
   c. Respiratory
      Pulmonary fibrosis
   d. Central nervous system

Confusion	Depression
Headaches	Dizziness
Weakness	Neurotoxicity

   e. Hematologic

Leukopenia	Anemia
Bleeding	Hyperuricemia
Thrombocytopenia	Electrolyte imbalances
Agranulocytosis	

   f. Gastrointestinal

Diarrhea	Enteritis
Anorexia	Intestinal ulcers
Vomiting	Paralytic ulcer
Mucositis	

    g. Hepatic

        Hepatotoxicity

    h. Genitourinary

Renal failure	Sterility
Amenorrhea	Hemorrhagic cystitis
Azoospermia	Renal calculi

3. Monitor for and reduce the severity of adverse effects.
   a. Document a baseline assessment of vital signs, cardiac rhythm, and weight.
      (This facilitates subsequent assessments for adverse reactions.)
   b. Ensure that baseline electrolyte, blood chemistry, bone marrow, and renal and hepatic function studies are done before administering the first dose.
      (This enables monitoring for adverse reactions.)
   c. Check the procedure for antineoplastic administration before administration.
      Stay with the client during initial administration.
      (Close monitoring can detect signs of hypersensitivity early.)
         Monitor for extravasation every 30 minutes.
      (Early detection enables prompt intervention to prevent tissue necrosis.)
         Follow protocol if extravasation occurs.
   d. Monitor temperature, vital signs, physical status, weight, and intake and output daily.
      (Frequent monitoring can detect adverse effects early.)
   e. Ensure adequate hydration, at least 2 L/day.
      (Good hydration can help prevent kidney damage from rapid destruction of cells.)
   f. Monitor for early signs of infection.
      (Bone marrow suppression increases the risk of infection.)
   g. Monitor for sodium, potassium, magnesium, phosphate, and calcium imbalances.
      (Electrolyte imbalances are commonly precipitated by renal injury, vomiting, and diarrhea.)
   h. Monitor for renal insufficiency: insufficient urine output, elevated specific gravity, elevated urine sodium levels.
      (Certain antineoplastics have toxic effects on renal glomeruli and tubules.)
   i. Monitor for renal calculi: flank pain, nausea, vomiting, abdominal pain; refer to *PC: Renal Calculi* if it occurs.
      (Rapid lysis of tumor cells can produce hyperuricemia.)
   j. Monitor for neurotoxicity: paresthesias, gait disturbance, disorientation, confusion, foot drop or wrist drop, fine motor activity disturbances.
      (Some antineoplastics impair neural conduction.)
4. Teach the client and family how to prevent or reduce the severity of adverse effects.
   a. Stress the importance of follow-up assessments and laboratory tests.
      (This can help detect adverse effects early.)
   b. Instruct to avoid crowds and people with infectious diseases.
      (A client receiving antineoplastic therapy is very susceptible to infectious diseases.)
   c. Teach to monitor weight and intake and output daily.
      (Regular monitoring can detect adverse effects early.)
   d. Instruct to consult with primary health care provider before taking any over-the-counter drugs.
      (Serious drug interactions can occur.)
   e. Advise to avoid vaccines.
      (A compromised immune system increases the risk for onset of disease.)
   f. Refer to appropriate nursing diagnoses for selected responses (*e.g., Altered Nutrition, Altered Oral Mucous Membranes*).
5. Instruct the client and family to report the following signs and symptoms:
   a. Fever (>100°F)

    b. Chills, sweating
    c. Diarrhea
    d. Severe cough
    e. Sore throat
    f. Unusual bleeding
    g. Burning on urination
    h. Muscle cramps
    i. Flu-like symptoms
    j. Pain, swelling at IV site
    k. Abdominal pain
    l. Confusion, dizziness
    m. Decreased urine output

PC: Anticonvulsant Therapy Adverse Effects

High-Risk Populations

- Hepatic insufficiency
- Renal insufficiency
- Coagulation problems
- Pregnancy or breast-feeding
- Hyperthyroidism
- Diabetes mellitus
- Older adult
- Debilitation
- Heart block
- Glaucoma
- Myocardial insufficiency

Nursing Goals

The nurse will manage or assist the client and family to manage and minimize adverse effects.

Interventions

Refer also to a pharmacology text for specific information on the individual drug.
1. Assess for contraindications to anticonvulsant therapy:
    a. Hypersensitivity
    b. Bone marrow depression
    c. Blood dyscrasias
    d. Porphyria
    e. Myasthenia gravis
    f. Respiratory obstruction

2. Explain possible adverse effects:
   a. Systemic
      Hypersensitivity (excessive side effects, rashes)
      Lupus-like reactions
   b. Central nervous system
      Depression   Personality changes
      Irritability   Tremors
      Ataxia
   c. Hematologic
      Leukopenia   Anemias
      Bone marrow suppression
   d. Gastrointestinal
      Gingival hyperplasia (with hydantoin)
   e. Hepatic
      Hepatitis
   f. Genitourinary
      Albuminuria   Impotence
      Urine retention
3. Monitor for and reduce the severity of adverse effects.
   a. Document baseline information on seizures: type, frequency, usual time, presence of aura, precipitating factors.
   b. Administer medication at regular intervals.
      (Regular administration helps prevent fluctuating serum drug levels.)
   c. Keep a flow record of serum drug levels; report levels outside the therapeutic range.
      (Seizures can occur with lower levels; higher levels can cause toxicity.)
   d. Monitor hepatic and blood count studies.
      (These studies can detect blood dyscrasias and hepatic dysfunction.)
   e. Monitor for sore throat, persistent fatigue, fever, and infections.
      (These signs and symptoms can indicate blood dyscrasias.)
   f. Take vital signs before and after parenteral drug administration.
      (Vital signs demonstrate the drug's effect on cardiac function.)
   g. When administering the drug IV, monitor vital signs closely and give the drug slowly.
      (Close monitoring can enable early detection of bradycardia, hypotension, and respiratory depression.)
4. Teach the client and family how to prevent or reduce the severity of adverse effects.
   a. Stress not to alter the dosage or abruptly discontinue the medication.
      (Changing the regimen can precipitate severe seizures.)
   b. Emphasize to take the medication on time, around-the-clock if needed.
      (Regular administration helps maintain therapeutic drug levels.)
   c. Instruct to consult with a pharmacist before taking any over-the-counter medications.
      (Certain medications reduce the effects of anticonvulsants.)
   d. Stress the importance of maintaining a proper diet; encourage to consult with a physician to determine the need for supplements.
      (Some anticonvulsants interfere with vitamin and mineral absorption.)

PC: Antidepressant Therapy Adverse Effects

High-Risk Populations

- Increased ocular pressure
- Impaired renal function
- Impaired hepatic function
- Urine retention
- Diabetes mellitus
- Seizure disorder
- Hyperthyroidism
- Parkinson's disease
- Pregnancy or breast-feeding
- Electroconvulsant therapy
- Cardiovascular disease
- Schizophrenia, psychoses
- Older adults

Nursing Goals

The nurse will manage or assist the client and family to manage and minimize adverse effects.

Interventions

Refer also to a pharmacology text for specific information on the individual drug.
1. Assess for contraindications to antidepressant therapy:
   a. Hypersensitivity
   b. Narrow-angle glaucoma
   c. Acute recovery phase postmyocardial infarction
   d. Severe renal impairment
   e. Severe hepatic impairment
   f. Prostatic hypertrophy
   g. Cerebrovascular disease
   h. Cardiovascular disease
   i. Schizophrenia (for monoamine oxidase [MAO] inhibitors)
   j. Anesthesia administration within the past 1–2 weeks (for MAO inhibitors)
   k. Hypertension (for MAO inhibitors)
   l. Concomitant use of MAO inhibitors and tricyclics
   m. Seizure disorder (for tricyclics)
   n. Ingestion of foods containing tyramine (for MAO inhibitors)
   o. Concomitant use of MAO inhibitors, sympathomimetics, narcotics, sedatives, hypnotics, barbiturates, phenothiazides, and antihypertensives
2. Explain possible adverse effects:
   a. Systemic
      Hypersensitivity (rash, petechiae, urticaria, photosensitivity)
      Diaphoresis
   b. Central nervous system
      Nightmares

       Delusions   Ataxia
       Agitation   Seizures
       Hypomania   Paresthesias
       Confusion   Extrapyramidal symptoms
       Hallucinations   Tremors

  c. Cardiovascular
       Orthostatic hypotension   Tachycardia
       Hypertension Dysrhythmias (with MAO inhibitors)

  d. Hematologic
       Blood dyscrasias
       Bone marrow suppression

  e. Gastrointestinal
       Paralytic ileus
       Vomiting
       Diarrhea

  f. Hepatic
       Hepatotoxicity

  g. Genitourinary
       Urine retention   Impotence
       Prostatic hypertrophy   Nocturia
       Acute renal failure

  h. Endocrine
       Altered blood glucose levels

3. Monitor for and reduce the severity of adverse effects.
  a. Consult with a pharmacist regarding potential interactions with the client's other medications.
    (MAO inhibitors cause many adverse interactions.)
  b. Document baseline pulse, cardiac rhythm, and blood pressure.
    (Antidepressants can seriously affect cardiac function; baseline assessment enables accurate monitoring during drug therapy.)
  c. Ensure that baseline blood, renal, and hepatic function studies are done.
    (Baseline values allow monitoring for changes.)
  d. Record signs and symptoms of depression before initiating therapy.
    (This information facilitates evaluation of the client's response to therapy.)
  e. Monitor weight, intake, and output and assess for edema.
    (Some antidepressants can cause fluid retention and anorexia.)

4. Teach the client and family how to prevent or reduce the severity of adverse effects.
  a. Stress that alcohol potentiates medication effects.
  b. Instruct the client to consult a pharmacist before taking any over-the-counter drugs.
    (Many medications interact with antidepressants.)
  c. Warn the client not to adjust dosage or discontinue medication without consulting a physician or nurse.
  d. For a client taking an MAO inhibitor, stress the importance of avoiding certain foods containing tyramine, such as avocados, bananas, fava beans, raisins, figs, aged cheeses, sour cream, red wines, sherry, beer, yeast, yogurt, pickled herring, chicken liver, aged meats, fermented sausages, chocolate, caffeine, soy sauce, licorice.
    (These foods have a pressor effect, which may cause a hypertensive reaction.)
  e. Instruct the client to continue to avoid hazardous foods and medications for several weeks after the medication is discontinued.
    (MAO enzyme regeneration takes several weeks.)
  f. Advise family members to watch for and report signs of hypomania or exaggerated symptoms in the client.
  g. Explain that MAO inhibitors must be discontinued 1 week before anesthesia administration.
    (MAO inhibitors can have serious interactions with anesthetics and narcotics.)

   h. For diaphoresis-related electrolyte depletion associated with selective serotonin reuptake inhibitors, instruct to
       Avoid caffeine
       Avoid activity in hot weather
       Drink 8 oz of fluids with electrolytes every 30 minutes
5. Instruct the client to report the following signs and symptoms:
   a. Hypertensive reaction (headache, neck stiffness, palpitations, sweating, nausea, photophobia)
   b. Visual disturbances
   c. Jaundice
   d. Rash
   e. Abdominal pain
   f. Pruritus
   g. Urinary problems
   h. Seizures
   i. Changes in mental status

PC: Antiarrhythmic Therapy Adverse Effects

High-Risk Populations

- Hypertension
- Diabetes mellitus
- Children
- Older adult
- Impaired hepatic function
- Impaired renal function
- Cardiomegaly
- Pulmonary pathology
- Thyrotoxicosis
- Peripheral vascular disease
- Atrioventricular conduction abnormalities
- Congestive heart failure
- Hypotension
- Digitalis intoxication
- Potassium imbalance

Nursing Goals

The nurse will manage or assist the client and family to manage and minimize adverse effects.

Interventions

Refer also to a pharmacology text for specific information on the individual drug.

1. Assess for contraindications to antiarrhythmic therapy:
   a. Hypersensitivity
   b. Cardiac, renal, or hepatic failure
   c. Heart block
   d. Thrombocytopenia purpura
   e. Myasthenia gravis
2. Explain possible adverse effects:
   a. Systemic
      Hypersensitivity (rash, difficulty breathing, heightened side effects)
      Lupus-like reaction
   b. Cardiovascular
      Worsening or new dysrhythmia
      Hypotension
      Cardiotoxicity (widened QRS complex greater than 25%, ventricular extrasystoles, absent P waves)
   c. Central nervous system
      Dizziness
      Apprehension
   d. Hematologic
      Agranulocytosis
3. Monitor for and reduce the severity of adverse effects.
   a. Establish a baseline assessment of blood pressure, heart rate, respiratory rate, peripheral pulses, lung sounds, and intake and output.
      (Baseline assessment facilitates evaluation for adverse reactions to drug therapy.)
   b. Report any electrolyte imbalance, acid–base imbalance, or oxygenation problems.
      (Dysrhythmias are aggravated by these conditions).
   c. Withhold the dose and consult the physician if the client experiences a significant drop in blood pressure, bradycardia, worsening dysrhythmia, or a new dysrhythmia after receiving the medication.
      (These signs may indicate an adverse reaction.)
   d. During parenteral administration, have emergency drugs (*e.g.*, vasopressors, cardiac glycosides, diuretics) available and resuscitation equipment on hand; use microdrip infusion equipment to ensure close regulation of IV flow rate.
4. Teach the client and family how to prevent or reduce the severity of adverse effects.
   a. Stress the importance of ongoing follow-up with the primary health care provider.
   b. Emphasize the need to take the medication on time and to avoid "doubling up" on doses.
      (A regular schedule prevents toxic blood levels.)
   c. Instruct to take the medication with food.
      (This can help minimize gastrointestinal distress.)
   d. Teach to monitor pulse and blood pressure daily.
      (Careful monitoring can detect early signs of adverse effects.)
   e. Advise to consult a pharmacist before taking any over-the-counter drugs.
      (Possible drug interactions may alter cardiac stability.)
5. Instruct the client and family to report the following signs and symptoms:
   a. Dizziness, faintness
   b. Palpitations
   c. Visual disturbances
   d. Hallucinations
   e. Confusion
   f. Headache
   g. 1- to 2-lb weight gain
   h. Coldness and numbness in extremities

PC: Antipsychotic Therapy Adverse Effects

High-Risk Populations

- Glaucoma
- Prosthetic hypertrophy
- Epilepsy
- Diabetes mellitus
- Severe hypertension
- Ulcers
- Cardiovascular disease
- Chronic respiratory disorders
- Hepatic insufficiency
- Pregnancy or breast-feeding
- Exposure to extreme heat, phosphorus insecticides, or pesticides

Nursing Goals

The nurse will manage or assist the client and family to manage and minimize adverse effects.

Interventions

Refer also to a pharmacology text for specific information on the individual drug.
1. Assess for contraindications to antipsychotic therapy:
   a. Bone marrow suppression
   b. Blood dyscrasias
   c. Parkinson's disease
   d. Hepatic insufficiency
   e. Renal insufficiency
   f. Cerebral arteriosclerosis
   g. Coronary artery disease
   h. Circulatory collapse
   i. Mitral insufficiency
   j. Severe hypotension
   k. Alcoholism
   l. Subcortical brain damage
   m. Comatose states
2. Explain possible adverse effects:
   a. Systemic
      Hypersensitivity (rash, abdominal pain, jaundice, blood dyscrasias)
      Photosensitivity
      Fever
   b. Cardiovascular
      Hypertension   Orthostatic hypotension
      Palpitations
   c. Central nervous system
      Extrapyramidal (acute dystonia, akathisia, pseudoparkinsonism)

Hyperreflexia	Tardive dyskinesia
Cerebral edema	Neuroleptic malignant syndrome
Sleep disturbances	Bizarre dreams

d. Gastrointestinal
  Constipation
  Paralytic ileus
  Fecal impaction

e. Hematologic

Agranulocytosis	Thrombocytopenia
Leukopenia	Purpura
Leukocytosis	Pancytopenia
Anemias	

f. Ophthalmic

Ptosis	Lens opacities
Pigmentary retinopathy	

g. Respiratory

Laryngospasm	Dyspnea
Bronchospasm	

h. Genitourinary

Urine retention	Incontinence
Enuresis	Impotence

i. Endocrine

Gynecomastia	Glycosuria
Altered libido	Hyperglycemia
Amenorrhea	

3. Monitor for and reduce the severity of adverse effects.

a. Document a baseline assessment of blood pressure (sitting, standing, and lying), pulse, and temperature.
   (Baseline assessment facilitates monitoring for adverse reactions.)

b. Ensure that baseline bone marrow, renal, and hepatic function studies are done before administering the first dose.
   (Results of these studies enable monitoring for changes.)

c. After parenteral administration, keep the client flat and monitor blood pressure.
   (These measures help reduce hypotensive effects.)

d. Monitor blood pressure during initial treatment.
   (Blood pressure monitoring detects early hypotensive effects.)

e. Assess bowel and bladder functioning.
   (Anticholinergic and antiadrenergic effects decrease sensory stimulation to the bowel and bladder.)

f. Observe for fine, wormlike movements of the tongue.
   (Early detection of tardive dyskinesia enables prompt intervention and possible reversal of its course.)

g. Monitor for acute dystonic reactions, neck spasms, eye rolling, dysphagia, convulsions.
   (Early detection of these signs may indicate the need for dose reduction.)

h. Ensure optimal hydration; evaluate urine specific gravity regularly.
   (Dehydration increases susceptibility to dystonic reactions.)

i. Monitor for signs and symptoms of blood dyscrasias: decreased white cells, platelets, and red cells; sore throat; fever; malaise.
   (Antipsychotic medication can cause bone marrow suppression.)

j. Monitor weight.
   (Antipsychotic medication can cause hypothyroidism, commonly marked by weight gain.)

k. Monitor for neuroleptic malignant syndrome; refer to *PC: Neuroleptic Malignant Syndrome* for interventions.
   (Neuroleptic malignant syndrome is a potentially dangerous adverse effect of antipsychotic drug therapy.)

4. Teach the client and family how to prevent or reduce the severity of adverse effects.
   a. Instruct to consult a pharmacist before taking any over-the-counter drugs.
      (Serious drug interactions can occur with various over-the-counter medications.)
   b. Stress the need to continue the medication regimen as prescribed and never abruptly to stop taking it.
      (Abrupt cessation can cause vomiting, tremors, and psychotic behavior.)
   c. Caution the client to protect himself from sun exposure with clothing, hat, sunglasses, and sunscreen.
      (Photosensitivity is a common side effect of antipsychotic therapy.)
   d. Warn against using alcohol, barbiturates, or sedatives.
      (Their effects are potentiated in combination with antipsychotic medication.)
5. Instruct the client and family to report the following signs and symptoms:
   a. Urine retention
   b. Visual disturbances
   c. Fever
   d. Sore throat
   e. Signs of infection
   f. Tremors
   g. Abdominal pain
   h. Fine, wormlike tongue movements
   i. Neck spasms
   j. Dysphagia
   k. Eye rolling
   l. Involuntary chewing, puckering
   m. Puffing movements

PC: Antihypertensive Therapy Adverse Effects

■ *Related to* **β-Adrenergic Blocker Therapy Adverse Effects**
■ *Related to* **Calcium Channel Blocker Therapy Adverse Effects**
■ *Related to* **Angiotensin-Converting Enzyme Therapy Adverse Effects**

Author's Note

Antihypertensive medications are classified into nine groups: central adrenergic agents, ganglionic blockers, peripherally acting catecholamine depleters, α-adrenergic blockers, calcium channel blockers, β-adrenergic blockers, vascular smooth muscle relaxants, angiotensin-converting enzymes, and diuretics. Because their sites of action differ greatly, it is not useful to present a generic collaborative problem of *PC: Antihypertensive Therapy Adverse Effects*. Instead, three classifications are addressed: β-adrenergic blockers, calcium channel blockers, and angiotensin-converting enzymes. For information on other classifications, consult a pharmacology text.

PC: β-Adrenergic Blocker Therapy Adverse Effects

High-Risk Populations

- Diabetes mellitus
- Severe liver disease
- Pregnancy or breast-feeding
- Chronic bronchitis, emphysema
- Peripheral vascular insufficiency
- Allergic rhinitis
- Renal insufficiency
- Hepatic insufficiency
- Myasthenia gravis

Nursing Goals

The nurse will manage or assist the client and family to manage and minimize adverse effects.

Interventions

Refer also to a pharmacology text for specific information on the individual drug.

1. Assess for contraindications to β-adrenergic blockers:
    a. Hypersensitivity
    b. Sinus bradycardia
    c. Second- or third-degree heart block
    d. PR interval greater than 0.24 second on ECG
    e. Severe congestive heart therapy
    f. Cardiogenic shock
    g. MAO inhibitor or tricyclic antidepressant therapy
    h. Bronchial asthma (for nonselective β-adrenergic blockers)
2. Explain possible adverse effects:
    a. Systemic
        Hypersensitivity (rash, pruritus)
    b. Central nervous system

Depression	Memory loss
Paresthesias	Bizarre dreams
Insomnia	Hallucinations
Behavior changes	Catatonia
Vertigo	

    c. Cardiovascular

Bradycardia	Cerebrovascular accident
Edema	Tachycardia
Hypotension	Peripheral arterial insufficiency
Congestive heart failure	

    d. Hematologic
        Agranulocytosis
        Thrombocytopenia
        Eosinophilia

    e. Gastrointestinal
        Diarrhea   Vomiting
        Ischemic colitis   Gastric pain
    f. Hepatic
        Hepatomegaly
    g. Respiratory
        Bronchospasm   Dyspnea
        Rales   Nasal congestion
    h. Endocrine
        Hypoglycemia or hyperglycemia
    i. Genitourinary
        Difficulty urinating
        Elevated blood urea nitrogen and serum transaminase
    j. Ophthalmic
        Blurred vision

3. Monitor for and reduce the severity of adverse effects.
    a. Establish a baseline assessment of pulse, blood pressure (lying, sitting, standing), lung fields, and peripheral pulses.
       (Baseline assessment facilitates monitoring for adverse reactions.)
    b. Ensure that baseline renal, hepatic, glucose, and blood studies are done before drug therapy begins.
       (Results of these studies enable monitoring for changes.)
    c. Establish with the physician the parameters (blood pressure, pulse) that call for withholding the medication.
       (Hypotension and bradycardia can reduce cardiac output.)
    d. Monitor intake, output, and weight and assess for edema.
       (Reduced cardiac output can cause fluid accumulation.)
    e. Monitor for congestive heart failure.
       (β-Adrenergic blockers can compromise cardiac function.)
    f. Monitor for hypoglycemia in a client with diabetes.
       (β-Adrenergic blockers interfere with the conversion of glycogen to glucose by occupying β-adrenergic receptor sites.)

4. Teach the client how to prevent or reduce the severity of adverse effects.
    a. Stress the importance of continuing the medication regimen as prescribed, and warn him never to discontinue the drug abruptly.
       (Abrupt cessation may precipitate dysrhythmias or angina.)
    b. Emphasize the need to monitor pulse and blood pressure daily. Explain the pulse and blood pressure values that indicate the need to withhold the medication.
    c. Instruct to weigh self daily, at the same time each day and wearing the same clothes every time; tell him to report any weight gain of 1 lb or more.
       (Weight gain may indicate fluid retention resulting from decreased cardiac output.)
    d. Explain the need to protect hands and feet from prolonged exposure to cold.
       (β-Adrenergic blockers decrease circulation in the skin and extremities.)
    e. Instruct to consult with his primary health care provider before exercising.
       (The medication impedes the body's adaptive response to stress.)
    f. Stress the importance of follow-up laboratory tests.
       (Significant abnormalities in liver or renal function studies and blood count may be seen.)

5. Instruct the client and family to report the following signs and symptoms:
    a. 1- to 2-lb weight gain
    b. Edema
    c. Difficulty breathing
    d. Pulse or blood pressure above or below preestablished parameters
    e. Dark urine
    f. Difficult urination
    g. Visual disturbances

h. Sore throat
i. Fever
j. Sleep disturbances
k. Memory loss
l. Mental changes
m. Behavioral changes

PC: Calcium Channel Blocker Therapy Adverse Effects

High-Risk Populations

- Renal insufficiency
- Hepatic insufficiency
- Hypotension
- Decreased left ventricular function
- Pregnancy or breast-feeding
- Digitalis therapy
- β-Adrenergic blocker therapy

Nursing Goals

The nurse will manage or assist the client and family to manage and minimize adverse effects.

Interventions

Refer also to a pharmacology text for specific information on the individual drug.

1. Assess for contraindications to calcium channel blocker therapy:
   a. Severe left ventricular dysfunction
   b. Sick sinus syndrome
   c. Second- or third-degree heart block
   d. Cardiogenic shock
   e. Systolic blood pressure greater than 90 mm Hg
   f. Acute myocardial infarction (with diltiazem)
   g. IV use of verapamil and β-adrenergic blockers
   h. Symptomatic hypotension
   i. Advanced congestive heart failure
2. Explain possible adverse effects:
   a. Systemic
      Hypersensitivity (rash, pruritus, extreme hypotension)
      Hair loss
      Sweating, chills
   b. Central nervous system
      Tremors   Insomnia

Confusion   Headache

Mood changes

c. Cardiovascular

Palpitations   Heart failure

Myocardial infarction   Bradycardia

Hypotension   Third-degree heart block (with verapamil)

d. Gastrointestinal

Diarrhea   Sore throat

Cramping

e. Hepatic

Elevated liver enzymes

f. Respiratory

Dyspnea   Pulmonary edema

Wheezing

g. Musculoskeletal

Muscle cramping   Inflammation

Joint stiffness

h. Genitourinary

Impotence

Menstrual irregularities

3. Monitor for and reduce the severity of adverse effects.

a. Establish a baseline assessment of pulse, blood pressure, cardiac rhythm, and lung fields.

(Baseline data facilitate detection of adverse reactions.)

b. Ensure that baseline hepatic function studies are performed before starting drug therapy.

(Calcium channel blockers can cause liver enzyme elevation.)

c. Carefully monitor blood pressure and heart rate during initial stages of therapy.

(Bradycardia and hypotension may occur.)

d. Monitor for congestive heart failure.

(Decreased cardiac output can compromise heart function.)

e. Establish with the physician the parameters (blood pressure, pulse) for withholding the medication.

(Hypotension and bradycardia can reduce cardiac output.)

f. Monitor intake, output, and weight and assess for edema.

(Reduced cardiac output can cause fluid accumulation.)

4. Teach the client and family how to prevent or reduce the severity of adverse effects. Refer to *PC: β-Adrenergic Blocker Therapy Adverse Effects* for specific interventions.

5. Instruct the client and family to report the following signs and symptoms:

a. 1- to 2-lb weight gain

b. Edema

c. Difficulty breathing

d. Pulse or blood pressure above or below preestablished parameters

e. Sleep disturbances

f. Mental changes

PC: Angiotensin-Converting Enzyme Therapy Adverse Effects

High-Risk Populations

- Severe renal dysfunction
- Systemic lupus-like syndrome
- Reduced white blood cell count
- Valvular stenosis
- Diabetes mellitus
- Pregnancy or breast-feeding
- Autoimmune disease (for captopril)
- Coronary disease (for captopril)
- Cerebrovascular disease (for captopril)
- Medication therapy that causes leukopenia or agranulocytosis
- Collagen vascular disease (for enalapril)

Nursing Goals

The nurse will manage or assist the client and family to manage and minimize adverse effects.

Interventions

Refer also to a pharmacology text for specific information on the individual drug.

1. Assess for contraindications to angiotensin-converting enzyme therapy:
   a. History of adverse effects
   b. Previous hypersensitivity
2. Explain possible adverse effects:
   a. Systemic
      Hypersensitivity (urticaria; rash; angioedema of face, throat, and extremities; difficulty breathing; stridor)
      Photosensitivity
      Alopecia
   b. Central nervous system

Vertigo	Insomnia
Fainting	Headache

   c. Cardiovascular

Tachycardia	Chest pain
Congestive heart failure	Palpitations
Hypotension	Flushing
Pericarditis	Raynaud's disease
Angina pectoris	

   d. Gastrointestinal

Loss of taste	Diarrhea
Vomiting	Peptic ulcer
Anorexia	

   e. Hematologic

Neutropenia	Eosinophilia

Agranulocytosis   Hyperkalemia
Hemolytic anemia
f. Musculoskeletal
Joint pain
g. Genitourinary
Proteinuria   Urinary frequency
Polyuria   Renal insufficiency
Oliguria
h. Respiratory
Cough

3. Monitor for and reduce the severity of adverse effects.
   a. Establish a baseline assessment of pulse, blood pressure (lying, sitting, and standing), cardiac rhythm, and lung fields.
      (Baseline assessment data are vital to evaluating response to therapy and identifying adverse reactions.)
   b. Ensure that baseline electrolyte, blood, and renal and hepatic function studies are performed.
      (The medication can cause liver enzyme elevation.)
   c. Carefully monitor blood pressure and heart rate during initial stages of therapy.
      (Bradycardia and hypotension may occur.)
   d. Monitor for congestive heart failure.
      (Decreased cardiac output can compromise heart function.)
   e. Establish with the physician the parameters (blood pressure, pulse) for withholding the medication.
      (Hypotension and bradycardia can reduce cardiac output.)
   f. Monitor intake, output, and weight and assess for edema.
      (Reduced cardiac output can cause fluid accumulation.)
4. Teach the client and family how to prevent or reduce the severity of adverse effects.
   a. Refer to *PC: β-Adrenergic Blocker Therapy Adverse Effects*, Interventions 4a–e.
   b. Stress the importance of follow-up laboratory tests.
      (Significant abnormalities in urinary protein and blood counts can occur.)
5. Instruct the client and family to report the following signs and symptoms:
   a. 1- to 2-lb weight gain
   b. Edema
   c. Difficulty breathing
   d. Pulse or blood pressure above or below preestablished parameters
   e. Dark urine
   f. Difficult urination
   g. Visual disturbances
   h. Sore throat
   i. Fever
   j. Sleep disturbances
   k. Memory loss
   l. Mental changes
   m. Behavioral changes

References/Bibliography

Adams, A. (1991). *Clinical drug therapy* (3rd ed.). Philadelphia: J. B. Lippincott.

Alfaro-LeFevre, R., Blicharz, M., Flynn, N., & Boyer, M. J. (1992). *Drug handbook: A nursing process approach.* Menlo Park, CA: Addison-Wesley Nursing.

DiPiro, J. Talbert, R. L., Hayes, P. E., Yee, G. C., Matzke, G., & Posey, L. M. (Eds.). (1995). *Pharmacotherapy* (2nd ed.). Norwalk, CT: Appleton & Lange.

Malseed, R. T. (1995). *Pharmacology: Drug therapy and nursing considerations* (4th ed.). Philadelphia: J. B. Lippincott.

McKenry, L., & Salerno, E. (1996). *Pharmacology in nursing* (17th ed.). St. Louis: C. V. Mosby.

Truhan, A. P., & Ahmed, A. R. (1989). Corticosteroids: A review with emphasis on complications of prolonged systemic therapy. *Annals of Allergy, 62,* 375–391.

Appendixes

Appendix I: Adult Assessment Guide

This guide directs the nurse to collect data to assess functional health patterns* of the individual and to determine the presence of actual, risk, or possible nursing diagnoses. Should the person have medical problems, the nurse will also have to assess for data to collaborate with the physician in monitoring for complications.

As with any printed assessment tool, the nurse must determine whether to collect or defer certain data. The symbol Δ identifies data that should be collected on hospitalized people. The collection of data in sections not marked with Δ probably should be deferred with most acutely ill people or when the information is irrelevant to the particular individual.

As the nurse interviews the person, significant data may surface. The nurse should then ask other questions (focus assessment) to determine the presence of a pattern. Each diagnosis in Section II has a focus assessment to help the nurse gather more pertinent data in a particular functional area.

For example, the client reports during the initial interview that she has a problem with incontinence. The nurse should ask specific questions using the focus assessment for *Altered Patterns of Urinary Elimination* to determine which incontinence diagnosis is present. After the nurse has identified the factors, the plan of care can be initiated.

Adult Data Base Assessment Format

1. Health Perception–Health Management Pattern
   a. Health management
      "How would you usually describe your health?"
         Excellent   Fair
         Good   Poor
      "How would you describe your health at this time?"
      Review the daily health practices of the individual
         Dental care   Leisure activities
         Food intake   Sun protection
         Fluid intake   Responsibility in the family
         Exercise regimen
      Use of
         Tobacco   Alcohol
         Salt, sugar, fat products
         Drugs (over-the-counter, prescribed)
      Knowledge of safety practices
         Fire prevention/smoke alarms
         Water safety   Children
         Automobile (maintenance, seat belts)
         Bicycle (helmets)
         Poison control
         Weapons in home
      Knowledge of disease and preventive behavior
         Specific disease (*e.g.,* heart disease, cancer, respiratory disease, childhood diseases, infections, dental disease)
         Susceptibility (*e.g.,* presence of risk factors, family history)

---

* The functional health patterns have been adapted from Gordon, M. (1982). *Nursing diagnosis: Application and process.* New York: McGraw-Hill.

"What do you do to keep healthy and to prevent disorders in yourself? In your children?"

Nutrition

Weight control

Exercise program

Self-examinations (breast, testicular)

Professional examinations (gynecologic, dental)

Immunizations

Stress management

b. Developmental history*

Family history

Maternal grandparents	Children
Mother	Paternal grandparents
Spouse	Father
Patient	Siblings

Assess for achievement of developmental tasks

Young adult

(Intimacy vs. isolation)

Accepting self and stabilizing self-concept

Establishing independence from parental home and financial aid

Becoming established in a vocation or profession that provides personal satisfaction, economic independence, and a feeling of making a worthwhile contribution to society

Learning to appraise and express love responsibly through more than sexual contexts

Establishing an intimate bond with another, either through marriage or with a close friend

Establishing and managing a residence/home

Finding a congenial social group

Deciding whether to have a family

Formulating a meaningful philosophy of life

Becoming involved as a citizen in the community

Middle age

(Generativity vs. stagnation)

Developing a sense of unity and abiding intimacy with mate

Helping growing and grown children become happy and responsible adults—relinquishing central position in their life

Taking pride in accomplishments of self and spouse

Finding pleasure in generativity and recognition in work

Balancing work with other roles

Preparing for retirement

Role reversal with parents/parental loss

Achieving mature social and civic responsibility

Developing or maintaining active organizational membership

Accepting and adjusting to changes of middle age (physical)

Socialization with new and old friends

Use of leisure time

Older adult

(Integrity vs. despair)

Deciding how and where to live out remaining years

Continuing supportive, close, and warm relationship with significant others, including a satisfying sexual relationship

Satisfactory living arrangements—safe, comfortable household routine

---

* Source: *Nursing history guide.* Nursing Department, Southeastern Missouri University, Cape Girardeau, Missouri.

Supplemental retirement income, if possible
Maintaining maximum level of self-health care
Maintaining interest in people outside of family
Maintaining social, civic, and political responsibility
Pursuing interests
Finding meaning in life after retirement
Facing inevitable illness and death of self and significant others
Formulating a philosophy of life
Finding meaning to life through philosophy/religion
Adjusting to death of spouse or loved one

c. Health perception
ΔReason for and expectations of hospitalization (and previous hospital experiences)
Δ"Describe your illness"
    Cause
    Onset
Δ"What treatments or practices have been recommended?"
    Diet   Surgery
    Weight loss   Cessation of smoking
    Medications Exercises
Δ"Are there any folk remedies that you have found helpful?"
Δ"Have you been able to follow the prescribed instructions?" If not,
    "What has prevented you?"
Δ"Have you experienced or do you anticipate a problem with caring for yourself (your
    children, a family member, your home)?"
    Mobility problems
    Sensory deficits (vision, hearing)
    Financial concerns
    Structural barriers (stairs, narrow doorway)

d. Safety
Δ"Are there any problems that could contribute to falls or accidents?"
    Unfamiliar setting
    Decreased sensorium (vertigo, confusion)
    Sensory deficits (visual, auditory, tactile)
    Motor deficits (gait, tremors, coordination)
    Urinary/bowel urgency

Δ2. Nutritional–Metabolic Pattern
"What is the usual daily food intake (meals, snacks)?"
"What is the usual fluid intake (type, amounts)?"
"How is your appetite?"
    Indigestion   Vomiting
    Nausea   Sore mouth
"What are your food restrictions or preferences?"
"Any supplements (vitamins, feedings)?"
"Has your weight changed in the last 6 months?" If yes, "Why?"
"Any problems with ability to eat?"
    Swallow liquids   Chew
    Swallow solids   Feed self
Skin
"What is the skin condition?"
    Color, temperature, turgor
    Lesions (type, description, location)
    Edema (type, location)
    Pruritus (location)
Are there any factors present that could contribute to pressure ulcer development?
    Immobility   Decreased circulation
    Dehydration   Sensory deficits
    Malnourishment

Δ3. Elimination Pattern

 a. Bladder

  "Are there any problems or complaints with the usual pattern of urinating?"

   Oliguria   Retention

   Polyuria   Burning

   Dysuria   Incontinence

   Dribbling

  "Are assistive devices used?"

   Intermittent catheterization Incontinence briefs

   Catheter (Foley, external)   Cystostomy

 b. Bowel

  "What is the usual time, frequency, color, consistency, pattern?"

  "Assistive devices (type, frequency)?"

   Ileostomy   Cathartics

   Colostomy   Laxatives

   Enemas   Suppositories

 4. Activity–Exercise Pattern

  "Describe usual daily/weekly activities of daily living"

   Occupation   Exercise pattern (type, frequency)

   Leisure activities Caregiving responsibilities

  Δ"Are there any limitations in ability?"

   Ambulating (gait, weight-bearing, balance)

   Bathing self (shower, tub)

   Dressing/grooming (oral hygiene)

   Toileting (commode, toilet, bedpan)

  "Are there complaints of dyspnea or fatigue?"

  ΔAre there factors present that could interfere with self-care after discharge?

   Motor deficits   Environmental barriers

   Cognitive/sensory deficits Lack of knowledge

   Emotional deficits   Lack of resources

Δ5. Sleep–Rest Pattern

  "What is the usual sleep pattern?"

   Bedtime   Sleep aids (medication, food)

   Hours slept   Sleep routine

  "Any problems?"

   Difficulty falling asleep Not feeling rested after sleep

   Difficulty remaining asleep Early awakening

Δ6. Cognitive–Perceptual Pattern

  "Any deficits in sensory perception (hearing, sight, touch)?"

   Glasses

   Hearing aid

  "Any complaints?"

   Vertigo

   Insensitivity to superficial pain

   Insensitivity to cold or heat

  "Able to read and write?"

 7. Self-Perception Pattern

  Δ"What are you most concerned about?"

  "What are your present health goals?"

  Δ"How would you describe yourself?"

  "Has being ill made you feel differently about yourself?"

  "To what do you attribute the following?"

   Becoming ill

   Getting better

   Maintaining health

8. Role–Relationship Pattern
    ΔCommunication
        Any hearing deficits? (hearing aids, lip-reading)
        What language is spoken?
        Is speech clear? Relevant?
        Assess ability to express self and understand others (verbally, in writing, with gestures)
    Relationships
        "Do you live alone?" "If not, with whom?"
        "To whom do you turn for help in time of need?"
        "Is there anyone who you are afraid of?"
    Assess family life (members, educational level, occupations)
        Cultural background   Decision-making
        Activities (lone or group)   Communication patterns
        Roles, discipline   Finances
    "Any complaints?"
        Parenting difficulties
        Difficulties with relatives (in-laws, parents)
        Marital difficulties
        Abuse (physical, verbal, substance)
9. Sexuality–Sexual Functioning Pattern
    "Has there been or do you anticipate a change in your sexual relations because of your condition?"
        Fertility   Pregnancy
        Libido   Contraceptives
        Erections   History
        Menstruation   Menopause
    "Have you ever been forced to have sexual relations?"
    "Have you ever experienced unwanted touching?"
    Assess knowledge of sexual functioning
10. Coping–Stress Management Pattern
    Δ"How do you make decisions (alone, with assistance, who)?"
    Δ"Has there been a change in your life in the past year (school, marital status, deaths, composition of family—moves, job, health)?"
    "What do you like about yourself?"
    "What would you like to change in your life?"
    "What is preventing you?"
    "What do you do when you are tense or under stress (*e.g.,* problem-solve, eat, sleep, take medications, seek help)?"
    Δ"What can the nurses do to provide you with more comfort and security during your hospitalization?"
11. Value–Belief System
    "With what (whom) do you find a source of strength or meaning?"
    "What are your religious practices (type, frequency)?"
    "Have your values or moral beliefs been challenged recently? Describe."
    Δ"Is there a religious person or practice (diet, book, ritual) that you would desire during hospitalization (institutionalization)?"
12. Physical Assessment (objective)
    a. General
        Age
        Height
        Weight (actual/approximate)
        General appearance
        Temperature, pulse, blood pressure, respirations

b. Cognitive–emotional

Language spoken	Ability to comprehend
Ability to read English	Level of anxiety
Ability to communicate	Interactive skills

c. Respiratory–circulatory
    Quality, cough, breath sounds
    Right/left pedal pulse

d. Metabolic–integumentary
    Skin
        Color, temperature, turgor, edema, lesions, bruises
        Tubes
    Mouth
        Gums, teeth
    Abdomen
        Bowel sounds, distended

e. Neurosensory
    Mental status
    Speech
    Pupils (size, reactivity to light)
    Eyes (appearance, drainage, ocular movements)

f. Muscular–skeletal
    Functional ability (mobility and safety)
        Dominant hand
        Use of right and left hands, arms, legs
        Strength, grasp
        Range of motion
        Gait (stability)
        Use of aids (wheelchair, braces, cane, walker)
        Weight-bearing (full, partial, none)

Appendix II: Adult Psychiatric Assessment Guide*

Bracketed Areas—To be completed by Admitting Nurse
Non-bracketed Areas—To be completed within 48 hrs of Admission by Primary Nurse

1. DEMOGRAPHIC INFORMATION

ADM/TRANS DATE / /	TIME am pm	AGE	SEX ☐ Male ☐ Female

HAIR COLOR: ☐ White ☐ Blond ☐ Brown ☐ Red ☐ Auburn
☐ Black ☐ Gray ☐ Other

EYE COLOR: ☐ Blue ☐ Brown ☐ Green ☐ Hazel ☐ Other

ETHNIC ORIGIN: ☐ Caucasian ☐ Am. Indian ☐ Hispanic ☐ Afr Amer ☐ Asian ☐ Other

ADMITTED FROM: ☐ Home ☐ Hospital ☐ Nursing Home ☐ Group Home ☐ Other

ADMITTED WITH: ☐ Family ☐ Friend ☐ Other

HOME CARE AGENCY PTA:

INFO OBTAINED FROM: ☐ Spouse ☐ Family ☐ Friend ☐ Patient ☐ Other

MARITAL STATUS: ☐ Single ☐ Married ☐ Divorced ☐ Separated ☐ Widow ☐ Widower

EMERGENCY CONTACT:
   Name   Address   Relationship   Telephone @ Home   @ Work

1.

2.

3.

PARENT/GUARDIAN:
   Name   Address   Relationship   Telephone @ Home   @ Work

REASON FOR ADMISSION:

PREVIOUS OR CURRENT HEALTH PROBLEMS ☐ No ☐ Yes. Describe: _____

---

* Developed by the Psychiatric Nursing Practice Council, Department of Pediatric, Perinatal, Psychiatric Nursing, University of Michigan Medical Center, Ann Arbor, Michigan. Used with permission.

PREVIOUS PSYCHIATRIC TX/HOSPITALIZATION: ☐ No ☐ Yes. Describe: _____

_____

_____

_____

2. ORIENTATION TO UNIT

☐ Patient Room　☐ Bathroom　☐ Showers　☐ Telephones　☐ Dining Room

☐ Community Rooms　　　☐ Staff Areas　　　☐ Other _____

EXPLANATION OF PATIENT'S RIGHTS BOOKLET

☐ Yes, by _____　☐ No. Explain why not. _____

BELONGINGS SEARCHED

☐ No　☐ Yes. By Whom? _____　Items Removed: _____

Articles were: ☐ Sent Home　☐ Stored

Money deposited in Cashier's Office ☐ No　☐ Yes Amount $ _____

EXPLANATION OF PROHIBITED ARTICLES

☐ Safety Razors　　☐ Razor Blades　☐ Scissors　　☐ Weapons

☐ Glass Articles　　☐ Other Sharps　☐ Cigarettes　☐ Pipe

☐ Chewing Tobacco　☐ Matches　　　☐ Lighter　　☐ Medications

☐ Drugs　　　　　　☐ Alcohol　　　☐ Cameras　　☐ Recording Devices

☐ Televisions

ORIENTATION TO UNIT COMPLETED BY R.N. Signature _____

3. HEALTH-PERCEPTION/HEALTH MANAGEMENT

HEIGHT	WEIGHT	TEMP	RESP	ALLERGIES

ALLERGIES

	Drugs	Food	Other

B/P　　　　　RIGHT　LEFT

☐ PCN　　☐ Chocolate　☐ Tape
☐ SULFA　☐ Shellfish　☐ Cosmetics
☐ ASA　　☐ Milk Products　☐ Wool

☐ Lying _____
☐ Sitting _____
☐ Standing _____

☐ Others _____

PULSE　　　　RIGHT　LEFT

ALLERGIC REACTIONS

☐ Lying _____
☐ Sitting _____
☐ Standing _____

☐ Rash　☐ N/V　　　　　　☐ Diarrhea

☐ Anaphylaxis ☐ Upper Respiratory

☐ Other _____

ALLERGY TREATMENT

_____

MEDICATIONS (Last 3 months)

NAME OF MEDICATION	DOSE	SCHEDULE	LAST DOSE	REASON	HOW LONG?

SUBSTANCES

Caffeine: ☐ No ☐ Coffee ☐ Tea ☐ Cola ☐ Chocolate

How much _____ How long? _____

Tobacco: ☐ No ☐ Cigarettes ☐ Cigars ☐ Pipe ☐ Chewing Tobacco

How much _____ How long? _____

DRUGS: ☐ No ☐ Marijuana ☐ Cocaine ☐ Heroin ☐ LSD
☐ Designer ☐ Amphetamines ☐ Barbiturates ☐ Other _____

How much/How long? _____

Last ingestion _____ How much? _____

Do you think you have a problem related to your drug intake? ☐ No ☐ Yes

ALCOHOL ☐ No ☐ Beer ☐ Liquor ☐ Wine

How much? _____

How long? _____ Frequency _____ Last drink _____ How much? _____

SYMPTOMS ☐ No ☐ Miss work ☐ Miss school ☐ Pass out
☐ Drink alone ☐ Drink with others ☐ Loss of memory

Family history of ETOH abuse? ☐ No ☐ Yes. Describe: _____

Do you think you have a drinking problem? ☐ No ☐ Yes. Describe: _____

KNOWN EXPOSURE TO COMMUNICABLE DISEASES: ☐ No ☐ Yes. Describe: _____

CURRENT ILLNESS/INFECTIONS: ☐ No ☐ Yes. Describe: _____

CHRONIC ILLNESS/INFECTION ☐ No ☐ Yes. Describe: _____

PAST ACCIDENT/INJURIES: ☐ No ☐ Yes. Describe: _____

GENERAL APPEARANCE:

☐ Clean ☐ Neat ☐ Unkempt ☐ Dirty ☐ Disheveled ☐ Odorous

☐ Well-nourished ☐ Obese ☐ Thin ☐ Emaciated

SELF-CARE (Dress/bathing)

☐ Independent ☐ Dependent ☐ Assistance. Describe _____

4. COPING/STRESS MANAGEMENT

What are the main concerns in your life right now? _____

How are you managing these concerns? _____

How do you manage your anger? _____

SIGNIFICANT/RECENT CHANGES	NO	YES	DESCRIBE
School			
Work			
Family Unit			
Health			
Finances			
Home			
Own illness			
Death of a significant other			
Marital status/relationship			
Retirement			

What makes you tense or nervous? _____

What do you do when you are feeling tense or nervous? _____

Does it help relieve your tension? ☐ No ☐ Yes   Are you impulsive? ☐ No ☐ Yes

Do you feel depressed? ☐ No ☐ Yes

Are you able to talk about your feelings? ☐ No ☐ Yes

SUICIDE POTENTIAL	NO	YES	DESCRIBE
1. Do you feel you have control over the events in your life?			
2. Feel like giving up?			
3. Feel guilty?			
4. Current thoughts of harming self?			

	NO	YES	DESCRIBE
5. Past attempts at harming self?			
6. Past thoughts of suicide?			
7. Past suicide attempts?			
8. Current thoughts of suicide?			
Plan for suicide?			
Ability to contract			
9. Recent suicide attempt?			
10. Attempt in the hospital?			
11. Family history of suicide?			
POTENTIAL FOR AGGRESSION	**NO**	**YES**	**DESCRIBE**
1. Have you ever hurt someone?			
2. Have you ever broken things/destroyed property?			
3. Are you having thoughts of hurting someone?			
4. Do you plan to hurt someone?			

5. NUTRITION-METABOLIC

TEETH   ☐ Normal   ☐ Dentures   ☐ Upper

                   ☐ Lower   ☐ Partial   ☐ Braces

ORAL
SYMPTOMS   ☐ None   ☐ Bleeding Gums   ☐ Sores/Patches

                   ☐ Swelling   ☐ Decay   ☐ Halitosis   ☐ Other

SKIN INTEGRITY   ☐ Intact   ☐ Turgor Normal   ☐ Diaphoretic   ☐ Turgor Poor

                   ☐ Cool   ☐ Hot   ☐ Moist   ☐ Dry

     Skin Breakdown. Describe: _____

     Reddened areas. Describe: _____

     Ecchymosis. Describe: _____

     Lesions. Describe: _____

     Warts. Describe: _____

MEAL PATTERN

     Number meals/day   1   2   3   4   5   Meal times _____

     With family   ☐ Yes   ☐ No   Meals include 4 basic food groups: ☐ Yes ☐ No

     Food restrictions/diet   _____

SELF-CARE
(feeding)   ☐ Independent   ☐ Dependent   ☐ Assistance. Describe: _____

PROBLEMS WITH EATING
OR WEIGHT   ☐ No   ☐ Yes. Describe _____

SYMPTOMS   ☐ No   ☐ Recent loss of appetite   ☐ Difficulty swallowing   ☐ Nausea   ☐ Vomiting

Describe problems: _____

FEEDING AIDS   ☐ No   ☐ Yes   ☐ Tubes   ☐ Special Utensils. Describe: _____

6. ELIMINATION

BOWEL HABITS: Last BM _____ # Stools/Day   0   1   2   3   4   ☐ Other _____

SYMPTOMS   ☐ No   ☐ Diarrhea   ☐ Constipation   ☐ Gas

☐ Cramping   ☐ Bleeding   ☐ Hemorrhoids   ☐ Involuntary stooling

☐ Use of laxatives   ☐ Other. Describe: _____

TREATMENT _____

BOWEL SOUNDS   ☐ Active   ☐ Inactive   ☐ Hyperactive   ☐ Sluggish

URINARY DIFFICULTIES   ☐ No   ☐ Yes

SYMPTOMS   ☐ Frequency   ☐ Burning   ☐ Pain   ☐ Bleeding

☐ Incontinence   ☐ Hesitancy   ☐ Dribbling   ☐ Urgency

☐ Stress

☐ Enuresis - Nocturnal - Daytime. Describe: _____

TREATMENT _____

ASSISTIVE DEVICES   ☐ No   ☐ Colostomy   ☐ Urinary Device

☐ Catheterizations   ☐ Other. Describe _____

Self Care: ☐ Independent   ☐ Dependent   ☐ With Assistance. Describe: _____

7. SEXUALITY/REPRODUCTION

ONSET OF MENARCHE/MENOPAUSE _____ LMP _____

SEXUALLY ACTIVE?   ☐ No   ☐ Yes   │ CURRENTLY PREGNANT? ☐ No ☐ Yes

SYMPTOMS   ☐ No   ☐ Dysmenorrhea   ☐ Heavy menstrual flow   ☐ Irregular cycle

CONTRACEPTIVES

☐ No   ☐ Yes   TYPE: ☐ Birth Control Pills   ☐ Vaginal Spermicides

☐ Condoms   ☐ Cervical cap   ☐ Diaphragm   ☐ Rhythm Method

☐ Other. Describe: _____

NUMBER: PREGNANCIES _____ LIVE BIRTHS _____ MISCARRIAGES _____ ABORTIONS _____

SELF BREAST EXAM   ☐ No   ☐ Yes   ☐ Deferred

SELF TESTICULAR EXAM   ☐ No   ☐ Yes   ☐ Deferred

SYMPTOMS   ☐ No   ☐ Painful intercourse   ☐ Open sores/lesions

☐ Drainage   ☐ Odor   ☐ Other _____

Recent change in sexual behavior?   ☐ No   ☐ Yes. Describe: _____

Have any sexual/reproductive concerns?   ☐ No   ☐ Yes. Describe: _____

KNOWN EXPOSURE TO STD?   ☐ No   ☐ Yes. See Below

☐ AIDS   ☐ Syphilis   ☐ Herpes   ☐ Gonorrhea   ☐ Chlamydia   ☐ Hepatitis B

☐ Other. Describe: _____

8. ACTIVITY/REST

ENERGY LEVEL ☐ Usual ☐ High ☐ Low
☐ Tires easily ☐ Lethargic ☐ Daily Variation

Describe _____

AMBULATION: ☐ Independent ☐ Dependent ☐ Assistance

CLIMB STAIRS: ☐ Independent ☐ Dependent ☐ Assistance

ASSISTIVE AIDS: ☐ No ☐ Cane ☐ Walker
☐ Crutches ☐ W/C ☐ Prosthesis

Describe problems: _____

ROM: ☐ Full ☐ Partial. Describe: _____

BALANCE/GAIT: ☐ Steady ☐ Unsteady. Describe: _____

ROUTINE EXERCISE PATTERN: Describe: _____

SYMPTOMS	NO	YES	WITH EXERTION	WITHOUT EXERTION	DESCRIBE
Chest pain					
Shortness of breath					
Coughing					
Palpitations					
Pedal edema					
Chest tightness					
Dizziness					
Joint pain					
High blood pressure					
Other					

ACTIVITY RESTRICTIONS ☐ No ☐ Yes. Describe: _____

HOBBIES/INTERESTS/EXTRA CURRICULAR ACTIVITIES Describe: _____

9. SLEEP/REST

Hrs. Sleep/Night _____ Hrs. Sleep/Daytime _____ Bedtime _____ Wake-up time _____

Feel rested? ☐ No ☐ Yes

BEDTIME RITUALS ☐ Reading ☐ Snacks ☐ T.V. ☐ Prayer ☐ Bath
☐ Exercise ☐ Nightlight ☐ Other. Describe: _____

SLEEPING AIDS
(Medications/Others) ☐ No ☐ Yes. Describe: _____

SYMPTOMS ☐ Awake easily ☐ Nightmares ☐ Night Sweats

☐ Insomnia - Early - Middle - Late   ☐ Recent Change   ☐ Fear Associated with sleep.

Describe: _____   ☐ Other. Describe: _____

10. COGNITIVE/PERCEPTUAL

EDUCATION   Last grade completed _____   College _____

Can patient read? ☐ No ☐ Yes   Can patient write? ☐ No ☐ Yes

PRIMARY LANGUAGE SPOKEN: ☐ English ☐ Other _____

VISION			HEARING		
R L		VISION CORRECTED WITH:	R L		PATIENT CAN:
☐ ☐ Normal	☐ Glasses		☐ ☐ Normal		☐ Use Sign Language
☐ ☐ Impaired	☐ Contacts		☐ ☐ Impaired		☐ Lip read
☐ ☐ Cataracts	☐ Prosthesis		☐ ☐ Deaf		☐ Other: _____
☐ ☐ Glaucoma	☐ Other. Describe: _____		☐ ☐ Hearing Aid		_____
☐ ☐ Blind	_____		☐ ☐ Other. Describe: _____		
☐ ☐ Blurred					_____
☐ ☐ Other. Describe: _____					

DISCOMFORT/PAIN ☐ No ☐ Yes. Location _____ Treatment _____

DISTRACTABILITY/ATTENTION SPAN

☐ Able to attend   ☐ Unable to attend   ☐ Easily distracted

☐ Other. Describe: _____

MOOD   *How would you describe your usual mood?*

☐ Pleasant	☐ Happy	☐ Shameful
☐ Irritable	☐ Euphoric	☐ Labile
☐ Recent change	☐ Anxious	☐ Helpless/Hopeless
☐ Calm	☐ Fearful	☐ Sad
☐ Guilty	☐ Other	

Describe: _____

AFFECT

☐ Appropriate	☐ Flat	☐ Restricted
☐ Blunted	☐ Expansive	

SPEECH RATE

☐ Normal	☐ Fast	☐ Slow
☐ Stutter	☐ Hesitant	☐ Pressured

SPEECH PRODUCTION

☐ Normal	☐ Loud	☐ Soft
☐ Clear	☐ Mumbling	☐ Slurred
☐ Monotone	☐ Mute	

COGNITION

Recent memory change? ☐ No ☐ Yes. Describe: _____

Persistent, bothersome or fearful thoughts that you cannot stop? ☐ No ☐ Yes.

Describe: _____

Rituals or practices that you feel compelled to do or cannot stop from doing? ☐ No ☐ Yes.

Describe: _____

THOUGHT CONTENT

DELUSIONS	NO	YES	DESCRIBE
Persecutory			
Grandiose			
Religious			
Self-accusatory			
HALLUCINATIONS			
Auditory			
Visual			
Tactile			
Olfactory			

ABSTRACTIONS (proverbs, similarity/differences) ☐ Within normal range

☐ Altered. Describe: _____

JUDGMENT (describe patient's answer)

1. "Stamped, addressed, sealed envelope" _____

2. "Smoke in theater" _____

INSIGHT

What is your understanding about why you are in the hospital? _____

MINI MENTAL STATUS EXAM

ORIENTATION   Score   Points

1. What is the   Year?   _____   1
                  Season? _____   1
                  Date?   _____   1
                  Day?   _____   1
                  Month?   _____   1
2. Where are we? State?   _____   1
                  County? _____   1
                  Town or
                    City? _____   1
                  Hospital? _____   1
                  Floor?   _____   1

REGISTRATION

3. Name three objects, taking
one second to say each. Then
ask the patient all three after
you have said them. Give one
point for each correct answer.
Repeat the answers until the
patient learns all three.   _____   3

ATTENTION AND CALCULATION

4. Serial sevens, give one
point for each correct answer.
Stop after 5 answers.
Alternate: Spell WORLD
backwards.   _____   5

RECALL

5. Ask for names of three ob-
jects learned in question 3.   _____   3

LANGUAGE   Score   Points

6. Point to a pencil and a
watch. Have the patient name
them as you point.   _____   2

7. Have the patient repeat
"No ifs, ands or buts."   _____   1

8. Have the patient follow a
three stage command: "Take
the paper in your right hand.
Fold the paper in half. Put the
paper on the floor."   _____   3

9. Have the patient read and
obey the following: "CLOSE
YOUR EYES."   _____   1

10. Have the patient write a
sentence of his/her choice.   _____   1

11. Have patient copy design.   _____   1

12. Total   _____ /30

THOUGHT FLOW

☐ spontaneous   ☐ sequential   ☐ appropriate   ☐ indecisive

☐ slowed response ☐ loose associations ☐ flight of ideas   ☐ thought blocking

☐ thought insertion ☐ thought withdrawal ☐ circumstantial   ☐ tangential

☐ poverty of thought ☐ illusion   ☐ Other. Describe: _____

11. SELF PERCEPTION

What do you like about yourself? _____

What don't you like about yourself? _____

Do you want to change?   ☐ No   ☐ Yes. Do you think you can change?   ☐ No   ☐ Yes

What do you think you will be doing in three years? Describe: _____

12. ROLE RELATIONSHIP

INTERACTIONS WITH SIGNIFICANT OTHERS:

Code:

SIGNIFICANT PEOPLE

A. Relaxed
B. Supportive
C. Tense
D. Argumentative
E. Abusive
F. Withdrawn
G. Other

NAME	AGE	RELATIONSHIP	INTERACTIONS (Use Code)

Who or what is your greatest support system? _____

Family concerns regarding your hospitalization: _____

13. VALUE/BELIEF

Is there a spiritual belief system that is important to you?

☐ No ☐ Yes. Describe: _____

Are there any practices within your spiritual system that are important for you during your hospitalization?

☐ No ☐ Yes. Describe: _____

Is your spiritual belief organized around a particular religion?

☐ No ☐ Yes. Describe: _____

What is most important to you in your life? Describe: _____

14. SIGNATURES

ADMITTING NURSE   R.N. SIGNATURE _____, R.N. _____
DATE/TIME

PRIMARY NURSE   R.N. SIGNATURE _____, R.N. _____
DATE/TIME

ADDITIONAL OBSERVATIONS: _____

R.N. SIGNATURE

© Copyright, 1988, Nurse Practice Committee, Department of Psychiatric Nursing, University of Michigan Hospitals

Appendix III: Pediatric Assessment*

This assessment tool contains questions useful for screening and for more specific focused questions. The focused questions should not be asked of all parents and children but are useful if indicated. The symbol Δ represents those questions that should be asked of most parents and children.

I. Identifying Information

Child's initials _____

Birthdate_____   Age _____

Sex _____

Weight _____   Percentile _____

Length or height _____   Percentile _____

Head circumference (if appropriate)_____   Percentile _____

Allergies _____

II. Data Base Assessment*

A. Health Perception–Health Management Pattern
   1. For all children
      a. How is your child's health in general?
      b. How is your child's health today?
      c. What do you do to keep your child well?
         Nutrition   Professional health care
         Opportunities for exercise and play   Immunization status
         Any regular medications? What are they? What is their purpose?
   2. For the hospitalized or ill child
      a. Why was your child admitted to the hospital?
         What caused the illness/injury?
         When did the illness begin?
      b. What treatment is your child receiving? What is your understanding of the purpose of the treatment? How do you think the treatment is working?
      c. Has your child ever been hospitalized before? For what reason? How did that go for you and the child?
      d. What expectations do you have about this hospitalization?
      e. Do you anticipate any problems in caring for your child when he goes home? What are the anticipated problems?
   3. For both well and ill children: complete for all children younger than 24 months of age and when appropriate because of related problems (*e.g.,* developmental disabilities, complications of prematurity).
      a. Did the mother have prenatal care? How long?
      b. Did the mother take any medications during pregnancy?
      c. Were there any complications during pregnancy?
      d. What were the infant's birth weight and length?
      e. What was the length of gestation?
      f. Were there any complications with the infant during the first month of life?

* Developed by Susan Ross, RN, MS, and Linda H. Snow, RN, MS, Assistant Professors, Department of Nursing, American International College, Springfield, Massachusetts, March, 1985. Used with permission. Adapted from Appendix I, Adult Assessment Guide.

B. Nutritional–Metabolic Pattern

Δ 1. How is the child's appetite?

Δ 2. Describe a typical day for your child in terms of what he eats and drinks at meals and snacks.

    a. Breast-fed

        How often?

        How long at each feeding?

        Any difficulties?

        Plans for continuing or weaning

    b. Formula-fed

        Name of formula

        Number of feedings in 24 hours

        Amount of formula at each feeding

        Any difficulties perceived

        Plans for continuing or weaning

    c. Solid foods

        When begun

        Food groups that child eats

        Approximate amounts at each meal

            Describe a typical after-school snack

Δ d. General

        Are there any food restrictions or special diet due to allergies, intolerances, other health problems, or religious practice?

        What vitamins and/or supplements does the child take?

        How much milk does the child drink in 24 hours?

        Does the child use a bottle or cup?

Δ 3. What are the child's special food likes and dislikes?

4. How often does the child go to "fast-food" restaurants? What does he usually order?

5. How much candy, other sweets, processed snack foods, and soda does your child eat/drink?

6. What, if any, concerns do you have about your child's appetite, feeding behavior, or diet?

C. Elimination Pattern

1. Bowel

Δ a. How many stools does your child have daily?

Δ b. What is the color, amount, and consistency?

Δ c. Is he toilet trained?

Δ d. Does he ever need laxatives, enemas, or suppositories? How often? How do you decide that one of the above is necessary?

Δ e. What is the usual colostomy/ileostomy care (if applicable)?

2. Bladder

Δ a. Does your child have any problems with urination?

        Bed-wetting (enuresis)   Oliguria

        Burning or other dysuria   Polyuria

        Dribbling   Urinary retention

b. Are any assistive devices used?

        Intermittent catheterization

        Indwelling catheter

    Stoma for urinary drainage—describe routine of care

Δ c. Is the child toilet trained?

        Daytime   Accidents?

        Nighttime

Δ 3. Skin—Does your child ever have any trouble with his skin (*e.g.,* itching, swelling, rashes, sores, acne, color, or temperature changes)? Describe.

D. Activity–Exercise Pattern

1. Gross motor abilities
   a. When did your child roll over? Sit unsupported? Walk alone? Climb stairs? Ride tricycle? (etc.) (Obtain information appropriate to child's age and developmental abilities.)
   b. What sports/exercise does your child enjoy and participate in?
   Δ c. What, if any, concerns do you have about your child's abilities in these areas?
2. Fine motor abilities
   a. Does your baby reach for things? Grasp? Transfer objects from one hand to another? Use his fingers to pick up objects? Feed himself a cracker? Use a spoon?
   b. What hobbies does your child have?
   c. What, if any, concerns do you have about your child's abilities to use his hands?
3. Self-care abilities or activities
   Δ a. How independent is your child in feeding himself? Describe the help he needs, if any.
   Δ b. How much help does your child need with toileting? If assistive devices are used, is child independent or does he need help? Describe. Does child use diapers, a potty chair, or toilet?
   Δ c. How much help does your child need with dressing (*e.g.*, buttons, ties, zippers)?
   Δ d. How much help does your child need with hygiene practices (*e.g.*, bathing, brushing teeth)? Does he prefer a shower or tub?

E. Sleep–Rest Patterns

Δ 1. How many hours does the child sleep each 24 hours?
   a. At night
   b. Naps
Δ 2. What is the child's usual sleep routine?
   a. Bedtime
   b. Naptime
   c. Rituals (*e.g.*, stories, drink)
   d. Security object(s)
Δ 3. Are there any problems related to sleep?
   a. Nightmares, night terrors
   b. Difficulty falling asleep
   c. Refusal at bedtime
   d. Waking up during night

F. Cognitive–Perceptual Pattern

Δ 1. Does the child have any sensory perception deficits (hearing, smell, sight, touch)? Describe.
2. What is child's grade level in school?
   a. How does he do in school?
   b. What, if any, problems are perceived by parent, teacher, or child relative to school achievement?

G. Self-Perception Pattern

Δ 1. How has your child's illness made you feel? What are you most concerned about?
Δ 2. For school-age and adolescent child: How does your illness (injury) make you feel? What are you most concerned about?
3. For well older school-age child and adolescent: How do you feel about yourself?

H. Role–Relationship Pattern

1. Communication
   a. Language development
      When did child coo? Babble? Say words? Phrases? Sentences? Use pronouns? (Use questions appropriate to child's age and developmental abilities.)

Δ Does the child use language appropriate for his age?

Δ What, if any, concerns do you have about your child's language development or characteristics of speech?

    b. What language is spoken at home?

  2. Relationships

    a. Describe family life

Δ Composition of household (family members, ages)

Δ Cultural background

Δ Roles

Δ Occupations and educational background of adults

Δ Decision-making patterns

Δ Communication patterns

Δ Discipline

Δ Problems (*e.g.*, finances, family violence, problems with parenting, marital problems)

    b. Peer relationships

Δ Does your child play with other children? Describe the quality of the child's play (*e.g.*, solitary, parallel, interactive, cooperative, aggressive).

Δ Does the child have a "best friend" of the same sex? Belong to a "gang"?

Δ Does your child prefer playmates who are older, younger, same age?

Δ Does your child have imaginary playmates?

Δ What concerns, if any, do you have about your child's relationships with others?

I. Sexuality–Sexual Functioning Pattern

Δ 1. What interest does your child show in sexuality/sexual function? How do you feel about this? How do you handle your child's curiosity and behavior?

  2. For adolescent, assess:

    a. Knowledge of sexual functioning

    b. Sexual activity (number of life-time partners)

    c. Knowledge of sexually transmitted diseases and risks

    d. Use of condoms

    e. Use of contraceptives

    f. History of pregnancy

    g. Sexual orientation

J. Coping–Stress Management Pattern

  1. How do you make decisions? (alone? with whom?)

Δ 2. Have there been any losses or changes in your life in the past year? In your child's? (*e.g.*, move, death of significant other or pet, loss of parental job)

Δ 3. To whom do you turn for support and help when you are feeling stressed?

  4. How do you manage child care, housework, and other responsibilities? For the teenager: How do you manage school work, sports and other activities, and work responsibilities?

  5. What can the nurses do to help you during this hospitalization?

K. Value–Belief System

Δ 1. What religious affiliation or preference do you hold?

Δ 2. Is there a religious person or practice (diet, book, ritual) that you desire during your child's hospitalization?

L. Physical Assessment (Objective)

  1. General appearance

  2. Temperature (note whether oral, rectal, or axillary)

  3. Skin

    a. Color

    b. Temperature

    c. Turgor
    d. Lesions
    e. Edema
    f. Excoriations
4. Head
    a. Size, shape
    b. Fontanelles and cranial sutures
5. Neck
6. Eyes (appearance, drainage)
    a. Pupils (size, equal, reactive to light)
    b. Vision
        Responds to visual stimulus   Wears glasses
7. Mouth and pharynx
    a. Mucous membranes (color, moisture, lesions)
    b. Teeth (number, primary and/or secondary, condition, orthodontic devices)
    c. Pharynx (redness, exudate, tonsils)
8. Ears (appearance, drainage)
    a. Tympanic membranes
    b. Responds to auditory stimulus
    c. Uses hearing aids
9. Pulses (radial, apical, peripheral)
    a. Rate
    b. Rhythm
    c. Quality
10. Blood pressure (note if by palpation, Doppler)
11. Respirations
    a. Rate
    b. Quality (include signs of respiratory distress)
    c. Breath sounds
12. Abdomen
    a. Bowel sounds
    b. Scars
    c. Prostheses
13. Genitalia
14. Functional ability (mobility and safety)
    a. Presence/absence of primary reflexes
    b. Gross and fine motor ability
    c. Dominant hand
    d. Mobility and use of four extremities
    e. Strength, grasp
    f. Use of aids (*e.g.*, wheelchair, braces, crutches)
    g. Weight-bearing
15. Mental status
    a. Orientation (time, person, place, events)
    b. Level of consciousness
    c. Pain (presence/absence, location, description)
    d. Affect
    e. Eye contact
    f. Use of language (ability and amount)
    g. Personal–social abilities (*e.g.*, self-care, nonverbal communication)
    h. Growth and development
        Cognitive development
          Objective data
          Stage of development according to Piaget
        Psychosocial development
          Objective data
          Stage of development according to Erikson

Appendix IV: Older Adult Assessment Guide*

Nursing Assessment Tool

Date: _____

Admitted from: ☐ Home alone ☐ Home with relative ☐ Long-term care facility
☐ Home with _____ ☐ Other _____

Mode of Arrival: ☐ Wheelchair ☐ Ambulance
Reason for Coming

_____

Past Medical History:

_____
_____

Medication (over the counter):	Dosage	Last Dose	Frequency

Health Maintenance Perception Pattern (from Resident's Viewpoint): "_____",

USE OF TOBACCO: ☐ None ☐ Quit (Date) _____ ☐ Pipe ☐ Cigar
☐ <1 pk/day ☐ 1 - 2 pks/day ☐ > 2 pks/day Pks/Year history _____

USE OF ALCOHOL: ☐ None Type _____ Amount _____ /day _____ /week ___/month

OTHER DRUGS: ☐ Yes ☐ No Type _____ Use _____

ALLERGIES (drugs, food, tape, dyes): ☐ Yes Type _____ Reaction _____

Activity/Exercise Pattern (from Resident's Viewpoint): "_____",

SELF-CARE ABILITY	Independent	Assistive Device	Assistance from Others	Assistance from Others & Equipment	Dependent/ Unable
Eating/Drinking					
Bathing					
Dressing/Grooming					
Toileting					
Bed Mobility					
Transferring					
Ambulating					
Stair Climbing					

Assistive Devices: ☐ None ☐ Crutches ☐ Walker ☐ Cane ☐ Bedside Commode
☐ Splint/Brace ☐ Wheelchair ☐ Other _____

Nutrition/Metabolic Pattern (from Resident's Viewpoint): "_____",
Special diet/supplements: _____
Previous Dietary Instructions: ☐ Yes ☐ No
Appetite: ☐ Normal ☐ Increased ☐ Decreased ☐ Decreased taste sensation ☐ Nausea
☐ Vomiting ☐ Stomatitis

CODE: (1) Non-applicable, (2) Unable to acquire, (3) Not a priority at this time, (4) Other - specify in notes.

* Used with permission of St. Joseph's Health Centre, London, Ontario, Canada. This form, which has since been integrated into the General Admission Data Base, was developed by Nancy A. Bols, RN, MSN, when a clinical specialist at St. Joseph's Health Centre.

_____

Weight Fluctuations last 6 months: ☐ None ☐ Gained ☐ Lost Lbs. _____
Swallowing Difficulty (Dysphagia): ☐ None ☐ Solids ☐ Liquids
Dentures: ☐ Upper ( ) Partial ( ) Full ☐ Lower ( ) Partial ( ) Full
History of Skin/Healing Problems: ☐ None ☐ Abnormal Healing ☐ Rash( ) ☐ Dryness
☐ Excess Perspiration

Elimination Pattern (from Resident's Viewpoint): "_____"

Bowel Habits: _____ # BMs/day _____ Date of last BM
☐ Within Normal Limits ☐ Constipation ☐ Diarrhea ☐ Incontinence
☐ Ostomy: Type:_____ Appliance _____ Self Care ☐ Yes ☐ No

Bladder Habits: ☐ WNL ☐ Frequency ☐ Dysuria ☐ Nocturia ☐ Urgency ☐ Hematuria
☐ Retention

Incontinency: ☐ Yes ☐ No _____ Total ☐ Daytime ☐ Nighttime ☐ Occasional
☐ Difficulty delaying voiding ☐ Difficulty reaching toilet

Assistive Devices: ☐ Intermittent catheterization ☐ Indwelling catheter ☐ External catheter
☐ Incontinent briefs ☐ Penile implant _____ Type

Sleep/Rest Pattern (from Resident's Viewpoint): "_____"

Habits: _____ hrs/night ☐ AM nap ☐ PM nap Feel rested after sleep ☐ No ☐ Yes
Problems: ☐ None ☐ Early waking ☐ Insomnia ☐ Nightmares

Cognitive-Perceptual Pattern (from Resident's Viewpoint): "_____"

Hearing: ☐ WNL ☐ Impaired ( ) Right ( ) Left ☐ Deaf ( ) Right ( ) Left
☐ Hearing Aid ☐ Tinnitus

Vision: ☐ WNL ☐ Eye Glasses ☐ Contact Lens
☐ Impaired ( ) Right ( ) Left ☐ Blind ( ) Right ( ) Left ☐ Cataract ( ) Right ( ) Left
☐ Glaucoma ☐ Prostheses ( ) Right ( ) Left

Vertigo: ☐ Yes ☐ No
Discomfort/Pain: ☐ None ☐ Acute ☐ Chronic ☐ Description _____
Pain Management:

Coping Stress Tolerance/Self-Perception/Self-Concept Pattern

_____

Major loss/change in past year: ☐ Yes ☐ No

_____

Affection/Reproduction Pattern
Are you an affectionate person? ☐ Yes ☐ No
Is your skin sensitive to touch? ☐ Yes ☐ No
Last Pap smear date: _____

Role/Relationship Pattern
What does your family think about your move?
_____

What do your friends think about your move?
_____

Are you afraid of anyone?
_____

CODE: (1) Non-applicable, (2) Unable to acquire, (3) Not a priority at this time, (4) Other - specify in notes.

_____

List Family Members:

_____   _____
_____   _____
_____   _____

List Friends:

_____   _____
_____   _____
_____   _____

Past Occupations:

_____   _____
_____   _____
_____   _____

Value/Belief Pattern

Religion: ☐ Roman Catholic ☐ Protestant ☐ Jewish ☐ Other (specify) _____

Religious Rituals: ☐ Yes ☐ No Contact: _____

Physical Assessment (Objective)

CLINICAL DATA Age _____ Height _____ Weight _____ (Actual/Approximate)

Temperature: _____

Pulse: ☐ Strong ☐ Weak ☐ Regular ☐ Irregular

Blood Pressure: Right Arm _____ Left Arm _____ Sitting _____ Lying _____

RESPIRATORY/CIRCULATORY

Rate:

Quality: ☐ WNL ☐ Shallow ☐ Rapid ☐ Labored ☐ Other _____

Cough: ☐ Yes ☐ No Describe _____

METABOLIC-INTEGUMENTARY

Skin Color: ☐ WNL ☐ Pale ☐ Cyanotic ☐ Ashen ☐ Jaundice ☐ Other

Temperature: ☐ WNL ☐ Warm ☐ Cool

Turgor: ☐ WNL ☐ Poor

Edema: ☐ Yes ☐ No Description/Location _____

Lesions: ☐ Yes ☐ No Description/Location _____

Bruises: ☐ Yes ☐ No Description/Location _____

Reddened: ☐ Yes ☐ No Description/Location _____

Pruritus: ☐ Yes ☐ No Description/Location _____

Tubes: Specify _____

Mouth Gums: ☐ WNL ☐ White plaque ☐ Lesions ☐ Other _____

Teeth: ☐ WNL ☐ Other _____

NEURO/SENSORY

Mental Status: ☐ Alert ☐ Receptive Aphasia ☐ Poor Historian ☐ Oriented ☐ Confused
☐ Combative ☐ Unresponsive

Speech: ☐ Normal ☐ Slurred ☐ Garbled ☐ Expressive Aphasia

Spoken Language: _____ Interpreter: _____

Pupils: ☐ Equal ☐ Unequal

Eyes: ☐ Clear ☐ Draining ☐ Reddened ☐ Other _____

MUSCULAR-SKELETAL

Range of motion: ☐ Full ☐ Other _____

Balance and Gait: ☐ Steady ☐ Unsteady

Hand grasps: ☐ Equal ☐ Strong ☐ Weakness/Paralysis ( ) Right ( ) Left

Leg Muscles: ☐ Equal ☐ Strong ☐ Weakness/Paralysis ( ) Right ( ) Left

Signature/Title _____ Date: _____

Appendix V: Maternal Assessment Guide*

This data base is divided into four sections. Section I directs the initial data collection on admission to the labor and delivery unit. Section II focuses on the collection of specific data during the immediate postdelivery period. Section III, organized under the functional health patterns, focuses on the collection of data on the family unit after the immediate postdelivery period. In Section III, the nurse can choose to defer the collection of certain data that are determined to be inappropriate. Section IV represents a Parental–Infant Interaction Assessment that is initiated during labor and delivery and is continued on the postpartum unit.

I. Intrapartal Assessment

1. Support person present
2. Childbirth preparation classes (type, location)
3. Prenatal history
   - Estimated date of confinement (EDC)
   - Past/present medical problems
     - Hospitalizations
     - Infections
     - Diabetes mellitus
     - Hypertension
4. Health history
   - History of communicable disease (gonorrhea, herpes, rubella, measles, hepatitis, mumps, acquired immunodeficiency syndrome)
   - Medications taken during pregnancy
   - Gravida, para (abortions, cesarean sections, miscarriages, premature)
   - Previous labor history (length, medications, problems)
   - Tobacco, alcohol, drug use
5. Labor history
   - When labor became apparent
   - Character and amount of show
   - Membranes (intact, ruptured, color)
   - Contractions (frequency, character)
6. Last food intake (time, type)
7. Last bowel movement
8. Present status

Rested	In control
Alert	Fearful
Tired	Out of control
Excited	Anxious
Exhausted	

9. Physical assessment
   - Vital signs
   - Cervix (effacement, dilatation)
   - Contractions (frequency, character)
   - Urine (glucose, acetone)
   - Fetal heart sounds

* Source: May, K. A., & Mahlmeister, L. (1994). *Maternal and neonatal nursing: Family-centered care* (3rd ed.). Philadelphia: J. B. Lippincott.

II. Immediate Postdelivery Assessment

1. Physical assessment
   Vital signs
   Uterine involution (position in cm)
   Lochia (amount, color)
   Perineal area (episiotomy, lacerations)
   Breasts
   Bowel sounds
   Bladder (voiding, distention, incontinence)
2. Present status (mother, significant other)
   Emotional status (describe)
   Discomforts (describe)

III. Postpartum Assessment

Assess each pattern for usual functioning and evaluate its impact on parenting, child care, and lactation as indicated. Proceed with health teaching under each pattern when indicated.

1. Health Perception–Health Maintenance Pattern
   "How would you usually describe your health?"
   "Do you have any chronic illness?"
   "How would you describe your health at this time?"
   Review the daily health practices of the individual (adults, children)

Dental care	Exercise regimen
Food intake	Leisure activities
Fluid intake	Responsibilities in the family

   Use of

Tobacco	Alcohol
Salt, sugar, fat products	Drugs (over-the-counter, prescribed)

   Knowledge of safety practices

Fire prevention	Poison control
Water safety	Automobile (maintenance, seat belts, infant seats)
Children/infants	Bicycle

   Knowledge of infant care

Nutrition (bottle, breast-feeding)	Sleep needs
Clothing needs	Developmental needs
Hygiene needs	

2. Nutritional–Metabolic Pattern
   "What is the usual daily food intake (meals, snacks)?"
   "What is the usual fluid intake (type, amounts)?"
   "How is your appetite?"

Indigestion	Vomiting
Nausea	Sore mouth

   "What are your food restrictions or preferences?"
   "Any supplements (vitamins, feedings)?"
   "Has your weight changed prior to pregnancy?" If yes, "Why?"

3. Elimination Pattern
   Bladder
   "Are there any problems or complaints with the usual pattern of urinating?"

Oliguria	Retention
Polyuria	Burning
Dysuria	Stress incontinence
Dribbling	

   Bowel
   "What is the usual time, frequency, color, consistency, pattern?"

"Assistive devices (type, frequency)?"

    Enemas   Cathartics

    Laxatives   Suppositories

4. Activity–Exercise Pattern

"Describe usual daily/weekly activities of daily living."

    Occupation

    Leisure activities

    Exercise pattern (type, frequency)

"Do you work outside the home?"

"Are there factors present that could interfere with activities at home (self-care, home care)?"

    Lack of knowledge

    Lack of resources

5. Sleep–Rest Pattern

"What is the usual sleep pattern?"

    Bedtime   Sleep aids (medication, food)

    Hours slept   Sleep routine

"Any problems?"

    Difficulty falling asleep

    Difficulty remaining asleep

    Not feeling rested after sleep

6. Cognitive–Perceptual Pattern

"Any deficits in sensory perception (hearing, sight, touch)?"

    Glasses

    Hearing aid

"Any complaints?"

    Vertigo

    Insensitivity to superficial pain

    Insensitivity to cold or heat

"Able to read and write?"

7. Self-Perception Pattern

"What are you most concerned about?"

"What are your present health goals?"

"How would you describe yourself?"

"How do you think your life will change with this baby?"

8. Role–Relationship Pattern

    Relationships

"To whom do you turn for help in time of need?"

Assess family life (members, educational level, occupations)

    Cultural background   Decision making

    Activities (lone or group)   Communication patterns

    Roles   Finances

"Any complaints?"

    Parenting difficulties

    Difficulties with relative (in-laws, parents)

    Marital difficulties

    Abuse (physical, verbal, substance)

9. Sexuality–Reproductive Pattern

    Age at menarche

    Contraceptive use (type, years of use)

    Leukorrhea, vaginal itching, postcoital bleeding, pain, or cystitis

    Sexual activities

"Have you been satisfied with the quality and quantity of your sexual activities (your partner)?"

"Any pain or discomfort with intercourse?"

"Has there been or do you expect a change in your sexual relations (related to pregnancy, child care, breast-feeding)?"

10. Coping–Stress Pattern

Δ "How do you make decisions (alone, with assistance, with whom)?"

Δ "Has there been a loss in your life in the past year (or changes—moves, job, health)?"

"What do you like about yourself?"

"What would you like to change in your life?"

"What is preventing you?"

"What do you do when you are tense or under stress (*e.g.*, problem-solve, eat, sleep, take medication, seek help)?"

11. Values–Belief Pattern

"With what (whom) do you find a source of strength or meaning?"

12. Physical Assessment

General appearance

Weight and height

Eyes (appearance, drainage)

　　Pupils (size, equal, reactive to light)

　　Vision (glasses)

Mouth

　　Mucous membrane (color, moisture, lesions)

　　Teeth (condition, loose, broken, dentures)

Hearing (hearing aids)

Pulses (radial, apical, peripheral)

　　Rate, rhythm, volume

Respirations

　　Rate, quality, breath sounds (upper and lower lobes)

Blood pressure

Temperature

Skin (color, temperature, turgor)

　　Lesions, edema, pruritus

Uterine involution (position in cm)

Lochia (amount, color)

Perineal area (episiotomy, lacerations)

Breasts

Bowel sounds

Bladder (voiding, distention, incontinence)

IV. Parental–Infant Interaction Assessment

Assess the quality of maternal–newborn acquaintance process.

A. Delivery Room Assessment

1. Attempts to see infant as soon as delivered
2. Response

Happy	Angry
Disappointed	Ambivalent
Apathetic	Sad

3. Holds and talks to infant
4. Uses baby's name
5. Response to partner

Happy	Angry
Ignores him	Indifferent

B. Postpartum Assessment

1. Verbal responses of mother

　　Verbalizes positive feelings

　　Seeks proximity by holding infant closely; touches and hugs

Smiles and gazes at infant; seeks eye-to-eye contact
Seeks family resemblance (*i.e.*, "has my eyes," "sleeps like his father")
Refers to infant by name and sex
Expresses interest in learning infant care
Performs nurturing behavior (*i.e.*, feeding, changing)
2. Requests that baby be taken to nursery
3. Complains about baby
4. Does not refer to baby by name
5. Nonverbal responses of mother

Looks, reaches out to baby	Tenses face, arms
Hugs, kisses baby	Turns head from baby
Smiles at baby	Unresponsive to partner/nurse
Positive eye contact with partner	Doesn't touch baby
Holds hand of partner	Doesn't look at baby
Breast-feeds baby	Pushes baby away
Sleepy, not drug-induced	Cries unhappily

Comments:
_____
_____

Appendix VI: Noninvasive Pain Relief Techniques

Noninvasive pain relief techniques are external measures that influence the person's internal response to pain.

General Principles
1. Convey to the person that you believe that the pain is present.
2. Explain the relationship of stress and muscle tension to pain.
3. Explain the various methods of relief and allow the person to choose one or two.
4. Attempt to teach the method when pain is absent or mild.
5. Perform the technique with the person to coach him and encourage him to focus on details of the distraction.
6. Encourage the person to practice the technique when the pain is mild.
7. Teach the person to use the technique before feeling pain (if the pain can be anticipated) and to increase the complexity of the distraction as the pain increases in intensity (*e.g.*, increase the volume of music through earphones as discomforts increase during a bone marrow aspiration).
8. Inform others (staff, family) about the technique and its purpose.
9. Explain that noninvasive pain relief can be used with medications and usually increases their effects.

Specific Techniques
- Distraction
- Cutaneous stimulation
- Relaxation

Distraction
Distraction is the deliberate focusing of attention on stimuli other than the pain sensation. The ability to be distracted from pain does not denote that the pain is nonexistent or mild. Even people with severe pain can choose to be distracted from their pain.

Distraction can be taught to children. (Caution parent not to confuse this therapeutic distraction technique that the child chooses to practice with the surprise distraction of a child before painful events. This latter technique serves only to produce feelings of mistrust and fear in children.)

Distraction cannot usually be practiced for very long periods. After the distraction ends, the person may have an increased awareness of the pain and fatigue.
1. Examples of distraction methods
    a. Visual distractions
        Counting objects (flowers on wallpaper, spots on wall, animals in picture, someone's blinks)
        Describe objects (pictures, slides)
    b. Auditory distractions (songs, tapes)
    c. Tactile kinesthetic distractions (holding, stroking, rocking, rhythmic breathing)
    d. Guided imagery (see Appendix X)
2. Breathing techniques
    a. Slow rhythmic
        Have person take slow, deep breaths through nose and exhale through mouth.
        Try to slow rate to nine breaths a minute, if possible.
        Instruct person to take extra breaths if needed.

   b. Heartbeat breathing (McCaffery & Beebe, 1989). Teach person to
      Take a slow deep breath.
      Count pulse on wrist.
      Inhale as you count two beats.
      Exhale as you count the next three beats.
   c. "He-who" breathing (McCaffery & Beebe, 1989). Instruct person to
      Take a slow deep breath.
      Inhale and say *he* on inhaling.
      Exhale and say *who* on exhaling.
      Rate can be increased (should not exceed 40/minute) if pain increases.

Cutaneous Stimulation

Cutaneous stimulation is stimulation of the skin's surface. Examples of methods follow.
1. Massage
   a. Rub with warm lubricant over painful part or over the opposite adjacent part if the actual painful part cannot be massaged (*e.g.*, if a fractured left leg is casted, the person can massage the fracture site on the right leg).
2. Application of cold
   a. The therapeutic effects of cold include:
      Reduces small-diameter nerve conduction, which lessens the perception of pain.
      Decreases the inflammatory response of tissues.
      Decreases blood flow.
      Decreases edema.
   b. The use of cold is indicated with
      Trauma (first 24–48 hours)
      Fractures
      Insect bites
      Hemorrhage
      Muscle spasms
      Rheumatoid arthritis (if relief is acquired)
      Pruritus
      Headaches
   c. The use of cold is contraindicated
      With Raynaud's disease
      With cold allergy
      48 hours after trauma
   d. Guidelines for use of cold
      Protect skin from cold burn (*e.g.*, layers of cloth between skin and cold source).
      Caution its use with people with limited communication ability or decreased sensorium (infants, sedated persons).
      Caution its use on areas with impaired sensation (*e.g.*, diabetic's foot).
   e. Examples of cold application methods
      Towel or washcloth soaked in ice water and wrung out
      Ice bags (Zip-loc plastic bag filled with ice water or frozen)
      Reusable gel pak (stored in refrigerator or freezer)
      Massage of painful site with ice
3. Application of heat
   a. The therapeutic uses of heat are
      Slows small-diameter nerve conduction, which lessens the perception of pain
      Increases the inflammatory response of stress
      Increases blood flow
      Increases edema
   b. The use of heat is indicated with
      Trauma (past 48 hours)
      Cystitis
      Hemorrhoids

Backache
Arthritis (if relief is attained)
Bursitis
c. The use of heat is contraindicated with
Trauma (first 24–48 hours)
Edema/hemorrhage
Vascular insufficiency
Malignant sites
Pruritus
d. Examples of heat application methods
Towel or washcloth soaked in warm water and wrung out (cover cloth with plastic around area to trap heat longer)
Heating pads (moist or dry)
Warm bath or shower
Sunbathing
Moist heat pack (commercially available)
4. External analgesic preparations (McCaffery & Beebe, 1989)
a. External analgesic preparations—ointments, lotions, liniments—produce a sensation (usually warmth) that may persist for several hours.
b. Guidelines for use
Do not use on broken skin.
Do not apply to mucous membranes (anus, vagina).
Always skin-test each product before using.
Follow directions and use sparingly, or painful burning may occur.
c. Examples of external analgesic preparations
Products with methyl salicylate (oil of wintergreen)
Products with menthol

Relaxation

Relaxation is a state of relief from skeletal muscle tension that the person achieves through the practice of deliberate techniques (Acute Pain Management Guideline Panel, 1992).
1. The therapeutic effects of relaxation are that it
Decreases anxiety
Provides the person with some control over pain
Decreases skeletal muscle tension
Serves as a distraction from pain
2. Examples of relaxation techniques
Biofeedback
Yoga
Meditation
Progressive relaxation exercises (see Appendix X)

References/Bibliography

Acute Pain Management Guideline Panel. (1992). *Acute pain management: Operative or medical procedures and trauma.* AHCPR Pub No 92-0032. Rockville, MD: Agency for Health Care Policy and Research.

Flynn, P. A. R. (1980). *Holistic health.* Maryland: Robert J Brady.

McCaffery, M. (1977a). Pain relief for the child: Problem areas and selected non-pharmacological methods. *Pediatric Nursing, 3*(4), 11–16.

McCaffery, M. (1977b). Technique to help a patient relax. *American Journal of Nursing, 77,* 794–795.

McCaffery, M. & Beebe, A. (1989). *Pain: Clinical manual for nursing practice.* St. Louis: C. V. Mosby.

Rancour, P. (1991). Guided Imagery: Healing when curing is out of the question. *Perspectives in Psychiatric Care, 27*(4), 30–33.

Shames, K. H. (1996). *Creative imagery in nursing.* Albany, NY: Delmar.

Appendix VII: Guidelines for Problem-Solving and Crisis Intervention

The two basic coping behaviors in response to problems are emotion-focused behaviors and problem-focused behaviors.*

Emotion-Focused Behaviors

1. *Minimization* occurs when the seriousness of a problem is minimized. This may be useful as a way to provide needed time for appraisal, but it may become dysfunctional when it precludes appraisal.
2. *Projection, displacement*, and *suppression of anger* occur when anger is attributed to or expressed toward a less threatening person or thing, which may reduce the threat enough to allow an individual to deal with it. Distortion of reality and disturbance of relationships may result, which further compound the problem. Suppression of anger may result in stress-related physical symptoms.
3. *Anticipatory preparation* is the mental rehearsal of possible consequences of behavior or outcomes of stressful situations, which provides the opportunity to develop perspective as well as to prepare for the worst. It becomes dysfunctional when the anticipation creates unmanageable stress, as, for example, in anticipatory mourning.
4. *Attribution* is the finding of personal meaning in the problem situation, which may be religious faith or individual belief. Examples are fate, the will of the divine, luck. Attribution may offer consolation but becomes maladaptive when all sense of self-responsibility is lost.

Problem-Focused Behaviors

1. *Goal-setting* is the conscious process of setting time limitations on behaviors, which is useful when goals are attainable and manageable. It may become stress-inducing if unrealistic or short-sighted.
2. *Information-seeking* is the learning about all aspects of a problem, which provides perspective and, in some cases, reinforces self-control.
3. *Mastery* is the learning of new procedures or skills, which facilitates self-esteem and self-control (*e.g.*, self-care of colostomies, insulin injection, or catheter care).
4. *Help-seeking* is the reaching out to others for support. Sharing feelings with others provides an emotional release, reassurance, and comfort, as, for example, with Weight Watchers and other self-help and support groups.

Problem-Solving Techniques

1. Identify the problem
   - What is wrong?
   - What are the causes?
   - Refer to pertinent literature, individuals, and organizations for more knowledge about the problem, if indicated.
2. Find the cause
   - Who or what is responsible for the problem?
   - How have you contributed to the problem?
   - Put yourself in the place of each person and consider the problem from his perspective.

---

* Lazarus, R. S., & Folkman, S. (1980). Analysis of coping in a middle-age community sample. *Journal of Health and Social Behavior, 21*(9), 219–239.

3. Discover the options
    What are your goals?
    What do you want to accomplish?
    What are the goals of the others involved in the problem?
    List all possible options for dealing with the problem (including not doing anything).
4. List advantages and disadvantages for each option
    What will happen if you do nothing?
    What is the worst thing that could happen with each option?
5. Choose an option and a plan
    What preparation do you need before implementing the plan?
    How do others fit into the plan?
    How will you know whether the plan is working?

Guidelines for Crisis Intervention

1. Assist the victim to confront reality (*e.g.*, encourage viewing of dead body).
2. Encourage people involved to display emotions of crying and anger (within limits).
3. Do not encourage the person to focus on all the implications of the crisis at once (*e.g.*, divorce, death) because they may be too overwhelming.
4. Avoid giving false reassurances, such as "It will be all right" or "Don't worry."
5. Clarify fantasies with facts; encourage verbalization to assist with catharsis and to identify misinformation.
6. Avoid encouraging person or family to blame others, but allow ventilation of anger (*e.g.*, rape).
7. Encourage person or family to seek help and validate its acceptability (*e.g.*, "A friend of mine found the American Cancer Society very helpful").
8. Assist person or family to identify resources (agencies, people) to help with everyday tasks of living until resolution is attained.

Appendix VIII: North American Nursing Diagnosis Association Guidelines for Nursing Diagnosis Submission

The North American Nursing Diagnosis Association (NANDA) solicits nursing diagnoses for review by the Association. Proposed diagnoses or revisions of diagnoses undergo a systematic review for determination of consistency with criteria for a nursing diagnosis. All submissions are subsequently staged according to evidence supporting either the level of development or validation (see Criteria for Staging Nursing Diagnoses and Definition of Terms).

You may submit at various levels depending on the level of completeness (*e.g.*, label and definition, label, definition, and defining characteristics, or all of the above with clinical research). Submit your work on the *Abstract of Nursing Diagnosis* form.

On receipt of your diagnosis, the Diagnostic Review Committee (DRC) will review and stage it. Diagnoses will be entered into the taxonomy at level 1.4. Before the development at level 1.4, you may seek consultation from the DRC and/or experts in the area of concern to assist you with further development and placement in the taxonomy.

Definition of Terms

Nursing diagnosis: a clinical judgment about individual, family, or community responses to actual or potential health problems/life processes. Nursing diagnoses provide the basis for selection of nursing interventions to achieve outcomes for which the nurse is accountable (approved at the 9th Conference, 1990).

Actual nursing diagnosis: describes human responses to health conditions/life processes that exist in an individual, family, or community. It is supported by risk factors that contribute to increased vulnerability.

Wellness nursing diagnosis: describes human responses to levels of wellness in an individual, family, or community that have a potential for enhancement to a higher state.

Components of a Diagnosis

Label: provides a name for a diagnosis; it is a concise term or phrase that represents a pattern of related cues. It may include qualifiers (see next section).

Definition: provides a clear, precise description, delineates its meaning, and helps differentiate it from similar diagnoses.

Defining characteristics: observable cues/inferences that cluster as manifestations of a nursing diagnosis. These are listed for actual and wellness diagnoses. A defining characteristic is described as "critical" if it must be present to make the diagnosis, and is described as "major" if it is usually present when the diagnosis exists. It is described as "minor" if it provides supporting evidence for the diagnosis but may not be present. Critical and major defining characteristics need to be substantiated by research.

Related factors: conditions/circumstances that contribute to the development/maintenance of a nursing diagnosis.

Risk factors: environmental factors and physiologic, psychological, genetic, or chemical elements that increase the vulnerability of an individual, family, or community to an unhealthful event.

Qualifiers for Diagnoses
(Suggested/not limited to the following)

Acute	severe but of short duration
Altered	a change from baseline
Chronic	lasting a long time, recurring, habitual, constant

Decreased	lessened, lesser in size, amount or degree
Deficient	inadequate in amount, quality or degree, defective, not sufficient, incomplete
Depleted	emptied wholly or in part, exhausted of
Disturbed	agitated, interrupted, interfered with
Dysfunctional	abnormal, incomplete functioning
Excessive	characterized by an amount or quantity that is greater than necessary, desirable, or useful
Increased	greater in size, amount or degree
Impaired	made worse, weakened, damaged, reduced, deteriorated
Ineffective	not producing the desired effect
Intermittent	stopping or starting again at intervals, periodic, cyclic
Potential for	(for use with wellness diagnoses)
Enhanced	made greater, to increase in quality or more desired

NANDA Developmental Stages for Nursing Diagnoses

1.0 Received for Development
   (DRC Consultation)
   1.1   Label Only
   1.2   Label and Definition
   1.3   Label and Defining Characteristics or Risk Factors
   1.4   Label, Definition, and Defining Characteristics or Risk Factors, References
2.0 Accepted for Clinical Development
   (Authentication/Substantiation)
   2.1   Label, Definition, Defining Characteristics and Literature Review
   2.2   Case Study
   2.3   Clinical Series
3.0 Clinically Supported
   (Validation and Testing)
   3.1   **
   3.2   **
   3.3   **
4.0 Revision
   (Refinement)
   4.1   **
   4.2   **
**Criteria Under Development

NANDA Criteria for Staging Nursing Diagnoses

1.0 Received for Development
   (DRC Consultation)
   1.1 Label Only
        This stage is primarily intended for submission by organized groups rather than individuals. The DRC will consult with and educate potential developers through distribution of printed guidelines for diagnostic development, telephone consultation, and referral to diagnostic development experts. At this stage, the label would be categorized as received for development.
   1.2 Label and Definition
        The label is clear and stated at a basic level. The definition is consistent with the label. The label and definition should be distinct and contrasted from other diagnoses. The definition differs from the defining characteristics and label, and these components should not be included in the definition. At this stage, the diagnosis must be consistent with the current NANDA definition of nursing diagnosis and is screened for meeting this criterion.

1.3 Label and Defining Characteristics or Risk Factors

The Defining characteristics or risk factors (for risk diagnoses) should be consistent with the label. The defining characteristics should be distinct, observable and measurable. The list of defining characteristics may include both major and minor characteristics. The number of major characteristics should be limited to five to seven.

1.4 Label, Definition, and Defining Characteristics or Risk Factors, References

The label, definition, and defining characteristics or risk factors are consistent. References are included. Criteria in 1.2 and 1.3 must be met. At this stage, the label will be forwarded to the Taxonomy Committee for classification. At stages 1.2, 1.3, and 1.4, the content will be examined for consistency with the current nursing knowledge base. The content should be consistent with the Definition of Terms. Collaboration with experts may be utilized. Consultation with the DRC is encouraged.

2.0 Accepted for Clinical Development
(Authentication/Substantiation)

2.1 Label, Definition, Defining Characteristics and Literature Review

A narrative review of relevant literature is required to demonstrate the existence of a substantive body of knowledge underlying the diagnosis. The literature review is consistent with the label and definition. Literature should include discussion and support of the defining characteristics or risk factors (for risk diagnoses), and related factors (for actual diagnoses).

2.2 Case Study

The criteria in 2.1 are met. The narrative includes the description of an actual case that exhibits the nursing diagnosis and includes defining characteristics or risk factors. Related factors, interventions and outcomes are optional.

2.3 Clinical Studies

The criteria for 2.1 are met. The narrative includes the description of a series of at least 10 cases that exhibit the diagnosis and includes defining characteristics or risk factors, related factors, interventions and outcomes.

3.0 Clinically Supported
(Validation and Testing)

3.1 **
3.2 **
3.3 **

4.0 Revision
(Refinement)

4.1 **
4.2 **

**Criteria Under Development

NANDA-Approved Nursing Diagnoses

This list represents the NANDA-approved nursing diagnoses for clinical use and testing (1994).

Pattern 1: Exchanging

1.1.2.1	Altered Nutrition: More than body requirements
1.1.2.2	Altered Nutrition: Less than body requirements
1.1.2.3	Altered Nutrition: Potential for more than body requirements
1.2.1.1	Risk for Infection
1.2.2.1	Risk for Altered Body Temperature
1.2.2.2	Hypothermia
1.2.2.3	Hyperthermia
1.2.2.4	Ineffective Thermoregulation
1.2.3.1	Dysreflexia
1.3.1.1	Constipation
1.3.1.1.1	Perceived Constipation

1.3.1.1.2	Colonic Constipation
1.3.1.2	Diarrhea
1.3.1.3	Bowel Incontinence
1.3.2	Altered Urinary Elimination
1.3.2.1.1	Stress Incontinence
1.3.2.1.2	Reflex Incontinence
1.3.2.1.3	Urge Incontinence
1.3.2.1.4	Functional Incontinence
1.3.2.1.5	Total Incontinence
1.3.2.2	Urinary Retention
1.4.1.1	Altered (Specify Type) Tissue Perfusion (Renal, cerebral, cardiopulmonary, gastrointestinal, peripheral)
1.4.1.2.1	Fluid Volume Excess
1.4.1.2.2.1	Fluid Volume Deficit
1.4.1.2.2.2	Risk for Fluid Volume Deficit
1.4.2.1	Decreased Cardiac Output
1.5.1.1	Impaired Gas Exchange
1.5.1.2	Ineffective Airway Clearance
1.5.1.3	Ineffective Breathing Pattern
1.5.1.3.1	Inability to Sustain Spontaneous Ventilation
1.5.1.3.2	Dysfunctional Ventilatory Weaning Response (DVWR)
1.6.1	Risk for Injury
1.6.1.1	Risk for Suffocation
1.6.1.2	Risk for Poisoning
1.6.1.3	Risk for Trauma
1.6.1.4	Risk for Aspiration
1.6.1.5	Risk for Disuse Syndrome
1.6.2	Altered Protection
1.6.2.1	Impaired Tissue Integrity
1.6.2.1.1	Altered Oral Mucous Membrane
1.6.2.1.2.1	Impaired Skin Integrity
1.6.2.1.2.2	Risk for Impaired Skin Integrity
1.7.1	Decreased Adaptive Capacity: Intracranial
1.8	Energy Field Disturbance

Pattern 2: Communicating

2.1.1.1	Impaired Verbal Communication

Pattern 3: Relating

3.1.1	Impaired Social Interaction
3.1.2	Social Isolation
3.1.3	Risk for Loneliness
3.2.1	Altered Role Performance
3.2.1.1.1	Altered Parenting
3.2.1.1.2	Risk for Altered Parenting
3.2.1.1.2.1	Risk for Altered Parent/Infant/Child Attachment
3.2.1.2.1	Sexual Dysfunction
3.2.2	Altered Family Processes
3.2.2.1	Caregiver Role Strain
3.2.2.2	Risk for Caregiver Role Strain
3.2.2.3.1	Altered Family Process: Alcoholism
3.2.3.1	Parental Role Conflict
3.3	Altered Sexuality Patterns

Pattern 4: Valuing

4.1.1	Spiritual Distress (distress of the human spirit)
4.2	Potential for Enhanced Spiritual Well-Being

Pattern 5: Choosing

5.1.1.1	Ineffective Individual Coping
5.1.1.1.1	Impaired Adjustment
5.1.1.1.2	Defensive Coping
5.1.1.1.3	Ineffective Denial
5.1.2.1.1	Ineffective Family Coping: Disabling
5.1.2.1.2	Ineffective Family Coping: Compromised
5.1.3.1	Potential for Enhanced Community Coping
5.1.3.2	Ineffective Community Coping
5.1.2.2	Family Coping: Potential for Growth
5.2.1	Ineffective Management of Therapeutic Regimen (Individuals)
5.2.1.1	Noncompliance (Specify)
5.2.2	Ineffective Management of Therapeutic Regimen: Families
5.2.3	Ineffective Management of Therapeutic Regimen: Community
5.2.4	Effective Management of Therapeutic Regimen: Individual
5.3.1.1	Decisional Conflict (Specify)
5.4	Health Seeking Behaviors (Specify)

Pattern 6: Moving

6.1.1.1	Impaired Physical Mobility
6.1.1.1.1	Risk for Peripheral Neurovascular Dysfunction
6.1.1.1.2	Risk for Perioperative Positioning Injury
6.1.1.2	Activity Intolerance
6.1.1.2.1	Fatigue
6.1.1.3	Risk for Activity Intolerance
6.2.1	Sleep Pattern Disturbance
6.3.1.1	Diversional Activity Deficit
6.4.1.1	Impaired Home Maintenance Management
6.4.2	Altered Health Maintenance
6.5.1	Feeding Self Care Deficit
6.5.1.1	Impaired Swallowing
6.5.1.2	Ineffective Breast-feeding
6.5.1.2.1	Interrupted Breast-feeding
6.5.1.3	Effective Breast-feeding
6.5.1.4	Ineffective Infant Feeding Pattern
6.5.2	Bathing/Hygiene Self Care Deficit
6.5.3	Dressing/Grooming Self Care Deficit
6.5.4	Toileting Self Care Deficit
6.6	Altered Growth and Development
6.7	Relocation Stress Syndrome
6.8.1	Risk for Disorganized Infant Behavior
6.8.2	Disorganized Infant Behavior
6.8.3	Potential for Enhanced Organized Infant Behavior

Pattern 7: Perceiving

7.1.1	Body Image Disturbance
7.1.2	Self Esteem Disturbance
7.1.2.1	Chronic Low Self Esteem
7.1.2.2	Situational Low Self Esteem
7.1.3	Personal Identity Disturbance
7.2	Sensory/Perceptual Alterations (Specify) (Visual, auditory, kinesthetic, gustatory, tactile, olfactory)
7.2.1.1	Unilateral Neglect
7.3.1	Hopelessness
7.3.2	Powerlessness

Pattern 8: Knowing

8.1.1	Knowledge Deficit (Specify)
8.2.1	Impaired Environmental Interpretation Syndrome
8.2.2	Acute Confusion
8.2.3	Chronic Confusion
8.3	Altered Thought Processes
8.3.1	Impaired Memory

Pattern 9: Feeling

9.1.1	Pain
9.1.1.1	Chronic Pain
9.2.1.1	Dysfunctional Grieving
9.2.1.2	Anticipatory Grieving
9.2.2	Risk for Violence: Self-directed or directed at others
9.2.2.1	Risk for Self-Mutilation
9.2.3	Post-trauma Response
9.2.3.1	Rape Trauma Syndrome
9.2.3.1.1	Rape Trauma Syndrome: Compound Reaction
9.2.3.1.2	Rape Trauma Syndrome: Silent Reaction
9.3.1	Anxiety
9.3.2	Fear

Appendix IX: Guidelines for Play Therapy

Play is a natural means of expression for children and is essential to their mental, emotional, and social well-being. The need for play during stress (*e.g.*, developmental, illness, treatments) is essential to provide the child with an outlet for emotional release and a sense of mastery over the situation. Play provides parents and professionals with opportunities to assess the mood, words, and actions of a child and identify the child's present perception of the situation.

A. General
  1. Professionals and parents use play to assist the child to
    a. Recognize feelings
    b. Cope with a new concept
    c. Identify fears
    d. Understand threatening or unknown events
    e. Clarify distortions received from others (parents, peers)
    f. Gain a sense of mastery
  2. Play can be used to diagnose the child's perception of the situation, perception of care-givers, and mental responses to events.
  3. Guidelines for therapeutic play
    a. Promote spontaneity by reflecting only what the child expresses.
    b. Avoid forcing the child to participate.
    c. Allow sufficient time without interruption.
    d. Identify when it is appropriate to encourage child to share concerns.
    e. Play for the child who cannot play for himself.
    f. Allow child to work freely on a project without direction or adult comment.
    g. Allow child to engage in violent nondestructive acts.

B. Types of Play
  1. Drawing and painting
    a. Supplies: Crayons, paint, brushes, paper
        Artwork usually requires little direction.
        Older children can be asked to draw what they like or do not like about the hospital.
        An old sheet can cover the bed clothes of a child confined to bed.
        Ask child to explain picture when it is done.
        Clarify misconceptions.
  2. Dramatic play
    b. Supplies: Puppets, dolls, stuffed animals, replicas of hospital equipment, actual hospital equipment, miniature hospital furniture
        Assign roles to the child and to the doll or puppet ("Mary, you are the nurse and the puppet is you.").
        Ask child to administer a treatment to the puppet or doll.
        Supervise the child when playing with equipment.
  3. Needle play (dramatic play)
    c. Supplies: Doll, stuffed animals, clean syringes and needles, alcohol wipes, water vial, Band-Aids, miniature IV sets (tubing, tourniquets, tongue blade for arm board)
        Introduce immediately after or in between the child's experiences.
        Expect reluctance to touch syringe.
        Demonstrate injection and ask the child to help you push the fluid in.

Allow child to give injections on the doll anywhere and however he wants to.
Make appropriate sounds of crying and protest to show the child that crying is permitted.
Show child how to give the doll love after the injection.
Encourage child to talk about why injections are needed.
Use group play to encourage participation.
Overly aggressive children should be shown acceptance.

Bibliography

Abbott, K. (1990). The therapeutic use of play in the psychological preparation of preschool children undergoing cardiac surgery. *Issues in Comprehensive Pediatric Nursing, 13*, 265–277.

Levinson, P., & Ousterhout, D. (1980). Art and play therapy with pediatric burn patients. *Journal of Burn Care and Rehabilitation, 1*, 42–46.

Petrillo, M., & Sanger, S. (1980). *Emotional care of hospitalized children* (2nd ed.). Philadelphia: J. B. Lippincott.

Smallwood, S. (1988). Preparing children for surgery. *AORN Journal, 47*(1), 177–182.

Taylor, M., & Williams, H. (1980). Use of therapeutic play in the ambulatory pediatric hematology clinic. *Cancer Nursing, 3*, 433–437.

Wong, D. (1995). *Nursing care of infants and children* (5th ed.). St. Louis: Mosby–Year Book.

Appendix X: Stress Management Techniques

The following techniques can be taught to provide an individual with an opportunity to control his response to stressors and, in turn, increase his ability to manage stress constructively. Suggested readings are listed at the end to provide more specific information.

Progressive Relaxation Technique

Progressive relaxation is a self-taught or instructed exercise that involves learning to constrict and relax muscle groups in a systematic way, beginning with the face and finishing with the feet. This exercise may be combined with breathing exercises that focus on inner body processes. It usually takes 15 to 30 minutes and may be accompanied by a taped instruction that directs the person concerning the sequence of muscles to be relaxed.

1. Wear loose clothing; remove glasses and shoes.
2. Sit or recline in a comfortable position with neck and knees supported; avoid lying completely flat.
3. Begin with slow, rhythmic breathing.
   a. Close your eyes or stare at a spot and take in a slow, deep breath.
   b. Exhale the breath slowly.
4. Continue rhythmic breathing at a slow, steady pace and feel the tension leaving your body with each breath.
5. Begin progressive relaxation of muscle groups.
   a. Breathe in and tense (tighten) your muscles and then relax the muscles as you breathe out.
   b. Suggested order for tension–relaxation cycle (with tension technique in parentheses):
      Face, jaw, mouth (squint eyes, wrinkle brow)
      Neck (pull chin to neck)
      Right hand (make a fist)
      Right arm (bend elbow in tightly)
      Left hand (make a fist)
      Left arm (bend elbow in tightly)
      Back, shoulders, chest (shrug shoulders up tightly)
      Abdomen (pull stomach in and bear down on chair)
      Right upper leg (push leg down)
      Right lower leg and foot (point toes toward body)
      Left upper leg (push leg down)
      Left lower leg and foot (point toes toward body)
6. Practice technique slowly.
7. End relaxation session when you are ready by counting to three, inhaling deeply, and saying, "I am relaxed."

Self-Coaching

Self-coaching is a procedure to decrease anxiety by understanding one's own signs of anxiety (such as increased heart rate or sweaty palms) and then coaching oneself to relax.

For example, "I am upset about this situation but I can control how anxious I get. I will take things one step at a time, and I won't focus on my fear. I'll think about what I must do to finish this task. The situation will not be forever. I can manage until it is over. I'll focus on taking deep breaths."

Thought Stopping

Thought stopping is a self-directed behavioral procedure learned to gain control of self-defeating thoughts. Through repeated systematic practice, a person does the following:

1. Says "Stop" when a self-defeating thought crosses the mind (*e.g.*, "I'm not smart enough" or "I'm not a good nurse")
2. Allows a brief period–15 to 30 seconds–of conscious relaxation (because of an increased focus on negative thoughts, it may seem at first that self-defeating thoughts increase; however, eventually the self-defeating thoughts will decrease)

Assertive Behavior

Assertive behavior is the open, honest, empathetic sharing of your opinions, desires, and feelings. Assertiveness is not a magical acquisition but a learned behavioral skill. Assertive people do not allow others to take advantage of them and thus are not victims. Assertive behavior is not domineering but remains controlled and nonaggressive. An assertive person
> Does not hurt others
> Does not wait for things to get better
> Does not invite victimization
> Listens attentively to the desires and feelings of others
> Takes the initiative to make relationships better
> Remains in control or uses silences as an alternative
> Examines all the risks involved before asserting
> Examines personal responsibilities in each situation before asserting

Refer to suggested readings for specific techniques or participate in an assertiveness training course led by a competent instructor. Assertive behavior is best learned slowly in several sessions rather than in one lengthy session or workshop.

Guided Imagery

This technique is the purposeful use of the imagination in a specific way to achieve relaxation and control. The person concentrates on the image and pictures himself involved in the scene. The following is an example of the technique.
1. Discuss with person an image he has experienced that is pleasurable and relaxing to him, such as
   a. Lying on a warm beach
   b. Feeling a cool wave of water
   c. Floating on a raft
   d. Watching the sun set
2. Choose a scene that will involve at least two senses.
3. Begin with rhythmic breathing and progressive relaxation.
4. Have a person travel mentally to the scene.
5. Have the person slowly experience the scene; how does it look? sound? smell? feel? taste?
6. Practice the imagery.
   a. Suggest tape-recording the imagined experience to assist with the technique.
   b. Practice the technique alone to reduce feelings of embarrassment.
7. End the imagery technique by counting to three and saying, "I am relaxed" (if the person does not use a specific ending, he may become drowsy and fall asleep, which defeats the purpose of the technique).

Bibliography

Alberti, R. E., & Emmons, L. (1974). *Your perfect right: A guide to assertive behavior* (2nd ed.). San Luis Obispo, CA: Impact.

Bloom, L., Coburn, K., & Pearlman, J. (1976). *The new assertive woman*. New York: Dell.

Chenevert, M. (1978). *Special techniques in assertiveness training for women in the health professions*. St. Louis: C. V. Mosby.

Chenevert, M. (1985). *Pro-nurse handbook*. St. Louis: C. V. Mosby.

Frisch, N. C., & Kelley, J. (1996). *Healing life's crisis: A guide for nurses*. Albany, NY: Delmar.

Gridano, D., & Everly, G. (1979). *Controlling stress and tension*. Englewood Cliffs, NJ: Prentice-Hall.

Herman, S. (1978). *Becoming assertive: A guide for nurses*. New York: Van Nostrand.

Hill, L., & Smith, N. (1985). *Self-care nursing*. Englewood Cliffs, NJ: Prentice-Hall (especially Part II, Self-care primarily associated with the mind).

McCaffery, M. (1979). *Nursing management of the patient with pain* (2nd ed.). Philadelphia: J. B. Lippincott (especially Chapter 9, Relaxation; Chapter 10, Imagery).

Rancour, P. (1991). Guided Imagery: Healing when curing is out of the question. *Perspectives in Psychiatric Care, 27*(4), 30–33.

Appendix XI: Conditions That Necessitate Nursing Care

Nursing Diagnoses*

1. Health Perception–Health Management
    Growth and Development, Altered
    Health Maintenance, Altered
    Health-Seeking Behaviors
    † Management of Therapeutic Regimen, Effective: Individual
    Management of Therapeutic Regimen (Individual), Ineffective
    † Management of Therapeutic Regimen, Ineffective: Community
    † Management of Therapeutic Regimen, Ineffective: Family
    Noncompliance
    Risk for Injury
        Risk for Suffocation
        Risk for Poisoning
        Risk for Trauma
    † Injury, Risk for Perioperative Positioning
2. Nutritional–Metabolic
    Body Temperature, Risk for Altered
        Hypothermia
        Hyperthermia
        Thermoregulation, Ineffective
    Fluid Volume Deficit
    Fluid Volume Excess
    Infection, Risk for
    △ Infection Transmission, Risk for
    Nutrition, Altered: Less Than Body Requirements
        Breast-feeding, Effective
        Breast-feeding, Ineffective
        Breast-feeding, Interrupted
        Feeding Pattern, Ineffective Infant
        Swallowing, Impaired
    Nutrition, Altered: More Than Body Requirements
    Nutrition, Altered: Risk for More Than Body Requirements
    Protection, Altered
        Tissue Integrity, Impaired
        Oral Mucous Membrane, Altered
        Skin Integrity, Impaired
3. Elimination
    △ Bowel Elimination, Altered
        Constipation
        Colonic Constipation
        Perceived Constipation

---

* The Functional Health Patterns were identified in Gordon, M. (1982). *Nursing diagnosis: Process and application.* New York: McGraw-Hill; with minor changes by the author.

† These categories were accepted by the North American Nursing Diagnosis Association in 1994.

△ These diagnoses are not currently on the NANDA list but have been included for clarity and usefulness.

　　　　　Diarrhea
　　　　　Bowel Incontinence
　　　Urinary Elimination, Altered Patterns of
　　　　　Urinary Retention
　　　　　Total Incontinence
　　　　　Functional Incontinence
　　　　　Reflex Incontinence
　　　　　Urge Incontinence
　　　　　Stress Incontinence
　　　△ Maturational Enuresis
4. Activity–Exercise
　　　Activity Intolerance
　　† Adaptive Capacity, Intracranial: Decreased
　　　Cardiac Output, Decreased
　　　Disuse Syndrome
　　　Diversional Activity Deficit
　　　Home Maintenance Management, Impaired
　　† Infant Behavior, Disorganized
　　† Infant Behavior, Risk for Disorganized
　　† Infant Behavior, Potential for Enhanced Organized
　　　Mobility, Impaired Physical
　　　Peripheral Neurovascular Dysfunction, Risk for
　　△ Respiratory Function, Risk for Altered
　　　　　Dysfunctional Ventilatory Weaning Response
　　　　　Ineffective Airway Clearance
　　　　　Ineffective Breathing Patterns
　　　　　Impaired Gas Exchange
　　　　　Ventilation, Inability to Sustain Spontaneous
　　△ Self-Care Deficit Syndrome
　　　　　(Specify) (△ Instrumental, Feeding, Bathing/Hygiene, Dressing/Grooming, Toilet-
　　　　　　ing)
　　　Tissue Perfusion, Altered (Specify Type) (Cerebral, Cardiopulmonary, Renal, Gas-
　　　　　trointestinal, Peripheral)
5. Sleep–Rest
　　　Sleep Pattern Disturbance
6. Cognitive–Perceptual
　　△ Comfort, Altered
　　　　　Acute Pain
　　　　　Chronic Pain
　　△ Confusion
　　　　　† Acute Confusion
　　　　　† Chronic Confusion
　　　Decisional Conflict
　　　Dysreflexia
　　† Environmental Interpretation Syndrome, Impaired
　　　Knowledge Deficit (specify)
　　　Risk for Aspiration
　　　Sensory–Perceptual Alterations: (Specify) (Visual, Auditory, Kinesthetic, Gustatory,
　　　　　Tactile, Olfactory)
　　　Thought Processes, Altered
　　　　　† Memory, Impaired
　　　Unilateral Neglect
7. Self-Perception
　　　Anxiety
　　　Fatigue
　　　Fear

Hopelessness
Powerlessness
△ Self-Concept Disturbance
    Body Image Disturbance
    Personal Identity Disturbance
    Self-Esteem Disturbance
        Chronic Low Self-Esteem
        Situational Low Self-Esteem
8. Role–Relationship
    △ Communication, Impaired
        Communication, Impaired Verbal
    Family Processes, Altered
        † Family Processes, Altered: Alcoholism
    △ Grieving
        Grieving, Anticipatory
        Grieving, Dysfunctional
    † Loneliness, Risk for
    † Parent–Infant Attachment, Risk for Altered
    Parenting, Altered
    Parental Role Conflict
    Role Performance, Altered
    Social Interaction, Impaired
    Social Isolation
9. Sexuality–Reproductive
    Sexual Dysfunction
    Sexuality Patterns, Altered
10. Coping–Stress Tolerance
    Adjustment, Impaired
    Caregiver Role Strain
    Coping, Ineffective Individual
        Defensive Coping
        Ineffective Denial
    Coping: Disabling, Ineffective Family
    Coping: Compromised, Ineffective Family
    Coping: Potential for Growth, Family
    † Coping, Ineffective Community
    † Coping, Potential for Enhanced Community
    † Energy Field Disturbance
    Post-trauma Response
        Rape Trauma Syndrome
    Relocation Stress Syndrome
    △ Self-Harm, Risk for
        Self-Abuse, Risk for
        Self-Mutilation, Risk for
        △ Suicide, Risk for
    Violence, Risk for
11. Value–Belief
    Spiritual Distress
    † Spiritual Well-Being, Potential for Enhanced

† These categories were accepted by the North American Nursing Diagnosis Association in 1994.
△ These diagnoses are not currently on the NANDA list but have been included for clarity and usefulness.

Collaborative Problems

1. Potential Complication: Gastrointestinal/Hepatic/Biliary
      PC: Paralytic Ileus/Small Bowel Obstruction
      PC: Hepatorenal Syndrome
      PC: Hyperbilirubinemia
      PC: Evisceration
      PC: Hepatosplenomegaly
      PC: Curling's Ulcer
      PC: Ascites
      PC: Gastrointestinal Bleeding
      PC: Hepatic Insufficiency/Failure
2. Potential Complication: Metabolic/Immune/Hematopoietic
      PC: Hypoglycemia, Hyperglycemia
      PC: Opportunistic Infections
      PC: Negative Nitrogen Balance
      PC: Electrolyte Imbalances
      PC: Thyroid Dysfunction
      PC: Hypothermia (Severe)
      PC: Hyperthermia (Severe)
      PC: Sepsis
      PC: Acidosis
      PC: Alkalosis
      PC: Anemia
      PC: Thrombocytopenia
      PC: Hypothyroidism/Hyperthyroidism
      PC: Allergic Reaction
      PC: Sickling Crisis
      PC: Adrenal Insufficiency
3. Potential Complication: Neurologic/Sensory
      PC: Increased Intracranial Pressure
      PC: Stroke
      PC: Seizures
      PC: Spinal Cord Compression
      PC: Autonomic Dysreflexia
      PC: Retinal detachment
      PC: Hydrocephalus
      PC: Microcephalus
      PC: Meningitis
      PC: Cranial Nerve Impairment
      PC: Paresis/Paresthesia/Paralysis
      PC: Neuroleptic Malignant Syndrome
      PC: Increased Intraocular Pressure
      PC: Corneal Ulceration
      PC: Neuropathies
      PC: Alcohol Withdrawal
4. Potential Complication: Cardiac/Vascular
      PC: Dysrhythmias
      PC: Congestive Heart Failure
      PC: Cardiogenic Shock
      PC: Thromboemboli/Deep Vein Thrombosis
      PC: Hypovolemic Shock
      PC: Peripheral Vascular Insufficiency
      PC: Hypertension
      PC: Congenital Heart Disease
      PC: Decreased Cardiac Output

PC: Cardiac Tamponade
PC: Air Embolism
PC: Disseminated Intravascular Coagulation
PC: Endocarditis
PC: Septic Shock
PC: Embolism
PC: Spinal Shock
PC: Ischemic Ulcers
PC: Angina
PC: Compartmental Syndrome
5. Potential Complication: Respiratory
PC: Atelectasis/Pneumonia
PC: Tracheobronchial Constriction
PC: Oxygen Toxicity
PC: Pulmonary Embolism
PC: Pleural Effusion
PC: Tracheal Necrosis
PC: Pneumothorax
PC: Laryngeal Edema
PC: Hypoxemia
6. Potential Complication: Renal/Urinary
PC: Acute Urinary Retention
PC: Renal Insufficiency
PC: Bladder Perforation
PC: Renal Calculi
7. Potential Complication: Reproductive
PC: Reproductive Tract Infections
PC: Fetal Distress
PC: Postpartum Hemorrhage
PC: Pregnancy-Associated Hypertension
PC: Prenatal Bleeding
PC: Preterm Labor
PC: Hypermenorrhea
PC: Polymenorrhea
PC: Intrapartum Hemorrhage
PC: Sexually Transmitted Disease
PC: Dystocia
8. Potential Complication: Musculoskeletal
PC: Pathologic Fractures
PC: Osteoporosis
PC: Joint Dislocation
PC: Osteomyelitis
9. Potential Complication: Medication Therapy Adverse Effects
PC: Adrenocorticosteroid Therapy Adverse Effects
PC: Antianxiety Therapy Adverse Effects
PC: Antiarrhythmic Therapy Adverse Effects
PC: Anticoagulant Therapy Adverse Effects
PC: Anticonvulsant Therapy Adverse Effects
PC: Antidepressant Therapy Adverse Effects
PC: Antihypertensive Therapy Adverse Effects
PC: β-Adrenergic Blocker Therapy Adverse Effects
PC: Calcium Channel Blocker Therapy Adverse Effects
PC: Angiotensin-Converting Enzyme Therapy Adverse Effects
PC: Antineoplastic Therapy Adverse Effects
PC: Antipsychotic Therapy Adverse Effects

Appendix XII: Self-Reporting Oncology Nursing Assessment*

This questionnaire is designed for the client or significant other to complete before an interview with the professional nurse. During the interview, the nurse reviews the answers with the client and significant other. Additional data obtained during the interview are recorded in the column on the right.

SELF-REPORTING PATIENT HEALTH QUESTIONNAIRE
(Please complete this questionnaire by checking off the appropriate word that fits your situation or writing in the information where space is provided. When you are not certain about a question put a "?" beside it. The nurse will discuss this with you privately during your interview.)

PART I: ADMISSION DATA	INTERVIEW INFORMATION
Date: __/__/__ Age: __ yrs. Male __ Female __ Name you prefer _____	
d m y	
If we are unable to reach you, whom could we contact on your behalf?	
1. _____ Phone (__) - ___	
2. _____ Phone (__) - ___	
What languages do you speak? _____	
Who is your family doctor? _____	
Which pharmacy/drugstore do you use? _____ Phone (__) - ___	

HEALTH MAINTENANCE

PART II: PATIENT HISTORY

1. What is the health problem that has brought you here today? _____

_____

2. What tests, surgeries or medical consultations have you had in the past 6 weeks?

_____

_____

3. What treatment(s) are you receiving at this time? _____

_____

(continued)

---

* Developed by Rosemary Allaster, RN, BA; Eunice Anderson, RN, MScN; Mary Liz Bland, RN, SBcN; Maureen Brock, RN, BScN; Gwen Flegel, RN; Bonnie Hall, RN, MScN; Maria Jefferies, RN, MSN; Sue Kudirka, RN; Marcia Langhorn, RN; Linda D. Riehl, RN; Heather Ryan, RN, MScN; and Marilyn Semple, RN, of the Nursing Department, London Regional Cancer Centre, London, Ontario, Canada. Used with permission.

		INTERVIEW INFORMATION

HEALTH PERCEPTION

4. List your past health history (major illness/operations/injuries/accidents with dates):

   _____

   _____

5. a. Do you smoke? Yes____ No____   b. Did you ever smoke? Yes____ No____

   If Yes, indicate type, amount, for how long, and when you quit: _____

   _____

6. Have you had any experience with cancer (yourself, relative, or a friend)?

   Yes____ No____

   If yes, specify person, relationship and type of cancer: _____

   _____

   _____

7. Do you take any medications? Yes____ No____ If yes, please list the prescription medications and over-the-counter medications you now take. Please include the dose—how many mg or mL you take, why you need to take the drug.

   _____

   _____

   _____

8. Do you have a drug plan? Yes____ No____

9. Do you have any ALLERGIES? Yes____ No____ If yes, please list the cause of your allergy and the allergic reaction that you have.

   _____

   _____

10. Please check the services you are now using: None____   Home Care____

    Visiting nurse ____ VON____ Public Health Nurse ____ Cancer Society ____

    Other (specify) _____

NUTRITION–METABOLIC

11. Please check the word to describe your diet: Regular____ Soft____ Liquid____

    Diabetic____ Other: _____

12. Do you take a diet supplement? Yes____ No____

    If yes, please specify: _____

13. Do you drink alcohol (beer, wine, liquor)? Yes____ No____

14. Place a check beside the word, if you are having problems with:

    Loss of appetite____ Nausea____ Vomiting____ Indigestion____

    Swallowing____ Chewing____ Meal preparation____ Mouth sores____

(continued)

		INTERVIEW INFORMATION
	Swelling (hands, ankles)___ Skin problems___ Dental problems___ Weight Loss___ Weight gain ___ 15. Do you have dentures? Yes___ No___ Upper___ Lower___ Partial___	
ELIMINATION	16. Place a check beside the word(s) if you are having problems with your urinary bladder: No problem___ Frequency___ Burning___ No control___ Not starting___ Other_____ 17. Are these problems new? Yes___ No___ If yes, explain _____ _____ 18. Place a check beside the word(s) if you are having problems with bowel function: No problem___ Constipation___ Diarrhea___ Hemorrhoids___ Other____ 19. Are these problems new? Yes___ No___ If yes, explain _____ _____	
ACTIVITY-EXERCISE	20. Place a check beside the word(s) if you are having any problems with: Bruising___ Bleeding___ Swelling___ Leg pain ___ Shortness of breath___ 21. Do you have a cough? Yes___ No___ Does your cough produce sputum? Yes___ No___ 22. Do you use oxygen? Yes___ No___ 23. Place a check beside the word(s) if you have noticed a change in your energy level when: Eating___ Bathing___ Dressing___ Walking___ Doing housework___ Preparing meals___ Shopping___ Doing your job___ Exercising___ Doing hobbies___ 24. Are these changes recent? Yes___ No___	
SLEEP-REST	25. Do you have any problems sleeping? Yes___ No___ If yes, explain _____ 26. Do you feel rested after sleep? Yes___ No___ If no, explain _____ 27. Do you take anything to help you sleep? Yes___ No___ If yes, explain _____	
COGNITIVE-PERCEPTUAL	28. Do you wear: Glasses? Yes___ No___ Contacts? Yes___ No___ Hearing Aid? Yes___ No___ 29. Place a check deside the word(s) if you are having problems with: Eyes___ Ears___ Nose___ Tongue___ Sight___ Hearing___ Smell___	*(continued)*

INTERVIEW INFORMATION

COGNITIVE–PERCEPTUAL

Taste___ Numbness___ Tingling___ Dizziness___ Seizures___ Headaches___

30. Are any of these problems new? Yes___ No___ If yes, explain:

_____

31. Do you have pain? Yes___ No___ If yes, where and when do you have pain? _____

_____

_____

Check the words that describe your pain: Piercing___ Shooting___ Burning___ Cramping___ Stinging___ Dull ache___ Constant___ Comes and goes___ Other___

32. Is your pain controlled? Yes___ No___

CONCEPT

33. Please check the words that describe how you are feeling.

Anxious___ Hopeful___ Content___ Angry___ Scared___ Depressed___ Other _____

ROLE–RELATIONSHIP

34. Marital status _____ Number of children _____

35. Do you live: Alone___ With spouse___ With family ___ Other___

36. What is your occupation? _____

Full time___ Part time___ Retired___ Student___

37. Are you working? Yes___ No___

If yes, where _____ Phone (___) ___ -

38. If you are not working, do you plan to return to work? Yes___ No___

39. Are you receiving sick benefits? Yes___ No___

SEXUALITY–REPRODUCTIVE

40. Do you use birth control? Yes___ No___

41. Are you planning to have a family in the future? Yes___ No___

FEMALE:

42. Are you still having menstrual periods? Yes___ No___

43. If yes, how long is your cycle? ___ days

If no, what age did you stop? ___ yrs

44. When was your last PAP test? _____

45. Do you practice breast self-examination? Yes___ No___

MALE:

46. Do you practice testicular self-examination? Yes___ No___

(continued)

		INTERVIEW INFORMATION
COPING STRESS–TOLERANCE	47. Have you experienced any recent stressful events in addition to your illness? Yes____ No____ If yes, explain _____ _____ 48. What helps you to manage when you feel stressed? _____ _____ 49. Who is most helpful in talking things over? _____ _____	
BELIEF VALUES	50. Do you have any religious or cultural beliefs that we should be aware of during your treatment? Yes____ No____ If you wish, please explain _____	
	51. Is there anything you wish to discuss while you are here? Yes____ No____ If you wish, please explain _____	

PATIENT'S SIGNATURE: _____

DATE: _____

NURSE'S SIGNATURE/INITIALS: _____

DATE: _____

IF COMPLETED BY SOMEONE OTHER THAN PATIENT:

_____

(Name and relationship to patient)

Index

Page numbers followed by *f* indicate figures; those followed by *t* indicate tables. Capitalized entries indicate nursing diagnoses.

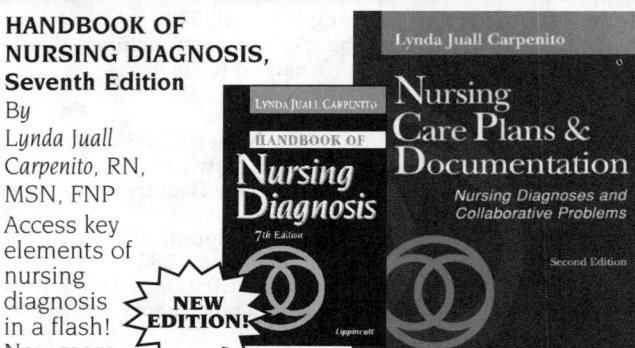
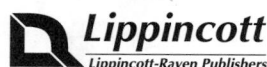